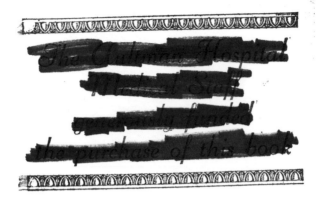
The Aultman Hospital
Medical Staff
generously funded
the purchase of this book

Reichel's Care of the Elderly
Clinical Aspects of Aging

FIFTH EDITION

Reichel's Care of the Elderly
Clinical Aspects of Aging
FIFTH EDITION

EDITORS

JOSEPH J. GALLO, M.D., M.P.H.

Assistant Professor, Department of Family Practice and Community Medicine, School of Medicine,
University of Pennsylvania, Philadelphia, Pennsylvania

JAN BUSBY-WHITEHEAD, M.D.

Associate Professor of Internal Medicine, Program on Aging,
University of North Carolina School of Medicine, Chapel Hill, North Carolina

PETER V. RABINS, M.D., M.P.H.

Professor of Psychiatry, Department of Psychiatry and Behavioral Sciences,
School of Medicine, The Johns Hopkins University, Baltimore, Maryland

REBECCA A. SILLIMAN, M.D., PH.D.

Associate Professor of Medicine and Public Health,
Geriatrics Section, Boston University Medical Center, Boston, Massachusetts

JOHN B. MURPHY, M.D.

Associate Professor and Residency Director, Department of Family Medicine,
Brown University School of Medicine, Pawtucket, Rhode Island

EDITOR EMERITUS

WILLIAM REICHEL, M.D.

Clinical Professor of Family Medicine, Georgetown University School of Medicine, Washington, D.C.
Adjunct Professor of Family Medicine, Brown University School of Medicine, Providence, Rhode Island

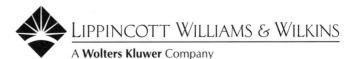

LIPPINCOTT WILLIAMS & WILKINS
A **Wolters Kluwer** Company
Philadelphia · Baltimore · New York · London
Buenos Aires · Hong Kong · Sydney · Tokyo

161004

Editor: Timothy Hiscock
Managing Editor: Grace Miller
Marketing Manager: Kathleen Neeley
Production Editor: Bill Cady
Design Coordinator: Mario Fernandez

351 West Camden Street
Baltimore, Maryland 21201-2436 USA

227 East Washington Square
Philadelphia, Pennsylvania 19106

Grateful acknowledgment is made for permission to use the following:

Final stanza from "Harvesting Mellow" by Helen Friedland, in *Threads of Experience,* edited by Sandra Haldeman Martz, fabric-and-thread images by Deidre Scherer, Papier-Mache Press, Watsonville, California, 1996.

The publisher is not responsible (as a matter of product liability, negligence or otherwise) for any injury resulting from any material contained herein. This publication contains information relating to general principles of medical care which should not be construed as specific instructions for individual patients. Manufacturers' product information and package inserts should be reviewed for current information, including contraindications, dosages and precautions.

Printed in the United States of America

First Edition, 1978　　　　　　　　　　Third Edition, 1989
Second Edition, 1983　　　　　　　　　Fourth Edition, 1995

Library of Congress Cataloging-in-Publication Data

Reichel's care of the elderly　:　clinical aspects of aging　/　Joseph J. Gallo . . . [et al.] editors.—5th ed.
　　p.　　cm.
　Rev. ed. of: Care of the elderly / editor, William Reichel. 4th ed. ©1995.
　Includes bibliographical references and index.
　ISBN 0-683-30169-1
　1. Geriatrics.　2. Aging　I. Gallo, Joseph J.　II. Reichel, William, 1937–　.　III. Care of the elderly.
　[DNLM: 1. Geriatrics.　2. Aging.　WT　100C271　1999]
　RC952.C53　1999
　618.97—dc21
　DNLM/DLC
　for Library of Congress　　　　　　　　　　　　　　　　　　　98-33917
　　　　　　　　　　　　　　　　　　　　　　　　　　　　　　　　CIP

The publishers have made every effort to trace the copyright holders for borrowed material. If they have inadvertently overlooked any, they will be pleased to make the necessary arrangements at the first opportunity.

To purchase additonal copies of this book, call our customer service department at **(800) 638-3030** or fax orders to **(301) 824-7390.** International customers should call **(301) 714-2324.**

99　00　01　02　03
1　2　3　4　5　6　7　8　9　10

*This book is dedicated to our older patients and their families,
from whom we learn so much about life.*

But harvesting now
from dwindling stores,
I taste each day
with a connoisseur's tongue
and slowly savor
rich, rare time
sweetened by so many suns.

—From "Harvesting Mellow" by Helen Friedland

Preface to the Fifth Edition

Readers of this book will be well aware that the projected growth of the world's aged population in the coming decades will be unprecedented. Population changes are occurring at the same time that health care systems all over the world are reinventing themselves; indeed, the demographic imperative is driving the reevaluation of how health care is organized. There is new emphasis on the role of the primary health care services, on the prevention of disability, on provision of services in the home and community, and on the use of health information systems that inform guidelines for care and monitor adherence to standards of care. Cost and ethical issues are thrust into the forefront of discussions about health care, especially health care for the elderly. Into this turbulent and uncertain context we step forward with this book.

Fortunately, we were able to build on the work of William Reichel, M.D. For more than 20 years and in four editions under his watchful eye, Williams & Wilkins has published this enduring textbook of geriatric medicine for the practitioner. William Reichel, a pioneer in American geriatrics, was advocating for geriatrics when there was much less awareness of the need for a special approach to the older patient. Under his able leadership the first edition was published in 1978 in response to the need for an American textbook of geriatric medicine that summarized clinical, social, and ethical differences in the approach to the health care of older adults. Subsequent editions appearing in 1983, 1989, and 1995 are a tribute to his vision.

Our new roles as Editors and Dr. Reichel's new role as Editor Emeritus are emphasized in the renaming of the book as *Reichel's Care of the Elderly: Clinical Aspects of Aging*. This fifth edition carries on the tradition of providing useful information written by leading practitioners, but with many new contributors and a number of new chapters that reflect the changing context of geriatric health care. We personally thank each contributor for a fine effort, and each of us is grateful for the opportunity to take this useful work into the 21st century.

Joseph J. Gallo, M.D., M.P.H.
Jan Busby-Whitehead, M.D.
Peter V. Rabins, M.D., M.P.H.
Rebecca A. Silliman, M.D., Ph.D.
John B. Murphy, M.D.

Acknowledgments

The editors gratefully acknowledge the helpful assistance of Carol Jean Gallo and JoAnn Romine in the many little tasks that went into the production of this book.

Editorial Board

Reviewers

The editors are indebted to the reviewers whose timely and thoughtful reviews have contributed to the quality of each chapter of this book.

LAWRENCE AWALT, M.D., Towson, Maryland

BETH CLINGMAN, M.S.W., Boston, Massachusetts

ELISE M. COLETTA, M.D., Providence, Rhode Island

MEL P. DALY, M.D., Baltimore, Maryland

RICHARD DeANDINO, M.D., San Juan, Puerto Rico

DAVID V. ESPINO, M.D., San Antonio, Texas

MADELINE FEINBERG, PHARM.D., Baltimore, Maryland

PHILLIP J. FERRIS, M.D., Baltimore, Maryland

CAROLE GARDNER, M.D., Atlanta, Georgia

ALAN GINSBURG, D.P.M., Baltimore, Maryland

JACK GURALNIK, M.D., Bethesda, Maryland

WILLIAM HAKKARINEN, M.D., Baltimore, Maryland

THOMAS C. HINES, M.D., Boston, Massachusetts

SAMUEL JONES, M.D., Fairfax, Virginia

MICHAEL KLAG, M.D., M.P.H., Baltimore, Maryland

ANDREW KLIPPER, M.D., Baltimore, Maryland

ANNE D. LAIDLAW, R.N., B.S.N., M.P.H., Baltimore, Maryland

VICKI L. LAMB, PH.D., Columbia, South Carolina

ANTHONY LEHMAN, M.D., M.S.P.H., Baltimore, Maryland

STEVEN A. LEVENSON, M.D., Baltimore, Maryland

ARLENE LOWNEY, R.N., Waltham, Massachusetts

RITA MITSCH, PHARM.D., Baltimore, Maryland

JANE NELSON, M.D., Alexandria, Virginia

J. MICHAEL NIEHOFF, M.D., Baltimore, Maryland

JAMES G. O'BRIEN, M.D., Louisville, Kentucky

JAMES J. PATTEE, M.D., Minneapolis, Minnesota

ALLAN PRISTOOP, M.D., Baltimore, Maryland

JAMES P. RICHARDSON, M.D., M.P.H., Baltimore, Maryland

THOMAS J. SCARAMELLA, M.D., Pawtucket, Rhode Island

RICHARD T. SCHOLZ, M.D., Towson, Maryland

COREY SMITH, M.A., M.H.S., Baltimore, Maryland

JERRY SOLON, PH.D., Silver Spring, Maryland

DONALD SPANGLER, M.D., Baltimore, Maryland

PHILLIP STONE, M.D., Baltimore, Maryland

MARTHA SWARTZ, M.S.S., J.D., Philadelphia, Pennsylvania

MARK R. TOLOSKY, M.H.A., J.D., FACHE, Springfield, Massachusetts

ANDREW A. WHITE, M.D., Winchester, Virginia

GEORGE A. XAKELLIS, M.D., Dearborn, Michigan

Contributors

REV. JOHN W. ABBOTT
Senior Advisor Emeritus
The Connecticut Hospice, Inc.
Branford, Connecticut

KATHLEEN ACKERMAN, M.D., M.P.H.
Director of Managed Care
Geriatrics Section
Boston University Medical Center
Associate Clinical Professor of Medicine
Boston University School of Medicine
Boston, Massachusetts

EMILY M. AGREE, PH.D.
Assistant Professor
Department of Population Dynamics
The Johns Hopkins University
Baltimore, Maryland

ANITA M. AISNER, M.D.
Assistant Professor of Medicine
Division of Geriatrics
Hospital of the University of Pennsylvania
Philadelphia, Pennsylvania

LODOVICO BALDUCCI, M.D.
Professor of Medicine
University of South Florida College of Medicine
Program Leader, Senior Adult Oncology Program
H. Lee Moffitt Cancer Center and Research Institute
Tampa, Florida

PATRICIA P. BARRY, M.D., M.P.H.
Chief, Geriatrics Section
Professor of Medicine
Boston University Medical Center
Boston, Massachusetts

B. LYNN BEATTIE, M.D., F.R.C.P.C.
Head, Division of Geriatric Medicine
Department of Medicine
The University of British Columbia Faculty of Medicine
Vancouver Hospital
Vancouver, British Columbia
Canada

MICHELE F. BELLANTONI, M.D.
Assistant Professor of Medicine
Division of Geriatric Medicine & Gerontology
School of Medicine
The Johns Hopkins University
Guest Scientist
Gerontology Research Center
National Institute on Aging
Baltimore, Maryland

MARK R. BELSKY, M.D.
Chief of Orthopedic Surgery
Newton-Wellesley Hospital
Newton, Massachusetts
Associate Clinical Professor of Orthopedic Surgery
Tufts University School of Medicine
Boston, Massachusetts

PATRICIA LANOIE BLANCHETTE, M.D., M.P.H.
Professor of Medicine and Public Health
Assistant Dean and Director, Geriatric Medicine Program
John A. Burns School of Medicine
Honolulu, Hawaii

MICHAEL B. BRAND, R.N., M.S.
Veterans Healthcare Administration
San Antonio, Texas

LOUIS C. BRESCHI, M.D.
Consultant in Urology
Department of Surgery
Franklin Square Hospital Center
Baltimore, Maryland

JOHN J. BRINK, PH.D.
Professor of Biology Emeritus
Department of Biology
Clark University
Worcester, Massachusetts

JAN BUSBY-WHITEHEAD, M.D.
Associate Professor of Internal Medicine
Program on Aging
University of North Carolina School of Medicine
Chapel Hill, North Carolina

DAVID B. CARR, M.D.
Assistant Professor of Medicine
Division of Geriatrics and Gerontology
Washington University
St. Louis, Missouri

LESLEY CARSON, M.D.
Assistant Professor of Medicine
Division of Geriatrics
Hospital of the University of Pennsylvania
Philadelphia, Pennsylvania

LISA B. CARUSO, M.D.
Fellow in Geriatric Medicine
Geriatrics Section, Boston Medical Center
Boston, Massachusetts

CHARLES A. CEFALU, M.D., M.S.
Professor and Chief of Geriatrics
Department of Family Medicine
Louisiana State University Medical Center
New Orleans, Louisiana

SUMANT S. CHUGH, M.D.
Renal Fellow
Division of Nephrology
Boston Medical Center
Boston, Massachusetts

MICHELLE CICILLINE, B.S.
Department of Family Medicine
Brown University School of Medicine
Pawtucket, Rhode Island

BARBARA A. CLARK, M.D.
Associate Professor of Medicine
Attending Nephrology
Allegheny University of the Health Sciences
Allegheny General Hospital
Pittsburgh, Pennsylvania

JACOB CLIMO, PH.D.
Professor
Department of Anthropology
Michigan State University
East Lansing, Michigan

ELISE M. COLETTA, M.D.
Chief of Gerontology
Memorial Hospital of Rhode Island
Pawtucket, Rhode Island
Assistant Professor of Family Medicine
Brown University School of Medicine
Providence, Rhode Island

JON PATRICK COONEY, M.D.
Clinical Assistant Professor of Medicine
Department of Medicine
Division of Geriatric Medicine
John A. Burns School of Medicine
University of Hawaii
Honolulu, Hawaii

DOROTHY H. COONS, B.S.
Research Associate Emeritus
Institute of Gerontology
Associate Professor Emeritus
The University of Michigan
Ann Arbor, Michigan

ROBERT S. CRAUSMAN, M.D., M.M.S., F.C.C.P.
Director, Internal Medicine Residency Program
Department of General Internal Medicine
Memorial Hospital of Rhode Island
Pawtucket, Rhode Island
Assistant Professor of Medicine
Brown University School of Medicine
Providence, Rhode Island

MEL P. DALY, M.B., B.CH., B.A.O.
Department of Medicine Greater Baltimore Medical Center
Associate Professor of Family Medicine
Internal Medicine
University of Maryland School of Medicine
Baltimore, Maryland

JANE F. DANAHY, M.D.
Department of Dermatology
Henry Ford Hospital
Detroit, Michigan

DAVID J. DOUKAS, M.D.
Associate Professor
Department of Family Medicine
Associate Director in Clinical Bioethics
The Program in Society and Medicine
University of Michigan Medical Center
Ann Arbor, Michigan

DAVID V. ESPINO, M.D.
Associate Professor & Director
Division of Community Geriatrics
Department of Family Practice
University of Texas Health Science Center at San Antonio
San Antonio, Texas

MARTINE EXTERMANN, M.D.
Assistant Professor of Medicine
University of South Florida College of Medicine
Senior Adult Oncology Program
H. Lee Moffitt Cancer Center and Research Institute
Tampa, Florida

FREDERICK A. FLATOW, M.D.
Medical Director
The Connecticut Hospice, Inc.
Branford, Connecticut

KEVIN C. FLEMING, M.D.
Assistant Professor
Department of Internal Medicine
Mayo Clinic
Rochester, Minnesota

JOHN A. FLYNN, M.D.
Assistant Professor of Medicine
Clinical Director
Division of General Internal Medicine
The Johns Hopkins University School of Medicine
Baltimore, Maryland

MARY ANN FORCIEA, M.D.
Assistant Professor of Medicine
Division of Geriatrics
Hospital of the University of Pennsylvania
Philadelphia, Pennsylvania

VICKI A. FREEDMAN, Ph.D.
Associate Social Scientist
RAND
Washington, D.C.

JOSEPH J. GALLO, M.D., M.P.H.
Assistant Professor
Department of Family Practice and Community Medicine
School of Medicine
University of Pennsylvania
Philadelphia, Pennsylvania

RAUL I. GARCIA, D.M.D., M.Med.Sc.
Professor and Chairman
Department of Health Policy and Health Services Research
Boston University Goldman School of Dental Medicine
Director, VA Dental Longitudinal Study
VA Outpatient Clinic
Boston, Massachusetts

LISA N. GELLER, Ph.D.
Fish & Richardson, P.C.
Boston, Massachusetts

BARBARA A. GILCHREST, M.D.
Professor & Chairman
Department of Dermatology
Boston University School of Medicine
Boston, Massachusetts

JAN S. GREENBERG, Ph.D.
Associate Professor
School of Social Work
University of Wisconsin-Madison
Madison, Wisconsin

RICHARD J. HAM, M.D.
Distinguished Professor of Geriatrics
SUNY Health Sciences Center
Program in Geriatrics
Syracuse, New York

ALFRED HANMER, M.D., F.A.C.S.
Orthopaedic Surgeon
Newton-Wellesley Hospital
Clinical Instructor in Orthopaedic Surgery
Tufts University School of Medicine
Newton, Massachusetts

WARREN L. HOLLEMAN, Ph.D.
Assistant Professor
Department of Family Medicine
Assistant Professor
Center for Ethics, Medicine, and Public Issues
Baylor College of Medicine
Houston, Texas

ANNE L. HUME, Pharm.D.
Professor of Pharmacy
University of Rhode Island
Kingston, Rhode Island
Adjunct Associate Professor of Family Medicine
Brown University School of Medicine
Providence, Rhode Island

ROSEMARY JOHNSON-HURZELER, R.N., M.P.H., H.A.
President & CEO
The Connecticut Hospice, Inc.
Branford, Connecticut

STEVE ILIFFE, M.R.C.G.P.
Reader in General Practice
Department of Primary Health Care
University College London Medical School
Whittington Hospital
London, United Kingdom

JERRY C. JOHNSON, M.D.
Associate Professor of Medicine
Institute of Aging and Geriatric Medicine Division
University of Pennsylvania
Philadelphia, Pennsylvania

THEODORE M. JOHNSON II, M.D., M.P.H.
Medical Director, Nursing Home Care Unit
Department of Extended Care
Atlanta VA Medical Center
Assistant Professor of Medicine
Division of Geriatrics
Emory University School of Medicine
Decatur, Georgia

FRAN E. KAISER, M.D.
Adjunct Professor of Medicine
St. Louis University School of Medicine
St. Louis, Missouri

ABDUL HAKIM KHAN, M.D., F.A.C.C.
Associate Professor of Medicine
Brown University, School of Medicine
Providence, Rhode Island
Director, Clinical Cardiac Pharmacology and
Continuing Medical Education
Memorial Hospital of Rhode Island
Pawtucket, Rhode Island

REVA B. KLEIN, M.D.
Assistant Clinical Professor of Neurology
Boston University
Medical Director, Adult Day Health Care
Boston Veterans Hospital
Boston, Massachusetts

JANICE E. KNOEFEL, M.D., M.P.H.
Associate Professor of Medicine & Neurology
University of New Mexico School of Medicine
Chief, Geriatrics/Extended Care
Department of Veterans Affairs
Albuquerque, New Mexico

MARTY WYNGAARDEN KRAUSS, Ph.D.
Associate Professor
Heller Graduate School
Brandeis University
Waltham, Massachusetts

RISA J. LAVIZZO-MOUREY, M.D., M.B.A.
Professor of Medicine
Chief, Division of Geriatrics
Hospital of the University of Pennsylvania
Director, Institute on Aging
University of Pennsylvania
Philadelphia, Pennsylvania

JEFFREY I. LEAVETT, M.D.
Assistant Professor of Medicine
Brown University School of Medicine
Director, Coronary Care Unit
Memorial Hospital of Rhode Island
Pawtucket, Rhode Island

SUSAN W. LEHMANN, M.D.
Assistant Professor
Department of Psychiatry and Behavioral Sciences
School of Medicine
The Johns Hopkins University
Baltimore, Maryland

STEVEN A. LEVENSON, M.D.
Multi-Facility Medical Director
Genesis Elder Care
Baltimore, Maryland

SUSAN M. LEVY, M.D.
Regional Director
Elderhealth Inc
Baltimore, Maryland

SHARI M. LING, M.D.
Assistant Professor of Medicine
Division of Geriatric Medicine and Gerontology
Division of Rheumatology
The Johns Hopkins University
Baltimore, Maryland

VICTORIA Y. LOUIE, M.Sc., R.D.N.
Consultant Dietitian
Royal Arch Masonic Home
Columbus Residence
Vancouver, British Columbia
Canada

ANDREA F. LUISI, Pharm.D.
Assistant Clinical Professor of Pharmacy
University of Rhode Island College of Pharmacy
Kingston, Rhode Island
Clinical Pharmacy Consultant
Eleanor Slater Hospital
Cranston, Rhode Island

CONSTANTINE G. LYKETSOS, M.D., M.H.S.
Associate Professor
Department of Psychiatry
School of Medicine
The Johns Hopkins University
Baltimore, Maryland

NANCY L. MACE, M.A.
Retired, Board of Directors for Alzheimer's Association
Chicago, Illinois
Former Assistant in Psychiatry
Johns Hopkins University
Baltimore, Maryland

VINCENT J. MARTORANA, D.P.M.
Section Chief
Division of Podiatry
Franklin Square Hospital Center
Baltimore, Maryland

CYNTHIA MATTOX, M.D.
Assistant Professor
Department of Ophthalmology
Tufts University School of Medicine
Boston, Massachusetts

LAURENCE B. McCULLOUGH, Ph.D.
Professor of Medicine, Community Medicine
    and Medical Ethics
Center for Ethics, Medicine, and Public Issues
Baylor College of Medicine
Houston, Texas

THOMAS D. McRAE, M.D.
Medical Director
Alzheimer's Disease Management Team
Pfizer Inc
Assistant Professor of Clinical Medicine
Division of Geriatrics
New York University School of Medicine
New York, New York

CHARLES P. MOUTON, M.D.
Assistant Professor
Department of Family Practice
University of Texas Health Science Center at San Antonio
San Antonio, Texas

CYNTHIA D. MULROW, M.D.
Professor of Medicine
University of Texas Health Science Center at San Antonio
Senior Research Associate
Audie L. Murphy Memorial Veterans Hospital
San Antonio, Texas

JOHN B. MURPHY, M.D.
Associate Professor and Residency Director
Department of Family Medicine
Brown University School of Medicine
Pawtucket, Rhode Island

JANE L. MURRAY, M.D.
Professor & Chair
Department of Family Medicine
University of Kansas
Kansas City, Kansas

TED D. NIRENBERG, PH.D.
Associate Professor
Department of Psychiatry and Human Behavior
Brown University
Department of Emergency Medicine
Rhode Island Hospital
Providence, Rhode Island

RICHARD A. NORTON, M.D.
Professor of Medicine
Tufts University School of Medicine
Boston, Massachusetts

JAMES G. O'BRIEN, M.D.
Professor of Geriatrics
Smock Endowed Chair in Geriatrics
University of Louisville
Louisville, Kentucky

NORMA J. OWENS, PHARM.D.
Professor of Pharmacy
University of Rhode Island College of Pharmacy
Kingston, Rhode Island
Geriatric Clinical Pharmacy Consultant
Rhode Island Hospital
Providence, Rhode Island

ROBERT PARIS, M.D.
Internist
Department of Internal Medicine
Winn Army Hospital
Hinesville, Georgia

NAVEEN S. PEREIRA, M.D.
Clinical Fellow
Division of Cardiology
Memorial Hospital of Rhode Island
Brown University School of Medicine
Pawtucket, Rhode Island

HELEN PETROVITCH, M.D.
Associate Professor of Medicine
University of Hawaii
John A. Burns School of Medicine
Honolulu, Hawaii

JAMES H. PIETSCH, J.D.
Associate Professor of Law
William S. Richardson School of Law
Adjunct Associate Professor of Medicine
John A. Burns School of Medicine
University of Hawaii
Honolulu, Hawaii

KENNETH POLIVY, M.D., F.A.C.S.
Orthopaedic Surgeon
Newton-Wellesley Hospital
Assistant Clinical Professor in Orthopaedic Surgery
Tufts University School of Medicine
Boston, Massachusetts

DAVID L. RABIN, M.D., M.P.H.
Professor and Associate Chair
Division of Community Health Care Studies
Department of Family Medicine
Georgetown University School of Medicine
Washington, D.C.

PETER V. RABINS, M.D., M.P.H.
Professor of Psychiatry
Department of Psychiatry and Behavioral Sciences
School of Medicine
The Johns Hopkins University
Baltimore, Maryland

GEORGE W. REBOK, PH.D.
Associate Professor
Department of Mental Hygiene
School of Hygiene and Public Health
The Johns Hopkins University
Baltimore, Maryland

ELIAS REICHEL, M.D.
Assistant Professor
Department of Ophthalmology
New England Eye Center
Tufts University School of Medicine
Boston, Massachusetts

WILLIAM REICHEL, M.D.
Clinical Professor of Family Medicine
Georgetown University School of Medicine
Washington, D.C.
Adjunct Professor of Family Medicine
Brown University School of Medicine
Providence, Rhode Island

REBECCA B. REILLY, M.D.
Clinical Geriatrician
Internal Medicine Midwest
Omaha, Nebraska

JILL A. RHYMES, M.D.
Professor of Medicine
Huffington Center on Aging
Baylor College of Medicine
Director, Geriatric Evaluation Unit
Department of Medicine
Houston VA Medical Center
Houston, Texas

JAMES P. RICHARDSON, M.D., M.P.H.
Chief, Division of Geriatric Medicine
Good Samaritan Hospital
Associate Professor
Department of Family Medicine and
     Epidemiology and Preventive Medicine
University of Maryland School of Medicine
Baltimore, Maryland

DUNCAN ROBERTSON, M.D., F.R.C.P., F.R.C.P.C.
Clinical Professor of Medicine
Department of Medicine, Faculty of Medicine
The University of British Columbia
Victoria, British Columbia
Canada

BRUCE E. ROBINSON, M.D., M.P.H.
Chief of Geriatrics
Sarasota Memorial Hospital
Professor of Medicine
University of South Florida College of Medicine
Tampa, Florida

G. WEBSTER ROSS, M.D.
Staff Neurologist
Outpatient Clinic
Associate Clinical Professor of Medicine
University of Hawaii
Honolulu, Hawaii

JOEL S. SCHUMAN, M.D.
Associate Professor of Ophthalmology
New England Eye Center
New England Medical Center
Boston, Massachusetts

EDNA P. SCHWAB, M.D.
Assistant Professor of Medicine
Division of Geriatrics
Hospital of the University of Pennsylvania
Philadelphia Veterans Administration Medical Center
Philadelphia, Pennsylvania

MARSHA MAILICK SELTZER, PH.D.
Professor
Waisman Center and School of Social Work
University of Wisconsin-Madison
Madison, Wisconsin

MARY C. SENGSTOCK, PH.D., C.C.S.
Professor
Department of Sociology
Wayne State University
Detroit, Michigan

REBECCA A. SILLIMAN, M.D., PH.D.
Associate Professor of Medicine and Public Health
Geriatrics Section
Boston University Medical Center
Boston, Massachusetts

RICHARD J. SORCINELLI, M.D.
Staff Physician
The Connecticut Hospice, Inc.
Branford, Connecticut

CYNTHIA D. STEELE, R.N., M.P.H.
Assistant Professor
Department of Psychiatry and Behavioral Sciences
School of Medicine
The Johns Hopkins University
Baltimore, Maryland

MICHAEL D. STEIN, M.D.
Associate Professor of Medicine
Divisions of Geriatrics and General Internal Medicine
Brown University School of Medicine
Director of HIV Activities
Rhode Island Hospital
Providence, Rhode Island

MARTIN STEINBERG, M.D.
Assistant Professor of Psychiatry
Department of Psychiatry and Behavioral Sciences
The Johns Hopkins University and Hospital
Baltimore, Maryland

JONATHAN TAYLOR, M.D.
Fellow in Gastroenterology
New England Medical Center
Boston, Massachusetts

THOMAS A. TEASDALE, DR.P.H.
Biostatistician
Department of Geriatrics and Extended Care
Veterans Affairs Medical Center
Houston, Texas

DOUGLAS THISTLE, R.PH., M.S.
Director of Pharmacy
The Connecticut Hospice, Inc.
Branford, Connecticut

ROY BURTON VERDERY, PH.D., M.D.
Associate Professor of Medicine
Arizona Center on Aging
University of Arizona School of Medicine
Tucson, Arizona

MICHAEL S. VERNON, M.D.
Vice-Chair
Department of Family Medicine
Carolinas Medical Center/Meyers Park
Charlotte, North Carolina

TOM J. WACHTEL, M.D.
Professor, Community Health and Medicine
Brown University School of Medicine
Physician in Charge of Geriatrics
Rhode Island Hospital
Providence, Rhode Island

GREGG A. WARSHAW, M.D.
Professor of Family Medicine
Department of Family Medicine
University of Cincinnati Medical Center
Cincinnati, Ohio

ALAN A. WARTENBERG, M.D., F.A.C.P.
Medical Director, Addiction Recovery Program
Faulkner Hospital
Assistant Professor of Medicine
Tufts University School of Medicine
Boston, Massachusetts

GILBERT L. WERGOWSKE, M.D.
Associate Professor of Medicine
Geriatric Medicine Program
John A. Burns School of Medicine
University of Hawaii
Honolulu, Hawaii

W. BRADLEY WHITE, M.D.
Orthopaedic Surgeon
Newton-Wellesley Hospital
Clinical Instructor in Orthopaedic Surgery
Tufts University School of Medicine
Newton, Massachusetts

FREDRICK M. WIGLEY, M.D.
Professor of Medicine
Department of Medicine
The Johns Hopkins University School of Medicine
Baltimore, Maryland

REV. SPENCER VAN B. WILKING, M.D.
Jewish Memorial Hospital
Geriatric Section
Boston, Massachusetts

LARRY A. WILSON, M.D.
Vice President for Medical Affairs
Franklin Square Hospital Center
Baltimore, Maryland

NANCY L. WILSON, M.A., A.C.S.W.
Instructor
Department of Geriatric Medicine
Assistant Director for Program Development
Huffington Center on Aging
Baylor College of Medicine
Houston, Texas

HELEN K. WU, M.D.
Assistant Professor of Ophthalmology
New England Eye Center
New England Medical Center
Boston, Massachusetts

HENRY M. YAGER, M.D.
Associate Chair, Department of Medicine
Newton-Wellesley Hospital
Newton, Massachusetts
Associate Professor of Medicine
Tufts University School of Medicine
Boston, Massachusetts

MILTON G. YODER, M.D., F.A.C.S.
Courtesy Staff
Clinical Instructor
Department of Otolaryngology and Head and Neck Surgery
School of Medicine
The Johns Hopkins University
Baltimore, Maryland

MASAKI YOSHIKAWA, M.D.
Professor Emeritus
University of Tokyo
Minato-ku, Tokyo, Japan

NIDAL A. YUNIS, M.D.
Internal Medicine Residency
Memorial Hospital of Rhode Island
Pawtucket, Rhode Island

Contents

SECTION I Care of the Elderly Patient
Evaluation, Diagnosis, and Management

SECTION II   Care of the Elderly Patient
Other Considerations

SECTION III Ethical Issues and the Elderly Patient

Care of the Elderly Patient
Evaluation, Diagnosis, and Management

CHAPTER 1

WILLIAM REICHEL AND JOSEPH J. GALLO

Essential Principles in the Care of the Elderly

We are witnessing a constant rise in the number of elders. The U.S. Bureau of the Census in 1995 found that persons 65 years or older number 33.5 million, or 12.8% of the U.S. population. The older population is expected to grow in future decades, with the most rapid increase between 2010 and 2030, when the baby boom generation reaches age 65 years. For years, the effect of an aging population was associated only with the developed nations. Over the next few decades we will witness a rise in the number and proportion of the elderly because of reduced infant mortality rates, increased life expectancy, and improved health status (1). A net gain of 800,000 persons over 65 years is noted each month, 70% in the developing world (1). The traditional family is also changing, with fewer young to take care of the old. Even Japan, with the world's longest life expectancy, is feeling the strain of caring for its aging population (2).

We certainly want good health care waiting for us in our golden years. But what is good care? In the care of the elderly patient, 11 essential principles should be considered: (1) the role of the physician as the integrator of the biopsychosocial-spiritual model; (2) continuity of care; (3) bolstering the family and home; (4) good communication skills; (5) building a sound doctor-patient relationship; (6) the need for thorough evaluation and assessment; (7) prevention and health maintenance; (8) intelligent treatment with attention to ethical decision making; (9) interdisciplinary collaboration; (10) respect for the usefulness and value of the aged individual; and (11) compassionate care. The embodiment of these 11 principles is a standard of excellence to which we can all aspire.

THE PHYSICIAN AS INTEGRATOR OF THE BIOPSYCHOSOCIAL MODEL

As medical care becomes more complex and specialized and as we place greater reliance on technology, good care requires a physician who provides leadership in the integration and coordination of the health care of the elderly patient. We have had a century of increasing advances in research and great accomplishments in diagnostic and curative medicine, but today we are realizing that scientific reductionism is not enough. The reforms in medical education, care, and research throughout this century have resulted in a tunnel vision of knowledge and skills about certain types of diseases and problems.

Society is calling out for a physician with a commitment to the person, not just to a specific disease state or mechanism. The person is part of a family and a larger community, or sadly, has no family and is isolated from the community. The first essential for the physician who cares for the elder is to act as an integrator of the biopsychosocial and spiritual model (3, 4). To accomplish this, the physician must know the patient thoroughly. This is not to denigrate the excellence of the specialties and subspecialties that have achieved much over the past few decades. But the ideal model of health care will exist when the patient is seen not from a single specialty point of view but with the full appreciation of other organ systems, emotional or psychosocial factors, information based on continuity over time, and knowledge of the patient's family and community.

We can expect more evidence to accumulate in a wide variety of areas that will illustrate the relation of the biological, psychological, social, and spiritual components in human problems. Mental stress during daily living, including reported awareness of tension, frustration, and sadness, more than doubled the risk of myocardial ischemia in one study (5). In a study of the relation of breast cancer survival and social ties, the absence of close personal ties and sources of emotional support was associated with an increased death rate (6). A study based on follow-up of the Baltimore cohort of the Epidemiologic Catchment Area Study suggested that a history of dysphoria or a major depressive episode increases the risk of myocardial infarction (7). In a study of both American and Finnish populations, hopelessness has been identified as a predictor of the progression of carotid atherosclerosis (8). We have much to learn about the dynamic relations between wellness and disease, psychosocial factors, and the spiritual state. The doctor practicing daily is aware of the higher mortality in the first year after widowhood, more pronounced in the surviving widower than in the widow, and the higher morbidity and mortality seen in the elderly on relocation.

CONTINUITY OF CARE

The ideal situation is a warm and supportive relationship, with the same personal physician serving as adviser, advocate, and friend as the patient moves through the labyrinth of medical care. It is unfortunate to see the many disruptions that take place in today's complex medical environment as the patient moves between office, home, hospital, specialized care units (coronary care units, intensive care units, stroke units, or oncology centers), nursing home, and hospice care.

The failure of physicians to make visits as necessary in the home and in the long-term care facilities is related to several factors in the United States, including training, physicians' attitudes, and reimbursement systems. Our medical school and residencies for generalist physicians have been doing an improving job of including the home and the nursing home as proper environments for medical education. The lack of reasonable reimbursement for visits to the home and nursing home remains a major problem. Physicians' attitudes have also been a problem, in that doctors in the health care system of the past few decades have been more interested in the acute aspects of care than in chronic and long-term care. These attitudes have been reinforced by the educational and reimbursement systems in place.

Wasson et al. (9) demonstrated that continuity of outpatient care for men aged 55 years and older resulted in more patient satisfaction, shorter hospitalizations, and fewer emergent hospital admissions. This carefully controlled study backs up, by rigorous research methodology, the value of continuity of care and its beneficial influence on medical care. In addition, one might envision improved critical care by having the same personal physician involved with the total health care team in specialized units. Communicating the substance of knowledge and understanding of the personal physician to other specialists is an important function of the personal physician. One might also anticipate that this role of continuity applies in general hospital care, in the home, in hospice care, and in the long-term care facility (10). Visits to the home and to the nursing home are absolutely indicated if we seek excellence in care of the elderly.

Many of our most serious problems in health care are related to failure in the continuity of care. With the population becoming older, with increasing specialization and emphasis on technology, and with the cost of care becoming very high, the greatest attention in the future must be given to the principle of continuity of care by a personal physician. We must be aware of new difficulties in our changing health care environment that affect continuity of care. Two examples are (*a*) changes of health insurance that interrupt established doctor-patient relationships and (*b*) the focus on higher physician productivity by managed and capitated care plans, which often makes it difficult for the patient to get a timely appointment.

BOLSTERING FAMILY AND HOME

Every physician should enlist means to keep an elderly person either in his or her own home or in an extended family setting. It should certainly be our goal as physicians to keep elderly persons functioning independently, preserving their lifestyles and self-respect as long as possible. The physician should use the prescription for a nursing home as specifically as a prescription for an antibiotic or an antihypertensive medication.

A number of forces have resulted in patients going to institutional settings when other arrangements might have been possible. Between 1960 and 1975, a massive push toward institutionalization created hundreds of thousands of nursing home beds. What are the forces that contributed to excessive institutional care? Funding mechanisms have been directed solely toward reimbursement for institutional care rather than for other arrangements. With the increased mobility of families, there simply may not be family members available in the community to participate in the elderly person's care. Houses are architecturally based on a small, nuclear family and do not permit housing an elderly patient. Finally, the increasing movement of women into the workforce has meant that fewer family members are available to remain home with the impaired or disabled elderly person.

What alternative can the physician recommend to these caregivers? A simple list includes homemakers, home health aides, other types of home care, day care, after care, specialized housing, visiting nurses, friendly visitors, foster home care, chore services, home renovation and repair services, congregate and home-delivered meal programs, transportation programs, and shopping services. Personal physicians should also understand and use legal and protective services for the elderly whenever indicated.

Who are the caregivers in American society? An examination of data from the 1982 National Long-Term Care Survey (11) revealed that caregivers to the disabled are predominantly women

and three quarters of them live with the person for whom they care. One third are themselves over 65 years old, poor or nearly poor, and in fair to poor health. Some caregivers face conflicts between their caregiving duties and the needs of other family members and jobs. More than 90% of the caregivers carry the burden without assistance from the formal health care system.

In the study by Stone et al. (11), 71.5% of caregivers to the functionally impaired elderly were women, daughters constituting 28.9%. Husbands accounted for 12.8% and sons for 8.5% of this population. In the case of sons, it is often the son's spouse, the daughter-in-law, who actually provides the care. The burden of caregiving is felt by many women today, sandwiched between the demands of their parents and of their children and grandchildren. It has been said that the empty nest syndrome has been replaced by a crowded nest syndrome. Many caregivers are under extreme burden and stress, and sometimes the question is, who is the real patient, the patient or the caregiver? The caregiver often is in more distress than the patient and develops serious physical and emotional problems as a result of the burden and stress.

The belief that old people are rejected by their families has been exploited as a social myth (12). Many families are struggling to cope with the needs of parents who are frail and debilitated. The family member, friend, or neighbor is often the crucial link in allowing the dependent elder to remain in the community. In repeated studies, the characteristics of the caregiver, more than those of the elderly patient, are essential in predicting institutional placement.

Even when adult children and elderly parents are separated by distance, their relationship may be unaffected, maintaining cohesion despite limited face-to-face contact. At a certain distance the telephone becomes an important substitute for visits (13). Nevertheless, for many adult children, separation by distance causes increased tension and difficulty in their efforts to care for their parents. Family connectedness in the case of geographically distant older parents may be reduced to telephone communication and visits for holidays and in the face of illness or crisis (14).

Cost containment today, particularly in the prospective payment system, will require greater reliance on alternatives to institutional care. We can expect to see many new resources and support systems, including more home-delivered care, innovative experiments in housing and transportation, a cadre of respite workers, and perhaps tax credits for family-oriented care. The personal physician in his or her community can be a significant advocate for the development of new resources and support systems that can help keep the elderly patient in his or her own home or in the home of a family member. We can also expect to see increased educational media (television programs, brochures, books, and courses not only at local hospitals and long-term care facilities but also at high schools, community colleges, and universities) that will provide information to the many families who are striving to keep an elderly member at home with a spouse, with family, or alone.

COMMUNICATION SKILLS

Specific communication skills are critical in good management of the elderly patient. Most important in good communication is listening and allowing patients to express themselves. The physician should use an open-ended approach, interpreting what the patient is saying and reading between the lines. The physician can use intuition in deciding what the patient means. Why did the patient really come to see the physician? The elderly patient complaining of headache or backache may be expressing depression or grief. We should not miss important verbal clues when the patient says, "I think these headaches started when I lost my husband."

It is helpful to leave the door open for other questions or comments by the patient, both at the conclusion of the visit and in the future. It is always helpful to say, "Do you have any other questions or concerns?" A physician anticipating a specific problem can make it easier for the patient to discuss this issue. For example, "You are doing well, but I know you are concerned about your arthritis and whether you will be able to climb the stairs in your home. At some point, we may want to discuss the various alternatives that are open to you."

Just as the physician providing care to children must deal with the parents, the physician providing care to the elderly must deal with their adult children. These children play a vital role in decision making and providing support, and the physician must therefore communicate with them and deal with their emotional reactions, such as guilt or grief. The physician taking care of an elderly patient with cancer must be prepared when the adult daughter tells the doctor, "Whatever you do, please don't tell my father he has cancer," especially when it is apparent that the parent is well aware of all aspects of his problem.

The physician should be careful when meeting with an elderly patient who discusses his or her absent spouse or child or when dealing with adult children or grandchildren in the absence of the patient. The physician should not necessarily accept everything that is said about the absent family member. Physicians must be able to listen carefully, ask questions, and collect information; our opinion of the situation might be entirely different if we had an opportunity to hear the view of the absent family member.

Peabody (15) in 1927 said, "The good physician knows his patients through and through, and his knowledge is bought dearly. Time, sympathy and understanding must be lavishly dispensed, but the reward is to be found in that personal bond which forms the greatest satisfaction of the practice of medicine." The physician who enters the patient's universe and understands the patient's perceptions, assumptions, values and religious beliefs is a tremendous advantage. Frankl (16) demonstrated how physicians can help patients understand the meaning and value of their lives. Of course, how elders find meaning in their lives is related to how they found meaning at other stages in their lives. It is therapeutic for the patient to feel that the physician cares enough about that individual to understand the patient's life, particularly the meaning and purposes of his or her present existence. Frankl (17) stated that human life can be fulfilled not only in creating and enjoying but also in suffering. He provides examples in which suffering becomes an opportunity for growth, an achievement, a means for ennoblement. Frankl's existential psychiatry or logotherapy is a useful psychologic method that helps the elderly patient appreciate the positive attributes, meanings, and purposes of his or her life.

Yalom (18) defines existential psychotherapy as "a dynamic approach to therapy which focuses on concerns that are rooted in the individual's existence." Many individuals are tormented by a crisis of meaning (19). Many suffer an existential vacuum, a lack of meaning in life (16–20). The patient in an existential vacuum may demonstrate many symptoms that rush in to fill it in the form of somatization, depression, alcoholism, and hypochondriasis. The physician recognizing an existential vacuum can help the patient find meaning. Frankl's main theme is that meaning is essential for life. Engagement or involvement in life's activities is a therapeutic answer to a lack of meaning in life. The physician can help guide the patient toward engagement with life, life's activities, other people, and other satisfactions.

Frankl (16, 17) advises all physicians to use hope as a therapeutic tool. The physician dealing with the elderly must focus on the significant role of hope in daily practice. As physicians, we must eventually understand the biologic basis of hope. We do not understand sufficiently the biochemical, neurophysiologic, and immunologic concomitants of different attitudes and emotions and how they are affected by the physician. Physicians can worsen panic and fear; they can also create a state of confidence, calm, relaxation, and hope.

In this day and age of increasing technology and subspecialization, the patient's recovery may still depend on the physician's ability to reduce panic and fear and to raise the prospect of hope. Cousins (21) describes the "quality beyond pure medical competence that patients need and look for in their physicians. They want reassurance. They want to be looked after and not just over. They want to be listened to. They want to feel that it makes a difference to the physician, a very big difference, whether they live or die. They want to feel that they are in the physician's thoughts." For example, in building the doctor-elderly patient relationship, nothing is more effective than the physician picking up the phone and calling the patient and saying: "I was thinking about your problem. How are you doing?" This expression of interest by telephone represents a potent method for cementing the relationship of doctor with patient.

Jules Pfeiffer's cartoon character the "modern Diogenes" carries on the following discourse upon meeting an inquisitive fellow traveler through the sands of time:

> Traveler: "What are you doing with the lantern?"
> Diogenes: "I'm searching."
> Traveler: "For an honest man?"
> Diogenes: "I gave that up long ago!"
> Traveler: "For hope?"
> Diogenes: "Lots of luck."
> Traveler: "For love?"
> Diogenes: "Forget it!"
> Traveler: "For tranquility?"
> Diogenes: "No way."
> Traveler: "For happiness?"
> Diogenes: "Fat chance."
> Traveler: "For justice?"
> Diogenes: "Are you kidding?"
> Traveler: "Then what are you looking for?"
> Diogenes: "Someone to talk to."

Help comes from feeling that one has been heard and understood (22).

DOCTOR-PATIENT RELATIONSHIP
What the Doctor and Patient Bring to Each Encounter

The physician must understand what both he or she and the patient bring to each interaction, including both positive and negative feelings. The patient's views of old age may be negative and fearful, believing illness signifies misery, approaching death, loss of self-esteem, loneliness, and dependency. The physician's own fears about aging and death may color the interview as well. The doctor may simply not view helping the older, impaired patient as worthwhile. The physician may have low expectations for success of treatment, writing off the elderly patient as senile, mentally ill, or hypochondriacal. The doctor may have significant conflicts in his or her own relationship with parent figures or may fear that the patient will die.

Knowing the Patient

Several recommended steps toward a sound doctor-patient relationship are particularly applicable to the elderly patient (15). The first is that the physician should know the patient thoroughly; the second is that the physician should know the patient thoroughly; and the third is that the physician should know the patient thoroughly. The interested physician performs the first step in building a sound doctor-patient relationship by gathering a complete history, including the personal and social history, and doing a complete physical. Ideally, the physician should be a good listener, warm and sensitive, providing the patient ample opportunity to express multiple problems and reflect upon his or her life history and current situation. Thus, the physician will be able to understand the meanings and purposes of the patient's present life.

As stated earlier, family and friends are the principal support system for the elderly, and usually nursing home placement is a last resort after all alternatives have failed. However, the physician must be able to recognize the dysfunctional family. Some elderly persons have been rejected by children. Like King Lear, these elderly may say, "How sharper than a serpent's tooth it is to have a thankless child." Some elderly persons have rejected a child for a variety of reasons. There are families with members estranged from each other for many years. The physician should understand what has happened over the years in the patient's marriage. Before the physician can hope to help families with such problems, it is important as a first step to recognize that these problems exist.

Creating a Partnership With the Patient

In all dealings with the patient, the physician should be frank and honest and share information truthfully. The patient should feel a sense of partnership with the physician. In this partnership, the doctor first reviews his or her perception of the patient's problems. Then for each problem the choices are considered, and decision making is shared with the patient. Although in some situations frankness is counterproductive, with most patients frankness is helpful. In some situations the elderly patient does not want to share in decision making but simply wants to surrender autonomy to a relative or to the physician. Again, in most cases, the physician should attempt to enter a partnership with the patient and share as much decision making as possible.

Discussions with the patient or family members should be presented in a hopeful manner. As discussed earlier, it is important to offer a positive approach whenever possible. The physician's infusion of optimism and cheerfulness is therapeutic. The physician should help patients appreciate such positive attributes or purposes as religious beliefs, relationships with children and grandchildren, the enjoyment of friends, and the enjoyment of the relationship with doctors, nurses, and other health professionals in the immediate therapeutic environment.

The physician should be careful that discussions with family members be held with the patient's consent. If the patient is sufficiently mentally impaired, it may be appropriate to deal with the closest relative. Complex ethical questions arise in the matter of confidentiality and decision making in regard to the elderly patient with partial mental impairment.

NEED FOR THOROUGH EVALUATION AND ASSESSMENT

The physician must avoid prejudging the patient. We must not allow preconceived notions of common patterns of illness to preclude the most careful individualized assessment of each patient. Conscientious history taking and physical examination are essential. Treatment choices should be considered only after a thorough evaluation. Judicious consideration of all factors may result in a decision to treat or not to treat certain problems in certain patients. Attention to lesser problems may be postponed according to the priorities of the moment rather than complicate an already variegated therapeutic program.

Physicians must avoid wastebasket diagnoses. The past concept of "chronic brain syndrome" or "arteriosclerotic brain disease" is one such example. Not all mental disturbance in the elderly is dementia; not all dementias in the elderly (in fact, only a minority) are arteriosclerotic. Neuropsychiatric disturbance in the elderly may be dropped into a wastebasket and casually accepted as both expectable and untreatable when a very treatable cause may be present. The physician must consider and seek out treatable disease.

For example, neuropsychiatric disturbance, including a dementia syndrome, may be caused by severe depression, a treatable disorder. The most common types of dementia are Alzheimer's disease and vascular dementia. Other forms of dementia, potentially reversible, include myxedema, chronic drug intoxication, pernicious anemia, folic acid deficiency, and chronic subdural hematoma. Neuropsychiatric disturbance may also include delirium or acute confusional state secondary to many types of medical illness or drug toxicity. Such delirious states can be helped if the primary disorder is recognized and treated.

It is often difficult to disentangle the physical from the emotional. Emotional disorder may manifest in the elderly as a physical problem, such as when musculoskeletal tension is the principal manifestation of depression. Conversely, physical disease in the elderly may manifest as a mental disorder: confusion, disorientation, or delirium often is the first sign of many common medical ailments, including myocardial infarction, pulmonary embolism, occult carcinomatosis, pneumonia, urinary tract infection, and dehydration (Table 1.1). For this reason it cannot be emphasized too many times that proper diagnosis is essential for specific treatment plans, such as for urinary tract infection causing an acute delirious state, folic acid deficiency causing a specific dementia, or depression. Each of these is highly specific. Treatment in each case is irrational if a specific diagnosis is not known.

It is often not sufficient to know the organic, anatomic, psychiatric diagnosis; rather we should seek a clearer understanding of the whole patient. At times it is more important to assess the elderly patient's functional status, which may have greater significance than the diagnostic or anatomic label. For example, in the case of a cerebrovascular accident, knowledge of the exact anatomic location as determined by arteriography may not help the patient as much as understanding the patient's functional state. It may

Table 1.1

Characteristics of Elderly Patients

1. Physical disease may present as a mental disorder, with confusion, disorientation, or delirium often being the first sign of many common medical ailments.
2. Functional or physiologic capacities are diminished. For example, creatinine clearance declines with age, although the rate of physiologic decline varies from person to person.
3. Adverse effects of drugs are more pronounced and more likely.
4. Typical signs and symptoms of disease may be hidden or slight. For example, pain may be absent in myocardial infarction, and fever may be minimal in pneumonia.
5. Multiple organic, psychological, and social problems are present.

be more important to know whether the patient can walk or climb stairs, can handle his or her own bathing, eating, and dressing; whether he or she can get out of bed and sit in a chair, can handle a wheelchair, or requires a cane or walker. All of these functional concerns must be considered in evaluating an elderly patient.

It is important to consider what is physiologic versus what is pathologic. Aging itself can be defined as the progressive deterioration or loss of functional capacity, which takes place in an organism after a period of reproductive maturity (Table 1.1). The Baltimore Longitudinal Study of Aging since 1958 has studied this decline in each of several specific functional capacities, such as glucose tolerance and creatinine clearance. There is a progressive deterioration of glucose tolerance with each decade of life. Indeed, hyperglycemia is so common in the elderly that to avoid labeling a disquietingly high proportion of people as diabetics, Elahi et al. (23) formulated a percentile system that ranks a subject with age-matched cohorts. (Some persons, however, show no evidence of deterioration of glucose tolerance or insulin tolerance to glucose with aging.) Although the accepted definitions allow the same diagnostic criteria to be applied at any age, it is often unclear who is truly diabetic. The rate of decline in creatinine clearance also accelerates with advancing age (24). This phenomenon appears to represent true renal aging, because it was seen in several hundred normal persons who were free of specific diseases and not taking medications that might alter glomerular filtration rate. The physician must not be quick in treating a laboratory value that simply may represent an altered physiologic state and not a true disease or pathologic disorder.

In fact, two major conclusions from the Baltimore Longitudinal Study of Aging emerge. Even when specific functional capacities change with age, health problems need not be a consequence of aging. Many of the most common disorders of old age result from pathologic processes and not from normal aging. The second important finding is that no single chronologic timetable of normal aging exists. Even within one person, the physiologic capacities of organs show aging at different rates. Between individuals, more difference is noted in older people than in younger people.

Increased adverse effects of drugs affect the elderly, who often tolerate medications poorly (Table 1.1). Polypharmacy is a major problem in the care of the elderly patient. Not only do psychotropic medications cause an altered response of the central nervous system, resulting in confusion and delirium, but also antibiotics or digitalis may cause these problems. Altered renal and hepatic functions may affect drug elimination. In general, the elderly demonstrate greater variability and idiosyncrasy in drug response than do younger persons.

Prudence is therefore extremely important in prescribing drugs for the elderly. The physician must determine whether the patient's complaint is justification for treatment. Is this medication absolutely necessary? The skill of the physician is required in weighing benefit versus risk. The benefit-risk balance is more important in the elderly patient than in younger ones. The physician must attempt to keep the total number of medications down to as small a number as possible.

Also affecting our diagnostic ability in the elderly is that signs and symptoms of disease in the aged may be slight or hidden. Pain, white blood cell response, and fever and chills are examples of defense mechanisms that may be diminished in older persons (Table 1.1). The aged person may have pneumonia or renal infection without chills or a rise in temperature. Myocardial infarction, ruptured abdominal aorta, perforated appendix, or mesenteric infarction may be present without pain in the elderly (25).

Multiple clinical, psychologic, and social problems (Table 1.1) are characteristic of the elderly (25). Clinically and pathologically, an elderly patient may have 10 or 15 problems. Geriatric patients should benefit from the use of a problem-oriented approach to medical records. Medical records not only should include the medical problem but should clearly indicate functional, psychologic, social, and family problems as well. The key feature of the problem-oriented record is the problem list, which serves as a table of contents to the patient's total medical history. It behooves us to use a problem list as a minimal or core component of a problem-oriented system in caring for the elderly patient. Without a problem list, we can easily lose track over time of the elderly patient's multiple problems; that, for example, the patient in 1953 was hospitalized for a psychiatric problem or in 1975 had a compression fracture of the T10 vertebra after slipping on ice. These problems may be lost to memory without some form of problem-oriented system. In addition, care is enhanced by maintaining a medication list that is updated each time the patient visits.

PREVENTION AND HEALTH MAINTENANCE

A tremendous revolution is taking place in the United States with emphasis on prevention, health maintenance, and wellness. Unfortunately, not all of the facts are in. For example, less is known about risk factors for heart disease and stroke for the elderly patient than for younger adults. However, enough is known about prevention that we are seeing a decline in the mortality rate from heart disease and cerebrovascular disease, which probably relates to increased preventive measures.

More and more physicians and nurses are emphasizing health maintenance and wellness in their practice and in their community education programs. However, the drive for wellness is coming not only from health professionals but also from the public itself. The personal physician has an opportunity to encourage preventive medicine and health maintenance at every age level and at each level of functional ability or disability.

A remarkable amount of new information about the role of exercise and strength training in the prevention or reversibility of frailty and physiologic decline is being discovered (26–28). It is expected that more will be learned and that the health of many elderly will be improved by exercise and physical activity. The next decade will see more advances in nutrition, exercise, and therapeutic measures to retard aging.

How do physicians and health professionals determine the standard for health screening and health promotion? *The Guide to Clinical Preventive Services* (29) is one standard for health screening guidelines. The second edition of the *Guide* is evidence based rather than expert based, as in the first edition. More and more evidence-based studies are under way.

Examples of two new conclusions in the new task force report include the following: screening is now recommended for all persons 50 years of age and older, with annual testing for fecal occult blood, periodic sigmoidoscopy, or both; and routine screening for prostate cancer with digital rectal examinations or serum tumor markers (e.g., prostate-specific antigen [PSA]) is not recommended for lack of evidence that early detection of prostate cancer improves survival. It is clear that each practicing physician must follow the medical literature and evaluate the algorithms and guidelines that unfold in the decade ahead. For each question, the evidence is being examined and reexamined.

We can expect that in any area of health screening and health promotion, the guidelines will not be written in stone but will be reconsidered and reevaluated according to the evidence that is examined. Physicians and health professionals caring for the elderly will witness tension and debate as new guidelines are written. But at any time, with the state of evidence-based knowledge that we do have in preventive medicine and health screening, there remains the differential between the physician's intellectual acceptance and awareness of these guidelines and the actual use of these guidelines on a regular, consistent basis. We can expect more societal pressure from hospitals, managed care organizations, and government health insurance programs to conform to guidelines that have been selected by each group as a standard of care.

INTELLIGENT TREATMENT WITH ATTENTION TO ETHICAL DECISION MAKING

The doctor should resist the temptation to treat with still more medications a new problem that is poorly understood. The question should be raised whether the present symptoms, such as confusion or depression, may be related to current drug use.

Therefore the aphorism "first do no harm." A similar concept was stated by Seegal (30) as the "principle of minimal interference" in the management of the elderly patient. "First do no harm" and the principle of minimal interference should be remembered when one reviews the abundant examples of iatrogenic problems among the elderly (31, 32).

The principle of minimal interference can be applied not only to drug therapy but to other decisions, including the use of diagnostic tests (the principle of diagnostic parsimony), surgical intervention, and decision making in regard to hospitalization or placement in a long-term care facility. The principle of minimal interference may result in decisions that are both humanistic and cost effective; e.g., a decision that the patient should remain in his or her own home, despite limited access to medical therapy, rather than reside in a long-term care facility; or the decision not to do a gastrointestinal workup in the evaluation of anemia when the patient is dying of malignant brain tumor.

In the care of the elderly, there are times for minimal interference and there are times for maximal intervention. Again, certainly the patient with dementia caused by myxedema deserves every effort to replace thyroid hormone carefully. The elderly patient with severe congestive heart failure secondary to rheumatic or congenital heart disease deserves full consideration for definitive treatment, including surgery, for his or her cardiac problems. The elderly patient with depression deserves specific treatment for this very treatable disorder.

In the future we will be faced with more and more difficult decisions of an ethical nature (see Section III, Ethical Issues and the Elderly Patient). For example, an 80-year old man may have a history of resection of an abdominal aneurysm in 1985, multiple myocardial infarctions, and multiple strokes causing severe dementia. His main problem on the current hospitalization is pneumonia causing a worsening of his confusion. Because of periods of sinus arrest, a pacemaker is considered. Should a pacemaker be used in patients with significant dementia? Should pneumonia be treated in patients with severe dementia or terminal carcinoma? Difficult and ambiguous clinical problems such as these will face the personal physician with increasing frequency. The physician in the future will be called upon to make complex decisions according to the accepted traditions and values of the specific religion, nation, and society or culture, with major guidance from the patient's stated wishes affirmed when the patient was fully competent. Section III of this text attempts to deal with the ethical dilemmas we face in daily practice in caring for the elderly.

In regard to all therapeutic decisions, a personal physician is at an advantage if his or her understanding of the patient is based on continuity of care. The physician then can consider the patient in totality, including psychologic, spiritual, social, family, and environmental factors. To recommend any treatment plan intelligently, it is beneficial to have the knowledge of home or institutional environment, the family constellation, the availability of friends, access to transportation, and the economic situation of the patient. Also, as the physician grapples with complex decisions of an ethical nature, specific knowledge of the patient's value systems and beliefs is critically important. Chapter 68 describes in detail the importance of eliciting a values history from patients not only when they are terminally ill but during the entire doctor-elderly patient relationship.

INTERDISCIPLINARY COLLABORATION

The physician must understand when to call upon other health professionals. One must know when to call upon visiting home nurses, social workers, psychologists, or representatives of community agencies. One must know when to call for legal or financial counseling. All physicians would do well to work in closer harmony with the patient's or family's clergyman or pastor.

The physician should know when to recommend specific rehabilitative therapies. Specific use of physical, occupational, recreational, and speech therapies is vital for the proper care of certain problems. For example, the elderly patient with diabetic neuropathy and flapping gait may benefit from bilateral leg braces. Another patient recovering from stroke may benefit from occupational therapy used to reintroduce the patient to the activities of normal daily living, not simply as a recreational or diversionary therapy.

The improvement of health care of the chronically ill elderly requires that health professionals work together for the best interest of the patient. That requires a genuine collaborative effort to bring about a system that will best meet the needs of the frail elderly. This collaboration will be even more important in new managed or capitated health care plans and community-based long-term care options involving home care, home hospice care, and other services.

RESPECT FOR THE USEFULNESS AND VALUE OF THE AGED INDIVIDUAL

Much in our society works to reject or devalue the aged. We are certainly living in a youth-oriented era, and a physician must guard against viewing the elderly as useless, insignificant, or worthless. This lack of respect and devaluation occurs in society at large, in the workplace, in the family, and in the entertainment media, but it should not occur in the doctor's office or other clinical settings. The anthropologist knows other cultures and societies in which the elders of the community are most valued. An hour of watching American television is instructive to witness the youth orientation of our society. Unfortunately, many elderly patients report that physicians have treated them poorly because the patient was old.

An exceptional book that is not actively directed to the elderly but that should be in the curriculum of medical students and residents is *Respectful Treatment: A Practical Handbook of Patient Care* (33). The author, Martin Lipp, describes the therapeutic benefit of respect in the doctor-patient relationship, especially in dealing with those we consider problem patients: the angry patient; the dependent, passive patient; the complaining, demanding patient; the denying patient; the overaffectionate patient; the mentally ill patient; and so on. Respect is therapeutic. Many patients feel weak and vulnerable, and they demonstrate low self-esteem because of age, illness, and various psychologic and personality factors. Respect is a message to the patient that quickly brings about a more sound doctor-patient relationship.

Discussions are held on the subject of calling patients, and elderly patients in particular, by their first name or by their last name preceded by Mr., Mrs., or Ms. An immediate demonstration of respect is to call elderly persons by their family name with Mr., Mrs., or Ms. used appropriately.

The next 20 years will see considerable social change, with redefinition of the age for retirement and other entitlement plans. We hope that social and economic changes will allow the elderly to function as a continuing resource in our society. We can expect to see reduced restrictions on older workers with particular reference to mandatory retirement. We can also expect to see more programs to provide skilled training, job counseling, and placement for older men and women, hence to initiate, enhance, and continue their voluntary participation in the workforce. We should anticipate the breakdown of stereotypes and greater recognition of the value of the elderly as a human resource.

There are many social forces at play. In 1930, 54% of men aged 65 and over were in the workforce. In 1960, 31% of that group were working. Compare this with 1996, when 17% of men and 9% of women over age 65 were working. Of 18 million Americans 65 to 74 who are not in hospitals or long-term care facilities, only 3 million are working. How many of these people want to work?

In following workers aged 51 to 61 in the 1992 Health and Retirement Study, a large majority of the groups studied indicated that they would prefer phasing down with continuing to do some paid work when they retire (34). Others approaching retirement or in retirement opt for a retirement career. Many have good health and financial stability or a satisfactory pension and would prefer to pursue a retirement career with passion. This may be part-time or full-time. The person retiring today at age 65 years or younger may enjoy a retirement career that may span 10 to 20 years. Society must allow elders to fulfill such roles and must retain the wisdom that has accumulated with time. At the same time, some who are approaching retirement do not want to or cannot continue employment, whether in their former role or in a new one. All of these variations should be considered in counseling our patients.

COMPASSIONATE CARE

In an increasingly technologic society, caring and compassion must be foremost in the practice of medicine. We must avoid the possible dehumanization that takes place when patients simply become subjects for study and treatment. Every year in the United States, we are seeing new accomplishments in medical technology and specialization. Computed tomography, computed nuclear medicine, magnetic resonance imaging, positron emission tomography, organ transplants, achievements in cardiovascular surgery, hemodialysis, and intensive and critical care all are becoming part of our routine medical environment. In such a new medical world, it is imperative that compassionate care not be lost in daily encounters between health professionals and elderly patients.

All of the great religions state some form of a Golden Rule: "You must love your neighbor as you do yourself" and "What you do not want done to yourself, do not do to others." The need to express compassion surpasses new technical achievements and new specialized knowledge (35). The physician's duty is to cure sometimes, to comfort always.

The attitude of the doctor toward the elderly patient is critically important. Is the physician willing to spend time with the patient? Is the physician willing to be involved in the chronic and long-term aspects of the patient's health as well as in acute illness? Is the physician concerned with the social, psychologic, and family aspects of the patient in addition to clinical and organic aspects?

Care and compassion demand that the physician dispense sufficient time in his or her encounters with elderly patients. There is evidence in one study (36) that physicians spend less time with elderly patients than with younger ones, but 15 to 20 minutes may be minimal time to carry out a visit in the office, home, hospital, or long-term care facility. An hour and a half, not necessarily in one sitting, may be required to complete an examination of a new patient, particularly in the presence of multiple complex problems. More time is required in each encounter if the various functions of counseling, psychologic support, health maintenance and prevention are to be carried out in addition to making decisions about treatment and possible rehabilitation.

Examples of failure in caring and compassion include the physician who waves from the door of the patient's room instead of going in; the physician who quickly resorts to psychotropic drugs in the office rather than taking the time to listen; and the physician on teaching rounds who never sees the patient and who limits his or her discussion to laboratory studies or some specific, interesting aspect of the case in a nearby conference room.

The physician should be a good listener and read between the lines what the patient is saying. Often the physician can express warmth, understanding, or sympathy by nonverbal means. Staying close to the patient and maintaining eye contact is helpful. Sitting next to the patient's bed or sitting on the edge of the bed in the hospital or long-term care facility brings the doctor right into the patient's small universe. The physician might put a hand on the patient's shoulder and pat or touch the patient or hold hands at appropriate points during the visit.

As the revered physician Eugene Stead Jr. would say: "What this patient needs is a doctor" (37). Our elderly patients, and in fact all of our patients, yearn for a physician who will listen and understand. Again, we remember Peabody's words (15), "The good physician knows his patients through and through, and his knowledge is bought dearly. Time, sympathy and understanding must be lavishly dispensed, but the reward is to be found in that personal bond which forms the greatest satisfaction of the practice of medicine. One of the essential qualities of the clinician is interest in humanity, where the secret of the care of the patient is in caring for the patient."

CHANGING TIMES IN HEALTH CARE

In the performance of these essential aspects of care of the elderly patient, the physician may be distraught that these are difficult times and a revolution in health care is taking place. The physician may feel discouraged during this period of cost containment, capitated health care for the elderly, increased competition, the malpractice threat, and other forces in health care reform taking place today. The physician may be disheartened by a system that provides financial incentives for saving money and that puts the physician at risk for spending; that excessively scrutinizes and profiles the physician in the hospital; and that may often seem to emphasize the financial bottom line rather than excellence of patient care. Despite this tug of war, the physician must simply have faith that excellence of patient care—care that is compassionate and humane, care that is characterized by continuity, care that is sensitive to psychosocial and family issues, and care that is characterized by all the other essential principles—will endure. Although the organization of health care delivery will undoubtedly change, we can expect society ultimately to demand a quality of care that we would each want for ourselves. We the authors can visualize that social pressure will enforce the maintenance of quality of care, patient satisfaction, and the fulfillment of the ethics of medicine and the other health care professions. The Federal Aviation Agency, which is characterized in this country by high standards of safety and quality, has been cited as one model that the U.S. health care system might follow.

OPPORTUNITIES FOR NEW DIRECTION AND CHANGE

As the primary care or generalist physician goes about his or her daily professional duties, situations in which there are no precise or clear answers arise. This circumstance was mentioned earlier, under prevention and health maintenance: the need for ongoing refinement of algorithms and guidelines for health promotion and health screening. But there are other areas that require reflection, research, and in some cases societal response.

Understanding Mental Disorders

Opportunities for understanding how to help older people remain independent and functioning are emerging in new studies of mental disorders. Much mental illness is poorly understood. Some elderly persons have atypical features, including paranoid ideation or eccentric behavior. We often lack the patient's full life history. In any case, the emotional disorder may not be easily classified. One elderly patient had fears of being watched by the CIA and the FBI, thinking they were saying he was masturbating and had bad body odor. Two attempts to arrange psychiatric consultation failed; the patient did not want to follow up with the psychotherapist. He appeared well in every other regard. After 6 months of office visits lasting 20 minutes each, his paranoid ideation improved and he was grateful that the treatment was helping tremendously. At a year he was free of paranoid thoughts. Was his behavior somehow related to depression, isolation, or loneliness? At 3 years he looks forward to his office visits and continues to express gratitude for the medical attention that cured him. There is much to learn about mental health disorders in the elderly who are living in the community.

We have discussed the work of Frankl (16, 17) and Yalom (18) and the existential vacuum. We have referred to existential psychotherapy and the use of hope as a therapeutic tool. The physician caring for 80- and 90-year-old patients must be prepared to hear the patient say, "I don't know why I'm still here" or "I don't know why God doesn't take me away. I have lived long enough." The physician must be alert to depression and suicidal ideation. But if the physician's assessment is that these statements do not represent suicidal thoughts, the physician must be prepared to respond to ruminations about death that are heard commonly in the very old. With-out entering too much into the world of theology, it might be appropriate for the physician to say such things as, "That's not for you to decide or ponder. There must be a reason you are still here. Apparently God must want you here for some reason. There is the friendship that you and I still enjoy and the friendship that you enjoy with the visiting nurse (or home health aide). There's your nephew in New Hampshire and his family. You may see him only 3 or 4 times a year, but I know that you both care about each other. Again, your being here is not really for you or me to decide. All of us must make the best of each day while we are still here."

What about the extraordinarily independent patient who is feisty and may be a bit eccentric? The patient does not accept what seems to be needed treatment or refuses home health aides or day care. Others have divorced themselves from the medical system, at least for the present, because of past treatment that was burdensome, expensive, and seemingly unnecessary. Some refuse supports such as health aides because they do not want the burden of strangers in the home or the expense of this assistance (even though they can afford it). They do not want to divert their savings in case they need it in the future or to preserve an inheritance for a loved one. They may recall bad experiences with a series of dentists whose bills ran into thousands of dollars. Or the patient may be wary because each time she has fractured a vertebra on account of her osteoporosis, she was kept in the hospital emergency room for 12 to 36 hours and underwent repeated bone scans and other seemingly needless tests. It seems prudent to state the case for what is reasonable but to allow as much self-determination and autonomous action as possible. This respect for the patient's autonomy may help cement or enhance the doctor-patient relationship. In fact, many elderly who exhibit extraordinary independence appear to do well despite their selective lack of participation in medical care or other support systems. Segerberg (38) anecdotally describes manifestations of exceptional independence in 1200 centenarians. Extraordinary independence should be studied more as a positive factor in successful aging, at least in some persons.

A reevaluation of mental health disorders is taking place, as seen not by the psychiatrist but rather by the primary care physician. This new perspective started with pioneering work from British general practitioners (39). Primary care physicians working with nurses, social workers, and others are managing depression in the elderly in primary care practice. New research from primary care is helping in redefining diagnostic criteria for many disorders in the elderly, including depression (e.g., depression without sadness) and dementia (40).

Helping the Disconnected Family

Climo (13, 14) critically examines the consequences of geographic separation when elders and adult children live at some distance from each other. American culture today fosters disconnectedness. Although some American families resemble the Norman Rockwell portrait, others do not. Many teenagers and young adults are thinking of the future and are not able to identify with their parents or grandparents. Many middle-aged persons are still thinking of the future and unable to identify with their elderly parents. Each is in a separate compartment and has difficulty with the cultural diversity between generations. The members of each generation may have their own dress and hair code, music, values, religious beliefs, friends, and traditions. If they gather for Thanksgiving or a wedding, it may be an ordeal. The parents may not want the grandparents to know that the grandchild is having problems with drugs. The parents may have moved away from a faith community that had great meaning to the grandparents. Secrets about marital status or financial problems may be commonplace between members or branches of a family. In fulfillment of independent living, with each generation determining its own existence, there is a disconnectedness, separation, isolation, and loneliness that each generation feels, particularly the elderly, who are not busy with work or child rearing and who are disappointed over their lack of connection with their children and grandchildren. Elders may feel dejected, wishing for more contact with their family members, their community or other people, and the elders simply may not be able to make these connections. They may especially be separated from young people who have chosen a new direction for their lives. The physician caring for the elderly must be prepared to deal with distant children, family estrangement, families rocked by divorce, and in general the lack of a support system. Understanding principles of family systems and family therapy is necessary. Whether it is in caring for the frail, disabled elder who suddenly cannot take care of herself or in providing end-of-life care, the physician must be able to deal with these complexities.

Successful Aging

We have already referred to the importance of meaning and value in the lives of elders. This may be heterogeneous, whether fulfillment in a family relationship, relationship with spouse, accomplishments in work past or present, helping someone or some cause, or spiritual or religious beliefs or values that provide fulfillment. We have already referred to the many approaching retirement who would like to work to continue the pleasure of exercising their knowledge and skill in an employment that brings pleasure. Many may find fulfillment in the arts and begin the writing or ceramics or painting that they always yearned to do.

The most successful aging would seem to be characterized by good health, but many with chronic disorders still age successfully. If health is not good, the elder should be free of some of the hardships of entering the medical or long-term care world, such as physical restraints that may be used unnecessarily in nursing homes. Financial stability ordinarily is a requirement, but some with meager incomes age successfully. As mentioned, some yearn for work, but there are barriers that prevent or obstruct the elder's fulfillment of these aspirations. Elders may embrace a course of volunteerism that brings great satisfaction. Although there is no financial reward, the elder may feel useful and find fulfillment in providing voluntary service to a cause. Spiritual participation or spiritual beliefs may bring the greatest satisfaction to many elders, and the physician should aim for an understanding of the elder's religious or spiritual perspective and beliefs. In many of the world's religions, to be old is associated with wisdom and great respect, but although our religious leaders and scriptures state that belief, it is often lost in American culture. Decades ago the extended family had great meaning in American culture and around the world. Not only has the extended family diminished in this country, but it is in transition around the world in less developed nations.

With more Americans living long, how do we promote successful aging? How do we allow more meaningful part-time or full-time work roles when desired? How do we encourage physical activity and exercise, good nutrition, and other measures of health maintenance? How do we reduce isolation and separateness from family and community? How do we create greater bonds of love and friendship for the elder? How do we aim for a society with financial or social security that will allow those approaching their older years not to worry about their future ability to exist comfortably and not to worry about the cost of future health care and long-term care? Not only should the elderly not have to worry about their future housing or health care, but they should be able to focus on their sources of greatest fulfillment: awaiting their grandson's college graduation; awaiting the birth of their great-granddaughter; attending the religious service that provides comfort and reassurance; or participating in the art or voluntary cause or job that they have sought. This is the challenge for America entering the new millennium, and we as physicians should be catalysts for bringing about those changes that would guarantee a successful aging for many, and not just for a few.

End-of-Life Care: Dying Well

As a society, we are beginning to realize that dying in America is often not optimal, and there is a crying out that end-of-life care must be improved. The negative aspects of the ways the dying process is handled by the medical profession and by families and their community has created a demand for assisted suicide. But there are many alternatives to assisted suicide that can improve the care of the dying patient. The greatest danger of assisted suicide or euthanasia in the era of cost cutting is that society or patients themselves will decide that their lives are not worth

living (41, 42). Woody Allen said, "Think of death as cutting down on your expenses." At a time when cost containment is paramount, we must fear for the frail, debilitated elderly, those who have been marginalized as a result of Alzheimer's disease and other major disorders.

Many initiatives in medical care, teaching, and research are focusing on improving the care of the dying (43). This has been called dying well (41, 44, 45), living while dying, and physician-assisted living. At first we thought that there was a rising interest in living wills and other advance directives (46) to be made with fully informed consent by a competent patient. Many elderly have witnessed burdensome, expensive, and apparently futile care provided to their friends and loved ones, and this has led to the importance of these health care directives, supported by the Cruzan Supreme Court decision and the Patient Self-Determination Act (46). In the last edition of this text, we wrote that the next decade will bring greater understanding and use of these advance directives, and thus the patient's preferences will be known and respected. But this has not happened (47). Only a minority of adult and older Americans have advance directives and the use of these instruments has not taken off.

Society is crying out for a paradigm shift in which people can die well, or continue to enjoy their family and loved ones and other treasures until their death. Pain must be alleviated, and we are near a point at which all pain in the dying will be manageable. All physicians should understand and use palliative care appropriately.

The paradigm shift calls for a change not only in physicians' practices but in the public's thinking. The patient dying well at home need not be required to go to the hospital for the final moments. We can expect that more terminally ill patients will choose to be at home to die with proper care from family, aides, caregivers, and volunteers, and as professionals we should respect and support the terminally ill patient's wish to die at home (45, 48). Doctors, health professionals, patients, and families will have to speak more openly about what is occurring and what options are available, particularly offering the possibility of comfort care and hospice principles. Home care, whether by the family or in a home hospice program, will be a choice that our patients will make with greater frequency, and we can anticipate a marked increase in attention to home care in our health care system in the years ahead.

Byock (45) speaks of the prospect for growth at the end of life. Dying can be a time of love and reconciliation, a time of transcendence of suffering. We can expect a new era in care at the end of life (45, 49). We must ensure greater continuity of care for dying patients. We must provide greater support to those caring for the dying and their family members. Again we must provide more and better information about treatment choices to dying patients and their families. As stated earlier, doctors and hospitals must treat their patients' pain. We must translate to the American people what Dyck, Lynn, Byock, and others have been proposing: that the possibility of dying well exists and that Americans should not be separated by a curtain from the dying process. Americans can more frequently die at home or in other care settings where they are surrounded by loved ones, and without the sword of pain as a threat. The patient's family and friends, the patient's faith community, the patient's doctor and the entire hospice team all can provide comfort, love, support, and spiritual counseling during the patient's life, and they will also be there in the bereavement period. America is crying out for this change to take place. We can expect that this will be the role of all primary care doctors as well as other health professionals in the years ahead.

REFERENCES

1. Holden C. New populations of old add to poor nations' burden. Science 1996;273:46–48.
2. Oshima S. Japan: feeling the strains of an aging population. Science 1996;273:44–45.
3. Engel GL. The need for a new medical model: a challenge for biomedicine. Science 1977;196:129–136.
4. Engel GL. How much longer must medicine's science be bound by a seventeenth century world view? Psychother Psychosom 1992;57:3–16.
5. Gulette EC, Blumenthal JA, Babyak M, et al. Effects of mental status on myocardial ischemia during daily life. JAMA 1997;277:1521–1526.
6. Reynolds P, Boyd PT, Blocklow RS, et al. The relationship between social ties and survival among black and white cancer patients. Cancer Epidemiol Biomarkers Prev 1994;3:253–259.
7. Pratt LA, Ford DE, Crum RM, et al. Depression, psychotropic medication, and risk of myocardial infarction. Prospective data from the Baltimore ECA follow-up. Circulation 1996;94:3123–3129.
8. Everson SA, Kaplan GA, Goldberg DE, et al. Hopelessness and 4-year progression of carotid atherosclerosis: The Kuopio Ischemic Heart Disease Risk Factor Study. Arterioscler Thromb Vasc Biol 1997;17:1490–1495.
9. Wasson JH, Sauvigne AE, Mogielnicki RP, et al. Continuity of outpatient medical care in elderly men: a randomized trial. JAMA 1984;2532:2413–2417.
10. Reichel W. The continuity imperative. JAMA 1981;246:2065.
11. Stone R, Cafferata GL, Sangl J. Caregivers of the frail elderly: a national profile. Gerontologist 1987;27:616–626.
12. Shanas E. Social myth as hypothesis: the case of the family relations of old people. Gerontologist 1979;19:3–9.
13. Climo J. Visits of distant living adult children and elderly parents. J Aging Studies 1988;2:57–69.
14. Climo J. Distant Parents. New Brunswick, NJ: Rutgers University Press, 1992.
15. Peabody FW. The care of the patient. JAMA 1927;88:877–882.
16. Frankl VE. Man's Search for Meaning. Boston: Beacon Press, 1959.
17. Frankl VE. The Doctor and the Soul. New York: Knopf, 1955.
18. Yalom ID. Existential Psychotherapy. New York: Basic Books, 1980.
19. Cassel EJ. The nature of suffering and the goals of medicine. N Engl J Med 1982;306:639–645.
20. Kushner H. When All You've Ever Wanted Isn't Enough. New York: Summit Books, 1986.
21. Cousins N. The physician as communicator. JAMA 1982;248:587–589.
22. Frank JD, Frank JB. Persuasion and Healing: A Comparative Study of Psychotherapy. 3rd ed. Baltimore: Johns Hopkins University Press, 1991.
23. Elahi D, Clark B, Andres R. Glucose tolerance, insulin sensitivity and age. In: Armbracht HJ, Coe RM, Wongsurawat N, eds. Endocrine Function and Aging. New York: Springer-Verlag, 1990:48–63.
24. Rowe JW, Andres R, Tobin JR, et al. The effect of age on creatinine clearance in men: a cross-sectional and longitudinal study. J Gerontol 1976;31:155–163.
25. Reichel W. Multiple problems in the elderly. In: Reichel W, ed. The Geriatric Patient. New York: Hospital Practice 1978:17–22.
26. Fiatarone MA, Evans WJ. The etiology and reversibility of muscle dysfunctions in the aged. J Gerontol 1993;48:77–83 (special issue).
27. Fiatarone MA, O'Neill EF, Ryan ND, et al. Exercise training and nutritional supplementation for physical frailty in very elderly patients. N Engl J Med 1994;330:1769–1775.
28. Lord SR, Ward JA, Williams P, Strudwick M. The effect of a 12-month exercise trial on balance, strength, and falls in older women. J Am Geriatr Soc 1995;43:1198–1206.

29. Guide to Clinical Preventive Services. Report of the U.S. Preventive Services Task Force. 2nd ed. Baltimore: Williams & Wilkins, 1996.

30. Seegal D. The principle of minimal interference in the management of the elderly patient. J Chron Dis 1964; 17:299–300.

31. Reichel W. Complications in the care of 500 elderly hospitalized patients. J Am Geriatr Soc 1965;13:973–981.

32. Steel K, Gertman PM, Crescenzi C, Anderson J. Iatrogenic illness on a general medical service at a university hospital. N Engl J Med 1981;304:638–642.

33. Lipp MR. Respectful Treatment: A Practical Handbook of Patient Care. 2nd ed. New York: Elsevier, 1986.

34. Ekerdt DJ, DeViney S, Kosloski K. Profiling plans for retirement. J Gerontol Soc Sci 1996;51B:S140-S149.

35. Glick S. Humanistic medicine in a modern age. N Engl J Med 1981;304:1036–1038.

36. Keeler EB, Solomon DH, Beck JC, et al. Effect of patient age on duration of medical encounters with physicians. Med Care 1982;20:1101–1108.

37. Wagner GS, Cebe B, Rozear MP, eds. What This Patient Needs Is a Doctor. Durham, NC: Carolina Academic Press, 1978.

38. Segerberg O. Living to Be 100. New York: Scribners, 1982.

39. Shepherd M, Cooper B, Brown AC, Kalton GW. Psychiatric Illness in General Practice. London: Oxford University Press, 1966.

40. Gallo JJ, Rabins PV, Lyketosos CG, et al. Depression without sadness: functional outcomes of nondysphoric depression in later life. J Am Geriatr Soc 1997;45:1–9.

41. Reichel W, Dyck AJ. Euthanasia: a contemporary moral quandary. Lancet 1989;2(8675):132–133.

42. Lynn J, Cohn F, Pickering JH, et al. The American Geriatrics Society on physician-assisted suicide: brief to the U.S. Supreme Court. J Am Geriatr Soc 1997;45:489–499.

43. Horgan J. Seeking a better way to die. Sci Am 1997; 276(5):100–105.

44. Dyck AJ. An Alternative to the ethic of euthanasia. In: Williams RH, ed. To Live and to Die: When, Why, and How? New York: Springer-Verlag, 1973:98–112.

45. Byock I. Dying Well: The Prospect for Growth at the End of Life. New York: Riverhead Books/Putnam, 1997.

46. Doukas DJ, Reichel W. Planning for Uncertainty: A Guide to Living Wills and Other Advance Directives for Health Care. Baltimore: Johns Hopkins University Press, 1993.

47. Siwek J. Decision-making in terminal care: four common pitfalls. Am Fam Physician 1994;50:1207–1208, 1211.

48. Sankar A. Dying at Home: A Family Guide for Caregiving. Baltimore: Johns Hopkins University Press, 1991.

49. Lynn J. Caring at the end of our lives. N Engl J Med 1996;335:201–202.

Multidimensional Assessment of the Older Patient

The cornerstone of the practice of geriatric medicine is the multidimensional assessment of the elderly. The term comprehensive geriatric assessment (CGA) refers to this process of evaluation and management of older patients. Although most people maintain good health and independent functioning as they age, multiple illnesses and their associated disabilities affect many seniors. The 1987 National Institutes of Health (NIH) consensus conference defined CGA as "a multidisciplinary evaluation in which the multiple problems of older patients are uncovered, described, and explained, if possible, and in which the resources and strengths of the person are catalogued, need for services assessed, and a coordinated care plan developed to focus interventions on the person's problems" (1). All definitions of CGA include emphasis on the multidisciplinary and interdisciplinary nature of this process. This approach is useful in all settings in which we encounter older patients, whether in the home, office, hospital, day facility, or institutional setting.

The traditional medical model for the care of patients focuses on the differential diagnosis of single symptoms. This process culminates in a specific organ system diagnosis and does not allow for the comprehensive evaluation of the typical geriatric patient who has multisystem disease complicated by other functional and psychosocial limitations. CGA allows us to focus on the disease and how it affects the person's ability to function successfully in his or her en-

vironment. Treatment plans can then be developed that emphasize functional independence as an important goal. A more holistic approach to the patient includes not only medical diagnostic accuracy but also optimal functioning within environmental limitations as a priority.

The roots of CGA are found in the British system of health care. In 1930, Marjory Warren developed geriatric assessment units in a large chronic care hospital (2). She recognized the importance of accurate diagnosis and assessment of older patients, who were often left neglected on chronic care wards. In the United States in the second half of this century we began to appreciate the effect of aging population trends on our health care system. It is now well recognized that persons over age 65 constitute a major segment of our population. The fastest-growing population in this country is the very old, over age 85, who have complex medical, functional, and psychosocial problems (3).

In the 1970s, the Department of Veterans Affairs (VA) recognized the growing aging veteran population and developed specialized geriatric research, education, and clinical centers (GRECCs) (4). These programs began to explore the benefits of CGA in the VA health care system.

In 1987, the NIH held its consensus development conference, which defined the goals, structure, process, and elements of geriatric assessment. Methods of assessment and their efficacy in various settings were reviewed by the consensus panel. Emphasis was placed on the need to incorporate CGA into the overall health care system for seniors and to identify areas for future research (1).

The past 10 to 15 years in this country has seen an expansion of the literature dealing with CGA. Additional texts include *Assessing the Elderly: A Practical Guide to Assessment* (6), the *Handbook of Geriatric Assessment* (7), and *Geriatric Assessment Technology: State of the Art* (8).

VALUE OF CGA

Determining the value of a given health care intervention requires that we examine the relation between quality and cost. The quality of a procedure is typically measured by its ability to produce desirable outcomes for the patient. The outcomes monitored in most studies addressing the effectiveness of CGA include mortality, hospital readmission and institutionalization rates, and level of physical and cognitive function. Cost effectiveness has not been well documented.

One of the first studies in this country to demonstrate the effect of an inpatient geriatric evaluation and management unit (GEMU) was published more than 10 years ago (9). It demonstrated improved 6-month survival in patients managed on an inpatient GEMU versus traditional VA hospital care. Since then a number of studies have addressed the role of CGA in inpatient GEMUs, inpatient geriatric consultation services, home assessment programs, posthospital services, and outpatient assessment services.

A recent meta-analysis identified more than 100 studies addressing CGA in various settings (10, 11). Of these, 28 studies were found to meet criteria for inclusion in the meta-analysis in that they truly examined the CGA intervention, were some form of a controlled trial, and provided usable information about outcomes. None of these studies demonstrated any negative influence on outcome by CGA. The strongest positive effects were found in the 6 inpatient GEMU studies. In this setting, there appeared to be a statistically significant 28% reduction in 6-month mortality, although this benefit diminished at 12-month follow-up. At 6 and 12 months, patients were 80% and 68%

more likely to be living at home than control populations. Hospital readmissions did not seem to be affected by the intervention.

The 8 studies of inpatient geriatric consult services demonstrated an effect on cognitive function but no influence on other outcome variables. The 7 in-home assessment programs showed a reduction in short-term mortality and institutional placement that was statistically significant. No consistent effect on hospitalization rates was demonstrated. The 4 outpatient CGA programs did not reveal any positive effect on the outcomes measured.

The variation in these results may, in part, be due to differences in program structure. The GEMU studies typically had control over the implementation of recommendations made by the assessment team. Inadequate provision for long-term outpatient follow-up was thought to be an important factor in the lack of benefit of outpatient, primarily consultative programs. The targeting of patients in some studies has also been problematic in that inclusion criteria for the assessment did not always focus on patients who would benefit from the intervention.

Another flaw may be the choice of traditional outcomes in the study evaluation process. Although a mortality benefit was demonstrated, death alone in a typically frail population may not be as important as quality of life. Patient and family satisfaction are also important outcomes. Although costly, institutionalization may be the best outcome for patients for whom life in a community setting is burdensome. Limited availability and cost of community programs such as day care may also adversely affect outcomes of CGA.

Finally, the success of CGA may be hindered by the fragmentation of information about individual patients across different levels of care. Repeated assessments in the hospital, outpatient, and long-term care settings are often performed without accurate transfer of information. These systems problems must be addressed to maximize the usefulness of the information and recommendations made in CGA. This will allow heath care providers to identify and respond to changes in functional level and psychosocial status in a timely and effective manner.

TARGETING

Identifying patients who will most likely benefit from a CGA is an important part of any effective program. Many criteria have been proposed (12). Any targeting criteria must be easy to use by patients, caregivers, and medical support staff, in the health care setting, or by phone. The criteria should take into account the goals of the program. The more intensive a program is in regard to time, cost, and overall difficulty of performance, the more restrictive the criteria should be. The selection of criteria is also based on our knowledge of the prevalence of the problem in a given population (12–14).

Health care usage indicators are often the focus for managed care organizations because of their concerns about managing health care costs for their enrollees (15). Such a strategy may not identify underusers of health care services who might benefit from assessment programs. This is a problem with screening programs that focus on self-reporting. A successful program must incorporate aggressive case finding as part of its screening process. The overall success of the targeting program depends on the development of criteria that are appropriate for the setting and the goals of the program. Table 2.1 lists recommended target criteria for patients who may be appropriate for CGA.

Exclusion criteria also should be considered. Patients who are too healthy or too sick are unlikely to benefit from CGA. Healthier patients are more likely to benefit from less intensive evaluations that focus on health care maintenance and disease prevention. Terminally ill and end-stage patients may be more likely to benefit from programs that focus on terminal and/or palliative care. However, even for these patients, CGA may be the process through which these care needs are identified.

The Short Form 36 questionnaire (SF-36) was developed for use in the Medical Outcome Study in the United States. The SF-36 detects differences in health status for patients with a variety of medical illnesses (16, 17). It includes questions on physical functioning, mental health, and general health perceptions. The abbreviated SF-12 has been developed for screening large populations. Such standardized tools may be useful to target patients who might benefit from CGA. These tools have been demonstrated to be useful in the elderly but are not without their problems.

THE CGA TEAM

By definition, comprehensive geriatric assessment is multidisciplinary and requires the expertise of multiple health care professionals. Traditional medical training emphasizes the physician-patient relationship. Many physicians have not been trained to function as members of a health care team. The composition of the team and the formality of the relations between the team members often vary with the setting in which the assessment is performed.

Typically the physician plays a central role, particularly in the initial assessment, accurate medical diagnosis being an important basis of the rest of the assessment. In acute care hospital settings the physician's role is pivotal, since the patient also has acute medical problems that must be accurately diagnosed and treated. The outcomes from that process affect the findings and recommendations of the assessment team.

Nurse practitioners and physician's assistants can often help gather medical information and

Table 2.1

Targeting Criteria for CGA

Age over 80
Geriatric syndromes
  Incontinence
  Confusion, dementia
  Impaired mobility, falls, fractures
  Malnutrition, weight loss
  Sensory impairment
  Pressure sores
Depression
Multiple chronic illnesses
Impaired activities of daily living
Polypharmacy
Support system problems
Hospital readmissions, health care usage information
  Frequent office and emergency room visits
Specific diagnoses, e.g., diabetes mellitus, congestive
   heart failure, coronary artery disease

Table 2.2

Geriatric Assessment Team

Core team
   Physician
   Geriatric nurse practitioner, physician's assistant
   Nurse
   Social worker
   Care manager
Extended team
   Physical therapist
   Occupational therapist
   Speech therapist
   Pharmacist
   Dietitian
   Psychologist
   Podiatrist
   Optometrist
   Audiologist
   Medical subspecialists
   Neurologist
   Physiatrist
   Psychiatrist
   Other subspecialists

can be important assets to a geriatric assessment team. Nursing traditionally provides input on functional assessment and patient care needs. Social work also plays an important role in the geriatric team.

Most outpatient programs have three primary team members, the physician, nurse, and social worker. Additional consultation may be requested from extended team members. Case managers or care managers are also playing an increasing role in CGA. Hospital inpatient and other institution-based teams are frequently larger and may include all of the disciplines in the initial assessment process. The role of different team members may vary according to the nature of the problems uncovered. Frequently the physician's role may be less important. Disciplines represented in the core and extended geriatric assessment team are listed in Table 2.2.

COMPONENTS OF GERIATRIC ASSESSMENT

The traditional domains of CGA are outlined in Table 2.3. Evaluation of physical health includes the gathering of information through the traditional history and physical examination and the development of a list showing the status and severity of acute and chronic medical problems. Assessment of vision and hearing is an important part of this process. The history and physical examination also focus on problems identified in other areas of the assessment. For example, the functional assessment may identify problems with gait and mobility that require more thorough neurologic and musculoskeletal assessment to determine causality. The assessment should also address appropriate health care maintenance and primary, secondary, and tertiary health care prevention. Because of the prevalence of poor nutrition, an appropriate nutritional evaluation should be part of the assessment. Additional testing may be done to diagnose the patient's medical problems.

Evaluation of functional status includes information on the patient's ability to perform basic and complex activities of daily living. Gait, balance, and risk of falls should also be assessed. The findings on functional assessment are often linked to the basic physical health assessment.

Table 2.3

Domains of Geriatric Assessment

Physical health
   Traditional history and physical examination
   Hearing and vision screen
Continence assessment
   Gait, mobility, and falls risk assessment
   Nutrition and dietary assessment
Functional ability
   Activities of daily living
   Instrumental activities of daily living
   Performance measures
Mental health
   Cognitive screening and assessment
   Depression screening and assessment
Social support
   Social history
   Values assessment and advance directive
     information
   Caregiver burden
   Finances
Environmental adequacy

Mental health evaluation should include the use of standardized cognitive screens and more thorough testing when indicated. Because of the atypical presentation of depression in this age group, screening for depression should also be included. Overall health satisfaction may be a reflection of psychologic health.

The social assessment should identify support network strengths and weaknesses. Some determination of the patient's values and the presence or absence of formal advance directives should be determined. Caregiver burden should be evaluated. Financial resources to meet current and future needs should also be assessed.

Environmental issues should be evaluated through patient and/or family reports or direct observation of the living situation. Accurate information allows for recommendations that may maximize functional independence in the individual's environment and address basic safety issues.

GERIATRIC ASSESSMENT TOOLS

Selecting appropriate tools for CGA requires consideration of the purpose, goals, and setting of the assessment. The literature is filled with scales and questionnaires that can be used to assess older patients. It is important to understand how a given tool has been developed and for what purpose it was designed. Although the value of standardized measurements cannot be overemphasized, there are also pitfalls in overreliance on the results (20). Whether the tool is based on self-report, caregiver report, or direct observation can influence the quality of the information obtained. The validity of self-reports may be affected by the patient's mood, cognitive abilities, and health care beliefs. The reliability of caregiver reports may reflect the caregiver's perception of a problem and its significance. Direct observation usually provides the most useful information and can often complement self- or caregiver reporting. The patient's performance may also be affected by the timing of the assessment. For instance, the performance on a mental status examination may be affected by the presence of an acute illness and not accurately reflect the patient's true baseline.

Understanding the sensitivity and specificity of a given assessment instrument is important to interpreting the results. It is important to know the populations on which a given tool was validated. Some tools may be appropriate for all patients; others may be used more selectively according to the presenting complaints at the time of the assessment. The administration of most tools requires some degree of training. It is important to know whether a given tool has been shown to have interrater reliability as well as test-retest reliability. All assessment tools have some limitations that should be considered in the overall final assessment of the patient and in developing recommendations from the assessment process.

MEDICAL HISTORY AND PHYSICAL ASSESSMENT

A thorough conventional medical history, physical examination, and diagnostic evaluation are critical to the assessment process. The process focuses on the definition of acute and chronic medical problems. This part of the evaluation often identifies areas that should have further assessment and/or diagnostic studies.

History taking from the older patient involves a unique interrelationship among the patient, a family member or caregiver, and the physician. The traditional interviewing process taught in medical training often does not address the additional skills needed in this triangular relationship. The skilled clinician quickly identifies the roles of the various parties in the interviewing process. Since the assessment typically deals with frail older patients, caregiver and/or family input is often needed to obtain accurate information or to confirm the patient's reports. However, it is also important to appreciate the different perceptions of a problem that the patient and his or her family member or caregiver may have. Other members of the interdisciplinary team may also provide insight into the validity of the history. Patients and their family members may share different information with different team members.

Most older patients have multiple complaints because they have multiple problems that require evaluation. Older patients tend to underreport symptoms, and careful questioning is necessary to evaluate the presence and seriousness of a complaint. Sensory problems, particularly difficulty hearing, can undermine the history taking. Access to augmentative hearing devices is important. Even if the patient's reliability is questioned because of cognitive problems, it is important to listen to the his or her description of symptoms. In most settings older patients try to present themselves in a very positive fashion. This may reflect their fear of an underlying serious medical problem or simply their desire to please the health care provider. Since the assessment is often initiated by another party or as a result of a recent change in condition, older patients are often fearful that the assessment may result in recommendations for further limitations of their functional independence. All of these factors need to be weighed in history taking.

It is always important to address patients in a professional manner and to request permission for inclusion of family members or caregivers in the assessment process. These efforts result in improved buy-in by the older person. Developing this mutually respectful relationship is also important to obtaining compliance with subsequent recommendations. It is helpful to explore the patient's perceptions of previous health care encounters and prior relations with physicians. Their basic health care belief systems should be explored and considered in the assessment and in subsequent recommendations.

In addition to the traditional chronicling of information about acute and chronic medical problems, information about health care maintenance status should be obtained. Although the value to a given patient of some of the standard preventive screenings may be questioned, it is important to evaluate each person's health care maintenance profile. In particular, many seniors are not adequately immunized. In spite of aggressive public health efforts, many do not receive annual flu vaccines and have not received recommended Pneumovax vaccination. Information on recent health assessments, including recent diagnostic tests and their results, should be obtained.

Past and current tobacco use should be noted. Alcohol abuse often goes undiagnosed in older patients, and screening with simple tools such as

the CAGE (need to cut down, annoyed by others' criticism of drinking, guilty feelings, eye opener) is often effective in identifying substance abuse problems (21). Documenting caffeine intake is also important, particularly since older patients may suffer from cardiovascular and sleep disorders in which caffeine may play a role. History of falls and injuries should be part of the assessment of risk of falls.

An accurate medication history must include current medications, prior treatment failures, and adverse drug reactions. Use of over-the-counter medications is important. True drug allergies should also be explored. Issues relating to medication compliance should also be addressed, recognizing that poor compliance or adherence to a medical regimen may reflect adverse reactions, cognitive problems, the person's health care beliefs, the complexity of the regimen, and cost concerns. Caregivers may have assumed some or all of the responsibility for obtaining and administering medications. Health care professionals may erroneously assume that they are complying with the prescribed regimen. In these instances, caregiver compliance should also be explored, as their compliance is often affected by the same limitations as the patient's.

The elderly patient's family history is frequently undervalued. There is often a concept that they have survived the risk of many illnesses, but even at a later age family history may identify an important risk factor.

The medical review of systems should focus on common geriatric syndromes such as continence, falls and mobility problems, sleep problems, cognitive problems, alterations in mood, and bowel dysfunction. Since cardiopulmonary disease is so prevalent in this population, a careful review is warranted.

The physical assessment should include an accurate general observation of the patient, which often provides clues to underlying problems. Poor hygiene may reflect other functional impairments that should be addressed in further assessment of the patient. Vital signs should include postural blood pressures and an accurate determination of the patient's height and weight. Height loss may indicate unrecognized osteoporosis. Weight loss may reflect undiagnosed nutritional problems. Simple screening of vision should be included, as this may affect many areas of function as well as performance on assessment instruments requiring visual acuity. Evaluation of hearing, which should be included, can be done with a simple whisper test, an audioscope, or more sophisticated testing (22). Further evaluation of the effect of hearing loss on the person's function can be obtained through screens such as the Hearing Handicap Inventory (23). An accurate dental assessment is important, as dentition may affect nutrition. If a patient has dentures, their fit should be assessed. The rest of a comprehensive physical examination should also be completed.

Laboratory studies are often ordered as part of the physical health assessment. Laboratory tests should be based on the specific symptom presentation (e.g., memory loss) or reflect appropriate monitoring of drug therapy.

FUNCTIONAL ASSESSMENT

Maintaining or improving functional status is at the core of geriatric medicine, and an accurate functional assessment is critical to CGA. Tools chosen to assist in functional assessment should be based on the purpose, setting, and timing of the assessment (20). Typically, function is measured in two areas: the activities of daily living (ADL) and the instrumental activities of daily living (IADL) (Table 2.4). The former refers to basic self-care activities. Most ADL measurement tools address some combination of dressing, toileting, transferring, feeding, bathing, continence, grooming, communication, and mobility. Typically ADL performance is lost in a predictable sequence. Skills for bathing and dressing are diminished before transferring, toileting, grooming, and eating. An atypical pattern of loss may have diagnostic significance. For example, early loss of continence may reflect a more localized problem with the genitourinary system. ADL deficits often indicate a need for in-home assistance in the community setting. The number and type of deficits suggest the amount of assistance needed. Problems with bathing alone may indicate a need for a home health aide 2 to 3 times per week, whereas dependence in more areas may require daily or 24-hour care.

Table 2.4

Common Tasks Included in ADL and IADL Scales

Katz Index of Activities of Daily Living
  Bathing
  Dressing
  Grooming
  Toileting
  Transfer
  Continence
  Feeding
  Communication
Lawton Instrumental Activities of Daily Living
  Shopping
  Cooking and meal preparation
  Laundry
  Using telephone
  Managing medication
  Transportation
  Household cleaning
  Managing finances

IADL includes the more complex functional activities generally required of a person independently living in the community. As these activities are often more complex than ADL, they may be more readily affected by mood and motivation. They are also affected by living arrangements (e.g., a nursing home resident does not use housekeeping skills). Activities typically measured are included in Table 2.4. The IADL items have a cultural and sex bias (24). Women are more likely to have skills in meal preparation, and men may have a more active role in managing finances. These more complex skills are usually impaired before basic ADL skills. Problems in these areas may be an early indication of cognitive or other mental health problems.

In most ADL and IADL scales, reported performance is rated for each activity. The rating may be as simple as independent versus dependent or may allow for various levels of assistance in performing the task. The goal of the test may be to measure performance or to measure the ability to perform. The latter may be adversely affected by problems with motivation, fear, or depression (25). Cognitive function may also influence results. Patients with dementia may require supervision to perform a task. For tools with either a dependent or independent rating, there should be a clear understanding of how tasks that require various levels of supervision but not actual physical assistance are to be rated (26). Many ADL scales do not take into account patients' preferences, as persons may not have skills in certain areas of their own choice. Most scales are limited in their ability to measure small changes over time that may actually indicate significant alteration in a patient's independence level. In scoring some tools, information regarding performance of specific tasks is lost. Therefore, it is important that not only total scores but also patterns of performance on those scales be examined (20, 25).

The Katz Index of Activities of Daily Living is a common ADL tool (27). The Katz Index was initially developed in a rehabilitation hospital to monitor patients' function over time. It has since been adapted for use in many settings. A commonly used measure of IADL was developed by Lawton and has since been adapted as a self-rated tool in the Duke University Multidimensional Functional Assessment Questionnaire (28, 29). Additional listings of functional assessment tools are available elsewhere (20, 25, 30).

Although there may be a role for developing new assessment tools, it would be better to focus efforts on refining the tools that have been developed. We should agree upon standards for measurement across the continuum of care. Different facilities within the same health care system often use different functional assessment tools, which may limit the value of the information.

To avoid some of the pitfalls encountered in the use of the traditional functional assessment measures, actual performance measures have been developed (31). The patient is typically asked to complete a specific task and is then evaluated by an objective observer to see whether the person meets criteria for accurate performance. The criterion may be the number of repetitions within a given time or the overall time needed to perform the activity. Many of these performance measures include tasks that are important components of ADL and IADL skills. Their role in CGA is not clear, and their superiority to other functional assessment tools has not been demonstrated. On the other hand, there are often significant differences between self-report and actual performance of an activity.

The Williams Timed Manual Performance Test has been used in the CGA setting; it seems to predict the need for additional services or actual institutional placement in the ensuing year (32). This test specifically involves the opening and closing of a number of fasteners followed by a series of activities including writing a sentence; turning over cards; picking up paper clips, pennies, and bottle caps and putting them in a can; stacking checkers; and transferring beans from a table to a coffee can. The activities are timed; individuals who take more than 350 seconds to complete the tasks are twice as likely to require services in the ensuing year as those who do not.

MENTAL HEALTH ASSESSMENT

Cognitive impairment and psychiatric illness are often inaccurately diagnosed in older patients. Conservative estimates indicate dementia in at least 5% of those over age 65 and in 20% over age 80. Estimates are that 50 to 80% of nursing facility residents have some degree of cognitive impairment. Depression as an isolated disorder or associated with other chronic medical problems is also prevalent. Many of the risk factors for depression occur with increased frequency as persons age. Late life is filled with many losses and major life stressors. Death of family and friends is increasingly common, as is the loss of one's physical health.

A formal mental status evaluation includes evaluation of multiple domains. Cognitive assessment includes evaluation of level of consciousness, attention, language skills, short-term and remote memory, orientation, abstract thinking, and performance on visuospatial tasks. A number of screening instruments help to identify problems with cognition (7). Various screening tools may concentrate on different aspects of cognition. For example, the Short Portable Mental Status Questionnaire consists of 10 questions that test orientation, memory, and calculation (33). The number of errors correlates with the degree of intellectual impairment. Up to two errors is considered normal. The score is also adjusted for lower levels of education. The specificity in community-dwelling elders is fairly high, although its sensitivity is fairly low. One major advantage is that this test is easy for clinicians to remember and simple to score (7). The fairly widely used Folstein Mini-Mental State Examination (MMSE) covers some additional areas of cognition (Table 2.5) (34). The MMSE is thought to be more sensitive than the Short Portable Mental Status Questionnaire. It tests delayed recall, written and spoken language, constructual abilities, orientation, and calculations. The maximum score is 30, and in general a score of 24 or below indicates cognitive impairment. The minimum acceptable score is reduced for persons with low levels of education. More highly educated patients may score normal and still have an underlying dementia (35, 36). It is important to remember that other disorders besides dementia may affect cognition. Patients who are delirious score poorly, as do patients with other brain disorders. Depressed patients may also score poorly on cognitive scales (34).

There are other useful assessment tools for patients who have been diagnosed as having dementia. The Hachinski Ischemic Score was developed to differentiate vascular dementia from degenerative dementia (37). Specific dementia rating scales often combine formal cognitive testing with functional variables. These tests, such as the Blessed Dementia Score (38) and the Functional Dementia Scale (39), assess the severity of the dementia. The Global Deterioration Scale, which has been further expanded into the FAST staging tool for Alzheimer's disease, has been found to correlate with scores on the MMSE (40, 41). Typically, Alzheimer's disease is divided into three stages: early, middle, and late. The Global Deterioration Scale identifies seven levels of progression, from no cognitive decline to end-stage disease. FAST staging adds levels to the later stages of the disease and relates functional deficits to the stages. Variation from the typical progression of dementia can suggest other diagnostic possibilities. For example, urinary incontinence in an early stage of the disease may suggest a urinary tract infection. These scales can also predict the need for additional supervision,

services, and even institutional placement, as well as mortality. They are most effective in programs geared to the evaluation of patients with cognitive dysfunction and for following these patients over time.

Depression is often underrecognized in the primary care setting, particularly in older patients. Depression may present atypically in older patients, sometimes with primarily cognitive problems, which has resulted in the term pseudodementia. Depressed older people may have a variety of somatic complaints rather than the typical mood symptoms of younger patients. Many physical illnesses and medications can be associated with depression and should be sought in the assessment process.

Routine screening for depression in CGA is important. Scales used to identify depression document depressive symptoms and their severity as derived from the criteria for major depression found in *Diagnostic and Statistical Manual of Mental Disorders,* 4th edition (DSM-IV) (42). Examples of such scales include the Zung Self-Rating Depression Scale, which consists of 20 statements the patient rates on a scale of 1 to 4 according to frequency of the symptoms (43). Elderly patients tend to score higher, which is probably related to the physical symptoms addressed in the scale (44). The Beck Depression Inventory is administered by an interviewer. It contains 21 statements related to depressive symptoms; the patient is asked to say whether he or she has these feelings rarely, sometimes, occasionally, or most of the time (45). A short self-administered version has also been developed (46).

The Geriatric Depression Scale (GDS) consists of a 30-item yes or no questionnaire (Table 2.6) (47). Higher scores reflect the presence and severity of underlying depression. The short form of the GDS consists of 15 questions. Although it has not been as well validated, it may be useful as a short screening tool (48, 49). The GDS is not very useful in dementia patients (50). The Cornell Scale of Depression and Dementia may be more sensitive in identifying depression in patients who are demented (51). Results of standardized assessment instruments should be weighed in the overall assessment process.

Table 2.5

Mini-Mental State Examination

Maximum Score	Score	
		ORIENTATION
5	( )	1. What is the (year) (season) (date) (day) (month)?
5	( )	2. Where are we: (state) (country) (town) (hospital) (floor)?
		REGISTRATION
3	( )	3. Name 3 objects: 1 second to say each. Then ask the patient all 3 after you have said them.
		Give 1 point for each correct answer. Then repeat them until he or she learns all 3. Count trials and record.
		Trials
		ATTENTION AND CALCULATION
5	( )	4. Serial 7s. 1 point for each correct. Stop after 5 answers. Alternatively, spell "world" backward if cannot subtract.
		RECALL
3	( )	5. Ask for 3 objects repeated above. Give 1 point for each correct.
		LANGUAGE
9	( )	6. Name a pencil and watch (2 points)
		7. Repeat the following: "No ifs, ands or buts." (1 point)
		8. Follow a 3-stage command: "Take a paper in your right hand, fold it in half, and put it on the floor." (3 points)
		9. Read and obey the following: "Close your eyes." (1 point)
		10. Write a sentence. (1 point)
		11. Copy design. (1 point)

TOTAL SCORE

1. 1 point for each correct answer.
2. 1 point for each correct answer.
3. 1 point for each of the 3 object names that is correctly repeated the first time. Then repeat them until all 3 are repeated but give no further points.
4. 1 point for each correct subtraction. If the patient does not or cannot make any subtractions, have him or her spell the word "world" backward. If an attempt at subtraction is made, this is the preferred task.
5. 1 point for each object.
6. 1 point for each correctly named object. Give no points if an approximate but incorrect word is used.
7. 1 point if completely and correctly completed.
8. 1 point for each command followed.
9. 1 point only if the patient carries out the activity. No points if the sentence is read correctly but the act is not done.
10. Sentence should be grammatically correct and have subject, verb, and predicate.
11. 1 point if each figure has 5 sides and the overlap is correct.

Reprinted with permission from Folstein MF, Folstein SE, McHugh PR. "Mini-mental state": a practical method for grading the cognitive state of patients for the clinician. J Psychiatr Res 1975;12:189. Copyright 1975, Pergamon Journals, Ltd. Courtesy of Dr. Marshal Folstein.

Table 2.6

Geriatric Depression Scale

1 Are you basically satisfied with your life? (no)
2 Have you dropped many of your activities and interests? (yes)
3 Do you feel that your life is empty? (yes)
4 Do you often get bored? (yes)
5 Are you hopeful about the future? (no)
6 Are you bothered by thoughts you cannot get out of your head? (yes)
7 Are you in good spirits most of the time? (no)
8 Are you afraid that something bad is going to happen to you? (yes)
9 Do you feel happy most of the time? (no)
10 Do you often feel helpless? (yes)
11 Do you often get restless and fidgety? (yes)
12 Do you prefer to stay home at night rather than do new things? (yes)
13 Do you frequently worry about the future? (yes)
14 Do you feel that you have more problems with memory than most? (yes)
15 Do you think it is wonderful to be alive now? (no)
16 Do you often feel downhearted and blue? (yes)
17 Do you feel pretty worthless the way you are now? (yes)
18 Do you worry a lot about the past? (yes)
19 Do you find life very exciting? (no)
20 Is it hard for you to get started on new projects? (yes)
21 Do you feel full of energy? (no)
22 Do you feel that your situation is hopeless? (yes)
23 Do you think that most people are better off than you are? (yes)
24 Do you frequently get upset over little things? (yes)
25 Do you frequently feel like crying? (yes)
26 Do you have trouble concentrating? (yes)
27 Do you enjoy getting up in the morning? (no)
28 Do you prefer to avoid social gatherings? (yes)
29 Is it easy for you to make decisions? (no)
30 Is your mind as clear as it used to be? (no)

Score one point for each response that matches the yes or no answer after the question.

Adapted from Yesavage JA. Brink TL. Development and validation of a geriatric depression screening scale: a preliminary report. J Psychiatr Res 1983;17:41. Copyright 1983, Pergamon Journals Ltd.

SOCIAL ASSESSMENT

Social assessment is another component of CGA. Information on family structure, available support systems, living arrangements, stressful life events, and basic financial resources is typically gathered.

Changes in basic family structure have affected the traditional support network available to many older patients. Many seniors have children over age 65. In the past women took on the role of caregiver for aging parents. As more women work and as many are themselves single parents, their ability to fulfill this role has been limited. Even an older child who is not working may have assumed another role for his or her own children or grandchildren that may lessen their ability to care for their parents. Smaller families means fewer adult children available to share the caregiving.

A person's informal support network may include neighbors and other lifelong friends. The presence of family members does not always correlate with healthy supportive relationships for the older person. Family members may have their own physical and/or mental health problems. A lifelong pattern of family dysfunction is not corrected by the stresses of caring for an aging relative. The majority of support for older patients in the community does come from this informal social support network. It is only when this support system fails or the person's needs overwhelm the ability of these care providers that more formal services are needed. These include mainly social welfare programs, which are available in many communities. Members of the assessment team, particularly the social worker, should be well acquainted with the services available in the community and the way they are accessed and financed. This information can often be obtained and updated from local offices on aging.

Since most patients presenting for a CGA have a physical or functional decline that precipitates the assessment, it is important to evaluate the patient's caregivers to determine their ability to participate in the ongoing support needed for the patient. Caregiver burnout may be one of the primary issues at hand. Structured questionnaires such as the Zarit Burden Interview (52) and the Caregiver Strain Index (53) help identify these issues in a structured manner. Recommendations from the assessment process may include a plan to lessen the caregiver's burden as well as recommendations for the caregiver to develop backup support for respite care to attend to his or her own physical and/or mental health needs. Linked with caregiver burden and stress is the concern for elder abuse or neglect. Clues may show up in the basic history and physical examination and may be further explored in the social assessment. The assessment may be requested by state or local adult protective service agencies, which may already be involved. Although the presence of actual abuse cannot be understated, the most common reason for referral to protective service agencies is self-neglect, often related to inadequate social support networks.

An understanding of the older person's financial situation is necessary to determine whether the person cane provide for his or her day-to-day needs. This includes day-to-day living expenses as well as health care costs. Financial limitations can result in medication noncompliance, failure to seek health care, and inability to hire additional help to meet care needs. Referral for financial planning may be part of the assessment process. Many seniors resist using outside support available through local, state, and federal programs.

The social assessment should also identify need for information about planning including wills, power of attorney, the need for guardianship, and medical advance directives. A values history has been suggested to complement formal advance directives (54). This tool allows persons to identify their basic quality of life values and indicate specific care preferences. It may be during CGA that these issues are first raised. The patient and/or the family should be provided with appropriate information to allow them to follow through on such recommendations.

In summary, the social assessment should provide an overall view of the social functioning of the person. This includes social interactions with family and friends and community involvement (church, social groups, hobbies, interests). Some seniors are working or only recently retired. Their basic coping skills and ability to manage life stresses should be determined. The social assessment should include a determination of the environmental fit of a person's living arrangement and/or recommendations for change to meet their physical, functional, and social needs. The current and future options for living, considering the patient's values and family needs and in keeping with the patient's overall well-being, should be determined.

ENVIRONMENTAL ASSESSMENT

Linked with the social assessment is the environmental assessment. An understanding of the living arrangements, including specific information about the physical layout of the home and environs, is important. Assessment of the environment focuses on areas that can improve the person's ability to function in that environment and addresses safety concerns that are often problematic in seniors' homes. The value of an in-home assessment is often emphasized. Comparison of the findings of an internist's office assessment with those of a geriatric nurse's home evaluation revealed that the nurse discovered more social, mental health, and medical problems (55). Many assessments rely on patient and family report of the home environment. Home hazards are often linked to falls. Home safety checklists may be reviewed in the home or provided to patients and their families so that they may evaluate the environment (56). General home evaluation should include assessment of lighting, flooring, furniture location, heating, and air conditioning. The kitchen, bathroom, and stairway should be carefully evaluated for safety issues, since these areas are common sites for falls and injuries. Recommendations for adaptive devices that may improve functional mobility should be made. Outside environment should also be examined. This includes access to the neighborhood, general safety, and a sense of the neighbors and their ages. Ease of access to the home should also be assessed. Basic home protection, such as locks on doors and windows, should be examined, since many seniors are vulnerable to crime.

SPECIAL ISSUES

Sleep

Difficulty sleeping is a common complaint in older patients and may be an indication of more serious underlying disease. Sleep disturbances can result in excessive napping during the day. It is important to obtain a thorough sleep history that addresses how long the patient sleeps, when he or she goes to sleep, whether there are frequent awakenings and what precipitates them, and the frequency of daytime napping. Recent changes in sleep cycle may indicate new physical or mental health problems or reflect the effect of medications, alcohol, or caffeine use. The prevalence of sleep apnea increases with age. Patients with dementia may have disturbances in the sleep cycle that create significant problems in the home. Sometimes this is related to inactivity or frequent napping during the day. Recommendations may be needed to correct this problem, a significant cause of caregiver strain.

Alcoholism and Abuse

It is estimated that about 5% of community elders have alcoholism (57). As in younger patients, alcohol abuse is a major factor in physical and mental health problems and may result in institutional placement and hospital admissions (58). Because of physiologic aging changes, the ability to tolerate a given amount of alcohol is diminished. Alcohol may also interfere with medications and cause problems with impaired balance, falls, and adverse cardiac effects.

The CAGE questionnaire has a fairly high predictive value in patients who answer more than two questions positively (21). The questions include the following: Has the person attempted to cut down on his or her drinking? Has anyone been annoyed or angered by his or her drinking? Has the person ever felt guilty about drinking? Has the person ever used alcohol to reduce the effects of a hangover or otherwise deal with early withdrawal symptoms? The Michigan Alcoholism Screening Test (MAST) is a 25-item questionnaire that evaluates the social and behavioral effects of alcohol use (59). Both of these tests have been used in older populations. These screening tools may be less sensitive in the el-derly because the symptoms of alcoholism they evaluate are less problematic in this age group. An older patient may not be working or may have stopped driving for other reasons. Alcoholism in elders may reflect a long-term problem or may have developed late in life as a response to various life stressors such as retirement or late-life losses.

Seniors may also abuse prescription medications. They may develop dependence on benzodiazepines and/or chronic pain medications. It is important to address how these medications may affect function. Use of these medications often causes depression. Accurate assessment of pain is also an important part of the assessment process. It is very unlikely that a patient will become addicted to pain medications that are being used to treat actual physical pain.

Pain

A variety of tools can help in the assessment of acute and chronic pain. Many of the chronic illnesses common to elders cause pain. Although the prevalence of pain increases with age, there has been little detailed study of pain in the elderly (60). Pain should be characterized to determine the causation. Most pain assessment tools rely on the patient's report for rating the severity of pain. The most commonly used are based on a visual analog, descriptive pain intensity, or numeric scale. These tools can be used in the initial assessment of pain and in monitoring the effectiveness of various interventions. Pain management strategies are discussed in a variety of guidelines, including National Guidelines for Acute and Chronic Pain Management (61, 62). Untreated pain can result in anxiety, depression, and malnutrition. It is always important to attempt to diagnose the cause of pain and to treat the underlying problem when possible.

Continence

Problems with urinary continence are prevalent in the aging population and are often underdiagnosed. About 5 to 10% of community-residing elders have incontinent episodes at least weekly (63). The prevalence increases with additional functional limitations and occurs in 40 to 60% of institutionalized elderly (64). Urinary incontinence is associated with an increased risk of infection, contributes to skin breakdown, and may create social isolation in community seniors. Urinary tract problems can result in sleep disturbance and increase the risk of falls.

Screening for urinary incontinence should be part of the CGA. During the physical examination, problems with hygiene that reflect urinary incontinence should be noted. Family members and caregivers should also be questioned about problems with continence. National guidelines for the evaluation and treatment of urinary incontinence have been developed (65).

Nutrition

Undernutrition is prevalent among elders in all settings. It is associated with increased morbidity, prolonged hospitalizations, increased risk of pressure ulcers, and increased mortality (66). A number of factors may influence the adequacy of oral intake. Meals are traditionally associated with a social environment, and the lack of such stimulation may result in loss of interest in food. Changes in taste, often related to xerostomia, can result in decreased food intake. Problems with oral hygiene, dentition, swallowing, or gastrointestinal disorders may be implicated. Loss of appetite may be related to specific diseases or medications. Depression, which is commonly associated with weight loss, may be the presenting feature in some elders. Functional limitations may limit access to food. Shopping and food preparation may become problematic, and many functionally impaired seniors depend on prepared foods or even food programs. The selection, seasoning, and method of preparation may not be their choice. Physical limitations may affect the actual eating process, which may become so time consuming that food is no longer palatable. Patients with memory problems may simply forget to eat. Financial limitations can result in poor food choices. Restrictive diets, particularly in institutional settings, are often inappropriately ordered, particularly when weight loss and nutritional deficits have been identified. In hospital settings acute illness and diagnostic and surgical procedures may result in limitations in food intake.

Nutritional screening is an important compo-

nent of CGA. The traditional dietary assessment includes a dietary history, anthropometric measurements, and evaluation of some basic laboratory parameters. Dietary intake is probably best measured, when possible, through a diet log, because recall of intake is often less reliable. It is important to find out about the quantity and type of food ingested, methods of food preparation, recent changes in dietary intake, dietary restrictions, and ability to obtain and purchase food.

Obtaining anthropometric measurements from older patients is often difficult (67). Accurate height and weight measurements may be difficult because of functional limitations. Low serum albumin and cholesterol levels have been associated with increased morbidity and mortality in older patients; however, other medical problems may affect the predictive value of these test results (68, 69). Prealbumin levels, because of the short half-life of this protein, are more sensitive to short-term nutritional deficits but are often not readily available.

In response to the concerns about nutrition, the U.S. National Screening Initiative developed a public awareness checklist that allows patients and their caregivers to rate their nutritional health (70). This 10-item scored questionnaire helps to identify those who have an adequate nutritional intake and those who are at moderate or high nutritional risk. Recommendations for intervention are based on the score. Those identified as being at increased risk are then screened at two levels. Level 1 collects additional data on weight, diet, and functional status, with recommendations for additional referral. Level 2 screening uses these data plus a determination of body mass index and laboratory data to address the nutritional problem further.

A newer nutritional assessment tool is the Mini-Nutritional Assessment (MNA), which targets frail elders (71). The assessment entails obtaining some basic anthropometric information, including body mass index, midarm circumference, and calf circumference. History of weight loss and answers to six general questions relating to levels of independence, polypharmacy, psychologic stress, memory loss, and any skin breakdown are obtained. There are also specific dietary questions related to food intake and self-assessment questions. The maximum score is 30 points; a score above 24 identifies a well-nourished person; a score less than 13 identifies those who are malnourished. Those with scores in between are considered at risk.

Mobility, Gait, and Balance

Mobility of an older patient is closely linked to his or her ability to perform ADLs. Therefore, assessment of mobility, including evaluation of gait and balance, is critical. Problems in these areas often result in an increased risk of falls, which are a major cause of morbidity and mortality in older age groups. About a third of community-dwelling persons over age 65 fall each year. About 2 to 3% of these falls result in hospitalization. Only about half of patients who are hospitalized are alive a year later. Accidents are a major cause of death in those over age 65, and falls account for about two thirds of these accidental deaths (72). The CGA should include a thorough history of any falls and their sequelae as well as an assessment of the risk of falling. Falls can result in significant physical injury that may lead to long-term disability from the acute injury. Fear of falling and consequent restriction of activity are also consequences of falls in elders. Recurrent falls may result in institutionalization. A significant number of falls are preventable if appropriate interventions are made, either to improve mobility or to address safety issues in the environment. Immobility results in deconditioning, which further heightens the risk of falls and leads to the development of contractures, functional incontinence, and pressure sores. Accurate assessment of mobility problems may identify medical conditions that appropriate treatment can ameliorate, improving function. It may also predict the adverse outcomes noted earlier. Traditional physical examination often underestimates mobility problems.

A simple performance measurement of gait and balance is the "get-up and go" test (73). Patients are scored qualitatively, with 1 as normal and 5 as severely abnormal, for standing from a chair, walking 3 meters, turning around, walking back to the chair, and sitting. A more quantitative rating via the "Up & Go" test is obtained by asking the patient to perform the same tasks

and scoring the time it takes to do them (74). The Tinetti Balance and Gait Evaluation scores performance on gait and balance maneuvers (75). Other useful tools include measurement of gait speed over a fixed course and modifications of the Romberg test that better evaluate balance. Patients who score poorly on these tests need more careful evaluation for the cause of their gait, balance, and/or mobility problems so that appropriate recommendations for intervention can be made.

Driving

The number of motor vehicle accidents per miles driven increases with age (76). During the CGA, information about driving should include any history of accidents or motor vehicle violations. Although most seniors limit their driving to familiar areas, they often suffer from multiple medical problems and functional limitations that may impair the skills needed for safe driving. Many cognition-impaired patients do not have insight into their limitations. Most localities do not have good alternative transportation systems that can easily replace driving. Family members may continue to support the elderly unsafe driver because they want to avoid the issue or are concerned that they will have to assume responsibility for transporting the senior relative. It is important that the geriatric assessment team understand local requirements for reporting impaired drivers. With the aging driving population, there is a clear need for programs that more thoroughly assess the older person's ability to drive safely.

Sexuality

An accurate sexual history also has its place in the evaluation of elderly patients. Many seniors remain sexually active or desire sexual activity. Health care providers are often uncomfortable discussing sexual activity with older patients. Family members may be uncomfortable with their relative's sexual interests. Identifying problems that may affect a satisfactory sexual relationship is important. Problems with male impotence may be amenable to treatment. Vaginal lubrication may be achieved through hormone replacement or the use of lubricants. For the sexually active senior, counseling about sexually transmitted diseases, including AIDS, should be addressed. Concerns about sexual interest and activity can be particularly problematic in demented patients. These problems should be discussed openly in the assessment.

GERIATRIC ASSESSMENT IN VARIOUS SETTINGS

CGA can be applied in a variety of settings. Specific recommendations for each setting and limitations are discussed next.

The Community

Many of the components of CGA can be incorporated into a generalist practice. Many of the screening and less time-consuming assessment tools can be included in the initial evaluation of an older patient or in serial follow-up visits. Many of the assessment tools can be administered by office staff with some limited degree of training. The patient's primary physician often has a unique perspective on the patient's overall health care status. Several references specifically address incorporating geriatric assessment in the traditional office practice (77, 78). This does require spending time to learn about community resources and to access other health care providers to assist in assessment.

In some cases, because of time, cost restraints, the complexity of problems, and the need for access to other team members, it is more appropriate to refer a patient for a formal outpatient assessment. A typical outpatient CGA, which takes 3 to 4 hours, offers a snapshot of the person. The value of consultative CGA programs in the outpatient setting is linked to follow-up and implementation of recommendations (10, 11).

Geriatric assessment can also be done in the home. These programs have demonstrated usefulness in older patients (10, 11). A home assessment may also be incorporated into an outpatient assessment. This allows for a more accurate environmental assessment and for evaluation of performance in the patient's own environment. Home assessments may be linked with formal home care programs in which skilled nurses and therapists can gather appropriate information and initiate interventions in the home environment.

Adult day care is increasingly available and is another area in which CGA can be performed. More day care programs are being structured to deal with complex medical patients in addition to their prior social role. Some programs provide on-site therapy in addition to skilled nursing interventions. These programs can often complement formal home care. Their value in delaying institutionalization requires more careful study. Obstacles to day care include transportation and reimbursement issues, since most insurance, except for medical assistance, does not cover day care. A CGA may also recommend day care as an alternative to institutional placement to address socialization concerns and monitor medical issues. In all of these community settings, it is important to target patients appropriately and provide a mechanism to follow up on the recommendations made.

The Hospital

Because of the increased prevalence of acute and chronic medical problems, older patients are a disproportionate share of patients in acute care. In addition, they are at higher risk for developing iatrogenic complications while hospitalized (79). There are two basic models for inpatient geriatric assessment, the acute care GEMU and geriatric consultation. As discussed in the section on the value of CGA, the former has been shown to improve some patient outcomes. Consultation services have had some effect on the number of new diagnoses but a less favorable effect on other outcomes measured (10, 11). There are various models for inpatient GEMUs. In some the attending physician remains in charge of the patient's care and the unit medical director-geriatrician provides consultative input along with other members of the health care team. In other programs the control of the patient's management reverts to the medical director-geriatrician. In most units, there is some targeting process to identify high-risk frail elders who are most likely to benefit from the specialized inpatient care. Discrete units also have a role for teaching health care professionals the principles of geriatric care in their specialties. Ideally, these principles can be applied in other areas of the acute care setting. Determination of the best models for inpatient care of older patients warrants ongoing study and will be affected by changes in health care and the role of acute-care hospitals.

The Institutional Setting

Institutional care is being provided in an increasing variety of settings, reflecting a continuum based on level of care needed. This includes formal comprehensive rehabilitation facilities, subacute care units, traditional skilled nursing care units, long-term care units, and an increasing number of assisted living facilities. Comprehensive assessment is an integral part of most formal rehabilitation programs, and the presence of a coordinated team is mandated for reimbursement. Subacute and skilled nursing facilities are taking on much posthospital rehabilitation as well as the care of complex medically stable patients who require ongoing active therapies. In these settings thorough and accurate assessment on admission and serially is critical to the overall care of the patient. With the implementation of the Omnibus Budget Reconciliation Act (OBRA) of 1987, long-term care facilities are required to assess patients in a comprehensive manner within 15 days of admission, quarterly, and whenever there is a significant change in the patient's overall condition (80). This is performed through completion of the Minimum Data Set (MDS), which requires input from a variety of health care professionals, including nurses, rehabilitation specialists, recreational therapists, and social workers. Accurate assessment by a physician on admission is also important. The MDS addresses all of the important components of CGA. Certain findings trigger resident assessment protocols (RAPs), which allow the nursing staff to assess changes in the patient's condition and deal with new problems. Serial measurements allow for early identification of functional decline and trigger appropriate interventions. It is important that physicians practicing long-term care be familiar with the process and review the findings. The physician should be notified of any significant change in the MDS, and the patient should be reassessed.

Over the past few years the number of assisted living facilities has increased dramatically as an alternative to nursing facilities and in response to the changing population demographics. Efforts to develop regulatory guidelines for these facilities are under way and presumably will include some standard for assessment of the patient on admission and periodically thereafter.

COST AND REIMBURSEMENT

Since CGA is a time-intensive process, it is costly to develop and maintain these programs. Cost has been an obstacle to their development in the traditional fee-for-service system. The cost for an inpatient GEMU is included in hospital costs. Physician reimbursement is the same as for other acute-care physician services. Similarly, the physician component in the long-term care or outpatient setting is reimbursed with appropriate codes for the level of service provided. Office-based programs in a fee-for-service setting usually cannot generate adequate reimbursement to cover the cost of assessment. Consequently, in this setting the assessment is often performed over a series of visits.

GERIATRIC ASSESSMENT IN A MANAGED CARE ENVIRONMENT

The managed care setting overcomes some of the obstacles, particularly reimbursement, to providing CGA. Since accurate assessment has improved some patient outcomes, CGA is a service to be valued in integrated health care delivery networks that are reimbursed through global capitation. Successful programs recognize the importance of early case identification and targeting of older patients who are at risk for functional decline and high use of costly health care resources.

REFERENCES

1. National Institutes of Health Consensus Development Conference Statement: geriatric assessment methods for clinical decision-making. J Am Geriatr Soc 1988;36: 342–347.
2. Matthews DA. Dr. Marjory Warren and the origin of British geriatrics. J Am Geriatr Soc 1984;34:253–258.
3. Campion EW. The oldest old. N Engl J Med 1994;330: 1819–1820.
4. Goodwin M, Morley JE. Geriatric research, education and clinical centers: their impact on the development of American geriatrics. J Am Geriatr Soc 1994;42:1012–1019.
5. Deleted in proof.

6. Kane RA, Kane RL. Assessing the Elderly: A Practical Guide to Assessment. Lexington, MA: Lexington Books, 1981.

7. Gallo J, Reichel W, Anderson LM. Handbook of Geriatric Assessment. 2nd ed. Gaithersburg, MD: Aspen, 1995.

8. Rubenstein LZ, Wieland D, Bernabei R. Geriatric Assessment Technology: The State of the Art. New York: Springer, 1995.

9. Rubenstein LZ, Josephson KR, Wieland D, et al. Effectiveness of a geriatric evaluation unit: a randomized clinical trial. N Engl J Med 1984;311:1664–1670.

10. Stuck AE, Siu AL, Wieland GD, et al. Effects of comprehensive geriatric assessment on survival, residence, and function: a meta-analysis of controlled trials. Lancet 1993:342:1031–1036.

11. Stuck AE, Wieland G, Rubenstein LZ, et al. Comprehensive geriatric assessment: meta-analysis of the main effects and elements enhancing effectiveness. In: Rubenstein LZ, Wieland D, Bernabei R, eds. Geriatric Assessment Technology: The State of the Art. New York: Springer, 1995.

12. Winagrad CH. Targeting strategies: an overview of criteria and outcomes. J Am Geriatr Soc 1991:39(suppl): 253–255.

13. Reuben DB. Defining and refining targeting criteria. In: Rubenstein LZ, Wieland D, Bernabei R, eds. Geriatric Assessment Technology: The State of the Art. New York: Springer, 1995. Geriatric Assessment Technology: The State of the Art. New York: Springer, 1995.

14. Winagrad CH, Gerety DB, Chun M, et al. Screening for frailty: criteria and predictors of outcomes. J Am Geriatr Soc 1991;39:778–784.

15. Boult C, Dowd B, McCaffrey D, et al. Screening elders for risk of hospital admission. J Am Geriatr Soc 1993;41:811–817.

16. Hayes V, Morris J, Wolfe C, Morgan M. The SF-36 health survey questionnaire: is it suitable for use with older adults? Age Aging 1995;24:120–125.

17. Lyons RA, Perry HM, Littlepage BN. Evidence for the validity of the short-form 36 questionnaire (SF-36) in an elderly population. Age Aging 1994;23:182–184.

18. Deleted in proof.

19. Deleted in proof.

20. Feinstein AR, Josephy BR, Wells CK. Scientific and clinical problems in indexes of functional disability. Ann Intern Med 1986;105:413–420.

21. Mayfield D, McLeod G, Hall P. The CAGE questionnaire: validation of a new alcoholism screening instrument. Am J Psychiatry 1974;131:1121–1123.

22. Murlow CD, Lichtenstein MD. Screening for hearing impairment in the elderly. J Gen Intern Med 1991;6: 249–258.

23. Ventry IM, Weinstein BE. Identification of elderly people with hearing problems. ASHA 1983;7:25–37.

24. Teresi JA, Crass PS, Golden RR. Some applications of latent trait analysis to the measurement of ADL. J Gerontol 1984;44:S196–S204.

25. Kovar MG, Lawton MP. Functional disability: activities and instrumental activities of daily living. In: Lawton MP, Teresi JA, eds. Annual Review of Geriatrics and Gerontology. New York: Springer, 1994.

26. Kane RL, Saslow MG, Brundage T. Using ADLs to establish eligibility for long-term care among the cognitively impaired. Gerontologist 1991;31:60–66.

27. Katz S, Ford AB, Maskowitz RW, et al. Studies of illness in the aged. The Index of ADL: a standardized measure of biological and psychosocial function. JAMA 1963; 185:914–919.

28. Lawton MP, Brody EM. Assessment of older people: self maintaining and instrumental activities of daily living. Gerontologist 1969;9:179–185.

29. Duke University Center for the Study of Aging. Multidimensional Functional Assessment: The OARS Methodology. 2nd ed. Durham, NC: Duke University, 1978.

30. Applegate WB, Blass JP, Williams TF. Instruments for the functional assessment of older patients. N Engl J Med 1990;322:1207–1214.

31. Guralmick JM, Branch LG, Cummings SR, et al. Physical performance measures in aging research. J Gerontol Med Sci 1989;44:M141-M146.

32. Williams ME. Identifying the older person likely to require long-term care services. J Am Geriatr Soc 1987;35: 761–766.

33. Pfeiffer E. A short portable mental status questionnaire for the assessment of organic brain deficit in elderly patients. J Am Geriatr Soc 1975;23:433–441.

34. Folstein MR, Folstein SE, McHugh PR. "Mini-mental state": a practical method for grading the cognitive state of patients for the clinician. J Psychiatr Res 1975;12: 189–198.

35. Tombaugh TN, McIntyre NJ. The Mini-Mental State Examination: a comprehensive review. J Am Geriatr Soc 1992;40:922–935.

36. Crum RM, Anthony JC, Bassett SS, Folstein MF. Population-based norms for the Mini-Mental State Examination by age and educational level. JAMA 1993;269: 2386–2391.

37. Hachinski VA, Iliff LD, Zilhka E, et al. Cerebral blood flow in dementia. Ann Neurol 1975;32:632–637.

38. Blessed G, Tomlinson BE, Roth M. The association between quantitative measures of dementia and of senile changes in the cerebral grey matter of elderly subjects. Br J Psychiatry 1968;114:797–811.

39. Moore J, Bobula JA, Short TB, et al. A functional dementia scale. J Fam Pract 1983;16:490–503.

40. Reisberg B, Ferns, SH, DeLeon MH, et al. The global deterioration scale for assessment of primary degenerative dementia. Am J Psychiatry 1982;139:1136–1139.

41. Reisberg B. Dementia: a systematic approach to identifying reversible causes. Geriatrics 1986;41:30–46.

42. American Psychiatric Association. Diagnostic and Statistical Manual of Mental Disorders. 4th ed. Washington: American Psychiatric Association, 1994.

43. Zung WW. A self-rating depression scale. Arch Gen Psychiatry 1965;12:63–70.

44. Zung WW. Depression in the normal aged. Psychosomatics 1967;8:287–292.

45. Norris JT, Gallagher D, Wilson A, Winograd CH. Assessment of depression in geriatric medical outpatients: the validity of two screening measures. J Am Geriatr Soc 1987;35:989–995.

46. Beck AT, Beck RW. Screening depressed patients in family practice: a rapid technique. Postgrad Med 1972; 52:81–85.

47. Yesavage JA, Brink TL. Development and validation of a geriatric depression screening scale: a preliminary report. J Psychiatr Res 1983;17:37–49.

48. Yesavage JA. The use of self-rating depression scales in the elderly. In: Poor LW, ed. Clinical Memory Assessment of Older Adults. Washington: American Psychological Association, 1986:213–217.

49. Alden D, Austin C, Sturgeon R. A correlation between the geriatric depression scale long and short forms. J Gerontol 1989;4:P124–P125.

50. Kafonek S, Ettinger WH, Roca R. Instruments for screening for depression and dementia in a long-term care facility. J Am Geriatr Soc 1989;37:29–34.

51. Alexopoulos GS, Abrams RC, Young RC, Shamoian CA. Cornell Scale for Depression in Dementia. Biol Psychiatry 1988;23:271–284.

52. Zarit SH. Relatives of the impaired elderly: correlates of feelings of burden. Gerontologist 1980;20:649–655.

53. Robinson BC. Validation of a Caregiver Strain Index. J Gerontol 1983;38:244–248.

54. Doukas DJ, McCullough LB. The values history: assessing patient values and directives regarding long-term and end-of-life care. In: Gallo JJ, Reichel W, Anderson LM, eds. Handbook of Geriatric Assessment. 2nd ed. Gaithersburg, MD: Aspen, 1995.

55. Ramsdell J, Swart J, Jackson E, Renvall M. The yield of a home visit in the assessment of geriatric patients. J Am Geriatr Soc 1989;37:17–24.

56. US National Safety Council and AARP. Falling—The Unexpected Trip: A Safety Program for Older Adults. Program leader's guide. Washington: 1982.

57. Brody JA. Aging and alcohol abuse. J Am Geriatr Soc 1982;30:123–126.

58. West LJ, Maxwell DS, Noble EP, Solomon DH. Alcoholism. Ann Intern Med 1984;100:405–416.

59. Selzer ML. The Michigan alcoholism screening test: the quest for a new diagnostic instrument. Am J Psychiatry 1971;127:1653–1658.

60. Ferrell BA. Pain management in elderly people. J Am Geriatr Soc 1990;38:408–414.

61. Agency for Health Care Policy and Research. Acute Pain Management: Operative or Medical Procedures and Trauma. Rockville, MD: US Department of Health and Human Services, Public Health Service, Agency for Health Care Policy and Research, 1992.

62. Agency for Health Care Policy and Research. Management of Cancer Pain. Rockville, MD: US Department of Health and Human Services, Public Health Service, Agency for Health Care Policy and Research, 1994.

63. Herzos AR, Fultz NH. Prevalence and incidence of urinary incontinence in community dwelling populations. J Am Geriatr Soc 1990;38:273–281.

64. Ouslander JG, Kane RL, Abrass IB. Urinary incontinence in elderly nursing home patients. JAMA 1982;248: 1194–1198.

65. Agency for Health Care Policy Research. Urinary Incontinence in Adults. Clinical Practice Guideline 2 (AHCPR 92–0038). Rockville, MD: US Department of Health and Human Services, Public Health Service, Agency for Health Care Policy and Research, 1992.

66. Reuben DB, Greendale GA, Harrison GG. Nutrition screening in older persons. J Am Geriatr Soc 1995;43: 415–425.

67. Chumlea WC. Status of anthropometry and body composition data in elderly subjects. Am J Clin Nutr 1989; 50:1158–1166.

68. Corti MC, Guralnik JM, Salive ME, et al. Serum albumin level and physical disability as predictors of mortality in older persons. JAMA 1994;272:1036–1042.

69. Noel MA, Smith TK, Ettinger WH. Characteristics and outcomes of hospitalized older patients who develop hypocholesterolemia. J Am Geriatr Soc 1981;39:455–461.

70. The Nutritional Screening Initiative. Report of Nutrition Screen: 1. Toward a Common View. Washington, 1991.

71. Guigoz Y, Vellas B, Garry P. Assessing the nutritional status of the elderly: the Mini Nutritional Assessment as part of the geriatric evaluation. Nutr Rev 1996;54:559–564.

72. Rubenstein LZ, Robbins AS, Schulman BC, et al. Falls and instability in the elderly. J Am Geriatr Soc 1988; 36:266–278.

73. Mathias S, Nayak US, Isaacs B. Balance in elderly patients: the "get-up and go" test. Arch Phys Med Rehabil 1986;67:387–389.

74. Podsiadlo D, Richardson S. The timed "Up & Go": a test of basic functional mobility for frail elderly persons. J Am Geriatr Soc 1991;38:142–148.

75. Tinetti ME. Performance-orientated assessment of mobility problems in elderly patients. J Am Geriatr Soc 1986;34:119–126.

76. Cerelli E. Older Drivers: The Age Factor in Traffic Safety. Washington: US Department of Transportation, National Highway Traffic Safety Administration, 1989.

77. Lachs MS, Feinstein AR, Cooney LM Jr, et al. A simple procedure for general screening for functional disability in elderly patients. Ann Intern Med 1990;112:699–706.

78. Fleming KC, Evans JM, Weber DC, Chutka DS. Practical functional assessment of elderly patients: a primary care approach. Mayo Clin Proc 1995;70:890–910.

79. Gorbien M, Bishop J, Beers M, et al. Iatrogenic illness in hospitalized elderly people. J Am Geriatr Soc 1992;40: 1031–1042.

80. Elon R, Pawlson LG. The impact of OBRA on medical practice within nursing facilities. J Am Geriatr Soc 1992; 40:958–963.

CHAPTER 3

JOHN B. MURPHY AND MICHELLE CICILLINE

Prevention for Older Persons

Health promotion and disease prevention targeted at older persons should be designed to maximize length of life, but as important or more so, should focus on improving or maintaining the quality of a person's remaining life. There are good data to demonstrate the efficacy of certain preventive health interventions, even for persons of advanced age, and thus a nihilistic approach to preventive health care for elderly persons is not justifiable. However, a cautious or skeptical approach is warranted. Far too frequently preventive health interventions of demonstrated efficacy in younger populations are presumed to be effective for older persons as well. Such presumptions disregard the unique qualities of older persons and the important balance between quality and quantity of life as well as running the risk of exposing older persons to ineffective and in some cases harmful interventions.

Primary and secondary prevention are the focus of this chapter. Primary prevention consists of efforts to prevent disease (e.g., counseling, immunizations, and chemoprophylaxis). Secondary prevention (also known as screening) is identification of a disease or disorder in the asymptomatic phase. The distinction between preventive interventions for asymptomatic persons and diagnosis in symptomatic persons cannot be overemphasized. The following discussion relates to asymptomatic persons without specific risk factors for the index disease or condition.

The research database that supports clinical decision making as it relates to prevention for older persons has numerous gaps and omissions. Because of the difficulty and cost of conducting large-scale trials to validate primary and secondary preventive health efforts for older persons, it is likely that many of the shortcomings in our existing database will persist for some time. Therefore, physicians are called upon to use their judgment about preventive health interventions. For informed judgments physicians must go beyond considering well-known risk factors (e.g., comorbid illness) and add the variables of active life expectancy, functional status, and the patient's preference.

Although the average life expectancy for a given person (Table 3.1) is an important variable, at least as important is the concept of active life expectancy (ALE), the probable period of life free of disability with independence in activities of daily living (1). The fundamental tenet of ALE as a measure of health status is that morbidity and mortality are not the only criteria for assessing health outcomes for older persons. Functional status and independence play important roles in defining both health and quality of life. Furthermore, functional status by itself (activities of daily living or instrumental activities of daily living) is a powerful predictor of mortality and other health outcomes. When the data are clear, the decision about which preventive health measures to offer a given patient is easy. When the data are conflicting or lacking, the clinician should incorporate his or her knowledge of a patient's comorbid illnesses, functional status, active life expectancy, and preferences into the decisions about which preventive health measures to offer a given patient.

Primary and secondary prevention recommendations vary greatly, depending upon the organization making the recommendation. It is not

Table 3.1

Total and Active Life Expectancy

Age	Total Life Expectancy (yrs)		Active Life Expectancy (yrs)	
	Men	Women	Men	Women
65	15–17	19–21	11–13	15–17
75	8–11	11–13	6–7	8–9
85	4–6	6	2–3	2–4
90+	1–2	<1	<1	

Adapted from Branch LG, Guralnik JM, Foley DJ, et al. Active life expectancy for 10,000 Caucasian men and women in three communities. J Gerontol 1991;46:M145–M150.

surprising that subspecialty societies and organizations such as the American Cancer Society have relatively extensive and/or aggressive recommendations for the diseases or conditions on which they focus. This undoubtedly stems, in part, from an honest zeal to do the most possible to minimize the effects of these diseases, but it also stems from selection bias. The patient population seen in the primary care physician's office clearly differs from that seen in the university hospital subspecialty clinic. There is no question that the prevalence of disease in the subspecialist's office is higher, and so it is the subspecialist's impression that yet unproven interventions have greater efficacy. It necessarily follows, however, that such potential for selection bias must not be incorporated into general screening recommendations. For this reason the recommendations of more broadly based groups, such as the U.S. Preventive Services Task Force and the Canadian Task Force on the Periodic Health Examination, probably hold greater validity for the family physician or general internist in clinical practice.

Older patients have many competing risks for death, and the absolute effect of a new diagnosis on life expectancy is often relatively small. Consequently, the potential gain in survival even from perfect therapy may also be small. Moreover, no therapy or intervention is perfect, and the risks of therapy often increase with age. In the elderly the combination of a high burden of competing risks and high rates of treatment-related complications conspires to reduce the net benefit of numerous interventions. As compared with younger patients, the elderly should be offered only the most clearly effective interventions.

The choice of preventive health interventions is important, but how one conducts prevention is probably more important to effective prevention programs. In clinical practice it is insufficient simply to decide what preventive health interventions to implement; one must be equally concerned about how to ensure that appropriate interventions are carried out. Nonetheless, a discussion of the important process of practicing prevention is beyond the scope of this chapter. This chapter focuses on prevention recommendations and the data supporting them.

PRIMARY PREVENTION
Counseling
Tobacco

Some 16.1% of men and 12.4% of women 65 years and older are cigarette smokers (2). These figures are much lower than those reported for other adult age groups. Nonetheless, the hazards of smoking extend well into late life, and the rates of total mortality among current smokers aged 65 and older are 2 to 10 times what they are for persons who have never smoked (3, 4). Even minimal counseling by health care providers has been shown to help the patient stop smoking, and the health benefits clearly extend to quitting in old age (5–13).

Exercise

Fewer than 20% of older persons regularly exercise at an intensity sufficient to improve cardiovascular fitness, and 40% of those aged 65 to 74 are overweight (2, 14, 16–18). Yet physical activity not only reduces coronary heart disease risk but also can improve musculoskeletal conditions, bone density, and risk of falls and fracture, and it enhances a sense of well-being for older persons (12, 19–23).

Although the evidence of the benefits of physical activity even in very old populations is incontrovertible, evidence is less convincing that counseling asymptomatic older adults to incorporate physical activity in their daily routines will affect their behavior. Nonetheless, increases in the duration, frequency, and intensity of activity that gradually progress over several months are safe for most older persons. There is very consistent consensus that counseling to promote regular physical activity is recommended for older adults (24).

Diet

A large proportion of community-dwelling elders consume diets that fail to meet the minimum recommended daily allowances (RDA) (25). Preliminary data suggest that daily supplementation with a multivitamin (approximating the U.S. RDA) or vitamin E in larger doses may improve immune function and result in fewer infection-related sick days for older persons (26–28). In men and women 65 years of age and older calcium intake of less than 600 mg per day is common, and intestinal calcium absorption may be reduced in older populations. Among homebound older persons and those living in long-term care facilities, vitamin D insufficiency has been detected and may contribute to reduced calcium absorption. Available information indicates that optimum calcium intake for men and women 65 years of age and older is 1500 mg a day (29), including both calcium from the diet and calcium taken in supplemental form. However, there is some reason to believe that dietary calcium is safer (30).

Any diet recommendation for an older population must be tempered by the concern that older persons have diminished nutritional reserve and are thus susceptible to malnutrition when embarking on stringent diets. Nonetheless, a prudent low-fat, high-fiber diet is a reasonable recommendation for older persons. One should not be deluded into thinking that a low-fat diet will have significant effect on coronary artery disease, but a low-fat, high-fiber diet may have more proximate benefit as it relates to constipation.

Alcohol

Counseling older primary care patients about their alcohol intake can result in changes in drinking behavior (31). The proportion of older persons who drink is increasing, with 14% of elderly men and 6% of older women being categorized as heavy drinkers (2). Furthermore, elders are felt to be at particularly high risk for alcohol abuse because of physiologic changes in alcohol distribution and metabolism, the concurrent use of prescription and nonprescription medications, the presence of comorbid illness, and an increased risk of falls and accidents. Thus, as recommended by the U.S. Preventive Services Task Force (USPSTF), it seems reasonable to inquire about a patient's alcohol intake and intervene when a concern is identified (32).

Accidental Injury

Accidents are the fifth most common cause of death for older persons in the United States (33). Preliminary data suggest that external hip protectors may prevent hip fractures in nursing home residents (34). Although a multifactorial intervention to reduce the risk of falling among elderly people living in the community has been demonstrated to be efficacious, the generalizability of this intervention remains to be demonstrated (35). Although data from controlled trials illustrating that counseling prevents accidents and injuries for persons 65 and older are lacking, it seems prudent to advise patients to use automobile safety belts and helmets when riding bicycles and to counsel them on abstinence from alcohol when driving and on home safety issues.

Medications

Three quarters of community-dwelling elders regularly use prescription medications and nonprescription medications; 15% take five or more prescription medications daily. The potential for adverse drug reactions and drug interactions clearly increases with the number of drugs taken and probably increases with age, and thus counseling to avoid unnecessary medications may be beneficial.

Immunoprophylaxis
Influenza Vaccine

More than 90% of deaths attributable to influenza occur among persons aged 65 or older. Influenza vaccination levels in this age group increased substantially from 1985 (23%) to 1994 (55%) (36). When a good match exists between the vaccine and circulating viruses, influenza vaccine has been demonstrated to prevent hospitalization for pneumonia and influenza in up to 70% of community-dwelling persons. In nursing home populations studies have indicated that the vaccine can be 50 to 60% effective in preventing hospitalization and pneumonia and 80% effective in preventing death. For these reasons, influenza vaccine is strongly recommended for all persons aged 65 and older.

Influenza vaccination is optimally administered from early October through mid-November, but starting in early September, one should immunize any person who should receive the vaccine when the opportunity arises. Furthermore, immunization of persons in risk groups should continue throughout the influenza season in a given community. It takes roughly 2 weeks for the influenza vaccine to become effective. Amantadine or rimantadine may be used to prevent influenza A illness in those who cannot receive vaccine. Although compliance with influenza vaccination guidelines has been affected by the concern about the perceived frequency of reactions, these concerns are not justified, as there is no difference in the frequency of adverse reactions between persons revaccinated with influenza vaccine and those receiving placebo (37).

Pneumococcal Vaccine

Streptococcus pneumoniae is the most common cause of community-acquired pneumonia and the second most common cause of bacterial meningitis in the United States (38). The 23-valent pneumococcal vaccine covers more than 85% of invasive infections and is recommended for all persons aged 65 or older. Among immunocompetent older persons vaccine efficacy is high and does not appear to decline with increasing intervals after vaccination.

Tetanus

Only 27% of those 70 years and older have protective levels of tetanus antibody, as compared with 88% of those 6 to 11 years (39). Although the occurrence of tetanus has decreased dramatically because of the use of the tetanus toxoid, most of the remaining tetanus illness and most of the mortality related to tetanus occur in older populations. Therefore, it is recommended

that older persons continue to receive booster vaccinations at mid decade every 10 years (e.g., 65, 75, 85). For those with no history of tetanus vaccination, a primary series of three doses is recommended. The first two doses should be given at least 4 weeks apart, and the third dose should be given 6 to 12 months after the first dose.

Chemoprophylaxis

Aspirin

The physicians health study demonstrated a conclusive reduction in the risk of myocardial infarction in men who took low-dose aspirin (325 mg every other day) (40). Subgroup analysis illustrated that men aged 60 to 69 and 70 to 84 received the most benefit. There was an insignificant increase in the risk of hemorrhagic stroke and an insignificant decrease in the risk of thrombotic stroke in men taking aspirin. An overview of the British Doctors' Trial and the Physicians' Health Study reported a 33% reduction in the risk of first myocardial infarction with the use of low-dose aspirin. Thus, it seems prudent that men aged 65 and older use low-dose aspirin for the primary prevention of heart disease. There is no randomized trial supporting the use of aspirin in women. However, the Nurses' Health Study (prospective cohort study) demonstrated a reduced risk of myocardial infarction in women using low-dose aspirin (235 mg 1 to 6 times a week) (41). In addition to cardioprotective benefits of aspirin, it may well be that regular aspirin use longer than 10 years substantially reduces the risk of colorectal cancer, but final conclusions await further study (42).

Estrogen Replacement Therapy

Postmenopausal hormone replacement therapy is a complex issue. Estrogen replacement therapy has been demonstrated to decrease risks of osteoporosis even when started in women over age 65, to decrease the risk of cardiovascular disease, and possibly to decrease the risk of colon cancer and Alzheimer's disease (43–46). In addition, estrogen replacement therapy can improve sexual function and cosmesis. It is also clear that estrogen replacement therapy without a progestin markedly increases the risk of endometrial cancer (47). However, a major concern regarding the use of estrogen replacement therapy is the risk of breast cancer (43, 48). Ongoing randomized placebo-controlled trials (e.g., the Women's Health Initiative) should clarify the magnitude of the risks and benefits, but until such time as data are available, physicians will have to use their judgment. Guiding principles should be that women who are at the greatest risk for coronary heart disease and osteoporosis should be strongly encouraged to consider estrogen replacement therapy and that for persons who are at very low risk for coronary heart disease and osteoporosis, the recommendations must be made more cautiously.

SECONDARY PREVENTION
Coronary Heart Disease

Coronary heart disease is the leading cause of death for Americans aged 65 and older. The primary emphasis on screening for coronary heart disease in the United States focuses on serum lipids. All patients with known coronary heart disease and at high risk for coronary heart disease should be screened for dyslipidemia. Intervention with these groups using cholesterol-lowering agents is widely recognized as efficacious. Although the hypothetical effect of cholesterol reduction on coronary heart disease end points in asymptomatic persons aged 65 and older is substantial, there is no direct evidence from clinical trials to support mortality benefit (49). In fact, the American College of Physicians recommends that evidence is insufficient to recommend or discourage screening for primary prevention for coronary heart disease in men and women aged 65 to 75 and that screening is not recommended for men and women 75 years of age and older (49, 50). Others acknowledge that this is very controversial but interpret the data differently and state that excluding older persons from cholesterol screening is inappropriate (51). Results from controlled trials are clearly needed to clarify whether or not to screen asymptomatic, low-risk older persons for coronary heart disease. In the absence of such data physicians must use their judgment, making individualized recommendations that should incorporate a patient's preference, functional status, comorbid illness, and active life expectancy.

Screening for asymptomatic coronary heart disease with resting electrocardiography (ECG), ambulatory ECG, or exercise ECG is not substantiated by available evidence (52).

Stroke

Cerebrovascular disease is the third leading cause of death for older persons. Carotid endarterectomy (CEA) offers documented benefit to patients with significant (at least 70%) symptomatic stenosis of the carotid artery (53, 54). Several randomized trials of carotid endarterectomy done in asymptomatic persons found that surgery reduced neither the incidence of stroke nor mortality rates. The results of the Asymptomatic Carotid Atherosclerosis Study (ACAS) challenged this view. This randomized controlled trial of carotid endarterectomy in asymptomatic patients with stenosis of the internal carotid artery of 60% or more found that carotid surgery done under carefully controlled conditions could decrease the risk for future stroke. However, it has been estimated that the cost of widespread screening for asymptomatic carotid disease is prohibitive, and the generalizability of this study with exceptionally low perioperative morbidity and mortality rates has been questioned (55). Furthermore, it has been estimated that screening of asymptomatic patients would result in only a small gain in quality-adjusted life years (4.75 days over 30 years). Thus, at present, screening of asymptomatic carotid disease does not appear supportable.

Hypertension is a major risk factor for stroke, and screening older persons for hypertension (isolated systolic or diastolic) has been demonstrated to be efficacious (56). The treatment of atrial fibrillation with warfarin has been conclusively shown to decrease risk of stroke in younger and older persons and thus screening for atrial fibrillation on physical examination is efficacious (57, 58).

Cancer
Cervical Cancer

Approximately 16,000 new cases of invasive cervical cancer are diagnosed each year, and about 5,000 women die of this disease annually; 40% are age 65 and older. Nonetheless, elderly women do not appear to benefit from Papanicolaou (Pap) testing if repeated cervical smears have been adequate and normal before age 65 (59). However, many older women have not previously been adequately screened. It is estimated that as many as 25% of women over age 65 have never had a Pap smear and up to 75% have not had regular screening. In addition to concerns about low levels of screening there are also questions related to the adequacy of sampling in older women. It is generally thought that the squamocolumnar junction is the site of optimal sampling for detecting cervical cancer. The squamocolumnar junction migrates rostrally with age, hence may be more difficult to sample in an older woman. The presence of endocervical cells is generally thought to be consistent with an adequate sample. Thus, screening for cervical cancer with Pap smears can be safely stopped in women aged 65 and older only in the absence of recent risk factors and previous cervical disease if the woman has had a minimum of three recent adequate (endocervical cells present) normal cervical smears. There is also clear evidence that it is unnecessary to perform Pap smears in women who have had a hysterectomy with removal of the entire cervix for benign gynecologic disease (60).

Breast Cancer

The incidence of breast cancer rises with age and does not level off until age 85 or later. Annual clinical breast examination in conjunction with mammography every 1 to 2 years has been unequivocally shown to be beneficial for women aged 50 to 69. For women aged 70 to 74 the data are limited and conflicting, and there are no data for women aged 75 and older. The American Geriatric Society recommended screening until age 85 and individualizing the decision after that age. The U.S. Preventive Services Task Force notes that screening beyond age 70 may be reasonable on other grounds. Again, the clinician should use the patient's preference and knowledge of the patient's comorbid illness, functional status, and active life expectancy to make an individualized recommendation.

Colon Cancer

Colorectal cancer increases in incidence throughout old age. A single randomized controlled trial has demonstrated efficacy of fecal occult blood testing (FOBT) as a screen for colon cancer (61). This trial, including more than 46,000 patients aged 50 and over found that the 13-year cumulative mortality from colorectal cancer was 33% lower among persons annually screened with FOBT than in a control group. There was no difference in overall mortality. Unfortunately, the report provided insufficient data to determine to what extent observed differences in outcome were attributable to FOBT as opposed to the large number of colonoscopies (40% of screened patients) that were performed because of frequent false-positive FOBT. Three large clinical trials of FOBT screening under way in Europe should help clarify the issue. Two case control studies have demonstrated efficacy of screening for colorectal cancer with a sigmoidoscopy (62, 63). On the basis of these studies it is reasonable to recommend screening with FOBT and/or sigmoidoscopy for relatively well and independent seniors.

Prostate Cancer

It was estimated that in 1996, approximately 317,000 men in the United States would receive a new diagnosis of prostate cancer and that of these 41,400 would die of it (64). However, whether early detection of this disease generally does more good than harm is a matter of great controversy. As a result, conflicting recommendations have been issued by various professional organizations. The debate is fueled by the absence of evidence from controlled studies showing that screening reduces mortality related to prostate cancer (65). Using a decision model that favors screening, men aged 50 to 69 appear to gain, on average, several weeks of life expectancy. Men in this age range who subsequently are diagnosed with cancer and have radical prostatectomy potentially add 3 or more years of life in their 50s; however, this decreases to 1.5 years for men in their 60s and 0.4 years in their 70s. Depending on age, 15 to 40% of persons screened require biopsy, and minor self-limiting complications have been reported in as many as 40% of men who have had biopsies. Radical prostatectomy for prostate cancer (curative therapy) carries a 50% chance of permanent sexual dysfunction, a 20 to 30% likelihood of some degree of urinary incontinence, and a 1% chance of perioperative death. Moreover, with assumptions that are less favorable to screening, the estimated net benefit to life expectancy decreases significantly. Similarly, the ratio of costs to health benefits escalates dramatically. Thus, men who are older than 69 generally increase life expectancy by only a few days with generous assumptions, and with less favorable assumptions screening may result in net harm in men 70 and older. For these reasons the American College of Physicians and the USPSTF do not recommend routine screening for prostate cancer with digital rectal exam or prostate-specific antigen (PSA). For men aged 50 to 69, physicians should describe the potential benefits and known harms of screening, diagnosis, and treatment and individualize the decision to screen. For men aged 70 and older, little is to be gained from screening, but the patient's preference should be considered (66).

Skin Cancer

Nonmelanoma skin cancers are the most common malignancies found in older persons. The incidence of basal and squamous cell carcinoma increases with age. When identified at early stage, both types of skin cancer are very treatable. There are no randomized trials demonstrating the efficacy of skin examination by a clinician. Nonetheless, given the high prevalence of these conditions, the low risk of false-positive screening skin examinations, and the availability of acceptable low-cost diagnostic and treatment options, routine examination of the skin as part of an annual examination for older persons is supportable.

Other Cancers

There are insufficient data to support screening for lung, ovarian, uterine (aside from asking about postmenopausal bleeding), or other malignancies in older persons who are asymptomatic and have no risk factors for these conditions.

Other Screening Maneuvers
Hearing

Hearing problems are one of the most prevalent conditions found in older Americans, with at least 36% of those age 75 and older affected. A single randomized controlled trial demonstrated the efficacy of screening older populations for hearing deficits with a hand-held otoscope. Assessment of efficacy was based on improvement in communication; social, emotional, and cognitive function; and mood in the group provided with hearing aids (67). These findings and the high prevalence of hearing problems in older populations indicate that a recommendation for routine screening with a desktop or hand-held audiometer is supportable. The frequency of screening is open to question.

Visual Acuity

The incidences of glaucoma, cataracts, and macular degeneration increase with age. Unfortunately, office glaucoma screening by primary care physicians has not been effective (68). Given that refractive problems are so common in older populations and the prevalence of these conditions increases with age, it is recommended that regular screening be conducted by an eye specialist for persons aged 65 and older. The frequency of screening is unclear.

Osteoporosis

There is insufficient evidence to recommend for or against screening for osteoporosis with densitometry in asymptomatic postmenopausal women. Recommendations against routine screening may be made on the grounds of the high cost, inconvenience, and lack of universally accepted criteria for initiating treatment based on bone density measurements. Selective screening may be appropriate for high-risk women who would consider hormone prophylaxis only if they know they were at high risk for osteoporosis or fracture.

Alzheimer's Disease

The relation between the APOE locus on chromosome 19 and the risk of late-onset familial and sporadic Alzheimer's disease has been confirmed in multiple clinical and population-based studies throughout the world. Unfortunately, APOE genotyping can never be expected to provide predictive certainty, and in fact some carriers have survived into their 90s without developing dementia. Furthermore, 40 to 50% of

Table 3.2

Screening: Age 60 and Older

NAME   Chart #

Date: _____

Age	60	61	62	63	64	65	66	67	68	69	70	71	72	73	74	75	76	77	78	79	80	81	82	83	84	85	85+
History																											
Complete H. & P.		once at entry																									
Functional status[a]											O					O					O					O	
Dietary intake[b]				O	O	O	O	O	O	O	O	O	O	O	O	O	O	O	O	O	O	O	O	O	O	O	O
Physical activity[c]		O	O	O	O	O	O	O	O	O	O	O	O	O	O	O	O	O	O	O	O	O	O	O	O	O	O
Tobacco, alcohol[d]		O	O	O	O	O	O	O	O	O	O	O	O	O	O	O	O	O	O	O	O	O	O	O	O	O	O
Medications[e]		O	O	O	O	O	O	O	O	O	O	O	O	O	O	O	O	O	O	O	O	O	O	O	O	O	O
Advanced directives[f]		O	O	O	O	O										O					O					O	
History of TIA		O	O	O	O	O	O	O	O	O	O	O	O	O													
Physical Examination																											
Height	O																										
Weight		O	O	O	O	O	O	O	O	O	O	O	O	O	O	O	O	O	O	O	O	O	O	O	O	O	O
Blood pressure		O	O	O	O	O	O	O	O	O	O	O	O	O	O	O	O	O	O	O	O	O	O	O	O	O	O
Pulse		O	O	O	O	O	O	O	O	O	O	O	O	O	O	O	O	O	O	O	O	O	O	O	O	O	O
Visual acuity						O	O	O	O	O	O	O	O	O	O	O	O	O	O	O	O	O	O	O	O	O	O
Audiometry[g]						O					O					O					O					O	
Clinical breast examination		O	O	O	O		O	●	O	O	O	O	O	O	O	O											
Mini-mental state examination[h]										O	O	O	O	O	O	O	O	O	O	O	O	O	O	O	O	O	O
Falls risk assessment[i]						O	O	O	O	O	O	O	O	O	O	O	O	O	O	O	O	O	O	O	O	O	O
Laboratory																											
Nonfasting cholesterol[j]		O	O	O	O		O	O	O	O	●					O											
Mammography[k]		O	O	O	O		O	O	O	O	O	O	O	O	O	O	◐	◐	◐	◐	◐	◐	◐	◐	◐	◐	
Pap test[l]			O	O	O	O																					
Fecal occult blood[m]	O	O	O	O	O	O	O	O	O	O	●	●	●	●	●												

O, perform; ● ●, see notes below.

[a]ADLs, IADLs, and mobility. [b]Fat, fiber, calories, protein and calcium. [c]Aerobic (pulse = 0.7[220-age], 20–30 min, 3 times/wk), and range of motion exercises. [d]CAGE (cut down, annoyed, guilty, eye opener). [e]Prescription medications (especially anxiolytics, and sedative/hypnotics), OTC medications and borrowed medications. [f]Durable power of attorney or living will depending on local statute. [g]Hand-held or desktop audiometry with a threshold of 40 dB. [h]Folstein Mini-Mental State Examination. [i]Get-Up and Go test (patient is observed as he or she rises from an armchair, walks 3 meters, and returns to sit in the chair). [j]● Perform only if patient is independent in IADLs and has no major illness. [k]● Continue to age 85 only if the patient has no major illness and is independent in IADLs. [l]Stop at age 65 if patient has at least three documented recent normal, adequate tests and no risk factors. [m]Stop at age 70 because active life expectancy is too short for a likelihood of benefit after age 70.

late-onset Alzheimer's patients have no allele. Consequently, the National Institute on Aging/Alzheimer's Association Working Group unanimously recommended against the use of APOE genotyping for predicting Alzheimer's disease in asymptomatic persons (69).

Functional Assessment

There are no controlled trials on the use of functional assessment as a screen for older populations. It has been posited that functional assessment of physical function (activities of daily living, instrumental activities of daily living, and mobility) and cognition is worthwhile. The rationale supporting screening is based on the notion that functional impairments (the result of unidentified diseases) and disease progression often go undetected and can be identified by a screening functional assessment. Many persons with cognitive deficits have irreversible dementias, but even in these cases, the primary care physician can substantially influence the quality of a patient's life by early identification. Thus, there may be grounds on which to recommend routine screening functional assessments.

SUMMARY

Table 3.2 summarizes the screening recommendations elaborated in this chapter. Some may find the recommendations parsimonious, and if they are, it is for two reasons. First, with asymptomatic older persons, who have many competing risks, one must exercise extreme caution in using unproven strategies no matter how promising. Second, even when there are effective screening strategies, many persons who should be screened are not. Thus it seems much wiser to invest our scarce resources in improving the screening rates for clearly efficacious interventions before investing in strategies whose efficacy is still in question.

REFERENCES

1. Katz S, Branch LG, Branson ML, et al. Active life expectancy. N Engl J Med 1983;309:1218–1224.
2. Hobbs F, Damon B. Sixty-five Plus in the United States: US Bureau of the Census Current Population Reports. Special Studies P23–190. Washington: US Government Printing Office, 1996.
3. LaCroix AZ, Lang J, Scheer P, et al. Smoking and mortality among older men and women in three communities. N Engl J Med 1991;324:1619–1625.
4. Bartecchi CE, MacKenzie TD, Schrier RW. The human costs of tobacco use: part 1. N Engl J Med 1994;330:907–912.
5. Vogt M, Cawley J, Scott J, et al. Smoking and mortality in older women. Arch Intern Med 1996;156:630–636.
6. Cummings SR, Reuben SM, Oster G, et al. The cost effectiveness of counseling smokers to quit. JAMA 1989;261:75–79.
7. Salive M, Coroni-Huntley J, LaCroix A, et al. Predictors of smoking cessation and relapse in older adults. Am J Public Health 1992;82:1268–1271.
8. Hermanson B, Omenn GS, Kronmal RA, et al. Beneficial six-year outcome of smoking cessation in older men and women with coronary artery disease: results from the Kass registry. N Engl J Med 1988;319:1365–1369.
9. Kiel D, Baron JA, Anderson JJ, et al. Smoking eliminates the protective effect of oral estrogen on the risk of hip fracture among women. Ann Intern Med 1992;116:712–716.
10. Kawachi I, Colditz GA, Stampfer MJ, et al. Smoking cessation and decreased risk of stroke in women. JAMA 1993;269:232–236.
11. Higgins MW, Enright PL, Kronmal RA, et al. Smoking and lung function in elderly men and women. The Cardiovascular Health Study. JAMA 1993;269:2741–2748.
12. Paffenbarger RS, Hyde RT, Wing HL. The association of changes in physical activity level and other lifestyle characteristics with mortality among men. N Engl J Med 1993;328:538–545.
13. Department of Health and Human Services. The Health Benefits of Smoking Cessation: A Report of the Surgeon General (DHHS [CDC] 90–8416). Rockville, MD: Department of Health and Human Services, 1990.
14. Elward K, Larson E, Wagner E. Factors Associated With Regular Aerobic Exercise in an Elderly Population. J Am Board Fam Pract 1992;5:467–474.
15. Healthy People 2000: National Health Promotion and Disease Prevention Objectives (DHHS (PHS) 91–50213, 1991:24). U.S. Department of Health and Human Services.
16. Morley MC, Cowper PA, Feussner JR, et al. Two-year trends in physical activity performance following supervised exercise among community-dwelling older veterans. J Am Geriatr Soc 1991;39:549–554.
17. Elward KS, Larson EB. Benefits of exercise for older adults: a review of existing evidence and recommendations for the general population. Clin Geriatr Med 1992;8:35–50.
18. Elder J, Williams SJ, Drew JA, et al. Longitudinal effects of preventive services on health behaviors among an elderly cohort. Am J Prev Med 1995;11:354–359.
19. Lee IM, Hsieh CC, Paffenbarger RS Jr. Exercise intensity and longevity in men: The Harvard Alumni Health Study. JAMA 1995;273:1179–1184.
20. Cummings SR, Nevitt M, Brower W, et al. Risk for hip fracture in white women. N Engl J Med 1995;332:767–773.

21. Cooper C, Barker D. Risk factors for hip fracture. N Engl J Med 1995;332:814–815.

22. Fiatarone M, O'Neill E, Ryan N, et al. Exercise training and nutritional supplementation for physical frailty in very old people. N Engl J Med 1994;330:1769–1775.

23. Jaglal SB, Kreiger N, Darlington G. Past and recent physical activity and the risk of hip fracture. Am J Epidemiol 1993;138:107–118.

24. Counseling to promote physical activity. In: Guide to Clinical Preventive Services. Report of the U.S. Preventive Services Task Force. 2nd ed. Baltimore: Williams & Wilkins, 1996:611–624.

25. Ryan AS, Craig LD, Finn SC. Nutrient intakes and dietary patterns of older Americans: a national study. J Gerontol Med Sci 1992;47:M145–M150.

26. Chandra RK. Effect of vitamin and trace element supplementation on immune response and infection in elderly subjects. Lancet 1992;340:1124–1127.

27. Bogden J, Bendich A, Kemp F, et al. Daily micronutrient supplements enhance delayed-hypersensitivity skin test responses in older people. Am J Clin Nutr 1994;60:437–447.

28. Meydanis S, Medani D, Blumberg J. Vitamin E supplementation and in vivo immune response in healthy elderly subjects. JAMA 1977;277:1380–1386.

29. Optimum calcium intake. NIH Consensus Development Panel on Optimum Calcium Intake. JAMA 1994;272:1942–1948.

30. Curhan G, Willett W, Speizer F, et al. Comparison of dietary calcium with supplemental calcium and other nutrients as factors affecting the risk for kidney stones in women. Ann Intern Med 1997;126:497–504.

31. Fleming MF, Barry KL, Manwell LB, et al. Brief physician advice for problem alcohol drinkers: a randomized, controlled trial in community-based primary care practices. JAMA 1997;277:1039–1045.

32. Screening for problem drinking. In: Guide to Clinical Preventive Services. Report of the U.S. Preventive Services Task Force. 2nd ed. Baltimore: Williams & Wilkins, 1996:567–582.

33. Parker S, Tong T, Bolden S, et al. Cancer statistics, 1997. CA Cancer J Clin 1997;47:5–27.

34. Lauritzen J, Petersen M, Lund B. Effective external hip protectors on hip fracture. Lancet 1993;341:11–13.

35. Tinetti M, Baker D, McEvay G, et al. A multifactorial intervention to reduce the risk of falling among elderly people living in the community. N Engl J Med 1994;331:821–827.

36. Prevention and control of influenza: recommendations of the Advisory Committee on Immunization Practices (ACIP). MMWR Morb Mortal Wkly Rep 1997;46:1–25.

37. Margolis KL, Nichol KL, Poland GA, Pluhar RE. Frequency of adverse reactions to influenza vaccine in the elderly: a randomized placebo-controlled trial. JAMA 1990;264:1139–1141.

38. Butler JC, Breiman RF, Campbell JF, et al. Pneumococcal polysaccharide vaccine efficacy: an evaluation of current recommendations. JAMA 1993;270:1826–1831.

39. Gergen PJ, McQuillan GM, Kiely M, et al. A population-based serologic survey of immunity to tetanus in the United States. N Engl J Med 1995;332:761–766.

40. Final report on the aspirin component of the Ongoing Physicians' Health Study. Steering Committee of the Physicians' Health Study Research Group. N Engl J Med 1989;321:129–135.

41. Manson JE, Stampfer MJ, Colditz GA, et al. A prospective study of aspirin use and primary prevention of cardiovascular disease in women. JAMA 1991;266:521–527.

42. Giovannucci E, Egan K, Hunter D, et al. Aspirin and the risk of colorectal cancer in women. N Engl J Med 1995;333:609–614.

43. Grodstein F, Stampfer M, Colditz G. Postmenopausal hormone therapy and mortality. N Engl J Med 1997;336:1769–1775.

44. Grodstein F, Stampfer M, Manson J, et al. Postmenopausal estrogen and progestin use and the risk of cardiovascular disease. N Engl J Med 1996;335:453–461.

45. Calle E, Miracle-McMahill H, Thun M, Heath C. Estrogen replacement therapy and risk of fatal colon cancer in a prospective cohort of postmenopausal women. J Natl Cancer Inst 1995;87:517–523.

46. Tang M, Jacobs D, Stern Y, et al. The effect of estrogen during menopause on risk and age at onset of Alzheimer's disease. Lancet 1996;348:429–432.

47. The effects of hormone replacement therapy on endometrial histology in postmenopausal women. The Postmenopausal Estrogen/Progestin Interventions (PEPI) Trial. The Writing Group for the PEPI Trial. JAMA 1996;275:370–375.

48. Stanford J, Weiss N, Voigt L, et al. Combined estrogen and progestin hormone replacement therapy in relation to risk of breast cancer. JAMA 1995;274:137–142.

49. Guidelines for using serum cholesterol, high-density lipid protein cholesterol and triglyceride levels as screening tests for preventing coronary heart disease in adults. American College of Physicians. Ann Intern Med 1996;124:515–517.

50. Garber A, Browner W, Hulley S. Cholesterol screening in asymptomatic adults, revisited. Ann Intern Med 1996;124:513–518.

51. Corti M, Guralnik J, Salive M, et al. Clarifying the direct relation between total cholesterol levels and death from coronary heart disease in older persons. Ann Intern Med 1997;126:753–760.

52. Screening for asymptomatic coronary artery disease. In: Guide to Clinical Preventive Services. Report of the U.S. Preventive Services Task Force. 2nd ed. Baltimore: Williams & Wilkins, 1996:3–14.

53. Beneficial effect of carotid endarterectomy in symptomatic patients with high-grade carotid stenosis. North American Symptomatic Carotid Endarterectomy Trial Collaborators. N Engl J Med 1991;325:445–453.

54. MRC European Carotid Surgery Trial: interim results for symptomatic patients with severe (70–99%) or with (0–29%) carotid stenosis. European Carotid Surgery Trialists' Collaborative Group. Lancet 1991;337:1235–1243.

55. Lee T, Solomon N, Heidenreich P, et al. Cost-effectiveness of screening for carotid stenosis in asymptomatic persons. Ann Intern Med 1996;126:337–346.

56. Prevention of stroke by antihypertensive drug treatment in older persons with isolated systolic hypertension. Fi-

nal results of the Systolic Hypertension in the Elderly Program (SHEP). SHEP Cooperative Research Group. JAMA 1991;265:3255–3264.

57. Petersen B, Boysen G, Godtfredsen J, et al. Placebo-controlled randomised trial of warfarin and aspirin for prevention of thromboembolic complications in atrial fibrillation. The Copenhagen AFASAK study. Lancet 1989; 1:175–179.

58. Preliminary report of the Stroke Prevention in Atrial Fibrillation Study. N Engl J Med 1990;322:863–868.

59. Screening for cervical cancer. In: Guide to Clinical Preventive Services. Report of the U.S. Preventive Services Task Force. 2nd ed. Baltimore: Williams & Wilkins, 1996:105–117.

60. Pearce K, Haefner H, Sarwar S, Nolan T. Cytopathological findings on vaginal Papanicolaou smears after a hysterectomy for benign gynecological disease. N Engl J Med 1996;335:1559–1562.

61. Mandel J, Bond J, Church T, et al. Reducing mortality from colorectal cancer by screening for occult blood. N Engl J Med 1993;328:1365–1371.

62. Selby J, Friedman G, Quesenberry C, Weiss N. A case-controlled study of screening sigmoidoscopy and mortality from colorectal cancer. N Engl J Med 1992;326: 653–657.

63. Newcomb P, Norfleet R, Storer B, et al. Screening sigmoidoscopy and colorectal cancer mortality. J Natl Cancer Inst 1992;84:1572–1575.

64. Parker S, Tong T, Wingo P. Cancer statistics, 1996. CA Cancer J Clin 1996;46:5–27.

65. Screening for prostate cancer. American College of Physicians. Ann Intern Med 1997;126:480–484.

66. Screening for prostate cancer. In: Guide to Clinical Preventive Services. Report of the U.S. Preventive Services Task Force. 2nd ed. Baltimore: Williams & Wilkins, 1996:119–134.

67. Mulrow C, Aguilar C, Endicott J, et al. Quality of life changes and hearing impairments: a randomized trial. Ann Intern Med 1990;113:188–194.

68. Tucker JB. Screening for open-angle glaucoma. Am Fam Physician 1993;48:75–80.

69. Post S, Whitehouse P, Binstock R, et al. The clinical introduction of genetic testing for Alzheimer's disease: an ethical perspective. JAMA 1997;277:832–836.

CHAPTER 4

EDNA P. SCHWAB, MARY ANN FORCIEA, LESLEY CARSON,
ANITA M. AISNER, AND RISA J. LAVIZZO-MOUREY

Clinical Practice Guidelines in Geriatrics

Clinical practice guidelines have existed for at least 50 years. Practice policies are an integration of information obtained from research, observations, clinical experience, and judgments of expert clinicians, scientists, and patients condensed into practical recommendations. Recently clinicians, health care agencies, researchers, insurers, policy makers, and health care administrators have used them as a standard for measuring the delivery of health care. Guidelines are developed for several purposes: to assist in medical decision making by practitioners and patients, to educate persons and groups, to improve quality of care, to control the cost of health care, and to reduce the incidence of negligent care. Guidelines help summarize current medical literature; they provide a blueprint for standardizing care and a mechanism for decreasing practice variability and medical costs.

The Institute of Medicine (IOM) has defined practice guidelines as "systematically developed statements to assist practitioner and patient decisions about appropriate health care for specific clinical circumstances." Guidelines are intended for use by practitioners, patients, families, and health care institutions. However, other users, such as payers, health benefit coordinators, public policy makers, and regulators, may refer to these guidelines and use them to determine which health care visits and procedures are appropriate for reimbursement.

The American Medical Association (AMA) has reported that more than 50 organizations are involved in guideline development. Professional societies have traditionally participated to ensure quality care based on professional standards, prevent intervention by non-health care agencies, and diminish the number of adverse outcomes that may lead to malpractice litigation. Other participating organizations include private research foundations, academic medical centers, health maintenance organizations (HMOs), hospitals, health associations, and other payer groups.

The federal government has supported practice guideline initiatives to promote public health, improve quality, and decrease the cost of federally funded health care programs. Support has come in the form of basic and applied research as well as funding and administration of projects. These activities primarily occur in several agencies run by the U.S. Public Health Service, including the Agency for Health Care Policy and Research (AHCPR), the National Institutes of Health (NIH), Food and Drug Administration, Centers for Disease Control, and Health Care Financing Administration. One of the missions of the AHCPR is to develop, review, and update relevant guidelines to be used by physicians, educators, and other health care professionals.

Policy makers and health care purchasers are keenly interested in guideline development, primarily because of escalating health care costs and concern for quality improvement. Health service research has consistently documented variations in physicians' practice patterns and inappropriate use of clinical services. It is anticipated that with development and implementation of clinical practice guidelines, changes in medical practice will lead to improved health outcomes and lower health care expenditures.

GUIDELINE DEVELOPMENT

There are various types of guidelines. Some target specific audiences, and others focus on specific problems or address prevention, rehabilitation, or technologies. Four approaches have been proposed in developing clinical practice guidelines: informal consensus, formal consensus, evidenced-based approaches, and explicit approaches. Informal consensus provides recommendation of experts based on subjective assessments of the evidence. Although this remains the most common method used to develop guidelines, it is difficult for users to assess its validity. Formal consensus conferences such as those developed by the NIH invite experts from various groups to discuss the evidence in an open forum. Again, scientific data supporting these recommendations may be lacking. Evidence-based approaches establish guidelines supported by scientific information. Recommendations are proposed according to the weight of the evidence, and areas of uncertainty and research are identified. Such guidelines have been used by the Canadian Task Force on the Periodic Health Examination and the AHCPR. This approach improves reliability and validity of guidelines. However, one major limitation is that frequently there are few well-designed clinical trials and data are inadequate. This is true especially in addressing elderly patient populations. The explicit approach uses the evidence-based approach but looks at effects on all important health outcomes. The strength of each recommendation is directly related to the strength of the evidence. Again, this approach is most consistently used in the AHCPR's guidelines.

Woolf (1) divides guideline development into four general steps: introductory decisions, assessment of clinical appropriateness, assessment of public policy issues, and guideline document development and evaluation. *Introductory decisions* include panel and topic selection, i.e., diseases, complaints, procedures, and so on, and the purpose of the guidelines. There is no formal mechanism for topic selection. Often topics are selected by interests of the specialty group. The IOM recommends that topics be selected on the basis of prevalence and burden of illness, cost of therapy, variability in practice, and potential for a guideline to improve health outcomes and to reduce cost. Once a topic is identified for development, a panel of 10 to 20 experts is selected to proceed with the draft. The panel may be composed of specialists, generalists, research methodologists, nonphysician health professionals, and patient or consumer representatives. The panel may function as a standing panel with expert consultants or an independent panel established with each topic selection.

Next, *clinical appropriateness* of the guidelines is assessed. The panel reviews clinical benefits of the proposed practice versus potential for an adverse event, extracting information from available scientific literature and expert opinion. Recommendations should reflect current literature and be justified with scientific evidence. When data are limited, weak, or nonexistent, professional judgments or expert panel conclusions are used. In these circumstances, explanations of the basis and evidence for the reasoning should accompany the recommendation. *Public policy issues* such as feasibility, resource allocation, and cost effectiveness should be considered. After *development* of a draft of recommendations, independent reviewers are selected to examine and revise them. Reviewers may consist of expert consultants, representatives of professional societies, government organizations, consumer groups, practicing clinicians, insurers, and other guideline users. The panel should define its target audience (practitioners and patients) and clinical setting and anticipate how to disseminate, implement, and evaluate the guidelines.

Content of guidelines should be specific, comprehensive, practical, and well supported by scientific research or expert opinion. Guidelines should be logical and unambiguous, should contain supporting evidence for their conclusions, and should state potential risks and benefits. Members of the development panel should also be listed. Guideline development as proposed by the IOM should contain eight key elements: validity (internal and external), reliability, clinical applicability, clinical flexibility, clarity, a multi-disciplinary approach, scheduled review, and documentation (Table 4.1). These elements of development distinguish guidelines from general medical textbook information and from cookbook medicine. Table 4.2 reviews criteria for evaluating guidelines.

Several obstacles to guideline development, implementation, and acceptance exist: There is a potential for lack of consensus on interpretation and conclusion of scientific data. Guideline development is extremely time consuming and expensive. No mechanisms exist to evaluate effec-

tiveness of guidelines in each phase of development. Acceptance by physicians and patients is not uniform. No mechanism exists to finance and disseminate guideline information or to measure compliance with practice guidelines by physicians and patients. Nevertheless, clinical practice guidelines can elevate the standard of medical care provided to various patient populations and curb the escalating costs of health care. Inclusions of scientific research, opinions of expert researchers and clinicians, and patients' preferences provide credibility and promote eventual acceptance of evidence-based practice guidelines.

Table 4.1

Desirable Attributes of Clinical Practice Guidelines

Attribute	Explanation
Validity	Valid guidelines lead to projected health and cost outcomes.
	Prospective assessment considers substance and quality of evidence, means used to evaluate evidence, and relation between evidence and recommendations.
Strength of evidence	Guidelines should be accompanied by descriptions of strength of evidence and expert judgment behind them.
Estimated outcomes	Guidelines should be accompanied by estimates of health and cost outcomes expected from interventions in question compared with alternative practices. Assessments of relevant outcomes consider patients' perceptions and preferences.
Reliability and reproducibility	Guidelines are reproducible and reliable if:
	• Given the same evidence and methods for development, another set of experts produces essentially the same statements.
	• Given the same clinical circumstances, guidelines are interpreted and applied consistently.
Clinical applicability	Guidelines should be as inclusive of appropriately defined populations as evidence and expert judgment permit and explicitly state the relevant population.
Clinical flexibility	Guidelines should identify specific known or generally expected exceptions to them and discuss how patients' preferences are to be identified and considered.
Clarity	Guidelines must use unambiguous language, define terms precisely, and use logical and easy-to-follow modes of presentation.
Multidisciplinary process	Representatives of key affected groups must participate in development of guidelines.
	Participation may include serving on development panels, providing evidence and viewpoints to panels, and reviewing draft guidelines.
Scheduled review	Guidelines must state when they should be reviewed for possible revisions, given new clinical evidence, professional consensus, or lack of it.
Documentation	Procedures used to develop guidelines, participants, evidence, assumptions, rationales, and analytic methods must be meticulously documented and described.

Reprinted with permission from Field MJ, Lohr KN, eds. Institute of Medicine Committee on Clinical Practice Guidelines. Guidelines for Clinical Practice: From Development to Use. Washington: National Academy Press, 1992.

Table 4.2

Criteria for Evaluating Guidelines

1. Is the guideline comprehensive as well as practical?
2. Does it contain scientific evidence to support its recommendations?
3. Does it include explanations when expert opinions or professional judgments are recommended?
4. Are the potential benefits and risks of the recommendation discussed?
5. Is it feasible and cost effective?
6. Does it target a specific audience or clinical setting?
7. Has it been developed and reviewed by a multidisciplinary panel of experts?
8. Has it been endorsed by a professional organization?
9. Has it been routinely reviewed and updated?

IMPLEMENTATION

No guideline, no matter how specific, important, or accurate, can change patient care unless the guideline is used. Implementation refers to actions taken to turn policies into desired results. Successful guideline implementation requires actions involving a variety of physicians, patients, insurers, and administrators. Guidelines developed to improve the care of geriatric patients may be the most difficult to apply to clinical practice because of variation among patients (e.g., a 75-year-old master athlete and a 75-year-old nursing home resident), nontraditional settings for care (home care, nursing homes, day hospitals), and cultural factors. The benefits of more rigorous strategies of patient care delivery may be highest in the elderly, where the prevalence of illness is highest.

Participants in Implementation Strategies

Factors from a variety of sources can influence outcomes of guideline initiatives. Some of these factors are as follows.

Patients and Families

The very illness addressed by the guidelines may limit the patient's compliance with guideline goals. Patients with dementia may have extreme difficulty complying with follow-up appointments and/or diagnostic tests, for example. Vision and hearing deficits and immobility may exclude patients from active participation in some guidelines. Sociocultural factors, such as literacy, familiarity with the biomedical model, health beliefs, gender, years out of training, and income, may be hurdles for patient-directed steps in the guidelines. Knowledge and expectations that patients bring to the physician may influence the degree to which patients are willing to allow their care to be directed by a guideline.

Practitioners

Provider characteristics may also influence the likelihood of acceptance of a guideline. Type, size, and setting of practice have been postulated to affect use of applications. In addition, the specialty of the physician has been said to affect attitudes toward guidelines in provision of good care. Eisenberg (2) has identified six activities which have been shown to change physician behavior: education, feedback, participation, administrative policies, incentives, and penalties. Modern HMOs commonly use most of these six strategies, with financial incentives and penalties felt to be the most powerful.

Institutions

The capacity of the practice site to manage information is the most critical feature of implementation. Comprehensive computerized record systems, which can offer reminders at the time of patients' visits and track outcomes, are ideal for initial application of guidelines and for modification. Other considerations, such as physical plant and institutional relations, are also important.

Economics

The participation of payers in guideline implementation is crucial in the current climate of medicine. The financial basis of the practice (capitated versus fee-for-service) affects attitudes of both patients and physicians as to quality of care. Provider ownership of affiliated diagnostic facilities may alter attitudes. Financial incentives and penalties are powerful shapers of behavior. Liability related to the use of guidelines is uncertain at present but in the future may influence adherence to guidelines.

Strategies to Improve Implementation

Successful application of clinical guidelines in real practices can be aided by a variety of strategies, as follows.

Education

The guideline may be simultaneously announced by a variety of techniques: a press conference given by the sponsoring agency, newspaper articles, and medical journal articles. Sharing the supportive material gathered in generation of the guideline with the practitioners who will be using the guideline is often helpful. This may include literature reviews, analyses of evidence, and information about benefits and costs of alternative therapies. The AHCPR has used this strategy, offering three levels of informative materials: a comprehensive analysis, a journal article-size review of the guidelines, and a pocket-size outline of the policy. Patients can learn about guidelines through articles in the lay press or by special materials developed for a variety of reading levels. Guidelines developed by specialty organizations are more likely to be accepted than those promulgated by governmental agencies.

Personal interactive strategies are the most effective means of dissemination to individual physician uses. Endorsement by locally recognized clinical leaders or authorities can also improve adherence. Health systems should not ignore the usefulness of informal encounters such as lunchtime conversations, bedside consultations, and hallway discussions in the efforts to alter physicians' behavior. Compliance with clinical guidelines (or documented reasons for divergence) may eventually be used as evidence for recertification. The Academy of Family Practice is using review of office records as one of the elements for recertification.

Feedback

As with any learning tool, feedback to providers and patients is critical for sustaining behavior change. Because the object of the guideline is to improve patients' outcomes, feedback to the physician should include outcome information. This information can be developed from chart reviews but is more completely gathered by computer systems.

Participation

Once the physician is aware of the existence of the guideline, any method that presents it at the time of decision making improves compliance. Although minor aids such as pocket guides and posted memoranda may induce minor alterations, the most efficient reminders are computer generated at the time of the visit. The best guidelines are formatted with simple logical steps that do not replace the individual history and physical examination of the patient by the physician and do not increase documentation required of the doctor.

Computer reminders can take a variety of forms: simple alerts (potassium under 3.5), embedded controls on orders (vancomycin orders must be approved by the infectious disease service), triggered advice (hemoccult positive, suggest x, y, z). These reminders can be structured to yield information rather than exert control (data on similar situations versus limits in ordering services). The most extensive programs can link the provider to sources of relevant information.

Administration

The successful implementation of most clinical guidelines requires administrative support. Information systems adequate to capture data, remind physicians and patients, and monitor adherence are fundamental. Personnel will be required to educate staff and patients about their objectives under the guidelines and to monitor actions and effects. The costs of many portions of the guidelines, such as nursing time for patient education, may not be immediately cost effective or may save costs of a different budget item. Administrative assistance in the dissemination of the guidelines themselves, such as funding for grand rounds speakers, luncheon seminars, and pocket guides, is often helpful.

Incentives

Better clinical outcomes are of course the best inducements to follow clinical guidelines. Since few health systems manage their information in ways that allow individual patients and physicians to analyze their outcomes, this altruistic incentive cannot be idealized. As better information technology develops, added incentive for documentation of adherence to or deviation from guidelines may become part of internal quality assurance programs, criteria for reappointment to hospital staff, and specialty recertification.

Penalties

Financial disincentives developed by the HMO industry have been among the most controversial aspects of their control of costs. Whenever penalties for nonadherence are considered, careful analysis of records is essential. Physicians may document completely valid reasons for deviation from recommendations. Such documented variations should not be categorized as noncompliance.

ETHICS OF CLINICAL GUIDELINES

The inherent value and justness of the clinical guideline are functions of its definition, mode of establishment, and clinical appropriateness. The ethical precepts of respect for autonomy, beneficence, nonmaleficence, and justice must be woven into formation of the guideline and its ultimate implementation. The complexity of geriatrics creates a special environment for the guideline that limits its effectiveness but emphasizes its usefulness.

A guideline can be variously defined; it can be considered a recommendation, clinical pathway, algorithm, standard, and so on. These definitions mirror degrees of flexibility from optional to mandatory. In geriatrics, branching nonlinear processes are the ideal for the most part. An 85-year-old community-dwelling man with an acute myocardial infarction, an 85-year-old nursing home resident with significant Alzheimer's dementia and acute myocardial infarction, and an 85-year-old man with a recent cerebral and acute myocardial infarction all require different treatments. Each of these scenarios demands critical examination of several suggested courses of action within not only the scientific but also the social constructs of care. Quality of life issues coupled with end of life issues become part of the clinical decisions. A rigid definition of clinical guideline is untenable; there is more than one acceptable course of action. A clinical guideline that demands a minimum consideration of social as well as medical factors is necessary to assure a certain quality of care. Ideally, the guideline's having flexibility as well as boundaries can improve the physician's ability to do good (beneficence) and enhance family-patient-physician communication and decision making (autonomy).

Geriatrics, with its all-encompassing focus and surfeit of information of variable quality, can benefit from well-researched recommendations but needs the freedom to incorporate new information, as it is a relatively new area of interest in research. Treatment areas ranging from osteoporosis to stroke are in flux. With the involvement of geriatric clinicians in guideline development, the guideline receives a measure of reality testing it might not otherwise have. As long as a guideline allows for change and is rigorously researched and regularly reviewed, the geriatrician's willingness to believe that improved care will result from certain practices and his or her ability to handle information overload will be enhanced.

The clinical appropriateness of the guideline not only is a function of purely clinical concern but also is affected by nonclinical measures. The community and particular population, especially in geriatrics, are difficult to define. For an influenza immunization guideline, gray areas of implementation are minimal. Public and personal health is enhanced by adherence to this guideline. However, algorithms for treatment of depression depend on background psychiatric illness, other medical problems, social milieu, medications, cost of medication, cost of therapy; the list is endless. A workable clinical guideline for depression at best can set criteria for minimal care and offer multiple approaches. Setting criteria for minimal care is very important and may at times suggest that community norms are not good enough. Value judgments in setting more than the criteria for minimal care are complicated; a guideline can only start the process. Nonclinical measures affect the implementation of guidelines. Guidelines for a given clinical problem are interpreted differently by different organizations, whether it be for utilization review, quality assurance, or resource containment. A guideline mandating a limitation on care must not be outside an accepted standard of care. Guidelines for treatment of pressure ulcers in various home and institutional settings are usable only if a variety of nutritional and treatment options are acceptable. Justice in terms of resource use can balance beneficence in the most complicated of geriatric issues only with the use of a very nonrestrictive guideline.

The U.S. Peer Review Improvement Act of 1982 set up peer organizations to ensure quality and cost efficiency by reviewing all Medicare inpatient treatment. The AHCPR was established in 1989 because of criticism of peer review organization criteria; a unit within the AHCPR commissions clinical guideline development, although these guidelines do not have legal force. In addition, clinical guidelines feature in actions involving medical negligence, although the courts critically evaluate their authority.

In summary, geriatrics can benefit from the flexible clinical guideline that recognizes its complexity and breadth; it is an area in which nothing is straightforward and ethical precepts of care are constantly assessed.

CURRENT SCOPE OF CLINICAL PRACTICE GUIDELINES

Today's milieu of clinical practice guidelines may be compared to the barrage of newly developed drugs to which physicians at all stages of their careers are regularly introduced. Whether a simple algorithm, critical pathway, newly published consensus statement, or formal evidence-based guideline, novel practice alternatives inundate us.

Because guideline development is spawned

Table 4.3

Clinical Topics Addressed by Guidelines of Varied Formats

Angina, chest pain
Anticoagulation, antithrombotic therapy
Atrial fibrillation
Alzheimer's disease
Benign prostatic hypertrophy
Carotid artery stenosis
Congestive heart failure, left ventricular systolic
    dysfunction
Depression
Dementia other than Alzheimer's
HIV infection
Hormone replacement
Immunizations
Myocardial infarction
Osteoarthritis
Osteoporosis
Pain management
Perioperative cardiovascular evaluation
Pressure ulcers
Stroke
Syncope
Use of various diagnostic procedures (e.g., ECG,
    cardiac catheterization)
Use of various laboratory tests (e.g., cardiac enzymes,
    thyroid function tests)
Use of various medications, treatments (e.g.,
    streptokinase, endarterectomy)
Urinary incontinence
Withdrawing and withholding life sustaining treatment

by the burden of illness, the growing elderly population is sure to be the targeted sector for future practice guidelines. To date, more than 1000 guidelines developed by national organizations are available, and countless others are being or have been developed at the regional or local level. Table 4.3 lists topics addressed in guidelines in varied formats.

Since the establishment of the U.S. Preventive Services Task Force in 1984, it has recommended screening tests for early detection of disease and other aspects of the periodic health examination. The AHCPR has sponsored development of various guidelines addressing topics of utmost interest in the geriatric population, including urinary incontinence, pressure ulcers, congestive heart failure, depression, dementia, and benign prostatic hypertrophy. Some of these guidelines have been modified and adapted to the long-term care setting by expert panels and committee members of the American Medical Directors Association.

Other health care professional organizations, from the Association of Consultant Pharmacists to associations of clinical laboratory specialists and various payers, are actively involved in development of practice guidelines. Hospitals and regional payer organizations incorporate practice guidelines in quality improvement programs. Our institution develops disease management protocols with active involvement of geriatricians in an effort to maximize early recognition, cost effective treatment, and quality of life in targeted populations while assessing improvement in quality of care.

The most salient feature of guideline development and implementation in the elderly population is dissemination of information about previously underrecognized and undertreated geriatric syndromes such as urinary incontinence, depression, and osteoporosis. Providers of care to the elderly should not feel overwhelmed by the various guidelines but should diligently assist in ensuring their appropriate use. In keeping with the momentum of the trend toward guideline development, Table 4.4 offers

some guidelines to the use of guidelines in the elderly. (Copies of Clinical Practice Guidelines from the AHCPR can be requested by calling 800-358-9295 or by writing to AHCPR Publications Clearinghouse, P.O. Box 8547, Silver Spring, MD 20907.)

This chapter is an overview of the status of clinical practice guidelines. We discuss development, implementation, and ethics of guidelines, with particular emphasis on their pitfalls in the complicated geriatric patient. Even though many guidelines are being adapted by the sundry stakeholders in care of the elderly, only time, extensive outcomes, and health services research will ultimately validate their pervasive use in the evolving health care environment.

REFERENCES

1. Woolf SH. Practice guidelines: a new reality in medicine. II. Methods of developing guidelines. Arch Intern Med 1992;152:946–952.
2. Eisenberg J. Doctor's Decisions and the Cost of Medical Care: The Reasons for Doctor's Practice Patterns and the Ways to Change Them. Ann Arbor, MI: Health Administration Press Perspectives, 1986.

BIBLIOGRAPHY

Battista RN, Hodge MJ, Vineis P. Medicine, practice and guidelines: the uneasy juncture of science and art. J Clin Epidemiol 1995;48:875–880.

Berg OH, Atkin D, et al. Clinical practice guidelines in practice and education. J Gen Intern Med 1997;12:S25–S33.

Berger JT, Rosner F. The ethics of practice guidelines. Arch Intern Med 1996;156:2051–2056.

Doyal L, Wilsher D. Withholding and withdrawing life sustaining treatment from elderly people towards formal guidelines. BMJ 1994;308:1689–1692.

Duff LA, Kitson AL, Seers K, Humphris D. Clinical guidelines: an introduction to their development and implementation. J Adv Nurs 1996;23:887–895.

Eddy DM. A Manual for Assessing Health Practices and Designing Practice Policies: The Explicit Approach. Philadelphia: American College of Physicians, 1992.

Ferguson JH. NIH consensus conferences: dissemination and impact. Ann N Y Acad Sci 1993;703:180–198.

Ferguson JH. The NIH Consensus Development Program. The evolution of guidelines. Int J Technol Assess Health Care 1996;12:460–474.

Field MJ, Lohr KN, eds. Institute of Medicine Committee on Clinical Practice Guidelines. Guidelines for Clinical Practice: From Development to Use. Washington: National Academy Press, 1992.

Fourth American College of Chest Physicians Consensus

Table 4.4

Guidelines for Using Guidelines in Care of the Elderly

Have guidelines been addressed with respect to your patient?

If addressed in past, has treatment been adequate or can you modify it?

If treatment can be modified, will it be to the satisfaction and/or benefit of your patient?

Is guideline appropriate for your specific patient? This decision varies with setting and with patient, family, caregiver wishes.

Is guideline based on best available scientific evidence?

Has guideline been endorsed by a national, regional, local organization with advocates for care of elderly?

Conference on Antithrombotic Therapy. Tucson, Arizona, April 1995. Proceedings. Chest 1995;108(4 suppl):225S–522S.

Hayward RSA, Wilson MC, Tunis SR, et al. Practice guidelines: what are we looking for? J Gen Intern Med 1996;11:176–178.

Iliffe S, Mitchley S, Gould M, Haines A. Evaluation of the use of brief screening instruments for dementia, depression and problem drinking among elderly people in general practice. Br J Gen Pract 1994;44:503–507.

Kelly JT. Role of clinical practice guidelines and clinical profiling in facilitating optimal laboratory use. Clin Chem 1995;41:1234–1236.

McDonald CJ, Overhage JM. Guidelines you can follow and can trust. An ideal and an example. JAMA 1994;271:872–873.

Miles A, Lugon M. Effective Clinical Practice. Cambridge, MA: Blackwell Scientific, 1996.

Murrey KO, Gottlieb LK, Schoenbaum SC. Implementing clinical guidelines: a quality management approach to reminder systems. QRB Qual Rev Bull 1992;18:423–433.

Overhage JM, Tierney WM, McDonald CJ. Computer reminders to implement preventive care guidelines for hospitalized patients. Arch Intern Med 1996;156:1551–1556.

Recommendations for the prevention and treatment of glucocorticoid-induced osteoporosis. American College of Rheumatology Task Force on Osteoporosis Guidelines. Arthritis Rheum 1996;39:1791–1801.

Report of the American College of Cardiology/American Heart Association Task Force on Practice Guidelines. Circulation 1996;93:1278–1317.

Rind DM, Safran C, Phillips RS, et al. Effect of computer-based alerts on the treatment and outcomes of hospitalized patients. Arch Intern Med 1994;154:1511–1517.

Weingarten SR, Riedinger MS, Conner L, et al. Practice guidelines and reminders to reduce duration of hospital stay for patients with chest pain: an interventional trial. Ann Intern Med 1994;120:257–263.

Woolf SH, DiGuiseppi CG, Atkins D, Kamerow DB. Developing evidence-based clinical practice guidelines: lessons learned by the US Preventive Services Task Force. Annu Rev Public Health 1996;17:511–538.

Woolf SH. AHCPR Interim Manual for Clinical Practice Guideline Development. Washington: US Department of Health and Human Services, May 1991.

CHAPTER 5

ANDREA F. LUISI, NORMA J. OWENS, AND ANNE L. HUME

Drugs and the Elderly

The elderly, particularly those over 80, are said to be the fastest-growing segment of the population. Because of the large burden of illness in many older persons, this age group tends to be the highest users of medication. However, there are still few data about specific drug use in the elderly. Most clinical trials published today focus on adults less than 70 years old. As geriatric health care providers, we often put our patients at risk by trying medications that have shown benefit in younger patients in hopes of similar results in our older patients.

This chapter reviews major issues associated with medication use in the elderly. It is divided into four sections: a review of the pharmacokinetic and pharmacodynamic changes that can affect drug therapy in the elderly; adverse drug reactions, underutilization of medications, and the appropriate use of drugs; a review of drug effects on mobility, urinary continence, and mental functioning; and an overview of common drugs used in the elderly and the recent literature that pertains to these agents.

PHARMACOLOGY AND AGING

Age-related physiologic changes as shown in Table 5.1 may alter the pharmacokinetic and pharmacodynamic properties of many drugs commonly prescribed to the elderly. This section is an overview of age-related physiologic changes in the pharmacokinetic and pharmacodynamic properties of drugs in the context of the potential effects of coexisting diseases and concomitant drug therapy. The contributions of diseases and drug therapy are considered because age-related physiologic changes may be most important in the frail older person with multiple chronic disorders and complex pharmacotherapy.

PHARMACOKINETICS
Absorption
Oral Absorption

The absorption of most drugs from the gastrointestinal (GI) tract is a passive process that can be influenced by several factors. Age-related physiologic changes may include increases in gastric pH and decreases in GI motility, splanchnic blood flow, and the mucosal surface area of the small intestine (1). An increase in the gastric pH may reduce the absorption of a few drugs, such as ketoconazole. Alternative agents that do not depend on an acidic pH are usually available. The absorption of alendronate may be doubled in the presence of a less acidic gastric pH (2). In general, drug absorption does not vary with age.

In addition to age-related physiologic changes, common coexisting diseases such as congestive heart failure may reduce the rate and extent of absorption (1). The concomitant use of some prescription and over-the-counter (OTC) drugs may also reduce absorption. For example, antacids and iron preparations may physically bind alendronate and ciprofloxacin, reducing or even preventing their systemic absorption. Drugs that stimulate gastric emptying, such as cisapride, may enhance systemic absorption of drugs such as levodopa.

Presystemic Clearance

Some drugs, as listed in Table 5.2, are well absorbed from the GI tract but are rapidly removed by the liver. This first-pass effect, or presystemic clearance, results in low systemic concentrations.

Table 5.1

Potential Age-Related Physiologic Changes Influencing Pharmacotherapy in the Elderly

Increases	Decreases
Gastric pH	Splanchnic blood flow
α_1-Acid glycoprotein concentrations	Surface area of the small intestine
Adipose tissue	Hepatic blood flow
	Total body water
	Hepatic metabolism (phase I)
	Renal tubular secretion
	Lean muscle mass
	Glomerular filtration rate

Age-related decreases in portal blood flow may increase the systemic bioavailability of these drugs. In addition to this age-related change, coexisting diseases and medications such as cimetidine may reduce hepatic blood flow, further decreasing presystemic clearance and potentially increasing the systemic concentration of these drugs.

Percutaneous Absorption

The absorption of drugs from transdermal preparations depends on their penetration through the epidermal layers and uptake by the dermal blood vessels. Age-related changes include atrophy of the epidermis, flattening of the junction between the dermis and the epidermis, and thinning of the dermis (3). The amount of lipids in the stratum corneum may be reduced and may directly affect its degree of hydration. Changes in the microcirculation have also been suggested, but findings are contradictory (3). In one of the few clinical studies available, the percutaneous absorption of highly lipid soluble drugs, such as estradiol and testosterone, was similar among young (18 to 40 years) and old (above 65 years) age groups, while more hydrophilic drugs, including hydrocortisone, were less well absorbed in the older group (4).

Distribution

Body Composition

Age-related physiologic changes affect body composition, plasma protein binding, and organ blood flow. Declines in lean muscle mass and total body water have been reported, and the percentage of adipose tissue may be doubled in older persons (1). Whether the latter change is truly age related is unclear, as one report indicated that the percentage of body fat does not increase significantly after age 40 except as the result of weight gain alone (5).

The importance of changes in body composition depends on the physiochemical properties of the individual drug. Water-soluble drugs such as digoxin may have a reduced volume of distribution, hence increased initial serum concentrations. Lipophilic drugs such as diazepam may have an increased volume of distribution and, when combined with decreases in certain components of metabolism, may result in substantial increases in their biologic half-life (1).

Protein Binding

While many drugs are bound to plasma proteins, this characteristic becomes important only when the degree of binding exceeds 90%, with 10% of the drug unbound and pharmacologically active. The major factors influencing protein binding include protein concentrations, concurrent diseases and drugs, and nutritional status. Basic drugs, such as lidocaine and propranolol, have a higher binding affinity for α_1-acid glycoprotein, which increases in response to inflammatory diseases. Whether the concentration of α_1-acid glycoprotein increases with age is unclear, but there may be potential for an increase in the protein binding of basic drugs in the older person and a reduction in the amount of the free, pharmacologically active drug (1, 6).

Acidic drugs such as phenytoin bind primar-

Table 5.2

Drugs With Extensive First-Pass Metabolism

Atenolol	Morphine
Desipramine	Nifedipine
Diltiazem	Nitroglycerin
Labetalol	Propranolol
Lovastatin	Simvastatin
Melatonin	Tacrine
Metoprolol	Verapamil

ily to albumin, which may decrease slightly in healthy older persons. In the frail elderly with multiple chronic diseases and poor nutritional status, the larger declines in albumin concentrations may result in clinically important increases in unbound phenytoin concentrations (1). Whenever feasible, a free, or unbound, drug concentration should be obtained so that the potential effects of altered protein binding can be avoided in interpreting the resulting value.

Metabolism

The clearance of drugs metabolized by the liver depends on hepatic blood flow and on the activity of different enzyme systems. Hepatic blood flow may decrease with advancing age such that a healthy 65-year-old person may have 40 to 45% lower blood flow than that of a young adult (1, 7). The hepatic metabolism of drugs has been classified into either the phase I enzymatic reactions of oxidation, reduction, and hydrolysis or the phase II enzymatic reactions of glucuronidation, acetylation, or sulfation. In general, phase I pathways exhibit greater age-related declines than do phase II reactions. Decreases in total liver mass and in the activity of the hepatic microsomal monooxygenase system have been associated with increased age (8).

Hepatic drug metabolism is also influenced by concomitant drug therapy, comorbid conditions, nutritional status, gender, genetics, and environmental factors. Concomitant drug therapy and genetics in particular may have a pronounced effect on drug metabolism, especially when combined with those associated with aging (1). Recent studies have improved our understanding of hepatic drug metabolism by identifying that the cytochrome P450 (CYP) system includes at least 12 isozyme families (9). Table 5.3 lists four isozymes responsible for the metabolism of many drugs and presents representative drugs as substrates, inhibitors, and inducers. Drugs that are enzyme inducers or inhibitors can increase or decrease, respectively, the metabolism of other drugs (the substrate). Some isozymes, such as CYP2D6, are under genetic control, with some persons (poor metabolizers) lacking the gene required for manufacturing the isozyme. As a result, these persons are unable to metabolize the drug (substrate) effectively. In addition, the activity of CYP3A differs by gender, with men having a greater metabolic capacity than women (10).

An improved understanding of drug metabolism is essential in caring for older persons for three reasons. First, the prevention of drug interactions, especially with newly released agents, may be easier if one knows the specific isozyme through which individual drugs are metabolized. Second, the identification of individual patients as being at particular risk for a serious drug interaction may become possible, as certain

Table 5.3

CYP Isozyme Families

	CYP1A2	CYP2C9/10	CYP2D6	CYP3A
Substrate	R-warfarin Theophylline	Phenytoin S-warfarin Tolbutamide	Codeine Desipramine Metoprolol Flecainide	Cyclosporine Diltiazem Lovastatin Terfenadine Verapamil
Inhibitor	Ciprofloxacin Erythromycin		Haloperidol Quinidine	Diltiazem Erythromycin Ketoconazole Grapefruit juice
Inducer	Phenytoin Smoking			Troglitazone

isozymes, such as CYP2D6, exhibit genetic polymorphism. It may become possible routinely to phenotype persons as rapid or poor metabolizers and better tailor their drug therapy.

Renal Elimination

The renal clearance of many drugs may be reduced in older persons. Declines in glomerular filtration rate, renal plasma flow, and tubular secretion have been associated with advancing age. Evidence from the Baltimore Longitudinal Study of Aging indicates that declines in renal function may not be an inevitable outcome of aging, as one third of persons had no change in their renal function over 23 years (11).

Serum creatinine concentrations from frail elderly patients frequently are within the normal range because of decreases in muscle mass and concomitant creatinine production. Creatinine clearance (Cl) may be estimated by this formula:

$$Cl = [(140 - age) \times weight\ (kg)] \div (72 \times serum\ creatinine)$$

For women, the resulting value should be multiplied by 0.85. While this formula and others have been validated in general medical patients, it may overestimate the actual creatinine clearance by 20% or more in very frail elderly women (12).

Drugs that are excreted principally by the kidney may accumulate in the presence of renal insufficiency and may increase the risk of toxicity unless their dosage is reduced. Renally eliminated drugs include many antibiotics, such as aminoglycosides and imipenem, and cardiovascular agents, such as digoxin and atenolol, among many other therapeutic classes. In addition, many drugs have active or toxic metabolites that are renally eliminated and that may accumulate as renal function declines. Common examples include procainamide, codeine, meperidine, allopurinol, and chlorpropamide. Other examples are listed in Table 5.4 (13, 14). A final consideration is that in the older person with end-stage renal disease many pharmacokinetic properties, including absorption, protein binding, volume of distribution, and hepatic metabolism, may be altered as a direct result of the renal disease.

PHARMACODYNAMICS

Pharmacodynamics is the study of the effects of drugs at the receptor level. Until recently, few clinical trials have investigated the effects of aging or, more specifically, "age" on the pharmacodynamics of different drugs. While studies have demonstrated decreased pharmacody-

Table 5.4

Some Drugs Cleared by the Kidney That Require Dosage Adjustment in the Elderly

Class	Drug
ACE inhibitors	Benazepril, lisinopril, quinapril, ramipril
Agents for gout	Allopurinol, colchicine
Antiarrhythmics	Digoxin, disopyramide, procainamide
Antibiotics	Aminoglycosides, penicillins, quinolones, cephalosporins, sulfonamides, vancomycin
Antihypertensives	Hydralazine, methyldopa
Antineoplastics	Methotrexate
Antivirals	Acyclovir, amantadine
β-Blockers	Acebutolol, atenolol, nadolol, sotalol
Calcium channel blockers	Verapamil
Gastrointestinal agents	Cimetidine, famotidine, metoclopramide, nizatidine, ranitidine
Opioid analgesics	Codeine, meperidine,[a] morphine
Oral hypoglycemics	Chlorpropamide

Adapted from Bennett WM. Guide to drug dosage in renal failure. Clin Pharmacokinet 1988;15:326–354; McEvoy GK, ed. American Hospital Formulary Service. Bethesda, MD: American Society of Health-System Pharmacists, 1997.
[a]Meperidine is metabolized to the renally excreted neurotoxin normeperidine.

namic responses to β-adrenergic agonists and antagonists, an increased responsiveness has been reported with drugs including verapamil (15), midazolam (16), and prazosin (17).

The effect of aging on the pharmacodynamic response to warfarin remains controversial. While some studies have reported an increased risk of bleeding among older patients, others have failed to find an association between bleeding and advanced age (18, 19). Data from a large cohort indicated that the relative risk of major bleeding with warfarin was 3.2 for patients aged 65 years or older (20). In addition, the risk for intracranial hemorrhage may be increased among patients aged 75 years and older who have atrial fibrillation (21, 22).

ENSURING OPTIMAL PHARMACOTHERAPY IN THE ELDERLY

This section reviews major content areas important for ensuring optimal pharmacotherapy in the elderly. Since the elderly are such large consumers of medication, it is important to recognize and prevent adverse drug reactions. With the traditional approach to pharmacotherapy in the elderly focused on decreasing medication use, inappropriate underuse of medication may occur. Finally, the development of a coordinated medication database is necessary to prevent medication-related problems. Ensuring that each drug is appropriate and that the patient adheres to the regimen is also crucial in ensuring optimal pharmacotherapy.

Adverse Drug Reactions

The high use of medications combined with the older person's comorbid conditions places them at greater risk for adverse drug reactions than other groups of people. Concern about adverse drug reactions and inappropriate prescribing in older people has resulted in legislative changes to force review of drug prescribing in nursing home patients and the publication of methods to foster appropriate prescribing. Two important publications highlight the adverse drug reaction risk of hospitalized persons.

In 1991, Leape et al. (23) published their findings on iatrogenesis in hospitalized patients. Complications from drug therapy were the most common cause of all adverse events, accounting for 19.4% of 1133 identified events. Age was associated with a higher rate of adverse events: 11.46 adverse events per 100 discharges in persons over age 65 versus 2.36 in persons less than 65. This rate of adverse drug events was verified recently in a prospective cohort study by Bates et al. (24). Over a 6-month period all adult admissions to two large urban teaching hospitals were prospectively reviewed for adverse drug events. Approximately 6.5 per 100 nonobstetric admissions were reported. The preventable events were most likely to be serious or life threatening. Patients in medical intensive care units had the highest rate of adverse events even after controlling for the number of medications prescribed; no particular medication class was identified as causing a disproportionate number of such events (24). Lack of knowledge about therapy (defined as errors in drug choice and inadequate knowledge of indications for use, appropriate dose or route, and available dosage forms) was identified as a common cause of error (25).

Published information about adverse drug reactions in the community is more difficult to evaluate. Some inference may be drawn from the reported rates of hospitalization caused by drug side effects. Grymonpre et al. (26) found that 19% of all nonelective medical admissions in persons over age 50 are associated with intentional medication noncompliance, treatment failure, alcohol, or medication error. The risk of a drug-associated problem increased with the numbers of diseases and was higher in women than in men. When evaluating readmission rates for hospitalization within 6 months in older persons, Bero et al. (27) showed that 20% of the readmissions were related to medication problems, including adverse drug reactions, noncompliance, overdose, lack of necessary drug therapy, and underdosage. Adverse events in this study included nonsteroidal anti-inflammatory-induced GI bleeds, diuretic-induced hyponatremia and hypokalemia, digitalis toxicity, and hypoglycemia from oral hypoglycemics.

The high rate of adverse reactions to certain medications in older patients has led to the publication of lists of so-called inappropriate medications (28). Certain medications have side effect profiles best avoided in older persons or elimination characteristics that are unsuitable for most older persons. Therefore, groups of experts in the use of drugs in older patients have developed consensus criteria for avoiding certain medications. These criteria have been applied to prescribing in the community-dwelling older person using national cross-sectional data (29). These data suggest that approximately 6 million older Americans are prescribed one of the consensus-defined contraindicated medications. These medications include drugs with questionable efficacy, such as dipyridamole and propoxyphene; drugs with a high side effect risk including amitriptyline and indomethacin; and drugs with unfavorable pharmacokinetic profiles coupled with high side effect risks, such as diazepam, chlorpropamide, and chlordiazepoxide. While these drugs are best avoided in most older persons, what is most needed to lessen adverse effects in the elderly is the appropriate use of only the most needed medications (30).

Underprescribing of Medications

Historically, the overuse of medications in the elderly has been a major focus of health care professionals. Several studies have described the negative outcomes resulting from the overuse of medication in this population (23, 31–33). However, recent studies have also reported that underprescribing of medications for the elderly may lead to negative health outcomes. Specifically, this refers to the use of β-blockers and thrombolytics in the treatment of a myocardial infarction (MI) and warfarin to prevent stroke in patients with atrial fibrillation (34–41).

β-Blockers are recommended for use in patients with acute MI both early, to reduce morbidity and mortality, and late, as secondary prevention, in the course of treatment (42). The several contraindications to β-blocker therapy do not include age. The results of a recent study, which examined β-blocker use and mortality rates over a 2-year postdischarge period in Medicare recipients who had had an MI, showed that only 21% of eligible patients received β-blocker therapy (34). Age greater than 75 years was associated with underuse of β-blockers. The

mortality rate was 43% less among β-blocker recipients than nonrecipients. Patients were nearly 3 times as likely to be prescribed a calcium channel blocker as a β-blocker, although the role of the former drugs in this setting is limited. Other studies have also reported the underuse of β-blockers in the elderly, with only 30 to 60% of eligible patients receiving this therapy (35–38).

Three studies have described the underprescribing of thrombolytic therapy (38–40). Age greater than 75 years was strongly associated with not receiving thrombolytic therapy in these reports. Krumholz et al. (39) found that 25% of eligible patients did not receive thrombolytics.

Physicians are hesitant to prescribe anticoagulant therapy for elderly patients despite compelling evidence that the use of anticoagulants reduces the risk of stroke from nonvalvular atrial fibrillation (22). Albers et al. (41) designed a study to assess the use of antithrombotic therapy (either warfarin or aspirin) for patients with nonvalvular atrial fibrillation in six academic hospitals. Use of these agents upon admission and at discharge were compared. Risk factors for stroke and contraindications to anticoagulation were also assessed to determine whether there was a relation to the choice of antithrombotic therapy. Some 83% of those enrolled in this study were older than 60 years. At discharge, more than 20% of patients with risk factors for stroke and no contraindications to anticoagulation were not receiving antithrombotic therapy. Of this group, 34% were prescribed aspirin, even though they did not have a contraindication to anticoagulation. This study also reported that patients older than 75 years with no contraindications were less likely to be prescribed anticoagulation than younger patients. However, the difference was not statistically significant. Finally, more than 50% of the patients admitted on warfarin had an international normalized ratio (INR) less than the recommended range of 2 to 3. Warfarin is recommended as a first-line agent in patients older than 75 years with atrial fibrillation because of the increased rate of stroke in this population. Warfarin is also recommended in those aged 65 to 75 years if risk factors for stroke are present (43). Risk factors for stroke include previous stroke, transient ischemic attack, or systemic embolism; advanced age; hypertension; cardiac disorders, including congestive heart failure, angina, and myocardial infarction; and diabetes (22).

Two studies show that physicians hesitate to prescribe anticoagulants in elderly patients and would use this treatment less intensively than is recommended (44, 45). An explanation for the underprescribing of warfarin in this population is the possible increased risk of bleeding. There have been conflicting reports about the risk associated with warfarin therapy in the elderly (20, 46–48). The evidence does suggest that there is an increased risk; however, careful patient selection and monitoring of therapy can minimize this risk. The potential for a decrease in the rate of thromboembolism must be compared with the increase in the bleeding risk.

McLaughlin et al. (35) and Ayanian et al. (49) have shown that practitioners are reticent to prescribe certain treatments. A factor that may contribute to the underprescribing of medications is lack of knowledge that the treatment may be beneficial in certain patient populations. Ayanian et al. (49) found that internists and family practitioners were less likely to prescribe certain treatments such as thrombolytics or β-blockers for MI than cardiologists. This study underscores an important point, that the dissemination of information from clinical trials may not be widespread or rapid. New and better techniques to educate health care professionals about the benefits of treating the elderly are needed.

All therapeutic interventions are associated with risks. Certainly, the therapies described here involve risk, potentially life threatening. However, not receiving appropriate treatment may also be a detriment to the elderly patient.

Coordinated Medication Database

The third major topic in ensuring optimal pharmacotherapy in the elderly is the most fundamental: the development of a coordinated medication database. All drugs, including prescription, OTC, natural or herbal products, and "borrowed" or saved medications should be included. The list is essential to prevent drug-induced disease and drug-food and drug-drug interactions. The following section focuses on two components of the comprehensive medication database.

Over-the-Counter Drugs

The use of OTC products should be thoroughly documented as more prescription drugs are switched to this class. Patients may not consider an OTC product to be a drug and may neglect to inform the physician or other provider about its use unless specifically prompted. When asking about the use of OTC products, reliance on a brand name identified by the patient is no longer sufficient. Increasingly, a new OTC drug is given an established product's name with a slight change such as Mylanta AR, which contains famotidine instead of the traditional aluminum-magnesium antacid.

Although OTC drugs were rarely associated with significant drug-induced disease or drug interactions in the past, the risk of developing medication-related problems has increased. A case control study has reported that the use of nonsteroidal anti-inflammatory drugs (NSAIDs) is correlated with initiation of antihypertensive therapy in the elderly population (50) In addition, a recent clinical trial demonstrates that the addition of ibuprofen to antihypertensive therapy with hydrochlorothiazide reduced blood pressure control (51). The OTC use of NSAIDs has also been recognized as an important cause of upper GI hemorrhage (52).

A final issue with OTC products should be considered. The use of these medications is frequently self-directed, and while they are generally very safe, patients may not recognize that ibuprofen, naproxen, and fenoprofen or famotidine, ranitidine, cimetidine, and nizatidine are from the same pharmacologic classes. Patients may use multiple products from within the same pharmacologic class unless they are specifically advised always to consult the pharmacist or physician.

Natural Products

Information should also be obtained about the use of natural products, as 28% of Americans aged 50 years or older reported the use of some type of alternative therapy such as herbal remedies, chiropractic, and massage therapy in a 1991 survey (53). Some 70% of respondents did not tell their physician that they were using an alternative therapy (53). Only 5% reported the use of herbal products in the study, but this figure may be much higher, since the widespread promotion and use of herbal and natural products, such as melatonin, began *after* the study.

Natural products may have benefits, side effects, and drug interactions. For example, feverfew has been shown to reduce the number and severity of migraine headaches (54), while half to one clove of garlic daily reduced elevated total cholesterol concentrations by 9% in a meta-analysis (55). St. John's wort may contain chemicals that act as monoamine oxidase inhibitors (56). While some clinical trials with natural products have been published, a key consideration remains whether the product from the local health food store is identical or even similar to the preparation used in a specific study. Content and bioavailability data on natural products are generally lacking. Table 5.5 lists selected herbal products by their common use or indication.

Toxicity from natural products may arise either from the product itself or from unlabeled components. For example, gingko, which is used for enhancing memory, may cause restlessness, nausea, and vomiting (56). Teas containing comfrey have been associated with hepatic failure (56). The presence of unlabeled ingredients, including diazepam and mefenamic acid, in pharmacologic doses was reported in a case series of four women who presented with symptoms consistent with NSAID toxicity after taking Chinese herbal products (57).

Table 5.5

Common Uses for Herbal Products

Antiaging agents	Benign prostatic hypertrophy
Gotu kola	Cucurbita
Royal jelly	Nettle
Antiarthritic and antiaging agents	Saw palmetto
Alfalfa	Diuretic agents
Arnica	Borage
Calendula	Broom
Capsicum	Buchu
Chamomile	Horsetail
Devil's claw	Juniper
Kelp	Nettle
Pokeroot	Hypotensive agents
Yucca	Garlic
Antidepressant agents	Ginseng
L-Tryptophan	Hawthorne
St. John's wort	Circulation improvers
Anti-infective, antiseptic, healing agents	Butcher's broom
Aloe	Gingko
Barberry	Lipid-lowering agents
Buchu	Alfalfa
Calendula	Bran
Comfrey	Garlic
Cranberry	Ginseng
Echinacea	Evening primrose
Goldenseal	Sedative, hypnotic
Aphrodisiac, sexual stimulant	Valerian root
Ginseng	
Royal jelly	
Saw palmetto	
Yohimbe	

Table 5.6

Evaluating the Appropriateness of Pharmacotherapy

Clinical Consideration	Example
Is there a specific indication for the drug, and is it effective?	"Unpaired" drugs such as digoxin and H_2 antagonists without a documented indication for use
Is the dosage appropriate, given renal and/or hepatic function?	Antibiotics and many other drugs
Are the duration of therapy and specific outcomes defined?	Short-term benzodiazepine use for acute grief vs. long-term indiscriminate use
Are the instructions for use practical and appropriate to the person?	Simple instructions for warfarin use
Are drug-drug, drug-disease, and drug-diet interactions avoided?	
Are drugs prescribed to treat the side effects of other medications?	Use of levodopa for drug-induced parkinsonian symptoms from metoclopramide
Are the most cost-effective drugs prescribed?	Multiple dose captopril for hypertension

The potential for drug interactions between natural products and prescription medications is a particular concern, but information on this topic is generally lacking. For example, sassafras tea contains safrole, a potent inhibitor of hepatic microsomal hydroxylating enzymes responsible for the metabolism of the active isomer of warfarin (56).

Appropriateness of Drug Therapy

In developing a coordinated medication database, the appropriateness of all drugs should be evaluated. Beers et al. (28) published a list of "inappropriate" medications that was developed according to consensus criteria. The fact that an elderly patient avoids these drugs does not necessarily mean that the rest of the patient's medications are appropriate. A medication appropriateness index has been developed to identify practical issues to consider in evaluating drug therapy (58). The following discussion focuses on several questions listed in Table 5.6.

Is there a specific indication for the drug, and is it effective? Every drug should be matched to a well-documented diagnosis. The use of drugs unpaired to a diagnosis should be carefully reevaluated and their use discontinued whenever possible. Cardiac medications, including digoxin and quinidine, frequently are found to

be unpaired in reviews of the nursing home resident's medical record. Histamine (H_2) receptor antagonists have also been identified as common unpaired drugs.

Is the dosage appropriate, given renal and hepatic function? Aging is a dynamic process. The presence of diseases such as diabetes mellitus or the use of drugs such as aminoglycosides may contribute to subtle declines in renal function over time. As many drug-induced diseases are dose-related, a simple reevaluation of the dosage may minimize problems.

Are the instructions for use practical and appropriate to the person? In the hospital, complicated dosing regimens for drugs such as warfarin permit the careful titration of therapy to the person. At home, dosing regimens should be as simple as possible. Whenever possible, doses should be linked to specific daily events such as bedtime to minimize problems.

Medication Counseling

Talking with older patients about their medications is low tech and frequently overlooked. Inadequate communication remains a major cause of noncompliance with prescribed regimens, treatment failures, medication misuse, and adverse reactions. Medication counseling usually occurs at the end of an office visit, when many patients, young and old, do not remember the precise details of what was discussed.

Counseling must be conducted in an atmosphere sensitive to the person's cultural or ethnic background, concomitant diseases, and age-related declines. The concept of chronic medication use may be new to certain cultural or ethnic groups. For example, if the chronic nature of hypertension has not been discussed, a person may assume that the disease is cured when the medication runs out. An effective counseling strategy must also acknowledge any visual, auditory, or cognitive impairments. While a spouse or other family member should be present during discussion of medications, the potential for subtle cognitive impairment in these persons should also be considered. The patient or caregiver should know the name and description of the drug, dosage, route, frequency, duration of therapy, special directions including those for a missed dose, side effects, food and drug interactions, disease state effects, storage and stability, refills, and self-monitoring techniques.

Promoting Adherence

The number of prescribed medications remains one of the most important determinants of compliance. Basic considerations in promoting adherence are listed in Table 5.7.

DRUGS AND FUNCTIONAL STATUS

Medications carry both a benefit and risk. Practitioners recognize the traditional risk of idiosyncratic adverse side effects in older persons and may alter their prescribing habits according to their experience with particular medications. For the frail older person, side effects

Table 5.7

Simple Strategies for Promoting Compliance

Reduce the number of prescribed drugs.
Simplify all dosage regimens.
Use the best-tolerated medications.
Evaluate the patient's functional ability to take
  medications.
Promote routine contact with single physician.
Promote routine contact with only one pharmacy.

that affect the ability to function may be important to the quality of life. Medications may affect a person's mobility, urinary continence, and mental functioning.

Mobility

Ray et al. (31) first demonstrated the association between the use of psychotropic medications and falls. In this now classic article, benzodiazepines with a long elimination half-life, tricyclic antidepressants, and typical antipsychotics were shown to be significantly associated with falls resulting in hip fracture. A strong dose-response effect was observed. While a causal relationship can not be claimed because of the study design used, many other investigators have confirmed this association.

New evidence suggests a biologic cause for benzodiazepine-associated falls. Assessment of cognitive and balance measures showed that one oral dose of diazepam in 10 healthy persons, average age 70 years, increased the anterior tibialis muscle's latency time and lowered neurocognitive tests in comparison with placebo (59). Use of antipsychotics or drugs in the anxiolytic-sedative-hypnotic group were shown to be independent risk factors associated with injurious falls (60).

The long-term use of oral corticosteroids leads to osteoporosis through an increase in bone resorption, a decrease in calcium absorption in the intestine, and an increase in calcium excretion in the kidneys. Efforts to prevent osteoporosis in patients who require oral treatment with corticosteroids have shown inconsistent results. One prospective trial showed that calcitriol 0.6 μg per day with 1 g of elemental calcium administered for a year prevented bone loss in the lumbar spine but not in the femoral neck or distal radius. Intranasal calcitonin may improve the protective effect (61). Patients with osteoporosis who are also receiving oral corticosteroids should be treated with bisphosphonates, nasal calcitonin, and calcitriol (62, 63).

Urinary Continence

Drugs may also impair a person's ability to control urination. Urinary retention may be caused by many medications, including anticholinergic agents, drugs with anticholinergic side effects, and smooth muscle relaxants, such as nifedipine (64, 65). Inhibiting the cholinergic pathways prevents the bladder from contracting, which may lead to overflow incontinence. This is especially troublesome in older men with prostatic hypertrophy. Additionally, the α-agonists, such as phenylpropanolamine, tighten the urinary sphincter, which can contribute to urinary retention in men. In women, however, who are more likely to have stress incontinence secondary to pelvic floor atrophy, α-agonists and estrogens may improve sphincter tone (66, 67). This is true for α-blockers such as prazosin, terazosin, and doxazosin. By relaxing the urinary sphincter, α-blockers may alleviate urinary retention in men suffering from prostatic hypertrophy; in women these drugs may worsen stress incontinence. Thus patients must be informed and questioned about changes in their ability to remain continent when such medications are added to their regimens.

Mental Functioning

Drug-induced changes in mental functioning remain a common clinical condition; the prevalence estimates of delirium in medical inpatients are reported to range between 10 and 30%. Some authors claim drug toxicity to be the most common cause of reversible delirium (68). Most studies evaluating drug-induced changes in mental functioning cite multiple risk factors including advanced age, comorbid diseases, postoperative states, and polypharmacy. While it may be difficult to isolate any particular causative factor in a patient, the maintenance of cognitive ability is vital for optimal patient functioning and independence. This must be a defined goal of any drug therapy.

Drugs most commonly cited as causative in drug-induced mental deterioration include those with psychiatric or neurologic effects, diuretics, centrally active antihypertensives, antiinfectives, anticholinergics, analgesics, corticosteroids, H_2 receptor antagonists, and opioids.

Anticonvulsants are reported to cause a wide range of mental state and behavior changes. Newer agents with pharmacologic action at the γ-aminobutyric (GABA) receptor, such as tiagabine, topiramate, and vigabatrin, may cause depression. Carbamazepine and valproate modulate mood and are successful therapies for bipolar disorders. In persons with treatment-resistant seizure disorders who were successfully controlled with newer anticonvulsants such as lamotrigine, tiagabine, topiramate, and vigabatrin, frank psychosis is reported to occur in approximately 2 to 3% (69). Older anticonvulsants, such as phenytoin and phenobarbital, are well documented in their effects to impair concentration, mental energy, mood, and memory. When treating older adults with seizure disorders, adherence to the recommendation for single-agent therapy should be followed.

Other drug classes frequently implicated as a cause of mental status changes include those with neurologic effects such as benzodiazepines, antipsychotics, anticholinergics, and some centrally acting antihypertensives. Benzodiazepines should be sparingly used, and when necessary for those in the 65 to 75 age group, reduction to half of the customary adult dosage is recommended. Specific dosage guidelines for those older than 75 years and for those with significant concomitant illness are not available. One quarter of the recommended adult dose is a conservative starting dose.

Medications with anticholinergic effects continue to be reported as a cause for mental status changes, along with other side effects such as chronic constipation, in older persons (70, 71). Diphenhydramine should be avoided as a hypnotic in older persons. Careful attention to the use of OTC medications is also needed, as anticholinergic antihistamines are often used in combination products promoted for sleep or analgesic plus sleep effects and in cough and cold products.

Treatment choices for hypertension are large, allowing practitioners to avoid the use of centrally active agents in older persons. The association between depression and the use of β-blockers continues to be controversial (72). The large-scale retrospective studies do not consistently show the association between the use of β-blockers and development of depression (73, 74). Certainly case reports of a compelling nature describe persons who develop depression after the initiation of a β-blocker. The presentation of depression may be atypical in an older person, with a predominance of vegetative symptoms such as sleeplessness, appetite suppression, and constipation, as well as lability of mood. The onset is usually insidious, occurring over months rather than abruptly after a medication is started (72).

SELECTED PHARMACOLOGIC GROUPS

Natural Products

Melatonin

Melatonin is a neurohormone secreted by the pineal gland at night, with peak production occurring between 2 and 4 AM (75). While it is recognized to control circadian rhythms, melatonin may also have other direct effects on sleep, mood disorders, cancer, immune disorders, and aging. Moderate decreases in the nighttime serum concentrations of melatonin have been associated with aging (76). A relation between low concentrations of melatonin and sleep disorders in the elderly may also exist (76, 77). Certain drugs, such as alcohol, caffeine, benzodiazepines, β-adrenergic blockers, and valproic acid, may reduce the production and release of melatonin, possibly explaining the drugs' varied effects on the central nervous system (78, 79).

Melatonin has been available as a food supplement for several years. In 1995, 20 million new consumers began taking it, although one report indicated that only 500 people had participated in clinical trials of it for disorders of biologic rhythms and sleep (80). The lack of information on the safety and efficacy of melatonin from randomized clinical trials has resulted in many unanswered questions. For example, the optimal dose, time of administration, duration, and preparation of melatonin for the elderly with insomnia is unknown. Doses of melatonin generally have been 0.3 to 2 mg daily, with the time of administration ranging from bedtime to 2 hours earlier (75). The bioavailability of melatonin preparations may vary widely. The side effect and drug interaction profiles of melatonin remain unknown.

Dehydroepiandrosterone

Dehydroepiandrosterone (DHEA) is a hormone synthesized primarily by the adrenal gland and partially metabolized into androgens, including testosterone and other androgenic compounds that can be further transformed into weakly estrogenic substances (81). DHEA may also increase concentrations of insulinlike growth factor 1 and affect neurotransmitter receptors (82). Concentrations of DHEA and its sulfate, DHEAS, peak in persons aged 25 and have been estimated to decline by 2% per year until the eighth and ninth decade, when residual concentrations are only 10 to 20% of the peak level (83).

While DHEA may have protective effects against colon cancer, diabetes mellitus, atherosclerosis, and viral infections, interest in the hormone has centered on its potential benefits against aging (79). Recently, the relationships between baseline DHEAS concentrations and declines in functional, psychological, and mental status were reported from a 4-year community-based cohort study of 622 persons over age 65 (82). Significantly lower baseline DHEAS concentrations were present in women with functional limitations and overall poor health status, but the relation did not achieve statistical significance in men.

Clinical studies with DHEA have included only small numbers of elderly persons for short periods with inconclusive results (84, 85). The long-term safety of DHEA remains unknown. Since DHEA may be metabolized to androgenic and estrogenic compounds, it may increase the risk of breast or prostate cancers when ingested for a long period.

Diuretics

Diuretics can be divided into three general groups: thiazides and related drugs, loop diuretics, and potassium-sparing agents. Thiazides include hydrochlorothiazide, chlorthalidone, metolazone, and indapamide among many others. Alone or in combination with potassium-sparing diuretics, hydrochlorothiazide remains the most commonly prescribed thiazide diuretic. Chlorthalidone has a half-life in excess of 40 hours and can result in significant hypokalemia. Metolazone differs from other thiazides in that its antihypertensive activity persists even as the creatinine clearance drops below 30 mL/min, while indapamide is lipid neutral.

Loop diuretics include furosemide, bumetanide, and torsemide. In general, loop diuretics are less effective than thiazides as antihypertensive agents. The use of loop diuretics as antihypertensive agents is limited primarily to patients who have a creatinine clearance below 30 mL/min or who have concomitant edema. Potassium-sparing diuretics include triamterene, amiloride, and spironolactone. They are used to minimize or correct the hypokalemia associated with thiazide diuretics, as amiloride and triamterene lack significant antihypertensive properties. Hyperkalemia secondary to potassium-sparing diuretics has occurred in the presence of concomitant renal insufficiency, diabetes mellitus, angiotensin-converting enzyme (ACE) inhibitors, and potassium supplementation. Although it is uncommon, older patients receiving triamterene may develop nephrolithiasis.

The use of thiazide diuretics in newly diagnosed elderly hypertensives has increased after the publication of three studies demonstrating the benefits of diuretics in older patients with hypertension (86–89). The results of these trials suggest that the use of a low-dose thiazide diuretic can reduce the risk of stroke and coronary heart disease in the otherwise healthy elderly. Subsequently, the Joint National Committee on the Detection, Evaluation, and Treatment of High Blood Pressure has recommended both diuretics and β-blockers as first-line agents in the treatment of hypertension. The newer agents, such as calcium channel blockers and ACE inhibitors, may have a role in particular settings (90).

Other results from the Systolic Hypertension in the Elderly Program (SHEP) trial have been published. The use of low-dose diuretics to treat isolated systolic hypertension (ISH) was shown to decrease the risk of developing heart failure, especially in patients with a history of electrocardiographic evidence of a prior myocardial infarction (91). The data from SHEP also show that the treatment of ISH does not cause deterioration in the quality of life. Mood, cognitive function, basic self-care skills, and moderate leisure activity remained stable in the participants of SHEP, regardless of treatment assignment (92). Finally, the data from SHEP were analyzed to determine whether outcomes would differ between diabetics and nondiabetics. The research group found that the absolute risk reduction was greater for diabetics who received treatment than for treated nondiabetics (93).

Higher doses of diuretics may worsen serum electrolyte, glucose, and lipoprotein concentrations. Monane et al. (94) have shown that the use of high-dose thiazides (at least 50 mg) is significantly associated with the initiation of lipid-lowering agents in older people.

In low doses and when carefully monitored, thiazide diuretics are safe, effective, and inexpensive first-line antihypertensive agents for otherwise healthy elderly persons (90). Doses should be limited to 12.5 to 25 mg of hydrochlorothiazide (or an equivalent thiazide) per day. Serum potassium concentrations should be monitored routinely, and supplementation should be initiated when levels approach 3.5 mEq/L. Persistent hypokalemia despite appropriate supplementation may suggest concomitant hypomagnesemia, which must be corrected first.

β-Blockers

β-Blockers can be differentiated on the basis of cardioselectivity, lipid solubility, intrinsic sympathomimetic activity, and presence of concomitant α-blocking activity. Cardioselective β-blockers such as atenolol exert most of their effects on cardiac β_1 receptors and less on β_2 receptors. Cardioselectivity is relative and disappears with increasing doses of a β-blocker. β-Blockers also differ in their lipid solubilities. Previously, only the highly lipid-soluble agents such as propranolol and metoprolol were believed to penetrate the central nervous system to a significant degree. It was thought that drowsiness and other central nervous system side effects could be minimized by choosing a hydrophilic drug such as nadolol. However, it is now recognized that all β-blockers cross the blood-brain barrier.

β-Blockers with intrinsic sympathomimetic activity (ISA), such as pindolol, may have slight agonist properties at low levels of sympathetic nervous system activity. This may produce less resting bradycardia. ISA is also associated with fewer adverse effects on lipid and lipoprotein concentrations. However, with the possible exception of acebutolol, β-blockers with ISA do not provide protection against recurrent myocardial infarction.

β-Blockers have been shown to decrease cardiovascular morbidity and mortality when used to treat elderly hypertensive patients (87, 88). These agents are recommended as first-line treatment of hypertension in older patients (90).

A common belief is that β-blockers impair psychologic functioning, including cognitive ability. This has been challenged in several studies of older hypertensives (95, 96). Drowsiness was no more common with atenolol or metoprolol than with placebo in 27 older patients with hypertension (95).

The other side effects of β-blockers are well-known extensions of their pharmacologic properties. The withdrawal syndrome following abrupt discontinuation is a final important consideration in using β-blockers in the elderly. Given the presence of silent coronary artery disease in older persons, β-blockers should be carefully tapered whenever possible in this population.

Angiotensin-Converting Enzyme Inhibitors

ACE inhibitors vary in their structure, pharmacokinetics, duration, and potency. Enalapril, fosinopril, moexipril, benazepril, quinapril, trandolapril, and ramipril are hydrolyzed into active compounds, resulting in a prolonged onset and duration of activity. All of the ACE inhibitors have recommended dosage reductions for patients with renal insufficiency.

ACE inhibitors are effective in the treatment of hypertension in older persons. However, these agents have not been shown to decrease morbidity and mortality, as have diuretics and β-blockers (90). All ACE inhibitors may produce hypotension within a few hours of the first dose (97). This is more likely to occur in patients who are volume-depleted, such as those receiving high-dose diuretic therapy. The risk may be reduced if a small dose of an ACE inhibitor is used to start therapy and the dosage is slowly titrated thereafter. Volume depletion and congestive heart failure also put a patient at risk for acute renal dysfunction when an ACE inhibitor is started.

Concomitant diuretic and NSAID use may also increase the risk of ACE inhibitor-induced renal dysfunction. The elderly are at more risk than younger patients. Dehydration should be corrected, and diuretics may have to be temporarily withheld if ACE inhibitor therapy is necessary and the risk of acute renal dysfunction seems high. If renal dysfunction does occur, decreasing the dose of the ACE inhibitor or concomitant diuretic may correct the abnormality. Finally, the possibility of bilateral renal artery stenosis should always be considered in any older person who has recently developed severe hypertension and develops acute renal failure from an ACE inhibitor (97).

A dry nonproductive cough is seen in as many as 20% of patients taking ACE inhibitors. While discontinuing the drug is always preferred, a reduction in the dose may lessen the coughing in some patients. Case reports have suggested that nifedipine or an NSAID may lessen the cough while continuing the ACE inhibitor (98, 99). However, the NSAID may blunt the antihypertensive activity of ACE inhibitors and in the setting of congestive heart failure may produce acute renal failure. Inhaled sodium cromoglycate has also been studied. Further studies are needed before this can be recommended as a definitive treatment (100).

A high incidence of skin rash has been noted to occur in the initial trials of captopril. However, this appears to have been related to the high dosages used at the time. Hyperkalemia can develop with all ACE inhibitors, usually in the presence of preexisting renal dysfunction or concomitant intake of potassium supplements, potassium-sparing diuretics, or a salt substitute. Angioedema of the face, lips, tongue, glottis, larynx, and mucous membranes, which has been reported with the first dose of all ACE inhibitors, can occur anytime during treatment and can be life threatening.

Several studies have shown that ACE inhibitors can decrease mortality in patients with heart failure (101–103). ACE inhibitors have also been shown to improve symptoms and quality of life in patients with congestive heart failure (103). A growing number of studies have shown that ACE inhibitor use after MI can improve survival and decrease the incidence of congestive heart failure (104–106). Contrary results were reported in the Cooperative New Scandinavian Enalapril Survival Study (CONSENSUS) II trial (107). However, CONSENSUS II was different in many ways from these other trials. For example, in CONSENSUS II, the ACE inhibitor was started acutely after the MI (versus waiting at least 3 days in other trials), and all patients with MI were randomized (versus only those with left ventricular dysfunction). Finally, ACE inhibitors appear to slow the progression of diabetic nephropathy (108–110).

Angiotensin-II Receptor Antagonists

Losartan and valsartan belong to a new class of drugs, the angiotensin-II receptor antagonists. These agents are effective in treating hypertension, are well tolerated, and have a lower incidence of cough than the ACE inhibitors (111, 112). The Evaluation of Losartan in the Elderly Study (ELITE) was a randomized trial of losartan versus captopril in 722 patients older than 65 years who had heart failure (113). The primary end point, the frequency of a persisting increase in serum creatinine of at least 0.3 mg/dL, was similar in the two groups. The secondary end point, death and/or hospital admission for heart failure, was also similar between the groups (9.4% for losartan versus 13.2% for captopril; p =.075). However, a greater decrease in all-cause mortality occurred in the losartan group (4.8% versus 8.7% for captopril; p =.035). Further study of this class of medications is needed to determine its place in the treatment of hypertension and heart failure.

Calcium Channel Blockers

Calcium channel blockers fall into five distinct pharmacologic groups, including the dihydropyridines (nifedipine, felodipine, isradipine, amlodipine, nicardipine, nimodipine), diltiazem, verapamil, bepridil, and mibefradil. Mibefradil is a new drug, and little information on its use in the elderly is available.

Vasodilation, negative inotropic effects, and cardiac conduction effects are three major properties of calcium channel blockers. Vasodilation is greatest with most of the dihydropyridines, while negative inotropic properties predominate with verapamil. Cardiac conduction disturbances are associated most frequently with verapamil, to a lesser extent with diltiazem, and rarely with the dihydropyridine calcium channel blockers. The hemodynamic effects of calcium channel blockers portrayed in comparison charts are derived from studies in normal healthy persons. Actual clinical responses among the elderly are the result of direct and indirect hemodynamic effects including age-related decreases in baroreceptor responsiveness and concomitant cardiovascular diseases.

Calcium channel blockers are effective antihypertensive agents in older persons, although their actual effects on morbidity and mortality are unknown. They do not adversely effect coexisting diseases such as chronic obstructive lung disease and gout. Adverse effects of calcium channel blockers usually are an extension of their pharmacologic properties. Constipation, also common with verapamil, can be minimized by the concomitant use of a stool softener. Pedal edema typically is associated with the dihydropyridines.

Calcium channel blockers have become one of the most commonly prescribed groups of drugs to treat hypertension (86). Several recent publications suggest that the use of these agents may be associated with an increase in the risk of myocardial infarction and mortality (114–116). There are several possible biases to these studies. Since the publication of these trials, the Food and Drug Administration (FDA) has concluded that calcium channel blockers are safe (117). However, the FDA did warn that the use of short-acting nifedipine may increase the risk of myocardial infarction in some patients, and the use of this agent to treat hypertension should be discouraged.

The Multicenter Isradipine Diuretic Atherosclerosis Study (MIDAS) was designed to compare isradipine, a short-acting dihydropyridine calcium channel blocker, with hydrochlorothiazide. The main outcome measure was the rate of progression in carotid artery intimal-medial thickness (IMT). Secondary outcomes included major vascular events, such as MI, stroke, congestive heart failure, angina, and sudden death, as well as nonmajor vascular events and procedures, such as transient ischemic attack, dysrhythmia, aortic valve replacement, and femoral popliteal bypass graft. Although no difference in IMT was found between the treatment groups over the 3-year study period, in the isradipine group there was a higher incidence of major vascular events (not statistically significant) and significantly more nonmajor vascular events and procedures than in the thiazide group (118).

In summary, more than one study has produced similar results: calcium channel blockers, short-acting dihydropyridines in particular, have adverse health effects in elderly hypertensives. In addition, a dose response was seen in these studies, with higher doses increasing the risk of a negative outcome. Finally, a large, randomized, controlled trial (MIDAS) supported the findings of the smaller epidemiologic studies. These studies suggest that the short-acting dihydropyridine calcium channel blockers should be used cautiously.

Additional concerns with the long-term safety of short-acting calcium channel blockers have been raised by three reports (119–121). The use of dihydropyridines was associated with increased perioperative bleeding (119) and an increased incidence of GI hemorrhage (120).

These data may not be applicable to the long-acting products, which are more commonly prescribed. The National Institutes of Health Antihypertensive and Lipid Lowering to Prevent Heart Attack Trial (ALLHAT) may answer some questions about the long-acting products. It seems prudent to restrict the use of short-acting dihydropyridines whenever possible.

Cholesterol-Lowering Drugs

Four major groups of cholesterol-lowering medications are available. The bile acid sequestrants include colestipol and cholestyramine; the fibric acid derivatives are gemfibrozil and clofibrate; the HMG-CoA reductase inhibitors, also known as the statins, include lovastatin, simvastatin, fluvastatin, pravastatin, and atorvastatin; and niacin is the fourth.

Few data on the use of cholesterol-lowering drugs in the elderly are available. More important, the association between elevated cholesterol and coronary heart disease in older populations remains unclear. Data from the Framingham Heart Study found the risk ratio for the development of coronary heart disease was less for those over age 50 than for those younger than 50 (122). Krumholz et al. (123) found no association between serum cholesterol and incidence of or death from coronary heart disease (CHD) in persons over age 70. However, two recent studies in older adults have found an association between increased serum cholesterol and the risk of CHD (124, 125).

Two recent secondary prevention studies included elderly subjects. The Scandinavian Simvastatin Survival Study (4S) and the Cholesterol and Recurrent Events trial (CARE) enrolled patients up to age 70 and 75 years, respectively (126, 127). Both studies found that drug treatment significantly decreased the risk of death (4S), death from CHD or nonfatal MI (CARE), and the risk of major coronary events (4S and CARE). Based on the results from these studies, secondary prevention in the elderly can now be recommended.

The results of the Antihypertensive and Lipid Lowering to Prevent Heart Attack Trial (ALLHAT) are expected in 2002. This study will compare the benefits of drug treatment (a statin) versus usual care in elderly men and women. Finally, the results of the Cholesterol Reduction in Seniors Program (CRISP) pilot study demonstrated the safety of lovastatin 20 to 40 mg in men and women over age 65 being treated for a year. Significant reductions in total cholesterol and low-density lipoprotein were observed in both treatment groups. This study was designed to also measure CHD risk reduction. However, the trial was prematurely stopped because of lack of funds (128).

Elderly patients who are otherwise in good health and are at increased risk for a myocardial infarction should be considered for treatment of hypercholesterolemia (129). Estrogen replacement therapy should be discussed with postmenopausal women.

Caution should be exercised in the use of these agents. A recent review of animal studies of carcinogenicity of lipid-lowering drugs suggested that long-term trials of these agents in humans are needed to determine whether they cause cancer in humans. These agents caused cancer in laboratory rats at levels of exposure that are equivalent to human doses (130).

Nitrates

Nitrates include nitroglycerin, isosorbide dinitrate, isosorbide-5-mononitrate, erythrityl tetranitrate, and pentaerythritol tetranitrate. Isosorbide mononitrate, the primary active metabolite of isosorbide dinitrate, differs from its parent compound and nitroglycerin in that it does not undergo significant first-pass metabolism.

Information comparing the pharmacokinetics and pharmacodynamics of nitrates across age groups is limited. Greater systemic bioavailability might be expected with the use of nitroglycerin or isosorbide dinitrate in elderly patients, as both drugs have a high degree of first-pass metabolism. In addition, it is unknown whether age-related differences occur in the percutaneous absorption of nitrates from transdermal preparations. In one study anginal symptoms among the elderly were relieved more rapidly with the use of an oral nitroglycerin spray than with sublingual tablets, possibly the result of dryness in the mouth, which may slow the dissolution of sublingual tablets (131).

Hemodynamic sensitivity to nitrates does not appear to change with age. However, baroreceptor activity can decline, and the elderly may not be able to increase their heart rate adequately in response to nitrate-induced vasodilation. Therefore, postural symptoms from nitrate administration may be greater in older patients.

A critical issue in the use of all nitrates is the development of tolerance. Nitrate tolerance is prevented by having a daily 10-hour nitrate-free interval, which can be during sleep, when sympathetic tone and myocardial oxygen demand are low, unless the patient is having anginal symptoms during REM sleep (132). With a nitroglycerin patch, applying it early in the morning and removing it in the early evening should be adequate. Recent claims about new nitrate dosage forms and their purported lack of tolerance simply indicate that the drug-free interval has been incorporated into the labeled prescribing directions; it is not an intrinsic advantage of the product.

Nonsteroidal Anti-inflammatory Drugs

NSAIDs can be divided into broad groups: acetic acids, propionic acids, oxicams, and salicylates. The drugs vary in their duration of action, dosing, potency, tissue penetration, and cost (133). Although they are effective in older populations, the use of NSAIDs has been associated with many side effects, including gastropathy and nephrotoxicity, in the elderly. Proposed risk factors for NSAID-induced gastropathy include a history of peptic ulcer disease or GI bleeding, advanced age, large doses, cigarette smoking, and concomitant ethanol and exposure to other ulcerogenic drugs.

Once an NSAID-induced ulcer has been identified, the need for continued therapy should be reevaluated. If the NSAID can be discontinued, ulcers heal rapidly with any standard therapy for peptic ulcer disease. When continued therapy is warranted, the choice of an ulcer treatment is more problematic. Studies with H_2-receptor antagonists and sucralfate have been conflicting, but ulcers less than 5 mm in diameter often heal spontaneously despite continued NSAID therapy (133). Omeprazole 40 mg per day was more effective than ranitidine 150 mg twice daily in healing large gastric ulcers, despite continued NSAID therapy (134).

Prevention of NSAID-induced gastropathy must begin with a reevaluation of the need for the drug. Acetaminophen or a nonacetylated salicylate may be as effective as an NSAID for osteoarthritis (135). While food or H_2-receptor antagonists may decrease dyspeptic symptoms, the risk of developing a gastric ulceration and clinically significant GI bleeding is not reduced.

The only drug approved for the prevention of NSAID-induced gastric ulceration is misoprostol, which has both antisecretory and mucosal protective properties (136). The recommended dose is 200 μg 4 times daily, with meals and at bedtime. Diarrhea and abdominal pain are common, with the diarrhea dose related and generally transient. The diarrhea may be lessened by starting at 100 μg 2 to 3 times daily and gradually increasing the dose as tolerated. While risk factors for NSAID-induced gastropathy have been proposed, identifying actual candidates for whom long-term prophylaxis with misoprostol would be cost-effective remains problematic. Studies of the cost-effectiveness of misoprostol have been conflicting as a result of major differences in the assumed risks associated with the use of NSAIDs (136).

NSAIDs may decrease the effectiveness of antihypertensive medication. A meta-analysis by Pope et al. (137) showed that indomethacin and naproxen increased the mean arterial pressure in hypertensive subjects by 3.59 mm Hg and 3.75 mm Hg, respectively. However, this was in a young group of patients, average age 46 years. As previously stated, Gurwitz et al. (50) found that current users of NSAIDs were more likely to initiate therapy with an antihypertensive than nonusers. This was a case-control study of Medicaid enrollees aged 65 years and older. The likelihood of starting antihypertensive medication increased with increasing doses of NSAIDs (50). Elderly patients taking NSAIDs should have their blood pressure monitored, whether or not they are on antihypertensive medication.

Oral Hypoglycemic Agents

First-generation sulfonylureas include tolbutamide, tolazamide, acetohexamide, and chlorpropamide. Their use has declined since the introduction of glyburide and glipizide, which offer potential advantages in terms of fewer drug interactions and side effects. Chlorpropamide should be avoided in elderly diabetics because of its prolonged half-life, which approaches 72 hours, and the accompanying risk of hypoglycemia. In addition, the use of chlorpropamide has been associated with the development of hyponatremia in older patients (138). Glyburide is metabolized by the liver to active metabolites that are cleared renally. Glipizide, which is metabolized to inactive metabolites, may be preferred in the elderly (139).

Both glyburide and glipizide can be administered once daily, depending on the total daily dose. Glipizide is available as a long-acting preparation that can also be administered once a day. For patients who are able to take the immediate-release product once daily, drug selection should be based on tolerability. Glipizide should

not be taken with food; the absorption of the drug may be reduced. The presence of food does not affect the absorption of glyburide.

Recently, three new agents have been approved for treatment. Metformin, a biguanide, has multiple mechanisms of action. It decreases hepatic glucose output by decreasing gluconeogenesis and increases glucose clearance in the muscle. Metformin has also been shown to decrease plasma insulin concentrations. It rarely results in hypoglycemia when used as monotherapy, but it can cause troublesome GI side effects, including diarrhea, discomfort, anorexia, and a metallic taste. A slow dosage titration can minimize these effects. The most serious side effect associated with biguanide therapy is lactic acidosis, but its overall incidence is low (0.027 to 0.06 cases per 1000 patient-years). Contraindications to therapy include conditions associated with increased production or decreased elimination of lactate, such as renal impairment, hepatic disease, congestive heart failure, and alcoholism. Metformin is as effective as the sulfonylureas. However, because of the contraindications, many elderly patients are not eligible for therapy (140).

Acarbose is an α-glucosidase inhibitor that slows down carbohydrate metabolism in the gut. This results in a lower postprandial concentration of blood glucose. GI intolerance, including flatulence (70%) and diarrhea is very common with acarbose but may be minimized by a slow titration of the dosage. The clinical efficacy of acarbose is less than that of the sulfonylureas or metformin (141). However, acarbose may be beneficial to patients with postprandial hyperglycemia. Acarbose is dosed 3 times a day, before each meal. Compliance may be difficult with this product. Contraindications to therapy with acarbose include inflammatory bowel disease, colonic ulceration or partial intestinal obstruction, chronic intestinal disease associated with marked disorders of absorption or digestion, conditions that may be exacerbated by increased gas formation (e.g. hernias), and impaired hepatic function (142). If patients have a hypoglycemic episode while taking acarbose, they should be warned to ingest oral glucose rather than a carbohydrate.

Troglitazone is the first of a new class of agents, the thiazolidinediones. It appears to prevent hyperglycemia primarily by decreasing insulin resistance. Although few studies in the elderly are available, age has not been shown to alter the drug's pharmacokinetics. Troglitazone has caused mild, reversible increases in serum aminotransferases. In some patients this has progressed to severe hepatocellular damage, hepatic necrosis, hepatic failure, liver transplantation, and death. The drug was withdrawn from the market in the United Kingdom on December 1, 1997. It may also cause edema and GI intolerance (143).

Thrombolytic Agents

Thrombolysis with streptokinase or tissue plasminogen activator (TPA) has been shown to decrease mortality in the elderly patient with an MI (144, 145). However, these agents have been associated with a high rate of intracerebral hemorrhage in the elderly (146, 147).

Recent guidelines published by the American College of Cardiology/American Heart Association Task Force on Practice Guidelines (42) recommend thrombolysis for those with ST segment elevation who present within 12 hours and are less than 75 years or who have bundle-branch block and history suggesting acute MI. These guidelines suggest there is evidence to support the use of thrombolytics in persons over 75 years. The overall risk of mortality in this age group is higher than among younger patients. The risk of cerebral hemorrhage from thrombolytics is also higher in this age group. Therefore, the relative benefit of therapy is reduced. However, there still is a benefit for a properly selected patient older than 75 years without contraindications.

Four recent clinical trials assessed the efficacy and safety of thrombolytics in acute ischemic stroke (148–151). The Multicenter Acute Stroke Trial-Europe (MAST-E) was stopped prematurely because of the increase in mortality in the streptokinase group, mainly due to hemorrhagic transformation of the stroke. The MAST-Italy trial also found increased mortality in patients randomized to streptokinase, alone or with aspirin. The European Cooperative Acute Stroke Study (ECASS) and the National Institute of Neurological Disorders and Stroke TPA Stroke Study Group (NINDS) trials evaluated TPA given within 6 or 3 hours of symptoms, respectively. Neither trial found a mortality difference between TPA and placebo. The dose of TPA was slightly lower in the NINDS trial (0.9 mg/kg versus 1.1 mg/kg). The ECASS trial also found no difference between groups in the rate of cerebral hemorrhage. Significantly more patients receiving TPA in the NINDS trial had symptomatic intracerebral hemorrhage than the placebo group (6.4% versus 0.6%). Both studies concluded that thrombolytic therapy improved some functional measures and clinical outcome at 3 months.

Which patients are the best candidates to receive thrombolytic therapy after an ischemic stroke? Although there are no clear guidelines, the patient must meet certain baseline criteria before eligibility is even considered: (1) early treatment, preferably within 3 hours of symptom onset; and (2) absence of any brain injury on a computed tomography (CT) scan. Most patients are ineligible for thrombolytic therapy because they do not meet the first criterion. A neurologic examination and CT scan must be performed before treatment can begin. Also, the CT scan must be examined very carefully to determine whether the patient is eligible for thrombolysis.

PSYCHOTROPIC AGENTS

Psychotropic agents are commonly used in the elderly. Even when used cautiously for an appropriate indication, psychotropic drugs may result in adverse effects on the functional status of many older persons, as discussed previously.

Antipsychotic Agents

Antipsychotic agents are effective for the treatment of psychiatric conditions, including schizophrenia and other diseases resulting in delusions or psychosis. Their use in the elderly, especially in nursing homes, has been much higher than necessary for the treatment of patients with a psychiatric diagnosis. Their increased use is primarily due to attempts to control behavioral problems in demented patients. However, few data document their efficacy for this purpose. In a meta-analysis of 33 studies of patients with primary dementia, the effectiveness of antipsychotic agents prescribed for agitation was recently evaluated (152). A statistically significant mean effect size of 0.18 was shown for the use of an antipsychotic versus placebo. No antipsychotic was more effective than another. Only 18 of 100 patients would be expected to respond on the basis of effect size.

Antipsychotic agents are also misused frequently when prescribed "as needed," or prn. They are not effective when used in this manner, and it is likely that the patient will experience only the acute sedative properties of these drugs (153).

Because of misuse of these drugs, regulations define appropriate and inappropriate indications for antipsychotic use (Omnibus Budget Reconciliation Act of 1987). These drugs have been associated with tardive dyskinesia and other movement disorders, dystonia, anticholinergic reactions, hypotension, and increased risk of falls and hip fractures in the elderly (31, 154, 155). Several recent trials have reported successful attempts to withdraw elderly nursing home residents from antipsychotic medication (156–159). Two of the trials (156, 157) focused on educational programs to reduce antipsychotic drug use. The trial by Rovner et al. (159) implemented a program that included education, structured activities for the patients, and guidelines for appropriate drug use. Finally, Semla et al. (158) reported the differences in antipsychotic drug use before and after OBRA 87 implementation. All of these trials resulted in significant decreases in antipsychotic drug use among the patients studied. Of trials that reported on patient behavior, no increases in behavior problems were noted in the groups with decreased drug use.

Benzodiazepines

Many benzodiazepines are available to treat anxiety and short-term insomnia in older persons. Problems with their use usually develop when predictable pharmacokinetic and pharmacodynamic changes are overlooked and when "normal" doses of long-acting agents are prescribed for an indeterminate course of therapy.

Benzodiazepines commonly cause sedation, ataxia, and impaired psychomotor performance. They also produce anterograde amnesia in which patients report inability to acquire or store information. While these effects are temporary, they may precipitate falls or delirium in susceptible persons. The use of benzodiazepines has been well established as a risk factor for falls and fractures in this population (31, 32, 160). A recent report suggests that the use of benzodiazepines with a short elimination half-life may also be associated with an increased risk of falls and hip fracture (161). Finally, a report describes the association between use of long-acting benzodiazepines and an increased risk of motor vehicle crashes in the elderly, in which at least one person sustained bodily injury (162). These authors found that more than 20% of the elderly population studied were current users of benzodiazepines. Accidents were more likely to occur with long-acting agents, either in the first week of use (rate ratio, 1.45; 95% CI, 1.04–2.03) or with continuous use (rate ratio, 1.26; 95% CI, 1.09–1.45).

Antidepressants

Unlike other psychotropic agents, antidepressants are probably underused in the elderly. As the number of drugs continues to increase, a comprehensive strategy for choosing among the various agents is essential. In general, if all antidepressants are equally effective, the goal should be either to avoid or to promote certain side effects for individual geriatric patients.

One strategy might be to focus only on antidepressants that lack major anticholinergic effects. Amitriptyline, imipramine, doxepin, and protriptyline possess significant anticholinergic properties. While these drugs have been used in older persons for many years, newer antidepressants may offer important advantages. The anticholinergic properties of antidepressants are well recognized to cause dry mouth, constipation, and urinary retention, which may already affect an older person. Confusion and delirium have also been associated with the use of highly anticholinergic antidepressants in older patients with preexisting cognitive impairment. However, the anticholinergic effect of blurring vision is easily overlooked. In the presence of age-related declines in vision or decreases in proprioception caused by disease, the potential for blurred vision to place a person at greater risk for falling must be considered and specifically avoided. The ability of antidepressants to produce orthostatic hypotension by α-adrenergic blockade should also be minimized, especially to lessen the risk of falls in older persons.

After considering these major factors, the preferred agents may be limited to desipramine, nortriptyline, trazodone, and the selective serotonin reuptake inhibitors (SSRIs), such as fluoxetine. From here the selection of an antidepressant may be based on the individual patient's characteristics. For example, an anxious patient unable to sleep may benefit from the use of trazodone, as it is very sedating. For the patient with psychomotor impairment who is withdrawn, the choice might be desipramine, which is not very sedating, or one of the SSRIs.

Trazodone has been used extensively in the elderly, especially before the availability of the SSRIs. It can cause orthostatic hypotension, arrhythmias, sedation, and confusion. Priapism has been associated with trazodone use, and on rare occasions surgical intervention has been required. It can be difficult to determine the optimal dose because of trazodone's wide dosage range (150 to 600 mg per day). Trazodone's sedative properties can be used to an advantage: a small dose can be added to treat insomnia associated with depression in conjunction with another agent for the depression itself (163).

Fluoxetine and the new SSRIs are also an important advance in the treatment of depression. Although as effective as the older drugs, their side effect profile is very different from those of traditional antidepressant agents. Anxiety, nervousness, insomnia, and tremor may occur with this class. The SSRIs are metabolized by the cytochrome P450 system in the liver. However, each SSRI inhibits this system to a different extent. A patient's drug regimen should be reviewed for potential interactions before starting an SSRI.

Methylphenidate has been studied, both retrospectively and prospectively, as an antidepressant in the elderly (164). Most studies enrolled small numbers of patients and were very short, no longer than 8 weeks. However, these studies have shown a benefit with the use of methylphenidate. Only one study compared methylphenidate with another agent, nortriptyline. This was a retrospective study in patients with a history of stroke who had been treated with either agent for at least 4 weeks. The researchers in this study found that response to methylphenidate was much quicker (2.4 days versus 27 days for nortriptyline). Dunner (165) reports that stimulants are not antidepressants but may "restore feelings of hopefulness, spontaneity, and zest for life." Methylphenidate should be avoided in those with a history of anxiety, nervousness, or psychosis; it may decrease the seizure threshold and cause tachyarrhythmias, and it has potential for abuse. Randomized, controlled comparison trials of longer duration must be completed before extensive use of this agent can be recommended.

Two new agents, venlafaxine and nefazodone, have been introduced over the last couple of years. Venlafaxine has been studied in more than 300 elderly patients, according to the manufacturer. These trials have not been published. The adverse effect profile was similar to that expected with younger patients. These side effects may include asthenia, sweating, nausea, constipation, vomiting, somnolence, dry mouth, dizziness, nervousness, tremor, and sexual dysfunction (impotence, abnormal ejaculation or orgasm). Nefazodone has been studied in approximately 500 patients older than 65 years. Adverse events were similar to those in younger patients, including somnolence, dry mouth, nausea, dizziness, constipation, asthenia, blurred vision, and confusion. Because of pharmacokinetic differences in older patients, the manufacturer recommends that patients over age 65 be started at half the usual dose (166, 167).

After selecting an antidepressant, careful attention to the proper dose is essential to the successful use of these drugs in older persons. Most antidepressants have prolonged half-lives, and some have long-acting active metabolites.

Finally, response to antidepressant therapy typically takes longer in older persons than in younger patients. About 6 to 12 weeks of therapy may be needed before a positive or negative response can be assessed. It has been recommended that treatment continue for 6 months after remission from a first episode of major depression. A minimum of 12 months of treatment should be used after a second or third episode to prevent recurrence (168).

COGNITION-ENHANCING MEDICATIONS

Alzheimer's disease is the most common dementia, affecting approximately 4 million Americans. While no cure is available, the Food and Drug Administration has recently approved two drugs for the treatment of mild to moderate Alzheimer's disease. In addition to the approval of two new medications, investigators have also recently published many provocative articles on the primary treatment or prevention of Alzheimer's disease with medications marketed for treatment of other conditions.

Cholinergic Therapy

Depletion of acetylcholine may be the most critical neurochemical loss in patients with Alzheimer's disease, and replacement of acetylcholine is the most investigated therapeutic approach at present. Cholinergic transmission can be improved in brain tissue by inhibiting acetylcholinesterase, the enzyme that metabolizes acetylcholine, through more direct replacement of choline or acetylcholine, and through direct receptor stimulation. The two drugs presently marketed for the treatment of mild to moderate Alzheimer's disease, tacrine and donepezil, both inhibit acetylcholinesterase.

Tacrine is the most widely studied drug for the treatment of Alzheimer's disease. The results of major large-scale placebo-controlled trials using appropriate measures of outcome show that mental decline in Alzheimer's disease is arrested by approximately 5 to 6 months. Long-term clinical trials are not being conducted because of ethical considerations, but follow-up in a small number of patients for an average of 72 weeks suggests that tacrine may delay the progression of Alzheimer's disease (169). Additionally, as a part of an earlier trial to evaluate tacrine, the concomitant use of hormone replacement therapy was assessed in a secondary retrospective analysis. Patients who received estrogen replacement

therapy and were randomized to receive tacrine treatment achieved significantly better outcomes in the Alzheimer's Disease Assessment Scale, the Clinician Interview Based Impression of Change, the Mini-Mental State Examination, and the Caregiver's Impression of Change than women who did not receive hormone replacement therapy (170). Limitations to the use of tacrine include gastric side effects and hepatotoxicity requiring frequent alanine aminotransferase monitoring. Tacrine must be dosed 4 times a day because of its poor pharmacokinetic profile and must be monitored for drug interactions when used in combination with cimetidine or theophylline products.

Donepezil is a piperidine-based noncompetitive inhibitor of acetylcholinesterase approved for the treatment of Alzheimer's disease by the FDA in December 1996. In a 12-week double-blind placebo-controlled trial, patients with mild to moderate probable Alzheimer's disease were randomized to receive donepezil or placebo. Donepezil 5 mg daily was significantly better than placebo in the ADAS-cog score and the MMSE. A correlation was found among donepezil serum concentrations, inhibition of acetylcholinesterase, and improvement in outcome measures (171). In long-term studies (2 years of treatment), use of donepezil at 5 or 10 mg per day was associated with a four-point improvement in the ADAS-cog score in comparison with expected outcomes in untreated patients (172). Donepezil has a favorable pharmacokinetic profile and has not been reported to cause hepatotoxicity, as do the acridine-based drugs.

Anti-inflammatory Therapy

Inflammation may contribute to neuronal loss in Alzheimer's disease. Evidence points to the presence of many inflammatory compounds, including acute-phase proteins, cytokines, complement, and activated microglial cells in histologic studies of neuritic plaques (173). There are also epidemiologic studies in twins to suggest that persons who use anti-inflammatory therapy are less likely to develop Alzheimer's disease (174, 175). Most of the published research to date suggests a positive effect of the use of NSAIDs in either slowing the progression of disease or lessening the symptoms of patients with Alzheimer's disease (176).

Corticosteroids and other anti-inflammatory agents are also under consideration for their possible role in the treatment of Alzheimer's disease. A prospective placebo-controlled trial now under way is evaluating the effect of 20 mg of prednisone per day for 1 month followed by 10 mg per day for 1 year (177). Colchicine and hydroxychloroquine penetrate the blood-brain barrier and may also prove to be candidates for clinical trials (173).

Antioxidants

Free radicals damage cells by altering the electron number of DNA, membranes, and enzymes and impair the function and structure of lipids, proteins, nucleic acids, and other cell components. Free radicals may play a role in neurodegeneration by either initiating or maintaining a cascade of events that antioxidants block. Compounds in this class include idebenone, lazaroids, and pyrrolopyrimidines (178).

Selegiline reduces the rate of free radical generation, and α-tocopherol (vitamin E), ascorbic acid, and retinol are vitamins with antioxidant activity. Recently, the use of selegiline and the use of α-tocopherol were evaluated singly and in combination for the treatment of patients with moderately severe Alzheimer's disease (179). Some 341 patients with moderately severe probable Alzheimer's disease were randomized to receive selegiline 5 mg twice a day, α-tocopherol 1000 IU twice a day, both, or placebo for 2 years. Outcome measures were functionally defined; the authors evaluated decline in the ability to provide self-care, discharge to a nursing home, death, or the development of severe dementia as measured by the Clinical Dementia Rating Scale. A significant improvement in the primary functional outcome measure in patients who received selegiline, α-tocopherol, or both drugs was demonstrated. The difference measured at 2 years was both clinically relevant and statistically significant—a risk ratio of 0.57 for selegiline, 0.47 for α-tocopherol, and 0.69 for the combination therapy.

Delayed onset of functional decline in areas such as self-care had never been demonstrated in a randomized trial in patients with Alzheimer's disease. It is interesting that sole therapy with either selegiline or α-tocopherol was no less effective than combined therapy with these two agents. The authors speculate that this may be due to the advanced condition of their study patients, to a similar mechanism of action of the two agents, or perhaps to a drug interaction resulting in an outcome that was not additive (179).

Ovarian Steroids

Research in recent years has begun to evaluate the effects of estrogen on cognition in women. The use of estrogen during menopause and the subsequent development of Alzheimer's disease years later were evaluated through retrospective case-control studies. In four epidemiologic studies the use of hormone replacement therapy was documented prior to the development of Alzheimer's disease (180–183). Three of these four studies reached positive conclusions regarding an association between hormone replacement therapy and a decreased likelihood of subsequently developing Alzheimer's disease. Investigation into a possible dose-response effect was undertaken in some of these studies, suggesting that use of higher doses of estrogen or use of estrogen longer than a year is associated with an even lower risk of subsequently developing Alzheimer's disease (180–182). In spite of methodologic problems in this area of research, there appears to be a collection of positive publications pointing out a consistent finding that women who use hormone replacement therapy may reduce their risk of developing Alzheimer's disease by approximately a third to a half.

Estrogen as a treatment for women with dementia has been studied in small randomized trials. One double-blind, randomized, placebo-controlled trial evaluated conjugated equine estrogens (CEE) in the treatment of Alzheimer's disease in women who were over age 70 and without symptoms of depression. CEE 0.625 mg daily was cycled every 3 months with a 2-week course of progestin for a total treatment period of 9 months. An interim analysis has demonstrated improvement in the Clinician Interview-Based Impression of Change (184). The Women's Health Initiative is investigating this hypothesis in a large-scale randomized, placebo-controlled primary intervention trial. If the risk reduction seen in the retrospective case control studies is a true estimate of an effect size, estrogen therapy for women with Alzheimer's disease will represent a significant public health finding.

REFERENCES

1. Mayersohn MB. Special pharmacokinetic considerations in the elderly. In: Evans WE, Schentag JJ, Jusko WJ, eds. Applied Pharmacokinetics. Vancouver: Applied Therapeutics, 1992:1–43.
2. Gertz BJ, Holland SD, Kline WF, et al. Studies of the oral bioavailability of alendronate. Clin Pharmacol Ther 1995;58:288–298.
3. Harvell JD, Maibach HI. Percutaneous absorption and inflammation in aged skin: a review. J Am Acad Dermatol 1994;31:1015–1021.
4. Roskos KV, Maibach HI, Guy RH. The effect of aging on percutaneous absorption in man. J Pharmacokinet Biopharm 1989;17:617–630.
5. Silver AJ, Guillen CP, Kahl MJ, Morley JE. Effect of aging on body fat. J Am Geriatr Soc 1993;41:211–213.
6. Veering BT, Burm AG, Souverijn JH, et al. The effect of age on serum concentrations of albumin and alpha-1-acid glycoprotein. Br J Clin Pharmacol 1990;29:201–206.
7. Wynne HA, Cope LH, Mutch E, et al. The effect of age upon liver volume and apparent liver blood flow in healthy man. Hepatology 1989;9:297–301.
8. Sotaniemi EA, Arranto AJ, Pelkonen O, Pasanen M. Age and cytochrome P450-linked drug metabolism in humans: an analysis of 226 subjects with equal histopathologic conditions. Clin Pharmacol Ther 1997;61:331–339.
9. Slaughter RL, Edwards DJ. Recent advances: the cytochrome P450 enzymes. Ann Pharmacother 1995;29:619–624.
10. Hunt CM, Westerkam WR, Stave GM, Wilson JA. Hepatic cytochrome P4503A (CYP3A) activity in the elderly. Mech Ageing Dev 1992;64:189–199.
11. Lindeman RD, Tobin J, Shock NW. Longitudinal studies on the rate of decline in renal function with age. J Am Geriatr Soc 1985;33:278–285.
12. Drusano GL, Muncie HL, Hoopes JM, Damron DJ, Warren JW. Commonly used methods of estimating creatinine clearance are inadequate for elderly debilitated nursing home residents. J Am Geriatr Soc 1988;36:437–441.
13. Bennett WM. Guide to drug dosage in renal failure. Clin Pharmacokinet 1988;15:326–354.
14. McEvoy GK, ed. American Hospital Formulary Service. Bethesda, MD: American Society of Health-System Pharmacists, 1997.
15. Abernethy DR, Schwartz JB, Todd EL, et al. Verapamil pharmacokinetics and disposition in young and elderly hypertensive patients. Ann Intern Med 1986;105:329–339.
16. Jacobs JR, Reves JG, Marty J, et al. Aging increases pharmacodynamic sensitivity to the hypnotic effects of midazolam. Anesth Analg 1995;80:143–148.
17. Andros E, Detmar-Hanna D, Suteparuk S, et al. The effect of aging on the pharmacokinetics and pharmacodynamics of prazosin. Eur J Clin Pharmacol 1996;50:41–46.
18. Gurwitz JH, Avorn J. The ambiguous relationship between aging and adverse drug reactions. Ann Intern Med 1991;114:956–966.
19. Levine MN, Raskob G, Landefeld S, Hirsh J. Hemorrhagic complications of anticoagulant treatment. Chest 1995;108:276S–290S.
20. Landefeld CS, Goldman L. Major bleeding in outpatients treated with warfarin: incidence and prediction by factors known at the start of outpatient therapy. Am J Med 1989;87:144–152.
21. Albers GW. Atrial fibrillation and stroke: three new studies, three remaining questions. Arch Intern Med 1994;154:1443–1448.
22. Risk factors for stroke and efficacy of antithrombotic therapy in atrial fibrillation. Analysis of pooled data from five randomized controlled trials. Arch Intern Med 1994;154:1449–1457.
23. Leape LL, Brennan A, Laird N, et al. The nature of adverse events in hospitalized patients. Results of the Harvard Medical Practice Study II. N Engl J Med 1991;324:377–384.
24. Bates DW, Cullen DJ, Laird N, et al. Incidence of adverse drug events and potential adverse drug events. JAMA 1995;274:29–34.
25. Leape LL, Bates DW, Cullen DJ. Systems analysis of adverse drug events. JAMA 1995;274:35–43.
26. Grymonpre RE, Mitenko PA, Sitar DS, et al. Drug-associated hospital admissions in older medical patients. J Am Geriatr Soc 1988;36:1092–1098.
27. Bero LA, Lipton HL, Bird JA. Characterization of geriatric drug related hospital readmissions. Med Care 1991;29:989–1003.
28. Beers MH, Ouslander JG, Rollingher I, et al. Explicit criteria for determining inappropriate medication use in nursing homes. Arch Intern Med 1991;151:1825–1832.
29. Wilcox SM, Himmelstein DU, Woolhandler S. Inappropriate drug prescribing for the community dwelling elderly. JAMA 1994;272:292–296.
30. Plushner S, Helling DK. Identifying inappropriate prescribing in the elderly: time to refocus. Ann Pharmacother 1996;30:81–83.
31. Ray WA, Griffin MR, Schaffner W, et al. Psychotropic drug use and the risk of hip fracture. N Engl J Med 1987;316:363–369.
32. Ray WA, Griffin MR, Downey W. Benzodiazepines of long and short elimination half-life and the risk of hip fracture. JAMA 1989;262:3303–3307.
33. Steele K, Gertman PM, Crescenzi C, Anderson J. Iatrogenic illness on a general medical service at a university hospital. N Engl J Med 1981;304:638–642.

34. Soumerai SB, McLaughlin TJ, Spiegelman D, et al. Adverse outcomes of underuse of beta-blockers in elderly survivors of acute myocardial infarction. JAMA 1997; 277:115–121.

35. McLaughlin TJ, Soumerai SB, Willison DJ, et al. Adherence to national guidelines for drug treatment of suspected acute myocardial infarction: evidence for undertreatment in women and the elderly. Arch Intern Med 1996;156:799–805.

36. Gurwitz JH, Goldberg RJ, Chen Z, et al. Beta-blocker therapy in acute myocardial infarction: evidence for underutilization in the elderly. Am J Med 1992;93:605–610.

37. Meehan TP, Hennen J, Radford MJ, et al. Process and outcome of care for acute myocardial infarction among Medicare beneficiaries in Connecticut: a quality improvement demonstration project. Ann Intern Med 1995;122:928–936.

38. Ellerbeck EF, Jencks SF, Radford MJ, et al. Quality of care for Medicare patients with acute myocardial infarction: a four-state pilot study from the Cooperative Cardiovascular Project. JAMA 1995;273:1509–1514.

39. Krumholz HM, Murillo JE, Chen J, et al. Thrombolytic therapy for eligible elderly patients with acute myocardial infarction. JAMA 1997;277:1683–1688.

40. Gurwitz JH, Gore JM, Goldberg RJ, et al. Recent age-related trends in the use of thrombolytic therapy on patients who have had acute myocardial infarction. Ann Intern Med 1996;124:283–291.

41. Albers GW, Yim JM, Belew KM, et al. Status of antithrombotic therapy for patients with atrial fibrillation in university hospitals. Arch Intern Med 1996;156:2311–2316.

42. Ryan TJ, Anderson JL, Antman EM, et al. ACC/AHA guidelines for the management of patients with acute myocardial infarction. A report of the American College of Cardiology/American Heart Association Task Force on Practice Guidelines (Committee on Management of Acute Myocardial Infarction). J Am Coll Cardiol 1996;28:1328–1428.

43. Laupacis A, Albers G, Dalen J, et al. Antithrombotic therapy in atrial fibrillation. Chest 1995;108(4 suppl):352S–359S.

44. McCrory DC, Matchar DB, Samsa G, et al. Physician attitudes about anticoagulation for nonvalvular atrial fibrillation in the elderly. Arch Intern Med 1995;155:277–281.

45. Kutner M, Nixon G, Silverstone F. Physicians' attitudes toward oral anticoagulants and antiplatelet agents for stroke prevention in elderly patients with atrial fibrillation. Arch Intern Med 1991;151:1950–1953.

46. Fihn SD, Callahan CM, Martin DC, et al. The risk for and severity of bleeding complications in elderly patients treated with warfarin. Ann Intern Med 1996;124:970–979.

47. Bleeding during antithrombotic therapy in patients with atrial fibrillation. The Stroke Prevention in Atrial Fibrillation Investigators. Arch Intern Med 1996;156:409–416.

48. Gurwitz JH, Goldbert RJ, Holden A, et al. Age-related risks of long-term anticoagulant therapy. Arch Intern Med 1988;148:1733–1736.

49. Ayanian JZ, Hauptman PJ, Guadagnoli E, et al. Knowledge and practices of generalist and specialist physicians regarding drug therapy for acute myocardial infarction. N Engl J Med 1994;331:1136–1142.

50. Gurwitz JH, Avorn J, Bohn RL, et al. Initiation of antihypertensive treatment during nonsteroidal anti-inflammatory drug therapy. JAMA 1994;272:781–786.

51. Gurwitz JH, Everitt DE, Monane M, et al. The impact of ibuprofen on the efficacy of antihypertensive treatment with hydrochlorothiazide in elderly persons. J Gerontol A Biol Sci Med Sci 1996;51:74–79.

52. Wilcox CM, Shalek KA, Cotsonis G. Striking prevalence of over-the-counter nonsteroidal anti-inflammatory drug use in patients with upper gastrointestinal hemorrhage. Arch Intern Med 1994;154:42–45.

53. Eisenberg DM, Kessler RC, Foster C, Norlock FE, Calkins DR, DelBanco TL. Unconventional medicine in the United States—prevalence, costs, and patterns of use. N Engl J Med 1993;328:246–252.

54. Murphy JJ, Heptinstall S, Mitchell JR. Randomised double-blind placebo-controlled trial of feverfew in migraine prevention. Lancet 1988;2:189–192.

55. Warshafsky S, Kamer RS, Sivak SL. Effect of garlic on total serum cholesterol. A meta-analysis. Ann Intern Med 1993;119:599–605.

56. Tyler VE. The honest herbal: a sensible guide to the use of herbs and related remedies. Binghamton, NY: Hawthorne Press, 1993.

57. Gertner E, Marshall PS, Filandrinos D, et al. Complications resulting from the use of Chinese herbal medications containing undeclared prescription drugs. Arthr Rheum 1995;38:614–617.

58. Hanlon JT, Schmader KE, Samsa GP, et al. A method for assessing drug therapy appropriateness. J Clin Epidemiol 1992;45:1045–1051.

59. Cutson TM, Gray SL, Hughes MA, et al. Effect of a single dose of diazepam on balance measures in older persons. J Am Geriatr Soc 1997;45:435–440.

60. Mustard CA, Mayer R. Case-control study of exposure to medication and the risk of injurious falls requiring hospitalization among nursing home residents. Am J Epidemiol 1997;145:738–745.

61. Sambrook P, Birmingham J, Kelly P, et al. Prevention of corticosteroid osteoporosis: a comparison of calcium, calcitriol, and calcitonin. N Engl J Med 1993;328:1747–1752.

62. Picado C, Luengo M. Corticosteroid-induced bone loss. Prevention and management. Drug Saf 1996;15:347–359.

63. Adachi JD, Bensen WG, Brown J, et al. Intermittent etidronate therapy to prevent corticosteroid-induced osteoporosis. N Engl J Med 1997;337:382–387.

64. Fantl JA, Newman DK, Colling J, et al. Managing Acute and Chronic Urinary Incontinence. Clinical Practice Guideline. Quick Reference Guide for Clinicians 2, 1996 Update (AHCPR 96–0686). Rockville, MD: US

Department of Health and Human Services, Public Health Service, Agency for Health Care Policy and Research, March 1996.

65. Agency for Health Care Policy and Research. Urinary Incontinence in Adults. Rockville, MD: US Department of Health and Human Services, Public Health Service, Agency for Health Care Policy and Research. Available at: http://text.nlm.nih.gov/ahcpr/ui/www/uitoc.html.

66. Walter S, Kjaergaard B, Lose G, et al. Stress urinary incontinence in postmenopausal women treated with oral estrogen (estriol) and an alpha-adrenoceptor-stimulating agent: a randomized double-blind placebo-controlled study. Int Urogynecol J 1990;1:74–79.

67. Hilton P, Tweddell AL, Mayne C. Oral and vaginal estrogens alone and in combination with alpha-adrenergic stimulation in genuine stress incontinence. Int Urogynecol J 1990;1:80–86.

68. Carter GL, Dawson AH, Lopert R. Drug-induced delirium. Incidence, management and prevention. Drug Saf 1996;15:291–301.

69. Trimble MR. Anticonvulsant induced psychiatric disorders. Drug Saf 1996;15:159–166.

70. Monane M, Avorn J, Beers MH, Everitt DE. Anticholinergic drug use and bowel function in nursing home patients. Arch Intern Med 1993;153:633–638.

71. Tejera CA, Saravay SM, Goldman E, et al. Diphenhydramine-induced delirium in elderly hospitalized patients with mild dementia. Psychosomatics 1994;35:399–402.

72. Ganzini L, Walsh JR, Millar SB. Drug-induced depression in the aged. What can be done? Drugs Aging 1993;3:147–158.

73. Thiessen BQ, Wallace SM, Blackburn JL, et al. Increased prescribing of antidepressants subsequent to beta-blocker therapy. Arch Intern Med 1990;150:2286–2290.

74. Bright RA, Everitt DE. Beta-blockers and depression. Evidence against an association. JAMA 1992;267:1783–1787.

75. Brzezinski A. Melatonin in humans. N Engl J Med 1997;336:186–195.

76. Waldhauser F, Weiszenbacher G, Tatzer E, et al. Alterations in nocturnal serum melatonin levels in humans with growth and aging. J Clin Endocrinol Metab 1988;66:648–652.

77. Haimov I, Laudon M, Zisapel N, et al. Sleep disorders and melatonin rhythms in elderly people. BMJ 1994;309:167.

78. Garfinkel D, Laudon M, Nof D, Zisapel N. Improvement of sleep quality in elderly people by controlled-release melatonin. Lancet 1995;346:541–544.

79. Monteleone P, Tortorella A, Borriello R, et al. Suppression of nocturnal plasma melatonin levels by evening administration of sodium valproate in healthy humans. Biol Psychiatry 1997;41:336–341.

80. Lamberg L. Melatonin potentially useful but safety, efficacy remain uncertain. JAMA 1996;276:1011–1014.

81. Baulieu E. Dehydroepiandrosterone (DHEA): A foun-

tain of youth? J Clin Endocrinol Metab 1996;81:3147–3151.

82. Berr C, Lafont S, Debuire B, et al. Relationships of dehydroepiandrosterone sulfate in the elderly with functional, psychological, and mental status and short-term mortality: a French community-based study. Proc Natl Acad Sci 1996;93:13410–13415.

83. Orentreich N, Brind JL, Vogelman JH, et al. Long-term longitudinal measurements of plasma dehydroepiandrosterone sulfate in normal men. J Clin Endocrinol Metab 1992;75:1002–1004.

84. Wolkowitz OM, Reus VI, Roberts E, et al. Dehydroepiandrosterone (DHEA) treatment of depression. Biol Psychiatry 1997;41:311–318.

85. Wolf OT, Neumann O, Hellhammer DH, et al. Effects of a two-week physiological dehydroepiandrosterone substitution on cognitive performance and well-being in healthy elderly women and men. J Clin Endocrinol Metab 1997;82:2363–2367.

86. Psaty BM, Koepsell TD, Yanez ND, et al. Temporal patterns of antihypertensive medication use among older adults, 1989 through 1992: an effect of the major clinical trials on clinical practice? JAMA 1995;273:1436–1438.

87. Prevention of stroke by antihypertensive drug treatment in older persons with isolated systolic hypertension. Final results of the Systolic Hypertension in the Elderly Program (SHEP). SHEP Cooperative Research Group. JAMA 1991;265:3255–3264.

88. Medical Research Council trial of treatment of hypertension in older adults: principal results. MRC Working Party. BMJ 1992;304:405–412.

89. Dahlof B, Lindholm LH, Hansson L, et al. Morbidity and mortality in the Swedish Trial in Old Patients with Hypertension (STOP-Hypertension). Lancet 1991;338:1281–1285.

90. The sixth report of the Joint National Committee on prevention, detection, evaluation, and treatment of high blood pressure. Arch Intern Med 1997;157:2413–2445.

91. Kostis JB, Davis BR, Cutler J, et al. Prevention of heart failure by antihypertensive drug treatment in older persons with isolated systolic hypertension. JAMA 1997;278:212–216.

92. Applegate WB, Pressel S, Wittes J, et al. Impact of the treatment of isolated systolic hypertension on behavioral variables: results from the systolic hypertension in the elderly program. Arch Intern Med 1994;154:2154–2160.

93. Curb DJ, Pressel SL, Cutler JA, et al. Effect of diuretic-based antihypertensive treatment on cardiovascular disease risk in older diabetic patients with isolated systolic hypertension. JAMA 1996;276:1886–1892.

94. Monane M, Gurwitz JH, Bohn RL, et al. The impact of thiazide diuretics on the initiation of lipid-reducing agents in older people: a population-based analysis. J Am Geriatr Soc 1997;45:71–75.

95. Gengo FM, Fagan SC, de Padova A, et al. The effect of

beta-blockers on mental performance in older hypertensive patients. Arch Intern Med 1988;148:779–784.

96. Skinner MH, Futterman A, Morrissette D, et al. Atenolol compared with nifedipine: effect on cognitive function and mood in elderly hypertensive patients. Ann Intern Med 1992;116:615–623.

97. Alderman CP. Adverse effects of the angiotensin-converting enzyme inhibitors. Ann Pharmacother 1996; 30:55–61.

98. Israili ZH, Hall WD. Cough and angioneurotic edema associated with angiotensin-converting enzyme inhibitor therapy: a review of the literature and pathophysiology. Ann Intern Med 1992;117:234–242.

99. Fogari R, Zoppi A, Tettamanti F, et al. Indomethacin or nifedipine for cough induced by captopril therapy. J Cardiovasc Pharmacol 1992;19:670–675.

100. Hargreaves MR, Benson MK. Inhaled sodium cromoglycate in angiotensin-converting enzyme cough. Lancet 1995;345:13–16.

101. Effects of enalapril on mortality in severe congestive heart failure. Results of the Cooperative North Scandinavian Enalapril Survival Study (CONSENSUS). The CONSENSUS Trial Study Group. N Engl J Med 1987;316:1429–1435.

102. Effect of enalapril on survival in patients with reduced left ventricular ejection fractions and congestive heart failure. The SOLVD Investigators. N Engl J Med 1991; 325:293–302.

103. Cohn JN, Johnson G, Ziesche S, et al. A comparison of enalapril with hydralazine-isosorbide dinitrate in the treatment of chronic congestive heart failure. N Engl J Med 1991;325:303–310.

104. Pfeffer MA, Braunwald E, Moye LA, et al. Effect of captopril on mortality and morbidity in patients with left ventricular dysfunction after myocardial infarction: results of the survival and ventricular enlargement trial. N Engl J Med 1992;327:669–677.

105. Effect of ramipril on mortality and morbidity of survivors of acute myocardial infarction with clinical evidence of heart failure. The Acute Infarction Ramipril Efficacy (AIRE) Study Investigators. Lancet 1993;342: 821–827.

106. Kober L, Torp-Pedersen C, Carlsen JE. A clinical trial of the angiotensin-converting enzyme inhibitor trandolapril in patients with left ventricular dysfunction after myocardial infarction. N Engl J Med 1995;333: 1670–1676.

107. Swedberg K, Held P, Kjekshus J, et al. Effects of the Early Administration of Enalapril on Mortality in Patients With Acute Myocardial Infarction. Results of the Cooperative New Scandinavian Enalapril Survival Study II (CONSENSUS II). N Engl J Med 1992;327: 678–684.

108. Mogensen CE. Renoprotective role of ACE inhibitors in diabetic nephropathy. Br Heart J 1994;72(3 suppl): S38–S45.

109. Ravid M, Lang R, Rachmani R, Lishner M. Long-term renoprotective effect of angiotensin-converting enzyme inhibition in non-insulin-dependent diabetes mellitus: a 7-year follow-up study. Arch Intern Med 1996;156:286–289.

110. Mathiesen ER, Hommel E, Giese J, Parving HH. Efficacy of captopril in postponing nephropathy in normotensive insulin dependent diabetic patients with microalbuminuria. BMJ 1991;303:81–87.

111. Schaefer KL, Porter JA. Angiotensin II receptor antagonists: the prototype losartan. Ann Pharmacother 1996;30:625–636.

112. Markham A, Goa KL. Valsartan. Drugs 1997;54: 299–311.

113. Pitt B, Segal R, Martinez FA, et al. Randomised trial of losartan versus captopril in patients over 65 with heart failure. Lancet 1997;349:747–752.

114. Psaty BM, Heckbert SR, Koepsell TD, et al. The risk of myocardial infarction associated with antihypertensive drug therapies. JAMA 1995;274:620–625.

115. Furberg CD, Psaty BM, Meyer JV. Nifedipine: dose-related increase in mortality in patients with coronary heart disease. Circulation 1995;92:1326–1331.

116. Pahor M, Guralnik JM, Corti MC, et al. Long-term survival and use of antihypertensive medications in older persons. J Am Geriatr Soc 1995;43:1191–1197.

117. Marwick C. FDA gives calcium channel blockers clean bill of health but warns of short-acting nifedipine hazards. JAMA 1996;275:423–424.

118. Borhani NO, Mercuri M, Borhani PA, et al. Final outcome results of the Multicenter Isradipine Diuretic Atherosclerosis Study (MIDAS). JAMA 1996;276:785–791.

119. Wagenknecht L, Furberg CD, Hammon J, et al. Surgical bleeding: an unexpected effect of calcium antagonists. BMJ 1995;310:776–777.

120. Pahor M, Guralnik JM, Furberg CD, et al. Risk of gastrointestinal hemorrhage with calcium antagonists in hypertensive patients over 67. Lancet 1996;347:1061–1066.

121. Pahor M, Guralnik JM, Ferucci L, et al. Calcium-channel blockade and incidence of cancer in aged populations. Lancet 1996;348:493–497.

122. Kannel WB, Castelli WP, Gordon T, et al. Serum cholesterol, lipoproteins, and the risk of coronary heart disease. The Framingham study. Ann Intern Med 1971;74:1–12.

123. Krumholz HM, Seeman TE, Merrill SS, et al. Lack of association between cholesterol and coronary heart disease mortality and morbidity and all-cause mortality in persons older than 70 years. JAMA 1994;272: 1335–1340.

124. Frost PH, Davis BR, Burlando AJ, et al. Serum lipids and incidence of coronary heart disease. Findings from the Systolic Hypertension in the Elderly Program (SHEP). Circulation 1996;94:2381–2388.

125. Aronow WS, Ahn C. Risk factors for new coronary events in a large cohort of very elderly patients with and without coronary artery disease. Am J Cardiol 1996;77:864–866.

126. Randomised trial of cholesterol lowering in 4444 patients

with coronary heart disease: the Scandinavian Simvastatin Survival Study (4S). Lancet 1994;344:1383–1389.

127. Sacks FM, Pfeffer M, Moye LA, et al. The effect of pravastatin on coronary events after myocardial infarction in patients with average cholesterol levels. N Engl J Med 1996;335:1001–1009.

128. LaRosa JC, Applegate W, Crouse JR III, et al. Cholesterol lowering in the elderly: Results of the Cholesterol Reduction in Seniors Program (CRISP) pilot study. Arch Intern Med 1994;154:529–539.

129. Summary of the second report of the National Cholesterol Education Program (NCEP) Expert Panel on Detection, Evaluation, and Treatment of High Blood Cholesterol in Adults. JAMA 1993;269:3015–3023.

130. Newman TB, Hulley SB. Carcinogenicity of lipid-lowering drugs. JAMA 1996;275:55–60.

131. Reisin LH, Landau E, Darawshi A. More rapid relief of pain with isosorbide dinitrate oral spray than with sublingual tablets in elderly patients with angina pectoris. Am J Cardiol 1988;61:2E.

132. Parker JO, Farrel B, Lahey KA, Moe G. Effect of intervals between doses on the development of tolerance to isosorbide dinitrate. N Engl J Med 1987;316:1440–1444.

133. Brooks PM, Day RO. Nonsteroidal antiinflammatory drugs—differences and similarities. N Engl J Med 1991;324:1716–1725.

134. Walan A, Bader JP, Classen M, et al. Effect of omeprazole and ranitidine on ulcer healing and relapse rates in patients with benign gastric ulcer. N Engl J Med 1989;320:69–75.

135. Bradley JD, Brandt KD, Katz BP, et al. Comparison of an antiinflammatory dose of ibuprofen, an analgesic dose of ibuprofen, and acetaminophen in the treatment of patients with osteoarthritis of the knee. N Engl J Med 1991;325:87–91.

136. Walt RP. Misoprostol for the treatment of peptic ulcer and antiinflammatory-drug-induced gastroduodenal ulceration. N Engl J Med 1992;327:1575–1580.

137. Pope JE, Anderson JJ, Felson DT. A meta-analysis of the effects of nonsteroidal anti-inflammatory drugs on blood pressure. Arch Intern Med 1993;153:477–484.

138. Ruoff G. The management of non-insulin dependent diabetes mellitus in the elderly. J Fam Pract 1993;36:329–335.

139. Mooradian AD. Drug therapy of non-insulin-dependent diabetes mellitus in the elderly. Drugs 1996;51:931–941.

140. Melchior WR, Jaber LA. Metformin: an antihyperglycemic agent for treatment of type II diabetes. Ann Pharmacother 1996;30:158–164.

141. The pharmacological treatment of hyperglycemia in NIDDM. American Diabetes Association. Diabetes Care 1995;18:1510–1518.

142. Balfour JA, McTavish D. Acarbose. Drugs 1993;46:1025–1054.

143. Spencer CM, Markham A. Troglitazone. Drugs 1997;54:89–101.

144. Randomised trial of intravenous streptokinase, oral aspirin, both, or neither among 17,187 cases of suspected acute myocardial infarction: ISIS-2. ISIS-2 (Second International Study of Infarct Survival) Collaborative Group. Lancet 1988;2:349–360.

145. Long-term effects of intravenous thrombolysis in acute myocardial infarction: final report of the GISSI study. Gruppo Italiano per lo Studio della Streptochinasi nell'Infarto Miocardico (GISSI). Lancet 1987;2:871–874.

146. Maggioni AP, Franzosi JG, Santoro E, et al. Analysis of the risk of stroke in 20,891 patients with acute myocardial infarction following thrombolytic and antithrombotic treatment. N Engl J Med 1992;327:1–6.

147. Krumholz HM, Pasternak RC, Weinstein MC, et al. Cost effectiveness of thrombolytic therapy with streptokinase in elderly patients with suspected acute myocardial infarction. N Engl J Med 1992;327:7–13.

148. Thrombolytic therapy with streptokinase in acute ischemic stroke. The Multicenter Acute Stroke Trial-Europe Study Group. N Engl J Med 1996;335:145–150.

149. Tissue plasminogen activator for acute ischemic stroke. The National Institute of Neurological Disorders and Stroke rt-PA Stroke Study Group. N Engl J Med 1995;333:1581–1587.

150. Multicentre Acute Stroke Trial-Italy (MAST-I) Group. Randomised controlled trial of streptokinase, aspirin, and combination of both in treatment of acute ischaemic stroke. Lancet 1995;346:1509–1514.

151. Hacke W, Kaste M, Fieschi C, et al. Intravenous thrombolysis with recombinant tissue plasminogen activator for acute hemispheric stroke. European Cooperative Acute Stroke Study (ECASS). JAMA 1995;274:1017–1025.

152. Schneider LS, Pollock VE, Lyness SA. A meta-analysis of controlled trials of neuroleptic treatment in dementia. J Am Geriatr Soc 1990;38:553–563.

153. Druckenbrod RW, Rosen J, Cluxton RJ. As-needed dosing of antipsychotic drugs: limitations and guidelines for use in the elderly agitated patient. Ann Pharmacother 1993;27:645–648.

154. Lantz MS, Marin D. Pharmacologic treatment of agitation in dementia: a comprehensive review. J Geriatr Psychiatry Neurol 1996;9:107–119.

155. Tinetti ME, Williams TF, Mayewski R. Fall risk index for elderly patients based on number of chronic disabilities. Am J Med 1986;80:429–434.

156. Thapa PB, Meador KG, Gideon P, et al. Effects of antipsychotic withdrawal in elderly nursing home residents. J Am Geriatr Soc 1994;42:280–286.

157. Ray WA, Taylor JA, Meador KG, et al. Reducing antipsychotic drug use in nursing homes: a controlled trial of provider education. Arch Intern Med 1993;153:713–721.

158. Semla TP, Palla K, Poddig B, et al. Effect of the Omnibus Reconciliation Act 1987 on antipsychotic prescribing in nursing home residents. J Am Geriatr Soc 1994;42:648–652.

159. Rovner BW, Steele CD, Shmuely Y, Folstein MF. A randomized trial of dementia care in nursing homes. J Am Geriatr Soc 1996;44:7–13.

160. Gales BJ, Menard SM. Relationship between the administration of selected medications and falls in hospitalized elderly patients. Ann Pharmacother 1995;29: 354–358.

161. Herings RM, Stricker BH, de Boer A, et al. Benzodiazepines and the risk of falling leading to femur fractures: dosage more important than elimination half-life. Arch Intern Med 1995;155:1801–1807.

162. Hemmelgarn B, Suissa S, Huang A, et al. Benzodiazepine use and the risk of motor vehicle crash in the elderly. JAMA 1997;278:27–31.

163. Rothschild AJ. The diagnosis and treatment of late-life depression. J Clin Psychiatry 1996;57(suppl 5):5–11.

164. Emptage RE, Semla TP. Depression in the medically ill elderly: a focus on methylphenidate. Ann Pharmacother 1996;30:151–157.

165. Dunner DL. Therapeutic considerations in treating depression in the elderly. J Clin Psychiatry 1994;55(12 suppl):48–58.

166. Scott MA, Shelton PS, Gattis W. Therapeutic options for treating major depression, and the role of venlafaxine. Pharmacotherapy 1996;16:352–365.

167. Cyr M, Brown CS. Nefazodone: its place among antidepressants. Ann Pharmacother 1996;30:1006–1012.

168. NIH consensus conference. Diagnosis and treatment of depression in late life. JAMA 1992;268:1018–1024.

169. Eagger SA, Richards M, Levy R. Long-term effects of tacrine in Alzheimer's disease: an open study. Int J Geriatr Psychiatry 199;9:643–647.

170. Schneider LS, Farlow MR, Henderson VW, Pogoda JM. Effects of estrogen replacement therapy on response to tacrine in patients with Alzheimer's disease. Neurology 1996;46:1580–1584.

171. Rogers SL, Friedhoff LT. The efficacy and safety of donepezil in patients with Alzheimer's disease: results of a US Multicentre, Randomized, Double-Blind, Placebo-Controlled Trial. Donepezil Study Group. Dementia 1996;7:293–303.

172. Bryson HM, Benfield P. Donepezil. Drugs Aging 1997;10:234–239.

173. Aisen PS, Davis KL. The search for disease-modifying treatment for Alzheimer's disease. Neurology 1997;48 (suppl 6):S35–S41.

174. Andersen K, Launer LJ, Ott A, et al. Do nonsteroidal anti-inflammatory drugs decrease the risk for Alzheimer's disease? The Rotterdam Study. Neurology 1995;45:1441–1445.

175. Breitner JC, Gau BA, Welsh KA, et al. Inverse association of anti-inflammatory treatments and Alzheimer's disease: initial results of a co-twin control study. Neurology 1994;44:227–232.

176. Breitner JC. Inflammatory processes and antiinflammatory drugs in Alzheimer's disease: a current appraisal. Neurobiol Aging 1996;17:789–794.

177. Aisen PS, Altstiel L, Marin D, Davis K. Treatment of Alzheimer's disease with prednisone: results of pilot studies and design of a multicenter trial. J Am Geriatr Soc 1995;43:SA27.

178. Parnetti L, Senin U, Mecocci P. Cognitive enhancement therapy for Alzheimer's disease: the way forward. Drugs 1997;53:752–768.

179. Sano M, Ernesto C, Thomas RG, et al. A controlled trial of selegiline, alpha-tocopherol, or both as treatment for Alzheimer's disease. N Engl J Med 1997;336:1216–1222.

180. Paganini-Hill A, Henderson VW. Estrogen replacement therapy and risk of Alzheimer's disease. Arch Intern Med 1996;156:2213–2217.

181. Brennan DE, Kukull WA, Stergachis A, et al. Postmenopausal estrogen replacement therapy and the risk of Alzheimer's disease: a population-based case-control study. Am J Epidemiol 1994;140:262–267.

182. Kawas C, Resnick S, Morrison A, et al. A prospective study of estrogen replacement therapy and the risk of developing Alzheimer's disease: the Baltimore Longitudinal Study of Aging. Neurology 1997;48:1517–1521.

183. Tang MX, Jacobs D, Stern Y, et al. Effect of oestrogen during menopause on risk and age at onset of Alzheimer's disease. Lancet 1996;348:429–432.

184. Birge SJ. The role of estrogen in the treatment of Alzheimer's disease. Neurology 1997;48:S36–S41.

Common Complaints of the Elderly

Although the HCFA guideline has broadened the concept of the word complaint (in that "chief complaint" is the term to be used for the main reason for the patient's visit, whether or not the patient is complaining) this chapter concerns itself with those troublesome or worrying symptoms of which an elderly patient may actually complain.

It could well be argued that the elderly do not complain enough. It is a principle of geriatric medicine that unpresented, unrecognized, and undiagnosed medical problems are common and must be carefully sought. Sometimes one must use family or other witnesses and a direct questioning approach (the review of systems) to find life-threatening and functionally impairing issues that must be addressed by the clinician. It is so frequent that the main management issue is not presented by the patient as a complaint that in geriatric medicine one must make a considerable effort to broaden the historical input, i.e., the subjective of a subjective, objective, assessment, (and) plan (SOAP) approach, using such techniques as preappointment and ongoing symptom questionnaires for the family and patient. Direct questioning, including reviewing the systems as the patient is examined (a sort of guided imagery approach), is one method to discover these unpresented, unrecognized issues.

However, such an approach is presumptuous and imposes the clinician's own set of medical values on the problems and their order of priority. So Osler's oft-quoted adage, "Listen to the patient; he is telling you the diagnosis," remains relevant, even though it may be only partially true in a patient whose perception is impaired.

What patients complain of is probably what is troubling them most, the symptom or issue that is most important to them personally, regardless of its medical significance. So the patient with multiple disabilities, life-threatening illness, or terminal illness may well be more concerned about apparently medically trivial issues such as oral dryness or skin irritation.

Between these two extremes are the issues that are not brought out because of fear, embarrassment, or negativity: sexual issues, bladder dysfunction, and sadness, for example, are areas in which one must practice gentle ways of expressing interest, of asking questions in a sufficiently open-ended way to define the patient's concerns.

Yet one of the most common faults of medicine as it is practiced is to focus *too much* on the patient's own complaint and perception. After all, one could argue that this emphasis has led to the relative neglect of common problems (among which are many of the major syndromes of geriatric medicine) in which the onset is insidious, the progression slow, and thus the patient's perception worn down, often regarding quite treatable illness as inevitable and unfixable. To reduce disability and improve health in old age, we must do more long-term prevention: improving nutrition, exercise, and hydration and in a broader sense facilitating involvement, motivation, and enjoyment—all essential aspects of a healthful life. But compliance with recommendations associated with chronic problems and prevention is often difficult. The route to involvement and compliance by the patient may well be to address his or her own concerns. Simply prescribing exercise rarely motivates a patient to do so, but if the complaint is, for example, constipation, edema of the ankles, or poor appetite, part of the response should be to recommend activity and exercise. And yet often we respond to such complaints with a medication.

As will become clear, symptoms of which the patient may truly complain often are the obscure presentations of underlying serious illness; yet the symptoms themselves must be addressed to satisfy the patient and to reduce their effect on function (the aim of good geriatric medical care). A reflex prescription of medication is almost never sufficient and can be harmful; yet a comprehensive workup is also generally inappropriate as an initial response. Watchful waiting is often the key to reasonable management, but there must be *scheduled* follow-up with specific inquiry. In this way excessive and unnecessary investigation can be safely avoided, and yet the symptom and patient are not lost to follow-up. Watchful waiting is a vital piece of the primary care physician's art, and we are losing track of it in our discontinuous system.

For most of these common complaints any decent clinician could come up with a wide differential diagnosis of medical conditions and quite often medication side effects that may be significant contributors to the problem. Yet often when these traditional medical routes have been investigated or tried, one is still left with the problem: the patient still has a dry mouth, a poor appetite, or musculoskeletal discomfort. It is the practical, symptomatic management, often a little beyond traditional medical approaches, on which these accounts concentrate.

ANKLE SWELLING

Ankle swelling is not only a common complaint, it is a very common phenomenon. Most cases are caused by venous stasis, and therefore medications (i.e., diuretics) are not indicated except in a tiny minority of cases. After a quick clinical hunt for fluid retention elsewhere and predisposers such as otherwise occult congestive failure, protein deficiency, or abdominal mass, treatment for this is an educational opportunity: exercise with proper support and footwear is the mainstay, and elevating the feet whenever sitting

down is essential. If the skin stays in good condition, no treatment may be needed. A commitment to long-term diuretics for this alone, with the consequent fluid and electrolyte concerns, should be a major step, not taken lightly.

POOR APPETITE

Any clinician can think of factors that may reduce appetite: medications, depression, upper gastrointestinal disturbance, cancer somewhere. But often one is left still with a patient who complains of poor appetite, and this must itself be addressed. In such circumstances any food the patient fancies should be used in moderation to get oral intake started. Easy-to-handle finger foods can help. Soups can be enriched with protein: a nutritionally dense meal or snack, whenever the patient can be persuaded to eat, is the vital principle. Increased frequency of meals and snacks, or a can of food supplement between meals, can all increase intake, and the latter can energize and stimulate the appetite when mealtime comes. Cuing and socialization may help; others prefer to eat unobserved. Rigid adherence to traditional meal schedules must be avoided: eat anytime is the rule. It is such dietary and behavioral techniques, rather than medication approaches, that will help, and a persistent approach is needed, recognizing that this is a serious problem that will cause poor health (and death) if left unaddressed (1).

CONSTIPATION

Kellogg and many other fanatics have left their mark: many elders (and younger patients) believe that constipation is the correct term when one simply fails to have daily bowel movements; much laxative abuse ensues. So simply defining constipation may help: constipation is the passage of uncomfortably hard stool and/or the inability to pass a stool even when the bowel is full and causing a sensation of the need to evacuate. However, constipation can be a real problem, and its complications (impaction, obstruction, and fecal leakage) are dreadful, so this complaint should be taken seriously and investigated, with the well-known proviso of considering changed bowel habit as a warning sign of colonic or rectal carcinoma. Many know about fiber, but *three* interventions (fiber, fluid, and exercise) are required to treat and prevent constipation. Some constipated immobile elders can benefit from using the so-called gastrocolic reflex, the sensation of fullness following a meal: the technique is that, following breakfast or lunch, a little light exercise is taken, even some abdominal massage in the unmuscled, and then the patient sits on the toilet—the optimal time to have a bowel movement. This is a type of bowel retraining for some who have persistently failed to answer the call to stool. Thus the complaint of constipation gives the opportunity to educate about diet, fluids, and exercise, three areas in which it is difficult to garner enthusiastic patient compliance (2).

DIZZINESS

Dizziness is one of the most common complaints in geriatric medicine. The differential diagnosis is very wide, but a careful history generally enables the clinician to distinguish the minority of patients with a classical dizziness-producing syndrome, such as Ménière's syndrome or benign positional vertigo (BPV). The hazards of symptomatic treatment for dizziness, such as vestibular sedatives (e.g., meclizine [Antivert]), are well recognized. Although occasionally useful, they are often continued over the long term in patients in whom benefit has not been shown. They must not be reflexively prescribed. They do *not* substitute for a simple history-based diagnostic investigation, which should focus especially on patient safety. As a complaint, dizziness opens up consideration of the person's whole situation in regard to balance, gait and mobility, and the environment. Dizziness is often the final expression of multiple small deficits in vision, postural control, sensation, and awareness. Whereas deficits that may contribute to dizziness must be sought and addressed, clinical pragmatism is essential: use of aids to stability and balance (walking aids if acceptable) and environmental modifications (lighting, grab bars) to make hazardous parts of the house, such as the stairs, safer (3).

UNCOMFORTABLE FEET

The range of foot discomfort that people chronically tolerate is astonishing, with the un-healthful consequences of reduced mobility and unnecessary stress on vulnerable hips and knees often provoking pain in those joints or the back when the feet are the cause. Consultation with a good podiatrist, preferably one who would consider orthotics or other shoe modifications, as well as traditional podiatric skills to cushion, soften, scale, and smooth, is invaluable. (Even if the patient does not complain about them, always look at the feet.)

HEARING LOSS

Hearing loss is so common and insidious that many accept it as inevitable. The patient almost always sees it as less of a problem than others do. So simple referral for a hearing aid or audiologic evaluation is not the complete answer; many patients won't wear an aid or even admit they have a problem. And after years of quiet, adapting to normal noise is a problem too. So one needs persistence and determination but mostly candor, not allowing the patient to deny a problem others have noted. However, many of the hearing problems of old age cannot be corrected by a hearing aid alone. The way generic background noise and background music can blot out word discrimination and the many people who partially rely on lip reading to understand the spoken word underscore the importance of environment and the skill of the conversant in helping elders with hearing loss to maintain optimal social functioning. So family members must be taught to ensure good lighting and full facial contact to allow the "amplification" of lip reading and advised to avoid quiet discussion in the company of the patient on the assumption that he or she can't hear; this feeds paranoia and suspiciousness and is humiliating.

INCONTINENCE

A major syndrome of geriatric medicine, incontinence is covered in much more detail elsewhere, and most are well aware that an actual complaint of incontinence should be taken very seriously, not so much as a sign of serious underlying disease as a distressing, humiliating symptom that needs a prompt and efficient response. The popularity and safety (in terms of skin health and hygiene) of modern diapering techniques make pads and diapers an excellent first aid remedy if acceptable to the patient: diapers are a quick remedy to the embarrassment of wetting floors, furniture, and clothing, with the inevitable immobility and withdrawal that this produces if unaddressed. However, diapering should not substitute for investigation appropriate to the overall status of the patient. An underrecommended but very simple technique is scheduled toileting, which aims to ensure that the bladder is emptied before leakage by evolving a schedule that keeps the person dry. If stress incontinence is the problem and there is a special occasion to be faced, a practical hint is to use a tampon temporarily: if it works, it does indicate that there is probably a problem with the vesicourethral angle. Again, this technique must not substitute for more definitive approaches if appropriate (and tampons can be forgotten). Double voiding can be a useful adjunct: in female patients, after the bladder appears to be emptied, the patient relaxes a little, and then tries to urinate again, thus ensuring that a constant residual sediment is not sitting on the trigone to cause irritation. But perhaps the most common piece of ungiven advice is *not* to restrict fluid intake: by increasing the concentration, irritability, and sediment in the urine, urinary irritability and therefore frequency and incontinence can actually be increased; yet patients often restrict fluid intake in hopes that they won't then have so many accidents.

INSOMNIA

Simply prescribing a hypnotic when a patient complains of inability to sleep is bad medicine for two reasons: first, a sleep disorder can be a symptom of depression and other disorders, as described in many sources; second, there are many misconceptions about what normal sleep is, particularly with increasing age. Whereas simple inability to fall asleep may be helped in the short term by any hypnotic (zolpidem [Ambien] is a favorite because of its short duration of action without hangover into the next day), there are many simple measures to facilitate sleep: exercise in the daytime until the midafternoon, a calm evening, calming music or a familiar book, and for some, a little activity (such as hospital-

ized patients who fall asleep out at the nurses' station but not in the gloom of their own rooms). In all patients a sense of security and comfort, familiarity, and the right environmental temperature are crucial components of good sleep. The fact that having physical exercise earlier in the day helps sleep should be emphasized: disordered sleep is often a symptom of disordered, underexercised lives in which boredom, inactivity, and daytime napping reduce the need and tendency to sleep at night. Underrecognized and undertreated are the sleep phase syndromes (advanced or late), in which the person falls asleep either much earlier or much later than everyone else and has a good night's sleep but at a socially inconvenient time. These disorders should be recognized early, when they are easy to correct, rather than allowing the patient to slide into full day-night reversal. Families may welcome the break of daytime napping at first, but inevitably the intolerable burden of an interrupted or at least excessively short night ultimately ensues (4).

INSTABILITY

Instability is not the word the patient uses: "unsteady on my feet," the common phase, describes a situation we all know too well: the patient looks unsafe walking, tentative and fragile, often won't accept help or a walking aid, and looks ready to fall at times, particularly when hurried, tired, or anxious. In our anxiety to figure out the medical reason, we may omit the simple remedies: appropriate footwear, a cane or other aid that increases proprioception and provides actual support, and the counsel to practice walking regularly, so as to maintain balance skills. Whereas there are classical altered gaits (e.g., parkinsonian, apraxic), often the gait is nonspecific but just does not look right; intellectual dissatisfaction at being unable to define what's wrong must not stop us from doing practical things about instability problems. Environment is a vital factor: surfaces, lighting, furniture arranged to allow patients to support themselves (this is what many patients do, as they will not use awkward or geriatric-looking walking frames around the house). Judiciously positioned grab bars, not just in the bathroom and toilet but on the stairs, in the living room, at awkward corners, and at steps, should also be considered. And of course, new-onset instability, like new-onset falling, is one of the classic geriatric prodromes, a sign of evolving possibly serious illness, such as congestive heart failure, anemia, pneumonia, or other infection.

ITCHING

Whereas the differential diagnosis of itching is very broad, including numerous metabolic, dermatologic, and iatrogenic causes (especially medications), the most common cause remains dryness of the skin (ichthyosis). And since scratching the skin, especially if the fingernails are unpared, damages it and causes histamine release, it produces more itching; a vicious circle of itching and scratching is quickly established. If scratching is a factor, nail care and mittens may be crucial. But if the skin is dry, the first step is to rehydrate the environment, as forced air systems and fans add greatly to drying. The second step is good skin care with emollients, avoiding both excessive drying and the irritation and maceration of sweat, urine, and other fluids. Allowing damp skin to air dry also causes excessive drying. Lac-Hydrin (ammonium lactate) can be helpful in rehydrating dry skin, but less expensive remedies may fix the problem. Chronic fungal infection can be a factor, and it is clinically worthwhile to treat a fungal-appearing rash empirically (since culture is expensive), especially if that is clearly the site of the itch. Over-the-counter medications, particularly the older antihistamines with their sedating, anticholinergic, and orthostatic properties, although sometimes symptomatically helpful, are fraught with hazard. The tricyclic doxepin is occasionally helpful though sedative. Persistent itching of undetermined cause mandates dermatologic and also psychiatric and/or psychologic consideration. Antipruritic medications are often continued chronically because nobody is clear whether they helped or not.

JOINT PAIN AND STIFFNESS

Osteoarthritis being the most common chronic illness in the world, many elders accept arthritis as an explanation of their pain and stiffness, assuming that this means nothing can be done, that it is an inevitable consequence of aging. The media tell patients and families that relief is available from medication, but too often we fall short of the many other methods available to reduce joint pain and discomfort: warmth, increased activity, exercise to increase muscular support and well-being, appropriate bracing to provide support, and properly used walking aids, including a cane of the correct length, can all reduce pain and stiffness. Restless, disturbed sleep (with its huge differential diagnosis) causes aches and pains in the day but is rarely considered as a cause. We sometimes undermedicate joint pain and stiffness. If pain relief allows the person to exercise more, improving muscular support and function and well-being, far more than just pain relief will be achieved. Some stoic patients who refuse pain medication benefit from being told that their function improves because of pain relief. We also underuse simple acetaminophen, an inexpensive and safe way to relieve musculoskeletal pain in many without the hazards of anti-inflammatory agents (which also have a crucial place and can be used in combination with acetaminophen as mentioned in the separate section on pain) (5).

LOW BACK PAIN

Once the serious things have been ruled out, and even after some degenerative or osteopenic changes have been identified, one may try simple analgesics or NSAIDs. Failing those, many other available methods are often not considered. Physicians are so bad at managing low-back pain that back manipulation is big business. Some patients do need back manipulation, but the great majority, young and old, can teach themselves back stretches, extensions, and exercises to increase flexibility and develop muscular support. Self-help books are available (6). Such simple exercises are well within the capacity of many elders, even the frail. Proper positioning in chairs, with low-back support (perhaps a lumbar pillow or roll) at the proper height, and a firm enough bed are also crucial. Many elders cannot tolerate a very hard mattress, simply because osteoarthritic joints and reduced subcutaneous muscle and fat make hard surfaces uncomfortable, but increasingly available are mattresses that are supportive but that have a soft surface so that the patient can sleep comfortably.

MEMORY LOSS

The significance of progressive memory loss—the possibility that it represents early Alzheimer's, particularly in the oldest old—is now widely recognized and emphasized in the media. Whereas controversy still reigns about whether age-associated memory impairment (AAMI) is a separate syndrome or simply an expression of early Alzheimer's, and whereas the complaint of memory loss (whether from the patient or a family member) must lead to searching questions to find other conditions that may cause it (particularly early dementias and depression but many other physical illnesses too), memory loss itself remains a common issue, something people have to cope with. There are many techniques for preventing memory loss in itself from ruining a person's ability to cope with life: Notices and reminders around the house, one notepad as a constant companion where reminders can be written down, telephone call prompts to remember appointments and medication doses for those living alone, and even computer-based reminder systems have all been shown to be helpful, but the patient needs help getting these things organized. Once memory loss is an issue in an older person, it is generally pointless to try to force memory to work: the "use it or lose it" philosophy may well be true earlier, but once memory loss is a problem, reminder techniques are the key to reducing its effect on the patient's life. Skinner (7) has written creatively about overcoming the embarrassment of forgetting people's names simply by introducing yourself, thus often prompting the person whose name has been forgotten to use his or her name in return.

DRY MOUTH

Undernutrition, from which the elderly often suffer but rarely complain, is a major consequence of oral discomfort, and dryness of the mouth is one of the most common symptoms noted by patients. It is an important factor in reducing the comfort of the terminally ill and chronically dependent patients. Many medica-

tions predispose to it, but so do mouth breathing, underhydration, and (least often considered) forced air and other heating systems that promote a dry environment. Poor teeth often add to overall discomfort too. The wise clinician therefore looks at the patient's whole situation when considering how to reduce this important complaint. Salivary replacements are available, but a combination of glycerine and traditionally lemon applications, ice chips, even hard candy to stimulate saliva, and room humidity often produce relief. Dry mouth is far more than a side effect of medications and reduced peripheral cholinergic activity; it is also a complaint that must be separately considered and managed.

CHRONIC PAIN

The patient specifies where the chronic pain is, and the clinician gets a history of its nature. A clinical hunt is needed, depending on the site, and bone scans have added to the capacity of radiographs to show unexpected bone changes as a cause. Often, however, the conclusion is that a combination of factors are producing a constant dull ache in some area; such pain is often a combination of immobility and bone and joint changes. The World Health Organization (WHO) stepladder approach should be used more frequently: a full trial of local and systemic methods concurrently, starting low and mild and often adding analgesics one to another until relief is obtained (8). Acetaminophen (underestimated by all, as it is so easily available) is underused: 4 g a day is safe even in cirrhotic patients under a clinician's supervision, and NSAIDs can sometimes be used simultaneously with effect. Adjunctive drugs, especially antidepressants, should be tried in combination with both, and local counterirritant and other therapies, including heat, massage, and more sophisticated methods such as transcutaneous nerve stimulation, should all be exhausted as therapeutic trials before moving up the stepladder even to codeine, an opioid that is terribly constipating in some and frequently cerebrally impairing.

IMPAIRED VISION

Many ophthalmologists and optometrists restrict themselves to correcting visual acuity, whereas there is much more to low vision in old age than lenses. There are some low vision programs, but often the personal physician must be prepared to discuss low vision methods: hand magnifiers, bright light for reading, avoidance of glare, and reduction of dazzle at night or in the dark, yellow lenses for night driving, reduction of daylight glare for some using tinted or ultraviolet-filtering lenses, and large-print books. Of course, in the elderly the classic cause of poor vision is presbyopia, in which the person cannot focus on things placed too close (and thus holds the newspaper at arm's length). Lenses can usually correct presbyopia.

SUMMARY

All of the common complaints described in this chapter have a broad differential diagnosis generally within the range of a good general physician. The consistent issue is that ruling in or out the medical causes often still leaves the patient with the complaint unrelieved. All these accounts emphasize that after suitable workup, the clinician must never fail to implement a prag-matic and practical approach to address the complaint, often going beyond traditional easy-to-prescribe management strategies. The emphasis—the core of geriatric medicine—is on maintaining function.

REFERENCES

1. Incorporating Nutrition Screening and Interventions Into Medical Practice: A Monograph for Physicians. Washington: Nutrition Screening Initiative, 1994.
2. Wieman HM. Constipation. In: Ham RJ, Sloane PD, eds. Primary Care Geriatrics: A Case-Based Approach. 3rd ed. St. Louis: Mosby-Year Book, 1997.
3. Sloane PD. Dizziness. In: Ham RJ, Sloane PD, eds. Primary Care Geriatrics: A Case-Based Approach. 3rd ed. St. Louis: Mosby-Year Book, 1997.
4. Dement WC, Miles LE, Carskadon MA. "White paper" on sleep and aging. J Am Geriatr Soc 1982;30:25–50.
5. Ham RJ. Arthritis. In: Mengel MB, Schwiebert LP, eds. Ambulatory Medicine: The Primary Care of Families. Norwalk, CT: Appleton & Lange, 1997.
6. McKenzie R. Treat Your Own Back. 7th ed. New Zealand: Spinal Publications, 1997 (distributed in United States).
7. Skinner BF, Vaughan ME. Enjoy Old Age. New York: WW Norton, 1983.
8. Cancer pain relief and palliative care. Report of a WHO Expert Committee. World Health Organ Tech Rep Ser 1990;804:1–75.

CHAPTER 7

ABDUL HAKIM KHAN, JEFFREY I. LEAVETT, NAVEEN S. PEREIRA, AND NIDAL A. YUNIS

Diagnosis and Management of Heart Disease in the Elderly

ISCHEMIC HEART DISEASE

Age-related atherosclerotic changes are common in the elderly, and they predispose the person to the development of coronary artery disease (1). These changes result from a combination of factors: aging, diet and other environmental factors, and probably genetic factors (2). The process is worsened by coronary risk factors such as smoking, hyperlipidemia, hypertension, and diabetes. Elderly people tend to gain weight, i.e., increase in fat body mass and decrease in lean muscle mass. Obesity, especially abdominal obesity, is associated with coronary artery disease. The prevalence of symptomatic coronary artery disease in people over age 75 is about 30% (3), while the prevalence from autopsy studies is about 60% (4). This variation reflects silent coronary artery disease or angina being attributed to noncardiac causes.

Clinical Features

Ischemic heart disease in the elderly is often diffuse and commonly manifests as typical angina; less commonly it presents as epigastric distress or indigestion, episodic dyspnea with exertion, or rarely as a feeling of fatigue and weakness. In addition, a history of claudication of the legs due to peripheral vascular disease, common in the elderly, may suggest coronary artery disease (5).

Diagnosis

The diagnosis of ischemic heart disease is confirmed by exercise stress test, preferably with myocardial nuclear imaging using thallium or sestamibi. Pharmacologic stress testing with dipyridamole, adenosine, or dobutamine is used in patients who cannot exercise because of coexisting illness such as arthritis. Dobutamine echocardiography is another option in which coronary artery disease is diagnosed on the basis of left ventricular wall motion abnormalities. A trial of sublingual nitroglycerin for angina may provide a useful clue to but is not diagnostic of coronary artery disease, and some elderly patients may choose to be treated medically without various testing procedures.

Treatment

Therapy is directed at correcting risk factors such as hyperlipidemia, hypertension, heart failure, and diabetes. Moderate exercise in the form of walking or other recreational activities has been noted to reduce cardiac risk factors and improve survival (5). Conditions that aggravate angina, such as anemia, hyperthyroidism, or fever, should be addressed. Pharmacologic therapy consists of nitrates, β-blockers, and calcium channel blockers (6). All patients with ischemic heart disease should take one adult aspirin a day, preferably enteric coated; those who are allergic to aspirin may use ticlopidine (7) or, better still, clopidogrel (8). Neutropenia is sometimes a side effect of ticlopidine but is very rare with clopidogrel. Nitrates play an important role in the management of angina. Venodilation, i.e., preload reduction that leads to a decrease in left ventricular (LV) wall stress, is the major mode of action of nitrates. In addition, nitrates relieve coronary spasm and dilate coronary arteries. Sublingual nitroglycerin 0.4 mg (1.3 to 1.6 mg) or nitroglycerin spray (one metered dose is 1.4 mg) is used to abort an acute attack of angina or is used prophylactically prior to activities that are known to precipitate angina. For an acute attack of angina, patients should be advised to repeat the dose every 2 to 5 minutes for up to three doses and to seek prompt medical attention if angina is not relieved, as this may herald the onset of acute infarction or unstable angina. A chronic oral nitrate, such as isosorbide dinitrate or isosorbide mononitrate, is used to prevent angina. Nitrate tolerance, which renders nitrate therapy less efficacious, can be avoided by observing an 8- to 12-hour nitrate-free interval during which no nitrate therapy is given except sublingual nitroglycerin if needed. The 24-hour nitroglycerin patch should be removed at bedtime to provide a nitrate-free period and a new one applied in the morning (9); for patients with nocturnal angina the nitrate-free time may be reversed. Isosorbide mononitrate preparations are less likely to cause tolerance if used appropriately, e.g., isosorbide mononitrate (Ismo) twice a day taken eccentrically, i.e., 7 hours apart, or isosorbide mononitrate (Imdur) taken once a day in the morning (10). Patients should be warned of potential side effects, including nitrate-induced headaches, dizziness, light-headedness and, rarely, syncope. Light-headedness can be relieved by lying down; aspirin or acetaminophen is helpful in controlling headaches, which tend to disappear with chronic nitrate therapy. Persistent headaches may necessitate downward dose titration or discontinuation of therapy. Sublingual nitroglycerin tablets deteriorate when exposed to light, and patients should be advised to carry them in colored bottles and to remove the cotton plug from the bottle for easy access to tablets. Intravenous nitroglycerin is used mainly in the acute setting, e.g., unstable angina or during surgery of patients with ischemic heart disease.

β-Blockers (propranolol, nadolol, metoprolol, atenolol), which have an additive effect in controlling angina, are commonly employed with nitrates (6). By blunting the catecholamine response, these agents reduce heart rate, blood pressure, and cardiac contractility and thus reduce myocardial oxygen needs. By reducing heart rate, they improve coronary (diastolic) blood flow. Side effects include symptomatic bradycardia, atrioventricular (AV) block, and hypotension. Other potential side effects include fatigue, depression, insomnia, and impotence. Precipitation or worsening of heart failure, claudication, and asthma are common in patients with these underlying conditions, and the use of β-blockers in these patients should be avoided or undertaken with precaution. For patients with asthma and claudication, selective $β_1$-agents such as metoprolol and atenolol, when used in low doses, may be better tolerated. At high doses, however, this advantage of selectivity is lost. β-Blockers are ideally suited for patients whose angina is precipitated by heightened catecholamine levels, such as with exercise, and for those who have concomitant conditions amenable to β-blocker therapy. The latter include hypertension, hypertrophic cardiomyopathy, hyperthyroidism for temporary control of symptoms, migraine prophylaxis, post-Q-wave myocardial infarction (MI), atrial fibrillation for rate control, and symptomatic ventricular arrhythmias. β-Blockers with intrinsic sympathomimetic activity (ISA) are less helpful in angina control but may be employed in patients in whom resting bradycardia is a limiting factor for β-blocker use. In these patients β-blockers with ISA may prevent worsening of resting bradycardia while blunting increase in heart rate that may follow physical or emotional stress. The dose of β-blocker should be titrated to obtain a resting heart rate of approximately 55 to 60 beats per minute provided that there are no associated side effects as noted earlier. β-Blocker therapy should not be stopped abruptly, as this may lead to rebound angina and rarely, MI.

Calcium channel blockers (e.g., amlodipine, felodipine, verapamil, and diltiazem) are another important class of drugs for the management of ischemic heart disease (6). Their mode of action derives from their ability to lower the intracellular concentration of calcium ion, which results in relaxation of smooth muscles of arterial walls, leading to vasodilation. In addition, certain agents in this class (verapamil and diltiazem) possess antiarrhythmic action against paroxysmal supraventricular tachycardia (PSVT) and slow ventricular rate in atrial fibrillation or flutter (11). Thus verapamil and diltiazem are ideal agents for patients with ischemic heart disease with concomitant supraventricular tachyrhythmias except in the setting of preexcitation syndrome (Wolff-Parkinson-White syndrome), in which they are contraindicated. In general, calcium channel blockers are employed when β-blockers are contraindicated or not tolerated and when angina remains refractory to combined treatment with nitrates and β-blockers. Calcium channel blockers are specifically indicated for patients with coronary artery spasm (Prinzmetal angina). They are fairly well tolerated and are safe for patients with asthma, diabetes, peripheral vascular disease, or systolic heart failure (amlodipine and felodipine but not verapamil or diltiazem). They should be avoided in patients with Q-wave acute MI except if ischemia is uncontrollable with nitrates and β-blockers. In non–Q-wave MI, diltiazem has been shown to reduce reinfarction rate. Verapamil and diltiazem should be avoided in those with systolic heart failure and patients with sick sinus syndrome (SSS) because of the danger of sinus node arrest or advanced AV block. All calcium channel blockers, especially verapamil, have the potential to cause constipation, particularly in the elderly, who are prone to this problem. Therapy may have to be discontinued if constipation persists despite the addition of a stool softener. Diuretic-resistant edema of legs is encountered more often with dihydropyridines (nifedipine, amlodipine, and felodipine) than with verapamil and diltiazem and should not be confused with edema due to heart failure.

Patients who continue to be symptomatic despite adequate medical therapy and those who have evidence of significant ischemia on noninvasive diagnostic studies should undergo cardiac catheterization to define the extent of coronary artery disease and determine whether they are candidates for coronary angioplasty or coronary artery bypass surgery. The risks of cardiac catheterization are increased in the elderly because of peripheral vascular disease, renal function impairment, and congestive heart failure, and therefore this procedure should be undertaken in properly selected patients who are can-

didates for angioplasty or bypass surgery. Recent data support the efficacy of angioplasty in the elderly, with success rates of about 85%; disadvantages include procedure-related complications noted earlier and higher (up to 35%) restenosis rate (12, 13). Mortality for those undergoing coronary artery bypass surgery is 2 to 3 times as high in elderly patients as in younger patients—about 5 to 6%. Surgery is associated with better angina control and quality of life (14). However, data from a recent study indicate a comparable quality of life and 5-year survival in the group randomized to coronary bypass surgery (CABG) or to percutaneous transluminal coronary angioplasty (PTCA) (15). This same study shows that diabetic patients do better with CABG than with PTCA (16). CABG is indicated for patients with left main coronary artery disease, patients with multivessel coronary disease and depressed LV function, and patients who remain symptomatic despite adequate medical therapy. Risk factors for operative mortality include age 70 years or above, female gender, emergency operation, and congestive heart failure. Operative mortality is also high for those undergoing repeat cardiac bypass surgery (17, 18). Internal mammary artery graft is preferred over saphenous vein graft because of its longer patency rate, i.e., a 10% occlusion rate compared with a 40 to 60% occlusion rate for saphenous vein graft at 10 years. With improved angioplasty techniques and use of stents, angioplasty may be preferred for carefully selected elderly patients, especially when the preoperative risk factors noted earlier are present (12, 13).

Patients with unstable angina and non–Q-wave MI should be managed in a monitored unit using aspirin, intravenous heparin, and nitrates, preferably intravenously. Most patients are also prescribed a β-blocker; calcium channel blockers are added if ischemia persists (19, 20). Thrombolytic therapy has not been shown to be effective in unstable angina or non–Q-wave infarction, and the risk of cerebral bleeding is increased in the elderly. Patients who have no contraindication to angioplasty or coronary bypass surgery and who are willing to undergo these procedures are evaluated by cardiac catheterization to determine further course of therapy. Catheterization is performed after 3 to 4 days of a cooling down period unless the patient has ongoing angina. Low molecular weight heparin given subcutaneously to patients with unstable angina or non–Q-wave MI has been shown to be superior to standard intravenous heparin with respect to combined end points of infarction, death, and revascularization and does not require monitoring of clotting parameters such as activated partial thromboplastin time (aPTT) (21). Low molecular weight heparin therefore may be preferred over unfractionated or standard intravenous heparin for ease of administration and because it does not require monitoring by blood tests. Trials evaluating the efficacy of oral IIb/IIIa platelet receptor antagonists for the management of acute coronary syndromes are in progress.

ACUTE MYOCARDIAL INFARCTION

Coronary artery disease, specifically acute myocardial infarction (AMI), is the leading cause of death in the United States. Elderly patients have a higher rate of mortality and complications associated with AMI, as well as more frequent comorbid conditions. Although most trials of AMI excluded patients more than 75 years of age, the weight of evidence suggests that therapies proven to reduce mortality in younger populations are at least as effective in the elderly.

Clinical Presentation

AMI is usually heralded by classic symptoms of chest pressure radiating to the left arm associated with dyspnea, diaphoresis, and nausea. This presentation is less common in the elderly because of factors such as altered pain threshold and cognitive deficits. Thus these patients may have atypical manifestations, such as epigastric distress, dyspnea, weakness, syncope, and even acute confusion.

Diagnosis

Diagnosis of AMI is made by a combination of history, electrocardiographic findings, and cardiac enzyme patterns. Due to a higher prevalence of severe coronary disease and prior MI, the elderly more frequently present with non–Q-wave MI. Non–Q-wave MI is associated with less extensive myocardial necrosis and lower peak crea-

tine kinase (CK) levels. Therefore it is important to follow the pattern of CK-MB isoenzymes. CK and CK-MB levels are usually normal at the onset of AMI, begin to rise 5 to 6 hours after symptom onset, and peak at about 18 to 20 hours. Because hospital presentation is often delayed in the elderly, this pattern may be altered. In a patient who presents late, i.e., after the CK has normalized, measurement of lactate dehydrogenase (LDH) is useful, as peak LDH levels do not occur until 3 to 4 days after symptom onset. Similarly, cardiac-specific troponins T and I remain elevated for a week or more after MI (22) and should be obtained, if available, in this situation.

Treatment

The main goals of therapy for AMI are to improve survival and preserve quality of life. There are two main phases in the treatment of AMI. The first is acute care and stabilization of the patient, which is generally accomplished within the first few hours to 24 hours of presentation (Table 7.1). The second phase is recovery, with therapy guided toward secondary prevention of recurrent events, risk stratification, and rehabilitation (Table 7.2). The recently published guidelines for the management of AMI by the American College of Cardiology and American Heart Association (ACC/AHA) (23) are highly recommended.

Summary of Acute Phase

To expedite evaluation and management of the patient with suspected AMI, several tasks must be completed within minutes of the patient's arrival. A targeted history, physical examination, and electrocardiogram (ECG) are performed to assess the likelihood of an acute coronary syndrome and any complications. Intravenous access (18 gauge or greater) is obtained. Oxygen is administered by nasal cannula, and aspirin is given to chew and swallow. If ongoing chest discomfort is present, sublingual nitroglycerin is given for pain relief. For continuing or refractory pain or if congestive heart failure is present, intravenous nitroglycerin is started. In the interim, morphine sulfate is administered if chest pain persists despite one or two sublingual nitroglycerin tablets. While these measures are being instituted, the emergency physician decides whether thrombolytic therapy or pri-

Table 7.1

Medications Indicated for Acute Phase of AMI

Medication	Route	Dosage	Indications	Contraindications	Side Effects
Thrombolytic agents					
t-PA	IV	15 mg bolus, then 0.75 mg/kg over 30 min, then 0.5 mg/kg over 60 min (total dose ≤ 100 mg)	Chest pain with ST elevation or LBBB for ≤ 12 hr (see Table 7.3)	See Table 7.3	Bleeding, any site, intracranial in 0.5–1% (reverse with cryo, FFP)
SK	IV	1.5 million U over 60 min	Same as for t-PA	See Table 7.3	Same as for t-PA
APSAC	IV	30 U bolus	Same as for t-PA	See Table 7.3	Same as for t-PA
r-PA	IV	Two 10 U boluses 30 min apart	Same as for t-PA	See Table 7.3	Same as for t-PA
Aspirin	po	160 mg (chew and swallow)	All patients	Allergy	Peptic ulcers
Nitroglycerin	IV	Begin at 5–10 μg/min, titrate by 5–10 μg/min q 5–10 min	Patients with ongoing or recurrent ischemia, CHF, HTN	SBP <100 HR <50, >110 RV infarct (use with caution)	Hypotension Headache Bradycardia (uncommon)
		Titrate dose to pain relief, MAP	Continue 24–48 hr		
Heparin	IV	70 U/kg bolus then 15 U/kg/hr	All t-PA patients, others Target PTT 50–75 Continue × 48 hr in stable patients, longer if high risk for emboli	Active bleeding at high risk	Bleeding, any site (reverse with protamine) Thrombocytopenia
	SC	7500 U q 12 hr	Low-risk patients. (optional with SK)	Same as for IV heparin	Same as for IV heparin
β-Blockade			All patients within 12 hr (esp HTN, tachycardia, ongoing ischemia)	Moderate or severe CHF Bronchospasm PR >0.24; 2° or 3° AV block HR <65, SBP <100	Worsened CHF Bronchospasm Heart block Bradycardia, hypotension
Metoprolol	IV	5 mg q 2 min × 3 doses			
Atenolol	IV	5 mg q 10 min × 2 doses			
ACE inhibitors			All patients (especially those with anterior MI, CHF, LV dysfunction)	SBP <100 Allergy Significant renal failure (creatinine>3) Bilateral renal a. stenosis	Hypotension Renal insufficiency Cough
Captopril	po	6.25 mg initially, aim for 50 tid			
Lisinopril	po	2.5–5 mg initially, aim for 10 qd			

Adapted from Leavitt JI, Khan AH, Demel K. Management of acute myocardial infarction. In: Khan AH, ed. Practical Cardiology: A Textbook for Primary Care Physicians. London: Edward Arnold Publishers (in press).

A, artery; APSAC, anisoylated plasminogen streptokinase activator complex; CHF, congestive heart failure; creat, serum creatinine; cryo, cryoprecipitate; FFP, fresh frozen plasma; HTN, hypertension; LBBB, left bundle branch block; MAP, mean arterial pressure; r-PA, recombinant plasminogen activator; RV, right ventricle; SBP, systolic blood pressure; SC, subcutaneous; SK, streptokinase; t-PA, tissue plaminogen activator.

Table 7.2

Medications Indicated for Secondary Prevention After AMI

Medication	Dosage[a]	Indications	Contraindications	Side Effects
Aspirin	160–325 mg	All patients	Allergy GI bleeding	Peptic ulcers GI blood loss
β-Blockade Metoprolol Atenolol	50–100 mg bid 100–200 mg/day	All patients (especially those with HTN, tachycardia, recurrent ischemia)	Moderate or severe CHF Bronchospasm PR >0.24; 2° or 3° AV block HR <65, SBP <100 mm Hg	Worsened CHF Bronchospasm Heart block Bradycardia, hypotension
Warfarin	Daily dose titrated to INR 2–3	Patients unable to take aspirin Atrial fibrillation Documented LV thrombus Severe wall motion abnormalities	Active bleeding Bleeding diathesis High risk for falls Pregnancy	Bleeding, any site
ACE inhibitors Captopril Lisinopril Ramipril	See Table 7.1 See Table 7.1 2.5 mg bid initially; aim for 5 bid	Patients with symptomatic (CHF) or asymptomatic LV dysfunction (EF ≤ 40%), especially if anterior infarct	SBP <90 mm Hg Allergy Significant renal failure (serum creatinine >3.0 mg/dL) Bilateral renal a. stenosis Pregnancy	Hypotension Renal insufficiency Hyperkalemia Cough
HMG-CoA reductase inhibitors Simvastatin Pravastatin	10–40 mg hs 20–40 mg hs	LDL > 125 mg/dL not responding to diet (target LDL < 100 mg/dL)	Liver disease Pregnancy	Elevated liver enzymes Myopathy (rare)
Ca²⁺ channel blockers Verapamil Diltiazem	360 mg/day 240–360 mg/day	Patients with ongoing ischemia or atrial fibrillation, nl LV function, no CHF, and contraindication to β-blockade	Decreased LV EF or CHF 2° or 3° AV block HR <65, SBP <100 mm Hg	Worsened CHF Heart block Bradycardia, hypotension

Adapted from Leavitt JI, Khan AH, Demel K. Management of acute myocardial infarction. In: Khan AH, ed. Practical Cardiology: A Textbook for Primary Care Physicians. London: Edward Arnold Pubishers (in press).

ACE, angiotensin converting enzyme; Ca²⁺, calcium; EF, ejection fraction; GI, gastrointestinal; HMG-CoA, 3-hydroxy-3-methylglutaryl Coenzyme A; INR, international normalized ratio; LDL, low-density liproprotein; LV, left ventricle; remainder of abbreviations per Table 7.1.

[a]Dosages shown are those used in clinical trials; no data are available for efficacy of lower dosages.

mary angioplasty is indicated and safe according to clinical and electrocardiographic criteria. If thrombolytic therapy is ordered, the infusion should begin ideally within 30 minutes of the patient's arrival at the hospital. Finally, the emergency physician should consider initiating treatment with β-adrenergic blocking agents. Intravenous heparin is mandatory when using tissue plasminogen activator (t-PA) but is optional if streptokinase is used. Patients presenting without ST segment elevation should be treated with all of these measures except thrombolytic agents (23).

Thrombolytic Therapy

Thrombolysis is indicated in patients presenting within 12 hours of the onset of chest pain with ST segment elevation or new left bundle-branch block (LBBB) pattern on the ECG (Table 7.3). Treatment with thrombolytic agents results in a highly significant 18% reduction in mortality (24). Randomized trials on more than 22,000 patients over age 65 demonstrate a significant benefit with thrombolytic therapy, even after adjusting for the higher rate of complications such as intracranial bleeding and other major bleeding in this age group. In fact, because of the higher mortality from AMI in this population (about 25 to 30% at 1 month in patients at least 75 years of age), elderly patients treated with thrombolytic therapy may derive a *greater* absolute benefit than do younger patients (24). Furthermore, thrombolytic therapy is cost effective in the elderly whether streptokinase (25) or t-PA (26) is used. Because of a higher rate of intracranial hemorrhage associated with t-PA than with streptokinase in patients over age 75, streptokinase may be safer (though possibly less effective) than t-PA in this age group.

Despite its proven benefit, thrombolytic therapy is underused, especially in the elderly (27–29). A recent study in the Medicare population found that only 44% of patients eligible for thrombolytic therapy actually received it (27). The 30-day mortality rate among eligible patients receiving thrombolytic therapy was only 11.7%, compared with 21.5% for eligible patients who were not treated. The elderly population has been shown to delay presentation to the hospital after symptom onset, thus limiting the

Table 7.3

Guidelines for Use of Thrombolytic Therapy

Indications

Chest pain or other symptoms consistent with AMI
ECG changes
  ≥1 mm ST elevation in ≥2 contiguous limb leads
  ≥1–2 mm ST elevation in ≥ 2 contiguous
    precordial leads
  New or indeterminate age left bundle branch block
Presentation within 12 hours of symptom onset

Contraindications

Absolute: Consider primary angioplasty
  Previous cerebral or spinal hemorrhage or known
    neoplasm
  Ischemic or embolic CVA or other cerebrovascular
    event within 1 year
  Intracranial or intraspinal surgery within 2 mo
  Active internal bleeding (not including menses)
  Suspected aortic dissection
  Previous allergy to SK or APSAC (but may use
    t-PA or r-PA)

Relative: Balance benefits vs. risk in individual patients
  Severe uncontrolled HTN on presentation (BP >
    180/110 mm Hg)
  History of ischemic or embolic CVA > 1 yr prior
    (absolute if within 1 yr) OR known intracranial/
    spinal aneurysm, AVM
  Major trauma or surgery within past 2–4 wk that
    could result in bleeding into a closed space,
    including head trauma
  Traumatic or prolonged (> 10 min) CPR within
    2–4 wk
  Subclavian or internal jugular cannulation OR
    recent puncture of a noncompressible vessel
  Serious gastrointestinal bleeding within 2–4 wk
  Known bleeding disorder, including severe hepatic
    or renal disease
  Current use of oral anticoagulants (INR ≥2)
  Hemorrhagic retinopathy
  Use of SK or APSAC, or streptococcal infection
    within 2 years (may use t-PA, r-PA)
  Pregnancy or 10 days postpartum
  History of chronic, severe HTN (diastolic > 100
    mm Hg), treated or untreated

Modified from Leavitt JI, Khan AH, Demel K. Management of acute myocardial infarction. In: Khan AH, ed. Practical Cardiology: A Textbook for Primary Care Physicians. London: Edward Arnold Publishers (in press).
AVM, arteriovenous malformation; BP, blood pressure; CPR, cardiopulmonary resuscitation; CVA, cerebrovascular accident; for remaining abbreviations, see Table. 7.1.

number of patients eligible for thrombolytic therapy (30). Greater efforts at educating this population about the need for prompt presentation, as well as improved identification of eligible patients and earlier administration of thrombolytic therapy in the hospital setting, should improve access to this life-saving treatment.

Primary Angioplasty

In patients with contraindications to thrombolytic therapy, primary angioplasty is a safe and effective alternative if access to facilities and experienced operators is immediately available. Some studies comparing primary angioplasty with thrombolytic therapy have indicated improved survival and lower risk of reinfarction and stroke with primary angioplasty (31), while other studies have shown survival to be similar for the two techniques (32). Thus, recommendations regarding primary angioplasty as the therapy of choice must await results of further trials.

Aspirin

Use of aspirin in the first 24 hours of AMI reduces short-term mortality and reinfarction in all age groups (33). Similarly, long-term aspirin use after AMI prolongs survival and prevents reinfarction and stroke. Thus, aspirin (160 mg chewed and swallowed initially, then 325 mg daily) should be given to all patients with suspected AMI soon after hospital presentation and continued indefinitely. Despite its efficacy, safety, and affordability, however, recent data show that aspirin is underused in patients with AMI (34–36).

Glycoprotein IIb/IIIa platelet receptor inhibitors are a new class of antiplatelet therapy. These agents have shown promise in preliminary trials in patients with acute coronary syndromes (37). Ongoing trials will clarify the role of these agents in AMI.

Heparin

Intravenous heparin is indicated in patients with AMI receiving t-PA, as it reduces coronary reocclusion and maintains vessel patency in such patients. In patients receiving streptokinase, however, intravenous heparin is not routinely indicated, as it has not been shown to improve angiographic or clinical outcomes. Patients with

AMI receiving streptokinase or no thrombolysis who are at high risk for systemic emboli (e.g., those with large or anterior MI, atrial fibrillation, or a prior embolic event) should receive intravenous heparin; all others should receive subcutaneous heparin 7500 U twice a day. For patients with non–Q-wave MI, as for patients with unstable angina, subcutaneous low molecular weight heparin, such as enoxaparin, may be used in place of standard heparin (see section on ischemic heart disease).

Use of a target PTT range of 50 to 75 seconds results in less bleeding and better clinical outcomes than the previous standard target PTT of 60 to 85 seconds (38). Efficacy and complication rates can be improved further by using a weight-adjusted heparin dosing nomogram and close monitoring of the PTT. Heparin should be continued for at least 48 hours after the MI. Subcutaneous heparin should be used until the patient is fully ambulatory. Intravenous heparin should be continued beyond 48 hours in patients at high risk for recurrent MI or systemic thromboembolism.

Nitroglycerin

By causing coronary and systemic vasodilation and improving collateral blood flow to ischemic myocardium, nitroglycerin is very useful for treating the pain associated with myocardial ischemia and infarction. While trials from the prethrombolysis era suggested that nitrates reduced mortality after AMI, recent trials have failed to show a significant effect of nitroglycerin preparations on survival (39, 40). While intravenous nitroglycerin need not be used routinely in all patients with AMI, it may be safely used at least for the first 24 hours of acute infarction, and longer if there is evidence of ongoing or recurrent ischemia, congestive heart failure, or hypertension.

The most important side effect of nitroglycerin therapy is systemic hypotension. Patients at highest risk for hypotension include those with right ventricular infarction, hypovolemia, borderline systolic blood pressure (90 to 100 mm Hg), or marked bradycardia or tachycardia. Because of its short half-life and ease of titration, nitroglycerin should be administered intravenously in the early phase of AMI; oral long-acting nitrates should not be used during this period.

β-Blockers

In AMI patients not receiving thrombolytic therapy, the use of early intravenous β-blockade reduces mortality by 13% by preventing cardiac rupture, ventricular fibrillation, and reinfarction (41). These beneficial effects appear to be even more striking in the elderly (42, 43). When used in patients receiving thrombolytic therapy, intravenous β-blockers reduce the incidence of nonfatal reinfarction and recurrent ischemia and may reduce mortality if given within 2 hours of symptom onset (44). Current guidelines recommend the use of intravenous β-blockade in all patients without contraindications who can be treated within 12 hours of the onset of AMI and at any time in patients with ongoing or recurrent ischemia or with tachyarrhythmias (23). Contraindications to intravenous β-blockade include hypotension (systolic blood pressure below 100 mm Hg), bradycardia (heart rate below 60 beats per minute), marked first-, second-, or third-degree heart block, bronchospasm, and moderate to severe congestive heart failure.

Oral β-blockers play an important role in the recovery phase of AMI, reducing long-term mortality by 22% overall through prevention of sudden cardiac death and recurrent MI (41). It is the highest-risk population after AMI (i.e., the elderly, those with LV dysfunction, and those with frequent ventricular ectopy) who derive the greatest benefit from treatment with β-blockers (45). Still, several studies show that β-blockers are underused after MI, especially in the elderly (36, 46). Treatment with β-blockers is recommended for all AMI survivors who do not possess clear contraindications to their use. The length of therapy may be individualized to each patient after at least 2 years of treatment (23).

Angiotensin-Converting Enzyme Inhibitors

When given within 24 hours of presentation to all AMI patients without contraindications to their use, angiotensin-converting enzyme (ACE) inhibitors provide a modest survival benefit (about 5 to 10%) (39, 40). The mechanism for this benefit appears to be prevention of deleterious ventricular remodeling and infarct expansion. Accordingly, patients with the largest infarcts derive the greatest benefit (about 20 to 25% mortality reduction) from ACE inhibitor therapy (47). Thus, patients with anterior MI, LV ejection fraction not more than 40%, congestive heart failure, or prior MI should be treated with ACE inhibitors, ideally within the first 24 hours. Therapy in these patients should be continued indefinitely. Patients initially treated with an ACE inhibitor who are found to have an ejection fraction above 40% and no evidence of congestive heart failure may stop taking this medication after 5 to 6 weeks.

The most serious side effect of ACE inhibitors is hypotension, which is especially dangerous early in AMI, as it may cause coronary hypoperfusion and infarct extension. Thus, therapy should be initiated with low doses of an oral agent and should not be started if the systolic blood pressure is less than 100 mm Hg. Other contraindications to ACE inhibitor use include clinically relevant renal failure (serum creatinine above 3 mg/dL, potassium above 5.5 mg/dL), bilateral renal artery stenosis, and known allergy to ACE inhibitors.

Warfarin

Warfarin is an excellent alternative for secondary prevention of recurrent events in patients unable to take aspirin. In patients not receiving antiplatelet therapy, anticoagulation with warfarin leads to about a 10 to 20% reduction in mortality after AMI, compared with placebo (48, 49). Warfarin also reduces recurrent MI and cerebrovascular events by a third to half. These benefits generally outweigh the risk of serious bleeding, which occurs in a minority of patients. The elderly are especially prone to bleeding complications on warfarin, however, and must be monitored closely.

Patients at high risk for arterial thromboembolism after AMI include those with LV thrombus, extensive wall motion abnormalities, or atrial fibrillation. These patients should take warfarin instead of aspirin after discharge (23). Recent data do not support the combined use of fixed low-dose warfarin and aspirin, which demonstrates an increase in bleeding and no improvement in outcomes (50).

Calcium Channel Blockers

Calcium channel blockers, especially nifedipine, are contraindicated in the acute phase of AMI. There may be a limited role for verapamil or diltiazem in patients with preserved LV systolic function and no evidence of congestive heart failure after AMI. However, even in this subgroup, β-blockers are the preferred therapy unless contraindicated. Verapamil and diltiazem have been shown to increase the coronary event rate in patients with heart failure or impaired LV function (51).

Lipid-Lowering Therapy

Recently completed randomized placebo-controlled trials of lipid-lowering drugs in patients after AMI have proved the importance of aggressive lipid management in this population at high risk for recurrent MI and coronary death. The Scandinavian Simvastatin Survival Study (4S) demonstrated a 34% reduction in major coronary events in hyperlipidemic patients treated with simvastatin (52). The Cholesterol and Recurrent Events (CARE) trial found similar results in patients with average cholesterol levels (53). Importantly, a similar statistically significant reduction in coronary events was seen in both trials in patients over age 60, and therefore, lipid-lowering therapy should not be avoided simply because of advanced age. Furthermore, all AMI survivors should be counseled regarding the importance of a low-cholesterol, low-fat diet as well as a supervised exercise program (discussed in next section).

Cardiac Rehabilitation

Cardiac rehabilitation programs provide structured support in a supervised setting during the difficult adjustment period after AMI, when depression, anxiety, and a decrease in functional capacity frequently become manifest. Cardiac rehabilitation programs lead to improved exercise tolerance, enhanced quality of life, and better adherence to risk factor modification. A meta-analysis of randomized trials of cardiac rehabilitation demonstrated a 25% reduction in mortality after AMI in younger patients enrolled in such programs (54). There are limited randomized data available for the elderly population.

Other Measures

The elderly patient is prone to disorientation and ICU psychosis in the hospital setting. Visual cues, such as clocks and calendars, and visits with family members are helpful in this regard. While anxiety is detrimental in this period, caution must be exercised with the use of anxiolytics in the elderly, particularly benzodiazepines, which may paradoxically worsen agitation. If agitation is present, a small dose of a neuroleptic agent, such as haloperidol, may be beneficial.

There is no role for lidocaine as prophylaxis for ventricular arrhythmias. If sustained ventricular tachycardia or ventricular fibrillation is present, however, lidocaine remains the drug of choice for treatment. Lidocaine must be used with caution in the elderly and those with hepatic dysfunction, as it may cause confusion and dysarthria, even at relatively low doses.

Complications

Detailed coverage is not possible in this section, and the reader is referred to the recent guidelines of the ACC/AHA Task Force (23). Recurrent post-MI pain may be due to recurrent ischemia, most often associated with ECG ST-T changes, which requires evaluation for prompt PTCA or CABG surgery. Alternatively, the pain may be due to pericarditis, which responds to nonsteroidal anti-inflammatory drugs such as aspirin 650 mg every 4 to 6 hours or ibuprofen 800 mg every 6 to 8 hours; steroids and indomethacin should be avoided. Congestive heart failure is managed as in other forms of heart failure, using ACE inhibitors, diuretics, digoxin, and nitrates (see section on congestive heart failure). Pulmonary edema is managed with intravenous furosemide, intravenous nitrates or nitroprusside, and if necessary, an inotropic agent such as dopamine, dobutamine, or milrinone. Heart failure or cardiogenic shock due to mechanical complications resulting from MI, such as papillary muscle infarction or rupture causing acute mitral regurgitation, or ventricular septal rupture, is managed initially by diuretics, intravenous nitrates or nitroprusside, and dobutamine followed by surgery. Diagnosis is suggested by a new systolic murmur and confirmed by echocardiogram or pulmonary artery catheterization. Patients in shock are managed additionally with an intra-aortic balloon pump and may benefit from angioplasty. Bradyarrhythmias and heart block in association with inferior infarction respond to atropine and when necessary, a temporary pacemaker; a permanent pacemaker is rarely required. On the other hand, bradyarrhythmias in association with anterior infarction usually require a temporary pacemaker followed by a permanent one (see section on arrhythmias).

CARDIAC ARRHYTHMIAS

Age-related degenerative changes of the sinus node lead to sinus node dysfunction commonly called the sick sinus syndrome (SSS); AV nodal disease often coexists in this syndrome. Similar degenerative changes may occur in the His-Purkinje system right bundle branch, left anterior, and left posterior fascicles of the left bundle branch. These conduction system diseases may lead to various degrees of AV block, bundle-branch blocks, and various cardiac arrhythmias. Ambulatory electrocardiography monitoring (Holter) indicates that bradyarrhythmias and tachyarrhythmias are common in elderly patients, especially those with underlying heart disease (55).

Sick Sinus Syndrome

SSS manifests itself as severe sinus bradycardia (heart rate less than 40 beats per minute), sinus node arrest, or pauses (55). These rhythm disorders may result in dizziness, near syncope, or syncope, i.e., Adam-Stokes attacks (55). Sinus pauses of more than 1.5 seconds are associated with increased mortality (56), while transient AV block is predictive of stroke but not mortality (57). Another manifestation of SSS is the bradycardia-tachycardia syndrome, in which bradycardia is interrupted by paroxysms of atrial tachyarrhythmias, such as atrial fibrillation or atrial tachycardia. When the tachycardia spontaneously terminates, there is a significant delay before the sick sinus node regains its function. During the long pause patients may have neurologic symptoms. In addition, tachycardia may provoke palpitations, angina, dizziness, hypotension, or dyspnea from heart failure. The treatment of SSS consists of implantation of a permanent demand pacemaker. In the case of the bradycardia-tachycardia syndrome, demand pacemaker therapy allows drug therapy to control the tachyarrhythmia without the danger of aggravating bradycardia, since the pacemaker kicks in to maintain the preset heart rate. In patients with AV block and preserved atrial contraction, the commonly used AV sequential or dual-chamber pacemaker allows AV synchrony and preserves the contribution of the atria to cardiac output (58).

Paroxysmal Supraventricular Tachycardia

PSVT is managed in the elderly by carotid sinus massage only if there is no evidence of occlusive carotid artery disease in the form of a carotid bruit, since syncope or stroke may be precipitated. Valsalva maneuver is preferred as initial therapy, and if that fails, intravenous adenosine 6 mg is given rapidly and repeated at double the dose after 5 minutes if there is no response (56). Alternatively, one may use intravenous verapamil 2.5 to 5 mg (57), which may be repeated at double the initial dose after 10 to 15 minutes if arrhythmia persists. Intravenous digoxin is the preferred agent (after adenosine) in patients with systolic heart failure. An initial dose of 0.5 mg in a previously nondigitalized patient is given over 5 to 10 minutes. Other useful intravenous agents include a β-blocker such as esmolol (half-life of 9 minutes) and diltiazem. If PSVT is associated with pulmonary edema, unstable angina, AMI, or severe hypotension, prompt cardioversion with 25 to 50 joules should be carried out if adenosine fails to convert the rhythm. Recurrent episodes may be prevented by chronic oral therapy with a β-blocker or a calcium channel blocker (verapamil or diltiazem) or by radiofrequency catheter ablation (59); chronic antiarrhythmic agents are preferably avoided.

Atrial Flutter

Atrial flutter in an elderly patient is most often due to underlying heart disease (hypertension, coronary artery disease, valvular disease); rarely noncardiac causes lead to atrial flutter, such as. pulmonary embolism. Untreated atrial flutter usually manifests as 2:1 AV conduction with an atrial rate of 300/minute and a ventricular rate of 150/minute. In the elderly this ratio may be 3:1 or greater because of associated AV nodal disease or concomitant therapy with digoxin, β-blocker, or calcium channel blocker. Therapy of atrial flutter is somewhat similar to the treatment of atrial fibrillation except that permanent cure may be achieved in selected cases with radiofrequency catheter ablation. Other therapeutic measures for restoration of sinus rhythm include the administration of intravenous ibutilide, as discussed under atrial fibrillation, or synchronized electrocardioversion using 25 to 50 joules, more if necessary. Alternatively, atrial pacing may be employed to terminate the flutter if these measures are not effective or are contraindicated. When cardioversion is not a consideration for any reason, ventricular rate control is achieved with a β-blocker, a rate-lowering calcium channel blocker, or digoxin, administered intravenously or orally as dictated by circumstances. Recurrent atrial flutter may be prevented by use of antiarrhythmic agents as discussed in atrial fibrillation. The role of chronic oral anticoagulation in atrial flutter is not as clearly established as it is in atrial fibrillation, but it may be appropriate, since some patients with atrial flutter manifest periods of atrial fibrillation.

Multifocal Atrial Tachycardia

Multifocal atrial tachycardia (MAT) most often occurs in the setting of chronic lung disease; heart failure and renal failure are less common causes. Therapy is directed at optimizing treatment of the underlying disease and correction of hypoxemia and electrolyte abnormalities. Drug therapy with verapamil or diltiazem is indicated for MAT with rapid rate. β-Blockers are effective and may be tried cautiously, since most patients have underlying cardiac or pulmonary disease. Intravenous magnesium may restore sinus rhythm or control ventricular rate, especially in the presence of hypomagnesemia (60).

Ventricular Arrhythmias

Chronic ventricular arrhythmias are common; they may be divided into benign, potentially lethal, and lethal categories. Management has recently been reviewed (61). Benign ventricular arrhythmias are encountered in patients without evidence of structural heart disease and are managed by removal of any offending factor such as caffeine, alcohol, cigarette smoking, or anxiety. Patients with troublesome palpitations are reassured, but if that fails, mild sedation or β-blocker therapy may be helpful. Potentially lethal arrhythmias occur in patients with underlying ischemic, valvular, or hypertensive heart diseases or cardiomyopathies. Ventricular arrhythmias in this category range from simple premature ventricular contractions to nonsustained ventricular tachycardia (NSVT). Unlike benign ventricular arrhythmias, potentially lethal ventricular arrhythmias are associated with higher risk of death. However, antiarrhythmic therapy has not been shown to reduce mortality in this group of patients and may be harmful, especially in the presence of ischemia or heart failure as was shown in the Cardiac Arrhythmia Suppression Trial (CAST). In this trial, postinfarction patients with low ejection fraction had an increased risk of death from antiarrhythmic drug-induced ventricular arrhythmias (i.e., proarrhythmia, such as torsades des pointes or sustained ventricular tachycardia). Therapeutic measures being tested in patients with NSVT include empiric therapy with amiodarone, use of an implantable cardioverter-defibrillator (ICD), and electrophysiologic guided antiarrhythmic therapy. Preliminary results of a recent trial favor the use of ICD over antiarrhythmic drug therapy in patients with NSVT with prior myocardial infarction and poor LV dysfunction (62). Malignant or lethal ventricular arrhythmias include sustained ventricular tachycardia; polymorphic ventricular tachycardia associated with long QT syndromes, such as torsades de pointes; ventricular flutter; and ventricular fibrillation. Patients resuscitated from ventricular tachycardia or ventricular fibrillation (VT/VF) not due to drug toxicity, accidental electrocution, cocaine, or other intravenous drug abuse or AMI are managed ideally with ICD. Other options include empiric therapy with amiodarone and the use of sotalol guided by Holter monitoring, as was shown in the electrophysiology study versus electrocardiographic monitoring (ESVEM) study. Any identifiable cause of VT/VF should be corrected. Causes include antiarrhythmic drugs, hypomagnesemia, hypokalemia, antidepressant drugs, and the combination of ketoconazole or erythromycin with terfenadine. Intravenous magnesium is the treatment of choice for acute management of torsades de pointes. Patients resuscitated from VT/VF who are found to have ischemic heart disease should be treated with PTCA or CABG if indicated. Subsequently, they should undergo electrophysiologic studies and be treated with antiarrhythmic drugs and/or implantation of ICD according to the results of these studies.

Patients with ventricular arrhythmias in the setting of AMI or unstable angina are managed with intravenous lidocaine or procainamide if lidocaine fails. The initial maintenance dose of lidocaine should be lower because of the potential for lidocaine toxicity in elderly patients: difficulty hearing, dizziness, seizures, and other neurologic symptoms. For sustained ventricular tachycardia unresponsive to these agents, intravenous amiodarone is the drug of choice (63).

Bradyarrhythmias

Sinus node and conduction system disease, as described earlier, account for most cases of bradyarrhythmias, including AV block of the Mobitz I and II variety or complete heart block. A permanent pacemaker is indicated for symptomatic patients. Patients with bifascicular block, i.e., right bundle-branch block with left anterior hemiblock, right bundle-branch block with left posterior hemiblock, or alternating right and left bundle-branch block, who are *symptomatic* (syncope, near syncope) should undergo evaluation for permanent pacemaker therapy. For acute emergencies an external transcutaneous pacemaker or transvenous pacemaker is used unless neither is easily accessible, in which case intravenous atropine or epinephrine therapy may be tried. Atropine is recommended for acute episodes of vagally mediated symptomatic bradycardia. Any known or suspected cause of symptomatic bradycardia, such as β-blockers, rate-lowering calcium channel blockers, or vagotonia associated with inferior myocardial infarction, should be looked for and managed appropriately. For detailed discussion of indications for permanent pacemaker, see the ACC/AHA Task Force report (64).

ATRIAL FIBRILLATION

Atrial fibrillation is one of the most common arrhythmias encountered in the elderly population. Various epidemiologic studies indicate a prevalence of 1.4 to 10% in the general population and 11 to 17% in the older population (65, 66). Therapy is aimed at control of symptoms and prevention of associated embolic complications. The issue of management, i.e., rate control, rhythm control, and anticoagulation, is being addressed in the ongoing Atrial Fibrillation Follow-up Investigation of Rhythm Management (AFFIRM) study sponsored by the National Heart, Lung, and Blood Institute. At present, selection of therapy is based on the nature and severity of underlying heart disease, patient compliance, and potential benefits and risks of chosen therapy.

Causation

Several conditions, both cardiac and noncardiac, are capable of precipitating atrial fibrillation (2). *Cardiac* conditions include ischemic heart disease, hypertensive heart disease, valvular heart disease, and cardiomyopathies. Rare causes in the elderly patient include atrial septal defect, left atrial myxoma, and so on. The postoperative course of patients undergoing cardiac surgery, including coronary artery bypass surgery, is often complicated by atrial fibrillation. *Noncardiac* causes include hyperthyroidism, chronic obstructive lung disease, pneumonia, and pheochromocytoma, and abnormalities of the autonomic nervous system (67).

Lone atrial fibrillation (68) is a term applied to describe atrial fibrillation occurring in the absence of detectable heart disease or hypertension. It is often precipitated by alcohol use, infection, anxiety, or electrolyte imbalance. While this condition is relatively benign in those below age 65, it increases the risk of stroke in the elderly.

Clinical Features

The clinical presentation of atrial fibrillation, which varies from patient to patient, includes palpitations, dizziness, syncope, anginal discomfort, dyspnea, and fatigue. Occasionally, patients with atrial fibrillation have pulmonary edema or an embolic complication such as stroke. Asymptomatic atrial fibrillation is diagnosed during routine evaluation or evaluation for causes unrelated to it. Persistent uncontrolled atrial fibrillation may lead to the development of *tachycardia-related cardiomyopathy,* which is reversible with rate control or restoration of sinus rhythm (68).

Physical examination reveals irregular jugular venous pulsations, variable S_1, and the absence of S_4, since there is no organized atrial contraction. Other features depend on the presence or absence of coexisting cardiac and noncardiac disorders. Mitral stenosis and hyperthyroidism should be specifically looked for in any patient with atrial fibrillation without a clear cause.

Diagnosis

The clinical diagnosis of atrial fibrillation is confirmed by *ECG.* Typical ECG features include irregular R-R intervals and P waves replaced by small undulations of the baseline, called fibrillatory (f) waves or simply by a nondescript baseline. In untreated atrial fibrillation the ventricular rate may range from 100 to 170 per minute. Faster rates are encountered in patients with hyperthyroidism or a high adrenergic state and in patients with preexcitation syndromes, such as Wolff-Parkinson-White syndrome. Slower ventricular rates are seen in patients receiving treatment with β-blockers, calcium channel blockers, and digitalis preparations and in patients with SSS. Atrial fibrillation with wide QRS complexes is encountered in patients with Wolff-Parkinson-White syndrome if ventricular conduction takes place via the accessory pathway or if there is functional (reversible) or permanent bundle-branch block. *Echocardiography* is an essential part of the evaluation of a patient with atrial fibrillation (68). It provides information relating to valves, heart function, and heart size, especially left atrial size, which can be useful in the selection of an appropriate course of therapy. *Transesophageal echocardiogram* offers an additional advantage in that the left atrial appendage, a common site for thrombus formation in patients with atrial fibrillation, can be visualized

(69, 70). *Thyroid function tests* should be done in patients without an obvious cause for atrial fibrillation. *Ambulatory electrocardiography* is helpful in monitoring the effects of rate-controlling measures and rhythm-controlling drugs and for the detection of drug-induced proarrhythmia. *An exercise stress test* may be performed for detection of underlying ischemic heart disease in patients with coronary risk factors. Performing *cardiac nuclear imaging studies, cardiac catheterization,* or *coronary angiographic studies* is indicated in selected cases according to clinical judgment and coronary risk factors.

Management
General

Patients should be encouraged to adopt a healthful lifestyle, refrain from smoking, and avoid or significantly curtail consumption of caffeinated drinks and alcohol. Congestive heart failure, ischemic heart disease, hypertension, and hyperthyroidism should be adequately treated, as should surgically correctable conditions such as mitral stenosis, aortic stenosis, and atrial septal defect, if appropriate.

Specific Therapy

Therapy of atrial fibrillation is aimed at controlling symptoms, improving cardiac hemodynamics, and reducing the risk of embolism, especially stroke (65, 68, 71, 72). This is achieved by using drugs to control heart rate or restore and maintain sinus rhythm (Table 7.4). Electrical cardioversion is used for elective or urgent restoration of sinus rhythm. Anticoagulation is used to reduce the risk of embolic stroke.

It is estimated that 50% of patients with a recent (less than 2 or 3 days) onset of atrial fibrillation convert spontaneously. Cardioversion therefore may be delayed for the first 24 hours, especially for lone atrial fibrillation, unless the patient is hemodynamically unstable. Patients with recent onset of atrial fibrillation, except those with lone atrial fibrillation who are under age 65, should receive intravenous heparin. At the same time, oral warfarin is initiated in anticipation of cardioversion or, if the patient is ineligible for cardioversion, for chronic prophylaxis against thromboembolic stroke.

Table 7.4

Atrial Fibrillation: Drugs Used for Controlling Ventricular Rate

Drug	Loading Dose	Maintenance Dose	Side Effects
Esmolol	500 μg/kg IV over 1 min	50 μg/kg IV for 4 min; maintenance dose 25–50 μg/kg/min q 5–10 min titrated to desired heart rate	Bronchospasm, CHF, AV block, hypotension
Metoprolol	5 mg IV q 5 min to total 15 mg	25–100 mg po bid	As above; also cool extremities, lethargy, depression, impotence
Atenolol	5 mg IV q 5 min to total 10 mg	50–100 mg po qd	Same as metoprolol
Diltiazem	1.25 mg/kg IV over 2 min; repeat if needed after 15 min as 0.35 mg/kg over 2 min	5–15 mg/hr IV or 90–360 mg po qd[a]	Hypotension, bradycardia, AV block, CHF, increased digoxin level
Verapamil	2.5–10 mg IV over 2 min	0.0005 mg/kg/min or 5–10 mg bolus q 30 min or 120–480 mg po qd[a]	Same as diltiazem; also constipation more frequent than diltiazem
Digoxin	0.25–0.5 mg IV; then 0.25 mg IV q 4 hr up to 1 mg in first 24 hr	0.125–0.375 mg po qd or 0.125–0.25 mg IV qd	Nausea, anorexia, ventricular arrhythmias, AV block; visual halos with chronic therapy

Adapted from Khan AH. Atrial fibrillation In: Khan AH, ed. Practical Cardiology: A Textbook for Primary Care Physicians. London: Edward Arnold Publishers (in press).

AV, atrioventricular; IV, intravenous; CHF, congestive heart failure.

[a]Sustained release preparation.

Restoration of Sinus Rhythm

It is generally accepted that cardioversion should be tried at least once in all patients with atrial fibrillation of less than 12 months' duration. The American College of Chest Physicians recommends that patients be anticoagulated with oral warfarin for 3 to 4 weeks (international normalized ratio [INR] of 2 to 3) prior to elective cardioversion (65, 68, 72). Restoration of sinus rhythm may be attempted with direct current (DC) electrical cardioversion. Alternatively, pharmacologic cardioversion using intravenous procainamide or intravenous ibutilide (a class III agent) may be attempted immediately prior to DC cardioversion (73–74). If pharmacologic cardioversion fails, DC cardioversion is carried out. After cardioversion, patients continue to receive oral anticoagulation for an additional 3 to 4

weeks, since atrial (mechanical) contraction may not resume for 2 to 4 weeks. This atrial stunning or paralysis may continue to predispose patients to thromboembolic risk; hence the need to maintain anticoagulation after cardioversion. A transesophageal echocardiogram performed immediately prior to cardioversion may avoid the need for the 3 to 4 weeks of precardioversion anticoagulation (69–70) if no clot or spontaneous echo contrast is detected. However, patients should receive intravenous heparin to obtain therapeutic aPTT prior to cardioversion. Warfarin is begun at the same time as heparin, and the latter is discontinued following cardioversion, when the INR is in the therapeutic range, i.e., 2 to 3. Oral anticoagulation is maintained for 3 to 4 weeks after cardioversion, as noted earlier. Transesophageal echocardiogram-guided cardioversion is being evaluated in trials. For the present, it is reserved for patients who are already in the hospital and in whom prolonged anticoagulation is considered risky.

Intravenous Agents Used for Restoration of Sinus Rhythm

Drugs used for restoration of sinus rhythm include procainamide, ibutilide, and amiodarone (73, 75). *Intravenous procainamide* is administered as a loading dose of 1g (or less if conversion is achieved) at less than 50 mg/minute, usually 20 to 30 mg/minute, while monitoring the ECG and blood pressure. The rate of administration is reduced if the QRS duration lengthens or if there is a significant drop in blood pressure. The intravenous class III agent *ibutilide,* which is preferred over procainamide, is administered as a 1-mg bolus over 10 minutes; if sinus rhythm has not been restored, another bolus is administered after 20 minutes (30 minutes from initial bolus). Proarrhythmia, i.e., drug-induced VT/VF, is a small but potentially serious complication of ibutilide as well as of intravenous procainamide. Patients should therefore be closely monitored for 4 to 6 hours after completion of intravenous antiarrhythmic therapy prior to discharge from the hospital. Patients with significant structural heart disease in whom maintenance therapy with oral antiarrhythmic drugs is contemplated should be hospitalized in a monitored unit for further observation for 2 to 3 days for proarrhythmic complications.

Cardioversion With Oral Antiarrhythmic Agents

Cardioversion with oral antiarrhythmic agents has the disadvantage of requiring hospitalization for cardiac monitoring of patients because of concern for proarrhythmia. Table 7.5 lists the drugs, dosages, and potential side effects of oral agents used for cardioversion. After cardioversion, these agents may be used to maintain sinus rhythm (68, 72) in patients at high risk for recurrence, such as those with frequent paroxysmal atrial fibrillation, and in those whose episodes of atrial fibrillation are accompanied by severe symptoms, such as syncope, angina, or pulmonary edema. Prior observations suggest that chronic antiarrhythmic therapy of patients with atrial fibrillation is associated with a higher death rate. Also,

the data from the Stroke Prevention in Atrial Fibrillation (SPAF) study suggest an increase in mortality in patients with heart failure receiving antiarrhythmic therapy (74). These agents, therefore, should be used only under circumstances mentioned earlier. Chronic oral amiodarone therapy is effective in maintaining sinus rhythm and is probably less proarrhythmic than other agents; it is a relatively safe agent in patients with heart failure or ischemic heart disease (75–76). However, noncardiac side effects should be monitored closely. Amiodarone and sotalol have yet to receive FDA approval for use in supraventricular tachyarrhythmias. Reference should be made to excellent reviews by Campbell (76) and Waldo (77).

Drugs for Controlling Ventricular Rate in Atrial Fibrillation

β-Adrenergic Receptor Blockers

Esmolol, a rapidly acting *intravenous* β-blocker with a half-life of 9 minutes, can be used when prompt control of ventricular rate is necessary. Other intravenous β-blocker preparations (metoprolol, propranolol, and atenolol) may be used as alternatives. For stable patients, *oral* β-blockers are effective in controlling heart rate, especially in situations associated with high adrenergic activity, such as exercise, emotional stress, and hyperthyroidism. Preoperative administration of β-blockers prior to cardiac surgery has been noted to decrease the incidence of atrial fibrillation in the postoperative phase.

Calcium Channel Blockers

Intravenous diltiazem is highly effective for prompt rate control; it is also safer than β-blockers in patients with bronchospasm (78). Intravenous verapamil may be used as an alternative to diltiazem. *Oral* diltiazem or verapamil is effective for chronic ventricular rate control in patients with atrial fibrillation (65, 68). These drugs are contraindicated in patients with atrial fibrillation and preexcitation syndromes.

Digoxin

Intravenous digoxin is the drug of choice for immediate rate control in patients with LV systolic dysfunction even though its onset of action

Table 7.5

Pharmacologic Cardioversion for Atrial Fibrillation

Drug	Oral Dose	Side Effects[a]	Avoid in
Class IA			
Quinidine gluconate	324–648 mg q 8–12 hr	Diarrhea, thrombocytopenia, cinchonism	CHF, long QT syndrome Liver failure Renal failure, lupuslike syndrome
Procainamide	0.5–1.5g q 6 hr	Nausea, lupuslike syndrome	CHF, long QT syndrome
Disopyramide	200–400 mg q 12 hr	Urinary retention, dry mouth, blurred vision	Older men at risk for urinary retention Glaucoma Renal failure
Class IC			
Flecainide	75–150 mg q 12 hr	Blurred vision	LV dysfunction, CAD
Propafenone	150–300 mg q 8 hr		LV dysfunction
Class III			
Sotalol	80–240 mg q 12 h	Bronchospasm, CHF, heart block, hypotension	CHF, bronchospasm Hypokalemia
Amiodarone	400–800 mg qd for 2–3 weeks then 200 mg qd	Thyroid, liver function abnormalities; photosensitivity, skin discoloration, pulmonary fibrosis Failure of other drugs CHF Renal failure	Pulmonary and liver disease

Adapted from Khan AH. Atrial fibrillation. In: Khan AH, ed. Practical Cardiology: A Textbook for Primary Care Physicians. London: Edward Arnold Publishers (in press).

LV, left ventricular; CHF, congestive heart failure; CAD, coronary artery disease; SVT, supraventricular tachycardia.

[a]Proarrhythmia is a potential complication of all of these agents.

is slower than β-blockers and calcium channel blockers. *Oral* digoxin is used for chronic rate control in patients with LV systolic dysfunction. In patients with atrial fibrillation and normal LV function, digoxin is less effective and is generally used only after (or in addition to) a β-blocker or a calcium channel blocker.

Combination Therapy

The intravenous administration of a combination of a β-blocker and a calcium channel blocker should be avoided or undertaken with great caution because of the danger of precipitating AV block or sinus node arrest, especially in patients with sick sinus syndrome. Moreover, the combination can lead to severe hypotension or heart failure in some patients. However, the cautious use of an *oral* combination of a β-blocker and a calcium channel blocker is fairly well tolerated. Digoxin added to a calcium channel blocker or to a β-blocker has also an additive effect in controlling ventricular rate and is less costly.

CONGESTIVE HEART FAILURE

Congestive heart failure is the most common diagnosis for patients above age 65 who are admitted to the hospital and is a frequent cause of rehospitalization, poor quality of life, and disability. The common causes of congestive heart failure in the elderly include coronary artery disease, hypertensive heart disease, valvular heart disease, cardiomyopathies, and rarely, adult congenital heart disease, such as atrial septal defect. It is important to separate systolic from diastolic heart failure for the purpose of management (79–81). Diastolic heart failure as a result of LV hypertrophy and myocardial infiltration with collagen and amyloid is common in the elderly. It should be suspected in patients with LV hypertrophy secondary to hypertensive heart disease, aortic stenosis, and hypertrophic cardiomyopathy. Ischemia impairs myocardial compliance and in combination with coronary artery disease may lead to transient or chronic diastolic heart failure. Patients with diastolic heart failure have a normal-sized heart on chest radiograph, accompanied by LV hypertrophy on the ECG. Patients with systolic heart failure have an enlarged heart. Common causes of systolic heart failure include MI, chronic coronary artery disease, dilated cardiomyopathies, and volume overload conditions such as aortic or mitral regurgitation. Echocardiogram is useful in separating diastolic from systolic heart failure (82). Main echocardiographic parameters that support diastolic heart failure include normal ejection fraction and reversal of the E-wave–to–A-wave ratio on mitral Doppler study. Echocardiographic findings in systolic heart failure include dilated cardiac chambers and a decrease in ejection fraction of up to 50%. Mitral regurgitation secondary to papillary muscle dysfunction and minimal LV hypertrophy are often found in the hearts of patients with systolic heart failure.

Clinical Features

Elderly patients may have dyspnea or undue fatigue with exertion. There may be elevation of jugular venous pressure, rales, third heart sound (S_3) and murmurs of mitral regurgitation or aortic stenosis. S_4 is a common finding in the elderly population but may be accentuated in diastolic heart failure. There may be hepatomegaly and peripheral pitting edema as well. Atypical presentations, which are fairly common, include dry hacking cough, change in mental status, and inability to sleep. Physical findings may be difficult to interpret because of chronic rales or edema from venostasis.

Diagnosis

Elderly patients with congestive heart failure should be evaluated with routine laboratory studies, ECG, chest radiograph, and echocardiogram. In a patient with heart failure of unclear causation or accompanied by atrial fibrillation, thyroid function tests should be obtained, as hyperthyroidism is a fairly common cause of heart failure and often presents in an atypical manner in the elderly patient (apathetic hyperthyroidism). Hypothyroidism is a rare cause of heart failure. Exercise tests, radionuclide imaging, and coronary angiography are obtained according to clinical presentation and guided by the results of previous studies.

Therapy

General measures include dietary control of sodium (up to 4 g per day). Correctable causes and conditions should be managed medically or if indicated, surgically (82). Some of these conditions include hypertension, anemia, thyroid function abnormalities, ischemic heart disease, valvular heart disease, and any infections, such as pneumonia. In patients with atrial fibrillation, either ventricular rate control or cardioversion should be considered if appropriate. Patients should be advised to avoid excessive fluid intake. In summer, fluid intake may be increased, but a better alternative is air conditioning, since hot and humid environments often worsen heart failure. Since alcohol is a myocardial depressant, alcoholic beverages should be discouraged or restricted to one or two drinks per day. Physical conditioning exercises, such as regular walking and working around the house, should be encouraged depending on the patient's tolerance. Some patients benefit from enrollment in a cardiac rehabilitation program. A nurse-directed multidisciplinary approach should be considered, as they have been shown to reduce hospitalization and improve the quality of life of elderly heart failure patients (83).

Medical therapy (Table 7.6) consists of diuretics for those who have evidence of peripheral

Table 7.6

Medications Commonly Used for Heart Failure

Drug	Initial Dose (mg)	Target Dose (mg)	Recommended Maximal Dose (mg)	Major Adverse Reactions
Thiazide diuretics				
Hydrochlorothiazide	25 qd	As needed	50 qd	Postural hypotension, hypokalemia, hyperglycemia, hyperuricemia, rash. Rash severe reaction includes pancreatitis, bone marrow suppression, and anaphylaxis.
Chlorthalidone	25 qd	As needed	50 qd	
Loop diuretics				
Furosemide	20–40 qd	As needed	240 bid	Same as thiazide diuretics.
Bumetanide	0.5–1 qd	As needed	10 qd	
Ethacrynic acid	50 qd	As needed	200 bid	
Thiazide-related diuretic				
Metolazone	2.5[a]	As needed	10 qd	Same as thiazide diuretics.
Potassium-sparing diuretics				
Spironolactone	25 qd	As needed	100 bid	Hyperkalemia, especially if administered with ACE inhibitor; rash; gynecomastia (spironolactone only).
Triamterene	50 qd	As needed	100 bid	
Amiloride	5 qd	As needed	40 qd	
ACE inhibitors				
Enalapril	2.5 bid	10 bid	20 bid	Hypotension, hyperkalemia, renal insufficiency, cough, skin rash, angioedema, neutropenia.
Captopril	6.25–12.5 tid	50 tid	100 tid	
Lisinopril	5 qd	20 qd	40 qd	
Quinapril	5 bid	20 bid	20 bid	
Digoxin	0.125 qd	As needed	As needed	Cardiotoxicity, confusion, nausea, anorexia, visual disturbances.
Hydralazine	10–25 tid	75 tid	100 tid	Headache, nausea, dizziness, tachycardiac, lupuslike syndrome.
Isosorbide dinitrate	10 tid	40 tid	80 tid	Headache, hypotension, flushing.

Reprinted from Konstam M, Dracup R, Baker D, et al. Heart Failure: Management of Patients With Left-Ventricular Systolic Dysfunction. Quick Reference Guide for Clinicians 11 (AHCPR 94-0613). Rockville, MD: US Department of Health and Human Services, Public Health Service, Agency for Health Care Policy and Research, 1994.

[a]Given as a single test dose initially.

edema or pulmonary congestion and an ACE inhibitor for those with low ejection fraction (79, 81). Digoxin is prescribed for those who remain symptomatic despite diuretics and an ACE inhibitor. For patients with mild to moderate heart failure a thiazide diuretic may suffice, but those with advanced heart failure or impaired renal function require a loop diuretic such as furosemide (79, 81). For patients who are refractory to large doses of furosemide, metolazone 1.5 to 5 mg followed by furosemide 40 to 60 mg an hour later often produces effective diuresis. Such therapy should be given intermittently, and the appropriate dose regimen should be established for each patient, since this combination sometimes leads to hypovolemia from severe diuresis. Patients in pulmonary edema or severe heart failure should be treated with intravenous furosemide, an intravenous inotrope (dobutamine, dopamine, or milrinone) and if tolerated, intravenous nitrates in a hospital setting. Once the patient's dry weight has been achieved, diuretic dose may be adjusted to a maintenance therapy, with diuretic holidays if possible to decrease interference with social activities. Serum sodium, potassium, uric acid, and magnesium should be monitored and corrected. Potassium supplementation may be necessary, but the use of potassium and potassium-sparing diuretics should be avoided or carefully monitored in patients receiving ACE inhibitors, which tend to conserve potassium, since additional potassium may lead to hyperkalemia with dangerous consequences. Similarly, patients with pure diastolic heart failure should be prescribed diuretics carefully (80), since aggressive diuresis in this setting may lead to hypotension and neurologic symptoms of dizziness or even syncope.

Angiotensin-Converting Enzyme Inhibitors

The standard of care today for the patients with low ejection fraction is an ACE inhibitor (see section on cardiomyopathies). Patients with ejection fraction less than 40%, whether or not symptomatic, should be treated with an ACE inhibitor (79, 81). For symptomatic patients, an ACE inhibitor improves symptoms and quality of life and prolongs survival (84). For asymptomatic patients ACE inhibitors have been shown to delay the on-

set of heart failure and decrease hospitalization for heart failure (85). Therapy should begin with a small dose that is increased every 4 to 5 days while the serum potassium and creatinine are monitored and the patient is observed for hypotension and cough. The cutoff for decreasing the dose or stopping the drug includes systolic blood pressure of 85 to 90 mm Hg or higher if symptomatic, serum creatinine rising above 2.5 mg/dL, or serum potassium rising above 5 mg/dL. For these patients alternative therapy includes the combination of isosorbide dinitrate and hydralazine (86). The initial dose of oral isosorbide dinitrate, 10 mg 3 times a day, may be gradually increased to the maximum tolerated dose, i.e., up to 40 mg 3 times a day. Hydralazine is prescribed beginning with 10 mg 3 times a day and gradually increased, if tolerated, up to 100 mg 3 times a day. Losartan is another suitable alternative (87). Side effects, precautions, and indications for losartan are similar to those for ACE inhibitors, except that losartan is less likely to cause cough. Losartan also possesses mild uricosuric action, which may benefit patients with heart failure and mild hyperuricemia who are receiving diuretics. Losartan may be initiated at 25 mg twice a day and increased to 50 mg twice a day if tolerated. The same parameters for monitoring ACE inhibitor therapy apply to angiotensin-II receptor antagonists with the exception of cough (losartan is approved by the Food and Drug Administration (FDA) for use in hypertension and is awaiting approval for congestive heart failure).

Digoxin

The recently completed Digitalis Investigation Group study of 6800 patients showed that chronic oral digitalis therapy in patients with congestive heart failure improved symptoms and decreased hospitalization for those with congestive heart failure but did not improve survival (88). Thus digoxin in patients with congestive heart failure should be restricted to those who remain symptomatic despite diuretics and vasodilator therapy and for those with New York Heart Association (NYHA) class IV heart failure. In addition, digoxin is administered to patients with atrial fibrillation, since it can control ventricular rate and not impair LV systolic function, as do β-blockers and calcium channel blockers (verapamil and diltiazem). Many older patients have decreased renal creatinine clearance and low muscle mass and are therefore prone to digitalis toxicity. Digitalis therapy therefore requires close monitoring of these patients. The physician should also be aware of drug interactions of digoxin with other drugs, such as quinidine and calcium channel blocking agents, which tend to raise digoxin levels. Hypokalemia, hypomagnesemia, hypothyroidism, and hypoxic lung disease all increase the risk of digitalis toxicity, and therefore these conditions should be appropriately managed (79).

Recently carvedilol, a nonselective β-blocker with mild vasodilatory and antioxidant properties, was noted to reduce long-term mortality by 65% in patients with congestive heart failure who had low ejection fraction and who were taking diuretics, ACE inhibitors, and digoxin (89). Carvedilol is started only when congestive heart failure has been relatively stabilized; it is not prescribed during decompensated congestive heart failure. (It is the only β-blocker approved by the FDA for use in congestive heart failure.) Starting dose is 3.125 mg twice a day, gradually increased to 25 mg twice a day over weeks. Patients should be closely followed for side effects, including possible worsening of heart failure.

Calcium channel blockers in patients with systolic heart failure have been noted to worsen heart failure and increase mortality, and they should be avoided. The newer agents amlodipine and felodipine are used when indicated (for ischemia or hypertension), as they are somewhat better tolerated than the older agents. In general calcium channel blockers are avoided in patients with systolic heart failure (81). For patients who remain refractory to these measures, intermittent inotropic therapy with dobutamine or milrinone given as an infusion in the hospital or in the outpatient heart failure clinic has been shown to improve symptoms but not survival.

VALVULAR HEART DISEASE
Epidemiology

Calcification and fibrosis of the valves are common in the elderly, mostly involving the aortic and mitral valves (90, 91). Aortic sclerosis is a relatively benign condition. It causes an ejection systolic murmur that often cannot be differentiated from the systolic murmur of aortic stenosis. Mitral valves undergo myxomatous changes leading to mitral valve prolapse. Mitral annular calcification, which may cause mitral regurgitation, is most common in the elderly woman.

Causation

The most common causes of valvular disease in the elderly are listed in Table 7.7. Rheumatic disease, which usually involves the aortic and mitral valve, is an unusual cause of isolated aortic stenosis. Aortic regurgitation can be classified as either acute or chronic. Chronic aortic regurgitation may be due to valvular disease or aortic root diseases. Aortic root dilation leading to aortic regurgitation may be secondary to long-

Table 7.7

Common Causes of Valvular Disease in the Elderly

Aortic stenosis
  Calcific
  Rheumatic
  Congenital
Aortic regurgitation
  Acute
    Aortic dissection
    Infective endocarditis
    Trauma
  Chronic
    Calcific
    Myxomatous
    Infective endocarditis
    Hypertension
    Syphilis
    Collagen-vascular diseases
Mitral regurgitation
  Acute
    Myocardial infarction
    Trauma
    Infective endocarditis
  Chronic
    Coronary artery disease
    Myxomatous degeneration
    Rheumatic heart disease
    Dilated cardiomyopathy
    Mitral annular calcification
    Mitral valve prolapse

standing hypertension, syphilis, aortic dissection, or collagen-vascular diseases. Acute mitral regurgitation is seen typically 3 to 5 days after an AMI or following trauma or infective endocarditis. Papillary muscle dysfunction or regional wall motion abnormality seen in coronary artery disease and mitral annular dilation in dilated cardiomyopathy can result in mitral regurgitation. Mitral annular calcification, which commonly involves the posterior annulus and subsequently the anterior annulus but rarely the mitral valve leaflets, is a common echocardiographic finding in elderly patients. Mitral annular calcification can cause mitral stenosis by mechanical impingement, mitral regurgitation by loss of annular elasticity, and conduction disturbances by myocardial infiltration and may be associated with the complications of atrial fibrillation, infective endocarditis, and thromboembolic phenomena (92).

Clinical Features

Echocardiography provides crucial information about the nature and severity of the valvular lesions, size of the left ventricle, and wall thickness and function. It also helps differentiate benign aortic ejection murmurs due to aortic sclerosis from valvular aortic stenosis. The carotid upstroke may be brisk even in severe aortic stenosis, and the pulse pressure may be normal because of loss of vascular elasticity in the elderly. The aortic ejection click frequently heard in younger patients with aortic stenosis is rarely heard in the elderly. The salient clinical features of the commonly encountered valvular lesions are outlined in Table 7.8.

Management

Management of valvular heart disease in the elderly depends on the type and severity of the valvular lesion, as outlined in Table 7.8. Echocardiography, including transesophageal echocardiography, is invaluable in characterizing the severity of the valvular lesion and is often an adequate diagnostic test for preoperative assessment. Cardiac catheterization usually is used to confirm the diagnosis, especially when echocardiography is poor in quality or confusing. Coronary angiography, which is essential in

elderly patients to detect concomitant coronary artery disease, identifies the need for CABG with valvular surgery. Common principles in management include prophylaxis of infective endocarditis, treatment of congestive heart failure with diuretics and digitalis, afterload reduction in aortic and mitral regurgitation, and surgery in aortic and mitral stenosis. Serial echocardiographic studies to monitor progression of severity and effect on LV function are important.

Surgery

Elderly patients undergoing valvular surgery have a higher mortality than younger patients, especially in the presence of certain risk factors, such as LV dysfunction and concomitant coronary artery disease (93). Aortic valve replacement in the symptomatic patient with severe aortic stenosis, however, even with an operative mortality of 5 to 11%, provides better quality of life and prolongs life expectancy compared with medical therapy (94, 95). Bioprosthetic valves are preferred in elderly patients because of increased durability and because the need for prolonged anticoagulation with its inherent risks is obviated. Morbidity and mortality are higher in mitral valve replacement than with aortic valve replacement. Operative mortality for mitral valve replacement ranges from 14 to 35%, with predictors of increased mortality being female gender, urgent surgery, impaired LV function, and coronary artery disease (96). In the elderly, mitral valve repair may be associated with a lower mortality than mitral valve replacement (97), although some studies have shown no difference in mortality (98). One study involving 50 consecutive patients 70 years and older revealed a mortality rate of 6%, with no patients requiring reoperation for mitral regurgitation (99). In North America in elderly patients with mitral stenosis, open mitral commissurotomy is more commonly performed than closed mitral commissurotomy. Many elderly patients require mitral valve replacement instead of mitral valve repair because they have calcific mitral disease, rigid leaflets, or thickening of the subvalvular apparatus (100). Cardiac rehabilitation is a critical component of postoperative care, and all patients should be encouraged to participate, especially in an outpa-

continued

Table 7.8

Summary of Clinical Features and Management

Valvular Lesion	Symptoms	Signs	Diagnosis	Management
Aortic stenosis	Dyspnea, chest pain, syncope	Delayed carotid upstroke, narrow pulse pressure, fixed or paradoxic S_2, harsh crescendo-decrescendo systolic murmur at 2nd right intercostal space radiating to neck	Echo: < 2 cm separation of aortic cusps and echodensities indicating calcification on M-mode echo; increased Doppler peak aortic velocities, mean pressure gradients, 2D images of thickened and immobile aortic cusps; cardiac catheterization: increased gradient across aortic valve, coronary artery disease	Mild: annual echocardiograms; moderate to severe: asymptomatic, echo follow-up; symptomatic or LV dysfunction: aortic valve replacement or aortic valvuloplasty
Aortic regurgitation	Dyspnea, fatigue	Wide pulse pressure, blowing diastolic murmur at left sternal border, Austin Flint murmur	Echo: M-mode reveals premature closure of mitral valve or diastolic opening of aortic valve; color flow imaging of width of AR jet relative to LVOT area in short axis indicates severity; shortened pressure half time by continuous-wave Doppler indicates severity; LV diastolic pressures elevated due to AR jet cardiac catheterization; aortography reveals severity of AR	Asymptomatic, mild to moderate: annual echo; severe: medical therapy with nifedipine or ACE inhibitors (11, 12) or aortic valve replacement,[a] especially with LV dysfunction; symptomatic: aortic valve replacement[a]
Mitral stenosis	Dyspnea, paroxysmal nocturnal dyspnea, orthopnea, hemoptysis dysphagia, hoarseness	Rumbling diastolic murmur at apex, opening snap, irregular rhythm (atrial fibrillation)	Echo: M-mode reveals thickened leaflets; 2D echo may show doming and diminished excursion of leaflets in diastole; valve area can be measured by direct planimetry or indirectly from mitral Doppler flow measurements Cardiac catheterization: pressure	Asymptomatic: no specific therapy; mild symptoms: diuretics, control atrial arrhythmias; moderate to severe symptoms or pulmonary hypertension: balloon

Table 7.8 (continued)

Summary of Clinical Features and Management

Valvular Lesion	Symptoms	Signs	Diagnosis	Management
			gradient between pulmonary capillary wedge pressures (LA pressure) and LV end diastolic pressures assesses degree of pulmonary hypertension	valvuloplasty or valvular surgery
Mitral regurgitation	Weakness, fatigue	Apical pansystolic murmur radiating to axilla	Echo: M-mode and 2D identify cause and estimate LV chamber dimensions and function. Color flow imaging reveals regurgitant jet into LA cardiac catheterization: left ventriculography can reveal severity of MR by opacification of LA due to regurgitant jet	Mild to moderate: annual echo; severe: symptomatic mitral valve repair vs. replacement before onset of LV dysfunction; if surgery contraindicated or as bridge to surgery, can reduce afterload with ACE inhibitor (13); asymptomatic: medical therapy if LV function not depressed and LV not dilated

AR, aortic regurgitation; 2D, two dimensional; echo, echocardiogram; LA, left atrial; LV, left ventricular; LVEDD, left ventricular end-diastolic dimension; LVEF, left ventricular ejection fraction; LVOT, left ventricular outflow tract; MR, mitral regurgitation.

[a]Predictors of success include LVEF > 55% and LVEDD < 1.5 cm.

tient program that offers exercise training, which facilitates functional recovery (101).

Valvuloplasty

The percutaneous approach to relieve stenosis in the mitral and aortic valves has been well described (102). The limitations to aortic valvuloplasty are the 50% restenosis rate at 6 months; a 3% operative mortality; 14% 30-day mortality; and an overall complication rate of 23%, including major complications such as cardiac perforation, severe aortic regurgitation, embolic phenomena, arrhythmias, myocardial infarction, and even death (103). Despite these limitations, selected patients who are poor candidates for surgery may benefit from this procedure for symptom relief, although survival is probably not improved. Preserved LV function is a strong predictor of event-free survival (104). Balloon *mitral valvuloplasty* for critical mitral stenosis has been used in the elderly with a success rate ranging from 46% to 68% (105). This rate is lower than that in younger patients because of the higher incidence of calcification of the valves and subvalvular apparatus in the elderly. It carries an overall operative mortality of 0.5 to 1% and major complications, including cardiac perforation (2%), severe mitral regurgitation (1.4%), cerebrovascular events, and perforation of interatrial septum (103). Higher operative mortality and complications have been reported in patients who are older than 70 years, those with severe LV dysfunction and severe pulmonary hypertension, and those requiring valvular or coronary surgery (105). Patients with calcified mitral valve apparatus have less symptomatic relief, more cardiac events, and a higher incidence of restenosis than do patients who have noncalcified valves (106). In summary, percutaneous mitral valvuloplasty is an attractive alternative to mitral valve replacement because it obviates general anesthesia and sternotomy and probably has a lower operative mortality rate, but the calcific valvular disease process in the elderly lowers the likelihood of a successful outcome.

CARDIOMYOPATHIES

According to the World Health Organization (WHO) and International Society and Federation of Cardiology, cardiomyopathies are classified as dilated, hypertrophic, or restrictive according to clinical presentation, pathophysiologic alterations, and morphologic findings (107).

Dilated Cardiomyopathy

Dilated cardiomyopathy is characterized by enlarged cardiac chambers with decrease in systolic function, i.e., low ejection fraction. It may be idiopathic or may follow viral myocarditis, commonly due to Coxsackie or echo viruses (108). Myocardial damage from chronic alcohol abuse or anthracycline myocardial toxicity accounts for some cases. In addition, features resembling idiopathic dilated cardiomyopathy may be seen in patients with coronary artery disease (ischemic cardiomyopathy), valvular heart disease (valvular cardiomyopathies), hypertensive heart disease (hypertensive cardiomyopathy), neuromuscular disorders, renal insufficiency, or endocrinopathies. Most persons with dilated cardiomyopathy seek medical attention for symptoms of congestive heart failure, but in others symptomatic arrhythmias such as atrial fibrillation or ventricular arrhythmias are presenting features. Physical examination may reveal evidence of biventricular failure, including elevated jugular venous pressure, pulmonary congestion, a third heart sound, hepatomegaly, and peripheral edema. In others these features may not be fully developed, so the diagnosis is established by echocardiographic examination. Mitral regurgitation and tricuspid regurgitation due to papillary muscle dysfunction or to tricuspid and mitral annular dilation are common. An ECG may reveal atrial fibrillation, left bundle-branch block, or sinus tachycardia. Chest radiograph may reveal cardiomegaly and pulmonary congestion. Cardiac catheterization should be considered for patients with risk factors for coronary disease. Similarly, myocardial biopsy is helpful in selected cases only, such as patients receiving anthracycline therapy or to detect early changes of rejection in those who have had cardiac transplantation.

The standard of care of patients with symptomatic or asymptomatic LV dysfunction (with an ejection fraction less than 40%) consists of an ACE inhibitor; other drugs, such as diuretics, nitrates, hydralazine, and digoxin, are used as needed (109). The use of these agents in patients with heart failure has been reviewed recently (110) and is discussed here in the section on congestive heart failure. ACE inhibitors given to patients with systolic failure have been shown to improve symptoms, prolong survival, reduce hospitalizations, and improve quality of life. As a general rule, therapy is started in low dosages, such as captopril 1.75 to 11.5 mg twice a day or enalapril 1.5 mg twice a day, and the dose is gradually titrated up over several days to weeks (see the section on congestive heart failure, Table 7.6). Patients who are intolerant of ACE inhibitor therapy because of cough or those whose therapy is limited by renal dysfunction or hyperkalemia may use a combination of nitrates and hydralazine. This form of therapy has been shown to improve symptoms and survival, although it may not be tolerated because of side effects, including palpitations, dizziness, or gastrointestinal symptoms. An alternative approach entails use of an angiotensin-II receptor antagonist, such as losartan (111). Diuretics are used for pulmonary congestion or peripheral edema. Digoxin is added in refractory and advanced cases (e.g., NYHA classes III and V) and in patients with atrial fibrillation to control ventricular rate. The β-blocker carvedilol, when added to an ACE inhibitor and diuretics, further improves symptoms and survival (109) of patients in NYHA classes II and III. Patients with atrial fibrillation are prescribed oral warfarin to maintain an INR of 2 to 3 to prevent thromboembolic complications.

Since cardiac transplantation is not an option for the elderly patient, refractory cases are treated by other therapeutic measures, such as intermittent intravenous dobutamine or milrinone once or twice a month for control of symptoms. However, this form of therapy has not been shown to prolong survival. Cardiomyoplasty, AV sequential pacing, and cardiac volume reduction surgery are all in the investigational stages and may be offered to patients on an individual basis. Sustained symptomatic ventricular tachycardia or patients resuscitated from cardiac arrest due to ventricular tachycardia may be evaluated and considered for chronic amio-

darone, sotalol, or implantation of a cardioverter defibrillator.

Hypertrophic Cardiomyopathy

Hypertrophic cardiomyopathy (HCM) can be an inherited form or sporadic form with diverse clinical features (111–113). In the young it is most often a genetic disease with autosomal dominant transmission, whereas in the elderly it is mostly acquired. Histologically, muscle fibers and muscle cells are noted to have an irregular arrangement, so that disarray and fibrotic changes are present in the myocardium. Symptoms consist of anginal chest pain, dyspnea, palpitations, dizziness, and syncope. Sudden death may be the first manifestation of the disease. The annual mortality rate in patients diagnosed young is about 6% per year, whereas it is 1.6% in those who are ages 45 to 60. Ventricular hypertrophy, especially involving the upper septum, characterizes the condition. There may be narrowing of the LV outflow tract (LVOT) caused by the protruding thick upper septum. Venturi forces created during systole cause anterior motion of the mitral valve toward the septum and contribute to the outflow tract narrowing. Mitral annular calcification, common in the elderly, also accentuates the LVOT obstruction (111). The LV chamber size is normal, and the LV systolic function is often hyperdynamic. Syncope may result from outflow tract obstruction during or following exercise, ventricular tachyarrhythmias, or rapid atrial fibrillation. Because of the noncompliant left ventricle, atrial contribution to ventricular filling is important in these patients, and the loss of atrial kick, which may happen with atrial fibrillation, may lead to severe hypotension and syncope.

Hypertension does not preclude hypertrophic cardiomyopathy. Older patients with hypertrophic cardiomyopathy may develop symptomatic hypotension following the use of diuretics and vasodilators. Antihypertensive therapy with these agents should be undertaken carefully. The prognosis of elderly patients with hypertrophic cardiomyopathy who are mildly symptomatic (NYHA class II) is fairly good, but those with advanced symptoms, i.e., NYHA class III, have a 36% 1-year mortality rate (113).

Treatment, as in younger patients, consists of using β-blockers or rate-controlling calcium channel blockers (verapamil or diltiazem) in those who are symptomatic (113). Therapy is not indicated for asymptomatic patients except those with massive (more than 35 mm) septal hypertrophy. Disopyramide is useful for prevention of recurrent atrial fibrillation, and its negative inotropic effect is beneficial for patients with an outflow tract gradient (112). Myomectomy is recommended for patients who remain symptomatic despite medical therapy. Novel approaches to therapy include AV sequential pacing and controlled septal infarction produced by injection of alcohol in the first septal perforator branch of the coronary artery supplying the septum (114).

Sudden death remains a major therapeutic challenge in patients with hypertrophic cardiomyopathy, including the elderly. Most often sudden death is due to ventricular tachycardia. Rarely, severe hypotension due to supraventricular tachycardia or bradyrhythmia (111) leads to sudden death. Evaluation with Holter monitoring or electrophysiologic testing may aid the selection of appropriate therapy. For patients who have symptomatic ventricular tachycardia or who have survived an episode of sustained ventricular tachycardia, an implantable cardioverter defibrillator is the therapy of choice. Alternatively, amiodarone therapy may be prescribed for these patients. Amiodarone is also very helpful in preventing recurrence of atrial fibrillation but is not yet FDA approved for this indication. Chronic oral anticoagulation to prevent thromboembolic complications is recommended for those with paroxysmal or sustained atrial fibrillation. Finally, prophylaxis against infective endocarditis is recommended whether or not patients have LVOT obstruction.

Restrictive Cardiomyopathy

Restrictive cardiomyopathy (115) in the elderly is often secondary to amyloidosis, which results in impaired diastolic relaxation; there may also be systolic dysfunction. Other causes include hemochromatosis and malignant (metastatic) heart disease. Amyloidosis should be suspected in elderly patients with unexplained heart failure, atrial fibrillation with slow ventricular response, low QRS voltage on an ECG, thick ventricular walls on echocardiogram that may reveal prominent echodensity (sparkling appearance), and normal or mildly dilated ventricles. The interatrial septum is thick, and the atria may be dilated. Therapy is usually directed at symptom control with judicious use of diuretics to relieve pulmonary congestion. Caution should be exercised in the use of digoxin or calcium channel blockers (verapamil, diltiazem) because these patients are sensitive to these agents. Phlebotomy is effective in controlling heart failure in patients with hemochromatosis.

PERICARDIAL DISEASES

The pericardium may be involved in inflammatory and noninflammatory conditions that may lead to pericardial effusion or pericardial constriction. The diagnosis of pericardial disease may also lead to the detection of a systemic disease in which the pericardium is involved as a bystander.

Causes of Pericarditis

Abnormalities of the pericardium may be encountered in several conditions (116, 117). Viral pericarditis can be due to cardiotropic viruses such as Coxsackie B, ECHO type 8, mumps, influenza, and Ebstein-Barr virus. These viruses may also be responsible for cases of idiopathic pericarditis. A history of a cold or influenzalike upper respiratory tract infection may precede the diagnosis of acute viral pericarditis.

Pericarditis due to other infective agents, such as bacteria, fungi, or rickettsiae, may be encountered in debilitated or immunocompromised patients and following thoracic surgery, pneumonia, or intravenous drug abuse. Common bacterial agents include *Staphylococcus aureus, Streptococcus pneumoniae, Haemophilus influenzae,* and less commonly Gram-negative rods. Rare causes of pericarditis in the elderly include immunologic and connective tissue disorders, such as systemic lupus erythematosus. Procainamide and hydralazine are known to cause a lupuslike syndrome with pericarditis that is reversible with cessation of the offending drug.

Pericarditis complicating AMI occurring within 24 to 48 hours of an infarction is generally benign and managed with nonsteroidal drugs, such as aspirin or ibuprofen, for relief of pain; indomethacin should be avoided because of its potential for aggravating myocardial injury in patients with coronary artery disease. Pericarditis, with or without effusion, occurring weeks to months after infarction is known as postmyocardial infarction syndrome or Dressler's syndrome and is characterized by chest pain, pericardial rub, fever, high sedimentation rate, pleuritis, and pulmonary infiltrates. An autoimmune process is most likely. A related condition, postcardiotomy syndrome, is seen in some patients after cardiac surgery. The term postcardiac injury syndrome is used to describe both entities (118). Neoplastic pericarditis due to primary malignant pericardial disease is very rare. More frequently, malignancy is secondary to a local spread from an adjoining structure, such as bronchogenic carcinoma, or metastatic spread via lymphatics or blood, such as with breast cancer. Effusions are hemorrhagic and tamponade is common. In some cases tumor encasement of the pericardium leads to constrictive pericarditis. Uremic pericarditis and pericardial effusion may be encountered in some patients with chronic renal failure, including those on hemodialysis. The causation of pericardial effusion in these patients is unclear but may be related to metabolic factors, infections, or bleeding in the pericardial space from low platelets or anticoagulation used during dialysis. The condition may progress to constrictive pericarditis after months or years. Increasing the frequency of dialysis may help to decrease pericardial effusion.

Clinical Features and Diagnosis

Features most commonly encountered include chest pain, fever, and pericardial rub. The chest pain is usually intense and anterior, over the precordium or the retrosternal area. It is pleuritic, i.e., aggravated by deep breathing, coughing, and movements of the trunk. Pain most often radiates to cervical areas and the trapezius ridge and less often to the posterior abdomen and the interscapular area (117). Pleuritic pain causes patients to breath fast and shallowly. Sitting up and leaning forward usually relieves pain, while lying down makes it worse.

These characteristics of the pain help differentiate pericarditis from angina but not from pneumonia or pulmonary infarction, since the latter conditions may also produce pleuritic pain. Pericardial rub confirms pericarditis. Rubs may be heard intermittently or continuously, and the detection of a rub therefore requires frequent auscultation. Pericardial rubs are commonly triphasic (117, 119); i.e., they have an atrial or presystolic component, a ventricular systolic component, and a ventricular diastolic component. The ventricular systolic component is most prominent.

The ECG in most leads typically shows ST-segment elevation that returns to baseline within weeks. This is followed by T-wave inversion that finally returns to normal baseline. PR segment depression representing atrial injury occasionally may be noted along with ST changes or rarely may be the only manifestation of acute pericarditis (117).

Other investigational tests are performed according to the clinical suspicion of a specific cause or to exclude certain causes. These include lupus erythematosus (LE), antinuclear antibody (for systemic lupus erythematosus), purified protein derivative skin test (for tuberculosis), chest radiograph, computed tomography scan (for malignancy), mammogram (for breast cancer), rheumatoid factor (for rheumatoid arthritis), and echocardiogram.

Treatment

Most cases of viral or postinfarction pericarditis resolve in 1 to 3 weeks. Treatment consists of analgesics and nonsteroidal agents such as aspirin for relief of pain. Steroids are avoided except in refractory cases (117, 118, 120). Other specific measures include drainage of purulent pericardial effusion and antibiotics for bacterial pericarditis, antituberculous therapy for tuberculous pericarditis, hemodialysis or drainage of effusion followed by local infiltration of steroids in the pericardial space for uremic pericarditis, irradiation and chemotherapy for pericarditis of malignancy, and pericardiectomy for recurrent pericarditis with effusion. A diagnostic pericardiocentesis may be necessary in some cases, and fluid is analyzed for cells, bacteria, glucose, protein, lupus erythematosus, and antinuclear antibody.

Pericardial Effusion (116, 117)

The mesothelial cells lining the pericardium secrete pericardial fluid, which normally amounts to less than 50 mL. Under pathologic conditions there is excessive production of fluid, which can have variable hemodynamic and clinical consequences. Any condition that causes acute pericarditis can lead to significant effusion. Other causes include trauma with bleeding in the pericardial space, congestive heart failure, hypothyroidism, cirrhosis, and obstruction of thoracic duct as a result of malignancy or damage during surgery.

Clinical Features and Diagnosis

A large amount of effusion, even in the absence of tamponade, may cause compression of adjoining structures and produce symptoms such as dysphagia from compression of the esophagus, hoarseness from compression of the recurrent laryngeal nerve, hiccups from compression of the phrenic nerve, and compression of the lung leading to an area of consolidation, detected as percussion dullness and bronchial breathing in the left infrascapular region (Ewart's sign) (116, 117).

When pericardial effusion is associated with an increase in intrapericardial pressure, it causes cardiac compression or cardiac tamponade. Tamponade may result from a sudden increase in intrapericardial volume,, such as 100 to 200 mL of blood in the pericardial space from puncture wound of the heart or from a large effusion increasing gradually, as in tuberculous pericarditis. In the latter situation, as much as a liter of fluid may accumulate before tamponade becomes evident.

Clinical features of tamponade include hypotension, tachycardia, distended jugular veins, and a significant pulsus paradoxus. The last is due to exaggeration of a fall in systolic blood pressure during inspiration from a normal of about 5 to 10 mm Hg to more than 10 mm Hg. Because right heart filling continues to be augmented during inspiration by a septal shift toward the left ventricle despite an increase in the intrapericardial pressure, this leads to an inspiratory decline in jugular venous pressure; i.e., Kussmaul's sign is absent. With progressive increase in the intrapericardial pressure, the patient develops cardiogenic shock. The ECG may show low voltage and electrical alternans, and the diagnosis is established by echocardiogram.

Treatment of Cardiac Tamponade

Pericardiocentesis with a long needle is performed for emergency relief of tamponade in a critically ill patient. It is preferably guided by echocardiography. Subxiphoid pericardiectomy with drainage in pleural space or peritoneum is used for large or recurrent effusions. Percutaneous balloon pericardiotomy is used in malignant or very frail patients. Other therapeutic measures, such as antibiotics and chemotherapeutic agents, are prescribed as indicated.

Constrictive Pericarditis

The hallmark of constrictive pericarditis is a thickened adherent pericardial sac that restricts filling of the heart. The condition is important, since with early recognition it is surgically treatable (121, 122). It can be confused with liver cirrhosis and with restrictive cardiomyopathy, with which it bears a close clinical resemblance (121–123).

Causation

The healing process associated with acute pericarditis, often with pericardial effusion, may result in constrictive pericarditis after weeks, months, or even years. Thus almost any condition that causes acute pericarditis may lead to constrictive pericarditis. Common causes of constrictive pericarditis include neoplastic diseases such as lymphoma, infectious diseases such as tuberculosis, bacterial infections, chronic renal failure, radiation therapy, and cardiac surgery. The process of healing associated with acute pericarditis leads to fibrosis, calcification, and adhesion of the two pericardial layers with obliteration of the pericardial space.

Clinical Features

Noncompliant pericardium interferes with diastolic filling of all cardiac chambers. Systolic function is normal. Decrease in cardiac output leads to poor perfusion of exercising muscles and causes fatigue, dyspnea, and sometimes syncope. Jugular veins are prominent, and hepatomegaly, ascites, and edema are noted. Auscultation of the heart may reveal a loud diastolic sound, pericardial knock, in timing like an early S_3, produced by abrupt cessation of the ventricular filling by the stiff pericardium. Kussmaul's sign is present and pulsus paradoxus is absent. The latter hemodynamic changes are due to inability of the right ventricle to increase its filling volume during inspiration because of the restraining effect of the rigid pericardium.

Diagnosis

Echocardiogram provides key hemodynamic findings. The presence of pericardial effusion indicates effusive constrictive pericarditis and may reveal thick pericardium. The ECG is abnormal but nonspecific. Chest radiograph may show evidence of pericardial calcification. Computed tomography and magnetic resonance imaging are most helpful in differentiating constrictive pericarditis from restrictive cardiomyopathy, which it resembles closely both hemodynamically and clinically. Cardiac catheterization shows typical dip-plateau pattern and equalization of diastolic pressures. Generally, the difference between left atrial mean and right atrial mean pressures, if present, amounts to less than 5 mm Hg, as opposed to more than 5 mm in patients with restrictive cardiomyopathy. Differential diagnoses include liver cirrhosis, cor pulmonale, and as noted earlier, restrictive cardiomyopathy.

Treatment

The definitive therapy is removal of the pericardium. Results are best when the procedure is done in the early stage of the disease; hence the importance of early recognition.

REFERENCES
Ischemic Heart Disease

1. Dormandy J, Mahir M, Ascady G, et al. Fate of the patient with chronic leg ischemia. J Cardiovasc Surg (Torino) 1989;30:50–57.
2. Nadelmann J, Frishman WH, Ooi WL, et al. Prevalence, incidence and prognosis of recognized and unrecognized myocardial infarction in persons aged 75 years and older: The Bronx Aging Study. Am J Cardiol 1990;66:533–537.
3. White NK, Edwards JE, Dry TJ. The relationship of the degree of coronary atherosclerosis with age in men. Circulation 1950;1:645–654.
4. Evelak L, Lie JT. Continued high incidence of coronary artery disease at autopsy in Olmsted County, Minnesota, 1950–1979. Circulation 1984;70:345–349.
5. Fries JF. Exercise and the health of the elderly. Am J Geriatric Cardiol 1997;6:24–32.
6. Management of stable angina pectoris. Recommendations of the Task Force of the European Society of Cardiology. Eur Heart J 1997;18:394–413.
7. Collaborative overview of randomised trials of antiplatelet therapy. I. Prevention of death, myocardial infarction, and stroke by prolonged antiplatelet therapy in various categories of patients. Antiplatelet Trialists' Collaboration. BMJ 1994;308:81–106.
8. A randomised, blinded, trial of clopidogrel versus aspirin in patients at risk of ischaemic events (CAPRIE). CAPRIE Steering Committee. Lancet 1996;348:1329–1339.
9. Parker JO, Amies MH, Hawkinson RW, et al. Intermittent transdermal nitroglycerin therapy in angina pectoris: clinically effective without tolerance or rebound. Circulation 1995;91:1368–1374.
10. Chrysant SG, Glasser SP, Bittar N, et al. Efficacy and safety of extended-release isosorbide mononitrate for stable effort angina pectoris. Am J Cardiol 1993;73:1249–1256.
11. Morris AD, Meredith PA, Reid JL. Pharmacokinetics of calcium antagonists: implications for therapy. In: Epstein M, ed. Calcium Antagonists in Clinical Medicine. Philadelphia: Hanley & Belfus, 1995:49–67.
12. Bonnier H, de Vries C, Michels R, el Gamal M. Initial and long-term results of coronary angioplasty and coronary bypass surgery in patients of 75 or older. Br Heart J 1993;70:122–125.
13. Metzger JP, Tabone X, Georges JL, et al. Coronary angioplasty in patients 75 years and older: a comparison with coronary bypass surgery. Eur Heart J 1994;15:213–217.
14. Erickson P. Coronary artery bypass surgery and health related quality of life: data from the National Health and Nutrition Examination Survey. Am J Geriatric Cardiol 1997;6:18–22.
15. Five-year clinical and functional outcome comparing bypass surgery and angioplasty in patients with multivessel coronary disease. A multicenter randomized trial. Writing Group for the Bypass Angioplasty Revascularization Investigation (BARI) Investigators. JAMA 1997;277:715–721.
16. Comparison of coronary bypass surgery with angioplasty in patients with multivessel disease. N Engl J Med 1996;335:217–225.
17. He Guo-Wei, Acuff TE, Ryan WH, et al. Influence of old age, gender and internal mammary artery grafting on

operative mortality and morbidity in coronary artery by-pass grafting. Am J Geriatric Cardiol 1996;5:22–35.

18. Buffolo E, Summo H, Aguiar L, et al. Myocardial revascularization in patients 70 years of age and older without the use of extracorporeal circulation. Am J Geriatric Cardiol 1997;6:7–15.

19. McClellan JR. Unstable angina: prognosis, noninvasive risk assessment and strategies for management. Clin Cardiol 1994;17:229–238.

20. Catherwood E, O'Rourke DJ. Clinical pathway management of unstable angina. Prog Cardiovasc Dis 1994;37:121–148.

21. Cohen M, Demers C, Gurfinkel EP, et al. A comparison of low-molecular-weight heparin with unfractionated heparin for unstable coronary artery disease. Efficacy and Safety of Subcutaneous Enoxaparin in Non–Q-Wave Coronary Events Study Group. N Engl J Med 1997;337:447–452.

Acute Myocardial Infarction

22. Van de Werf F. Cardiac troponins in acute ischemic syndromes. N Engl J Med 1996;335:1388–1389.

23. Ryan TJ, Anderson JL, Antman EM, et al. ACC/AHA guidelines for the management of patients with acute myocardial infarction. A report of the American College of Cardiology/American Heart Association Task Force on Practice Guidelines (Committee on Management of Acute Myocardial Infarction). J Am Coll Cardiol 1996;28:1328–1428.

24. Indications for fibrinolytic therapy in suspected acute myocardial infarction: collaborative overview of early mortality and major morbidity results from all randomised trials of more than 1000 patients. Fibrinolytic Therapy Trialists' (FTT) Collaborative Group. Lancet 1994;343:311–322.

25. Krumholz HM, Pasternak C, Weinstein MC, et al. Cost Effectiveness of thrombolytic therapy with streptokinase in elderly patients with suspected acute myocardial infarction. N Engl J Med 1992;327:7–13.

26. Mark DB, Hlatky MA, Califf RM, et al. Cost effectiveness of thrombolytic therapy with tissue plasminogen activator as compared with streptokinase for acute myocardial infarction. N Engl J Med 1995;332:1418–1424.

27. Krumholz HM, Murillo JE, Chen J, et al. Thrombolytic therapy for eligible elderly patients with acute myocardial infarction. JAMA 1997;277:1683–1688.

28. Translation of clinical trials into practice: a European population-based study of the use of thrombolysis for acute myocardial infarction. European Secondary Prevention Study Group. Lancet 1996;347:1203–1207.

29. Gurwitz JH, Gore JM, Goldberg RJ, et al. Recent age-related trends in the use of thrombolytic therapy on patients who have had acute myocardial infarction. Ann Intern Med 1996;124:283–291.

30. Gurwitz JH, McLaughlin TJ, Willison DJ, et al. Delayed hospital presentation in patients who have had acute myocardial infarction. Ann Intern Med 1997;126:593–599.

31. Weaver WD, Simes RJ, Betriu A, et al. Comparison of primary coronary angioplasty and intravenous thrombolytic therapy for acute myocardial infarction: a quantitative review. JAMA 1997;278:2093–2098.

32. Every NR, Parsons LS, Hlatky M, et al. A comparison of thrombolytic therapy with primary coronary angioplasty for acute myocardial infarction. N Engl J Med 1996;335:1253–1260.

33. Randomised trial of intravenous streptokinase, oral aspirin, both, or neither among 17,187 cases of suspected acute myocardial infarction: ISIS-2. ISIS-2 (Second International Study of Infarct Survival) Collaborative Group. Lancet 1988;2:349–360.

34. Saketkhou BB, Conte FJ, Noris M, et al. Emergency department use of aspirin in patients with possible acute myocardial infarction. Ann Intern Med 1997;127:126–129.

35. Krumholz HM, Radford MJ, Ellerbeck EF, et al. Aspirin in the treatment of acute myocardial infarction in elderly Medicare beneficiaries. Patterns of use and outcomes. Circulation 1995;92:2841–2847.

36. Ellerbeck EF, Jencks SF, Radford MJ, et al. Quality of care for Medicare and patients with acute myocardial infarction: A four-state pilot study from the Cooperative Cardiovascular Project. JAMA 1995;273:1509–1514.

37. Randomised placebo-controlled trial of abciximab before and during coronary intervention in refractory unstable angina: the CAPTURE Study. The CAPTURE Investigators. Lancet 1997;349:1429–1435.

38. Granger CB, Hirsh J, Califf RM, et al. Activated partial thromboplastin time and outcome after thrombolytic therapy for acute myocardial infarction: results from the GUSTO I Trial. Circulation 1996;93:870–878.

39. GISSI-3: effects of lisinopril and transdermal glyceryl trinitrate singly and together on 6-week mortality and ventricular function after acute myocardial infarction. Gruppo Italiano per lo Studio della Sopravvivenza nell'infarto Miocardico. Lancet 1994;343:1115–1122.

40. ISIS-4: a randomised factorial trial assessing early oral captopril, oral mononitrate, and intravenous magnesium sulphate in 58,050 patients with suspected acute myocardial infarction. ISIS-4 (Fourth International Study of Infarct Survival) Collaborative Group. Lancet 1995;345:669–685.

41. Yusuf S, Peto R, Lewis J, et al. Beta blockade during and after myocardial infarction: an overview of the randomized trials. Prog Cardiovasc Dis 1985;27:335–371.

42. Randomised trial of intravenous atenolol among 16,027 cases of suspected acute myocardial infarction: ISIS-1. First International Study of Infarct Survival Collaborative Group. Lancet 1986;2:57–66.

43. Metoprolol in acute myocardial infarction (MIAMI). The MIAMI Trial Research Group. Am J Cardiol 1985;56:1G–57G.

44. Roberts R, Rogers WJ, Mueller HS, et al. Immediate versus deferred beta-blockade following thrombolytic therapy in patients with acute myocardial infarction. Results

of the Thrombolysis in Myocardial Infarction (TIMI) II-B Study. Circulation 1991;83:422–437.

45. A randomized trial of propranolol in patients with acute myocardial infarction. I. Mortality results. JAMA 1982; 247:1707–1714.

46. Soumerai SB, McLaughlin TJ, Spiegelman D, et al. Adverse outcomes of under use of beta-blockers in elderly survivors of acute myocardial infarction. JAMA 1997; 277:115–121.

47. Pfeffer MA, Braunwald E, Moye LA, et al. Effect of captopril on mortality and morbidity in patients with left ventricular dysfunction after myocardial infarction. Results of the survival and ventricular enlargement trial. The SAVE Investigators. N Engl J Med 1992;327:669–677.

48. Smith P, Arnesen H, Holme I. The effect of warfarin on mortality and reinfarction after myocardial infarction. N Engl J Med 1990;323:147–152.

49. Effect of long-term oral anticoagulant treatment on mortality and cardiovascular morbidity after myocardial infarction. Anticoagulants in the Secondary Prevention of Events in Coronary Thrombosis (ASPECT) Research Group. Lancet 1994;343:499–503.

50. Randomised double-blind trial of fixed low-dose warfarin with aspirin after myocardial infarction. Coumadin Aspirin Reinfarction Study (CARS) Investigators. Lancet 1997;350:389–396.

51. The effect of diltiazem on mortality and reinfarction after myocardial infarction. The Multicenter Diltiazem Postinfarction Trial Research Group. N Engl J Med 1988;319:385–392.

52. Randomised trial of cholesterol lowering in 4444 patients with coronary heart disease: the Scandinavian Simvastatin Survival Study (4S). Lancet 1994;344: 1383–1389.

53. Sacks FM, Pfeffer MA, Moye LA, et al. The effect of pravastatin on coronary events after myocardial infarction in patients with average cholesterol levels. N Engl J Med 1996;335:1001–1009.

54. O'Connor GT, Buring JE, Yusuf S, et al. An overview of randomized trials of rehabilitation with exercise after myocardial infarction. Circulation 1989;80:234–244.

Cardiac Arrhythmias

55. Podrid PJ. Arrhythmias in the elderly subject. Cardiol Elderly 1997;5:18–21.

56. Raiha V, Piha SJ, Seppanen A, et al. Predictive value of continuous ambulatory electrocardiographic monitoring in elderly people. BMJ 1994;309:1263–1267.

57. Frishman WH, Heiman M, Karpenos A, et al. Twenty-four hour ambulatory electrocardiography in elderly subjects: prevalence of various arrhythmias and prognostic implications (report from the Bronx Longitudinal Aging Study). Am Heart J 1996;132:297–302.

58. Gonzalez R. Pacemakers in the elderly: selection of pacing systems. Am J Geriatric Cardiol 1997;6:16–19.

59. Jazayeri M, Hempe SL, Sra JS, et al. Selective Transcatheter ablation of the fast and slow pathways using radiofrequency energy in patients with atrioventricular

nodal reentrant tachycardia. Circulation 1992;85: 1318–1328.

60. Moran JL, Gallagher J, Peake SL, et al. Parenteral magnesium sulfate versus amiodarone in the therapy of atrial tachyarrhythmias: a prospective, randomized study. Crit Care Med 1995;23:1816–1824.

61. Khan AH. Management of chronic ventricular arrhythmias. Am Fam Physician 1994;49:1805–1811.

62. Moss AJ, Hall WJ, Cannom DS, et al. Improved survival with an implanted defibrillator in patients with coronary disease at high risk for ventricular arrhythmia. N Engl J Med 1996;335:1933–1940.

63. Desai AD, Sung C, Sung RJ. The role of intravenous amiodarone in the management of cardiac arrhythmias. Ann Intern Med 1997;127:294–303.

64. Dreifus LS, Fisch C, Griffin JC, et al. Guidelines for implantation of cardiac pacemakers and antiarrhythmia devices. A report of the American College of Cardiology/American Heart Association Task Force on Assessment of Diagnostic and Therapeutic Cardiovascular Procedures (Committee on Pacemaker Implantation). J Am Coll Cardiol 1991;18:1.

Atrial Fibrillation

65. Reardon M, Camm JA. Atrial fibrillation in the elderly. Clin Cardiol 1996;19:765–775.

66. Cairns JA, Connolly SJ. Nonrheumatic atrial fibrillation. Risk of stoke and antithrombotic therapy. Circulation 1991;84:469–481.

67. Coumel P. Neurogenic and humoral influences of the autonomic nervous system in the determination of paroxysmal atrial fibrillation. In: Ateul P, Coumel P, Janse MJ, eds. The Atrium in Health and Disease. Mount Kisco, NY: Futura, 1989:213–232.

68. Gilligan DM, Ellenbogen KA, Epstein AE. The management of atrial fibrillation. Am J Med 1996;101:413–421.

69. Manning WJ, Silverman DI, Gordon SPF, et al. Cardioversion from atrial fibrillation without prolonged anticoagulation with use of transesophageal echocardiography to exclude the presence of atrial thrombi. N Engl J Med 1993;328:750–755.

70. Kamensky G, Drahos P, Nadezda P. Evaluation of embolic risk in patients with atrial fibrillation using transesophageal echocardiography. J Noninvasive Cardiol 1997;1:40–46.

71. Orsinelli DA. Current recommendations for the anticoagulation of patients with atrial fibrillation. Cardiovasc Dis 1996;39:1–20.

72. Golzari H, Randall DC, Bahler RC. Atrial fibrillation: restoration and maintenance of sinus rhythm and indications for anticoagulation therapy. Ann Intern Med 1996;125:311–323.

73. Waldo AL, Pratt CM. Introduction: acute treatment of atrial fibrillation and flutter—ibutilide in perspective. Am J Cardiol 1996;78:1–2.

74. Stevenson WG, Ganz LI. Atrial fibrillation in heart failure. Heart Failure 1997;13:22–29.

75. Gold RL, Haffajee C, Sloan K, et al. Amiodarone for re-

fractory atrial fibrillation. Circulation 1990;82:1932–1939.

76. Campbell RW. Atrial fibrillation: steering a management course between thromboembolism and proarrhythmic risk. Eur Heart J 1995;16(suppl G):28–31.

77. Waldo AL. An approach to therapy of supraventricular tachyarrhythmias: an algorithm versus individualized therapy. Clin Cardiol 1997;17(suppl 2); II-21–II-26.

78. Ellenbogen KA, Dias VC, Plumb VJ, et al. A placebo-controlled trial of continuous intravenous diltiazem infusion for 24-hour heart rate control during atrial fibrillation and atrial flutter: a multicenter study. J Am Coll Cardiol 1991;18:891–897.

Congestive Heart Failure

79. Konstam M, Dracup K, Baker D, et al. Heart Failure: Management of Patients With Left Ventricular Systolic Dysfunction. Quick Reference Guide for Clinicians 11 (AHCPR 94–0613). Rockville, MD: US Department of Health and Human Services, Public Health Service, Agency for Health Care Policy and Research, 1994: 1–21.

80. Gaasch WH. Diagnosis and treatment of heart failure based on left ventricular systolic or diastolic dysfunction. JAMA 1994;271:1276.

81. Guidelines for the evaluation and management of heart failure. Report of the American College of Cardiology/American Heart Association Task Force on Practice Guidelines (Committee on Evaluation and Management of Heart Failure). Circulation 1995;92:2764–2784.

82. Aronow WS, Tresh D. Congestive heart failure in older persons. J Am Geriatr Soc 1997;45:1252–1258.

83. Rich MW, Beckham V, Wittenberg C, et al. A multidisciplinary intervention to prevent the readmission of elderly patients with congestive heart failure. N Engl J Med 1995;333:1190–1195.

84. Garg R, Yusuf S. Overview of randomized trials of angiotensin-converting enzyme inhibitors on mortality and morbidity in patients with heart failure. JAMA 1995;273:1450–1456.

85. Effect of enalapril on survival in patients with reduced left ventricular ejection fractions and congestive heart failure. The SOLVD Investigators. N Engl J Med 1991;325:293–302.

86. Cohn JN, Archibald DG, Ziesche S, et al. Effect of vasodilator therapy on mortality in chronic congestive heart failure. Results of a Veterans Administration Cooperative Study. N Engl J Med 1986;314:1547–1552.

87. Pitt B, Segal R, Martinez FA, et al. Randomised trial of losartan versus captopril in patients over 65 with heart failure. Lancet 1997;349:747–752.

88. The effect of digoxin on mortality and morbidity in patients with heart failure. The Digitalis Investigation Group. N Engl J Med 1997;336:525–533.

89. Packer M, Bristow MR, Cohn JN, et al. The effect of carvedilol on morbidity and mortality in patients with chronic heart failure. N Engl J Med 1996;334:1349–1355.

Valvular Heart Disease

90. Rose AG. Etiology of valvular heart disease. Curr Opin Cardiol 1996;11:98–113.

91. Lindroos M, Kupari M, Heikkila J, et al. Prevalence of aortic valve abnormalities in the elderly: an echocardiographic study of a random population sample. J Am Coll Cardiol 1993;21:1220–1225.

92. Aronow WS. Mitral annular calcification: significant and worth acting upon. Geriatrics 1991;46:73–75, 79–80, 85–86.

93. Edmunds LH, Stephenson LW, Edie RN, et al. Open heart surgery in octogenarians. N Engl J Med 1988;319:331–336.

94. Olsson M, Janfjall H, Orth-Gomer K, et al. Quality of life in octogenarians after valve replacement due to aortic stenosis: a prospective with younger patients. Eur Heart J 1996;17:583–589.

95. Logeais Y, Roussin R, Langanay T, et al. Aortic valve replacement for aortic stenosis in 200 consecutive octogenarians. J Heart Valve Dis 1995;4(suppl 1):S64–S71.

96. Freeman WK, Schaff HV, O'Brien PC, et al. Cardiac surgery in the octogenarian: perioperative outcome and clinical follow-up. J Am Coll Cardiol 1991;18: 29–35.

97. Scott ML, Stowe CL, Nunnally LC, et al. Mitral valve reconstruction in the elderly population. Ann Thorac Surg 1989;48:213.

98. Fremes SE, Goldman BS, Ivanov J, et al. Valvular surgery in the elderly. Circulation 1989;80(suppl): 1–77.

99. Azar H, Szentpetery S. Mitral valve repair in patients over the age of 70 years. Eur J Cardiothorac Surg 1994;8:298–300.

100. Craver JM, Cohen C, Weintraub WS. Case-matched comparison of mitral valve replacement and repair. Ann Thorac Surg 1990;49:964.

101. Bethel HJ, Mullee MA. A controlled trial of community-based coronary rehabilitation. Br Heart J 1990;64:370.

102. Cribier A, Savin T, Berland J, et al. Percutaneous transluminal balloon valvuloplasty of adult aortic stenosis: report of 92 cases. J Am Coll Cardiol 1987;9:381.

103. Berman AD, McKay RG, Grossman W. Balloon valvuloplasty. In: Cardiac Catheterization, Angiography, and Intervention. 5th ed. Baltimore: Williams & Wilkins, 1996:659.

104. Rodriguez AR, Kleiman NS, Minor ST, et al. Factors influencing the outcome of balloon aortic valvuloplasty in the elderly. Am Heart J 1990;120:373–380.

105. Lefevre T, Bonan R, Serra A, et al. Percutaneous mitral valvuloplasty in surgical high risk patients. J Am Coll Cardiol 1991;17:348.

106. Zhang HP, Allen JW, Lau FY, Ruiz CE. Immediate and late outcome of percutaneous balloon mitral valvotomy in patients with significantly calcified valves. Am Heart J 1995;129:501–506.

Cardiomyopathies

107. Richardson P, McKenna W, Bristow M, et al. Report of

the 1995 World Health Organization/ International Society and Federation of Cardiology Task Force on Definition and Classification of Cardiomyopathies. Circulation 1996;93:841–842.

108. Dec GW, Fuster VF. Idiopathic dilated cardiomyopathy. N Engl J Med 1994;331:1564–1575.

109. Konstam M, Dracup R, Baker D, et al. Heart Failure:
Evaluation and Care of Patients With Left Ventricular
Systolic Dysfunction. Clinical Practice Guideline 11
(AHCPR 94–0612). Rockville, MD: US Department of
Health and Human Services, Public Health Service,
Agency for Health Care Policy and Research, 1994:1–21.

110. Struthers AD. Rationalizing the heart failure trials: from
theory to practice. Eur Heart J 1997;18(suppl E):
E5–E8.

111. DeFranco AC, Lever HM. Changing concepts in hypertrophic cardiomyopathy. Contemp Intern Med
1992;Sept:106–127.

112. Wigle ED, Rakowski H, Kimball BP, et al. Hypertrophic
cardiomyopathy: clinical spectrum and treatment. Circulation 1995;92:1680–1692.

113. Spirito P, Seidman CE, McKenna WJ, Maron BJ. The
management of hypertrophic cardiomyopathy. N Engl
J Med 1997;336:775–785.

114. Knight C, Kurbaan AS, Seggewiss H, et al. Nonsurgical
septal reduction for hypertrophic obstructive cardiomyopathy. Circulation 1997; 95:2075–2081.

115. Kushiwaha SS, Fallon JT, Fuster VF. Medical progress:
restrictive cardiomyopathy. N Engl J Med 1997;336:
267–276.

Pericardial Diseases

116. Shabetai R. Diseases of the pericardium. Cardiol Clin
1990;8:579.

117. Spodick DH. Pericardial effusion. In: Spodick DH, ed.
The Pericardium: A Comprehensive Textbook. New
York: Marcel Dekker, 1997:126–152.

118. Khan AH. The postcardiac injury syndromes. Clin Cardiol 1992;15:67–72.

119. Spodick DH. The pericardial rub: a prospective study
of one hundred consecutive cases. JAMA 1976;
235:39.

120. Spodick DH. Pericarditis. In: Rekel RE, ed. Conn's
Current Therapy. Philadelphia: Saunders, 1995;289–
292.

121. Hancock RW. Constrictive pericarditis: modern view
of diagnosis and management. J Cardiovasc Med
1980;41:367.

122. Spodick DH. Constrictive pericarditis. In: Spodick DH,
ed. The Pericardium: A Comprehensive Textbook.
New York: Marcel Dekker, 1997:214–259.

123. Nashimura RA, Connolly DC, Parkin TW, Stanson
AW. Constrictive pericarditis: assessment of current
diagnostic procedures. Mayo Clinic Proc 1985;60:397.

CHAPTER 8

CYNTHIA D. MULROW AND MICHAEL B. BRAND

Hypertension in the Elderly

PREVALENCE

Prevalence estimates of hypertension vary widely with the number of blood pressure measurements taken and the cut point used to define systolic and diastolic hypertension. The National Health and Nutrition Examination Survey from 1988 to 1991 (NHANES III) defined hypertension as average systolic measurements of at least 140 mm Hg and/or diastolic measurements of at least 90 mm Hg based on the average of three blood pressure measurements (1). This survey showed that the prevalence of hypertension varies by age, ethnicity, and gender (Fig. 8.1). Non-Hispanic black men and women in the United States had a higher prevalence of hypertension than their non-Hispanic white or Mexican-American counterparts in all but the oldest range for men (above 80 years), in which Mexican-Americans had the highest prevalence. In general, men had higher age-specific rates of hypertension than women until 60 years of age, at which time non-Hispanic black and Mexican-American women had higher rates than male counterparts. By age 70, prevalence among non-Hispanic white women exceeded that in their male counterparts.

Figure 8.2 from the NHANES III shows that average systolic blood pressure tends to rise in both men and women throughout adult life, whereas average diastolic blood pressure peaks about age 55 (1). After the seventh decade, average systolic blood pressures are as high or higher in women than in men because of a sharper rise in systolic blood pressure with age in women. In both men and women, pulse pressure rises with age. Percentages of persons with severe hypertension also rise with age. For example, 4% of non-Hispanic black men aged 18 to 49 have stage 2 to 4 hypertension compared with 12% of those aged 50 to 69 and 20% of those aged 70 and older.

Isolated systolic hypertension is essentially a condition of older adults defined as average systolic blood pressure greater than 160 mm Hg from two measurements with diastolic blood pressures not more than 90 mm Hg. The Systolic Hypertension in the Elderly Program (SHEP) estimated its prevalence ranged from approximately 5% in those aged 60 to 69 years to approximately 10% in those more than 70 years of age to 20% in those more than 80 years of age (2). Using a definition with a lower systolic cut point, at least 140 mm Hg, increases prevalences to as high as 50% among the oldest old.

PATHOPHYSIOLOGY

A variety of pathophysiologic changes are related to hypertension in the elderly (3). Theoretically, some of these changes may have management implications. Older persons have less compliant blood vessels than younger persons; such decreases in vessel compliance are correlated with systolic pressure rises. The decreased compliance is related to loss of connective tissue elasticity and an increase in the prevalence of atherosclerosis, both of which raise peripheral vascular resistance.

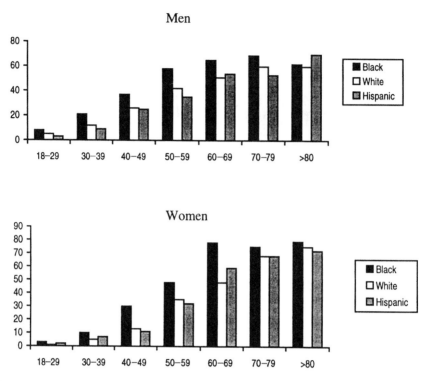

Figure 8.1.   Prevalence of hypertension by age, gender, and ethnicity for U.S. adults (NHANES III survey).

Older persons may also have age-related changes in vascular function, such as diminished β-adrenergic responsiveness of vascular smooth muscle, with resultant decreases in smooth muscle relaxation. Baroreceptor sensitivity is reduced. Plasma renin levels and renin responses to sodium depletion and upright posture decline with age, as do renal blood flow, glomerular filtration rate, and creatinine clearance. Elderly persons are less able to retain or excrete sodium maximally. Finally, older persons, particularly those with hypertension, have higher left ventricular mass and lower left ventricular early diastolic filling than younger persons with hypertension.

SCREENING AND DIAGNOSIS

The U.S. Preventive Services Task Force recommends periodic screening for hypertension in all adults (4). The optimal interval for screening has not been determined, but the Joint National Committee on Detection, Evaluation, and Treatment of High Blood Pressure suggests that persons with normal blood pressure have their blood pressure rechecked every 2 years and that persons with high normal levels be rechecked annually (5). The classification system used by the Joint National Committee to define hypertension is presented in Table 8.1 (5). When systolic and diastolic blood pressures fall into different categories, the higher category is used. Isolated systolic hypertension is defined as a systolic blood pressure of 140 mm Hg or more and a diastolic blood pressure below 90 mm Hg. It is staged according to the table. For example, an elderly person with an average blood pressure of 176/86 would be diagnosed as having stage 2 isolated systolic hypertension.

Blood pressure status is generally based on the average of two or more readings taken at each of two or more visits. It should not be diagnosed on the basis of a single measurement unless systolic blood pressure is greater than 210 mm Hg or diastolic blood pressure is greater than 120 mm Hg. Ensuring multiple readings (six to nine) before diagnosis is particularly important in the elderly because their blood pressure varies more

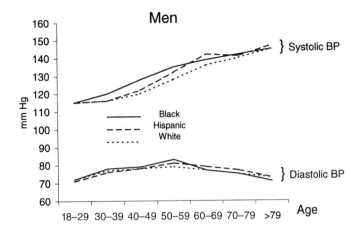

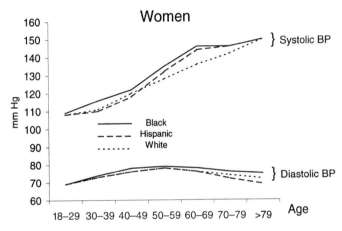

Figure 8.2.   Mean blood pressure values by age and ethnicity.

widely than that of middle-aged and younger adults (6). Blood pressure measurement is recommended with the patient seated with arm bared, supported, and at heart level. In elders it is recommended that blood pressure also be measured supine 1 to 3 minutes after standing to discover systolic blood pressure drops of 20 mm Hg or more, as they are likely to develop postural hypotension if antihypertensive drug therapy or other medications are prescribed (3, 6).

A mercury sphygmomanometer, calibrated aneroid manometer, or calibrated electronic device can be used to measure blood pressure. Several factors related to equipment, observers, and patients can result in inaccurate blood pressure readings. Measurement devices should be routinely calibrated and checked for pressure leaks. The bladder of the blood pressure cuff should wrap around at least 80% of the arm. Providers responsible for measuring blood pressure should be trained and checked in appropriate tech-

Table 8.1

Classification of Blood Pressure for Adults

Category	Systolic (mm Hg)	Diastolic (mm Hg)
Normal	<130	<85
High normal	130–139	85–89
Hypertension		
Stage 1	140–159	90–99
Stage 2	160–179	100–109
Stage 3	≥180	≥110

niques. They should use the first appearance of sound (phase I) to define systolic pressure and the disappearance of sound (Phase V) for definition of diastolic pressure and should try to avoid digit and artificial cutoff preferences. Finally, any of several factors having to do with the patient may lead to inaccurate blood pressure measurement, some of which may be more pronounced in elders (6). Ideally, measurement is done after 5 minutes of rest and half an hour to an hour after meals, smoking, and alcohol or caffeine intake.

PSEUDOHYPERTENSION AND WHITE-COAT HYPERTENSION

Older persons may have falsely high sphygmomanometer readings due to decreased arterial wall compliance and excessive vascular stiffness of upper extremity vessels. This condition is commonly termed pseudohypertension. Its actual prevalence is unknown, but experts recommend that clinicians have increased suspicion of pseudohypertension in elders with consistently elevated blood pressures and no evidence of target organ damage and in patients with nearly syncopal types of symptoms during therapy (5, 7). Unfortunately, there are not simple noninvasive mechanisms for establishing the diagnosis of pseudohypertension. Osler's maneuver of assessing the palpability of the radial artery after making it pulseless by compressing the brachial artery with sphygmomanometer cuff pressure greater than systolic readings is associated with significant observer variability and inaccuracy (7, 8). Intra-arterial or automatic infrasonic blood pressure measurements are accurate; they may be warranted in some cases to avoid erroneously labeling persons as having pseudohypertension and not treating them appropriately.

White-coat hypertension refers to high blood pressure readings when persons attend clinics and medical facilities but normal blood pressure readings outside of the office or at home. Older persons, particularly older women, have white-coat hypertension more commonly than younger persons (6, 9). Frequent measurement of blood pressure outside the clinician's office is recommended to determine any white-coat hyperten-

sion. Occasionally, ambulatory blood pressure monitoring may be used.

ASSESSING RISKS IN HYPERTENSIVE ELDERS

All hypertensive elders should have their overall risk of cardiovascular disease assessed. In general, systolic more than diastolic hypertension, higher pulse pressures (systolic minus diastolic blood pressure), a higher stage or level of hypertension, presence of target organ damage such as left ventricular hypertrophy, and presence of multiple risk factors such as dyslipidemia, diabetes, and obesity are all associated with higher risk of cardiovascular disease. An exception to this may be that level of blood pressure is not a risk indicator for cardiovascular or total mortality in men over age 75 and women over age 85 (10). The prevalence of most comorbid risk factors, excepting tobacco use, increases with age. Classic cardiovascular risk factors act in a synergistic and multiplicative manner in increasing the probability of cardiovascular disease (Fig. 8.3) (11). For example, a woman with systolic hypertension, dyslipidemia, and diabetes has approximately a 28% probability of having a coronary heart-related event in 10 years, compared with a probability of only 10% if she did not have diabetes and dyslipidemia. Thus, as elders generally have greater prevalences of risk factors, they are at much higher risk for cardiovascular disease than younger and middle-aged persons.

Assessment of risk has direct therapeutic implications (Table 8.2) (5). First, persons with concomitant risk factors such as obesity, sedentary lifestyle, and tobacco use should have those risk factors addressed directly. Second, as patients with multiple risk factors have associated higher baseline risks for cardiovascular disease, they can be expected to benefit more from antihypertensive therapy than persons without any risk factors (12). In the latter patient, initial therapy with nonpharmacologic interventions alone may be considered, whereas more aggressive initial therapy is appropriate in patients with multiple risk factors.

Many elders may have significant competing risks for death other than cardiovascular risks.

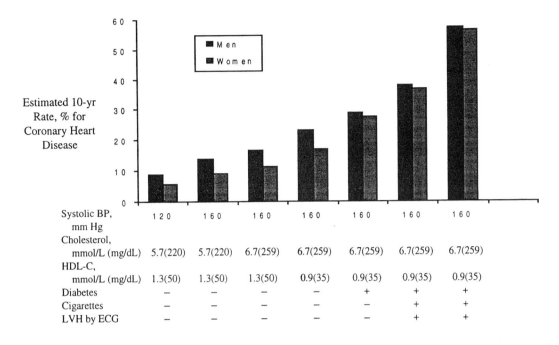

Figure 8.3.   Multiplicative risks for coronary heart disease.

For example, some elders have late-stage cancer, severe liver disease, or Alzheimer's disease. The benefits of treating hypertension in the face of these competing risks are not known. In such instances clinicians must rely solely on their own best judgments and patients' preferences regarding the need for and desirability of hypertension treatment.

SECONDARY HYPERTENSION

Secondary causes of hypertension occur in approximately 5% of persons with hypertension. They should be considered in elders (*a*) whose blood pressure is responding poorly to multiple drug therapy; (*b*) with stage 3 hypertension; (*c*) with previously well-controlled hypertension whose blood pressure becomes difficult to control; and (*d*) whose history, physical examination (abdominal bruit), or laboratory tests (unprovoked hypokalemia, hypercalcemia, elevated creatinine, or abnormal urinalysis) suggest such causes. Renal artery stenosis from atherosclerotic disease is one of the more common causes of secondary hypertension in elders, particularly in those with a history of heavy smoking or coexisting diffuse atherosclerotic vascular disease (13). Noninvasive tests that can be used to work up such patients include a captopril-enhanced radionuclide renal scan, duplex Doppler flow studies, and magnetic resonance angiography. Definitive diagnosis requires renal angiography.

TREATMENT
Drug Therapy

The efficacy of antihypertensive drug therapy in the elderly is supported by a meta-analysis of 14 randomized controlled trials of at least 1 year's duration (14). The trials included a total population of 17,213 elderly subjects with nearly 81,000 patient-years of follow-up. Most subjects were 60 to 80 years old and living in Western industrialized countries. Most trials evaluated diuretic and β-blocker therapies in a stepped-care approach. Diuretics were usually thiazides with addition of amiloride or triamterene. The β-blocker was usually atenolol or metoprolol. The average prevalence of cardio-

Table 8.2

Risk Stratification and Treatment[a]

	Risk Group A	Risk Group B	Risk Group C
	No risk factors; no TOD/CCD	At least one risk factor, not including diabetes; no TOD/CCD	TOD/CCD and/or diabetes, with or without other risk factors
Blood Pressure Stages (mm Hg)			
High normal (130/85–139/89)	Lifestyle modification	Lifestyle modification	Drug therapy[b]
Stage 1 (140/90–159/99)	Lifestyle modification (up to 12 months)	Lifestyle modification[c] (up to 6 months)	Drug therapy
Stages 2 and 3 (≥160/≥100)	Drug therapy	Drug therapy	Drug therapy

For example, a patient with diabetes, blood pressure of 142/94 mm Hg, and left ventricular hypertrophy falls into stage 1 hypertension with target organ disease (left ventricular hypertrophy) and another major risk factor (diabetes). This patient is stage 1, risk group C, and recommended for immediate pharmacologic treatment.

TOD/CCD, target organ disease/clinical cardiovascular disease.
[a]Lifestyle modification should be adjunctive therapy for all patients recommended for pharmacologic therapy.
[b]For those with heart failure or renal insufficiency or those with diabetes.
[c]For patients with multiple risk factors, clinicians should consider drugs as initial therapy plus lifestyle modifications.

vascular risk factors, cardiovascular disease, and competing comorbid diseases was lower among trial participants than the general population of hypertensive elderly persons.

Aggregate results of these trials showed that for every 1000 patients treated over a 5-year period, cardiovascular events (cerebrovascular or cardiac) were prevented in 63 subjects (95% confidence interval [CI] 36 to 91). Cerebrovascular and coronary heart disease events were prevented in 25 persons (95% CI 17 to 32) and 15 persons (95% CI 1 to 24), respectively, for every 1000 persons treated for 5 years. Data from the two trials restricted to persons with isolated systolic hypertension indicated that cardiovascular events were prevented in 83 persons (95% CI 56 to 100) for every 1000 patients treated for 5 years.

Existing trial data suggest that 5-year absolute morbidity and mortality benefits of antihypertensive therapy are greater for older than younger adults (12, 15, 16). However, trials generally show that benefits of antihypertensive treatment increase over time. Long-term cumulative benefits in younger persons with greater remaining life expectancy and fewer competing risks may exceed those in older persons. Whether benefits can be generalized to the oldest old (age over 85 years) and classes of antihypertensive agents such as ACE inhibitors is not yet established (12, 16).

Data on adverse effects of medical therapy in elders suggest that many regimens are well tolerated. The Medical Research Council's trial of hypertension in older adults (MRCOA) and SHEP showed no substantive differences between treatment and control groups for measures of cognitive, physical, or emotional function (2, 17). Systematic reviews assessing multiple drug trials of shorter duration found no consistent deleterious adverse effects on quality of life or neuropsychologic function (18, 19).

If there are no specific indications for another type of drug, a low-dose thiazide diuretic should be chosen because of the numerous trials showing improvements in morbidity and mortality with these agents and their low cost. β-Blockers and long-acting dihydropyridine calcium antagonists (nitrendipine) are appropriate alternatives because they lower blood pressure in elders and have been shown to decrease fatal and nonfatal cardiovascular events (20–22). Short-acting calcium antagonists should not be used (23–26). Indications for consideration and avoidance of other initial therapies are given in Table 8.3.

Persons who do not achieve blood pressure control with single agents can have a second agent added or a drug from another class substituted. If a diuretic was not the first drug, it is usually indicated as a second step because diuretics are often synergistic with other agents.

Nonpharmacologic Therapies

There are various nonpharmacologic antihypertensive therapies (Table 8.4). Most evaluations of the effectiveness of such therapies have been carried out in middle-aged persons, though there is evidence that nonpharmacologic therapy in elders is feasible (27). Evaluations of nonpharmacologic therapies have focused primarily on blood pressure reductions; no trials have evaluated long-term effects on morbidity or mortality.

Salt Restriction

Modest blood pressure-lowering effects of salt restriction are demonstrated by a meta-analysis of 28 randomized controlled trials in hypertensive persons (28). The trials included 1131 persons aged 8 to 73 years (mean age 47). The mean decrease in sodium excretion achieved across trials was 95 mmol/day (95% CI 71 to 119). This level of decrease is unrealistic in the general population (29, 30). A 60-mmol/day decrease in sodium intake is more realistic and would correspond to a reduction of the general population's sodium intake to the current daily recommended goal of 2.4 g (104 mmol).

Regression analysis showed that such a 60-mmol/day decrease in sodium intake would, on average, decrease blood pressure in hypertensive persons by 2.2 mm Hg systolic and 0.5 mm Hg

distolic. A subgroup analysis found blood pressure response to sodium reduction considerably larger in trials of hypertensive persons with a mean age greater than 45 years. These data suggest that salt restriction is more beneficial for older than younger hypertensive persons.

Potassium Supplementation

A meta-analysis of 21 randomized controlled trials established the benefits of potassium supplementation for treatment of hypertension (31). The trials included 1560 persons ranging in age from 19 to 79 years. The intervention consisted of either potassium chloride supplementation or high-potassium foods (average 60 mmol/day). The average decrease in blood pressure of those receiving potassium compared with controls was 4.4 mm Hg systolic and 2.5 mm Hg diastolic. Two small trials assessing potassium supplementation in elderly persons reached results generally consistent with the remainder of the trials (32, 33). The evidence suggests that for hypertensive persons an increase in potassium consumption of approximately 60 mmol/day (equivalent to 60 mEq or 2 g—roughly the amount in five bananas) over the typical person's consumption produces a significant decrease in blood pressure.

Calcium Supplementation

A meta-analysis of 19 randomized controlled trials concluded that evidence is suggestive but not conclusive regarding the utility of calcium supplementation for decreasing blood pressure (34). Most of the trials were small and short. Results in 11 of the trials showed no significant effect on blood pressure. Pooled results found that, on average, blood pressure decreased by 1.8 mm Hg systolic and 0.7 mm Hg diastolic. No data from randomized trials specifically addressing calcium supplementation in the elderly were reported. At this point the evidence does not support recommending calcium supplementation for the treatment of hypertension in persons with normal calcium levels (34, 35).

Magnesium Supplementation

A few short-term small randomized controlled trials address the effectiveness of magnesium supplementation as an antihypertensive

Table 8.3

Indications for Individualizing Antihypertensive Drug Therapy to Comorbid Conditions

Compelling Indications Based on Known Symptom, Morbidity, Mortality Benefits	May Have Favorable Symptom and/or Physiologic Effects on Comorbid Conditions	May Have Unfavorable Effects on Comorbid Conditions
Diabetes mellitus type I with proteinuria — ACEI	Angina — β-Blockers, CA	Bronchospastic disease — β-Blockers
Left ventricular dysfunction — ACEI, Diuretics	Atrial tachycardia and fibrillation — β-Blockers CA (non-DHP)	2nd- or 3rd-degree heart block — β-Blockers, CA (non-DHP), clonidine
Myocardial infarction — Non-ISA β-blockers	Diabetes mellitus type I & II with proteinuria — CA	Dyslipidemia — β-Blockers (non-ISA)
	Diabetes mellitus type II / Dyslipidemia — Low-dose diuretics, α-blockers	Gout — High-dose diuretics
	Essential tremor — β-Blockers (non-CS)	Heart failure — CA (except amlodipine)
	Left ventricular dysfunction — β-Blockers (use with caution) Losartan	Liver disease — Labetalol, methyldopa
	Hyperthyroidism — β-Blockers	Peripheral vascular disease — β-Blockers
	Migraine — β-blockers (non-CS) CA (non-DHP)	Renal insufficiency — Potassium-spring agents
	Osteoporosis — Thiazides	Renovascular disease — ACEI Angiotensin II receptor blockers
	Symptomatic Benign prostatic hypertrophy — α-Blockers	Type I and II diabetes — β-Blockers High-dose diuretics

ACEI, ACE inhibitors; CA, calcium antagonists; ISA, intrinsic sympathomimetic activity; DHP, dihydropyridine; non-CS, noncardioselective.

Table 8.4

Nonpharmacologic Antihypertensive Therapy

For overall cardiovascular health:
  Stop smoking
  Reduce intake of dietary saturated fat and
    cholesterol
  Limit intake of alcohol to no more than 2 drinks
    per day for men, 1 for women
Adjust cation intake:
  Reduce sodium intake to 100 mmol/day (2.4 g)
  Ensure potassium intake through supplements if
    necessary of 100 to 150 mmol (4 to 6 g)
  Consume US RDA of calcium (800 mg) and
    magnesium (350 mg for men, 280 mg for
    women)
Increase physical activity (minimum of 30 minutes/day
  at least 3 days/week)
If overweight, reduce caloric intake with goal of
  reducing body weight at least 10%

therapy (36–40). The study results are mixed and have not been assessed with a formal meta-analysis. For persons with normal magnesium levels, the available evidence does not warrant recommendation of magnesium supplementation as antihypertensive therapy.

Fish Oil Supplementation

The ability of fish oil (omega-3 polyunsaturated fatty acid) supplementation to decrease blood pressure in hypertensive persons was demonstrated by a meta-analysis of 6 randomized controlled trials (41). The trials included 291 mostly middle-aged white men and were generally short (average, 11 weeks). The average decrease in blood pressure in the treatment group (net of control group) was 5.5 mm Hg systolic and 3.5 mm Hg diastolic. The doses of fish oil supplementation used in the trials were generally greater than can be expected to be maintained by the typical person for prolonged periods (200 g of fish high in omega-2 PUFA or 6 to 10 capsules of commercially available fish oil supplements per day). It is unclear to what degree a benefit would be achieved at lower doses. Available evidence does not address elderly persons specifically, though the evidence does suggest a benefit from fish oil supplementation for those interested in this therapy.

High-Fiber, Reduced-Fat Diet

The Dietary Approaches to Stop Hypertension (DASH) trial found that a change in participants' dietary composition lowered their blood pressure (42). DASH enrolled 459 mostly middle-aged nonobese persons with an average blood pressure of 131/85 mm Hg. For 8 weeks participants followed a control diet, a diet rich in fruits and vegetables, or a combination diet rich in fruits, vegetables, and low-fat dairy products and with reduced total fat. Sodium intake and body weight were maintained at constant levels. The combination diet reduced blood pressure by 5.5/3 mm Hg more than the control diet. The fruit and vegetable diet reduced systolic blood pressure by 2.8 mm Hg more than the control diet (changes in diastolic blood pressure were not significant). Among the 133 subjects with hypertension, the combination diet reduced blood pressure by 11.4/5.5 mm Hg. DASH suggests that changing to a reduced-fat diet rich in fruits and vegetables and low-fat dairy products can lower blood pressure independently of weight loss or sodium restriction.

Weight Loss

A meta-analysis of five randomized controlled trials found that weight loss decreased blood pressure in obese hypertensive adults (43). The trials included 327 mostly middle-aged persons. Interventions consisted of calorie-restricted diets followed for 6 to 12 months. The average decrease in blood pressure as compared with control was 1.2/1 mm Hg diastolic per kilogram of body weight lost. A modest 5-kg (11 lb) weight loss, typical of the outcomes seen in the trials, translates to a decrease in blood pressure of 6/5 mm Hg. Blood pressure reductions generally occurred before normal weight was attained. Decreases in blood pressure were generally maintained in the absence of marked weight regain. Since the publication of the meta-analysis, a further eight randomized controlled trials corroborate these findings. None of the reported trials assessed elderly persons specifically. For obese hypertensive persons, weight loss can be an effective first-line treatment for hypertension if they are motivated to follow a long-term weight loss regimen.

Exercise

The beneficial effects of lower extremity aerobic exercise on hypertension was demonstrated by a meta-analysis of nine randomized controlled trials (44). The trials included 245 mostly white men ranging in age from 29 to 72 years. The average length of intervention programs was 18 weeks; average exercise frequency was 3 days per week; average duration of training was 47 minutes per session; and average intensity was 60% of VO_{2max}. All trials employed walking/jogging, cycling, or both. The average decrease in resting blood pressure of the exercisers compared with controls was approximately 7/5 mm Hg. None of the reported data specifically addressed elderly persons. Though many elderly persons cannot be expected to follow the relatively vigorous training programs assessed in these trials, the evidence suggests that barring contraindications to exercise, elderly persons with hypertension would benefit from even modest increases in aerobic activity.

Combined Drug and Nondrug Therapies

A few trials have investigated the effects of combining drug and nondrug therapies. Persons receiving antihypertensive drug therapy in combination with nonpharmacologic therapy achieved greater blood pressure reductions than those receiving nonpharmacologic therapy alone (45). Weight reduction in combination with drug therapy has been demonstrated to be especially effective (46). However, sodium restriction in combination with drug therapy was no more beneficial than drug therapy alone and resulted in lower quality of life measures than drug therapy alone (46).

TARGET BLOOD PRESSURES

Typical recommended target blood pressures are systolic blood pressure below 140 mm Hg and diastolic blood pressure below 90 mm Hg. Many authorities recommend lower targets for persons with diabetes (5). These targets are to a large extent based on artificial cut points chosen for study purposes rather than a specific biologic cut point defining increased risk. Coronary heart disease mortality risk associated with blood pressure occurs on a continuum that extends well below the arbitrarily defined level for abnormal blood pressure, beginning for systolic blood pressure about 110 mm Hg and for diastolic pressure above 70 mm Hg. In trials of isolated systolic hypertension in elders, no increases in cardiovascular morbidity or mortality have been seen with drops of diastolic blood pressure lower than 80 mm Hg (2). A trial involving 18,790 patients with average age of 62 years and diastolic blood pressures between 100 and 115 mm Hg evaluated target diastolic blood pressures of ≤90 mm Hg, ≤85 mm Hg, and ≤80 mm Hg (47). Most patients received a long-acting dihydropyridine calcium antagonist, felodipine (78%), and an ACE inhibitor (41%). There were no differences in major cardiovascular events between the three groups. The subset of diabetic patients randomized to the ≤80 group had half the rate of major cardiovascular events than those randomized to the ≤90 group (RR < 90 versus < 80 2.1 CI 1.2 to 3.4).

PATIENTS' GOALS AND NEGOTIATION

Goals of hypertension therapy should be negotiated individually with patients. In most instances the ideal goal is to reduce blood pressure to normal levels with minimal adverse effects. Teaching patients about their condition, necessary medications and adverse effects, and how to measure their blood pressure away from the office is desirable. Reasonable lifestyle modifications should be encouraged. Ideal antihypertensive therapy should be inexpensive and simple, with the aim of favoring long-acting formulations and integrating pill taking into routine activities of daily living. Strategies that improve compliance include access to convenient care, easily available information, counseling, reminders, self-monitoring, reinforcement, family therapy, and other forms of supervision or attention (48). Blood pressure should be monitored frequently; delays in changing the approach if therapy is unsuccessful should be avoided. Use of telecommunication and ancillary health care providers is encouraged to maintain frequent supportive contact and improve adherence to therapeutic regimens.

REFERENCES

1. Burt VL, Whelton P, Roccella EJ, et al. Prevalence of hypertension in the US adult population. Results from the Third National Health and Nutrition Examination Survey, 1988–1991. Hypertension 1995;25:305–313.
2. Prevention of stroke by antihypertensive drug treatment in older persons with isolated systolic hypertension. Final results of the Systolic Hypertension in the Elderly Program (SHEP). SHEP Cooperative Research Group. JAMA 1991;265:3255–3264.
3. Applegate WB. Hypertension in elderly patients. Ann Intern Med 1989;110:901–915.
4. Screening for hypertension. In: Guide to Clinical Preventive Services. Report of the U.S. Preventive Services Task Force. 2nd ed. Baltimore: Williams & Wilkins, 1996;39–52.
5. The sixth report of the Joint National Committee on prevention, detection, evaluation, and treatment of high blood pressure. Arch Intern Med 1997;157:2413–2446.
6. National High Blood Pressure Education Program Working Group. National High Blood Pressure Education Program Working Group Report on Hypertension in the Elderly. Hypertension 1994;23:275–285.
7. Zuschke CA, Pettyjohn FS. Pseudohypertension. South Med J 1995;88:1185–1190.
8. Belmin J, Visintin JM, Salvatore R, et al. Osler's maneuver: absence of usefulness for the detection of pseudohypertension in an elderly population. Am J Med 1995;98:42–49.
9. Wiinberg N, Hoegholm A, Chirstensen HR, et al. 24-h ambulatory blood pressure in 352 normal Danish subjects, related to age and gender. Am J Hypertens 1995;8:978–986.
10. Bulpitt CJ, Fletcher AE. Aging, blood pressure and mortality. J Hypertens 1992;10(suppl 7):S45–S49.
11. Alderman MH. Blood pressure management: individualized treatment based on absolute risk and the potential for benefit. Ann Intern Med 1993;119:329–335.
12. Gueyffier F, Boutitie F, Boissel JP, et al. Effect of antihypertensive drug treatment on cardiovascular outcomes in women and men: a meta-analysis of individual patient data from randomized, controlled trials. Ann Intern Med 1997;126:761–767.
13. Rimmer JM, Gennari FJ. Atherosclerotic renovascular disease and progressive renal failure. Ann Intern Med 1993;118:712–719.
14. Mulrow C, Lau J, Cornell J, Brand M. Antihypertensive drug therapy in the elderly. Cochrane Library, May 1997 at www.cochrane.org.
15. Collins R, Peto R, MacMahon S, et al. Blood pressure, stroke, and coronary heart disease. Part 2. Short-term reductions in blood pressure: overview of randomised drug trials in their epidemiological context. Lancet 1990;335:827–838.
16. Mulrow CD, Cornell JA, Herrera CR, et al. Hypertension in the elderly: implications and generalizability of randomized trials. JAMA 1994;272:1932–1938.
17. Medical Research Council trial of treatment of hypertension in older adults: principal results. MRC Working Party. BMJ 1992;304:405–412.
18. Muldoon MF, Waldstein SR, Jennings JR. Neuropsychological consequences of antihypertensive medication use. Exp Aging Res 1995;21:353–368.
19. Beto J, Bansal V. Quality of life in treatment of hypertension: a meta analysis of clinical trials. Am J Hypertens 1992;5:125–133.
20. Materson BJ, Reda DJ, Cushman WC, et al. Single-drug therapy for hypertension in men. A comparison of six antihypertensive agents with placebo. The Department of Veterans Affairs Cooperative Study Group on Antihypertensive Agents. N Engl J Med 1993;328:914–921.
21. Dahlof B, Lindholm LH, Hansson L, et al. Morbidity and mortality in the Swedish Trial in Older Patients with Hypertension (STOP-Hypertension). Lancet 1991;338:1281–1285.
22. Staessen JA, Fagard R, Thijs L, et al. Randomised double-blind comparison of placebo and active treatment for older patients with isolated systolic hypertension. Systolic Hypertension in Europe (Syst-Eur) Trial Investigators. Lancet 1997;350:757–764.
23. Psaty BM, Heckbert SR, Koepsell TD, et al. The risk of myocardial infarction associated with antihypertensive drug therapies. JAMA 1995;274:620–625.
24. Pahor M, Guralnik JM, Corti MC, et al. Long-term survival and use of antihypertensive medications in older persons. J Am Geriatr Soc 1995;43:1191–1197.
25. Pahor M, Guralnik JM, Furberg CD, et al. Risk of gastrointestinal haemorrhage with calcium antagonists in hypertensive persons over 67 years old. Lancet 1996;347:1061–1065.
26. National Heart, Lung, and Blood Institute. NHLBI Panel Reviews Safety of Calcium Channel Blockers. Bethesda, MD: US Department of Health and Human Services, August 31, 1995 (press release).
27. Applegate WB, Miller ST, Elam JT, et al. Nonpharmacologic intervention to reduce blood pressure in older patients with mild hypertension. Arch Intern Med 1992;152:1162–1166.
28. Midgley JP, Matthew AG, Greenwood CMT, Logan AG. Effect of reduced dietary sodium on blood pressure: a meta-analysis of randomized controlled trials. JAMA 1996;275:1590–1597.
29. The effects of nonpharmacologic interventions on blood pressure of persons with high normal levels. Results of the Trials of Hypertension Prevention, Phase I. JAMA 1992;267:1213–1220.
30. Kumanyika SK, Hebert PR, Cutler JA. Feasibility and efficacy of sodium reduction in the Trials of Hypertension Prevention, Pase I. Trials of Hypertension Prevention Collaborative Research Group. Hypertension 1993;22:502–512.
31. Whelton PK, He J, Cutler JA, et al. Effects of oral potas-

sium on blood pressure: meta-analysis of randomized controlled clinical trials. JAMA 1997;277:1624–1632.

32. Smith SR, Klotman PE, Svetkey LP. Potassium chloride lowers blood pressure and causes natriuresis in older patients with hypertension. J Am Soc Nephrol 1992;2:1302–1309.

33. Fotherby MD, Potter JF. Potassium supplementation reduces clinic and ambulatory blood pressure in elderly hypertensive patients. J Hypertens 1992;10:1403–1408.

34. Cutler JA, Brittain E. Calcium and blood pressure: an epidemiologic perspective. Am J Hypertens 1990;3:137S–146S.

35. Cappuccio FP, Siani A, Strazzullo P. Oral calcium supplementation and blood pressure: an overview of randomized controlled trials. J Hypertens 1989;7:941–946.

36. Witteman JC, Grobbee DE, Derkx FH, et al. Reduction of blood pressure with oral magnesium supplementation in women with mild to moderate hypertension. Am J Clin Nutr 1994;60:129–135.

37. Widman L, Wester PO, Stegmayr BK, Wirell M. The dose-dependent reduction in blood pressure through administration of magnesium: a double blind placebo controlled cross-over study. Am J Hypertens 1993;6:41–45.

38. Sanjuliani AF, de Abreu Fagundes VG, Francischetti EA. Effects of magnesium on blood pressure and intracellular ion levels of Brazilian hypertensive patients. Intern J Cardiol 1996;56:177–183.

39. Wirell MP, Wester PO, Stegmayr BG. Nutritional dose of magnesium in hypertensive patients on beta blockers lowers systolic blood pressure: a double-blind, cross-over study. J Intern Med 1994;236:189–195.

40. Ferrara LA, Iannuzzi R, Castaldo A, et al. Long-term magnesium supplementation in essential hypertension. Cardiology 1992;81:25–33.

41. Appel LJ, Miller ER III, Seidler AJ, Whelton PK. Does supplementation of diet with 'fish oil' reduce blood pressure? A meta-analysis of controlled clinical trials. Arch Intern Med 1993;153:1429–1438.

42. Appel LJ, Moore TJ, Obarzanek E, et al. A clinical trial of the effects of dietary patterns on blood pressure. DASH Collaborative Research Group. N Engl J Med 1997;336:1117–1124.

43. Staessen J, Fagard R, Amery A. The relationship between body weight and blood pressure. J Hum Hypertens 1988;2:207–217.

44. Kelley G, McClellan P. Antihypertensive effects of aerobic exercise: a brief meta-analytic review of randomized controlled trials. Am J Hypertens 1994;7:115–119.

45. The treatment of mild hypertension study. A randomized, placebo-controlled trial of a nutritional-hygienic regimen along with various drug monotherapies. The Treatment of Mild Hypertension Research Group. Arch Intern Med 1991;151:1413–1423.

46. Wassertheil-Smoller S, Oberman A, Blaufox MD, et al. The Trial of Antihypertensive Interventions and Management (TAIM) Study. Final results with regard to blood pressure, cardiovascular risk, and quality of life. Am J Hypertens 1992;5:37–44.

47. Hansson L, Zanchetti AZ. Carruthers SG, et al. Effects of intensive blood pressure lowering and low-dose aspirin in patients with hypertension; principal results of the Hypertension Optimal Treatment (HOT) trial. Lancer 1998;351:1755–1762.

48. Haynes RB, McKibbon KA, Kanani R, et al. Intervention to assist patients to follow prescriptions for medications. Cochrane Library, May 1997 at www.cochrane.org.

Exercise for Older Patients

The hallmark of aging is a structural and functional decline in the cells and tissues of all organs. The resulting physiologic changes include decreased muscle mass and strength; decreased maximal heart rate, exercise tolerance, and aerobic capacity; and increased body fat. Functional status is quite heterogeneous among older persons of similar chronologic age; therefore, other factors in addition to genetic processes must contribute to this variation. The development of subclinical and overt disease processes such as atherosclerotic coronary artery disease may adversely affect cardiac and physical function and promote sedentary behavior. Lifestyle behaviors such as cigarette smoking, imprudent diet, and physical inactivity may also contribute directly to the age-related decline in functional status (1–3).

Exercise may help prevent or slow the progression of functional loss. Numerous scientific studies provide evidence that physical activity leads to better mental and physical health (4). Exercise may have an important role as a therapeutic agent for the prevention and treatment of various diseases such as coronary artery disease, hypertension, non–insulin-dependent diabetes mellitus (NIDDM), obesity, osteoporosis, colon cancer, and possibly depression (5). Current evidence also suggests that regular physical activity may increase longevity in middle-aged and older men and women (6, 7). A graded inverse relation has been demonstrated between total physical activity and mortality in men (8).

This chapter briefly reviews the relation of physical activity to disease, possible mechanisms by which exercise promotes beneficial changes, the benefits and risks of exercise, the evaluation of older people for exercise programs, and guidelines for exercise prescriptions.

PHYSICAL ACTIVITY AND DISEASE
Coronary Artery Disease

Many epidemiologic studies have shown that low levels of cardiorespiratory fitness and physical activity are independent risk factors for coronary artery disease (CAD) in men. In the British Civil Servant Study, only strenuous physical activity was associated with a decreased risk of CAD (9). However, in the Multiple Risk Factor Intervention Trial, U.S. Railroad Study, and the Kuopio Ischemic Heart Disease Risk Factor Study, activity of low to moderate intensity was associated with reduced mortality from CAD (10–12). In the Kuopio study, 2 hours of conditioning exercise weekly was sufficient to reduce the risk of acute myocardial infarction.

In Paffenbarger's study of leisure-time activity in Harvard alumni, the relative risk for all-cause mortality was related to physical activity in a dose-dependent way (6). The greatest risk was found for those who expended fewer than 500 kcal/week, intermediate risk for those expending between 500 and 1999 kcal, and the least risk for those expending more than 2000 kcal per week. The figure of 2000 kcal weekly represents the energy expended in walking 3 miles daily for 7 days. In this study, the most active participants also had the lowest risk of cardiac events.

Mechanisms by which aerobic exercise may reduce the risk of cardiovascular disease include improvement of balance between myocardial oxygen demand and supply, reduced risk of lethal ventricular arrhythmias and development of eccentric ventricular hypertrophy, decreased blood coagulability by reducing adhesiveness of platelets and increased fibrinolysis, and improved plasma lipid and lipoprotein profile (4).

Hypertension

Population studies have also found an inverse correlation between physical activity and blood pressure. Clinical trials show that chronic aerobic training lowers systolic and diastolic blood pressure modestly in both normotensive and hypertensive people independent of weight loss or reduced body fat (13). A meta-analysis of 25 longitudinal studies reported average reductions in systolic pressure of 10.8 mm Hg and in diastolic pressure of 8.2 mm Hg (14). Moderate-intensity exercise was as effective as high-intensity exercise in achieving lower pressures. Possible mechanisms by which repeated physical activity affects blood pressure include a decline in resting cardiac output, a decline in sympathetic nervous system activity, and a decline in total peripheral resistance. Concomitant weight loss and dietary changes such as decreased sodium or alcohol intake may be contributing factors (15).

Diabetes Mellitus

Cross-sectional and longitudinal studies show an inverse relation between physical activity and the prevalence of NIDDM (16). Regular aerobic exercise combined with proper diet may prevent NIDDM and improve glycemic control in patients who have it. Insulin sensitivity is improved in skeletal muscle and other tissues with a single session of aerobic exercise, reducing blood glucose levels in diabetic patients. This effect is thought to occur because of an increase in cell membrane glucose transporter number and activity (17).

Obesity

People who are obese tend to be less active physically. Regular exercise contributes to maintenance of ideal body weight through caloric expenditure. In addition, exercise may improve body fat distribution, as some training studies suggest that upper abdominal subcutaneous fat is mobilized in preference to peripheral subcutaneous fat (18).

Osteoporosis

Peak bone mass occurs by the third decade and declines gradually throughout middle and old age, with an accelerated loss occurring in postmenopausal women. Although bone clearly responds to the physical stress of weight-bearing exercise, the amount and type necessary to attenuate bone loss is unclear (19).

Colon Cancer

Case control studies generally show a significant positive relation between exercise and decreased risk of colon cancer. Seven of nine prospective studies in men but only one of three in women were positive (20). However, only one of the positive studies controlled for dietary fat intake, possibly a confounding variable (21). Decreased intestinal transit time and decreased prostaglandin E are two possible mechanisms by which exercise may decrease the risk for colon cancer (20).

Depression

Most older persons who exercise regularly enjoy an improved sense of well-being and self-efficacy. However, a significant relation between levels of physical activity and the incidence of depression has not been proved (22).

EVALUATION OF OLDER PATIENTS PRIOR TO CONDITIONING

An older person should undergo a complete medical evaluation before beginning an exercise program. The history and physical examination should be targeted to the cardiovascular, pulmonary, musculoskeletal, and neurologic systems, as the presence of comorbid disease is common in this population. Laboratory tests should be performed to rule out impaired renal or liver function, anemia, and diabetes mellitus. In addition, a resting 12-lead electrocardiogram (ECG) should be performed. Many authorities believe that older persons should undergo a physician-monitored exercise treadmill test to screen for cardiac ischemia, exercise-induced arrhythmias or asthma, exaggerated hypertensive response, and other abnormalities that preclude participation in an exercise training program (23). Others believe that asymptomatic healthy older persons without major risk factors for CAD, diabetes mellitus, or hypertension and no history of these conditions are at low risk for CAD and therefore do not require testing (24).

Exercise tolerance testing also permits assessment of maximal aerobic capacity, which can be used to determine exercise goals and monitor progress. The test is performed with a bicycle or treadmill according to a standard multistage protocol (25). Disadvantages include the cost and the lack of availability of equipment and trained personnel. Contraindications to exercise stress testing include unstable angina, recent myocardial infarction, uncontrolled arrhythmias, severe aortic stenosis, third-degree heart block, dissecting aneurysm, myocarditis or pericarditis, recent pulmonary embolism or other thromboembolic disease, congestive heart failure, significant emotional disturbance, and neurologic or musculoskeletal limitations. Physicians performing the test should also be familiar with the indications for stopping a test and the criteria for an abnormal test. Persons with abnormal tests should be referred to the appropriate specialist for further evaluation.

THE EXERCISE PRESCRIPTION

The exercise prescription, tailored to the individual patient, describes the type, frequency, duration, and intensity of the proposed activity. It should include information on the warm-up, conditioning, and cool-down components of each exercise session. Various activities may be prescribed for improving aerobic fitness. Activities that involve a large proportion of the total muscle mass, maximize the use of large muscles and dynamic muscle contraction, and minimize the work of the heart per unit training effect will be most effective. Walking may be the most beneficial exercise for the older person in terms of safety, effectiveness, and simplicity. Cardiac patients generally require a supervised exercise program,

and those at highest risk also require ECG monitoring (26).

For all persons, the exercise session should begin with 5 minutes of walking followed by stretching exercises. This warm-up, designed to bring about gradual increases in blood flow as well as increases in tissue and general body temperatures, may prevent muscle aches, pains, and injuries and possibly reduce the incidence of cardiac rhythm abnormalities during the conditioning period. A rule of thumb is that mild perspiration should appear before the person begins vigorous activity.

Frequency is an important component of the exercise prescription. Most studies report little change in physical fitness if exercises are done fewer than 3 times a week and no added benefit if training is done more than 5 days weekly (26). The duration of the exercise sessions is usually set at 20 minutes initially and advanced to 30 to 60 minutes as the person progresses with training. Early studies reported that 20 to 30 minutes of continuous aerobic exercise was necessary to achieve a cardiovascular training effect. DeBusk et al., however, have shown that three 10-minute walks during the same day have the same fitness effect as one 30-minute walk (27). This finding may have important implications for compliance.

A minimum intensity is thought to be required for a person with a low fitness level to achieve a cardiovascular training effect. This level, as determined by the American College of Sports Medicine (ACSM), has decreased from 70% of maximal aerobic capacity in 1975 to 50% in 1986 and 40 to 50% in 1990. Low intensity is generally defined as less than 50%, moderate intensity as 50 to 70%, and high intensity as above 70% of maximal aerobic capacity. The intensity may be determined in one of two ways. If maximal aerobic capacity was measured during an exercise stress test, exercise intensity can be related to the maximal heart rate.

Alternatively, the maximal heart rate predicted by age can be determined by a formula: $220 - \text{age} = \text{maximal predicted heart rate}$. The target heart rate is calculated as percentage of maximal exercise capacity; i.e., $40\% \times (\text{maximal heart rate} - \text{resting heart rate}) + \text{resting heart rate}$. For example, for a 70-year-old patient with a resting heart rate of 72 and predicted maximal heart rate of 150 (220 − 70) who will be exercising at 40% of maximal exercise capacity, the target heart rate would be 40% × (150 − 72) + 72 = 103 beats per minute.

Because there is a linear relation between oxygen consumption and heart rate during submaximal work loads, the target heart rate can be monitored during exercise as an indication of training intensity. Exercise may also be prescribed in terms of metabolic equivalents (METS), which is the oxygen consumption during rest, or 3.5 mL O_2/kg per minute. METS have been determined for most activities. The usual safe range of exercise intensity is 4 to 7 METS for older persons with normal exercise stress tests (26).

Many older persons benefit from supervision of the initial physical activity to confirm that exercise capacity is not exceeded. If the program is unsupervised, persons should be carefully instructed on how and when to take their pulse to ensure that they are exercising at an appropriate level. Training duration and intensity should progress slowly, in a stepwise fashion, usually over 6 months or longer as needed. Depending on the initial exercise capacity, persons should begin at 40 to 50% of their maximal aerobic capacity for 10 to 20 minutes of continuous exercise. The duration of the session should be gradually increased to 30 to 45 minutes. Intensity may then be increased, usually not more than 10% per month.

A 10-minute cool-down session of slow walking and stretching exercises should conclude each exercise session. Older persons should be counseled to wear appropriate supportive footwear and loose clothing and to consult a physician if they develop pain in the chest, arm, neck, or jaw; severe shortness of breath; fainting or dizziness; irregular heartbeat during or after exercise; and injury or joint swelling.

RISKS OF EXERCISE

The possible adverse effects of exercise that are most worrisome are sudden death, injury, and osteoarthritis. The most serious but least common of these is sudden death, defined as death occurring either during the actual activity or within 1 hour after it. Although reported rates of sudden death vary from 4 to 56 times greater than chance, the absolute risk is low: one cardiac death per 396,000 hours of jogging or one death per 15,000 to 18,000 exercisers per year (28). In most documented cases of sudden death in older persons, overt CAD or identifiable risk factors were present prior to the event (29).

There are few data on the risks of injury associated with the physical activities performed by older people, such as walking and gardening. Injuries sustained by participants in organized exercise programs, which are primarily due to overuse, are relatively common. The ankle is the joint most likely to be injured. Most nontraumatic musculoskeletal injuries in runners are directly related to distance run and increasing mileage. Age and obesity do not appear to be contributing factors in current studies. There are no good studies of nontraumatic musculoskeletal injuries related to walking or cycling or gardening (30).

Preexistent musculoskeletal problems may be a deterrent to beginning an exercise regimen. One study reported that more than 50% of older persons involved in a variety of new activities developed injuries that were exacerbations of prior conditions (31). For previously healthy persons, injury rates ranging from 10 to 50% for both novice and experienced exercisers have been reported. Significantly lower rates of injury are associated with low-impact exercise, such as walking, than with higher-impact activities, such as aerobic dance and jogging. Almost all organized walk/jog exercise programs reporting injuries cite the primary involvement of the lower extremities. Because most participants recover from the injury and maintain training intensity by substituting an uphill treadmill walk for jogging, high impact rather than intensity has been implicated as the cause of injury. Older women seem to be more susceptible to lower extremity injury during jogging than are men (32).

The fear that the physical activity may stimulate osteoarthritis or exacerbate a preexisting condition has kept some patients from participating in an exercise program and may prevent physicians from recommending that they do so. Because osteoarthritis affects 85% of all persons 70 years or older, it is important to know whether activities should be limited in this population. Cross-sectional studies found no difference in the prevalence of musculoskeletal complaints, symptomatic osteoarthritis, or radiographic evidence of osteoarthritis in long-distance runners compared with nonrunners (33). A 2-year longitudinal study also showed no difference in the progression of osteoarthritis between runners and controls (34). In a recent randomized 18-month clinical trial of 439 community-dwelling adults aged 60 or older with radiographically evident knee osteoarthritis, pain, and self-reported disability, modest improvements in measures of disability, physical performance, and pain occurred with participation in either an aerobic or resistance exercise program (35).

Physical inactivity may in fact promote osteoarthritis through repetitive stress placed on joints supported by weak muscles and stiff tendons. Regular weight-bearing exercise may help prevent osteoarthritis by improving muscle strength, increasing bone density, and reducing obesity. For patients with early arthritis, regular weight-bearing exercise may halt disuse atrophy and stimulate cartilage growth.

STRENGTH TRAINING

A decrease in functional mobility and recurrent falls are associated with the well-documented decline in muscle strength in older people. This age-related muscle weakness may be related to physical inactivity (disuse syndrome), nutritionally inadequate diet, comorbid disease, and the biologic aging process. Several clinical trials of healthy community-dwelling men and women under 80 years of age have reported increases of 17 to 72% over baseline maximum isometric strength after 6 weeks of static exercise (36). Also, significant gains in muscle strength and mass with resistive exercise have been shown in a group of frail institutionalized nonagenarians (37). However, a long-term program of strength training appears to be necessary to sustain improvements in muscle function. Strength training appears to be well accepted by both men and women and to date has proved to be a safe intervention with appropriate supervision.

COMPLIANCE

Dropout rates as high as 50% from recommended exercise programs have been documented (38). Studies show that patients are more likely to participate in such a program if advised to do so by their physicians. Defining clearly the expected health benefits of exercise, such as lowering blood pressure and improving longevity, improves compliance. Older persons are also more likely to participate in activities that easily fit into their daily schedule. Any proposed activity that requires transportation, someone to exercise with, special equipment, or high cost will limit participation. Regular stepwise low-level exercise is preferable to infrequent bouts of strenuous physical activity. Encouragement by the physician or staff members by telephone at biweekly or monthly intervals may promote compliance with an exercise regimen. Visits at 6 months and 1 year to assess improvement in fitness are encouraged.

SUMMARY

Regular physical exercise has beneficial effects on many of the chronic diseases that burden the elderly. In addition, aerobic exercise reduces morbidity and mortality from cardiovascular disease, the primary cause of death for older men and women in the United States. A combined program of aerobic and strength training has great potential for preventing the functional decline associated with aging and preserving an active, independent lifestyle for older people.

REFERENCES

1. Schoenborn CA. Health habits of U.S. adults, 1985: the "Alameda 7" revisited. Public Health Rep 1986;101: 571–580.
2. Pollock M, Wilmore J. Exercise in Health and Disease: Evaluation and Prescription for Prevention and Rehabilitation. 2nd ed. Philadelphia: Saunders, 1990.
3. King AC, Blair SN, Bild DE, et al. Determinants of physical activity and interventions in adults. Med Sci Sports Exerc 1992;24:S221–S236.
4. Blair SN, Kohn LW III, Gordon NF. How much physical activity is good for health? Annu Rev Publ Health 1992;13:99–126.
5. Harris SS, Caspersen CJ, DeFriese GH, Estes H. Physical activity counseling for healthy adults as a primary preventive intervention in the clinical setting. JAMA 1989;261:3590–3598.
6. Paffenbarger RS Jr, Hyde RT, Wing AL, Hsieh CC. Physical activity, all-cause mortality and longevity of college alumni. N Engl J Med 1986;314:605–613.
7. Sherman SE, D'Agostino RB, Cobb JL, Kannel WB. Does

exercise reduce mortality rates in the elderly? Experience from the Framingham Heart Study. Am Heart J 1994;128:965–972.

8. Lee IM, Hsieh C, Paffenbarger RS. Exercise intensity and longevity in men. JAMA 1995;273:1179–1184.

9. Morris JN, Everitt MG, Pollard R, et al. Vigorous exercise in leisure-time: protection against coronary heart disease. Lancet 1980;2:1207–1210.

10. Leon AS, Connett J, Jacobs DR Jr, Rauramaa R. Leisure-time physical activity levels and risk of coronary heart disease and death. The Multiple Risk Factor Intervention Trial. JAMA 1987;258:2388–2395.

11. Slattery ML, Jacobs DR Jr, Nichaman MZ. Leisure time physical activity and coronary heart disease death. The US Railroad Study. Circulation 1989;79:304–311.

12. Lakka TA, Venalainen JM, Rauramaa R, et al. Relation of leisure-time physical activity and cardiorespiratory fitness to the risk of acute myocardial infarction in men. N Engl J Med 1994:330:1549–1554.

13. Gordon NF, Scott CB, Wilkinson WJ, et al. Exercise and mild essential hypertension: recommendations for adults. Sports Med 1990;10:390–404.

14. Hagberg JM. Exercise, fitness, and hypertension. In: Bouchard C, Shephard RJ, Sutton J, McPherson B, eds. Exercise, Fitness, and Health: A Consensus of Current Knowledge. Champaign, IL: Human Kinetics, 1990; 445–466.

15. Duncan JJ, Farr JE, Upton J, et al. The effects of aerobic exercise on plasma catecholamines and blood pressure in patients with mild essential hypertension. JAMA 1985;254:2609–2613.

16. Helmrich SP, Ragland DR, Leung RW, Paffenbarger RS. Physical activity and reduced occurrence of non-insulin dependent diabetes mellitus. N Engl J Med 1991; 325:147–152.

17. King P, Hirshman M, Horton Ed, Horton ES. Glucose transport in skeletal muscle membrane vesicles from control and exercised rats. Am J Physiol 1989;257: C1128–1138.

18. Troisi RJ, Heinold JW, Vokonas PS, Weiss ST. Cigarette smoking, dietary intake, and physical activity: effects on body fat distribution—the Normative Aging Study. Am J Clin Nutr 1991;53:1104–1111.

19. Snow-Harter C, Marcus R. Exercise, bone mineral density and osteoporosis. In: Holloszy JO, ed. Exercise and Sport Sciences Reviews. Baltimore: Williams & Wilkins, 1991;19:351–388.

20. Thompson WG. Exercise and health: fact or hype? South Med J 1994;87:567–574.

21. Gerhardsson M, Floderus B, Norell SE. Physical activity and colon cancer risk. Int J Epidemiol 1988;17:743–746.

22. Hughes JR. Psychological effects of habitual aerobic exercise: A critical review. Prev Med 1984;13:66–78.

23. Fleg JL, Goldberg AP. Exercise in older people: cardiovascular and metabolic adaptations. In: Hazzard WR, Andres R, Bierman EL, Blass J, eds. Principles of Geriatric Medicine and Gerontology. 2nd ed. New York: McGraw-Hill, 1989;85–100.

24. Kligman EW, Pepin E. Prescribing physical activity for older patients. Geriatrics 1991;47:33–47.

25. Bruce RA. Exercise testing of patients with coronary artery disease: principles and normal standards for evaluation. Ann Clin Res 1971;3:323–332.

26. American College of Sports Medicine. Guidelines for Exercise Testing and Prescription. 4th ed. Philadelphia: Lea & Febiger, 1991;314.

27. DeBusk RF, Stenestrand U, Sheehan M, Haskell WL. Training effects of long versus short bouts of exercise in healthy subjects. Am J Cardiol 1990;65:101–113.

28. Johnson RJ. Sudden death during exercise. Postgrad Med 1992;92:195–206.

29. Amsterdam EA. Sudden death during exercise. Cardiology 1990;77:411–417.

30. Pollack ML, Carroll JF, Graves JE, et al. Injuries and adherence to walk/jog and resistance training programs in the elderly. Med Sci Sports Exerc 1991;2: 1194–1200.

31. Matheson GO, McIntyre JG, Taunton JE, et al. Musculoskeletal injuries associated with physical activity in older adults. Med Sci Sports Exerc 1989;21:379–385.

32. Thompson PD. Cardiovascular hazards of physical activity. Exerc Sport Sci Rev 1982;10:208–235.

33. Panush RS, Stemmed C, Caldwell JR, et al. Is running associated with degenerative joint disease? JAMA 1986;255:1152–1154.

34. Lane NE, Bloch DA, Hubert HB, et al. Running, osteoarthritis and bone density: initial 2-year longitudinal study. Am J Med 1990;88:452–459.

35. Ettinger WH Jr, Burns R, Messier SP, et al. A randomized trial comparing aerobic exercise and resistance exercise with a health education program in older adults with knee osteoarthritis. The Fitness, Arthritis and Seniors Trial. JAMA 1997;277:25–31.

36. Nichols JF, Omize DK, Peterson KK, Nelson KP. Efficacy of heavy-resistance training for active women over sixty: muscular strength, body composition, and program adherence. J Am Geriatr Soc 1993;41:205–210.

37. Fiatarone MA, Marks EC, Ryan ND, et al. High-intensity strength training in nonagenarians: effects on skeletal muscle. JAMA 1990;263:3029–3034.

38. Buskirk ER. Exercise, fitness, and aging. In: Bouchard C, Shepard RJ, Stephens T, et al., eds. Exercise, Fitness, and Health: A Consensus of Current Knowledge. Champaign, IL: Human Kinetics, 1990;687–695.

CHAPTER 10

G. WEBSTER ROSS, ROBERT PARIS, AND HELEN PETROVITCH

Stroke Prevention and Management

Stroke is the third largest cause of death in the United States and the leading cause of serious long-term disability among the elderly. The estimated direct and indirect cost of stroke in the United States for 1997 is $40.9 billion (1). Improved risk factor control and better care of patients are probably related to the 4% per year steady decline in mortality from stroke that occurred in the United States between the mid-1960s and late 1980s (2). This decline, however, seems to have leveled off (3, 4). The public health effect of stroke is, on the other hand, beginning to increase as the proportion of elderly persons in the United States and other developed countries rises.

Fortunately, stroke research in recent years has helped to clarify pharmacologic and surgical issues related to stroke prevention. This chapter focuses on prevention of stroke, both primary and secondary, and on management of stroke during the acute and rehabilitation phases. The study of stroke prevention and management is complicated by the fact that there are several subtypes of stroke, each having different mechanisms and risk factor profiles. The underlying mechanism must be sought with a thorough clinical history, physical examination, and appropriate diagnostic tests (Table 10.1). Distinguishing between brain hemorrhages, comprising approximately 25% of strokes, and infarctions, which make up the remaining 75%, is important for management decisions. Infarction can be subclassified by the mechanism of ischemia. Cardioembolic strokes secondary to emboli originating in the heart constitute approximately 20% of infarctions. Some 15% are related to atherothrombo-

sis of the extracranial or intracranial large cerebral vessels or to emboli arising from an atherosclerotic source in these arteries. Lacunar infarctions (approximately 25% of infarctions) are caused by occlusion of arterioles supplying the basal ganglia, thalamus, periventricular white matter, and brainstem. The cause of the remaining 40% of infarctions cannot be determined, attesting to the fact that subclassification remains imprecise (5).

PRIMARY PREVENTION

The public health goal of primary stroke prevention is to decrease the incidence of first-ever stroke by modifying factors that increase risk of stroke. While increasing age, male gender, nonwhite race, and family history of stroke are all unmodifiable stroke risk factors, they can be used to identify the stroke-prone patient for further counseling and intervention.

Treatment of Modifiable Risk Factors
Hypertension

Hypertension, defined as blood pressure of 140/90 mm Hg or greater, is the most important of the modifiable risk factors. In fact, it is estimated that half of the 500,000 new stroke cases per year in the United States might be prevented with adequate control of hypertension (6). Reduced stroke risk has been demonstrated with treatment of mild, moderate, and severe hypertension (7) and for adults of all ages. Drug therapy has been shown to reduce incidence of stroke by 45% among older persons with diastolic hypertension (8, 9) and by 36% in men and women aged 65 years or more with isolated

Table 10.1

Diagnostic Tests for the Evaluation of Stroke

Diagnostic tests for emergency management
  Brain computed tomographic scan
  Chest radiograph
  Electrocardiogram
  Lumbar puncture
  Blood tests
    Complete blood and platelet count,
      prothrombin time, partial thromboplastin time
    Serum glucose and electrolytes, hepatic and
      renal function tests
Diagnostic tests for underlying mechanism and
    definitive management in selected patients
  Brain magnetic resonance image
  Magnetic resonance angiography
  Carotid duplex
  Echocardiography
    Transesophageal
    Transthoracic
    Contrast echocardiography
  Holter monitor
  Cerebral angiography
  Blood tests
    Erythrocyte sedimentation rate, antinuclear
      antibodies
    Antiphospholipid antibodies, VDRL/RPR

systolic hypertension (10). It has been suggested that a reasonable target for adequate hypertension control be considered a blood pressure at or below 125/85 mm Hg (11). However, there is disagreement regarding the lowest acceptable levels. It is probably best to treat only patients with blood pressure above 140/90 mm Hg and to bear in mind that overtreatment of hypertension may have an adverse effect on stroke risk.

Dietary and Lifestyle Factors

Cigarette smoking may be the second most important risk factor for stroke (12). As many as 61,500, or 12.3%, of new strokes occurring in the United States every year could be prevented by discontinuing smoking (6). Moreover, by 5 years after smoking cessation, stroke risk of ex-smokers is at the same level as that of non-smokers (13).

Elevated serum cholesterol is a risk factor for ischemic stroke, although the evidence is not as conclusive as it is for coronary artery disease (14, 15). A negative association of serum cholesterol with hemorrhagic stroke has been reported (16). Results of clinical trials examining the effect of cholesterol-lowering agents on stroke incidence are mixed (17, 18). However, the most recent evidence demonstrates that using 3-hydroxy-3-methylglutaryl coenzyme A reductase inhibitors (HMG CoA, or statin drugs) results in large reductions in serum cholesterol with concomitant significant reduction in stroke risk in middle-aged patients (18). The routine use of cholesterol-lowering agents in the elderly for reducing stroke risk cannot be recommended until clinical trials demonstrate safety and efficacy of these medications in persons over age 65.

Obesity affects one third of adults in the United States. Epidemiologic evidence supports obesity as an independent risk factor for ischemic stroke (19, 20). Although there have been no trials to assess the effect of weight reduction on stroke incidence, known overall health benefits make it reasonable to recommend weight reduction to reduce stroke risk in obese patients.

A physically active lifestyle has been found to be associated with a decreased risk of both ischemic and hemorrhagic stroke (21, 22). This is in part mediated by the beneficial effects of exercise on weight, blood pressure, high density lipoprotein levels, and insulin sensitivity (23).

Cardiac Conditions

The most important cardiac risk factor for stroke is atrial fibrillation (AF). Both the prevalence of AF and the number of strokes related to it increase with age. The attributable risk of stroke from AF rises from 1.5% during the sixth decade of life to 23.5% during the ninth decade (24). Acute myocardial infarction (MI), especially of the anterior wall, is associated with stroke, as are chronic congestive heart failure, valvular heart disease, and sick sinus syndrome. Abnormal ventricular wall motion or dysrhythmias lead to the formation of thrombi that can break off as emboli and occlude the cerebral vessels.

Pooled data from five large clinical trials comparing warfarin with placebo in patients aged 67 to 73 years with AF indicate that warfarin prevents stroke. There was a 65% reduction in stroke in the warfarin-treated groups over 1.2 to 2.3 years of follow-up (25). In addition, warfarin was more effective than aspirin in patients with AF and was safe for most patients. Only 1% of warfarin-treated patients had major bleeding, compared with 0.9% of controls, and the rate of major bleeding was related to the intensity of anticoagulation (especially with an international normalized ratio [INR] above 3) and uncontrolled hypertension (26). Guidelines from the American Heart Association for the use of warfarin in patients with AF have been developed. Patients below age 65 with AF and no other risk factors (lone AF) have a low risk of stroke not significantly lowered by warfarin and should take one aspirin a day (27). Warfarin at a dose to maintain the INR at 2 to 3 should be strongly considered for patients below age 65 who have other risk factors, including previous stroke, transient ischemic attack (TIA), hypertension, or congestive heart failure, and for any patient aged 65 years or above with AF (27). The benefit of warfarin for patients over age 75 remains uncertain. Evidence suggests that in this group warfarin is associated with a greater risk of intracerebral hemorrhage and may not be more effective than aspirin (26, 28). Aspirin may be the most reasonable choice for stroke prevention in these patients, especially if they are frail or prone to falls.

Diabetes Mellitus

Persons with diabetes or glucose intolerance have a risk of thromboembolic stroke 1.5 to 4 times that of persons with normal glucose tolerance. This effect is independent of other risk factors and is thought to be related to accelerated atherosclerosis and an increase in intracerebral small vessel disease. (29–31). There is no evidence thus far that strict glucose control reduces the risk of stroke (32).

Surgical Management

Carotid Artery Stenosis

Carotid artery stenosis is another important risk factor for stroke. Internal carotid artery stenosis of 50% or more is present in approximately 5% of the elderly population (33). The rate of TIA and stroke in patients with asymptomatic stenosis above 75% is more than 3% annually compared with slightly more than 1% for those with less than 75% stenosis (34). Recent evidence from the Asymptomatic Carotid Atherosclerosis Study shows that patients with asymptomatic carotid artery stenosis of 60% or more who undergo carotid endarterectomy (CEA) have a statistically significant 50% 5-year risk reduction for ipsilateral stroke, compared with those treated medically (35). The generalizability of the study findings has been questioned because of the stringent eligibility criteria and strict selection of surgical centers with low rates (below 2.3%) of perioperative stroke or death (36). The cost effectiveness of CEA for asymptomatic carotid stenosis has likewise not been proved (37). Treating physicians, however, must independently evaluate each patient with asymptomatic stenosis greater than 60% and base judgments of potential benefits and risks of surgery on the patient's general health and access to surgical centers with expertise in this procedure (38). For patients ineligible for surgery, risk factor control and one aspirin a day are reasonable options. Screening the general population for carotid stenosis is thought to be not a wise use of public health resources (36, 39).

Pharmacologic Management

Aspirin

Two trials have found no benefit of aspirin for the primary prevention of stroke (40, 41). In fact, there was a modest increase in intracerebral hemorrhage among those taking aspirin in the Physician's Health Study (40). A recent review of randomized trials of antiplatelet therapy found that high-risk patients (those with MI, angina, vascular surgery, angioplasty, peripheral vascular disease, or diabetes) treated with aspirin have a significantly lower rate of nonfatal stroke, while no decrease in stroke occurrence was found in low-risk patients receiving aspirin (42). The routine use of aspirin for the primary prevention of stroke, therefore, cannot be recommended for patients who have no other vascular risk factors.

Hormone Replacement Therapy

The favorable effect of estrogen on serum lipoproteins and fibrinogen provides biologic plausibility for estrogen having a protective effect against stroke (43); however, longitudinal studies of stroke risk show mixed results. Some show no association between stroke risk and current use of estrogen (44),and others demonstrate a reduction in stroke incidence and mortality in postmenopausal women taking either estrogen replacement alone or estrogen plus progestin (45, 46).

SECONDARY PREVENTION OF STROKE
Antiplatelet Medications

Aspirin and ticlopidine are inhibitors of platelet aggregation. It has been clearly shown that aspirin reduces the risk of recurrent stroke among patients with a history of TIA or stroke by more than 20% (42). Doses as low as 75 mg and as high as 1300 mg have been reported to be effective, with no clear evidence that high doses are more effective than low doses (42). Low doses seem preferable to minimize the gastrointestinal side effects and risk of serious bleeding. A reasonable dose is 325 mg per day. For patients who have persistent cerebral ischemic events while taking aspirin or who are aspirin intolerant, ticlopidine 250 mg twice daily should be considered (47). Ticlopidine is the only approved platelet inhibitor other than aspirin that has been proved to reduce risk of recurrent stroke (48, 49). Although it is slightly more effective than aspirin, it is not recommended as a first-line agent because of gastrointestinal side effects, a 2% incidence of reversible neutropenia requiring frequent monitoring of blood count, and rare death from aplastic anemia.

Carotid Endarterectomy

For patients with a history of TIA or nondisabling stroke who have ipsilateral internal carotid artery stenosis of 70% or more, CEA plus best medical care has been proved superior to best medical care alone (including aspirin therapy) (50, 51). The mean ages of patients for the two major trials examining CEA for symptomatic carotid stenosis were 62 and 65, and those above age 80 were excluded from one trial (50, 51). Data regarding the beneficial effects of CEA for the oldest old, therefore, are lacking. The surgical referral center should have experience performing the procedure and a low perioperative stroke and death rate. Patients with moderate stenosis (30 to 69%) have not been clearly shown to benefit from CEA.

MANAGEMENT OF ACUTE STROKE

Management of stroke during the acute phase is focused on minimizing the size of the infarction, reestablishing cerebral perfusion, and preventing new events and complications. Evidence suggests that stroke patients have lower mortality and improved functional outcome when hospitalized in specialized stroke units where care is coordinated by a multidisciplinary team of trained physicians, nurses, and rehabilitation therapists (52–54).

Initial supportive measures for acute ischemic stroke require close attention to blood pressure, oxygenation, and temperature. High blood pressure is often present during the first few days following a stroke, and it is tempting for clinicians to reduce blood pressure with medication to the "normal" range below 140/90. This may cause a decrease in cerebral perfusion and extension of the infarct because of impaired cerebral autoregulation, which worsens the neurologic deficit. In patients with chronic hypertension, autoregulation is altered, leading to brain hypoperfusion at low blood pressure levels that would be well tolerated in normotensive individuals (55). During acute stroke, higher blood pressure levels may help maintain cerebral perfusion. Recommendations are to not treat hypertension during acute ischemic stroke unless the systolic blood pressure exceeds 220 mm Hg, the calculated mean blood pressure exceeds 130 mm Hg, or there is acute hemorrhagic transformation of the infarct, MI, hypertensive encephalopathy, or aortic dissection (56). An exception to these guidelines is when recombinant tissue plasminogen activator (r-TPA) is used for thrombolysis. In that case blood pressure should be maintained below 185/110. Fever during the acute stroke phase has been associated with worsening outcome; therefore, it should be treated with antipyretics (56).

Complications such as deep vein thrombosis, pulmonary embolism, dysphagia and concomitant aspiration, skin breakdown, and falls are causes of significant morbidity and mortality in stroke patients. The use of low-dose subcutaneous heparin or low molecular weight heparin prevents deep vein thrombosis (57). Additional recommendations include early assessment of swallowing and initiation of a compensatory feeding program in patients with swallowing disorder, daily inspection and gentle cleansing of skin, and avoidance of skin injury through proper positioning and frequent turning when necessary to prevent skin breakdown. Use of chronic indwelling urinary catheters, which increase risk of urinary tract infection and sepsis, should be avoided. Early mobilization provides positive psychologic reinforcement for the patient and helps to prevent deep vein thrombosis and skin breakdown (52).

The management of acute stroke is changing dramatically. Thrombolytic therapy is becoming an accepted treatment to reestablish cerebral flow. Thrombolytic agents promote clot lysis by enhancing the conversion of plasminogen to plasmin, leading to fibrin degradation. A recent National Institute of Neurological Disorders and Stroke (NINDS)-sponsored trial shows that patients with acute stroke who receive r-TPA within 3 hours of onset have a better functional outcome than those treated with placebo, although r-TPA treatment is associated with an increased risk of symptomatic brain hemorrhage (58). This evidence led the U.S. Food and Drug Administration (FDA) to approve the drug for use in stroke in June 1996. Published guidelines for the use of this agent include patient selection criteria adopted from the NINDS study (Table 10.2) (58–60). Facilities with intensive care units or acute stroke units where bleeding and other complications may be managed promptly are crucial to optimal management.

Table 10.2

Recommendations for Selecting Patients for the Use of Intravenous Recombinant Tissue Plasminogen Activator (58)

Diagnosis is made by physician with expertise in diagnosing stroke

Brain CT is read by physicians with expertise in CT interpretation and shows no evidence of hemorrhage or early signs of large infarction

Treatment initiated within 3 hours of symptom onset

Exclusion criteria

  Previous stroke or head trauma within preceding 3 months

  Major surgery within 14 days

  History of intracranial hemorrhage

  Current use of oral anticoagulants or PT $>$ 15 seconds

  Use of heparin in the previous 48 hours

  Platelet count $<$ 100,000/mm^3

  Pretreatment systolic blood pressure $>$ 185 mm Hg or diastolic blood pressure $>$ 110 mm Hg

  Blood glucose $<$ 50 mg/dL or $<$ 400 mg/dL

  Seizure at the onset of stroke

  Gastrointestinal or urinary bleeding within preceding 21 days

  Recent myocardial infarction

  Rapidly improving neurologic signs

  Minor or isolated neurologic deficits

STROKE REHABILITATION

According to the Agency for Health Care Policy and Research clinical practice guideline *Post-Stroke Rehabilitation*, stroke rehabilitation includes prevention of secondary complications, treatment to reduce neurologic deficits, compensatory training to adapt to residual disabilities, and maintenance of function over the long term. To accomplish these goals rehabilitation should begin as soon as the diagnosis of stroke has been made and life-threatening complications resolved. The best candidates for admission to stroke rehabilitation programs are medically stable with one or more persistent disabilities and with preserved ability to learn and stamina to participate actively in the program (52). Upon admission to a rehabilitation program, a patient should have a baseline assessment, including standard measurement instruments for cognitive and communicative function, motor function, and disabilities in basic activities of daily living.

Attention to the neuropsychiatric complications of stroke are important not only for the patient but also for the family and other caregivers. Appropriate management of depression and other disturbances of behavior can improve the quality of life for the patient and enhance chances for a successful transition from hospital to home. Depression, which affects 30 to 50% of stroke patients, is most likely to occur in the first 2 years after stroke. It occurs most commonly in patients with left frontal strokes and in those with a history of psychiatric disease. The clinical syndrome is identical to idiopathic major depression, and patients respond to antidepressants as well as do those with major depression (61). Poststroke mania, which is much less common than depression (0.5%), is associated with right posterobasilar lesions. Conventional treatment with lithium, anticonvulsants, and neuroleptics is effective (61). Approximately 25% of stroke patients develop vascular dementia. Prevention and treatment of this complication are based on preventing recurrent stroke.

CONCLUSIONS

Primary prevention of stroke depends on risk factor control. Treatment of hypertension and cessation of smoking prevent stroke in the elderly. Weight loss in the obese patient and physical activity may lower stroke risk and improve general health, and hormone replacement therapy in postmenopausal women may also reduce stroke incidence. Warfarin should be considered for patients with AF who are age 65 and over or for those of any age who have other stroke risk factors. The excess risk of cerebral hemorrhage may preclude the use of warfarin in patients over age 75. Aspirin can be used when warfarin is contraindicated. Although there is evidence that CEA lowers stroke risk in patients with asymptomatic carotid stenosis greater than 60%, clinicians should consider the surgical risk of the patient as well as the experience of the surgical referral center prior to recommending CEA. Screening the general public for carotid artery stenosis is not thought to be a cost-effective strategy. Cholesterol-lowering agents look promising

for reducing stroke risk, but more research is needed to clarify the efficacy of these agents in the elderly.

Patients with a history of mild stroke or TIA and no indications for warfarin therapy should be treated with one aspirin a day to prevent recurrence. If aspirin is contraindicated or ineffective, ticlopidine can be substituted. Carotid endarterectomy should be considered for symptomatic patients with ipsilateral stenosis greater than 70%. More research is needed to define indications for this procedure in the oldest old.

The management of acute stroke is becoming more like that of acute MI, emphasizing early, aggressive intervention with clot-lysing agents for cerebral infarction. Experienced clinicians and facilities capable of quickly evaluating the patient on presentation as well as managing the complications of thrombolytic therapy (preferably in specialized stroke units) are essential for the safe and successful use of r-TPA.

Rehabilitation of stroke patients is aimed at preventing complications and maximizing functional outcome. Stroke patients with adequate cognition who are medically stable can best be treated in rehabilitation centers with access to physical, occupational, and speech therapy and programs to assist with return to the community.

REFERENCES

1. American Heart Association. Heart and Stroke Facts 1997. Statistical Update. Dallas, Texas: American Heart Association, 1997.
2. Vital Statistics of the United States, 1989. Vol 2: Mortality, Part A. Hyattsville, MD: National Center for Health Statistics, 1993.
3. Broderick JP, Phillips SJ, Whisnant JP, et al. Incidence rates of stroke in the eighties: the end of the decline in stroke? Stroke 1989;20:577–582.
4. Kagan A, Popper J, Reed DM, et al. Trends in stroke incidence and mortality in Hawaiian Japanese men. Stroke 1994;25:1170–1175.
5. Sacco RL, Ellenberg JH, Tatemichi TK, et al. Infarcts of undetermined cause: the NINCDS Stroke Data Bank. Ann Neurol 1989;25:382–390.
6. Gorelick PB. Stroke prevention: an opportunity for efficient utilization of health care resources during the coming decade. Stroke 1994;25:220–224.
7. Collins R, Peto R, MacMahon S, et al. Blood pressure, stroke, and coronary heart disease. Part 2. Short-term reductions in blood pressure: overview of randomised drug trials in their epidemiological context. Lancet 1990;335:827–838.

8. Five-year findings of the hypertension detection and follow-up program. III. Reduction in stroke incidence among persons with high blood pressure. Hypertension Detection and Follow-up Program Cooperative Group. JAMA 1982;247:633–638.

9. Curb JD, Borhani NO, Schnaper H, et al. Detection and treatment of hypertension in older individuals. Am J Epidemiol 1985;121:371–376.

10. Prevention of stroke by antihypertensive drug treatment in older persons with isolated systolic hypertension. Final results of the Systolic Hypertension in the Elderly Program (SHEP). SHEP Cooperative Research Group. JAMA 1991;265:3255–3264.

11. Fletcher AE, Bulpitt CJ. How far should blood pressure be lowered? N Engl J Med 1992;326:251–254.

12. Abbott RD, Yin Y, Reed DM, Yano K. Risk of stroke in male cigarette smokers. N Engl J Med 1986;315:717–720.

13. Wolf PA, D'Agostino RB, Kannel WB, et al. Cigarette smoking as a risk factor for stroke. The Framingham Study. JAMA 1988;259:1025–1029.

14. Benfante R, Yano K, Hwang LJ, et al. Elevated serum cholesterol is a risk factor for both coronary heart disease and thromboembolic stroke in Hawaiian Japanese men: implications of shared risk. Stroke 1994;25:814–820.

15. Lindenstrom E, Boysen G, Nyboe J. Influence of total cholesterol, high density lipoprotein cholesterol, and triglycerides on risk of cerebrovascular disease: the Copenhagen City Heart Study. BMJ 1994;309:11–15.

16. Yano K, Reed DM, MacLean CJ. Serum cholesterol and hemorrhagic stroke in the Honolulu Heart Program. Stroke 1989;20:1460–1465.

17. Atkins D, Psaty BM, Koepsell TD, et al. Cholesterol reduction and the risk for stroke in men: a meta-analysis of randomized, controlled trials. Ann Intern Med 1993;119:136–145.

18. Hebert PR, Gaziano JM, Chan KS, Hennekens CH. Cholesterol lowering with statin drugs, risk of stroke, and total mortality: an overview of randomized trials. JAMA 1997;278:313–321.

19. Abbott RD, Behrens GR, Sharp DS, et al. Body mass index and thromboembolic stroke in nonsmoking men in older middle age. The Honolulu Heart Program. Stroke 1994;25:2370–2376.

20. Rexrode KM, Hennekens CH, Willett WC, et al. A prospective study of body mass index, weight change, and risk of stroke in women. JAMA 1997;227:1539–1545.

21. Abbott RD, Rodriguez BL, Burchfiel CM, Curb JD. Physical activity in older middle-aged men and reduced risk of stroke: the Honolulu Heart Program. Am J Epidemiol 1994;139:881–893.

22. Kiely DK, Wolf PA, Cupples LA, et al. Physical activity and stroke risk: the Framingham Study. Am J Epidemiol 1994;140:608–620.

23. Bronner LL, Kanter DS, Manson JE. Primary prevention of stroke. N Engl J Med 1995;333:1392–1400.

24. Wolf PA, Abbott RD, Kannel WB. Atrial fibrillation as an independent risk factor for stroke: the Framingham Study. Stroke 1991;22:983–988.

25. Risk factors for stroke and efficacy of antithrombotic therapy in atrial fibrillation. Analysis of pooled data from five randomized controlled trials. Arch Intern Med 1994;154:1449–1457.

26. Albers GW. Atrial fibrillation and stroke: three new studies, three remaining questions. Arch Intern Med 1994;154:1443–1448.

27. Prystowsky EN, Benson DW Jr, Fuster V, et al. Management of patients with atrial fibrillation. A Statement for Healthcare Professionals. From the Subcommittee on Electrocardiography and Electrophysiology, American Heart Association.. Circulation 1996;93:1262–1277.

28. Warfarin versus aspirin for prevention of thromboembolism in atrial fibrillation: Stroke Prevention in Atrial Fibrillation II Study. Lancet 1994;343:687–691.

29. Burchfiel CM, Curb JD, Rodriguez BL, et al. Glucose intolerance and 22-year stroke incidence. The Honolulu Heart Program. Stroke 1994;25:951–957.

30. Abbott RD, Donahue RP, MacMahon SW, et al. Diabetes and the risk of stroke. The Honolulu Heart Program. JAMA 1987;257:949–952.

31. Currie CJ, Morgan CL, Gill L, et al. Epidemiology and costs of acute hospital care for cerebrovascular disease in diabetic and nondiabetic populations. Stroke 1997;28:1142–1146.

32. Alter M, Lai SM, Friday G, et al. Stroke recurrence in diabetics: does control of blood glucose reduce risk? Stroke 1997;28:1153–1157.

33. Pujia A, Rubba P, Spencer MP. Prevalence of extracranial carotid artery disease detectable by echo-Doppler in an elderly population. Stroke 1992;23:818–822.

34. Norris JW, Zhu CZ, Bornstein NM, Chambers BR. Vascular risks of asymptomatic carotid stenosis. Stroke 1991;22:1485–1490.

35. Endarterectomy for asymptomatic carotid artery stenosis. Executive Committee for the Asymptomatic Carotid Atherosclerosis Study. JAMA 1995;273:1421–1428.

36. Perry JR, Szalai JP, Norris JW. Consensus against both endarterectomy and routine screening for asymptomatic carotid artery stenosis. Arch Neurol 1997;54:24–28.

37. Frey JL. Asymptomatic carotid stenosis: surgery's the answer, but that's not the question. Ann Neurol 1996;405–406.

38. Toole JF. Quality-based medicine. Arch Neurol 1997;54:23–24.

39. Lee TT, Solomon NA, Heidenreich PA, et al. Cost-effectiveness of screening for carotid stenosis in asymptomatic persons. Ann Intern Med 1997;126:337–346.

40. Final report on the aspirin component of the ongoing Physicians' Health Study. Steering Committee of the Physicians' Health Study Research Group. N Engl J Med 1989;321:129–135.

41. Peto R, Gray R, Collins R, et al. Randomised trial of prophylactic daily aspirin in British male doctors. BMJ 1988;296:313–316.

42. Collaborative overview of randomised trials of an-

tiplatelet therapy. I. Prevention of death, myocardial infarction, and stroke by prolonged antiplatelet therapy in various categories of patients. Antiplatelet Trialists' Collaboration. BMJ 1994;308:81–106.

43. Effects of estrogen or estrogen/progestin regimens on heart disease risk factors in postmenopausal women. The Postmenopausal Estrogen/Progestin Interventions (PEPI) Trial. The Writing Group for the PEPI Trial. JAMA 1995;273:199–208.

44. Grodstein F, Stampfer MJ, Manson JE, et al. Postmenopausal estrogen and progestin use and the risk of cardiovascular disease. N Engl J Med 1996;335:453–461.

45. Finucane FF, Madans JH, Bush TL, et al. Decreased risk of stroke among postmenopausal hormone users: results from a national cohort. Arch Intern Med 1993; 153:73–79.

46. Falkeborn M, Persson I, Terént A, et al. Hormone replacement therapy and the risk of stroke: follow-up of a population-based cohort in Sweden. Arch Intern Med 1993;153:1201–1209.

47. Haynes RB, Sandler RS, Larson EB, et al. A critical appraisal of ticlopidine, a new antiplatelet agent: effectiveness and clinical indications for prophylaxis of atherosclerotic events. Arch Intern Med 1992;152:1376–1380.

48. Hass WK, Easton JD, Adams HP Jr, et al. A randomized trial comparing ticlopidine hydrochloride with aspirin for the prevention of stroke in high-risk patients. N Engl J Med 1989;321:501–507.

49. Gent M, Easton JD, Hachinski VC, et al. The Canadian American Ticlopidine Study (CATS) in thromboembolic stroke. Lancet 1989;1:1215–1220.

50. MRC European Carotid Surgery Trial: interim results for symptomatic patients with severe (70–99%) or with mild (0–29%) carotid stenosis. European Carotid Surgery Trialists' Collaborative Group.. Lancet 1991; 337:1235–1243.

51. Beneficial effect of carotid endarterectomy in symptomatic patients with high-grade carotid stenosis. North American Symptomatic Carotid Endarterectomy Trial Collaborators. N Engl J Med 1991;325:445–453.

52. Gresham GE, Duncan PW, Stason WB, et al. Post-Stroke Rehabilitation. Clinical Practice Guideline 16 (AHCPR 95-0662). Rockville, MD: US Department of Health and Human Services, Public Health Service, Agency for Health Care Policy and Research, 1995.

53. Kalra L, Dale P, Crome P. Improving stroke rehabilitation: a controlled study. Stroke 1993;24:1462–1467.

54. Jorgensen HS, Nakayama H, Raaschou HO, et al. The effect of a stroke unit: reductions in mortality, discharge rate to nursing home, length of hospital stay, and cost: a community-based study. Stroke 1995;26: 1178–1182.

55. Powers WJ. Acute hypertension after stroke: the scientific basis for treatment decisions. Neurology 1993; 43:461–467.

56. Adams HP Jr, Brott TG, Crowell RM, et al. Guidelines for the management of patients with acute ischemic stroke. A statement for healthcare professionals from a special writing group of the Stroke Council, American Heart Association. Stroke 1994;25:1901–1914.

57. Clagett GP, Anderson FA, Levine MN, et al. Prevention of venous thromboembolism. Chest 1992;102:391S–407S.

58. Tissue plasminogen activator for acute ischemic stroke. The National Institute of Neurological Disorders and Stroke r-TPA Stroke Study Group. N Engl J Med 1995;333:1581–1587.

59. Practice advisory: thrombolytic therapy for acute ischemic stroke—summary statement. Report of the Quality Standards Subcommittee of the American Academy of Neurology. Neurology 1996;47:835–839.

60. Adams HP Jr, Brott TG, Furlan AJ, et al. Guidelines for Thrombolytic Therapy for Acute Stroke: a supplement to the Guidelines for the Management of Patients with Acute Ischemic Stroke. A statement for healthcare professionals from a Special Writing Group of the Stroke Council, American Heart Association. Stroke 1996;27:1711–1718.

61. Beckson M, Cummings JL. Neuropsychiatric aspects of stroke. Int J Psychiatry Med 1991;21:1–15.

Pulmonary Problems in the Elderly

Pulmonary disease is a common cause of morbidity and mortality in the elderly. However, it is not inevitable, and despite an age-related decline in pulmonary function, it is never normal for a person to have to curtail normal levels of activity because of a pulmonary limitation. Thus the development of symptoms referable to the respiratory system, such as the subjective sensation of dyspnea, should always prompt a medical evaluation.

The various pulmonary diseases and symptoms that occur in aging populations are not unique to the elderly, but they do differ in prevalence and commonly in natural history from their manifestations in younger populations. This chapter is an overview of the common pulmonary symptoms and specific diseases that are particularly relevant to clinical practice in elder populations.

PULMONARY SIGNS AND SYMPTOMS

Pulmonary disease or insufficiency is associated with a variety of signs and symptoms. Many symptoms, such as fatigue, weakness, and weight loss, are nonspecific, but others, such as dyspnea, cough, wheezing, pleuritic chest discomfort, and hemoptysis, most often indicate pulmonary disease.

Dyspnea (shortness of breath or breathlessness) is a common clinical symptom. It is often precipitated by primary respiratory system abnormalities but can also be due to cardiac (e.g., pulmonary edema), systemic (e.g., deconditioning or anemia) or psychogenic (e.g., anxiety) factors. A thorough history, which is essential,

should include the acuity of the complaint and its severity. A positional component, such as orthopnea or platypnea, often suggests a specific cause, as can associated signs and symptoms. Dyspnea absent at rest may be present or exacerbated with exertion. The cause of dyspnea can generally be determined with minimal investigation beyond a detailed history and physical examination, and diagnostic testing is often limited to a standard chest radiograph (preferably both posteroanterior (PA) and lateral projections), a 12-lead electrical cardiogram, an objective measure of airflow (e.g., spirometry) and an objective assessment of gas exchange (pulse oximetry for screening or an arterial blood gas analysis) (1).

Cough is a common pulmonary complaint in elder patients. A cough with expectoration of purulent material suggests inflammation, possibly due to infection with bacteria, viruses, or *Mycobacterium;* chronic irritation from noxious agents such as cigarette smoke; or asthmatic inflammatory airway disease. A nonproductive or dry cough has a much broader differential diagnosis. Acute cough is more likely to be due to infection than chronic cough. Chronic cough, lasting more than a month, is most often due to postnasal drip, viral airway hyperactivity, cough-variant asthma, or gastroesophageal reflux (2). Furthermore, several pharmacologic agents, most notably the ACE inhibitors, can produce chronic cough. Congestive heart failure, bronchogenic lung cancer, recurrent aspiration, and interstitial lung disease (ILD) are less common causes, together accounting for fewer than 10% of cases (2). Cough should be considered a symptom, and therapy is best directed at the presumed diagnosis (e.g., decongestants, bronchodilators, or antacid treatments) rather than at cough suppression with antitussive agents (dextromethorphan or codeine).

Wheezing can be an isolated auscultatory finding on lung examination, may be audible to an examiner without a stethoscope, and frequently is first noted by patients. It is important not to confuse wheezing with stridor, as stridor indicates upper airway pathology (i.e., obstruction from tumor, vocal cord paralysis, or angioedema) and wheezing indicates lower airway pathology. Wheezing can be focal, as in the case of a localized obstruction (tumor or foreign body), or diffuse. Pleuritic or respirophasic chest discomfort indicates inflammation of the pleura and is often accompanied by a pleural friction rub on examination. The pulmonary parenchyma itself has no pain receptors, so pulmonary disorders such as pneumonia and pulmonary embolism do not cause pain unless they involve the pleura. Respirophasic chest discomfort should prompt an evaluation for infectious or other inflammatory causes, such as pneumonia, pulmonary thromboembolism, pneumothorax, and malignancy.

Hemoptysis is almost always due to an abnormality in the airways. It is critical to distinguish this complaint from both hematemesis and bleeding from above the larynx (e.g., epistaxis). In patients with hemoptysis the primary considerations include lower respiratory tract infection (i.e., bronchitis or pneumonia), bronchiectasis, bronchogenic cancer, and pulmonary tuberculosis (TB). Less common causes of hemoptysis are coagulopathy, pulmonary thromboembolism, and pulmonary alveolar hemorrhage syndromes (e.g., pulmonary vasculitis). The volume of hemoptysis is of little value in determining its cause, and bronchoscopic evaluation is often required.

CHRONIC OBSTRUCTIVE PULMONARY DISEASE AND ASTHMA

Chronic obstructive pulmonary disease (COPD) affecting the elderly comprises a group of disorders: emphysema, chronic bronchitis, bronchiectasis, and asthma. These disorders are related and are rightly considered together (3). Clinically, the term COPD is often used interchangeably with both chronic bronchitis and pulmonary emphysema. In the United States it is estimated that between 10 and 20% of the adult population is affected, with more than 3 million having severe impairment (4). These two conditions generally coexist to varying degrees in the same patients, are related to cigarette smoking, and respond to the same treatments, so this use of the term is justified. Chronic bronchitis is defined by the clinical findings of a productive cough for at least 3 months in each of 2 consecutive years. Hypertrophy of the mucous glands and mucous hypersecretion are the primary pathologic abnormalities. Pulmonary emphysema is characterized by diffuse parenchymal destruction, hyperinflation, and loss of alveolar surface area. Until recently, emphysema could be suspected clinically but only diagnosed pathologically. Most experts now accept high-resolution chest computed tomography (CT), which characteristically demonstrates widespread cystic dilation of terminal airspaces, thin-walled cysts and bullae, as diagnostic in the appropriate clinical context. Patients with COPD are prone to hypoventilation (CO_2 retention) and can develop either hypercarbic or hypoxemic respiratory failure. Bronchiectasis, the irreversible dilation and destruction of airways, is much less common in recent decades because of the appropriate use of antibiotics to treat respiratory infection. It frequently coexists with COPD and is characteristically associated with copious sputum production.

Patients with COPD come to medical attention in a variety of ways. Some develop disease insidiously, with a chronic cough, progressive dyspnea, weight loss, or fatigue. Poor nutritional status is common. Others develop respiratory failure (hypoxic or hypercarbic) in an exacerbation due to superimposed infection. Significant bronchospasm is common. Alternatively, in relatively asymptomatic persons, diagnosis can be incidental after a suggestive chest radiograph or screening spirometry. Unfortunately, many elder patients go undiagnosed, with pulmonary symptoms being falsely attributed to aging (5).

Asthma can appear at any age and may persist for a lifetime. It can best be described by its clinical features, airway inflammation with mucous hypersecretion and reversible airflow limitation (reactive airway disease). Patients may have either long-standing or new-onset disease (5–7). Asthma is very common in the general population, with a prevalence of 7 to 8% (5). This prevalence likely increases with age. Although the incidence is thought to decrease after childhood, there is a second peak in the elderly. Elders, however, are less likely to exhibit overt symptoms and frequently have more subtle and less specific manifestations. As with COPD, the high level of comorbidity in elder populations and the tendency for care providers falsely to ascribe many less specific respiratory symptoms to aging have led to underappreciation of this problem.

A true assessment of the epidemiology of asthma in elders over age 65 is complicated by the high prevalence of a cigarette smoking and concurrent cardiac disease, but estimates for reactive airways range as high as 10%. Mortality in older asthmatic populations is eightfold higher than that of younger populations. The overall mortality for asthmatics is 0.6 per 100,000 popluation, but in those over 65 with asthma the mortality is 4.9 per 100,000 population (5). Unlike younger patients, who die of their asthma, older patients generally die of a comorbidity and only uncommonly of asthma per se.

The evaluation requisite to make the diagnosis of COPD, asthma, or asthmatic bronchitis need not be extensive but should include some objective physiologic assessment of pulmonary function to complement a compatible clinical history and physical examination. In most cases simple office spirometry suffices. Patients with COPD characteristically demonstrate airflow limitation (a reduced ratio of forced expiratory volume in 1 second (FEV_1) to forced vital capacity (FVC); FEV_1/FVC less than 70%), which may be partially reversed after the administration of a bronchodilator if there is coexistent reactive airway disease (i.e., asthmatic bronchitis). Full pulmonary function testing characteristically shows gas trapping manifested by increased total lung capacity, functional residual capacity, and residual volume. The diffusing capacity for carbon monoxide, DL_{CO}, is typically reduced, and exercise capacity is generally diminished. Patients with untreated asthma characteristically demonstrate a limitation in airflow (reduced FEV_1, FEV_1/FVC, and peak expiratory flow) that is improved (15% improvement in FEV_1) after the administration of an inhaled β_2-agonist, which in the appropriate clinical context is diagnostic (8). Some patients have normal pulmonary function during asymptomatic periods. Full pulmonary function testing and bronchial challenge with methacholine are available for cases that are more difficult to diagnose.

The treatments of COPD and asthma are similar and are considered together. For both, principles of therapy are the same as with younger patients, but the dosing of medications must take into account diminished creatinine clearance, reduced hepatic functioning, and the increased incidence of untoward effects. The regimen should be individualized and works best if the patient is well informed about it. A stepped-care therapeutic approach should be aimed at the maintenance of stable, normal pulmonary function. The first treatment step after diagnosing COPD or asthma should be the recognition and elimination of precipitating and aggravating factors such as cigarette smoking, allergen exposure, sinusitis, and gastroesophageal reflux. Careful history taking and skin testing may reveal causative antigens in asthmatics, although elder patients are less often atopic. Medications such as β-blockers, frequently prescribed for coexisting cardiac disease, can exacerbate COPD or asthma, and other medications, such as aspirin and nonsteroidal anti-inflammatory drugs (NSAIDs), can precipitate bronchospasm in sensitive persons. A detailed occupational and recreational history is important, as occupational asthma is a possibility. In all cases, exposure to cigarette smoke should be minimized.

In COPD, smoking cessation is not likely to result in significant recovery of pulmonary function, but it does decrease the accelerated rate of decline in pulmonary function. An oxygen needs assessment is important for patients with COPD, since the life expectancy of hypoxemic patients is substantially improved with the institution of continuous supplemental oxygen therapy (9).

Supplemental oxygen should be reserved for those with a PaO_2 less than 55 torr, a hemoglobin-oxygen saturation less than 88%, or a reduced PaO_2 of less than 59 torr with an increased hematocrit or cor pulmonale. Those who desaturate with activity or with sleep may also benefit from supplemental oxygen. Periodic reassessment after the implementation of therapy is useful, since many patients only temporarily require oxygen therapy. Recent attention has been given to the potential role of lung volume reduction surgery in severely affected patients with emphysema. At present it is unclear which subset of patients is best suited to such treatment, and clinical trials are under way.

When prescribing medications, attention should be paid to the considerable cost of non-generic bronchodilators and the utility of a spacer or Aerochamber in improving medication delivery. β_2-Agonists are the mainstay of therapy for COPD and asthma in all age groups, and the increased concern over the possible association between β-agonist use with mortality in asthmatics is probably overrated. Available β-agonists include both nonselective (β_{1+2}; e.g., isoproterenol) and bronchial selective (β_2; metaproterenol, terbutaline, salbutamol, and fenoterol) adrenergic stimulants. Although adverse effects appear more closely related to the route of administration than to the β-adrenergic receptor selectivity, the wide availability of selective agents make them the agents of choice in the elderly. Bronchodilator aerosols can be administered via metered dose inhalers (MDI) or nebulizers, but the fact that the two systems are equally effective would seem to limit the role of nebulizers. The relatively poor side effect profile of oral preparations (e.g., metaproterenol) and recent availability of inhaled preparations (salmeterol) with a long duration of action make oral preparations inappropriate for most elderly patients.

The emerging view of asthma is that it is an inflammatory condition, and many experts now believe anti-inflammatory drugs should also be considered as first-line medical treatment. Corticosteroids are the most effective anti-inflammatory agents available for routine use, but the many side effects of systemic steroids, which include immunosuppression, osteoporosis, myopathy, glucose intolerance, cataract formation, and adrenal suppression, greatly limit their use in the aged. Many elders with asthma or COPD become steroid dependent (7). The advent of inhalational steroids (e.g., beclomethasone, triamcinolone, and flunisolide) has provided a relatively safe and effective alternative to systemic administration. Like oral steroids, they have a dose-dependent effect and reduce the frequency of asthmatic exacerbations, the need for concurrent medications and in particular, the need for systemic steroids (10). They do require several weeks of use before patients derive maximal benefit and therefore are not very useful in an acute exacerbation. They also are associated with local side effects, which include dysphonia due to laryngeal muscle myopathy, oropharyngeal candidiasis, chronic cough, and increased intraocular pressure; these effects are generally reversed with cessation of therapy. Although they are effective in asthmatics, only a minority (10%) of patients with stable COPD demonstrate improvement in pulmonary function with systemic steroid use (11, 12). Those with asthmatic bronchitis may, however, benefit. Physicians' practice has been to overprescribe corticosteroids for patients with COPD and thus subject patients to considerable risks of side effects without any clear benefit. It is therefore important to document objective improvement if steroids are to be part of a chronic medical regimen. Sodium cromoglyconate and nedocromil sodium are two other anti-inflammatory agents that improve lung function in asthmatics. The role of the newly available leukotriene receptor antagonists (zafirlukast) and 5-lipoxygenase enzyme inhibitors (zileuton) in the treatment of elderly patients with asthma or COPD remains to be determined but will likely be useful in reducing systemic steroid use.

Theophylline, a drug with bronchodilatory effects and potential effects on respiratory muscle strength, continues to be used in the treatment of asthma and COPD (13). It is orally available, and the routine monitoring of levels has greatly reduced the incidence of toxicity, but the potential for untoward effects and many drug-drug interactions make its routine use in the elderly problematic. Furthermore, the additional benefit to a patient who is using inhaled bronchodilators optimally is minimal. Inhalational anticholinergics, such as ipratropium bromide, are effective in a minority of patients with pure asthma but generally offer substantial benefit to those with COPD. There are minimal side effects. Antibiotics rarely have a role in the treatment of asthma and should be reserved for those with systemic manifestations of infection or a focal infiltrate on chest radiograph. They are beneficial for a COPD exacerbation and should be promptly initiated and either empirically directed toward likely pathogens or aimed at those demonstrated in sputum. Prophylactic antibiotic therapy with broad-spectrum antibiotics on a regular schedule of 1 week per month may be appropriate for some patients. Available mucolytic agents are generally less effective then adequate hydration (2 L of fluid per day). Finally, pulmonary rehabilitation with exercise and ventilatory training is an underused and potentially effective therapy in COPD for improving a patient's exercise tolerance and functional status.

PNEUMONIA

Infectious disease is a leading cause of death in the United States and the leading cause of death worldwide. It is estimated that in the United States 1.25 million patients are hospitalized each year for respiratory tract infections. The elderly are much more frequently hospitalized for pneumonia and have a markedly increased mortality. Pneumonia, the most common infectious cause of death in the elderly, has an attributable mortality of 198 per 100,000 population, accounting for 90% of all deaths from pneumonia (14). Age itself may not be a major risk factor in determining severity of pneumonia or mortality when other factors, such as functional status, medical comorbidity, nutritional status (e.g., serum albumin), immunosuppression, clinical presentation, and specific high-risk pathogens are considered (14, 15), but in practice it is a useful predictor of poor outcome (16).

The diagnosis of pneumonia in an elder can be difficult. A classic presentation with fever, dyspnea, productive cough, and pleuritic chest pain is relatively uncommon. Many are afebrile and have nonspecific symptoms such as fatigue, confusion, or general functional decline. Physical examination findings are often obscured by poor respiratory effort and comorbid illness. Pneumonia is thought to be a consequence of microaspiration of oral pathogens. When the inoculum of bacterial pathogens is sufficient to overcome host defenses, pneumonia ensues. This microaspiration has been shown to occur in 45% of healthy adults and 70% of those with impaired consciousness (17). Thus, a patient's oral microflora, whose composition varies dramatically between community and institutional living elders, plays a major role in determining the character of a pneumonia.

Much has been made of the distinction between typical and atypical pneumonia. Those labeled as typical usually are caused by bacterial pathogens that tend to produce segmental or lobar pulmonary consolidation with a productive cough and a sputum Gram stain generally demonstrating the infecting organism. These pneumonias have an increased propensity to develop parapneumonic pleural effusions, which may progress into empyema and require tube thoracostomy drainage. In contrast, the atypical pneumonias, most commonly *Mycoplasma pneumoniae, Legionella pneumoniae,* or a virus, tend to produce more diffuse pulmonary involvement with a nonproductive cough. This separation, however, is indistinct and often leads to erroneous clinical reasoning. A better distinction when considering pneumonia in an elder is between a community-acquired and an institutionally acquired infection.

Community-acquired pneumonia in the elderly is most often caused by *Streptococcus pneumoniae* (40 to 60% of cases; also known as *Pneumococcus*), *Haemophilus influenzae,* a virus, or *Legionella* (18). *Mycoplasma* is also a consideration if the elder has exposure to young adults and children. Community-acquired pneumonia can be severe, with the worst cases typically occurring as a result of *Legionella, Staphylococcus aureus,* or penicillin-resistant *Pneumococcus.* Gram-negative bacteria are also potential pathogens, particularly if the patient has a history of chronic pulmonary disease or alcohol abuse. If significant aspiration is a possibility, infection with oral anaerobes or a frank abscess can occur. Influenza infection is an important cause of respiratory disease in the elderly, and it predisposes to secondary bacterial infection 5 to 10 days later with *Pneumococcus, H. influenzae,* or *S. aureus* (14). Thus, pneumococcal and yearly influenza vaccinations are important preventative measures in the elderly. During an influenza outbreak, chemoprophylaxis (e.g., amantadine 100 mg/day) is warranted for debilitated persons.

Nursing home-acquired and nosocomial pneumonia, which develops after more than 72 hours in a hospital, is generally due to a different spectrum of pathogens. Pneumonia accounts for 18% of nosocomial infections and is second only to urinary tract infections (44%) in terms of frequency; it accounts for the highest mortality (19, 20). At any moment 3.2% of nursing home residents may have pneumonia (20). In these settings a number of factors further predispose to the development of pneumonia: coexisting acute illness, the use of nasogastric or endotracheal tubes, the use of pharmacologic agents that impair consciousness or gastric acidity, and the use of antibiotics, which alter a patient's usual bacterial flora. The most common pathogens in institutionally acquired pneumonia remain *Pneumococcus, H. influenzae, Legionella,* and influenza virus and also include *S. aureus,* aerobic Gram-negative organisms such as *Klebsiella pneumoniae, Escherichia coli,* and *Pseudomonas aeruginosa,* and anaerobes (20).

The evaluation and treatment of patients with suspected pneumonia must take into account the underlying health status, available support from friends and family, possible causes, and severity of illness. Although elders do tend to have more severe disease and poorer outcomes than younger adults, it is reasonable to treat less severe disease in healthier hosts in the outpatient setting with close clinical follow-up. It is often possible to treat nursing home residents without transfer to an acute-care hospital. Absolute indications for hospital admission do not exist, but multilobar involvement, alterations in consciousness, tachypnea (respiratory rate greater than 25 to 30), tachycardia, extremes of temperature (less than 35°C or greater than 40°C), leukocytosis, renal failure, hypotension, hypoxemia, hyponatremia, hyperglycemia, and recent

hospitalization are all important considerations (16). The laboratory evaluation of patients with suspected pneumonia should include standard PA and lateral chest radiographs, a complete blood count with differential, serum electrolytes, blood urea nitrogen, and glucose. Some assessment of oxygenation (pulse oximetry or arterial blood gas analysis) and blood cultures are prudent in patients who seem very ill. More controversial is the role of specific diagnostic testing with sputum Gram stain and culture to guide therapy. Given the limitations of current diagnostic techniques, the American Thoracic Society has recently issued recommendations for empiric therapy based on likely pathogens for community-acquired pneumonia (18). For elders with outpatient pneumonia they recommend treatment with a second-generation cephalosporin, trimethoprim-sulfamethoxazole, or a β-lactam with a β-lactamase inhibitor, with or without a macrolide. For hospitalized patients with a community-acquired pneumonia they recommend treatment with either a second-generation cephalosporin or a β-lactam with a β-lactamase inhibitor, with or without a macrolide. For severely affected hospitalized patients they recommend treatment with a macrolide and either a third-generation cephalosporin with anti-*Pseudomonas* activity or another antibiotic with anti-*Pseudomonas* activity. Many experts, however, disagree with empiric treatment and recommend basing therapy on appropriately collected sputum Gram stain and blood culture data when available.

Effective therapy for pneumonia is based on the prompt institution of appropriate antibiotics, adequate hydration, good pulmonary toilet with deep breathing and coughing, and general supportive care. Attention must be paid to potential drug interactions and toxicity (e.g., renal toxicity with aminoglycosides), which are increased in the elderly who are often taking multiple medications. In patients with poorly resolving pneumonia, it is necessary to consider the possibility of resistant organisms, TB or fungal infection, bronchogenic cancer, lymphoma, aspirated foreign bodies, chronic aspiration (e.g., lipoid pneumonia due to mineral oil aspiration), and pulmonary vasculitis (e.g., Wegener's granulomatosis) (21). In these cases, fiberoptic bronchoscopy with biopsy, computed tomography-guided needle biopsy, and serologic studies (e.g., ANCA, ANA, RF) are often useful.

PLEURAL EFFUSIONS

Pleural effusions result from a wide variety of disorders. In the elderly, congestive heart failure, the most common cause, typically presents as a transudative bilateral process. When unilateral, it is almost invariably right sided. Other likely causes in elder patients include exudative processes such as malignancy and infection (parapneumonic effusions). Hemothorax should prompt consideration of pulmonary thromboembolism, TB, occult trauma (e.g., rib fracture), and malignancy. Accurate diagnosis depends on a careful history, examination, and pleural fluid analysis. Three separate specimens taken for cytologic analysis have more than 90% sensitivity for malignancy. Pleural fluid cultures for TB have a low sensitivity, so pleural biopsy is indicated for suspected TB.

TUBERCULOSIS

TB, which steadily declined in incidence after the introduction of effective antimycobacterial chemotherapy in the 1950s, is now having an epidemic resurgence. The reasons for this resurgence include the AIDS epidemic, an aging population, and decreased vigilance of public health agencies and the medical community. The elderly, a large population at risk, have the highest incidence of any age group (22). The case rate for elders over 65 is 150 to 200 per 100,000 population compared with 4 to 6 per 100,000 in 15- to 44-year-olds (23). In Arkansas more than 50% of TB cases occur in elders, who constitute only 14% of the total population (23). As compared with young adults, the diagnosis is more often delayed, fairly commonly until after death, in the elderly (24). Cognitive impairment and medical comorbidity often combine to mask the typical history and symptoms associated with this disease (25).

Elders more frequently live in close quarters in nursing homes, retirement homes, and other assisted living settings and thus represent a major public health concern for institutional spread

(26). Many instances of institutional spread have been reported. Earlier in the century the prevalence of TB infection was 90%; hence many elders may still harbor viable bacilli. Some 20 to 25% of the elderly remain infected with TB, as evidenced by positive tuberculin skin reactions (greater than 10 mm) (23). Fortunately, most infected persons never develop active disease, and the positive skin test is due to remote exposure that has been successfully controlled by the subject's immune system. Fewer than 5 to 10% of nursing home residents with a positive skin test, or 2 to 3% of all nursing home residents, develop active disease (27). The risk of developing active disease is highest in the first 2 years following infection (skin test conversion) and then decreases with time. This risk is increased in those with diabetes mellitus, prior gastrectomy, immunosuppressive therapy, and general infirmity.

Skin test conversion (i.e., a positive tuberculin skin reaction) is a good marker for recent infection but is really useful only in the context of an ongoing surveillance program. Waning immunity to old infection can lead to a false-negative skin test, and therefore a repeat test after a week or two is recommended to take into account the boosting effect of sequential testing in those with ancient infection. Care must be taken to avoid misinterpreting this booster reaction as a new conversion (28, 29). It is recommended that all patients with known new skin test conversions be considered for prophylactic therapy with isoniazid (INH) (30). The risk-benefit ratio for treatment of elders with positive tests from presumed ancient infection, however, is not favorable because of the increased risk of hepatitis from INH. When INH is prescribed, pyridoxine supplementation (25 mg/day) may limit the development of neuropathy. All persons with positive skin tests should be evaluated with a chest radiograph to exclude active disease. Those with findings or symptoms suggesting active disease should be evaluated with microbiologic studies. Three negative acid fast stained and cultured morning sputum samples are generally sufficient to rule out pulmonary disease. If further evaluation is needed, bronchoscopic cultures and transbronchial lung biopsy or transthoracic needle biopsy can improve the yield.

Active disease in the elderly is usually a recrudescence of old infection and so is generally drug sensitive. Elders are also subject to a markedly increased incidence of nonpulmonary TB. TB meningitis occurs most commonly in elders and often signifies newly acquired disease. The kidneys are a common extrapulmonary site of disease that may manifest as sterile pyuria. Vertebral TB (Potts disease), also frequent, may present as back pain. The elderly are also at increased risk for miliary disease. Elder patients with pulmonary TB manifest cough, fever, hemoptysis, night sweats, and weight loss with about half the frequency of younger subjects with active disease (25), and they are less often correctly diagnosed and treated. It is therefore important to maintain a high level of suspicion for TB. Treatment with multidrug antituberculous therapy is effective and usually well tolerated, although the elderly require close monitoring for adverse reactions.

BRONCHOGENIC LUNG CANCER

Bronchogenic lung cancer is a geriatric disease. Half of patients diagnosed with this disease are over age 65, and the peak incidence is in the eighth decade of life (31). Lung cancer was uncommon until the early part of this century but now accounts for 18% of cancer deaths in men and 12% in women. It is now more common for women to die of lung than of breast cancer. Nearly all lung cancer can be directly attributed to cigarette smoking, and the change in the epidemiology of this disease reflects the demographics of tobacco use (32). Some 96 to 99% of men and 82 to 95% of women with lung cancer, depending on cell type, have a history of cigarette smoking (31). Approximately 170,000 cases of lung cancer are diagnosed each year in the United States, and 150,000 patients die of this disease. The estimated yearly cost to the U.S. health care system exceeds $10 billion (33).

Cigarette smokers have a tenfold risk of disease, but there is a dose-response relationship, with heavy smokers having a risk as much as 25 times that of nonsmokers. A newly recognized solitary pulmonary nodule in an elderly smoker proves to be cancer 70% of the time. The risk of cancer declines steadily in former smokers and

approaches that of nonsmokers after 8 to 10 years (33). Other causative agents, such as asbestos, uranium, radon, silica, beryllium, and nickel, are much less important, although patients with these exposures should be additionally cautioned about the potential synergistic effects of cigarette smoking on cancer development.

Bronchogenic lung cancer is divided histologically into small cell and non-small cell types. Small cell lung cancer, previously called oat cell cancer, is very aggressive and is assumed to be metastatic at the time of diagnosis. Surgical resection is therefore not generally considered as a curative option. Small cell cancer, although regarded as incurable, is sensitive to chemotherapy, the mainstay of treatment. In contrast, non-small cell cancer may be curable with surgical resection if identified at an early stage. Later-stage disease is not, and the role of radiation and chemotherapy is primarily palliative. In general, the elderly have the highest incidence of disease but tend to present with earlier-stage disease (34) and thus may be more likely to benefit from curative therapy.

The long natural history of bronchogenic cancer occurs predominantly in a clinically undetectable state. This is followed by a relatively short period when the patient remains asymptomatic, with a pulmonary lesion that could theoretically be detected on chest radiograph. Finally, patients who are not diagnosed incidentally come to medical attention with a variety of symptoms that include cough, a localized wheeze, hemoptysis, or dyspnea as the most common complaints. Chest wall pain may suggest a peripheral lesion. Patients may develop paraneoplastic syndromes. Most are associated with small cell carcinoma; they include ectopic adrenocorticotropic hormone (ACTH) production, syndrome of inappropriate antidiuretic hormone secretion (SIADH), and Eaton-Lambert syndrome (a syndrome of motor weakness). Hypercalcemia is an exception, being more frequently associated with squamous cell carcinoma. Clubbing can occur with any tumor cell type. Horner's syndrome, the combination of enophthalmos, miosis, ptosis, and anhydrosis, results when a tumor at the apex of the lung (superior sulcus) extends into the neck and destroys regional sympathetic ganglia. Bone pain suggests metastatic spread, and lung cancer is the most frequent malignant cause of superior vena cava syndrome.

Primary prevention of lung cancer through smoking cessation and reducing the number of new smokers is the most effective intervention. However, in the elderly, in whom primary prevention may not be possible, early detection is another important goal, since there is a poor cure rate for advanced disease. Mass screening strategies with chest radiography and sputum cytology have been attempted with only marginal benefits. The National Cancer Institute Cooperative Early Lung Cancer Detection Program, a multicenter study examining mass screening (35–37) led to the conclusion that it is not cost effective and attributed observed survival benefits to lead time bias (38). However, 90% of the subjects of this study were under 65 and were at less risk to develop cancer than older persons. Elderly populations have been shown to have an increased incidence of all types of bronchogenic lung cancer with an increased proportion of earlier stage of disease at the time of detection. Thus it may be reasonable to screen older high-risk patients (34).

INTERSTITIAL LUNG DISEASE

The diffuse interstitial diseases of the lung (ILD) are, generally, an insidious group of disorders that can present difficult diagnostic and therapeutic challenges. There are numerous specific entities, but fortunately, most are sufficiently uncommon in the elderly so as not to warrant consideration in each case. Several disorders, however, are common in aging populations (39), either as primary pulmonary disease (e.g., idiopathic pulmonary fibrosis or cryptogenic organizing pneumonitis) or as a manifestation of a more general disease process, such as rheumatoid arthritis or progressive systemic sclerosis. Patients usually come to medical attention because of subjective complaints of dyspnea or fatigue or after an incidental abnormal routine chest radiograph. Congestive heart failure, atypical pneumonia, lymphangitic spread of cancer, and chronic aspiration pneumonitis should be included in the differential diagnosis of ILD.

The pathology associated with ILD occurs primarily in the interstitial compartment of the lung and affects the alveolar septa, peribronchovascular space, and pulmonary microvasculature. These disorders frequently, though not invariably, manifest radiographically with a reduced lung volume and reticular and/or nodular (reticulonodular) pulmonary densities. Pulmonary function testing typically demonstrates a restrictive pattern of abnormality with reduced lung volumes (total lung capacity, functional residual capacity and residual volume), decreased airflow (FEV_1 and FVC) and a preserved or elevated FEV_1/FVC ratio. The diffusing capacity for carbon monoxide (DL_{CO}) is characteristically diminished, and gas exchange is often impaired, with an elevated alveolar to arterial oxygen difference (Aa gradient). It must, however, be emphasized that these physiologic tests are insensitive for detecting ILD, can be difficult to interpret in a patient with comorbid conditions such as smoking-related COPD, and only crudely correlate to disease severity. Unfortunately, more sophisticated physiologic testing has not been shown to be superior to routine testing in assessing the severity or progression of ILD. Histologic examination of lung tissue, obtained from a transbronchial or transthoracic needle or thoracoscopic or open procedure, is usually required for definitive diagnosis.

Idiopathic pulmonary fibrosis is the most common ILD that affects older populations. It has a mean age of onset of 55 years, and many present after age 65. Men are affected somewhat more commonly than women. Its prevalence in the very elderly (age over 75) is 8 times as high as in those aged 65 to 74 (22.4 versus 189.3 per 100,000 population) (39). Older patients tend to present to medical attention with a shorter duration of symptoms than younger patients (15 versus 29 months) (40), although the presentation is otherwise similar. Inspiratory rales are commonly present. Clubbing may be less common in older patients. The prognosis for this disease in elder patients is poor, with a median survival of only 3.7 years as compared with 7 years in younger patients (40). Death is most commonly due to progression of disease. The risk of bronchogenic cancer is increased, with an incidence of 10%. Treatment recommendations must be tempered with the understanding that there are limited data to support a survival advantage with immunosuppressive therapy. Therapy with corticosteroids and cytotoxic agents are the standard of care. There is growing experimental support for therapies with less toxic drugs, such as colchicine.

Many drugs, particularly those routinely used for cancer chemotherapy as well as some antibiotics, antiarrhythmic agents, anti-inflammatory agents, and antihypertensive agents; external beam radiation therapy; and many collagen-vascular diseases, such as rheumatoid arthritis and systemic lupus erythematosus, can produce pulmonary disease with a histopathology indistinguishable from that of idiopathic pulmonary fibrosis (40).

Cryptogenic organizing pneumonitis (COP, or idiopathic bronchiolitis obliterans organizing pneumonia) is another idiopathic disorder that can affect elderly patients. The mean age of presentation is 58 years, but it affects all age groups. Patients most often present with or after a flulike illness. Chest radiographic abnormalities commonly described include a ground-glass appearance, faint fluffy infiltrates that do not obscure underlying lung markings, and mixed interstitial and alveolar infiltrates. Inspiratory rales are common and digital clubbing is rare. The disease may resolve spontaneously and is very responsive to steroid therapy, which dramatically speeds resolution. Most patients recover fully, although they may relapse when steroid therapy is withdrawn (40).

Occupational or environmental interstitial lung disease should be considered in geriatric patients with compatible pulmonary function and chest radiographic abnormalities. There is generally a lag of years between the occupational exposure and the development of fibrotic lung disease, which may be silicosis, asbestosis, or coal workers pneumoconiosis. A detailed history should focus on possible asbestos, silica, or mixed-dust exposure. Hypersensitivity lung disease, which can also resemble idiopathic pulmonary fibrosis, is due to protein antigen exposure and is most often encountered in farmers and bird fanciers.

ACUTE RESPIRATORY DISTRESS SYNDROME

The adult respiratory distress syndrome (ARDS), which is frequently encountered in critically ill elderly patients, is the most severe form of noncardiogenic pulmonary edema (41). The clinical and radiographic manifestations are the same across all age groups, with affected persons developing diffuse pulmonary infiltrates seen on chest radiography, hypoxemia requiring high concentrations of inspired oxygen with normal cardiac filling pressures, and decreased pulmonary compliance (i.e., stiff lungs). Patients often need mechanical ventilation. It is difficult to predict which patients will develop ARDS, but its many risk factors include trauma, pneumonia, multisystem organ failure, sepsis syndrome, and massive blood transfusions. The role of aging on the development and resolution of ARDS is unknown, but elders have a higher mortality, which may be as much as 2 or 3 times as high as that of younger cohorts (41, 42). Current management strategies are primarily supportive and directed toward correcting underlying medical illness. Specific ventilator approaches using positive end expiratory pressure (PEEP) to maintain oxygenation at lower, less toxic concentrations of inspiratory oxygen, neuromuscular blockade, pressure control ventilation, inverse ratio ventilation, permissive hypercapnia, and prone ventilation have all been advocated, although none have any proven mortality benefit.

OBSTRUCTIVE SLEEP APNEA

Obstructive sleep apnea is a common form of sleep disordered breathing that is associated with serious medical problems: systemic hypertension, pulmonary hypertension, daytime somnolence, chronic headaches, and even cognitive impairment (43). Unfortunately, although this disorder has received much attention in younger populations, its has not been well studied in the elderly. In this age group, its true incidence, prevalence, and clinical significance are uncertain. Incidence rates of sleep disordered breathing in the elderly vary dramatically according to the definition used by investigators; the range is 10 to 40% of those over age 70 (44, 45). Using a stringent threshold of more than five apneas per hour, Hoch et al. (45) demonstrated an incidence of 12% in the eighth decade of life and 19% in the ninth decade of life. Assessment is further complicated by the frequency of insomnia, nocturnal awakening, and comorbid medical illness, which can interfere with a patient's sleep quality. It does appear, however, that sleep-disordered breathing with associated hemoglobin desaturation below 85% does occur with increasing frequency with age (44).

There are no data to support either mass screening for this disorder in the elderly or for the treatment of asymptomatic persons with sleep disordered breathing (46). The significance of the finding of sleep disordered breathing in apparently healthy elders is uncertain. This diagnosis should therefore be pursued only in those with compatible clinical presentations. Treatment recommendations are the same as with younger patients, with nasal continuous airway pressure and weight loss as the preferred first line of therapy.

CONCLUSION

Despite the broad variations in ethnicity, lifetime experience, occupational and recreational exposure, behavior, and medical comorbidity, a number of common symptoms and pulmonary diseases affect elderly patients. Clinicians caring for the elderly should be familiar with the meaning of these symptoms, the nature of these diseases, and common therapeutic principles. Symptoms and findings are often subtle and nonspecific. Historical findings usually associated with particular diseases may be lacking or difficult to obtain. Coexistent illness can often affect the physical examination and obscure specific pulmonary signs, which can make diagnosis difficult. Treatment is complicated by an increase in adverse drug reactions and medication interactions. Unfortunately, many patients afflicted with treatable pulmonary disease go undiagnosed and consequently untreated. It is therefore vital that clinicians consider pulmonary disease when caring for elder patients.

REFERENCES

1. Silvestri GA, Mahler DA. Evaluation of dyspnea in the elderly patient. Clin Chest Med 1993;14:393–404.
2. Irwin R, Corrao W, Pratter M. Chronic persistent cough in the adult: the spectrum and frequency of causes and successful outcome of specific therapy. Am Rev Respir Dis 1981;123:413.
3. Clausen JL. The diagnosis of emphysema, chronic bronchitis, and asthma. Clin Chest Med 1990;11:405–416.
4. Luce J. Long-term oxygen therapy: physiologic and economic considerations. Respir Care 1983;28:866–875.
5. Braman SS. Asthma in the elderly patient. Clin Chest Med 1993;14:413–422.
6. Bauer B, Reed C, Yunginger J, et al. Incidence and outcomes of asthma in the elderly. Chest 1997;111:303–310.
7. Braman SS, Kaemmerlen JT, Davis SM. Asthma in the elderly: a comparison between patients with recently acquired and long-standing disease. Am Rev Respir Dis 1991;143:336–340.
8. McFadden E Jr, Gilbert IA. Asthma. N Engl J Med 1992;327:1928–1937 (erratum, N Engl J Med 1993; 328:1640).
9. Continuous or nocturnal therapy in hypoxemic chronic obstructive lung disease. Nocturnal Oxygen Therapy Trial Group. Ann Intern Med 1980;93:391–398.
10. Barnes P. Drug Therapy: Inhaled glucocorticoids for asthma. N Engl J Med 1995;332:868–875.
11. Callahan C, Dittus R, Katz B. Oral corticosteroid therapy for stable chronic obstructive pulmonary disease: a meta-analysis. Ann Intern Med 1991;114:216–223.
12. Jackevicius C, Joyce D, Kesten S, Chapman K. Prehospitalization inhaled corticosteroid use in patients with COPD or asthma. Chest 1997;111:296–302.
13. Jenne JW. Theophylline use in asthma: some current issues. Clin Chest Med 1984;5:645–658.
14. Granton JT, Grossman RF. Community-acquired pneumonia in the elderly patient: clinical features, epidemiology, and treatment. Clin Chest Med 1993;14:537–553.
15. Manton KG. Cause specific mortality patterns among the oldest old: multiple cause of death trends 1968 to 1980. J Gerontol 1986;41:282–289.
16. Fine M, Auble T, Yearly D, et al. A prediction rule to identify low-risk patients with community acquired pneumonia. N Engl J Med 1997;336:243–250.
17. Huxley E, Viroslav J, Gray W, Pierce A. Pharyngeal aspiration in normal adults and patients with depressed consciousness. Am J Med 1978;64:564–567.
18. Niederman M, Bass J Jr, Campbell G. Guidelines for the initial management of adults with community-acquired pneumonia: diagnosis, assessment of severity, and initial antimicrobial therapy. Am Rev Respir Dis 1993; 148:1418–1426.
19. Emori T, Banerjee S, Culver D, et al. Nosocomial infections in elderly patients in the United States, 1986–1990. Am J Med 1991;91(suppl 3B):289S–293S.
20. Niederman MS. Nosocomial pneumonia in the elderly

patient: chronic care facility and hospital considerations. Clin Chest Med 1993;14:479–90.

21. Fein AM, Feinsilver SH, Niederman MS. Nonresolving and slowly resolving pneumonia: diagnosis and management in the elderly patient. Clin Chest Med 1993;14:555–569.

22. Couser J Jr, Glassroth J. Tuberculosis: an epidemic in older adults. Clin Chest Med 1993;14:491–499.

23. Stead WW. Special problems in tuberculosis: tuberculosis in the elderly and in residents of nursing homes, correctional facilities, long-term care hospitals, mental hospitals, shelters for the homeless, and jails. Clin Chest Med 1989;10:397–405.

24. Bobrowitz ID. Active tuberculosis undiagnosed until autopsy. Am J Med 1982;72:650–658.

25. Alvarez S, Shell C, Berk S. Pulmonary tuberculosis in elderly men. Am J Med 1987;82:602–606.

26. Stead WW, Lofgren JP, Warren E, Thomas C. Tuberculosis as an endemic and nosocomial infection among the elderly in nursing homes. N Engl J Med 1985;312:1483–1487.

27. Stead WW, To T. The significance of the tuberculin skin test in elderly persons. Ann Intern Med 1987;107:837–842.

28. Stead WW, Steiner P. Second-strength PPD test. N Engl J Med 1971;285:294–295.

29. Van den Brande P, Demedts M. Four-stage tuberculin testing in elderly subjects induces age-dependent progressive boosting. Chest 1992;101:447–450.

30. Stead WW, To T, Harrison RW, Abraham J III. Benefit-risk considerations in preventive treatment for tuberculosis in elderly persons. Ann Intern Med 1987;107:843–845.

31. Greenberg ER, Korson R, Baker J, et al. Incidence of lung cancer by cell type: a population-based study in New Hampshire and Vermont. J Natl Cancer Inst 1984;72:599–603.

32. Loeb L, Ernster V, Warner K, et al. Smoking and lung cancer: an overview. Cancer Res 1984;44:5940–5948.

33. Lee CT Jr, Matthay RA. Lung cancer in the elderly patient. Clin Chest Med 1993;14:453–478.

34. O'Rourke MA, Feussner JR, Feigl P, Laszlo J. Age trends of lung cancer stage at diagnosis: implications for lung cancer screening in the elderly. JAMA 1987;258:921–926.

35. Fontana RS, Sanderson DR, Taylor WF, et al. Early lung cancer detection: results of the initial (prevalence) radiologic and cytologic screening in the Mayo Clinic study. Am Rev Respir Dis 1984;130:561–565.

36. Flehinger BJ, Melamed MR, Zaman MB, et al. Early lung cancer detection: results of the initial (prevalence) radiologic and cytologic screening in the Memorial Sloan-Kettering study. Am Rev Respir Dis 1984;130:555–560.

37. Frost JK, Ball W Jr, Levin ML, et al. Early lung cancer detection: results of the initial (prevalence) radiologic and cytologic screening in the Johns Hopkins study. Am Rev Respir Dis 1984;130:549–554.

38. Eddy DM. Screening for lung cancer. Ann Intern Med 1989;111:232–237.

39. Coultas D, Zumwalt R, Black W, Sobonya R. The epidemiology of interstitial lung disease. Am J Respir Crit Care Med 1994;150:967–972.

40. Wade J III, King T Jr. Infiltrative and interstitial lung disease in the elderly patient. Clin Chest Med 1993;14:501–521.

41. Griffith D, Idell S. Approach to adult respiratory distress syndrome and respiratory failure in elderly patients. Clin Chest Med 1993;14:571–582.

42. Gee M, Gottlieb J, Albertine K. Physiology of aging related to outcome in adult respiratory distress syndrome. J Appl Physiol 1990;69:822–829.

43. Findley L, Barth J, Powers D, et al. Cognitive impairment in patients with obstructive sleep apnea and associated hypoxemia. Chest 1986;90:686–690.

44. Feinsilver SH, Hertz G. Sleep in the elderly patient. Clin Chest Med 1993;14:405–411.

45. Hoch C, Reynolds C, Monk T, et al. Comparison of sleep-disordered breathing among healthy elderly in the seventh, eighth and ninth decades of life. Sleep 1990;13:502–511.

46. Phillips B, Berry D, Schmitt F, et al. Sleep disordered breathing in the healthy elderly. Chest 1992;101:345–349.

Peripheral Vascular Disease in the Elderly

Peripheral vascular disease (PVD) affects approximately 20% of men and women after age 65 years (1, 2). At younger ages PVD affects men more frequently than women (3). PVD usually is related to the development of atherosclerosis (1), a slow and insidious process beginning with damage to the endothelial lining of the artery. Damage varies by location but primarily affects specific arteries and bifurcations (3, 4), locations that may be subject to greater degrees of stress or wear and tear such as torsion, elevated pressure, or turbulent flow (3). Specifically, early damage usually occurs at the orifices of the intercostal and lumbar arteries and the distal segments of the superficial femoral artery and common iliac artery.

PATHOPHYSIOLOGY AND RISK FACTORS

The initial damage caused by these stressors is followed by disruption of the endothelial lining, leading to adhesion of platelets to the wall of the vessel. Platelets subsequently aggregate and then release factors that cause smooth muscle cells and macrophages to move to the injured area, producing a lipid and connective tissue matrix. Repeated injury leads to thickening, hardening, and the development of calcium and cholesterol deposits in the process of atherosclerotic plaque formation. In addition to the sites of early damage already indicated, plaque formation may lead to occlusion of major arteries, most commonly at bifurcations with acute angles (1).

These include the distal superficial femoral artery lying in Hunter's canal, the common femoral artery extending into the superficial femoral artery, the distal abdominal aorta, and the aortic bifurcation (1).

Risk factors associated with PVD include cigarette smoking; hypertension; hyperlipidemia, especially disorders of high-density lipoprotein (HDL) and triglycerides; diabetes; family history of atherosclerosis; obesity; and stress (1, 2, 4). A recent study discounts obesity as a risk factor for vascular complications in patients with diabetes (5). Advanced or occlusive peripheral arterial disease is significantly and inversely correlated with HDL cholesterol and significantly positively correlated with advancing age, smoking, and elevated blood glucose (6). Camargo et al. (7) recently studied 22,071 male physicians queried about alcohol use and followed for 11 years. Men who drank one to six drinks per week had an 18% lower risk, and those who drank seven or more drinks per week had a 26% lower risk of PVD, after adjusting for other risk factors. The protective effect of alcohol is thought to be secondary to its beneficial effect on the lipid profile. Risk factors may act by increasing the risk of vessel injury or by retarding healing after injury. Specifically, elevated blood pressure may cause initial endothelial injury, elevated lipid levels may speed up plaque formation, and smoking may cause artery spasm and promote platelet aggregation (3). A study by Graham et al. (8) evaluated plasma homocysteine levels of 750 patients with various forms of atherosclerotic vascular disease, including PVD, with 800 control subjects from 9 European countries. The highest levels were associated with more than a doubling of the risk for all forms of vascular disease independent of hypertension, serum cholesterol, and smoking.

Symptoms of PVD occur when the artery cannot adequately provide for the metabolic needs of the limb (4). This usually occurs on exertion, but in severe cases metabolic needs may outstrip supply at rest. At rest the cross-sectional area of the artery must be reduced by 75% before a decrease in pressure and flow occurs (4). A 75% reduction corresponds to a reduction in diameter of approximately 50% (9). Even without total occlusion of the artery, blood flow can be maintained above these levels at rest with the development of collateral circulation. Rarely, acute symptoms (discussed later) occur in patients with or without a history of PVD when total occlusion of an arterial segment occurs. This may occur by three possible mechanisms or a combination thereof: embolism, thrombosis, or trauma (4).

Emboli most commonly arise from an enlarged chamber of the heart in a patient with chronic congestive heart failure with or without an arrhythmia such as acute or chronic atrial fibrillation or supraventricular or ventricular tachycardia (4, 10). In these instances, the emboli are large and may occlude large arterial vessels, such as the superficial femoral artery or aortic bifurcation, which are severely affected by the atherosclerotic process. Occlusion of the aortic bifurcation, or saddle embolus, is a surgical emergency. When the obstruction is complete, the clinical symptoms typically include severe leg, thigh, and buttock pain with gradual onset of cyanosis, numbness, and coolness over the area. An abrupt loss of pulses from the femoral area distally accompanies these findings, all evolving over several hours (11).

The second most common source of emboli may be from an ulcerated atherosclerotic plaque at a smaller segment of a peripheral artery. The most common site for an embolus from an atherosclerotic process is first at the carotid bifurcation and second in the limbs (4). A rare complication involves the fragmentation of microemboli from a nonoccluding atherosclerotic plaque that lodges in a distal pedal or digital artery, leading to complete arterial obstruction and gangrene. The initial presentation may be a vesicular lesion on the tip of the toes. This is called the blue toes syndrome (11, 12). An occlusion secondary to a thrombus is not likely to occur in the limb arteries because of collateral circulation and relatively low metabolic requirements.

CLINICAL PRESENTATION AND EVALUATION

A thorough history and physical examination are sufficient to make the presumptive diagnosis of PVD. Noninvasive testing gauges the severity and extent of disease to help in selecting therapy (1). The practitioner must be able to distinguish chronic from acute physical findings that require immediate attention. Delay or misdiagnosis can lead to irreversible ischemia and amputation.

The clinical presentation of potentially serious ischemia can best be remembered in terms of the six Ps, pain, paresthesia, pulselessness, paralysis, poikilothermia, and pallor (13). The first P, pain, specifically is muscle pain secondary to ischemia, usually and initially occurring on exertion and relieved at rest. This pain, called intermittent claudication, is the most common initial symptom (4), although claudication itself does not imply impending occlusion.

The severity and the distribution of signs and symptoms depend on the particular arterial segment compromised or occluded, the size of the thrombus or embolus, and the extent of the collateral circulation to the affected muscle group (1, 3, 4). Classic patterns of pain associated with specific arterial segments include the following: pain in the calf secondary to ischemia of the superficial femoral artery; hip and back pain secondary to obstructive ischemia of the aortoiliac artery; calf and thigh pain associated with ischemia of the iliac arteries; buttock pain on exertion associated with erectile dysfunction in a man; buttock, thigh, and calf pain associated with ischemia distal to the common iliac artery or abdominal aorta; and foot pain occurring at rest and usually associated with the ischemia secondary to severe obstruction (1, 4).

Rest pain, regardless of whether in the foot solely or the lower extremities in general, is usually a sign of severe ischemia secondary to arterial insufficiency (12). This may also occur when more than one named artery is obstructed or severely affected by the atherosclerotic process. The pain may also occur on minimal exercise (4, 12). The pain occurs because the ischemia is made worse by lack of gravity and blood flow when lying flat. Pain also occurs because cardiac output, hence blood flow, decreases with sleep. The pain may not be relieved by opioids, often is worse at night, and frequently wakes the patient. Measures that may relieve the pain during the early stages of severe ischemia include analgesics, rubbing the foot, sleeping in a recliner, dangling the leg while standing or sitting, hanging the foot over the bed, and walking (1, 4, 12). The second P is paresthesia or numbness secondary to death of nerve tissue supplying the diseased segment (4). This is particularly common in diabetics, as is discussed later in this chapter.

The third and fourth Ps are pulselessness and paralysis of a lower extremity, usually occurring in the late process of peripheral vascular insufficiency (4). Though the determination of the strength of the pulse (absent, diminished, normal, or hyperactive) is important in determining the severity and extent of disease, the presence of pulses does not always indicate the absence of disease. This is true especially if the disease process is not too severe (11).

Palpation of pulses simultaneously at equidistant points on both lower extremities is recommended to evaluate strength and symmetry of the pulses. To avoid palpating your own pulse, use light pressure and a digit other than the index finger. Auscultation over the pulse using the bell of the stethoscope helps to detect bruits. Bruits are noted by hearing a squeaking or swooshing sound that may indicate turbulent blood flow past a narrowed or diseased segment. However, a bruit by itself is not sufficient evidence of PVD (12). Lastly, bruits may disappear at a certain point beyond critical stenosis of an arterial segment because of the severe reduction of blood flow.

The fifth P, poikilothermia, is a change in temperature between the proximal (unaffected) and distal (diseased) segments of the lower extremity or between an affected and unaffected leg or foot. Poikilothermia can best be assessed by touching the skin with the palm of the hand or fingers. Cold or cool toes or feet, however, do not necessarily indicate PVD when unaccompanied by other symptoms. The temperature of the environment and that of the patient should be kept in mind when evaluating coolness of an extremity (12).

The sixth P is pallor or paleness in color of the affected muscle, adjacent subcutaneous tissue, and skin due to lack of blood supply (4), which can best be appreciated by eliciting elevation pallor and dependent rubor. Note skin color changes on repositioning the lower extremity: (a) pale color that develops after elevating the affected extremity to 45° for several minutes, related to inability of the diseased arterial system to pump sufficient blood into the arteriolar and capillary systems against gravity; and (b) a dark red color to the lower extremity after it is placed in a dependent position for several minutes, indicating pooling of blood in the arterioles and capillaries secondary to arterial vascular incompetence. Arterial vascular insufficiency can also be appreciated by a determination of adequacy of capillary refill. This can be elicited by pressing on the tip of one of the toes and observing a normal blanching response followed by return of color. If return to normal color takes more than 3 seconds, there is delayed refill and evidence of inadequate circulation (12).

Physical findings elsewhere that may indirectly suggest PVD include bruits in the carotid or flank area, physical findings of an old stroke, retinal vascular changes seen on funduscopic examination, difference in blood pressure between the two upper extremities, asymmetry or atrophy of the pelvic girdle and lower extremity musculature, and left ventricular hypertrophy as evidenced by an S_4 sound, shift of the point of maximal impulse on palpation of the chest, or electrocardiographic or echocardiographic evidence (3). Other more subtle findings of the extent of peripheral vascular disease include loss of hair; thin, shiny, or scaly skin; and thickened or brittle nails on the affected leg or foot (3, 11, 12).

Late complications of PVD include ulceration and gangrene. Fortunately, these complications are rare with chronic aortoiliac occlusion. Ulceration and gangrene usually indicate distal disease (11). When the blood flow to the foot is marginal, acute ischemic ulceration and gangrene may also be precipitated by minimal trauma (4). This occurs because reduced clearance of endogenous toxins produces an anaerobic environment for surface bacteria and a reduced ability to fight infection (4).

Older patients with symptoms of PVD commonly develop functional decline as the sole manifestation of ischemia. However, a deterioration in the status of the peripheral arterial supply may not diminish functional status (2). In lieu of painful walking, older patients may elect to use a wheelchair or not walk at all, leading to functional incontinence. Older patients may fail to report symptoms because of fear and anxiety. Older patients with symptomatic PVD also become socially isolated and depressed because of the chronic pain of ischemia. They may give up dancing, walks, or other social activities outside the home. Particularly in diabetics, late complications of the associated loss of sensation or peripheral neuropathy can lead to disequilibrium and falls (1, 2).

Underserved minority older adults or those with financial or transportation barriers to receiving health care may be especially reluctant to report symptoms. They frequently initially present to the emergency room rather than a clinic setting with late complications of the disease such as ulceration, cellulitis, or gangrene, requiring in many cases multiple hospitalizations and amputations.

Atypical presentation of PVD may occur in the frail or demented nursing home elderly, who have long since lost their ability to walk and therefore do not have exercise-related ischemia. The only symptom in these cases may be acute agitation or worsening evening confusion secondary to night rest pain that occurs when the lower extremity is elevated and blood flow is not assisted by gravity. The only direct indications of PVD may be subtle physical changes discussed earlier (3).

Clinically significant PVD occurs typically in three clinically distinct patterns. Two of these are relevant to older patients. The first involves the most common presentation: the 65- to 75-year-old patient of either sex with several known risk factors for the disease and with a history of either coronary or cerebral vascular disease. Pain usually occurs initially on walking certain distances or climbing stairs. Though disease may be diffuse throughout the lower extremities, the major pathology and subsequent atherosclerotic lesions occur in the femoral and popliteal arteries. Physical examination commonly shows bruits over these areas, with reduced pulses distal and at the level of the popliteal, posterior tibial, and dorsalis pedis arteries (3).

The second scenario involves the person with a long history of poorly controlled diabetes mellitus. The patient initially complains of aching pain on exertion in the lateral leg and foot, particularly the dorsal aspect. Rest pain may also occur at night. Disease occurs extensively in the distal tibial, popliteal, profundus femoris, and peroneal arteries, sparing the aorta and iliac arteries (1, 3). Other common physical signs of vascular insufficiency are thin atrophied skin, lack of hair, pallor alternating with rubor, thickened and brittle nails, muscle wasting, and ulcerations. Physical examination commonly reveals good popliteal pulses but weak to absent posterior tibial and dorsalis pedis pulses (3). Diabetic patients with peripheral vascular disease characteristically have more extensive disease below the knee, typically have the associated pain of peripheral neuropathy, and are more susceptible to infection than nondiabetics (Table 12.1) (4).

DIFFERENTIAL DIAGNOSIS

The differential diagnosis of chronic leg pain also includes the pain of pseudoclaudication, peripheral neuropathy, chronic venous insufficiency, restless legs syndrome, and muscular pain. The typical muscle pain secondary to the ischemia caused by PVD is frequently mistaken for the pain caused by the compression of the spinal nerve by hypertrophic ridging of the vertebrae or protruded lumbar discs in patients with lumbar spinal stenosis: pseudoclaudication. Though the character and intensity of the pain are generally the same, precipitating and relieving factors differ. In contrast to the pain of

Table 12.1

Common Clinical Patterns of Peripheral Vascular Disease

	Elderly	Diabetic
Age group	65–75 years	40 and older
Frequency	Very common	Common
Risk factors	History of smoking, obesity, hypertension, coronary artery disease, hyperlipidemia, diabetes, family history of atherosclerotic disease, stress, cerebrovascular disease	Long-standing poorly controlled diabetes
Clinical presentation	Calf pain initially on claudication or walking up stairs; reduced pulses and possible bruits at the popliteal, posterior tibial, and dorsal pedis arteries	Aching pain initially on exertion in the lateral leg and dorsal foot; subsequent rest pain at night; atrophied skin, lack of hair, pallor alternating with rubor, thickened nails, muscle wasting, ulcerations, weak to absent posterior tibial and dorsalis pedis pulses
Anatomic lesions	Femoral and popliteal arteries	Distal tibial, popliteal, profunda femoris, peroneal arteries
Progress of disease	Stable over 5–10 yr	Dry and wet gangrene; amputation

PVD that is initiated by exercise and relieved by rest, the pain of pseudoclaudication is usually precipitated by extension of the spinal cord. Other positions that cause the pain of pseudoclaudication include prolonged standing or other back movements. Alternatively, the pain is relieved by flexing the spinal canal, as in sitting, leaning forward, and lying flat. Like intermittent claudication, however, the aching pain of pseudoclaudication is usually associated with a late finding of numbness and weakness of the legs (1, 4). Specifically, pulses may be present in a patient with severe vascular disease at rest but may disappear with exertion. Observation of the loss of pulses in combination with pain on exertion may be very helpful in distinguishing true vascular pain from pseudovascular pain or pain of neurologic origin (11).

The pain of chronic venous insufficiency is also a dull aching or throbbing pain that occurs below the knee and tends to be bilateral and symmetric. It characteristically occurs on standing, especially after long periods, allowing grav-itational pooling of the venous blood in small veins and venules. Chronic venous insufficiency can also cause an aching or cramping pain at night. In contrast to the ischemic pain of vascular insufficiency, the pain of venous insufficiency may improve with exercise. This is because the massaging motion of the muscles of the calf and lower leg force the blood into the central venous circulation. Even though edema is commonly a presenting sign of chronic venous insufficiency that is made worse by prolonged standing, pulses are present unless obscured by obesity or severe edema. In addition, in long-standing cases, the skin of the lower legs and feet has a characteristic thickening and dark appearance secondary to chronic thrombosis of the subcutaneous venous supply. The pain of chronic venous insufficiency is usually relieved by elevation and support stockings. Weight loss is also therapeutic (3, 14).

The leg pain of peripheral neuropathy typically produces a sharp throbbing or burning and intermittent pain and is typically not affected by exertion, rest, or position. The pain tends to occur mainly at night (3). Restless legs syndrome causes a tingling, prickly, or crawling pain that wakes the patient up at night when the legs are immobile. The syndrome is characterized by uncontrollable movements of the patient's legs, usually relieved by walking. The cause of restless legs syndrome is unknown. However, aspirin and short-acting benzodiazepines (lorazepam) taken before bedtime relieve symptoms. The physical examination of the lower extremities is usually normal in patients with restless legs syndrome (14). Muscular pain classically produces a cramplike pain that wakes the patient and may be preceded by an unusual amount of exercise. Walking usually relieves the pain and is usually followed by soreness of the muscle group. The pain of muscle strain usually occurs in the calf but may also occur in the foot or toes. Pulses and skin examination are normal (14).

The differential diagnosis of leg ulcers in a new patient with leg pain of undetermined origin can be confusing. However, the site and characteristics of the ulcer can be helpful in differentiating between venous and arterial origin. Ischemic arterial ulcers tend to be well demarcated and circular or punched out in appearance, although the borders may initially appear irregular. The color of the ulcer is a gray base with a pale area of skin surrounding the borders. Ischemic arterial ulcers are usually very painful and do not bleed when touched (12). Venous ulcers tend to occur after chronic thickening of the skin with hyperpigmentation and to have a more irregular border than arterial ulcers. Venous ulcers are found typically on the medial aspect of the leg (15, 16). They are usually associated with a constant aching pain that is relieved or improved with leg elevation (16). Ulcerations secondary to PVD in diabetics often develop at pressure points. These include the heels, dorsa of the toes, and medial and lateral malleoli.

After a thorough history and physical examination, the physician should have formulated an opinion as to the presence of PVD, its extent, and the suspected location of occlusion (1, 4). The physician can use specific diagnostic noninvasive and invasive procedures to confirm the diagnosis for decision making regarding medical or surgical management. Nonspecific signs of PVD that may not necessarily correlate with the degree or severity of disease include calcification of the walls of the arteries seen on routine radiographic examination of the extremity or abdomen (11). The noninvasive tests mentioned in the next section are best used in the absence of complete obstruction.

NONINVASIVE ASSESSMENT

The Doppler probe offers a noninvasive accurate assessment of the presence and extent of the disease, using sound waves (ultrasound) bounced off tissues of varying density and measured in megahertz. A low frequency, in the order of 5 MHz, is required to evaluate superficial vessels, and a frequency of 8 to 10 MHz is necessary to evaluate deep arteries (12). The Doppler examination is useful for evaluating symmetry of arterial pressure between the two lower extremities, for detecting the loss of a previously detected signal (13), and for direct measurement of arterial pressure in millimeters of mercury (mm Hg) (12).

The Doppler test can quantify the degree of stenosis of an arterial segment through calculation of the ankle-brachial index (ABI). The ABI is defined as the ratio of ankle systolic blood pressure to arm systolic blood pressure (12). Calculation of ABI is useful because obstruction of an arterial segment typically reduces pressure at or beyond the involved segment. The ABI normally is greater than or equal to 1 (4). In general, if only one artery is obstructed, the index is typically greater than 0.5, but if several arteries are obstructed, the index is usually less than 0.5 (12, 17). Patients with ischemic pain on exertion (claudication) typically have an ABI between 0.5 and 0.95. This is equivalent to mild to moderate arterial disease. Patients with ischemic pain at rest have an ABI less than 0.5. Patients with severe PVD have an ABI below 0.25 (12, 17).

Several recent studies indicate the prognostic value of the ABI. Vogt et al. (18) showed an increase in cardiovascular mortality, cancer, and short-term mortality (4 years) with low ABI in elderly white women. Newman et al. (19) showed an increase in adverse outcomes, including stroke, angina, myocardial infarction, congestive heart failure, and mortality in older hypertensive men and women with reduced ABI. After adjusting for cardiovascular disease, patients with diabetes, smoking, older age, hypertension, elevated serum creatinine, reduced lung function, abnormal electrocardiograms, abnormal echocardiograms, and increased fibrinogen levels had lower ABIs (20). Diagnoses of cancer, congestive heart failure, renal failure, chronic lung disease, and age over 65 but not a history of limb salvage procedure were found to be independently associated with mortality according to a study by Mc-Dermott et al. (21).

The ABI can also be used in conjunction with a supervised exercise protocol in a vascular laboratory to detect intermittent claudication, specifically for evaluation of functional capacity. New technology combining Doppler ultrasound (determining blood flow) and imaging ultrasound (determining anatomy) has made possible visual images of the specific location and severity of lower extremity vascular disease (3). Imaging ultrasound can also detect false aneurysms or periarterial hematomas, which may occur as a complication of arterial catheterization procedures such as contrast angiography and angioplasty (12).

INVASIVE ASSESSMENT

Angiography is usually reserved for evaluating the patient with severe PVD who has incapacitating claudication or pain at rest for whom loss of limb is a real possibility and for whom surgery is being planned (1). These patients characteristically are unable to carry out their usual activities of daily living (4). Catheterization is performed through the common femoral or axillary artery via the percutaneous technique (9). Angiography confirms the clinical findings and determines the site of the obstruction (11).

Though intraoperative angiography has been considered the gold standard for definitive evaluation of PVD, magnetic resonance imaging (MRI) has been used as a safer noninvasive alternative to traditional angiography in recent years to avoid the risks accompanying use of intravenous contrast agents. A study by Owen et al. (22) compared angiography and MRI in 23 patients with symptomatic PVD. They showed that

magnetic resonance angiography (MRA) was more sensitive for identifying cases treatable with bypass grafting, preventing amputation. In a multicenter trial, the two techniques had similar sensitivity in discriminating between nearly occluded vessels and patent segments. However, MRA was more sensitive but less specific than contrast angiography for detecting nearly normal segments (23).

It is important for physicians and patients to understand the natural history and treatment options for PVD, since its prognosis is relatively good when neither diabetes nor the familial variety described previously is involved. In more than three quarters of patients who develop the pain of claudication on exertion, the disease is benign and the symptoms usually remain stable for 5 years; fewer than 1 in 10 eventually require surgery (namely, amputation) (4, 11). Two thirds of patients affected with PVD can be treated medically without surgical intervention. However, symptoms may significantly deteriorate rapidly, depending on the number of the following risk factors: the progression of the atherosclerotic process; other complicating conditions (hypotension secondary to acute myocardial infarction, chronic hypoperfusion secondary to chronic left ventricular dysfunction, acute or chronic arrhythmias); and drugs that may worsen cardiac function, such as propranolol (11). Figure 12.1 shows the fate of 104 patients with symptomatic PVD (claudicators) followed for 8 years.

MEDICAL TREATMENT

Initial treatment of PVD usually entails a trial of medical management for at least 6 months to 1 year. This entails prevention, including modification of risk factors, exercise, and good foot care. The goals of therapy for patients with chronic PVD are twofold: preventing limb loss and enhancing quality of life (12). Modification of risk factors can slow the atherosclerotic process, including weight reduction, control of blood pressure and blood sugar as it relates to diabetics, smoking cessation, diet modification (reduction of saturated fats and cholesterol), and treatment of lipid disorders (3, 4, 11, 12). Smoking cessation is associated with an increased walking distance, a reduced incidence of ampu-

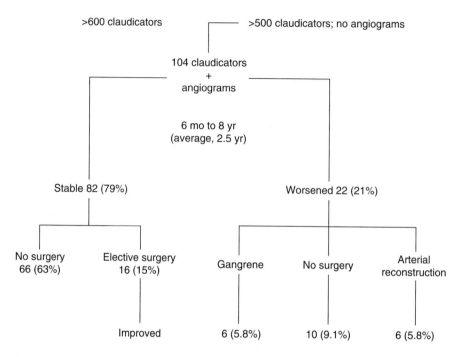

Figure 12.1. Fate of 104 claudicators. Three patients who had arteriograms were followed for 6 months to 8 years (average 2.5 years) in an attempt at nonsurgical management. (Reprinted with permission from Imparato AM, Riles TS. Peripheral arterial disease. In: Schwartz SI, Shires GT, Spencer FC, eds. Principles of Surgery. 5th ed. New York: McGraw-Hill, 1989.)

tation, and decreased mortality (9). Treatment of lipid abnormalities with lipid-lowering drugs results in angiographically proven regression of femoral artery plaques (9). Medical management is especially beneficial, since claudication usually progresses to gangrene at a rate of 2.3% per year—only in patients with severe claudication or marked or trophic physical findings (i.e., rubor, absence of hair, and brittle nails) (11). On the other hand, persistent smoking can reduce the time to gangrene and limb loss (4).

A regular tailored program of exercise reduces the frequency and intensity of claudication. Improvement is thought to occur by increasing collateral circulation and muscle efficiency (3). Exercise produces a gradual increase in walking tolerance before claudication occurs, improves mobility and overall function, and promotes a feeling of well-being for the elderly patient (11, 12). For patients who are unable to walk, an alternative exercise is having the patient stand on his or her toes and rock back

and forth until calf pain develops. This exercise should be repeated as often as possible, as much as 20 times per day (11). Concurrent or associated illness, severity of disease, and location of disease realistically affect a patient's ability to undergo exercise rehabilitation (11).

The physician should take time to explain and reinforce to the patient the benefits of risk factor modification and regular exercise, especially to allay the fear that exercise may cause further damage to the patient's feet or legs (12). Equally important to prevention is avoiding trauma, tight shoes, and walking barefoot. Other measures include daily visual inspection of feet and toes, wearing cotton socks, having calluses and corns removed as soon as possible, and avoiding agents of thermal injuries, including sunburn, very hot water, heating pads, and hot water bottles (12). Though the effect of trauma may be insignificant on a lower extremity with normal circulation, the effect may be devastating in one with impaired circulation. The associated abnormal anaerobic metabolism may result in gangrene. Superficial fungal infections may also become more serious when circulation is poor, especially in patients with long-standing diabetes (11).

In general, drug therapy for PVD is limited to a few agents. Only one vasodilator, pentoxifylline, is clinically useful in patients with PVD. It reduces the frequency of claudication and increases walking distances (1, 4). This occurs by increasing red blood cell flexibility, improving cell membrane permeability, promoting fibrinolytic action, and reducing fibrinogen levels and platelet aggregation (12). Vasodilators such as isoxsuprine are ineffective, since they do not affect the disease segment of the artery. Instead they may cause vasodilation of the unaffected segment, diverting blood from the diseased segment (steal syndrome) (3). Drugs of this type may also cause cerebral vasodilation, leading to postural hypotension and falls in older people (24).

Verapamil, a calcium channel blocker, increased pain-free and total walking distance significantly compared with placebo in a double-blind, crossover study of 44 patients with PVD, with no differences in side effects between the treated and untreated groups (25). Though anecdotal evidence suggests β-blockers have a detrimental effect on patients with PVD, the results of various clinical trials do not support this (26, 27). Chelating agents (i.e., EDTA, or ethylenediaminetetraacetic acid) have been touted as useful in preventing the atherosclerotic process by chelating free radicals and calcium and relieving symptoms of PVD. However, clinical trials have not shown them to be effective (28).

Aspirin, an antiplatelet drug, at 325 mg every other day compared with placebo has been shown to reduce the incidence of thrombosis requiring peripheral vascular surgery in patients with or without intermittent claudication (29). An overview of 60 randomized trials of antiplatelet therapy and 12,000 patients showed that antiplatelet therapy significantly reduced the risk of vascular reocclusion after peripheral arterial procedures compared with placebo (30). Antiplatelet therapy is most effective in the first year of treatment, less effective but still significant in the second year, and insignificant there-

after. The protective effect is independent of sex, age, blood pressure, comorbid disease, and type of antiplatelet therapy (9).

Dipyridamole 75 mg 3 times per day has been used as an alternative to aspirin as an antiplatelet drug for PVD and is sometimes used in combination with aspirin. However, few data indicate that this drug has any beneficial effect (31). Anticoagulation therapy with heparin or warfarin sodium for PVD has not been shown to be effective (11).

SURGICAL TREATMENT

Surgery for PVD is indicated for the patient who is disabled and unable to carry out daily activities, who is unresponsive to medical treatment, or who has ischemic rest pain and ulceration. Severe cases are ultimately unresponsive to medical measures, and loss of limb is inevitable unless the circulation is restored promptly (1, 4). Surgery is indicated in only about 10 to 20% of patients. The morbidity and mortality associated with the elective procedures (bypass or angioplasty) are 11% and 2 to 4%, respectively (2).

Surgical options include direct (bypass or endarterectomy) reconstruction, indirect revascularization, and angioplasty (11). Percutaneous transluminal balloon angioplasty, performed under fluoroscopy, entails dilation of the stenotic or focal portion of the affected artery with a percutaneous balloon-tipped catheter (4, 12). Angioplasty is best for short proximal segmental obstructions in the iliac arteries, with success rates of 85%, and may be as effective as bypass surgery (3, 4). Angioplasty of the femoropopliteal artery is less useful, with success rates of 70% at 3 years (1). Lesions that are longer or more distal are better treated with bypass (3). Since angioplasty is less invasive, the mortality and morbidity are lower; however, the restenosis rates are higher (2). Angioplasty is also less costly. Because of the high restenosis rate, vascular surgeons have begun placing stents in the diseased segments with or without balloon dilation. Complications include stent dislodgement, intimal damage, and distal embolization (12). The bypass entails the use of autologous grafts taken from the patient's greater saphenous vein or from an upper extremity vein if the saphenous vein is damaged. Autologous grafts are preferred because of the lower risk of infection and higher patency rate. If autologous grafting is not possible, synthetic grafts (Dacron or polytetrafluoroethylene) are used (13).

There has been a 24-fold growth in the use of angioplasty for PVD since the 1980s with the expectation that it would replace bypass surgery and subsequent amputation. However, the actual rates of bypass surgery doubled and the rates of amputation have remained the same during the period (32). Because angioplasty is more cost effective, less invasive, and associated with less morbidity and mortality, the American Heart Association has issued guidelines for its use. The use of invasive treatment is recommended for patients who are "truly incapacitated by their exercise limitations, be it for recreational, vocational. or personal reasons" (33). Data on end points such as quality of life, walking ability, and community activity for angioplasty and bypass surgery are lacking (2). Newer technology using a laser technique for angioplasty is in development and may be useful for more distal lesions (3).

An interesting association exists between PVD and coronary artery disease. In patients with PVD and coronary artery disease, perioperative and 5-year mortality is 2 to 3 times that of patients with PVD without coronary artery disease, with most of the mortality secondary to myocardial infarction. Studies have shown an improved survival rate in selected patients who have had peripheral vascular surgery after coronary artery bypass (34). Several factors have been identified in the assessment of patients with coronary artery disease and PVD who might benefit from coronary artery bypass. Historically, advancing age, a history of recent myocardial infarction, and congestive heart failure can identify patients at high risk for poor outcomes, while hypertension, diabetes, angina, and dysrhythmia are controversial predictors. Other independent predictors of postoperative cardiac events include an abnormal resting electrocardiograph, inability to complete a treadmill exercise test because of severe calf pain, poor left ventricular function, abnormal dipyridamole-thallium-201 scintigraphy, and periods of ischemia on ambulatory electrocardiographic monitoring (34). Any patient with a history of cardiac disease, an abnormal electrocardiogram, and abnormal cardiac perfusion and function testing should proceed to coronary angiography (9).

COMPLICATIONS ASSOCIATED WITH PVD

The diabetic patient with PVD deserves special consideration in evaluation, monitoring, and treatment for the following reasons: a predilection for specific sites of involvement below the knee; the associated peripheral neuropathy of the leg or foot translating into inability to appreciate pain, leading further to a slow or nonhealing state; and development of anaerobic infections that may be difficult or impossible to treat effectively. Treatment measures include local debridement of necrotic tissue surrounding the ulcer and judicious yet aggressive treatment with antibiotics. Deep infection such as osteomyelitis should be suspected if healing of infections and ulcers is delayed more than a couple of months. If osteomyelitis or wet gangrene develops, an amputation is often necessary (4). A 1991 health report from Washington state indicates that diabetics' risk of lower-extremity amputation is 40 times that of nondiabetics, with men more commonly affected than women (35).

Amputations primarily occur in the elderly population, with 75% in those aged 65 and older. Most of them are below the knee, with the major cause being PVD. Between 30 and 60% of patients who require an initial unilateral amputation for PVD and gangrene require an amputation of the other lower extremity in 5 years (1). Amputation below the knee is preferable to above the knee, since studies show improved postoperative mortality, lower energy requirements, and improved chances of walking. Though insignificant at younger ages, the extra energy cost associated with amputation above the knee can play havoc with the older patient, often precipitating angina and possibly a worsening of symptoms of chronic obstructive lung disease. The shift of the center of gravity and consequent disequilibrium caused by amputations in general, especially above the knee, can be a major contributor to falls in the elderly (36). For this reason, those with unilateral amputations below the knee have a 75% chance of independent walking. Those with bilateral amputation below the knee have a 50% chance, and unilateral amputation above the knee carries a 50% chance (4). Additionally, prostheses are used more frequently when the knee is retained than when it is not. Older patients in need of an amputation and prosthesis are more likely to have weak upper extremities and impaired skin integrity. An integral part of the postoperative training of the patient is instruction on proper stump care, including regular evaluation of skin integrity, massage, proper wrapping, and hygiene. Because a wheelchair may be necessary for the elderly patient with a prosthesis for traveling long distances, training in the use of this device at the same time is also recommended (4).

A complication of PVD is peripheral aneurysm. Especially in the popliteal segment, a peripheral aneurysm should be resected or bypassed unless medically contraindicated. Rupture or thrombosis of a particular aneurysm can lead to limb loss. The mortality and morbidity associated with elective surgery are about the same as for surgical treatment of peripheral vascular disease in general (4).

Abdominal aneurysms present a particularly difficult problem for the primary care physician regarding diagnosis, monitoring, and treatment. These subtle ticking time bombs can usually be appreciated only by careful abdominal palpation for a pulsating mass as well as listening for abdominal bruit. The strongest predictor of these lesions has been found to be smoking. Others include family history, old age, atherosclerosis, hypertension, and elevated cholesterol. Protective factors include diabetes, black race, and female sex (37). The most common presenting symptoms of impending rupture are abdominal, back, or flank pain; leukocytosis; abdominal tenderness; and a pulsatile mass on physical examination. Patients are frequently misdiagnosed as having urinary tract infection or obstruction, spinal disease, or diverticulitis. Abdominal sonogram is the initial diagnostic test recommended (38). For aneurysms less than 6 cm in diameter, the mainstays of treatment are control of hypertension, close clinical monitoring, and ultrasonography at 3- to 6-month intervals. Elective surgical intervention (resection followed by

grafting) is indicated if the aneurysm is larger than 6 cm in diameter, since there is a 50% chance of rupture and the mortality is lower than for emergency surgery (2.5% versus 15 to 80%). An aggressive surgical approach is also indicated for the patient with an abdominal aneurysm that continues to enlarge. The decision for surgery also depends on the presence or absence of cardiac, renal, or lung disease (4). Stent grafts are an alternative to open surgical correction, although long-term outcomes (after a year) are unknown (39, 40).

In conclusion, the primary care physician should clearly understand the pathophysiology, associated risk factors, subtypes and associated ages of onset, signs and symptoms, and physical findings of PVD. Thoroughly understanding the available noninvasive and invasive procedures is important for making the diagnosis of PVD. Understanding the medical and surgical treatment options available and prognoses associated with each is essential for providing quality care.

REFERENCES

1. American Geriatrics Society. Geriatric Review Syllabus. 3rd ed. Dubuque, IA: Kendall/Hunt Publishing, 1996: 97, 233.
2. Hiatt WR, Regensteiner JG. Nonsurgical management of peripheral arterial disease. Hosp Pract 1993;28: 53–72.
3. Woolley DC. Peripheral vascular disease. In: Ham RJ, Sloane PD, eds. Primary Care Geriatrics: A Case-Based Approach. 2nd ed. St. Louis: Mosby-Year Book, 1992: 578–583.
4. Hazzard WR, Andres R, Bierman EL, Blass JP. Peripheral Vascular Disease: Principles Of Geriatric Medicine And Gerontology. 2nd ed. New York: McGraw-Hill, 1990: 328,476–481.
5. Klein R, Klein BE, Moss SE. Is obesity related to microvascular and macrovascular complications in diabetes? The Wisconsin Epidemiologic Study of Diabetic Retinopathy. Arch Intern Med 1997;157:650–656.
6. Drexel H, Steurer J, Muntwyler J, et al. Predictors of the presence and extent of peripheral arterial occlusive disease. Circulation 1996;94(suppl 2):II199–II205.
7. Camargo CA, Stampfer MJ, Glynn RJ, et al. Prospective study of moderate alcohol consumption and risk of peripheral vascular disease. Circulation 1997;95:577–580.
8. Graham IM, Daly LE, Refsum HM, et al. Plasma homocysteine as a risk factor for vascular disease. JAMA 1997; 277:1775–1781.
9. Green RM, Ouriel K. Peripheral arterial disease. In: Schwartz SI, Shires GT, Spencer FC, eds. Principles of

Geriatric Surgery. 5th ed. New York: McGraw-Hill, 1994:927–937.

10. Creager MA, Dzau VJ. Vascular diseases of the extremities. In: Isselbacher KJ, Harrisons' Principles of Internal Medicine. 13th ed. New York: McGraw-Hill, 1994: 1138.

11. Imparato AM, Riles TS. Peripheral arterial disease. In: Schwartz SI, Shires GT, Spencer FC, eds. Principles of Surgery. 5th ed. New York: McGraw-Hill, 1989:957–916.

12. Cantwell-Gab K. Identifying chronic peripheral arterial disease. Am J Nurs 1996;96:40–48.

13. Fellows E, Jocz AM. Getting the upper hand on lower extremity arterial disease. Nursing 91 1991;21:34–42.

14. Herr KA. Night leg pain. Geriatr Nurs 1992;13:13–16.

15. Callam MJ, Lunch DJ. Preventing and treating leg ulcers. Patient Care 1992;26:118–145.

16. Habif TP. Clinical Dermatology: A Color Guide to Diagnosis and Therapy. 3rd ed. St. Louis: Mosby-Year Book, 1996:76–77.

17. Plummer ES, Albert SG. Focused assessment of foot care in older adults. J Am Geriatr Soc 1996;44:310–313.

18. Vogt MT, Cauley TA, Newman AB, et al. Decreased ankle/arm blood pressure index and mortality in elderly women. JAMA 1993;270:465–469.

19. Newman AB, Sutton-Tyrell K, Vogt MT, Kuller LH. Morbidity and mortality in hypertensive adults with a low ankle/arm blood pressure index. JAMA 1993;270: 487–490.

20. Newman AB, Siscovick DS, Manolio TA, et al. Ankle-arm index as a marker of atherosclerosis in the cardiovascular health study. Circulation 1993;88:837–845.

21. McDermott MM, Feinglass J, Slavensky R, Pearce WH. The ankle-brachial index as a predictor of survival in patients with peripheral vascular disease. J Gen Intern Med 1994;9:445–449.

22. Owen RS, Carpenter JP, Baum RA, et al. Magnetic resonance imaging of angiographically occult runoff vessels in peripheral arterial occlusive disease. N Engl J Med 1992;326:1577–1581.

23. Baum RA, Rutter CM, Sunshine JH, et al. Multicenter trial to evaluate vascular magnetic resonance angiography of the lower extremity. JAMA 1995;274:875–880.

24. Willcox SM, Himmelstein DU, Woolhandler S. Inappropriate drug prescribing for the community-dwelling elderly. JAMA 1994;272:292–296.

25. Bagger JP, Helligsoe P, Randsbaek F, et al. Effect of verapamil in intermittent claudication: a randomized, double-blind, placebo-controlled, cross-over study after individual dose-response assessment. Circulation 1997; 95:411–414.

26. Radack K, Deck C. B-Adrenergic blocker therapy does not worsen intermittent claudication in subjects with

peripheral arterial disease: a meta-analysis of randomized controlled trials. Arch Intern Med 1991;151:1769–1776.

27. Solomon SA, Ramsey LE, Yeo WW, et al. Beta blockade and intermittent claudication: placebo controlled trial of atenolol and nifedipine and their combination. BMJ 1991;303:1100–1104.

28. Van Rij AM, Solomon C, Packer SG, Hopkins WG. Chelation therapy for intermittent claudication. A double-blind, randomized, controlled trial. Circulation 1994;90:1194–1199.

29. Goldhaber SZ, Manson JE, Stampfer MJ, et al. Low-dose aspirin and subsequent peripheral arterial surgery in the physicians' health study. Lancet 1992;340:143–145.

30. Collaborative overview of randomised trials of antiplatelet therapy. II. Maintenance of vascular graft or arterial patency by antiplatelet therapy. Antiplatelet Trialists' Collaboration. BMJ 1994;308:159–168.

31. Green D, Miller V. Role of Dipyridamole in the therapy of vascular disease. Geriatrics 1993;48:46.

32. Tunis SR, Bass EB, Steinberg EP. The use of angioplasty, bypass surgery, and amputation in the management of peripheral vascular disease. N Engl J Med 1991;325: 556–562.

33. Pentecost MJ, Criqui MH, Dorros G, et al. Guidelines for peripheral percutaneous transluminal angioplasty of the abdominal aorta and lower extremity vessels. A statement for health professionals from a special writing group of the Councils on Cardiovascular Radiology, Arteriosclerosis, Cardio-Thoracic and Vascular Surgery, Clinical Cardiology, and Epidemiology and Prevention, the American Heart Association. Circulation 1994;89: 511–531.

34. Gajraj H, Jamieson CW. Coronary artery disease in patients with peripheral vascular disease. Br J Surg 1994; 81:333–342.

35. Lower Extremity amputations among persons with diabetes mellitus—Washington, 1988. MMWR Morb Mortal Wkly Rep 1991;40:737–739.

36. Baloh RV. Dizziness in older people. J Am Geriatr Soc 1992;40:713–721.

37. Lederle FA, Johnson GR, Wilson SE, et al. Prevalence and association of abdominal aneurysm detected through screening. Ann Intern Med 1997;126:441–449.

38. Lederle FA, Parenti CM, Chute P. Ruptured abdominal aortic aneurysm: the internist as diagnostician. Am J Med 1994;96:163–167.

39. Dake MD, Miller DC, Semba CP, et al. Transluminal placement of endovascular stent-grafts for the treatment of descending thoracic aortic aneurysms. N Engl J Med 1994;331:1729–1734.

40. Blum U, Voshage G, Lammer J, et al. Endoluminal stent-grafts for infrarenal abdominal aortic aneurysms. N Engl J Med 1997;336:13–20.

CHAPTER 13

SUSAN W. LEHMANN AND PETER V. RABINS

Clinical Geropsychiatry

While most older people are mentally healthy, persons over age 65 are vulnerable to the same spectrum of psychiatric disorders as are younger people (1). Community epidemiologic studies indicate that prevalence rates for major depressive disorder, panic disorder, and substance use disorders are lower in the elderly. However, the prevalence of phobic disorders does not change with age, and the prevalence of cognitive disorders and their associated psychiatric morbidity sharply increase with age (2).

Psychiatric problems in the elderly are more common in certain settings. For instance, anxiety and depressive disorders are common among patients in medical clinics, while confusional states (delirium) are seen in approximately 25% of hospitalized patients on medical and surgical services (3). In nursing homes and long-term care facilities, more than 50% of residents have been found to suffer from some sort of psychiatric problem, most commonly dementia, and behavioral problems and depression are common (4). In all, there is a need for careful attention to psychiatric symptoms in the elderly, since compassionate and appropriate treatment improve both overall functioning and quality of life.

EVALUATION
History

The evaluation of the older adult with a possible mental disorder begins, as does any medical evaluation, with a careful history. If the patient is accompanied by family members, it is helpful to meet with them too, to facilitate obtaining a complete history and database. The history should focus on a thorough assessment of the reason for the appointment, including a careful determination of when symptoms first appeared, how they have progressed over time, and accompanying features. In addition, the complete history should include the following:

1. *Family psychiatric history.* The clinician should inquire whether any blood relatives, especially first-degree relatives, have ever suffered from a mental disorder or alcoholism or have been hospitalized in a psychiatric facility.
2. *Psychiatric history of the patient.* This should include any prior contact with psychiatrists or therapists, prior psychiatric hospitalizations, or previous treatment by any medical professional for mood problems or bad nerves.
3. *Medical history.* It is important to detail all prior hospitalizations and surgeries and any current medical conditions that continue to be a focus of treatment.
4. *Medications.* This should be a complete list of all medications, both prescription drugs and over-the-counter medications being taken by the patient, including dosages. Because many medications prescribed for a variety of medical conditions have psychiatric side effects, it is helpful to inquire about the length of time the patient has taken the medication and to pay particular attention to changes in medications prescribed shortly before the onset of the presenting psychiatric symptoms.
5. *Personal history.* This includes information about the patient's family of origin, siblings,

childhood history, schooling (especially level of education), work history, adjustment to retirement, sexual history, marital history, and children. It is also important to inquire about the patient's living situation, including with whom he or she lives and the type of home (i.e., house or apartment, rented or owned). This is also a good time to ask about any structural aspects of the home that may pose problems for the patient, such as stairs, second floor bathrooms, tub, and showers.

6. *Patterns of alcohol use.* Problems of alcohol use and abuse occur in the elderly, as in younger persons, and may underlie symptoms of anxiety, depression, irritability, memory loss, sleep disturbance, sexual dysfunction, and paranoia. It is necessary to obtain information on the type of alcohol consumed, how frequently, and how much and to inquire about early-morning shakes, blackouts, alcohol-induced seizures, and prior episodes of detoxification or treatment.

Mental Status Examination

The heart of the psychiatric evaluation is the mental status examination, the here-and-now data gathering equivalent of the physical examination. It allows a systematic examination of the major aspects of the patient's mental state. Depending on the nature of the presenting complaint and the cooperativeness of the patient, certain areas of the mental status examination may be emphasized, while others may be only touched on briefly. The complete mental status examination, however, always includes attention to the following areas.

1. *General appearance.* This includes observation of neatness and personal hygiene, eye contact during the interview, and any abnormal movements, tremors, tics, or unusual behaviors.
2. *Speech.* This refers to the form and structure of the patient's verbal language. It includes attention to the rate, rhythm, and loudness of the patient's speech and whether the patient's use of language is coherent, goal-directed, logical, and easy to follow. Does the patient seem to jump from one idea to another with

little connection between ideas? This is described as loose associations and in an extreme form may be called flight of ideas. Some patients may have trouble sticking to the topic at hand and exhibit a tendency to wander off track (tangentiality) but can be redirected to the issue being discussed. Obsessional patients may be inclined to be overinclusive in detail (circumstantiality), sometimes losing sight of the forest for the trees. Aphasic patients have word-finding difficulty, paraphasias (made-up words), and nonfluent or fluent but content-free speech.

3. *Mood.* The assessment of mood involves both ascertainment of the patient's subjective description of his or her mood state and the clinician's objective observations of the patient's mood. Some depressed elderly patients report that they don't feel depressed yet appear tense, anxious, sad, or withdrawn.
4. *Suicidal ideation.* It is important to ask any patient with a sad mood about suicidal thoughts. Contrary to popular myths, asking about suicidal thoughts does not increase the likelihood that a patient will follow through on such ideas. We distinguish between passive suicidal ideation (i.e., wishing one were dead or would die) and active suicidal ideation (i.e., planning self-harm). Many depressed patients express passive wishes for death but are adamant that they would never attempt suicide for personal, religious, or family reasons.
5. *Abnormal thought content.*
   a. Hallucinations are sensory experiences that are perceived in the absence of a sensory stimulus. Auditory and visual hallucinations are most common, but tactile and olfactory hallucinations also occur in some disorders.
   b. Delusions are idiosyncratic fixed false beliefs that are not culturally determined or shared. Paranoid delusions and delusions of persecution are most common. Manic patients may have grandiose delusions about themselves and their abilities. Other types of delusions that may develop in older patients are delusional jealousy (falsely believing one's spouse has been un-

faithful) and delusions of parasitosis (believing one's skin to be infested with worms or insects). Often the delusion seems plausible until further medical or social investigation reveals it to be unfounded. A distinguishing feature of delusions is that the patient cannot be persuaded that the belief is false despite evidence to the contrary.

c. Obsessive thoughts are intrusive, repetitive, unwanted ideas that a person cannot stop from coming to mind.

d. Compulsions are intrusive, repetitive, unwanted behaviors that a person cannot stop, although they seem unnecessary, excessive, or foolish. Some examples are compulsive hand washing and checking behaviors.

e. Phobias are excessive specific fears that cause a person to avoid the dreaded situation.

6. *Cognitive assessment.* Every psychiatric evaluation of the older patient should include an assessment of cognitive functioning. Depending on the nature of the initial presenting complaint and the cooperativeness of the patient, this assessment may be fairly brief or very detailed and focused. A basic cognitive screening should include the following areas of assessment: level of alertness, attentiveness, orientation, short- and long-term memory, attention and concentration, naming ability and language comprehension, and abstract reasoning. If significant cognitive impairment is detected in one or more of these areas, further neuropsychologic testing and/or laboratory testing may be warranted.

SPECIFIC CONDITIONS

Anxiety Disorders

Anxiety is feelings of tension and distress that are distinct from sadness and that usually lack a stressful stimulus of such severity as to explain the feeling. It often has both somatic (physical) and psychologic components. *Generalized anxiety disorder* is a condition marked by excessive worry and anxiety persisting for 6 months or more. It is accompanied by signs and symptoms of motor tension, including muscle aches or soreness; a feeling of restlessness; a feeling of shakiness; and reports of easy fatigability. In addition, there are feelings of being on edge, having difficulty concentrating and falling asleep, and being unusually irritable. At least three of these additional symptoms of motor tension must be present along with the subjective distress of constant worry to make the diagnosis of generalized anxiety disorder. *Panic disorder* is diagnosed when the patient reports discrete episodes (attacks) of intense fear and somatic anxiety symptoms that are both unprovoked and unexpected. The associated somatic symptoms include palpitations, sweating, trembling, shortness of breath, chest discomfort, light-headedness, and abdominal distress. It is common for panic attacks to occur repeatedly in certain circumstances, e.g., in a grocery store. Specific phobias are clearly delineated fears of objects of situations that a person realizes are unrealistic but can nevertheless not resist. They sometimes occur in concert with panic attacks.

The anxiety disorders are among the most common psychologic problems identified in mental health surveys. Nonpharmacologic and pharmacologic therapies are usually used. Desensitization (gradually exposing the patient to the source of distress) coupled with relaxation is often effective. The most effective pharmacologic therapy is the use of antidepressants. There is no evidence that one antidepressant is better than another. While drugs with high anticholinergic properties, such as imipramine, are often used in the young, medications with less anticholinergic activity, such as nortriptyline, are suggested for the elderly. In addition to tricyclic antidepressants (e.g., nortriptyline, desipramine), selective serotonin reuptake inhibitors (SSRIs), such as paroxetine, sertraline, and fluoxetine, are effective for anxiety disorders. SSRIs are often better tolerated with fewer side effects than tricyclic antidepressants.

Benzodiazepine compounds are also effective for anxiety disorder. Because of their addictive potential, however, they are generally not prescribed as a first-line therapy. Short-acting benzodiazepines (e.g., alprazolam) have more abuse and addiction liability than longer-acting compounds (e.g., clonazepam), but the longer-acting compounds are more likely to accumulate and lead to sedation, functional impairment, and drowsiness. Buspirone is nonaddicting but appears to be less effective in the treatment of anxiety than benzodiazepines or antidepressants. If symptoms are severe and immediate relief desirable, the clinician may choose to initiate treatment with both an antidepressant and benzodiazepine and taper the benzodiazepine several weeks after the antidepressant begins to work.

Mixed Anxiety and Depression

Symptoms of anxiety and depression frequently affect the patient simultaneously. The clinician should make an effort to determine which is primary and to focus treatment on that set of symptoms. In our experience, depression is more frequently the primary disorder, but this is controversial. Features in the history suggesting that depression is primary include a history of a depressive episode, a family history of depressive episodes, diurnal mood variation (i.e., a tendency for symptoms to be worse in the morning) self-blame, guilt, and hopelessness and mental somatization. While anxiety disorders can begin de novo in late life, it is much more common for a depressive episode to appear for the first time in an older person. Because antidepressants are effective in both, they should be the first-line treatment when the clinician is unsure which is primary.

Mood Disorders

Mood disorders are the most frequently clinically diagnosed and the most treatable psychiatric disorders in older people (5, 6). They encompass a spectrum of disorders ranging from adjustment disorder (in which an identified psychosocial stressor provokes a mild depressive reaction that impairs functioning) to psychotic major depression with hallucinations and/or delusions to mania.

Major depression is characterized by a persistent diminution in three spheres of functioning: (*a*) mood, (*b*) vital sense (a measure of one's sense of well-being and energy), and (*c*) attitude toward oneself (self-confidence). Depressed patients

tend to have a more negative self-assessment than is usual for them, may be self-blaming, or can have excessive feelings of guilt, regret, or worthlessness. Patients with major depression experience loss of energy, disturbed sleep (usually insomnia and early morning awakening), diminished appetite and weight loss, difficulty thinking and concentrating, and a loss of interest or pleasure in activities that were once enjoyed. Ruminant thoughts of death and suicidal thoughts may occur during the course of a major depression. Elderly patients who are depressed often complain of physical rather than psychologic distress. Up to a third of older people who suffer from major depression do not describe their mood as depressed. Rather they focus on feelings of weakness, lack of energy, and lack of motivation. Somatic complaints, including headaches, gastrointestinal disturbances, and body aches, are common. Occasionally, hallucinations and delusions occur. Such hallucinations and delusions tend to have a depressive theme and are consistent with a low mood, e.g., the persecutory delusion that one deserves punishment; the delusion that one has no money, clothes, or insurance; and the delusion that one has a terrible illness that doctors cannot find.

Major depression can first occur at any point in the life span. It may occur as a single episode, but recurrence is common. The causation of major depression is complex, involving genetic, neurochemical, and psychologic factors. While genetic transmission is poorly understood, it is clear that affective (mood) disorders tend to run in families and that there is a higher prevalence of affective disorders among first-degree relatives of depressed individuals. The neurochemistry of depression is an active area of research focusing on abnormalities in adrenergic and serotonergic neurotransmissions in the brain. Many commonly prescribed medications, including steroids, reserpine, methyldopa, antiparkinsonian drugs, and β-adrenergic blockers, can cause depression. Depression is especially common in diseases of the brain. For example, 30 to 60% of poststroke patients have a clinically significant episode of depression within 6 months to 2 years of the stroke. The incidence of poststroke depression has been found to be greatest among patients with strokes affecting the left anterior cerebral hemisphere (7). While major depression can occur in the absence of any precipitating event, psychologic issues such as recent loss (i.e., job, independence, social supports) and chronic medical illness play a contributing role in many cases (8). Regardless of whether psychologic factors provoke a depressive episode, they clearly can affect its course and outcomes. Supportive psychotherapy is an important part of the treatment of depression in conjunction with appropriate pharmacotherapy.

The psychopharmacologic treatment of major depression has advanced considerably in recent years, and many effective antidepressant medications are available. Tricyclic antidepressants are older drugs with well-established efficacy. Older persons do best when given antidepressants with the least anticholinergic activity; therefore, nortriptyline and desipramine are favored for older people. Many of the newer SSRIs, fluoxetine, sertraline, and paroxetine, are well tolerated by older patients. They have minimal anticholinergic effects and are not associated with blood pressure and heart rate changes. However, SSRIs can impair sleep even when taken in the morning. If this occurs, adding trazodone at bedtime can improve sleep. Nausea, another common side effect, may be dose related. Monoamine oxidase inhibitors can be given to older patients if prescribed cautiously; they may be indicated for difficult cases when other medications have failed.

A number of newer antidepressants deserve mention: Bupropion is a novel antidepressant with mild central nervous system-activating effects whose mechanism of action is still unclear. It has minimal anticholinergic effects and few cardiovascular side effects but has a higher risk of inducing seizures at higher doses. Venlafaxine is a new antidepressant that inhibits both norepinephrine and serotonin reuptake and has a side effect profile similar to those of the SSRI agents, but it may also increase blood pressure. Nefazodone, another new antidepressant, is a selective $S-HT_2$ receptor antagonist. It is well tolerated in older patients but must be used cautiously because of potential drug interactions.

At this writing the newest antidepressant to be approved by the U.S. Food and Drug Administration (FDA) is mirtazapine. It has nonadrenergic and serotonergic pharmacologic action and is not structurally related to any other available antidepressants. Published studies of drug interactions with mirtazapine and studies of its effectiveness in elderly patients are lacking.

All antidepressants must be taken for a minimum of 6 to 8 weeks at appropriate dosages before efficacy can be determined. To prevent relapse they should be prescribed for a minimum of 6 to 12 months once the right dose and therapeutic response have been achieved.

Another effective treatment for serious depression is electroconvulsive therapy (ECT) (9, 10). ECT may be the first-line treatment of choice if the patient cannot eat or is refusing to eat and is at risk for dehydration. It may be used as a second-line treatment after one or two antidepressant trials have failed to improve symptoms adequately. There is no age limit to ECT, although several medical conditions are relative contraindications that must be evaluated case by case. These include recent myocardial infarction, coronary artery disease, hypertensive cardiovascular disease, bronchopulmonary disease, and venous thrombosis. The only absolute contraindication for ECT is increased intracranial pressure, since ECT causes a rise in cerebrospinal fluid pressure that may lead to herniation. Relapse of major depression after ECT is high, and therefore it must be followed by maintenance antidepressant treatment.

Bipolar disorder is a lifelong recurrent disorder characterized by one or more manic episodes. There is often at least one prior episode of major depression. Recurrence can take the form of either polarity, mania or depression. While most patients with bipolar disorder have their first episode of illness before age 50, late-onset mood disorder does occur (11). Most patients with late-onset mania have had at least one episode of major depression, often 10 to 15 years earlier. There is a tendency for patients with late-onset bipolar disorder to have a lower incidence of positive family history of mood disorders. In addition, a number of studies of late-onset mania reveal a high rate of secondary mania, in which there seems to be association between onset of mania and known brain injury, especially affecting the right side of the brain, or another medical problem such as thyrotoxicosis or hypercortisolemia.

Patients having a manic episode usually have little need for sleep, are talkative, and may have loose associations in their speech. Hyperactivity, hypersexuality, overspending, and involvement in foolish or unwise endeavors are frequently seen. Patients usually have an inflated self-esteem and increased sense of well-being but may also be irritable and demanding to those around them. Frank grandiose delusions may develop, such as believing oneself to be chosen by God for a special mission.

The mainstay of treatment for mania is lithium pharmacotherapy, sometimes in combination with low-dose antipsychotic medication. For patients who cannot tolerate lithium because of sensitivity to side effects or impaired renal function, valproic acid and carbamazepine are alternative mood-stabilizing agents. While many patients enjoy long periods of remission, it is typical for episodes of illness to become more frequent with age. In addition, complicated clinical conditions such as mixed episodes, in which symptoms of mania and depression coexist, and rapid cycling, in which four or more mood episodes occur within 12 months, may develop. Because of its high recurrence rate, patients with bipolar disorder often require life-long pharmacologic treatment and regular psychiatric monitoring.

Dysthymic disorder is a chronic depressive condition lasting 2 years or longer and marked by a persistently low mood more days than not and at least two of the following: appetite change, insomnia, low energy, low self-esteem, poor concentration or difficulty making decisions, and hopelessness. It may be a milder depressive disorder than major depression in severity of individual symptoms, but the chronicity of the depressive symptoms can be disabling and demoralizing to the patient and may contribute to lowering functional capacities (12). In addition, some patients with dysthymic disorder go on to develop a major depressive episode. In older people, dysthymic disorder often develops in the setting of physical disability, multiple medical problems, isolation, and loneliness. Many patients with a dysthymic disorder respond to treatment with an antidepressant. Supportive psychotherapy is a vital component of treatment, the goals being to increase social contacts and activity level and to improve self-esteem and outlook through an empathic therapeutic relationship.

Grief is not a mental disorder, and depressive symptoms are considered to be part of the normal bereavement process. While persons vary in their response to losing a loved one, there are common predictable phases to grieving (13). The initial response, which lasts several days, is characterized by shock, disbelief, and emotional numbing. This is often followed by anger and frustration. Usually these initial reactions give way to a long period of fluctuating despair, mourning, and wishing to be with the deceased. During the first 3 to 6 months following the death of a loved one, insomnia is common, as are frequent episodes of tearfulness, anxiety, and a loss of interest or pleasure in activities once enjoyed. Usually the intensity of symptoms begins to remit after the first 6 to 12 months; strong feelings of loss and mourning continue for 1 to 2 years, longer for some people. In addition, intense emotional feelings tend to return on the anniversary of the loved one's death and birthday and at holiday times.

It is unclear at what point a bereaved person should be referred for professional help or counseling. The support of family, friends, and clergy are sufficient to help most bereaved persons through the grieving process. Widow and widower support groups can also be helpful in adjusting to life without a spouse and increasing social contacts. When the bereaved person is overwhelmed by grief and unable to begin to return to usual activities or if grief is complicated by panic attacks, delusions, or suicidal thoughts, referral for psychiatric evaluation is indicated. Grief may trigger a full major depressive episode. While sadness, disruption of sleep, and loss of motivation and interest may be part of an uncomplicated grief syndrome, feelings of guilt, worthlessness, and hopelessness are not part of grief and should signal concern that a major depression has developed and should be treated as outlined earlier.

Suicide

Suicide is the third leading cause of death due to injury among persons over age 65, after unintentional falls and motor vehicle accidents. Age-specific rates for suicide have consistently been higher among the elderly than for any other age group. Of particular concern are recent data from the National Center for Health Statistics (NCHS) of the Centers for Disease Control and Prevention that indicate that after decades of declining rates, the period from 1980 to 1992 saw a marked increase in the rate of suicide among persons aged 65 and older (14). Of persons 65 and older, men accounted for 81% of the suicides. Rates were highest for divorced or widowed men. Other risk factors include depression, alcoholism, chemical dependency, physical illness, and social isolation. Older persons make fewer attempts per completed suicide than other age groups and tend to use violent means of suicide. Indeed, firearms were the most common method of suicide by both men and women over age 65.

While suicide cannot be predicted with complete accuracy, the potential for suicide must be considered seriously by all health providers who care for the elderly. Particular attention must be paid to patients who are despondent, overwhelmed by the burdens of physical illness or disability, lack social support, drink alcohol excessively, or have made previous suicide attempts. Clinicians must become comfortable about asking their older patients about suicidal ideation and should not hesitate to seek psychiatric consultation for any patient who seems at high risk.

Personality Disorder

Personality is the set of enduring traits that makes each person unique. Traits are universally shared characteristics on which persons differ. They include patterns of perceiving and relating to one's self and one's social environment. For example, all people can be rated on their tendency for tidiness. People vary widely in this tendency, but for each person a certain degree of tidiness or lack thereof is characteristic. Personality disorders are diagnosed when a person falls at the extreme end of the normal distribution on a set of traits that commonly occur together. Personality disorders reflect enduring, inflexible, and maladaptive patterns of inner experience and behavior. For example, *histrionic personality disorder* is diagnosed when a person exhibits provocativeness, self-dramatization, emotional lability, and self-centeredness and frequently engages in attention-seeking behaviors. *Antisocial personality disorder* is associated with repeated illegal actions, impulsivity, frequent lies, consistent irresponsibility, lack of remorse, and lack of concern toward others. *Obsessive-compulsive personality disorder* is characterized by extreme perfectionism, rigidity, emotional inexpressiveness, excessive preoccupation with rules and details, and inflexibility. *Dependent personality behavior* is characterized by an excessive need to be taken care of by others, which leads to difficulty making independent everyday decisions. These persons lack confidence in their own judgment or abilities to do things on their own, and they often go to excessive lengths to obtain reassurance or support. To satisfy a diagnosis of personality disorder, problems in these realms must be lifelong. Thus in the elderly a diagnosis of a personality disorder must reflect a pattern of behavior that has been present throughout adulthood and has caused problems for the person throughout his or her life.

Personality disorders complicate the care of the medically ill. Patients with histrionic personality disorder or prominent histrionic traits are likely to present physical symptoms in a dramatic fashion, to demonstrate marked emotional lability, and to be provocative and demanding. Conversely, patients with obsessive-compulsive personality disorder may underreport symptoms, have very high expectations of their physicians, be inflexible, be unable to make decisions, and have difficulty accepting the lack of clear guidelines that sometimes occurs in medical conditions.

The physician who is aware that a personality disorder is underlying a problematic patient's behavior can avoid or alleviate problems by considering the patient's predispositions. Patients with prominent obsessional traits often need detailed discussions of proposed procedures and an extensive and specific discussion regarding the steps that are to be taken, the order in which they are to be taken, and the implications of the most likely outcomes. For the histrionic patient, on the other hand, an extensive detailed discussion is often overwhelming. While all patients need options and clear descriptions, patients with histrionic features often do best when information is presented with a reassuring, calm tone, a concise description of alternatives, a direct acknowledgment of emotional distress ("I know this is upsetting, but let me present the alternatives before we discuss them") and frequent short visits. Patients with dependent personality disorder have difficulty following through with recommendations on their own and do better if important persons in their social support network are part of the treatment process.

Psychotic Symptoms

Hallucinations (perceptions without a stimulus occurring in any of the five senses) and delusions (false ideas that are unshakable and persistent) occur in many medical and psychiatric disorders. The first step in their assessment is to determine whether a cognitive impairment (delirium or dementia) is present. The importance of this step is twofold. First, cognitive disorder is a common cause of hallucinations and delusions, and second, this recognition leads to the appropriate medical evaluation.

Hallucinations and delusions can also be caused by depression, schizophrenia, and delusional disorder. After a primary cognitive disorder has been ruled out, the next step is to assess for mood disorder. Self-deprecation, self-blame, hopelessness, loss of interest in usually enjoyed activities, somatic preoccupations, and complaints of sad mood all suggest the possibility that major depression is the cause of the psychotic symptoms.

Schizophrenia and *delusional disorder* are uncommon conditions, occurring in fewer than 1% of the population. They can present to medical practitioners with isolated somatic delusions (e.g., belief that someone is sending an electrical shock into the body or belief in a physical illness for which there is no evidence). By definition a *delusional disorder* is characterized by a single delusion occurring in the absence of cognitive impairment, mood impairment, and other psychiatric symptoms. *Schizophrenia* is an illness in which symptoms are present for at least 6 months, hallucina-

tions and social dilapidation are predominant, and mood disorder criteria are not met. While schizophrenia most commonly begins in early adulthood, it can begin in late life. Patients with late-onset schizophrenia frequently have paranoid delusions, social isolation, and hearing impairment (15).

Psychotic symptoms may arise from toxic effects of prescribed medication, such as carbidopa with levodopa (Sinemet) or steroids. In addition, isolated visual hallucinations (i.e., not accompanied by delusions, cognitive impairment, or mood disorder) sometimes occur in patients with a wide variety of visual disorders, such as glaucoma, cataracts, and retinal degeneration (16). Finally, hallucinations and delusions may develop in the course of several neurologic diseases such as dementia, Huntington's disease, and Parkinson's disease.

The treatment of psychotic symptoms depends, in part, on the diagnosis of the underlying disorder. If the patient is delirious, all attempts should be made to correct the underlying abnormality and to avoid pharmacotherapy unless there are clear indications. So-called neuroleptic, psychotropic, or antipsychotic drugs are the treatment of choice when pharmacotherapy is necessary. In dementia, reorientation and activity therapy should be tried first. Pharmacotherapy is appropriate when these symptoms increase the likelihood of danger of harm to the patient or others or cause emotional distress to the patient. For mood disorder several studies demonstrate that delusional major depression responds better to the combination of an antidepressant and neuroleptic than to an antidepressant alone.

Psychiatric Treatment of Irreversible Cognitive Disorders

Dementia and delirium are discussed in detail in Chapters 15, 16, and 17. About 60% of patients with dementia have psychotic symptoms sometime in the course of a dementing illness. These noncognitive symptoms, which can interfere with the quality of life of the patient and caregiver, are often amenable to treatment. When appropriate, nonpharmacologic environmental therapy is most desirable because of the potential side effects of drugs. Nondrug treatments include providing a structured environment, stimulating the patient at an appropriate level, and providing the level of care that that person needs. When hallucinations and delusions interfere with function, become distressing to the patient, or are dangerous to others, cautious low-dosage neuroleptic therapy is appropriate.

Some 15 to 30% of patients with dementia also suffer from depression that interferes with function. Antidepressant drugs with low anticholinergic properties (e.g., nortriptyline, desipramine, SSRIs) are recommended. Emotional support for both patient and caregiver is indicated in all cases. The physician should play an important role in educating the family, in managing specific behavioral and noncognitive symptoms, and in helping the families address their social, legal, and financial concerns.

OVERVIEW OF TREATMENT ISSUES
Pharmacotherapy

While older patients can benefit from the same psychopharmacologic agents as younger ones, the clinician must be aware both of changes in physiology and pharmacokinetics with age and of potential interactions with other medications. Prescribing psychotropic medication for older patients requires special considerations discussed in detail in other sources (3). However, some important principles are outlined here.

Perhaps the most familiar axiom in prescribing for older adults is "start low and go slow." This means that for just about every medication, be it an anxiolytic, antipsychotic, or antidepressant, one should start at a low dose and titrate the dose up to a therapeutic dose slowly and gradually. A good rule of thumb is to allow at least five days between each dosage increase. This allows the patient to adjust to a new medication and to report any troublesome side effects before they become problematic.

Older patients are more sensitive to the anticholinergic effects of medication and therefore more likely than younger patients to develop delirium, constipation, urinary retention, dry mouth, and orthostatic hypotension. For these reasons medications with the least anticholinergic effects are preferred when a choice of several agents is available.

Another important principle is to choose medications with shorter half-lives. Because of the changes in hepatic metabolism that occur with aging, the half-lives of most pharmacologic agents are prolonged in older people. This increases the likelihood that psychologically active metabolites will accumulate over time and cause toxicity. Obviously this problem is worsened if the original drug and/or its active metabolite or metabolites have long half-lives to begin with. Among benzodiazepines, for instance, lorazepam (half-life 16 hours) and oxazepam (half-life 8 hours) are better tolerated in older people than is diazepam (half-life 3 to 4 days). If a longer-acting benzodiazepine is required to manage severe anxiety or withdrawal from benzodiazepines, clonazepam (half-life 1 to 2 days) is useful.

Lithium carbonate deserves special mention, since it is nearly totally excreted by the kidneys. Because glomerular filtration rate and creatinine clearance decrease steadily with age, older patients are likely to develop lithium-induced tremor and delirium at low doses. Furthermore, recent studies seem to indicate that the therapeutic effects of lithium occur at lower blood levels in older patients than in younger ones. For all of these reasons older patients require lower doses of lithium than younger patients, usually 150 mg daily to 300 mg twice a day (1).

In general the lowest dose of antipsychotic medication needed to control symptoms should be prescribed. In addition to their extrapyramidal and anticholinergic side effects, neuroleptics are likely to cause tardive dyskinesia in the elderly.

For most antidepressants, on the other hand, patients do best if the medication is within the therapeutic range regardless of age. Low-dose antidepressant treatment is likely to be inadequate to treat a major depressive episode. Because of wide variations in older persons' hepatic metabolism, it is impossible to predict the dose of antidepressant needed to achieve a therapeutic level, but often it is the same as for much younger persons. It is important to give an antidepressant an adequate trial length (4 to 6 weeks minimum) at a therapeutic dose before deciding that the medication trial was a failure and changing to another antidepressant. Indeed, there is evidence that for some antidepressants, such as fluoxetine, a longer trial period, 6 to 8 weeks, may be necessary to establish maximum therapeutic benefits. Furthermore, to prevent relapse it is important that full-strength antidepressant therapy continue for 6 to 12 months once a therapeutic response has begun. Long-term antidepressant therapy is indicated for patients with recurrent depression.

Finally, as with all medications, it is important to consider drug interactions. Fluoxetine, for example, increases serum levels of digoxin, warfarin, and other protein-bound drugs. Tricyclic antidepressants and neuroleptics have hypotensive effects that can compound the effects of antihypertensive medications. Nonsteroidal anti-inflammatory drugs increase the plasma level of lithium and put an older patient at risk for lithium toxicity. Thus, the older patient must be carefully monitored while being treated with psychotropic medications to avoid both undertreatment and toxicity. Monoamine oxidase inhibitors should not be prescribed concomitantly with SSRIs or venlafaxine, and to avoid serotonin syndrome there should be a minimum 2- to 5-week washout period after one agent has been discontinued and the other type of antidepressant started. Serotonin syndrome is a serious, sometimes fatal, condition that is characterized by hyperthermia, rigidity, myoclonus, autonomic instability, and mental status changes. Because of interactions with the cytochrome P450 IIIA$_4$ isozyme, nefazodone is contraindicated in patients who are also taking cisapride, astemizole, terfenadine, or triazolam. Adverse reactions may also develop if nefazodone is prescribed with alprazolam (Xanax). Nefazodone has also been found to increase the peak and trough plasma concentrations of digoxin.

Psychotherapy

Individual Psychotherapy

Contrary to many prevailing myths, older patients do benefit from psychotherapy in the treatment of a variety of disorders (17). For patients with depression, anxiety, and bereavement, psychotherapy is an important part of treatment even when pharmacotherapy is indicated. Through psychotherapy older people can im-

prove significantly in self-esteem, self-awareness, adaptation, and personal satisfaction. No one psychotherapeutic method works best with older people. We recommend a pluralistic approach that emphasizes life review and focuses on specific issues of concern. Many persons benefit from a focus on the development of problem-solving skills. Some patients benefit from a return to an active, creative life. Also, patients with anxiety disorders and phobias may benefit from a more cognitive-behavioral approach that stresses the importance of positive problem solving and teaches relaxation techniques.

Marital Therapy

Marital or couples therapy is helpful for older people in several circumstances. Retirement and late-life illnesses can dramatically alter the dynamics of a marriage. Spouses who were used to busy but relatively independent work lives may find it an adjustment to be home together most of the time. Roles may change as one spouse does more or less of the cooking, shopping, and housekeeping. If one spouse is unable to drive because of health problems, this can put limitations on the lifestyles of both partners. Retirement also means living on a fixed income for most people, and these new financial constraints may pose an additional burden. In short, the reality of living "the golden years" often does not meet the expectations for this time of life. This may result in disappointment or resentment, especially if one spouse blames the other for preventing the fulfillment of the retirement dream. In addition, problems can develop between widowed or divorced elders involved in new relationships. Issues such as whether to live together or marry, how to combine finances, and how to deal with each other's adult children can put a strain on the relationship. While couples issues may be the presenting focus for treatment, usually they are not. Rather, these issues may emerge as the patient is beginning treatment for depression or anxiety. Short-term marital therapy can be very useful in defusing stressful situations, improving communications between partners, and fostering a more healthful adaptation to the couples' changing way of life.

Family Assessment

Often other family issues come to light during the course of assessment and treatment of the older patient. For some, decreased functional abilities or illness raises dependence on adult children. This may necessitate moving in with adult children or moving closer geographically. When an elderly person develops dementia and/or other disabling medical illness, the spouse or adult child may become a primary caregiver and have to assume new responsibilities for the impaired person's personal and financial care. Older patients may find that their grown children need them in new or different ways, e.g., because of illness or divorce on the part of the adult children.

These and other situations can produce family conflict and stress. It is very helpful to meet with all involved family members at least once to assess how various family members relate to one another, solve problems, deal with their changing family dynamics, and address the needs of the impaired elder person. These meetings can also be useful for teaching the family about the impaired older person's medications and illness, for mobilizing family and community resources, and for identifying others in the family who need support or counseling.

Barriers to Treatment

There are many reasons older people often do not get the psychologic treatment they need (18). One common reason is that older people themselves are reluctant to see a psychiatrist because of embarrassment and negative attitudes. While education is slowly changing society's outlook on mental illness and mental health care, older people who grew up in the Depression or earlier may still believe one should solve one's own problems and "pick oneself up by the boot straps." To such persons, seeking help for psychologic problems is viewed as a sign of personal weakness. Other contributors to elders not receiving care for emotional problems include the negative attitude of their physician; the focus by patient, family, or physician on medical issues; and lack of transportation. These issues are best overcome by discussing them openly and reviewing the reasons a person is reluctant to seek help.

REFERENCES

1. Jenike MA. Geriatric Psychiatry and Psychopharmacology: A Clinical Approach. Chicago: Year Book Medical, 1989.
2. Regier DA, Boyd JH, Burke JD Jr, et al. One-month prevalence of mental disorders in the United States. Arch Gen Psychiatry 1988;45:977–986.
3. Lipowski ZJ. Delirium (acute confusional state). JAMA 1987;258:1789–1792.
4. Rovner BW, Kafonek S, Filipp L, et al. Prevalence of mental illness in a community nursing home. Am J Psychiatry 1986;143:1446–1449.
5. Blazer DG. Depression in Late Life. 2nd ed. St. Louis: Mosby-Year Book, 1993.
6. Blazer DG. Is depression more frequent in late life? J Geriatr Psychiatry 1994;2:193–199.
7. Lipsey JR, Robinson RG, Pearlson GD, et al. The dexamethasone suppression test and mood following stroke. Am J Psychiatry 1985;142:318–323.
8. Roberts RE, Kaplan GA, Shema S, Strawbridge WJ. Does growing old increase the risk for depression? Am J Psychiatry 1997;154:1384–1390.
9. Philibert RA, Richards L, Lynch CF, et al. Effect of ECT on mortality and clinical outcome in geriatric unipolar depression. J Clin Psychiatry 1995;56:390–394.
10. Cattan RA, Barry PP, Mead G, et al. Electroconvulsive therapy in octogenarians. J Am Geriatr Soc 1990;38:753–758.
11. Shulman KI. Recent developments in the epidemiology, co-morbidity and outcome of mania in old age. Rev Clin Gerontol 1996;6:249–254.
12. Blazer D, Hughes, DC, George LK. The epidemiology of depression in an elderly community population. Gerontologist 1987;27:281–287.
13. Bruce ML, Kim K, Leaf PJ. Depressive episodes and dysphoria resulting from conjugal bereavement in a prospective community sample. Am J Psychiatry 1990;147:608–611.
14. Meehan PJ, Saltzman LE, Sattin RW. Suicides among older United States residents: epidemiologic characteristics and trends. Am J Public Health 1991;81:1198–1200.
15. Jeste DV, Harris MJ, Krull A, et al. Clinical and neuropsychological characteristics of patients with late-onset schizophrenia. Am J Psychiatry 1995;152:722–730.
16. Holroyd S, Rabins PV, Finkelstein D, et al. Visual hallucinations in patients from an ophthalmology clinic and medical clinic population. J Nerv Ment Dis 1994;182:272–276.
17. Myers WA. New Techniques in the Psychotherapy of Older Patients. Washington: American Psychiatry Press, 1991.
18. Waxman HM, Carner EA, Klein M. Underutilization of mental health professionals by community elderly. Gerontologist 1984;24:23–30.

CHAPTER 14

ALAN A. WARTENBERG AND TED D. NIRENBERG

Alcohol and Other Drug Abuse in Older Patients

The abuse of alcohol and other drugs in Western society is extremely common, with prevalence rates of approximately 15% for alcohol abuse and 5% for other drugs (1, 2). It is clear that such use is only occasionally detected by physicians, although abusers are more likely than nonabusers to be seen in the medical setting, whether inpatient (3) or outpatient (4). In older persons, the diagnosis is even more rarely suspected, diagnosed, treated, or referred (5, 6). While there is a tendency for drinking to decrease with age (7, 8) and although estimates of the prevalence of alcoholism or problem drinking among older persons range between 2 and 10%, studies of elderly hospital patients find much higher rates, ranging from 8 to 70%, depending on diagnostic criteria used and the subpopulation under study (9–11). A recent report indicated that among elderly who have used alcohol in the past year, more than 25% have responses suggesting or establishing alcoholism on a reliable screening instrument (12). A study showed that the national prevalence of alcohol-related hospitalizations of elderly persons was 54.7 per 10,000 men and 14.8 per 10,000 women, with an estimated total cost of more than $233 million (13).

Recently, there has been significantly increased attention to the problems of chemical dependency in the elderly. The American Medical Association has issued a special communication of guidelines for primary care providers in the prevention, treatment, and diagnosis of alcoholism in older adults (14), and its journal has published a council report on the same topic (15). A recent extensive review of substance use disorders (16) includes a section on the elderly (17).

Physicians, nurses, and other health care professionals have received little training in the recognition and management of patients with alcohol and other drug abuse (18). We are particularly unlikely to entertain these diagnoses when the patients do not fit our stereotypic view of an alcohol or other drug abuser. We are also rarely trained in issues of prescription drug abuse and in judicious prescribing when alcohol and other drug abuse can or should be suspected.

The older patient presents special issues in the recognition and management of alcohol and other drug abuse. There have been few studies of treatment efficacy in this population (19, 20), and many treatment recommendations are based on studies on younger persons, which may not be applicable to the older patient. Presentation may be atypical, and management decisions may be affected by the other medical and/or psychiatric issues common in the elderly.

NATURAL HISTORY
Alcohol

Clinical observations have led to the classification of elderly problem drinkers and alcoholics on the basis of whether alcohol problems began early or late in their life: early versus late onset (21, 22). Efforts at classification attempt to capture more variation in drinking patterns by including categories for drinkers whose problems are transient or intermittent throughout their lifetime or those that vary over time with respect to the quantity and consequences of drinking (23).

Dunham has argued that at least four distinct drinking patterns may pose problems for elderly drinkers—heavy, moderate, light, and infrequent—and that there is considerable movement in and out of drinking patterns throughout a drinker's lifetime (24). The age cutoff used to delineate late-onset alcohol problem drinking typically ranges from 40 to 60 years (25). Late-onset problem drinking has been reported to account for 28 to 40% of elderly problem drinkers found in clinical samples (26). Early-onset drinkers frequently have had medical problems related to their drinking, and many have had hospitalizations for treatment of medical sequelae, detoxification, or rehabilitation. There is often a strong family history of alcohol abuse, and both the first use of alcohol and the onset of problematic use may have been early in life. Such persons may have episodes of intoxication, a withdrawal syndrome, or serious medical sequelae, including trauma. The family is often devastated by extreme dysfunction, with resentment of years of abuse on the part of spouse or caretaker, siblings, children, and friends.

Alcohol and other drug abuse may be problematic on the part of other family members as well. The patient is likely to minimize or deny problems and resist help. The addition of an organic brain syndrome, generally secondary to alcohol abuse but possibly other causes (e.g., multiple infarctions, hypothyroidism, vitamin B_{12} deficiency, syphilis, or Alzheimer's disease), may further complicate management. Patients may be incapable of understanding their situation and of accepting the necessary help but be competent enough to make decisions regarding their care.

The epidemiologic literature on risk factors predicting vulnerability to late-onset alcohol problems is limited (11). Several studies report that late-onset alcoholics are less likely to have a family history of alcohol abuse and alcohol-related legal or social problems than early-onset alcoholics (27, 28) and that early alcohol problems are not good predictors of later alcohol abuse (29).

Some evidence suggests that late-onset alcohol problems are a maladaptive response to common personal, social, and environmental stressors that are correlates of aging. For example, the loss of self-image associated with cessation of employment, either inside or outside the home, and/or loss of youth, health, and mobility may leave the older person with significant feelings of anxiety and depression and with an inadequate support system to deal with the losses. Crises such as bereavement, social isolation, unwanted residential change, death of a spouse or child, financial distress, fear of crime, loneliness, and even pressure from peers in some retirement communities to increase alcohol intake all have been posited as plausible causal factors for late-onset alcohol problems (30). Fear of physical abuse and abandonment by caregivers may particularly affect women and be a factor in their alcohol and other drug abuse. Depression and anxiety may lead to use of alcohol to self-medicate (31), which may ultimately lead to increasing tolerance, withdrawal, and continued use of alcohol to avoid withdrawal. Alcohol may be used by the patient who finds that it decreases the severity of an essential or head-bobbing tremor or that it allows him or her to sleep. Continued use in this setting may again lead to problematic use.

In the person with late-onset alcohol problems, the family may be functional and able and willing to assist in treatment. It is relatively unlikely that other members of the family have been adversely affected by the alcohol abuse, and they are likely to enter into a therapeutic alliance with the physician or therapist. The patient may be willing to admit that the alcohol use has become problematic and to accept help.

Although metabolism of alcohol is not particularly affected by age, the volume of distribution may change because of reduction in body fat, allowing more of a dose of alcohol to reach the brain (32, 33). In addition, the aging brain may be more susceptible to the effects of alcohol (34). Older persons may find that the amount of alcohol that they could easily tolerate when they were young results in adverse effects. The older patient may present because of such adverse consequences as falls, with increased incidence of fracture and subdural hematoma, anemia, gastritis with and without hemorrhage, alcoholic liver disease, pancreatitis, alcohol amnestic syndrome, and early dementia. Alcohol use may increase blood pressure, and the patient may have late-onset or labile hypertension or hypertension that is difficult to control. The reader is referred to reviews of the medical consequences of using alcohol and other drugs (35, 36).

Sedative-Hypnotics

Anxiety disorders and insomnia are common in older persons, and a substantial number of prescriptions for anxiolytic and soporific drugs are used in this population. Normal changes in sleeping patterns may be troublesome, and the physician who fails to take a complete sleep history or inquire into sleep hygiene may prescribe hypnotics inappropriately. While benzodiazepines have become the primary class of prescribed agents, use of barbiturates, meprobamate, chloral hydrate, and other barbituratelike drugs is not uncommon (37).

While most patients for whom sedative-hypnotics are prescribed take them safely and effectively over a long time, abuse and dependence occur in some patients, particularly those with underlying alcohol abuse or personality disorders. The person abusing such drugs may develop tolerance over time, gradually increasing the number of doses per day or the amount of each dose. This often results in calls to physicians' offices for refills of prescriptions prior to visits and ultimately may result in claims of lost prescriptions, stolen pills, loss of pills in the toilet, and so on. Patients seeking additional drugs may visit several physicians, emergency departments, or walk-in clinics. Increasing use of sedatives may result in retrograde or anterograde amnesia, deterioration of personal hygiene, confusion, lethargy, and obtundation. Automatic behavior, in which the patient does not remember taking the medication because of its amnestic effects, may result in multiple doses taken with serious adverse consequences.

Other central nervous system depressants, such as alcohol or opioids, may have additive or synergistic effects with sedatives, and greater caution should be exercised in prescribing them. In the alcohol-abusing patient, the concomitant use of benzodiazepines or other sedatives may result in more rapid deterioration and can have serious effects, including risks of respiratory depression, aspiration, pneumonia, falls, and motor vehicle and other accidents. As with alcohol, some patients who develop sedative-hypnotic abuse have a long-standing history of chemical dependency, while others develop abuse later in life, secondary to other problems associated with aging or losses in their lives. The natural history and presentation vary considerably with the nature of onset and medical and psychiatric comorbidities.

Opioids

Abuse of illicit opioids, particularly heroin, is extremely rare in patients over 60, although patients with long-standing opioid abuse occasionally survive into old age. Opium smoking may be seen in older persons from Asian cultures. However, licit opioid abuse is more common in the elderly. The increase in painful conditions, particularly arthritis and low back pain, may result in prescriptions for oral opioids with abuse potential. As with sedative-hypnotics, abuse occurs in a minority of patients, but the results of such abuse may be serious for patients and family. Fear of abuse often leads to underprescribing of opioids for painful conditions, particularly cancer and other intractable pain. The patient with a history of alcohol or other drug abuse and patients with certain psychiatric syndromes may be particularly likely to abuse opioids and other drugs.

Clinicians working with chronic pain patients usually find that patients can be maintained on a stable dose of opioids for long periods with little or no escalation of dose or problematic use (38). There appears to be relatively little tolerance to the analgesic effects of opioids; dose increases of 10 to 20% per year are common. On the other hand, tolerance to the mood-altering or euphoriant effects of opioids occurs rapidly, causing the need to escalate the dose. Patients may believe that they are increasing the dose to combat pain, but it is more likely that they are receiving relief of psychic rather than somatic pain.

Increases in doses lead to the same issues as with sedative-hypnotics, including frequent refills, excuses of lost pills or prescriptions, and doctor shopping. In addition, since the dominant form of opioid prescription is for combinations containing aspirin or acetaminophen, toxicity from these agents may occur. High-dose opioids may result in personality changes, irritability, sedation, and accidental trauma. Central nervous system stimulation with seizures and delirium may occur with propoxyphene, pentazocine, and meperidine.

Other Drugs

Abuse of cocaine and other stimulants is extremely rare in the elderly, as is abuse of psychotomimetic drugs and inhalants. Prescription of amphetamines or methylphenidate for depression rarely results in abuse and toxicity. Use of cannabis may occur, particularly by persons with histories of such use, and occasionally cannabis is self-prescribed to combat nausea from chemotherapy or to treat glaucoma. The elderly may take high-dose aspirin or nonsteroidal anti-inflammatory drugs without medical supervision to treat pain, sometimes with serious medical consequences, including gastrointestinal hemorrhage, acid-base disturbances, confusion, and delirium (39). Use of multiple medications with anticholinergic effects is common in the elderly, and while not generally related to abuse, it may result in behavioral changes and presentations with memory impairment, agitation, confusion, or delirium.

Drug-drug interactions, as well as interactions with alcohol, tobacco, and even food products, are very common, particularly in the elderly, among whom polypharmacy is common. Reduction in renal and/or hepatic clearance, decrease in body weight and/or fat, displacement of one drug from protein binding sites by another, and other factors may make such interactions common and problematic (40, 41). A careful history of drugs prescribed by all of the patient's physicians, as well as prescribed drugs obtained from other sources (a family member's or friend's medication), over-the-counter drug use, tobacco use, and dietary history, including recent gain or loss of weight, may be required in detecting problems related to drug-drug interaction.

DIAGNOSIS

The diagnosis of chemical dependency, like most others in clinical medicine, should be largely based on history. The criteria in the *Diagnostic and Statistical Manual of Mental Disorders*, fourth edition (DSM-IV), are widely accepted (42). Three of seven criteria are required for a diagnosis of a substance dependence disorder, but patients having one or two criteria should be closely monitored (Table 14.1).

The CAGE questionnaire (*c*ut down on use; *a*nger if use brought up; *g*uilt over use; need for *e*ye opener) (43) may be helpful. Although it has

---

Table 14.1

Diagnostic Criteria for Substance Dependence

Three or more of the following:
(1) Tolerance, as defined by either of the following:
   (a) A need for increased amounts of substance to achieve intoxication or desired effects
   (b) Diminished effect with continued use of same or cross-tolerant substance
(2) Withdrawal, as manifested by either of the following:
   (a) The characteristic withdrawal syndrome
   (b) The same or cross-tolerant drug taken to relieve or avoid withdrawal[a]
(3) Substance often taken in larger amounts or over longer period than intended
(4) Persistent desire or unsuccessful efforts to cut down or control use
(5) Great deal of time spent in activities necessary to obtain, use, or recover from the effects of the substance
(6) Important social, occupational, or recreational activities given up or reduced because of substance use
(7) Use continued despite knowledge of having a persistent or recurrent physical or psychologic problem likely to have been caused or exacerbated by use

Modified from American Psychiatric Association. Diagnostic and Statistical Manual of Mental Disorders. 4th ed. Washington: American Psychiatric Association, 1994:181.
[a]May not apply to cannabis, phencyclidine, hallucinogens.

not been specifically validated in older populations, there is evidence that it may be at least a useful screening tool in older populations (44). A positive response to two of the CAGE questions is associated with sensitivity and specificity in the 90% range in the younger patients, but it must be stressed that this is a screening instrument, and definitive diagnosis should be based on more comprehensive evaluation. Positive responses to these following questions may add to the positive predictive value of the CAGE questions (45): Was your last drink with 24 hours of the interview? Do you think you have ever had a drinking problem? The Michigan Alcoholism Screening Test (MAST), which is widely used, may have less utility than the CAGE in the elderly (46). One group has found that the short MAST (sMAST) may be more sensitive as a screening tool than the CAGE or standard MAST in older persons (47).

A complete substance use history should be obtained, asking questions in a calm, nonjudgmental, and open-ended way. Emphasis should be on specific questions about quantity and frequency of use, including problematic binge drinking. Specific questions such as "What day did you last drink alcohol?" and "How much did you drink that day?" may be useful. Asking whether the number of drinking occasions per week or month and the amount of drinks per occasion are typical or have changed over time may also be informative. Specific questions regarding doses of prescribed drugs and whether such doses are ever exceeded, as well as asking about frequency of refills, should be part of the history. A recent study found that asking specific questions regarding quantity and frequency of alcohol use improved detection of problem drinking (48).

Many, if not most, patients will be quite open about their substance use when asked directly about their history. For patients who seem evasive, it may be very useful and even essential to obtain information from significant others, whether family, friends, or neighbors. The patient may minimize or categorically deny problems, while others in a patient's system may be in a better position to give accurate information. Resistance on the part of the patient to answer questions or allow interviews of significant others should raise the clinician's level of suspicion and should be met with persistent efforts to obtain the needed information. Confidentiality issues may limit the ability to obtain needed information, and the clinicians should be sure of their legal footing in problematic cases.

A history of certain medical and social problems should prompt the physician to explore the possibility of substance abuse further, even though the patient may deny such a problem. For example, a history of gastrointestinal hemorrhage, unexplained abdominal pain, pancreatitis, liver dysfunction, or frequent unexplained somatic complaints, anxiety, or affective disorders may be suggestive of substance use and should lead the clinician to obtain a comprehensive substance use history.

Mental status changes, a history of family dysfunction, divorce, and frequent job changes or geographic moves should alert the clinician further to assess the possibility of substance abuse. One of the most immediate and clinically convenient ways of assessing a person's blood alcohol concentration (BAC) is to use a breath alcohol test. A reliable and valid measure of alcohol and/or drug use is essential, since clinicians' judgment of patients' states of intoxication is poor, probably because of drug tolerance. A BAC of more than 100 mg/100 mL in a person who shows no signs of inebriation (sustained nystagmus, dysarthria, ataxia, lability of mood, sedation) or a BAC of 250 mg/100 mL in a conscious patient indicates significant tolerance and suggests a diagnosis of alcohol dependence, as well as predicting the likelihood of a significant abstinence syndrome.

Sedative-hypnotics produce a picture similar to that of alcohol, but blood levels are more difficult to obtain. Benzodiazepine and barbiturate levels can be measured in serum but may not be immediately available. Patients who state that they are taking medications as prescribed but have serum levels far above expected levels are probably taking medication beyond the prescribed dose. Similarly, high serum levels in a patient showing no signs of toxicity suggest dependency. Abuse of butabarbital-containing drugs for headache has become quite common; measurement of butabarbital serum levels and/or acetaminophen or salicylate levels may be definitive.

The patient who abuses opioids may show considerable tolerance and have few or no signs of toxicity. However, pupillary miosis should be seen if the drug was recently used. While levels of most opioids cannot be easily measured in serum, urine toxicology studies can provide a qualitative result. Serum salicylate or acetaminophen levels can be useful in the patient taking combination analgesic products, alerting the clinician to the need for separate treatment. Patients with sedation or obtundation or with pupillary miosis and slowed respiration must be assumed to have opioid intoxication. Abuse of mixed agonist-antagonists, such as pentazocine, propoxyphene, and meperidine, may cause central nervous system stimulation, including seizures and delirium.

Because polysubstance use has become so common, it is advisable to obtain a qualitative urine toxicology screen in any patient suspected of chemical dependency. This should be done before treatment with any psychoactive drug. Clinicians should familiarize themselves with the use and limitations of toxicology studies (49), particularly if there are any legal ramifications to the urine drug testing. Drug testing should be used as one component of the comprehensive assessment, because false-positive and false-negative results are possible. The patient's use may be in amounts below the limits of detection; he or she may use a prescribed medication with metabolites that cross-react as other drugs on assays; or the patient may adulterate or substitute the urine sample. While positive urine toxicology studies may alert the clinician to unsuspected use of sedative-hypnotics, opioids, or other drugs, a negative study does not exclude such use.

TREATMENT
Role of the Primary Care Provider

If a diagnosis of chemical dependency is made or suspected, it is incumbent on the clinician to determine the risk of an abstinence or withdrawal syndrome (50, 51). Well-intentioned advice to a patient to cut down or quit alcohol or abrupt discontinuation of a benzodiazepine prescription af-

ter evidence of misuse or abuse may result in a patient suffering withdrawal symptoms such as seizures, delirium, and/or a hyperautonomic syndrome, which in many patients, particularly the elderly, may have disastrous consequences. The level of tolerance and the patient's previous experiences in discontinuing drug use are good predictors of the likelihood of an abstinence syndrome.

The older patient may have fewer hyperautonomic signs and symptoms, leading to diagnostic confusion when a seizure or delirium supervenes. When a hyperautonomic state occurs, it may result in angina or myocardial infarction in patients with preexisting coronary heart disease, exacerbation of hypertension with possibility of stroke, diabetes going out of control, or hypoxia and collapse in the patient with underlying chronic obstructive pulmonary disease. Withdrawal of short-acting benzodiazepines or other sedative hypnotics may be similar to alcohol withdrawal syndrome. With barbiturates and barbituratelike drugs, status epilepticus may occur, and delirium may be particularly severe. Opioid withdrawal also may cause a hyperautonomic state, although generally less severe than that with alcohol or sedative hypnotics.

In general, the older patient should be treated in a medically managed or monitored setting, since morbidity and mortality may be high. A complete medical evaluation must be done, with laboratory studies appropriate to the clinical setting: complete blood count, electrolytes, blood sugar, blood urea nitrogen and creatinine, chemistry panel with liver function tests, total protein and albumin, uric acid, calcium, and phosphorus. Serum magnesium levels should be obtained in most cases, since hypomagnesemia is common and predisposes to seizures and cardiac arrhythmias. All patients should be given adequate doses of thiamine; generally 100 mg intramuscularly should be given initially, and then similar doses intramuscularly should be given daily until the patient is taking oral medication. Failure to give adequate thiamine supplementation may result in irreversible Wernicke-Korsakoff syndrome, with permanent neurologic and/or cognitive disability. Supplementation of other vitamins and minerals may be needed, and other nutritional supplementation should be considered in the debilitated elderly patient.

An electrocardiogram and chest radiograph may be obtained if not done recently, particularly if underlying coronary disease is a concern or if tuberculosis or aspiration is a possibility. Tuberculosis skin tests and controls should be done for patients at risk who have not been recently tested. Further studies, including B_{12} and folic acid levels, computed tomography or magnetic resonance imaging, and electroencephalography, may be needed if a seizure has occurred or to exclude intercurrent problems. Human immunodeficiency virus disease may occur in the elderly, and risk behaviors should be discussed, including blood transfusion and organ (including cornea) transplantation done before widespread HIV antibody testing.

Abstinence syndromes should be treated in consultation with those with experience, such as someone with pain management and/or substance abuse expertise, particularly with older patients. Benzodiazepines are generally equally effective in the treatment of withdrawal, but because of concerns about drug accumulation, long-acting drugs should be used cautiously, since they may result in protracted toxicity, including respiratory depression, aspiration, pneumonia, or intoxication with mood lability, combative behavior, confusion, and injury to self or others.

Short-acting drugs, particularly lorazepam, are preferred. Oxazepam, with a longer latency, produces a choppier course. If short-acting drugs are not given with adequate frequency, breakthrough withdrawal, with serious consequences, may occur (52, 53). If shorter-acting drugs are used, the drug should be initially given as often as every 3 to 4 hours and generally not less than every 6 hours. The drug should be tapered over 5 to 7 days. Care should be taken to reduce the dose of the drug rather than the interval, to decrease the likelihood of long periods of reduced drug levels. A recently published meta-analysis of alcohol withdrawal treatments supports the use of benzodiazepines (54).

Patients using sedative-hypnotics should have the dose tapered over 10 to 21 days, depending on the dose and duration of use. Since this withdrawal may have severe consequences and since many clinicians have little experience with its management, referral to a chemical dependency program where there is more experience is recommended. A variety of regimens may be used (50, 51, 55, 56). Conversion to the equivalent dose of a long-acting benzodiazepine such as chlordiazepoxide, diazepam, or clonazepam is generally recommended, with careful observation and withholding of doses if there is evidence of oversedation. If the patient is using a barbiturate or barbituratelike drug, conversion to phenobarbital in divided doses with a gradual taper is recommended (56). While there has been recent enthusiasm for the use of carbamazepine and valproic acid in the treatment of sedative-hypnotic withdrawal, there are few studies, and none have been reported in older adults. Such treatment should not be undertaken outside of a specialty setting and should be done with great caution if at all, since the potential for seizures, delirium, and hyperautonomic symptoms is high.

Patients using minor opioids can generally be treated in a supervised setting by tapering the dose of the medication they are taking. Short-acting drugs, such as codeine, hydrocodone, or oxycodone, can generally be tapered over 5 to 10 days. Combination products may have to be avoided because of their salicylate or acetaminophen. The patient with high-dose use or use of major opioids (e.g., hydromorphone, oxymorphone) may be switched to a longer-acting drug, such as methadone or morphine sulfate (MS-Contin), and tapered over a longer period. This should be done in consultation with someone with pain management and/or substance abuse expertise and again is preferably done in a specialized setting. Rapid or ultrarapid opioid detoxification (ROD and UROD), using general anesthesia, has been the subject of media attention, but there are no adequately controlled trials reported. Treatment of older adults using such techniques should await further study.

For patients who use opioids for pain reduction, effective treatment of the underlying pain problem with alternative therapies must be undertaken or it is unlikely that the detoxification will be successful. Use of nonsteroidal anti-inflammatory drugs; antidepressants; anticonvulsants; physical measures such as heat, ultrasound, or diathermy; and special procedures such as nerve blocks, transcutaneous electrical nerve stimulation (TENS), and acupuncture may be needed. In some cases provision of adequate opioid analgesia in less abusable forms, such as transdermal fentanyl patches, may be appropriate.

Psychosocial Treatment

Most studies of treatment have been carried out with younger patients; there have been few systematic studies of treatment in the elderly. Overall, the elderly receive a disproportionately large number of prescriptions for psychoactive drugs. When they present at the physician's office with psychosocial issues, the elderly receive less counseling than other age groups, and they are more likely to receive psychoactive medications. Psychosocial issues must be addressed with patients whose alcohol or other drug abuse began late in life, often as a response to life stresses or losses, and treatment should concentrate on improvement in their social support network. Increased family visits, reentry into the job market, use of elder cabs to provide transportation to organized activities, volunteer activities (e.g., teaching their skills to younger unemployed or those starting businesses, involvement in child day care), and visiting nurse and homemaker services may all decrease the chance of returning to chemical dependency or help to detect relapse early, so that it may be promptly addressed.

The traditional forms of treatment in younger patients, including techniques to decrease denial, minimization, and rationalization, generally entail group techniques that are quite confrontational. Such techniques may not be appropriate for older persons. Putting older persons with late-onset dependency together with younger patients may both frighten and alienate them; hearing information on illicit drugs, criminal activities, domestic violence, acquired immunodeficiency syndrome, and other issues may increase their conviction that they are in the wrong place and do not share a problem with many others in the group.

One-to-one therapy, groups consisting of older persons, resocialization efforts, and consid-eration of psychopharmacologic measures (e.g., antidepressants) may all be useful for the older patient (57). Family therapy is particularly important, since family members may be dismayed by the appearance of chemical dependency in an older relative and may feel guilty or project blame. In the patient with long-standing chemical dependency who has survived to old age, there may be very significant family issues; treatment approaches for such patients may have to be more like those used in a younger population.

While in many cases patients do well with social referral and/or one-to-one therapy, in some cases self-help or mutual-help programs are useful for both patients and family. Al-Anon, Families Anonymous, and Narcanon are groups for the significant others of patients with chemical dependency. It should be stressed to family and friends that their involvement in such groups is for their own benefit, not necessarily the recovery of the affected relative. Alcoholics Anonymous may be a source for individual and group support, and the 12 steps of the recovery program, as well as its spiritual nature, may appeal to many older persons. The primary care provider may help with locating appropriate meetings and sponsors and encourage involvement in non-12-step recovery programs such as SMART recovery (formerly Rational Recovery), Women for Sobriety, and others, when appropriate.

There is always a role for brief advice by the provider, and such advice may be very effective. A study that included some older adults found that brief physician advice significantly reduced both alcohol use and use of health resources, at minimal cost and with minimal training of the providers (58). In addition, the physician may consider the use of anticraving drugs such as naltrexone, which may be useful in decreasing both alcohol and opioid use (59, 60).

Prevention and Early Intervention

Health care professionals have an important role to play in the prevention of chemical dependency, both in the patient population at large and in the elderly (61, 62). The clinician should have a complete history, regularly updated, that includes information on the use of alcohol and other drugs and on the medical, psychiatric, and social problems that may be related to substance abuse. Early intervention may allow resolution of the problem before severe comorbidities and individual and social dysfunction occur. The clinician can also suggest more functional coping strategies, such as stress reduction techniques, proper diet, exercise, and recreational activities. Availability of substance abuse educational material in the physician's waiting area may give patients permission to discuss their own personal issues with the clinician. Physicians should be particularly careful in their prescribing practices so as not facilitate or even create iatrogenic chemical dependencies.

REFERENCES

1. Knupfer G. The prevalence in various social groups of eight different drinking patterns, from abstaining to frequent drunkenness: analysis of ten U.S. surveys combined. Br J Addict 1989;84:1305–1318.
2. Myers JK, Weissman MM, Tischler GL, et al. Six-month prevalence of psychiatric disorders in three communities. Arch Gen Psychiatry 1984;41:959–967.
3. Bristow MF, Clare AN. Prevalence and characteristics of at-risk drinkers among elderly acute medical inpatients. Br J Addict 1992;87:291–294.
4. Cleary PD, Miller M, Bush BT, et al. Prevalence and recognition of alcohol abuse in a primary care population. Am J Med 1988;85:466–471.
5. Finlayson RD, Hurt RD, Davis LJ, Morse RM. Alcoholism in elderly persons: a study of the psychiatric and psychosocial features of 216 inpatients. Mayo Clin Proc 1988;63:761–768.
6. Miller F, Whitcup S, Sacks M, Lynch PE. Unrecognized drug dependence and withdrawal in the elderly. Drug Alcohol Depend 1985;15:177–179.
7. Barnes GM. Alcohol use among older persons: findings from a western New York state general population survey. J Am Geriatr Soc 1979;27:244–250.
8. Adams WL, Garry PJ, Rhyne R, et al. Alcohol intake in the healthy elderly: changes with age in a cross-sectional and longitudinal survey. J Am Geriatr Soc 1990;38:211–216.
9. Atkinson RM. Aging and alcohol use disorders: diagnostic issues in the elderly. Int Psychogeriatr 1990;2:55–72.
10. Gomberg ESL. Drugs, alcohol and aging. In: Kozowski LT, Annis HM, Cappel HD, et al., eds. Research Advances in Alcohol and Drug Problems. New York: Plenum, 1990:171–213.
11. Douglas R. Aging and alcohol problems: opportunities for socioepidemiological research. In: Galanter M, ed.
12. Laforge RG, Nirenberg TD, Lewis DC, Murphy JB. Problem drinking, gender and stressful life events among hospitalized elderly drinkers. Behav Health Aging 1993;3:129–138.
13. Adams WL, Yuan Z, Barboriak JJ, Rimm AA. Alcohol-related hospitalizations of elderly people: prevalence and geographic variation in the United States. JAMA 1993;270:1222–1225.
14. Steindler EM, Atkinson RM, Beresford TB, et al. Alcoholism in the Elderly: Diagnosis, Treatment and Prevention; Guidelines for Primary Care Physicians. Chicago: American Medical Association, 1996.
15. Alcoholism in the elderly. Council on Scientific Affairs, American Medical Association. JAMA 1996;275:797–801.
16. Samet JH, O'Connor PG, Stein MD. Alcohol and other substance abuse. Med Clin North Am 1997;81:4.
17. Reid MC, Anderson PA. Geriatric substance use disorders. Med Clin North Am 197;81:999–1016.
18. Lewis DC, Niven RG, Czechowicz D, Trumble JG. A review of medical education in alcohol and other drug abuse. JAMA 1987;257:2945–2948.
19. Schuckit MA, Atkinson JH, Miller PL, Berman J. A three-year follow-up of elderly alcoholics. J Clin Psychiatry 1980;41:412–416.
20. Miller NS, Belkin BM, Gold MS. Alcohol and drug dependence among the elderly: epidemiology, diagnosis, and treatment. Comprehens Psychiatry 1991;32:153–165.
21. Zimberg S. Two types of problem drinkers: both can be managed. Geriatrics 1974;29:135–138.
22. Hartford JT, Samorajski T. Alcoholism in the geriatric population. J Am Geriatr Soc 1982;30:18–24.
23. Atkinson RM. Alcohol and Alcohol Abuse in Old Age. Washington: American Psychiatric Press, 1984.
24. Dunham RG. Aging and changing patterns of alcohol use. J Psychoact Drugs 1981;13:143–151.
25. Rosin AJ, Glatt MM. Alcohol excess in the elderly. Q J Stud Alcohol 1971;32:53–59.
26. Atkinson RM, Turner JA, Kofoed LL, Tolson RL. Early versus late onset alcoholism in older persons: preliminary findings. Alcoholism 1985;9:513–515.
27. Bienenfeld D. Alcoholism in the elderly. Am Fam Physician 1987;36:163–169.
28. Vaillant GE. The Natural History of Alcoholism: Causes, Patterns and Paths to Recovery. Cambridge, MA: Harvard University Press, 1983.
29. Institute of Medicine. Prevention and Treatment of Alcohol Problems: Research Opportunities. Report of a Study by a Committee of the Institute of Medicine Division of Mental Health and Behavioral Medicine. Washington: National Academy Press, 1989.
30. Alexander F, Duff RW. Social interaction and alcohol use in retirement communities. Gerontologist 1988;28:632–638.

31. Liepman MR, Nirenberg TD, Porges R, Wartenberg A. Depression associated with substance abuse. In: Cameron OG, ed. Presentations of Depression. New York: Wiley, 1987:131–167.

32. Gambert S. Substance abuse in the elderly. In: Lowinson JH, Ruiz P, Millman RR, Langrod JG, eds. Substance Abuse: A Comprehensive Textbook. 2nd ed. Baltimore: Williams & Wilkins, 1992;843–851.

33. Vogel-Sprott M, Barrett P. Age, drinking habits and the effects of alcohol. J Stud Alcohol 1984;45:517–521.

34. Lister RG, Eckardt MJ, Weingartner H. Ethanol intoxication and memory: recent developments and new directions. In: Galanter M, ed. Recent Developments in Alcoholism. New York: Plenum, 1987:111–126.

35. Wartenberg AA. Medical complications of addiction. Section V. Chapter 1, General approach to the patient. Chapter 2, Medical syndromes associated with specific drugs. Chapter 3, Management of common medical problems. In: Miller NS, ed. Principles of Addiction Medicine. Washington: American Society of Addiction Medicine, 1994.

36. Novick DM. The medically ill substance abuser. In: Lowinson JH, Ruiz P, Millman RR, Langrod JG, eds. Substance Abuse: A Comprehensive Textbook. 2nd ed. Baltimore: Williams & Wilkins, 1992:657–674.

37. Closser MH. Benzodiazepines and the elderly: a review of potential problems. J Substance Abuse Treat 1991; 8:35–41.

38. McGivney WT, Crooks GM. The care of patients with severe chronic pain in terminal illness. JAMA 1984;251: 752–757.

39. Hoppman RA, Peden JG, Ober SK. Central nervous system side effects of non-steroidal anti-inflammatory drugs: aseptic meningitis, psychosis and cognitive dysfunction. Arch Intern Med 1991;151:1309–1313.

40. Miller NS. The pharmacology of interactions between medical and psychiatric drugs. In: Miller NS, ed. The Pharmacology of Alcohol and Drugs of Abuse and Addiction. New York: Springer-Verlag, 1991:279–289.

41. Wartenberg AA. Drug-drug interactions in pharmacological therapies. In: Miller NS, Gold MS, eds. Pharmacological Therapies for Drug and Alcohol Addictions. New York: Marcel Dekker, 1994:101–126.

42. American Psychiatric Association. Diagnostic and Statistical Manual of Mental Disorders. 4th ed. Washington: American Psychiatric Association, 1994.

43. Ewing JA. Detecting Alcoholism: the CAGE questionnaire. JAMA 1984;252:1905–1907.

44. Jones TV, Lindsey BA, Yount P, et al. Alcoholism screening questionnaires. J Gen Intern Med 1993;8:674–678.

45. Cyr MG, Wartman SA. The effectiveness of routine screening questions in the detection of alcoholism. JAMA 1988;259:51–54.

46. Sobell LC, Cellucci T, Nirenberg TD, Sobell MB. Do quantity-frequency data underestimate drinking-related health risks. Am J Public Health 1982;72:823–828.

47. McGann KP, Marion GS. Screening for alcoholism in the elderly: the validity of the brief screening measures. Substance Abuse 1992;13:188–195.

48. Adams WL, Barry KL, Fleming MF. Screening for problem drinking in older primary care patients. JAMA 1996;276:1964–1967.

49. Schwartz RA. Urine testing in the detection of drugs of abuse. Arch Intern Med 1988;148:2407–2412.

50. Kasser C, Geller A, Howell E, Wartenberg A. Detoxification: Principles and Protocols. Principles of Addiction Medicine Update Series. Washington: American Society of Addiction Medicine, 1997:1–51.

51. Sellers EM, Naranjo CA. New strategies for the treatment of alcohol withdrawal. Psychopharmacol Bull 1988;22:88–92.

52. Hill A, Williams D. Hazards associated with the use of benzodiazepines. J Substance Abuse Treat 1993;10: 449–452.

53. Mayo-Smith MF, Bernard D. Late onset seizures in alcohol withdrawal. J Addict Dis 1993;12:188 (abstract 34a).

54. Mayo-Smith MI and American Society of Addiction Medicine Working Group on Pharmacological Management. Pharmacological management of alcohol withdrawal: a meta-analysis and evidence-based practice guideline. JAMA 1997;278:144–151.

55. Smith DE, Wesson DR. A phenobarbital technique for withdrawal of barbiturate abuse. Arch Gen Psychiatry 1971;24:56–61.

56. Sullivan JT, Sellers EM. Treating alcohol, barbiturate and benzodiazepine withdrawal. Rational Drug Ther 1986;20:1–9.

57. Curtis JR, Geller G, Stokes EJ, et al. Characteristics, diagnosis, and treatment of alcoholism in elderly patients. J Am Geriatr Soc 1989;37:310–316.

58. Fleming MF, Barry KL, Manwell LB, et al. Brief physician advice for problem alcohol drinkers. JAMA 1997; 277:1039–1045.

59. Volpicelli JR, Alterman AI, Hayashida M, O'Brien CP. Naltrexone in the treatment of alcohol dependence. Arch Gen Psychiatry 1992;49:876–880.

60. O'Malley SS, Jaffe AJ, Chang G, et al. Naltrexone and coping skills therapy for alcohol dependence. Arch Gen Psychiatry 1992;49:881–887.

61. Wallack L. Practical issues, ethical concerns and future directions in the prevention of alcohol-related problems. J Primary Prevent 1984;4:199–224.

62. Noel NE, McCrady BS. Target populations for alcohol abuse prevention. In: Miller PM, Nirenberg TD, eds. Prevention of Alcohol Abuse. New York: Plenum, 1984:55–94.

Evaluation and Management of Delirium and Dementia

Loss of memory and other types of cognitive dysfunction are very common among the elderly. This chapter addresses the evaluation and management of the two major syndromes that describe these disorders: delirium or acute cognitive dysfunction; and dementia or chronic cognitive dysfunction. It is important to distinguish these syndromes when evaluating the confused elderly patient because the treatment and prognosis are dramatically different.

DELIRIUM

The hallmarks of delirium are acute onset, alterations in level of consciousness, deficits in attention, and potential reversibility. The fourth edition of *Diagnostic and Statistical Manual of Mental Disorders* (DSM-IV) of the American Psychiatric Association (APA) defines delirium on the basis of key criteria and on evidence of cause (e.g., general medical condition, substance intoxication) (1). See Table 15.1 for a representative example (1).

The prevalence of delirium varies from less than 1% to more than 50% (2). This variation is explained primarily by the population being studied and the study methodology. Delirium is relatively uncommon in purely community-residing ambulatory elders. It is much more common in hospitalized elderly, but postoperative and intensive care patients are more likely to be delirious than are general medical patients. Delirium is also relatively common among nursing home residents.

The underlying causes of delirium are not well understood, primarily because of the difficulties in studying such acutely ill and widely varying patients. There is some evidence for cholinergic dysfunction (2). Indeed, the side effects of anticholinergic medications can mimic delirium. There is also evidence for dysregulation of the hypothalamic-pituitary-adrenal axis and elevations of cortisol (3).

Many different proximate causes can trigger delirium. These may be broadly divided into localized central nervous system (CNS) conditions and non-CNS systemic conditions. The CNS conditions include infections, such as meningitis and encephalitis; trauma, such as that resulting in subdural hematoma; tumors, either primary or metastatic; and drugs, including anesthetics, neuroleptics, antidepressants, sedative-hypnotics, anticonvulsants, opioids, and alcohol. The non-CNS systemic conditions include infections, such as sepsis, pneumonia, urinary tract infection, subacute bacterial endocarditis, and osteomyelitis; cardiopulmonary disorders, including acute myocardial infarction, decompensation of congestive heart failure, and exacerbation of chronic obstructive pulmonary disease; endocrine and metabolic disorders, including vitamin B_{12} or folic acid deficiency and abnormal glucose or electrolytes; tumors anywhere other than the CNS; sensory deprivation due to impaired hearing or vision; environmental disruption such as is seen in hospitals, intensive care, and nursing homes; and drugs, including anti-inflammatories (both

Table 15.1

Diagnostic Criteria for Delirium Due to . . .
[Indicate the General Medical Condition]

Disturbance of consciousness (i.e., reduced clarity of awareness of the environment) with reduced ability to focus, sustain, or shift attention

A change in cognition, such as memory deficit, disorientation, language disturbance, or a perceptual disturbance that is not better accounted for by a preexisting, established, or evolving dementia

Disturbance developing over a short period, usually hours to days, and tending to fluctuate during the day

Evidence from history, physical examination, or laboratory findings that disturbance is caused by direct physiologic consequences of a general medical condition

Modified from American Psychiatric Association. Diagnostic and Statistical Manual of Mental Disorders. 4th ed. Washington: American Psychiatric Association, 1994:129.

steroids and nonsteroidals), antihistamines, and H_2-blockers.

The risk factors for delirium are also not completely understood; a preexisting dementia, however, is probably the greatest risk (4). Advancing age and medical frailty also appear to increase risk of delirium, but how much of this risk is actually due to subclinical or unrecognized dementia is not known. Delirium itself is clearly a marker for poor outcome, with reported mortality ratios varying from 1.6 to 19.7 (2, 4). Whether better recognition and more aggressive treatment of the causes underlying delirium would improve these statistics remains to be seen.

Recognition of delirium is critical but often neglected. Usually the problem is an all-too-ready tendency to attribute the patient's symptoms to dementia and to assume a nihilistic attitude in this regard. Almost equally common is the tendency to attribute the symptoms to normal aging, i.e., to ignore the symptoms. One way to avoid these pitfalls to differential diagnosis is to use a standardized evaluation instrument with any patients who have any symptoms. One such instrument that has gained wide acceptance is

that of Inouye et al. (5), the confusion assessment method, or CAM. See Table 15.2 for this algorithm (5).

Treatment of Delirium

Once delirium has been diagnosed, the key is to identify and treat the cause. Often this resolves the delirium. Frequently, however, some residual impairment remains or an underlying dementia is unmasked. Little is known about direct treatment of the symptoms of the syndrome, such as with the newer cholinergic-enhancing drugs. This area requires active investigation.

Table 15.2

The Confusion Assessment Method (CAM)
Diagnostic Algorithm

Feature 1 *Acute onset and fluctuating course* is usually obtained from a family member or nurse and is shown by positive responses to the following questions: Is there evidence of an acute change in mental status from the patient's baseline: Did the (abnormal) behavior fluctuate during the day, that is, tend to come and go, or increase and decrease in severity?

Feature 2 *Inattention* is shown by a positive response to the following question. Did the patient have difficulty focusing attention, for example, being easily distractible or having difficulty keeping track of what was being said?

Feature 3 *Disorganized thinking* is shown by a positive response to the following question: Was the patient's thinking disorganized or incoherent, such as rambling or irrelevant conversation, unclear or illogical flow of ideas, or unpredictable switching from subject to subject?

Feature 4 *Altered level of consciousness* is shown by any answer other than "alert" to the following question: Overall, how would you rate this patient's level of consciousness? (alert, [normal], vigilant [hyperalert], lethargic [drowsy, easily aroused], stupor [difficult to arouse], or coma [unarousable])

The diagnosis of delirium by CAM requires the presence of features 1 and 2 and either 3 or 4.

Adapted from Inouye SK, van Dyck CM, Aleissi CA, et al. Clarifying confusion: the Confusion Assessment Method. A new method for detection of delirium. Ann Intern Med 1990;113:941–948.

DEMENTIA

As already noted, dementia is a syndrome of chronic cognitive impairment. Its hallmarks are a gradual, insidious onset, no alteration of consciousness except in the final stages, and sufficient memory and other cognitive impairment to impair social or occupational function. This requirement for functional impairment is important because it allows one to distinguish dementia from memory complaints associated with normal aging and from mild cognitive impairment, a condition many believe is a prodrome to dementia, especially Alzheimer's disease. As with delirium, DSM-IV now defines dementia on the basis of key criteria as well as evidence of a specific cause (e.g., Alzheimer's disease, vascular causes, head trauma) (1). See Table 15.3 for the DSM-IV criteria for dementia of the Alzheimer's type (1). As already noted, it is important for the clinician to make the differential diagnosis between delirium and dementia; the comparisons listed in Table 15.4 should help with this. Sometimes the diagnosis is delirium in the setting of

dementia (not too rare, given the significant risk of delirium that dementia carries).

Reversible Dementia

Once the differential diagnosis between delirium and dementia has been made, the next consideration is whether the dementia is reversible. This classic concept in geriatric medicine has come more into question in recent years. In 1988, Clarfield (6) published the results of a meta-analysis that suggested that rather than a prevalence as high as 20% of all dementias, the prevalence of reversible dementia in academic settings was more like 8%, and the percentage of these patients properly treated whose dementia actually reversed was 3%. Also in 1988, Hector and Burton (7) suggested that vitamin B_{12} deficiency, a common cause of reversible dementia, actually causes delirium.

Nonetheless, the concept remains useful because a variety of diseases and conditions cause the sort of cognitive symptoms that meet the criteria for dementia in at least some elderly people,

Table 15.3

Diagnostic Criteria for Dementia of the Alzheimer's Type

A. Multiple cognitive deficits manifested by both of the following:
  1. Memory impairment (impaired ability to learn or recall information)
  2. One or more of the following cognitive disturbances:
      a. Aphasia (language disturbance)
      b. Apraxia (impaired ability to carry our motor activities despite intact motor function)
      c. Agnosia (failure to recognize or identify objects despite intact sensory function)
      d. Disturbance in executive functioning (i.e., planning, organizing, sequencing, abstracting)
B. The cognitive deficits in criteria A1 and A2 each cause significant impairment in social or occupational functioning and represent a significant decline from a previous level of functioning
C. Course characterized by gradual onset and continuing cognitive decline
D. The cognitive deficits in criteria A1 and A2 are not due to any of the following:
  1. Other central nervous system conditions that cause progressive deficits in memory and cognition (e.g., cerebrovascular disease, Parkinson's disease, Huntington's disease, subdural hematoma, normal-pressure hydrocephalus, brain tumor)
  2. Systemic conditions that are known to cause dementia (e.g., hypothyroidism, vitamin B_{12} or folic acid deficiency, niacin deficiency, hypercalcemia, neurosyphilis, HIV infection)
  3. Substance-induced conditions
E. The deficits not occurring exclusively during delirium
F. The disturbance not better accounted for by another axis I disorder (e.g., major depressive disorder, schizophrenia)

Modified from American Psychiatric Association. Diagnostic and Statistical Manual of Mental Disorders. 4th ed. Washington: American Psychiatric Association, 1994:142–143.

Table 15.4

Differentiating Delirium From Dementia

Delirium	Dementia
Abrupt, precise onset	Gradual, ill-defined onset
Altered level of consciousness	Normal alertness until end stage
Short attention span	Normal attention span until late stages
Hallucinations common	Hallucinations uncommon until late stages (except Lewy body dementia)
Loss of orientation early	Orientation preserved in early stages
Psychomotor changes common (agitation or lethargy)	Psychomotor changes uncommon until late stages
Usually reversible if cause found and treated	Usually irreversible

and prompt recognition and treatment of such conditions can improve the person's cognitive function. The next question is what should the work-up for dementia include? The answer, of course, can be debated, but almost no one would disagree with the Agency for Health Care Policy and Research (AHCPR) guidelines, which recommend a focused history and physical and functional and mental status assessments with standardized instruments (8). These steps allow the detection of several of the most common causes of possibly reversible dementia: drugs (toxicity, side effects, or interactions), depression, alcohol abuse, and normal-pressure hydrocephalus. The other common cause, endocrine and metabolic disorders, may be suspected on this basis but requires laboratory confirmation (9).

Cognitive symptoms in the clinical setting of depression that resolve with antidepressant treatment have been termed pseudodementia. As the APA practice guideline points out, as many as half of these patients may go on to develop a full-blown dementia within 5 years (10). Classically, such patients are said to have don't-know rather than near-miss answers, and they tend to highlight their disability. However, patients with mild dementia often have depressive symptoms thought to be due to recognition of their impairment. Thus the APA guidelines recommend a low threshold for antidepressant treatment whenever depressed mood or other depressive symptoms coexist with cognitive symptoms (see treatment section).

The debate about the dementia work-up actu-

ally centers on laboratory tests and brain scans; it is mainly driven by the increasing cost consciousness in medicine and by an increasing emphasis on evidence-based medicine. Of four recently published consensus-derived practice guidelines (8–11), the one from the American Academy of Neurology tackles the issue in detail (9). While cautioning that testing should be guided by clinical suspicions derived from history and physical examination, this document recommends the following tests as routine: complete blood count, serum electrolytes (including calcium), glucose, blood urea nitrogen and creatinine, liver function tests, thyroid function tests (free thyroxine index and thyroid-stimulating hormone), serum vitamin B_{12}, and syphilis serology (rapid plasma reagin or Venereal Disease Research Laboratory). The following tests are described as helpful in certain cases but optional: sedimentation rate, serum folate, human immunodeficiency virus (HIV) testing, chest radiograph, urinalysis, 24-hour urine for heavy metals, toxicology screen, computed tomography (CT) or magnetic resonance imaging (MRI) of the brain, neuropsychologic testing, lumbar puncture, electroencephalography, positron emission tomography (PET), and single photon emission computed tomography (SPECT).

Treatment of Reversible Dementia

Once a reversible dementia has been diagnosed, one must treat the underlying cause. This should result in at least some improvement in the patient's cognitive function. Prompt treatment appears to be crucial. Clinical experience suggests that the longer the treatment delay, the more likely is some residual impairment, but perhaps this is the unmasking of an underlying irreversible dementia.

Irreversible Dementias

Underlying the irreversible dementias are various forms of neuronal degeneration that are progressive and so far apparently permanent. These may be grouped by causation: vascular disease, genetic disorders (e.g., Huntington's disease), infections (e.g., Creutzfeldt-Jakob disease), and trauma (e.g., dementia pugilistica). The largest category, however, is that of dementias due to as yet unknown causes: Alzheimer's disease, Pick's disease, diffuse Lewy body disease, and progressive supranuclear palsy are chief examples. Prevalence data for these various types of irreversible dementia vary from study to study and from country to country. In the United States Alzheimer's disease is the most common, accounting for up to about 50 to 75% of dementias. Most would agree that vascular dementia, either alone or in combination with Alzheimer's disease, is next most common (10). In Japan, vascular dementias appear to be more common, perhaps even surpassing Alzheimer's disease. Whether this is due to true national differences or to variation in study methodology is not clear (12).

Alzheimer's Disease

The biology of Alzheimer's disease is discussed in detail in Chapter 17. The disease was first described by Alois Alzheimer in 1906 and for most of this century was thought to be a rare disorder of middle age. In the 1970s, however, researchers began to describe the same hallmark pathologic changes noted by Alzheimer—neuritic plaques and neurofibrillary tangles—in the brains of elderly demented persons (13).

Until that time, most dementia in the elderly was attributed either to a presumed vascular process, "hardening of the arteries," or to aging itself. Since that time a tremendous amount has been learned, and Alzheimer's disease is now classified as early onset (before age 60) or late onset (after 60). Its underlying cause or causes still

remain to be discovered. Single-gene defects have been implicated in some early-onset cases (14). None have been found so far in late-onset cases, although apolipoprotein E type 4 genotype has been demonstrated to increase risk of late-onset disease (14). It may increase the risk for other dementias as well (15). Age is probably the single greatest risk factor for Alzheimer's disease. The prevalence is 5 to 10% in persons over 65 but increases to 25 to 50% in those over 85 (10).

There is still no direct diagnostic test for Alzheimer's disease in the living, despite many attempts to develop one. There are two commercial tests, but their use remains controversial and so far they have not gained widespread acceptance. Because of this lack of a diagnostic test, the diagnosis of Alzheimer's disease has traditionally been regarded as relying on exclusion. Thinking has changed, however, and most experts prefer that Alzheimer's disease be a diagnosis of inclusion based on characteristic history, physical examination, and disease course (11).

The most important aspect of the diagnosis of Alzheimer's disease is that the patient meet the criteria for dementia. Memory impairment is, of course, key, with immediate and short-term recall affected initially and long-term, i.e., distant past events, affected eventually. Language deficits are common, usually word-finding difficulty but occasionally marked aphasia. Insidious onset and gradual progression are also features. In addition, careful neurologic examination reveals no focal findings. As the disease progresses, neurologic signs emerge, although they are still nonfocal. These include symmetrically increased deep tendon reflexes, paratonia, and primitive reflexes such as palmomental, grasp, and suck reflexes. Behavioral symptoms, which are also common, are discussed in detail in Chapter 16.

The characteristic progression of Alzheimer's disease has been described by a number of staging systems. The two most widely used are the Global Deterioration Scale and the Clinical Dementia Rating scale (16–18). The primary advantage of these scales is that they facilitate communication among professionals regarding the condition of a patient and the anticipation of needs, which vary from stage to stage. In addition, when patients of a known stage have symptoms not characteristic of the stage, it can serve as a flag that another process, such as an acute medical illness, may be going on. Finally, these scales may also have some prognostic value, letting families know what to expect.

For practitioners who do not see large numbers of Alzheimer's disease patients, learning one of these staging systems may not be practical. Even so, it is important to stage the patient, and the simplest system is to classify the patient's condition as mild, moderate, or severe. Patients with mild dementia have difficulty functioning, particularly with complex tasks such as paying bills and preparing an elaborate meal, but generally can survive on their own. Patients with moderate dementia have difficulty with simpler tasks, including some basic activities of daily living such as bathing and dressing, and for these patients, survival without significant assistance is hazardous. Patients with severe dementia lose the ability to do even the most basic of activities, including feeding and toileting themselves. Eventually, the ability to walk and even speech are lost. Severely demented patients require continuous supervision, and for most patients and families, nursing home placement is the only possibility.

Vascular Dementia

As previously noted, vascular disease is the second most common cause of dementia in the elderly in the United States. Criteria for making this diagnosis have been developed by the NINDS-AIREN working group (19). A useful screening tool, the Rosen-modified Hachinski Ischemia Scale, is shown in Table 15.5 (20). Recent expert consensus is that this condition is overdiagnosed in primary care (11). The reason for this is likely the overreading of CT and MRI studies showing white matter changes likely due to microvascular disease but not likely to cause dementia. Another contributing factor may be that physicians are more comfortable conveying a diagnosis of vascular dementia than Alzheimer's disease.

Key features of vascular dementia are cognitive deficits temporally related to strokelike episodes, which result in the classically described

Table 15.5
Modified Hachinski Ischemia Score

	Score If Present (absent = 0)
1. Abrupt onset	2
2. Stepwise deterioration	1
3. Somatic complaints	1
4. Emotional incontinence	1
5. History of hypertension	1
6. History of stroke	2
7. Focal neurologic signs	2
8. Focal neurologic symptoms	2

Total ≤ 4, dementia not likely due to vascular causes.
Total ≥ 7, dementia likely due to vascular causes.

stepwise decline, and focal neurologic findings. Patients may also show more emotional lability, and interestingly enough, insight may be preserved. Vascular disease risk factors, including hypertension, diabetes, hyperlipidemia, cardiac arrhythmias, and smoking, are usually present and long-standing.

Other Dementias

Detailed discussion of the many other types of irreversible dementia is beyond the scope of this chapter. The prevalence of these conditions varies from relatively uncommon to very rare. Most are associated with distinctive neurologic abnormalities (e.g., the choreoathetoid movements of Huntington's disease and the upward gaze paralysis of progressive supranuclear palsy). Others have features atypical of Alzheimer's disease (e.g., the social disinhibition of Pick's disease and the relatively rapid progression of Creutzfeldt-Jakob disease). One of these bears particular mention: the dementia associated with Lewy body disease. These patients have dementia and at least one of three core symptoms early in the disease course: detailed visual hallucinations, parkinsonian signs, or alterations of alertness or attention (21). It is important to consider this diagnosis because many of these patients are hypersensitive to neuroleptic drugs that might ordinarily be prescribed for their psychotic symptoms but are in fact contraindicated.

Treatment of Irreversible Dementias

The most important thing to remember about irreversible dementias is that they are treatable. Many symptoms can be ameliorated, and in many cases function can be improved and/or prolonged. Unfortunately, to date, a sort of therapeutic nihilism regarding these conditions is widespread among physicians. This is understandable, given that in the past no medications were effective in any of these conditions. Fortunately, this situation is changing, and there is hope that physicians' attitudes will change as well.

General Treatment Considerations

Before discussing specific treatments, one must consider several general treatments that can apply to any of the irreversible dementias. First and foremost is to ensure the patient's safety. The steps necessary to do this vary from patient to patient and as the disease progresses. All patients should have an identification bracelet that notes their condition and that cannot be easily removed. It may be necessary to disconnect the kitchen stove to prevent fires or to lower the temperature of the water heater to prevent scalding. Special locks may have to be installed to prevent wandering. This is one of many areas in which caregivers can get advice from the Alzheimer's Association. In some cases, a home visit by a trained nurse or occupational therapist can be particularly valuable to identify and implement recommendations.

The next consideration is to keep the patient as mentally and physically active as possible within the limits of his or her present ability. There is a growing amount of anecdotal evidence that much of the disability associated with severely ill patients stems from disuse and neglect rather than from the neurologic defects of the disease itself. Patients should be encouraged to take walks daily (with a caregiver if necessary). They may also enjoy other forms of exercise, such as dancing. Mental exercise should be tailored to the patient's interests as well as ability. Mildly affected patients might try writing, perhaps reading a paragraph in the newspaper and writing what they remember, keeping a journal of the day's events, or recording stories from the past. Patients who are uncomfortable or have difficulty with writing can do the same exercises orally, either with a tape recorder or talking to a caregiver. Patients who like puzzles can be given simple ones. Likewise, simple versions of previously enjoyed crafts may be available. Patients who can no longer read may still enjoy looking at pictures in books or magazines. Other options include more formally structured activities. Most communities now have activity programs for demented patients, and in a few communities the Alzheimer's Association has started support groups for mildly affected patients. These both provide caregivers with much-needed respite and offer potential benefits to patients.

The third general principle is to maintain adequate nutrition. Mildly affected patients who are still living on their own are at particular risk. They may have trouble with choosing the appropriate foods when shopping or with preparing foods (most sources of protein require cooking), or they may simply forget to eat. These patients require that someone look in regularly to ensure that they have appropriate food in the house and are eating properly. Severely ill patients cannot feed themselves and many eventually have difficulty swallowing. Pureed or liquid foods may help, especially if presented through a straw or a nipple so as to take advantage of the suck reflex. Patients' and families' wishes regarding feeding tubes should be discussed as early as possible in the disease course so that those wishes can be honored if the need for such intervention arises. If such discussions are left until the patient is severely affected, his or her wishes cannot be known and the stress on the family may be such that it causes great difficulties in making a decision. It should be considered that a feeding tube at this stage may prolong the terminal phase of the illness rather than provide any real benefit.

The fourth general treatment concern is to be alert for concomitant medical illnesses. Acute cognitive decline or new disruptive behaviors should prompt a careful medical evaluation to look for acute problems, such as a urinary tract infection. A corollary is that medications should be kept to a minimum because of an increased likelihood of side effects.

The fifth general treatment area is to encourage planning. As soon as a dementia diagnosis is made, the patient and family should be directed to consider the future. Wills should be in order, financial planning should take place, power of attorney should be completed, advance directives (living wills or health care proxies) should be executed, and considerations should be given to future caregiving needs, perhaps even visiting nursing homes and choosing one if beds are in short supply and waits are long in the area. The need to do this early is mandated by the progressive nature of these diseases and the desire to have the patient participate in decisions as much as possible. Even moderately demented patients may still have decision-specific capacity. For example, a patient may no longer be able to understand a complex financial document but be able to sign a power of attorney and know that he or she wants the spouse to make financial decisions.

The final general treatment consideration is to monitor and maintain caregiver health and well-being. There are probably no other adult chronic diseases that put such great stress and strain on family member caregivers for such long periods. Often, caregivers are reluctant to share their burdens with others, even close family members, because of the perceived stigma attached to dementia. And too, demented patients often look well and hence fail to elicit natural sympathy from friends and family who don't live with the patient. The primary care physician should watch for symptoms of depression and be aware of signs of caregiver burnout such as anger, lashing out at the patient, or substance abuse (caffeine, nicotine, alcohol, prescription drugs). There are many strategies to help caregivers. Probably the single most important is referral to the local Alzheimer's Association chapter. Through the Alzheimer's Association, caregivers can join support groups and learn about the disease and referral to community resources. Another important way to help caregivers is to encourage respite. This should occur for short periods every day or at least several times a week and for longer periods as well. Brief respite can be provided by family members, paid caregivers, or Alzheimer's day programs. Longer-term respite, such as a 1-

or 2-week vacation, may be available through local nursing homes. A recent study found that intensive support of spouse caregivers through support groups, family counseling, and the availability of a counselor 24 hours a day for emergency telephone advice was able to delay the patients' institutionalization by nearly a year (22).

Specific Disease Treatments

TREATMENT OF ALZHEIMER'S DISEASE. The cholinergic hypothesis in Alzheimer's disease states that loss of cholinergic function in the brain correlates directly with memory loss (23). Over the past 20 years or so, a large variety of evidence has been gathered to support this hypothesis (13), and this has led to the pursuit of a variety of treatments. These include trying to enhance brain acetylcholine synthesis by providing precursors (choline or lecithin), supplying direct cholinergic agonists (intrathecal bethanechol), and using acetylcholinesterase inhibitors to block the breakdown of acetylcholine. So far, only this last strategy has had any success (12).

The prototype cholinesterase inhibitor is tacrine, an acridine derivative that was initially tested in the 1940s as an adjunct to anesthesia. In 1986, Summers et al. (24) published a study showing remarkable success with this drug in treating a small group of patients with Alzheimer's disease. This led to a number of studies around the world that tried to duplicate their work. Some were positive and others were not (25). Eventually, in part because of strong grass roots pressure, the National Institute on Aging organized a large multicenter trial (26); a second trial was organized by the Parke-Davis division of Warner-Lambert (27). Both of these trials showed improvements in memory using the Alzheimer's Disease Assessment Scale's cognitive subscale (ADAS-cog), and the latter also showed global improvement using the Clinician's Interview-Based Impression of Change (CIBIC). The results of these trials led to the approval of tacrine (Cognex) as the first drug specifically for the treatment of Alzheimer's disease.

Tacrine was marketed in 1993, but it never gained widespread use for a variety of reasons. First, it requires a prolonged titration scheme and dosing 4 times a day. Second, it requires frequent liver function test monitoring because of a high incidence of elevated liver enzymes. These reverse when the drug is stopped and generally do not recur when the patient is rechallenged, but many physicians and families find this too difficult. Third, there are drug interactions, notably with theophylline, requiring dosage lowering and careful monitoring of theophylline levels. Finally, it has a high incidence of peripheral cholinergic side effects (nausea, vomiting, and diarrhea). These seem to be dose-related, but unfortunately, so is efficacy. On top of all of this, the efficacy for most patients is modest at best (25).

In 1997, the first of the next generation of cholinesterase inhibitors arrived on the market. Donepezil (Aricept) is a piperidine-based reversible cholinesterase inhibitor without the drawbacks of tacrine. It does not require titration. It comes in 5- and 10-mg doses, and both are effective. However, because some patients derive additional benefit from the higher dose, physicians may decide to increase the dose from 5 to 10 mg after 4 to 6 weeks of therapy. In the pivotal clinical trials, 10 mg showed a strong trend toward greater efficacy than 5 mg, but the studies were not powered to confirm this statistically. In these trials, patients who were increased from 5 to 10 mg after only a week of therapy had a higher incidence of gastrointestinal side effects; in patients whose dose was increased after 4 to 6 weeks, the incidence was comparable with that of 5 mg and placebo (28).

Donepezil is given once a day. It does not cause liver enzyme elevations or other laboratory abnormalities. It is metabolized by the cytochrome P450 system, but because its serum concentrations are so low, drug interactions do not appear to be a problem. It has been shown not to have any significant interactions with theophylline, warfarin, digoxin, or cimetidine (28). Even though peripheral cholinergic effects appear to be low with donepezil, physicians should still be cautious in prescribing this drug to patients with conditions that might worsen with increased peripheral cholinergic stimulation, such as peptic ulcer disease and sick sinus syndrome. In the pivotal trials, 2% of donepezil patients had syncope compared with 1% of placebo patients (28).

In terms of efficacy, in both the 3- and 6-month pivotal trials, donepezil-treated patients showed statistically significant mean improvements compared with placebo-treated patients on both ADAS-cog (the primary memory measure) and CIBIC-plus (a global function measure that includes caregiver input) (29, 30). These effects were lost over 3 to 6 weeks in placebo washout phases, but the patients did not show rebound worsening. Patients in these trials also showed a range of responses. For example, in the 6-month trial best response on ADAS-cog, 26% of patients treated with 10 mg showed a robust improvement (more than 7 points) from baseline ADAS-cog; 32% showed a modest improvement (4 to 7 points); 24% showed small or no change (0 to 4 points) from baseline. Because Alzheimer's disease is progressive, one way to consider a treatment's efficacy is to look at the cumulative percentage of patients who showed either improvement or no decline from baseline scores over the course of a trial. In this study, those numbers were 82% for 10 mg-treated patients, 83% for 5 mg-treated patients, and 59% for placebo-treated patients. The converse of this is that 17 to 18% of actively treated patients actually declined over 6 months, while 41% of placebo-treated patients declined.

For most clinicians not familiar with the ADAS-cog, translating these results into clinically meaningful terms can be difficult. A retrospective analysis of data from this same 6-month trial looked at time to loss of function according to Kaplan-Meier analysis and the three function subscales from the Clinical Dementia Rating scale (31). This analysis showed that patients treated with 10 mg maintained baseline level of functioning for 123 weeks. The figure for 5 mg-treated patients was 92 weeks and for placebo-treated patients was 68 weeks. Thus, at 10 mg per day, donepezil treatment was projected to maintain the patient's function about a year longer than placebo. Interestingly, a retrospective analysis of tacrine patients treated for long term found a delay of nursing home placement of about a year (32).

Regrettably, there are no prospective long-term (more than 6 months) randomized, double-blind, placebo-controlled data available for donepezil. Nor are there data yet on severely ill patients. (The range of Mini-Mental State Examination scores in the pivotal trials, and hence in the approved indications for the drug, was 10 to 26.) There are anecdotal reports of severely ill patients showing noticeable improvement. Also, ongoing phase IIIb studies will eventually provide some of this information. To date, there is no evidence that donepezil or any cholinesterase inhibitor alters the underlying course of Alzheimer's disease. As the disease progresses, cholinergic neurons continue to die, and indeed, other neurotransmitter systems also appear to be disrupted (13). Long-term open-label data show that, on average, donepezil-treated patients decline below baseline ADAS-cog scores at about 40 weeks, but throughout the course of therapy their scores are higher than would be projected for untreated patients (33). Given the current state of knowledge, a logical approach to stopping donepezil is to discontinue therapy when the patient declines to the severe stage of the disease, when there are no longer enough cholinergic neurons functioning for the drug to make a difference. Objectively this probably corresponds to MMSE scores in the range of 0 to 5.

The recommended starting dose of donepezil is 5 mg. It may be given with or without food. It is recommended that it be given at bedtime to minimize the gastrointestinal side effects, but if insomnia is a problem, it may be given in the morning. The patient should be evaluated at 4 to 6 weeks, using an objective measure of cognitive function such as the MMSE as well as caregiver impressions, which they should be encouraged to record. At this point, if the patient is tolerating the drug well, the dose should probably be increased to 10 mg. (Both doses cost the same in the United States.) The drug should probably be continued for at least 6 months. This is the minimum amount of time during which one can expect to see decline in untreated patients. Thus, if the patient has improved or at least showed no decline from baseline, it is reasonable to assume that the drug is providing benefit in this progressive disease. If the patient has declined significantly at 6 months, the drug should probably be stopped. If the drug's benefit or lack thereof is unclear, stopping donepezil and reevaluating at 6 weeks should reveal whether it was helping or not.

No one thinks that cholinesterase inhibitors are a cure for Alzheimer's disease. For most patients, however, they do seem to maintain cognitive and other function longer than not treating. This has significant implications for patients and caregivers and probably for society as well. At this writing, donepezil is the only viable drug therapy approved for Alzheimer's disease, although rivastigmine (Exelon, ENA-713) is soon likely be on the market in the United States. Several other compounds, including metrifonate (already marketed as an antihelminthic), eptastigmine, huperazine, and galanthamine, are in various stages of approval. Efficacy of all of these compounds is likely to be similar; therefore, physicians' choices are likely to be based on drug safety, tolerability, and convenience. In the near future, until a cure is found, cholinergic enhancement will likely remain a major part of the treatment regimen for Alzheimer's disease.

Vitamin E. Alzheimer's disease may involve the accumulation of free radicals and the damage they may cause to nerve cells. Vitamin E (α-tocopherol) is a lipid-soluble vitamin that traps free radicals. This may reduce the damage to nerve cells and thus delay the progression of the disease.

In a multicenter placebo-controlled double-blind clinical trial conducted by the Alzheimer's Disease Cooperative Study group, the effects of vitamin E were evaluated in patients with moderate Alzheimer's disease (34). The objective was to determine whether vitamin E 2000 IU/day alone or in combination with selegiline 10 mg/day would slow the deterioration associated with Alzheimer's disease. Selegiline, also known as deprenyl (Eldepryl), was included in the study because it has the dual properties of being an antioxidant, somewhat similar to vitamin E, and an inhibitor of monoamine oxidase (MAO). As an MAO-B inhibitor with some degree of selectivity, it increases the levels of certain neurotransmitters in the brain, particularly dopamine, and to a lesser extent norepinephrine and serotonin.

A total of 341 patients were treated for up to 2 years. The objective of the study was to determine whether treatment would slow the progression of the disease as measured by the time to reach one or more of the following four clinical end points: death, institutionalization (placement in a skilled nursing facility), loss of the ability to perform two of three basic activities of daily living (eating, grooming, using the toilet), or an overall increase in the severity of the dementia from moderate to severe according to a standard rating instrument. The ADAS-cog and the MMSE were secondary end points.

The time to reach at least one of the four primary end points was increased by vitamin E alone or in combination with selegiline; it was also increased by selegiline alone. The effect of each of the three treatments was significant compared with placebo *only* after a statistical adjustment was made for baseline MMSE score. The adjusted time to reach at least one of the four possible outcomes was 440 days for placebo, 670 days for vitamin E alone, 655 days for selegiline alone, and 585 days for the combination of vitamin E and selegiline.

There were no significant effects on cognition as measured by the ADAS-cog or the MMSE by any of the treatments. For the MMSE the degree of decline from baseline was identical for the vitamin E- and placebo-treated groups (−4.6 points). For the ADAS-cog the mean change from baseline was a worsening of 8.3 points for the vitamin E group compared with a worsening of 6.7 points for the placebo group. These differences were not statistically significant. Although falls and syncope were more frequent in the treatment groups (especially the group receiving combined treatment) than in the placebo group, these events did not lead to discontinuation of treatment. The authors concluded that vitamin E treatment was relatively well tolerated.

These results, while encouraging, must be viewed with caution for several reasons. First, additional studies must be performed to replicate these findings. Second, significance was obtained only after statistical adjustment was made for one of the baseline variables. Third, the results are not internally consistent because no effect was obtained on cognitive performance yet positive effects were reported for the clinical end points. Finally, the results also lack internal consistency because the combined treatment group did worse than the groups taking vitamin E or selegiline alone.

The 2000-IU dose of vitamin E used in this trial is considerably higher than either the U.S. Recommended Daily Allowance of 30 IU contained in several multivitamin preparations or the dose of 400 IU contained in some high-potency preparations. Although approximately 30% of patients in the donepezil clinical trials were taking vitamins concomitantly, there are no data on the relatively high dose of vitamin E used in this trial in combination with donepezil. It is probably advisable that these two medications not be started at the same time. The reason for this is that the toxic side effects that may be seen with high doses of vitamin E are gastrointestinal (nausea, vomiting, cramping, and diarrhea), headache, and fatigue. Since some of these may also be seen with donepezil, if the two are started together and one or more of these side effects occurs, determining which is causing the side effect may be difficult.

The APA guidelines state that vitamin E "may be used in moderately impaired patients with Alzheimer's disease in order to delay the progression of the disease" (10). They also state that vitamin E "might be considered for use in combination with a cholinesterase inhibitor." However, the authors note that efficacy has not been studied in mildly affected patients, there is no clinical experience of use in combination with a cholinesterase inhibitor, and the relatively high dose studied in the moderately affected patients may worsen the coagulation defects in patients with a vitamin K deficiency or those taking warfarin. Other authors have also expressed caution (35).

Anti-inflammatory Drugs. A number of studies suggest that inflammation may play a role in the pathogenesis of Alzheimer's disease. In addition to amyloid protein, neuritic plaques have been found to contain such markers of inflammation as complement and cytokines. In the brain these proteins are secreted by microglial cells, the cerebral counterparts of macrophages. Microglia themselves are often found in association with neuritic plaques, and the proteins they secrete may contribute to the disease process. These findings have led to the hypothesis that anti-inflammatory drugs, both steroids and non-steroidal anti-inflammatory drugs (NSAIDs), may slow the progression or delay the onset of the Alzheimer's disease.

A recent study performed by researchers from Johns Hopkins University sought to determine whether NSAID usage was associated with a reduced risk of Alzheimer's disease (36). Results revealed that the overall risk of Alzheimer's disease was significantly reduced by 50% for people who had ever taken NSAIDs. The amount of risk reduction depended on the estimated duration of use, with those taking NSAIDs for more than 2 years having a risk reduction of 60% compared with a 35% risk reduction in those taking NSAIDs for less than 2 years. Although the risk of Alzheimer's disease was slightly reduced among those who had taken aspirin (26%), this was not significantly different from placebo. There was no evidence of risk reduction among those who had taken acetaminophen, which was expected, since it has little or no anti-inflammatory activity. The inconsistent findings for aspirin were explained by the possibility that low doses of aspirin were taken to prevent heart disease, which may be inadequate for anti-inflammatory effects in the CNS.

There have been other studies in the literature investigating the role of NSAIDs in Alzheimer's disease (37). Virtually all are prevention studies, which are typically case-control in design and often small in sample size. These studies have reported varying reductions in risk. No large placebo-controlled studies of NSAIDs have been reported in the treatment of patients diagnosed with Alzheimer's disease. There is one double blind, placebo-controlled study of indomethacin in 44 patients (38). The results were reported as positive but were not widely accepted because of methodologic problems. In addition, nearly 42% of the actively treated patients discontinued the trial early, most because of gastrointestinal side effects. Chronic use of NSAIDs carries the potential for serious adverse events, including nephrotoxicity, gastric irritation and bleeding, and peptic ulcer disease, and some, including indomethacin, have been associated with cognitive impairment in the elderly. These risks and the limited nature of the data so far should temper any decision regarding their use for either prevention or treatment of Alzheimer's disease. Particular caution should be exercised in regard to concomitant use with a cholinesterase inhibitor, given the possibility for synergy in gastric irritation. At least one group does not recommend their use at this time. Patients treated with such combinations should be carefully monitored for safety and tolerance, and expectations of enhanced efficacy should be tempered by the absence of available evidence.

Estrogen. The situation with regard to the use of estrogen in Alzheimer's disease is similar to that for NSAIDs. There is basic research showing positive effects on neurons (39). Estrogen has the potential for both preventive and acute treatment, albeit only in women. A variety of epidemiologic studies support the possibility of prevention or at least delay of onset of disease (40). Unfortunately, none of these studies is convincing enough to make it clear that benefits outweigh risks (41). There are also no large-scale, double-blind, placebo-controlled trials with positive results, though one such trial organized by the Alzheimer's Disease Cooperative Study Units is nearing completion. Although it had several limitations, a retrospective study of the tacrine data found better cognitive performance in women taking both tacrine and estrogen than in those taking tacrine alone (42). The APA guidelines suggest that estrogen use should be considered in postmenopausal women (10).

Ginkgo Biloba. A recent large-scale, double-blind, placebo-controlled 1-year trial of ginkgo found very modest positive results (43). There were several methodologic problems with this trial, the most important being that very mildly affected patients were probably overrepresented. Nonetheless, ginkgo biloba did appear safe and well tolerated. Since it may help and probably won't hurt, cost is probably the deciding factor for its use.

Antidepressants. The use of antidepressants in Alzheimer's disease has not been well studied. Early in the course of the disease, patients may develop depressive symptoms in reaction to their perceived loss of function or to the diagnosis itself. In some patients it may not be clear whether the cognitive loss is due to depression or the reverse. In either of these cases a trial of an antidepressant is probably warranted. The agent of choice is a selective serotonin reuptake inhibitor. Tricyclic antidepressants with anticholinergic side effects should be avoided.

Neuroleptics. Neuroleptics are frequently prescribed for the behavioral symptoms of Alzheimer's disease. A meta-analysis of their use by Schneider et al. (44) showed similar efficacy for haloperidol (Haldol) and thioridazine (Mellaril). Their efficacy was very modest, and side effects were common. The newer agents, so-called atypical antipsychotics such as risperidone (Risperdal), may show a somewhat greater efficacy with fewer side effects at low doses, but detailed results must be published, and more prospective controlled studies are needed in this area.

TREATMENT OF VASCULAR DEMENTIA. Treatment of vascular dementia has received far less attention from researchers and the pharmaceutical industry than has Alzheimer's disease. This is in part because it is less common and in part because it is harder to identify pure cases. The thrust of treatment, of course, is to control any other conditions that contribute to the vascular disease in the hope of preventing further vascular insults. While this is intuitively obvious, actual efficacy in altering the course of vascular dementia has not been documented and because of ethical considerations probably will not be. Most clinicians would also recommend an aspirin per day, though more aggressive anticoagulation with warfarin is probably not wise because of the increased risk of falls in these patients. Whether cholinesterase inhibitors benefit these patients is not known, though studies with donepezil are under way. No cholinergic deficit has been demonstrated in these patients, but a general enhancement of memory by increasing cholinergic function may be beneficial. Another drug, propentofylline, is in phase III trials.

TREATMENT OF OTHER IRREVERSIBLE DEMENTIAS. There are no specific treatments for the other irreversible dementias. The drugs already described, especially cholinesterase inhibitors, may be useful for some conditions. Unfortunately, more specific treatment necessitates a better understanding of the pathology underlying each condition, and some conditions are so rare that it will be many more years before this is accomplished.

CONCLUSION

Loss of memory and other cognitive function is probably the disability that most people fear the most as they get older, and the increasing prevalence of these conditions with aging gives a basis to such fears. Fortunately, in the past 2 decades or so, we have learned a lot about the diseases that cause these problems. In recent years this research has begun to pay off in terms of specific treatments for some diseases, and this progress is likely to continue. Now more than ever it is incumbent on physicians working with the elderly to recognize cognitive impairment, to understand its evaluation and differential diagnosis, and to begin appropriate treatment.

REFERENCES

1. American Psychiatric Association. Diagnostic and Statistical Manual of Mental Disorders. 4th ed. Washington: American Psychiatric Association, 1994.
2. Francis J, Kapoor WN. Delirium in hospitalized elderly. J Gen Intern Med 1990;5:65–79.
3. McIntosh TK, Bush HL, Yeston NS, et al. Beta-endorphin, cortisol and post-operative delirium: a preliminary report. Psychoneuroendocrinology 1985;10:303–313.
4. Pompei P, Foreman M, Rudberg MA, et al. Delirium in hospitalized older persons: outcomes and predictors. J Am Geriatr Soc 1994;42:809–815.
5. Inouye SK, van Dyck CH, Alessi CA, et al. Clarifying confusion: the confusion assessment method, a new method for detection of delirium. Ann Intern Med 1990; 113:941–948.
6. Clarfield AM. The reversible dementias: do they reverse? Ann Intern Med 1988;109:476–486.
7. Hector M, Burton JR. What are the psychiatric manifestations of vitamin B-12 deficiency? J Am Geriatr Soc 1988;36:1105–1112.
8. Costa PT Jr, Williams TF, Somerfield M, et al. Recognition and Initial Assessment of Alzheimer's Disease and Related Dementias (AHCPR 97–0702). Rockville, MD: US Department of Health and Human Services, Public Health Service, Agency for Health Care Policy and Research, 1996.
9. Practice parameter for diagnosis and evaluation of dementia (summary statement). Report of the Quality Standards Subcommittee of the American Academy of Neurology. Neurology 1994;44:2203–2206.
10. Practice guideline for the treatment of patients with Alzheimer's disease and other dementias of late life. American Psychiatric Association. Am J Psychiatry 1997;154(suppl):1–39.
11. Small GW, Rabins PV, Barry PP, et al. Diagnosis and treatment of Alzheimer's disease and related disorders: consensus statement of American Association for

Geriatric Psychiatry, Alzheimer's Association, and American Geriatrics Society. JAMA 1997;278:1363–1371.

12. Hendrie HC. Epidemiology of Alzheimer's disease. Geriatrics 1997;52(suppl 2):S4–S8.

13. Green RC. Alzheimer's disease and other dementing disorders. In: Joynt RJ, ed. Clinical Neurology. Philadelphia: Lippincott-Raven, 1995.

14. Goate AM. molecular genetics of Alzheimer's disease. Geriatrics 1997;52(suppl 2):S9–S12.

15. Slooter AJ, Tang MX, van Duijn CM, et al. Apolipoprotein E epsilon4 and the risk of dementia with stroke. JAMA 1997;277:818–821.

16. Reisberg B, Ferris SH, deLeon MJ, Crook T. The Global Deterioration Scale for the assessment of primary degenerative dementia. Am J Psychiatry 1982;139:1136–1139.

17. Hughes CP, Berg L, Danziger WL, et al. A new clinical scale for the staging of dementia. Br J Psychiatry 1982;140:566–572.

18. Morris JC. The Clinical Dementia Rating (CDR): current version and scoring rules. Neurology 1993;43:2412–2414.

19. Roman GC, Tatemichi TK, Erkinjuntti T, et al. Vascular dementia: diagnostic criteria for research studies. Report of the NINDS-AIREN International Workshop. Neurology 1993;43:250–260.

20. Rosen WG, Terry RD, Fuld PA, et al. Pathological verification of ischemic score in differentiation of dementias. Ann Neurol 1980;7:486–488.

21. McKeith LG, Galasko D, Kosaka K, et al. Consensus guidelines for the clinical and pathologic diagnosis of dementia with Lewy bodies (DLB): Report of the Consortium on DLB international workshop. Neurology 1996;47:1113–1124.

22. Mittelman MS, Ferris SH, Shulman E, et al. A family intervention to delay nursing home placement of patients with Alzheimer's disease: a randomized, controlled clinical trial. JAMA 1996;276:1725–1731.

23. Perry EK. The cholinergic hypothesis: ten years on. Br Med Bull 1986;42:66–69.

24. Summers WK, Majovski LV, Marsh GM, et al. Oral tetrahydroaminoacridine in long-term treatment of senile dementia, Alzheimer's type. N Engl J Med 1986; 315:1241–1245.

25. Davis KL, Powchik P. Tacrine. Lancet 1995;345:625–630.

26. Davis KL, Thal LJ, Gamzu ER, et al. A double-blind, placebo-controlled, multicenter study of tacrine for Alzheimer's disease. N Engl J Med 1992;327:1253–1259.

27. Farlow M, Gracon SI, Hershey LA, et al. A controlled trial of tacrine in Alzheimer's disease. JAMA 1992;268:2523–2529.

28. Aricept (donepezil hydrochloride) package insert. Teaneck, NJ: Eisai, 1997.

29. Rogers SL, Doody RS, Mohs RC, et al. Donepezil improves cognition and global function in Alzheimer's disease: a 15-week, double-blind, placebo-controlled study. Donepezil Study Group. Arch Intern Med 1998; 158:1021–1031.

30. Rogers SL, Farlow MR, Doody RS, et al. A 24-week, double-blind, placebo-controlled trial of donepezil in patients with Alzheimer's disease. Neurology 1998;50: 136–145.

31. Friedhoff L, Rogers SL. Donepezil lengthens time to loss of activities of daily living in patients with mild to moderate Alzheimer's disease: results of a preliminary evaluation. Neurology 1997;48:A100 (abstract).

32. Knopman D, Schneider L, Davis K, et al. Long-term tacrine (Cognex) treatment effects on nursing home placement and mortality. Tacrine Study Group. Neurology 1996;47:166–177.

33. Rogers SL, Friedhoff LT. Long-term efficacy and safety of donepezil in the treatment of Alzheimer's disease: an interim analysis of the results of a us multicentre open label extension study. Eur Neuropsychopharmacol 1998;8:67–75.

34. Sano M, Ernesto C, Thomas RG, et al. A controlled trial of selegiline, alpha-tocopherol, or both as treatment for Alzheimer's disease. N Engl J Med 1997;336:1216–1222.

35. Drachman DA, Leber P. Treatment of Alzheimer's disease: searching for a breakthrough, settling for less. N Engl J Med 1997;336:1245–1247.

36. Stewart, WF, Kawas, C, et al. Risk of Alzheimer's disease and duration of NSAID use. Neurology 1997;48:626–632.

37. McGeer PL, Schulzer M, McGeer EG. Arthritis and anti-inflammatory agents as possible protective factors for Alzheimer's disease: a review of 17 epidemiologic studies. Neurology 1996;47:425–432.

38. Rogers J, Kirby LC, et al. Clinical trial of indomethacin in Alzheimer's disease. Neurology 1993;43:1609–1611.

39. McEwen BS, Alves SE, Bulloch K, Weiland NG. Ovarian steroids and the brain: implications for cognition and aging. Neurology 1997;48(suppl 7):S8–S15.

40. Henderson VW. The epidemiology of estrogen replacement therapy and Alzheimer's disease. Neurology 1997; 48(suppl 7):S27–S35.

41. Barret-Connor E, Kritz-Silverstein D. Estrogen replacement therapy and cognitive functioning in older women. JAMA 1993;269:2637–2641.

42. Schneider LS, Farlow MR, Henderson VW, Pogoda JM. Effects of estrogen replacement therapy on response to tacrine in patients with Alzheimer's disease. Neurology 1996;46:1580–1584.

43. LeBars PL, Katz MM, Berman N, et al. A placebo-controlled, double-blind, randomized trial of an extract of ginkgo biloba for dementia. JAMA 1997;278:1327–1332.

44. Schneider LS, Pollock VE, Lyness SA. A metaanalysis of controlled trials of neuroleptic treatment in dementia. J Am Geriatr Soc 1990;38:553–563.

CHAPTER 16

CONSTANTINE G. LYKETSOS, CYNTHIA D. STEELE, AND MARTIN STEINBERG

Behavioral Disturbances in Dementia

BACKGROUND AND DEFINITIONS

Dementia is a syndrome defined by a global decline in cognitive capacity occurring in clear consciousness. Most dementia is a chronic illness that is typically progressive and irreversible and that is associated with a range of behavioral and mental disturbances. In this chapter we use the term behavioral disturbances to refer to all noncognitive disturbances in mental life or behavior that may afflict a patient with a dementing illness. Depression, anxiety, fearfulness, delusions, and apathy are all examples of mental disturbances. Similarly, aggression, explosive outbursts, wandering, repetitive calling out, and inappropriate sexual advances are all behaviors that dementia patients may exhibit.

The behavioral disturbances of dementia have considerable importance. These disturbances increase the morbidity of the dementia patient by adding mental suffering and further impairing function. Moreover, these disturbances adversely affect those around the patient, particularly the patient's caregivers. They add to the complexity of caregiving and increase the time required for it. Behavioral disturbances in dementia are associated with depression, functional impairment, and burnout among caregivers. Additionally, they are associated with a greater likelihood of nursing home placement for the patient with dementia.

While in some cases the behavioral disturbances of dementia have been associated with the brain damage brought on by the dementing disease, this relation is neither completely proved nor the only cause of behavioral disturbance. Dementia patients, by the nature of their condition, are vulnerable to stressors and often respond to such stressors by exhibiting a behavioral disturbance. Thus, for example, aggression in a dementia patient may be the consequence of brain damage to inhibitory brain centers, the result of an otherwise hidden urinary tract infection, or the consequence of an abusive caregiver. Therefore, behavioral disturbance in dementia is not a single entity. Nor do these disturbances have a single cause; rather they are influenced by a range of variables with synergistic effects. For a more thorough discussion of behavioral disturbance in dementia, refer to the report of a recent consensus conference (1). Additionally, a guideline to the treatment of Alzheimer's disease and related disorders (2) provides an overview of all aspects of the treatment of dementia.

EPIDEMIOLOGY OF BEHAVIORAL DISTURBANCES IN DEMENTIA

The cumulative prevalence of behavioral disturbances in dementia patients is on the order of 60 to 70% over the course of most dementing illness. The cumulative prevalence of the more serious disturbances, those which involve considerable mental suffering (such as major depression), or some form of dangerousness (such as aggression), is on the order of 40 to 50% over the course of the illness. The prevalence of behavioral disturbances tends to be lower among community-residing patients and more common among patients who attend specialty dementia and Alzheimer clinics at academic medical centers.

The prevalence is even higher among institutionalized patients, such as in nursing homes and psychiatric inpatient units. As expected, the type and the severity of behavioral disturbances differ across these three settings because of selection bias. Table 16.1 is a summary of the cumulative prevalence (i.e., over the course of a dementing illness) of several specific behavioral disturbances.

Incidence estimates of the onset of new cases of behavioral disturbance in patients with dementia on an annual basis have rarely been published. With regard to major depression, one study reports a 2-year incidence of approximately 1% in patients with Alzheimer's disease (3). A different 5-year cohort study suggests that the incidence of depressed mood with vegetative signs is 5% every 6 months and of depressed mood alone, about 14% every 6 months for patients with Alzheimer's disease (4). The incidence of delusions has been estimated at 17% every 6 months, and the incidence of hallucinations at 9% every 6 months in Alzheimer's disease (4). Also in Alzheimer patients, the incidence of other behavioral disturbances, such as wandering and aggression, has been estimated at 36% every 6 months (4). Whether these estimates generalize to patients with other types of dementia is unknown.

The persistence of behavioral symptoms over time in dementia patients has been the subject of considerable debate. Few empiric studies have been published. From these it appears that unless treated, behavioral disturbances in dementia are persistent. In a three-site longitudinal study of 335 patients with mild to moderate Alzheimer's disease there was a high likelihood of persistence of individual behavioral disturbances over 5 years (4). For delusions the probability of persistence every 6 months was 60%. For hallucinations the estimate was 52%. For wandering, physical aggression, and similar behavioral disturbances the estimate was 80%. For depressed mood the estimate was 47%, and for depressed mood with vegetative signs the estimate was 28%. While this was a volunteer clinical sample restricted to Alzheimer's disease, it is the best study to date and provides good evidence that over time behavior disturbances do not spontaneously remit.

Table 16.1

Cumulative Prevalence Estimates for Behavioral Disturbances in Dementia Patients

Disturbance Home (%)	Community (%)	Outpatient (%)	Nursing
Delirium	N/A	N/A	N/A
Major depressive episode	7–15	20–25	30–40
Other (minor) depression	25–30	25–40	N/A
Manic episode	1–2	2	N/A
Delusions	15–20	40–45	40–50
Hallucinations	8–15	15	20–25
Sleep disorders	10–15	50–60	N/A
Inappropriate sexual behaviors	7	10–15	15–20
Apathy	N/A	14	N/A
Any aggression	50–65	40–50	45–50
Unprovoked aggression	6–10	17	20–25
Calling out	N/A	33	11
Disinhibition	20–35	35–50	40–45
Other aberrant motor behaviors	10	15–20	17–20

N/A, not applicable.

APPROACHING THE BEHAVIORALLY DISTURBED DEMENTIA PATIENT

There are several principles important to the assessment and treatment of behavioral disturbances associated with dementia (5). Behavioral disturbances are diverse in presentation and causation, so distinguishing one from another is both possible and necessary. Behavioral disturbances in dementia do not always have a single cause. A variety of contributing causes in predictable domains should be considered case by case. When a new behavioral disturbance occurs, it is necessary to work it up systematically by classifying it and by investigating possible contributing causes *before* embarking on treatments.

There is no single or universal treatment for behavioral disturbances. Continuing with general supportive patient care and providing a wide range of interventions is critical. Patients must be monitored for response to treatment as well as for side effects, particularly when medicines are used. Side effects tend to occur more often, to last longer, and to take longer to resolve than in elderly patients who do not suffer from dementia.

We propose a systematic four-step approach to any new behavioral disturbance in dementia. The first step, describing the disturbance, has as its main outcome a decision about how to classify the behavioral disturbance. Description begins with the observable phenomena of the disturbance, the behaviors the patient is exhibiting, and places them in the context of the patient's circumstances, mental state, and physical state of health. This phase requires a careful history from the patient and from one or more collateral sources, typically the primary caregiver. Important factors are the behaviors observed, their temporal onset, course, associated circumstances, and relation to key environmental factors, such as caregiver status and recent stressors. History taking is followed by a careful examination, both physical and neurologic. The mental status of the patient is assessed in detail by an experienced examiner. Laboratory studies may also be needed.

The next goal is to decide whether the behavioral disturbance fits a recognizable pattern. De-

termining which pattern best describes the situation depends on the clinical circumstance and requires clinical judgment about which aspects of the situation to emphasize. In some cases the clinician emphasizes recognition of a mental syndrome, such as delirium, major depression, minor depression, apathy, or mania, and associates the entire disturbance with this syndrome. In other cases certain disruptive behaviors are being driven by a particular mental state, such as a delusion or a hallucination. Sometimes the disturbance is primarily a disruption in one of the primary drives of sleep, sexuality, or feeding. In yet others the primary emphasis is on the observed behaviors as consequences of behavioral dyscontrol brought about by brain damage from the dementing disease. Finally, some disturbances have the characteristics of a catastrophic reaction (an excessive outburst of emotion and/or disruptive behavior precipitated by the patient's being confronted with a cognitive impairment) or of an adjustment reaction (such as with a change in routine, a move to a new residence, or the introduction of a new caregiver).

After describing the behavioral disturbance and classifying it, the next step is to decode it. Decoding is looking for causes that may contribute to the onset or continuation of the disturbance. Table 16.2 lists the domains to consider in this process. Medications and general medical conditions have been associated with all types of behavioral disturbance through two additional mechanisms. If the observed pattern most closely resembles delirium, medications and general medical conditions are most likely to be the cause. Particular attention should be paid

Table 16.2

Contributing Causes to a Behavioral Disturbance in Dementia

Medication (any type)
Medical condition (new or recurrent)
Psychiatric disorder (new or recurrent)
Cognitive disorder
Recognizable mental or behavioral syndrome
Environment
Caregiver approach or impairment

to the possible effects of medication accumulation; all medications ought to be considered as possible causes of a new behavioral disturbance.

The most common medical conditions associated with behavioral disturbance are a urinary tract infection (both in men and women), dehydration, constipation, pain (such as from osteoarthritis or dental carries), visual impairment, hearing impairment, a viral syndrome (respiratory or gastrointestinal infection), and skin breakdown (particularly in nursing home or in institutionalized patients). Less common are stroke, pneumonia, deep venous thrombosis, and cardiac disease. Additionally, neglect of basic physical needs (leading to hunger, sleepiness, thirst, boredom, or fatigue) that the patient cannot adequately communicate is a cause of behavioral disturbance. In patients who have known chronic medical problems, such as diabetes, hypertension, or cardiac disease, a relapse of one of these conditions should be considered. The next issue is whether the patient is suffering from a new or recurrent psychiatric disorder. In some patients the psychiatric disorder is primary (i.e., not caused by the dementing disease), the recurrence of a lifelong psychiatric disorder, such as major depressive disorder, bipolar disorder, panic disorder, or schizophrenia. All of these may recur in the context of dementia and appear as a behavioral disturbance. In other patients the disorder is secondary to a factor other than the dementing disease, typically a general medical problem (e.g., hypothyroidism, a medication). The disorder may also be due to the brain damage caused by the dementing disease. This is discussed further later in this chapter.

The next part of decoding is to determine whether the behavioral disturbance is related to the cognitive disorder. For example, is the patient irritable because he or she is forgetting things or getting frustrated because he or she can't talk? Is the patient forgetful enough to believe that he or she is living in a different period of his or her life and therefore believe that some persons are alive (typically parents or spouses) who are dead? A dementia patient may thus look at himself or herself in the mirror believing that he or she is young and not recognize the person who is there. Most of the behavioral disturbances directly linked to the cognitive disorder present

as catastrophic reactions, acute behavioral, physical, or verbal reactions out of proportion to seemingly minor stressors. These include anger, emotional lability, and at times aggression.

The next question is whether there is evidence that the dementing disease has involved brain areas other than the ones associated with the cognitive disorder. Involvement of other brain areas may lead to characteristic behavioral or mental syndromes or secondary and/or organic disorders. Most often these occur with involvement of the frontal lobes, the temporal lobes, and certain subcortical regions.

There are several examples. Disinhibition, expressed in inappropriate social behavior, pacing, wandering, or perseveration may be related to damage to select frontal lobe and basal ganglia areas. Another syndrome consists of exploratory curiosity with hyperphagia and hypersexuality. In animals this is called the Klüver-Bucy syndrome; it is associated with damage to the temporal poles and the amygdala. Damage to anterior frontal and subcortical structures may lead to atypical mood syndromes, both depressivelike and maniclike states. Apathy (6), a state of passive lack of interest, has been associated with damage to the temporal lobes, the cingulum, the dorsolateral frontal lobes, and the caudate nucleus.

Brain damage has been associated with unprovoked aggression, particularly if there is disturbed (usually increased) noradrenergic or dopaminergic neurotransmission. Repetitive or compulsive behaviors have been associated with brain injury to orbitofrontal areas and the cingulum. Delusions and hallucinations have also been related to injury to the limbic system. Finally, disturbances of the basic drives, namely, sleep, sex, and feeding, may appear as the dementing disease spreads to relevant brain areas.

The next component of decoding is to determine whether there is something in the environment that is affecting the behavioral disturbance. Common environmental stressors include disruption of routines, overstimulation (too much noise or too many people), understimulation (few people, with the patient spending much time alone), and other upset peers (patients).

The final consideration should be given to caregiver-patient relations. Almost all patients with dementia have caregivers. Many of them have more than one at a time. Caring for dementia patients is difficult and requires a degree of sophistication that almost any caregiver is capable of acquiring with proper guidance. However, inexperienced caregiving, dominating caregivers, and caregivers who themselves are impaired through medical or psychiatric disturbances may interact with patients in such a way as to exacerbate or cause a behavioral disturbance. When evaluating a new behavioral disturbance, the clinician should consider the caregiver's understanding of the patient's level of condition, whether the caregiver is new to the patient (as is common in nursing homes and with agency nurses), whether the caregiver is approaching the patient properly, and whether there are too many caregivers involved in the patient's care. Most of these sorts of problems occur in nursing homes. However, many occur in private homes, particularly if patients do not have established routines or the caregiver is impaired by a physical or mental disorder.

Once a behavioral disturbance has been classified and decoded, the stage is set for devising interventions to treat it. There are several types of interventions. First are preventive interventions, which include the development and maintenance of daily routines, the provision of routine primary medical care, attention to the patient's sleep and eating patterns, safety measures to prevent accidents, teaching caregivers about the practical aspects of dementia care and behavioral disturbances, and linkage with experienced and accessible professionals to help assess and treat a behavioral disturbance. Second are interventions that address and remove the cause of behavioral disturbances, such as the discontinuation of an offending medication or the treatment of a bladder infection. Third are attempts to apply behavior management techniques (7) or special programs for dementia patients with disruptive behaviors in nursing homes (8). Finally, there are specific or empiric interventions targeted at particular disturbances. These may include psychotropic medications, electroconvulsive therapy (ECT), or bright light therapies.

A single intervention rarely makes a dramatic difference in a patient's condition. A variety of concurrent interventions are usually necessary. *Most of these involve changing the patient's environment (rather than changing the patient) to fit the state of impairment or to meet needs.* Decoding provides clues on interventions that may be tried. If recent medicines seem temporally related to the onset of the problem, these ought be stopped or reduced. If the patient has a large medication burden, efforts should be made to reduce the burden. If the evaluation reveals a medical problem such as constipation or a urinary tract infection, this should be treated as soon and as effectively as possible, and time should be allowed for the patient to recover fully.

Dementia patients may require a week longer to recover from routine medical problems than nondemented elderly. If a patient has a recurrent psychiatric disorder, it should be treated in standard ways. (An exception to this is the limited ability of dementia patients to engage in insight-oriented psychotherapy.) If a patient's behavioral disturbance appears closely linked to the cognitive disorder itself, efforts should be made to reduce the likelihood that he or she will face these deficits. If a patient becomes lost and confused in a familiar environment in the evening, the caregiver should attempt to structure the patient's time more in the evening and to provide more one-on-one attention at that time. If the problem is a specific mental syndrome associated with damage to particular brain areas, it should be treated specifically, often with a pharmacologic agent.

If the problem is linked to the patient's routine, appropriate changes should be made. Patients may need more frequent meals and snacks so that they are less likely to be hungry; they may require more personal attention from caregivers; or they may need simpler levels of activity. If the problem relates to the caregiver's approach, caregivers should be taught how to approach patients and manage their behavior by sophisticated clinicians. Such education is best provided through modeling by an experienced clinician in the environment in which the problem is occurring during the time of day the problem is most likely to occur and with regular repeat teaching sessions to reinforce the lesson.

Once a set of interventions for a particular behavioral disturbance has been planned, specific implementation plans should be mapped out to determine whether they work. This map ought to include who shall do what intervention when, how long it is expected for individual interventions to take effect, and what will be done if interventions fail. When mapping out a treatment approach, fallback plans are very important, as it may be necessary to attempt several interventions before a patient improves. A fallback plan also gives caregivers, who are with the disturbed patient day in and day out, a sense that something is being done and helps maintain their morale. A fallback plan should provide for an intervention if a crisis occurs (e.g., if the patient becomes unmanageable, hospitalization should be available). In our experience hospitalization on an inpatient geropsychiatric unit benefits many seriously behaviorally disturbed dementia patients.

An important consideration in determining the outcome of treatment is the use of standardized assessment scales. Several such scales have good reliability, validity, and clinical utility. These may be used to describe the type and severity of a behavioral disturbance as well as to assess response to interventions. Four scales are recommended for their wide availability and relative ease of use. The Neuropsychiatric Inventory (9) quantifies 10 types of behavioral disturbance in dementia, each on a 10-point scale, assessing both frequency and severity of disturbance. It is most useful when clinicians are interested in a broad set of disturbances, as it is short and can be administered by a clinician who is not a physician. The Dementia Signs and Symptoms Scale (10), which assesses 6 types of behavioral disturbances, is most effective in quantifying mania and irritability. Finally, the Cornell Scale for Depression in Dementia (11) and the Apathy Evaluation Scale (12) may be used to quantify depressive disturbances or apathy.

It is important to sustain the treatment plan once it is initiated. Many times the onus to sustain the plan is on the caregivers. The clinician should be sensitive to this and make it easy for the caregivers to implement the plan. Also, when using medicines, clinicians should be alerted to the fact that side effects occur more often, last longer, and take longer to remit than in the general population, so that as few medicines as possible should be used as briefly as possible and at as low a dose as possible. The rule "start low and go slow" applies. Adjustments of medicines should be made over periods that are longer than routinely practiced with other elderly patients. In this era of managed care pressures, it is always tempting to adjust medicines rapidly. This may lead to short-term benefits, and the patient may seem quieter or less explosive, but it may lead to side effects associated with rapidly escalating medication doses.

SPECIFIC BEHAVIORAL DISTURBANCES

See Table 16.3 for pharmacologic treatment options. For more detail on the use of psychopharmaceuticals in general, see Hyman et al. (13).

Delirium

Clinical Features

The hallmark of delirium is impairment in sensorium. Patients whose sensorium is impaired are distractible, inattentive, disoriented, and hard to engage in a conversation. Most develop a range of mental symptoms, such as irritability, visual or auditory hallucinations, misperceptions, delusions, affective lability, depression, euphoria, and social withdrawal. Some patients are hypervigilant, active, and easily startled. Others are lethargic, withdrawn, or hard to arouse. Most cases of delirium develop suddenly and are reversible after treatment of the causes, often an acute general medical problem. In patients with dementia, particularly moderate to severe dementia, the assessment and recognition of delirium are complicated, since the level of impairment in cognition makes it difficult to determine whether the sensorium is impaired. The cognitive impairment may wax and wane and give the impression of fluctuations in sensorium. Certain dementing diseases, such as cerebrovascular dementia and diffuse Lewy body disease, are accompanied by chronic delirium. In these patients the waxing and waning in sensorium can occur at any point through the day and intermittently throughout the course of the week.

Table 16.3

Medications to Treat Depressive and Other Behavioral Syndromes in Dementia

Agent	Starting Dose	Weekly Dose Increase	Peak Effective Dose
SSRIs			
Sertraline	25 mg in AM	25 mg qd	175–200 mg qd
Fluoxetine	10 mg in AM	10 mg qd	60–80 mg qd
Paroxetine	10 mg at bedtime	10 mg qd	30–40 mg qd
Tricyclics			
Nortriptyline	10 mg at bedtime	10 mg qd	50–150 ng/dL
Desipramine	10 mg at bedtime	10 mg qd	150–200 ng/dL
Other agents			
Venlafaxine	25 mg bid	25 mg bid	400 mg qd
Bupropion	75 mg bid	50 mg bid	400 mg qd
Nefazodone	50 mg bid	50 mg bid	500 mg qd
Antipsychotics			
Haloperidol	0.5 mg at bedtime	0.5 mg qd	6–10 mg qd
Thioridazine	10 mg at bedtime	10 mg qd	60–80 mg qd
Thiothixene	1 mg at bedtime	1 mg qd	8–10 mg qd
Trifluoperazine	1 mg at bedtime	1 mg qd	8–10 mg qd
Newer antipsychotics			
Risperidone	0.5 mg at bedtime	0.5 mg qd	6 mg qd
Olanzapine	2.5 mg at bedtime	2.5 mg qd	15 mg qd
Clozapine	25 mg bid	25 mg bid	100 mg qd

Treatment

The deliria that accompany dementia are hard to treat, particularly if they are chronic. Environmental modifications to improve orientation, such as good lighting, one-on-one attention, supportive care, and attention to the patient's personal needs and wants, are central aspects of treatment. If delirium is chronic and consistently accompanied by a sleep disturbance, efforts may be made to stabilize the sleep disturbance through the use of bright lights (14) or medications (see sleep under the section on drives). Pharmacologic intervention is warranted if patients are aggressive, engaging in other dangerous behaviors, or having delusions or hallucinations. Neuroleptic therapy is preferred. Haloperidol 0.25 to 0.5 mg before bed is a first-line treatment option. Alternatives include risperidone 0.25 to 0.5 mg before bed or any other high potency neuroleptic, such as thiothixene or trifluoperazine. Patients with Lewy body dementia often develop parkinsonism on low doses of neuroleptics. In that case a nontra-

ditional neuroleptic, such as risperidone, olanzapine, clozapine, or quetiapine, may be tried first. Patients should be monitored carefully for side effects, in particular sedation, dry mouth, blurred vision, constipation, urinary retention, worsening of delirium, orthostatic hypotension, parkinsonism, dystonia, and akathisia, all of which may occur with neuroleptics. Other alternatives are the benzodiazepines, such as lorazepam 0.25 to 0.5 mg 1 to 3 times per day, although these should be used infrequently and in extreme situations. Trazodone 25 to 75 mg may calm anxious, confused patients for a short time, until behavioral strategies take hold.

Mood Disturbances

Clinical Features

A wide range of mood *symptoms* have been described in dementia patients, including irritability, anxiety, and dysphoria. Irritable or anxious patients are upset, emotionally aroused, explosive, and at times hostile. They often can be redirected and calmed down. Others are emotionally labile, with moods ranging from sadness to irritability to explosiveness over short periods with or without environmental provocation. These symptoms are typically nonspecific and rarely require pharmacologic treatment. More often they are best dealt with by reassuring, distracting, and spending time with the patient.

A variety of mood *syndromes* have been described in dementia patients. The most common is minor depression, in which patients have mild anhedonia, social withdrawal, and occasional sadness. They may feel depleted and exhibit mild neurovegetative change. Rarely are patients with minor depression self-deprecating; rarely do they show other cognitive symptoms of depression, such as guilt, self-blame, hopelessness, or low self-esteem. The syndrome of major depression is characterized by anhedonia or sadness accompanied by impaired vital sense (insomnia, anorexia, low libido, fatigue) and the feeling of being a burden on others, decreased confidence, decreased hope, and decreased self-esteem. Many depressed dementia patients deny feeling sad or depressed but acknowledge anhedonia or mental depletion or are reported by their caregiver to be sad or to cry at home. Minor and major depression are most common in patients whose dementing disease first affects frontal-subcortical circuits, such as Parkinson's disease, Huntington's disease, and stroke. A significant number of patients with Alzheimer's disease and other dementias, however, have major or minor depressive syndrome.

Mania and manialike episodes also affect dementia patients. Classic mania with euphoria, increased talkativeness, increased energy, decreased sleep, flight of ideas, and grandiose ideas is seen occasionally. More often in dementia, manic syndromes take on atypical presentations with irritability, explosiveness, mood lability, decreased sleep, increased pacing, and overconfidence. Some patients develop delusions of grandeur, although these are not common. Maniclike states may be most common in advanced dementia patients.

Treatment

All treatments for the depressed, irritable, maniclike, and anxious states should be preceded by a workup as discussed in the decoding section. This should be followed by efforts to provide the patient with routines, distraction, predictability in the environment, and optimal physical health. Most cases of major depression and many cases of minor depression require antidepressant therapy. Although the use of antidepressants in dementia is *not* well established through placebo-controlled trials, there is evidence from case reports and series to support their use. First-line agents are the selective serotonin reuptake inhibitors (SSRIs) and the tricyclic antidepressants. The SSRIs are preferred because they have a lower side effect profile. Sertraline is probably the best starting agent, given its shorter half-life than fluoxetine and a lower likelihood of anticholinergic side effects than paroxetine. An alternative starting agent is nortriptyline. Table 16.3 lists the antidepressants most commonly used to treat depressive symptoms in dementia, including starting doses, weekly dose increases, and peak doses, beyond which additional benefits are unlikely.

Persistence in the treatment of depression is important. After a first agent has failed at an adequate therapeutic dose for 6 to 8 weeks, an alternative agent should be tried. Venlafaxine, bupropion, nefazodone, and the monoamine oxidase inhibitors may be considered. For patients who are partial responders to an antidepressant, boosting strategies using lithium carbonate 150 to 600 mg a day, fluphenazine 0.25 mg a day, or thyroxin 50 to 100 μg a day may be considered. The advantage of boosting strategies is that the patient may respond within a week or two. If he or she does not respond, the booster ought to be discontinued. If a patient continues to be depressed after several antidepressant trials, particularly if there is danger, such as with serious weight loss or suicidal ideas, ECT should be considered. This is the fastest and most efficacious treatment for major depression, and it has a favorable safety profile in dementia (15) despite the stigma associated with it.

Treatment of mania and of emotional lability or irritability typically begins with the use of mood-stabilizing agents followed by neuroleptics. Given its low side effect profile, divalproex sodium (DVS) is the first choice. In dementia patients, the starting dose is 125 mg twice a day.

The dose should be titrated up slowly to a blood level as close to 100 ng/dL as possible. A good way of monitoring for the side effects of DVS in dementia patients is to check for nystagmus and ataxia, which reflect the concentration of free drug in the serum. To prevent rare but serious liver or bone marrow toxicity, liver tests (primarily transaminases) and complete blood counts must be monitored. Alternatives to DVS are carbamazepine, lithium carbonate, gabapentin and the neuroleptics (Table 16.3). Carbamazepine, starting at 100 mg twice a day and increasing to a blood level between 8 and 10 ng/dL if tolerated, with monitoring of liver tests and complete blood count, is an acceptable alternative for mania, maniclike states, lability, or irritability in dementia. As with DVS, the complete blood count must be monitored. Lithium carbonate starting at 150 mg a day and increasing to a blood level between 0.5 and 0.8 mEq/dL is usually tolerated by dementia patients and can have good therapeutic effects, although it has a low therapeutic index and must be used with caution. Patients taking lithium must have serum creatinine and thyroid functions checked quarterly. There is also clinical evidence that gabapentin starting at 300 mg twice daily and increasing to 2 g daily in divided doses has efficacy in treating these disturbances.

Any one of the neuroleptics in Table 16.3 may also be used. Combination therapies of neuroleptics and mood stabilizers or combinations of mood stabilizers may also be considered. The latter are best used only by experienced clinicians. Side effects of mood stabilizers include tremors, gait instability, falls, sleep disturbances, slurred speech, other cerebellar signs, bone marrow suppression, and hepatotoxicity, particularly with DVS.

Psychotic Disturbances

Clinical Features

Delusions are fixed, false idiosyncratic beliefs. The most common dementia-associated delusions have persecutory themes and are not greatly elaborated. For example, patients may insist that they are not in their home when they are. They may also believe that others are stealing their belongings or their spouse is unfaithful. As a result they may try to leave and go home, hit their spouse, or hide their belongings. However, they are unable to elaborate the delusions further, although they may be quite fearful. Significant minorities of dementia patients exhibit delusional misidentifications, hypochondriacal delusions, or grandiose delusions. Bizarre delusions, such as of extraterrestrials, or delusions of passivity, such as those seen in schizophrenia, are extremely rare in dementia patients. Mood-congruent delusions associated with depression, such as delusions of poverty or body rotting, or those associated with mania, such as grandiose delusions, are also seen in dementia patients in the context of these mood syndromes.

It is easy to explain away a delusion in a dementia patient by attributing it to the cognitive impairment. However, most dementia patients do not have delusions. Also, delusions are fixed, and patients cannot be talked out of them even with contravening evidence. Delusions may direct behavior, such as driving patients to aggression, to elopement, or to other actions, such as barricading themselves in their rooms.

Hallucinations are perceptions without a stimulus. Visual and auditory hallucinations are equally likely to occur in dementia. Some patients develop olfactory, gustatory, or tactile hallucinations. Patients with dementia and coexisting visual disturbances may manifest the Charles Bonnet syndrome, in which they hallucinate small people, children, or other live creatures. Similarly, patients with auditory impairments may exhibit auditory hallucinations. Hallucinations are very real and extremely distressing to patients. They may also lead to aggression.

Treatments

Delusions or hallucinations, whether occurring independently or in association with mood syndromes, typically require pharmacologic treatments. However, sometimes pharmacologic treatments are not indicated, particularly if patients are not disturbed by these experiences or if the experiences do not lead to disruptions in the patient's environment that cannot otherwise be controlled. The preferred pharmacologic treatments are neuroleptics, which are listed in Table 16.3. Their use has been supported by clinical trials, case series, and case reports. Low-potency agents, such as thioridazine, are more likely to cause sedation, orthostatic hypertension, constipation and urinary retention, and other anticholinergic side effects than strong neuroleptics, such as haloperidol. The latter are more likely to cause extrapyramidal side effects, such as parkinsonism, akathisia, and dystonia. All neuroleptics have been associated with neuroleptic malignant syndrome and all except clozapine, with tardive dyskinesia. Tardive dyskinesia is most likely in patients who are brain injured, female, or elderly.

The choice of first-line agent to treat delusions and hallucinations in dementia depends on side effect profile. Low-potency medications are preferred because patients with dementia are more susceptible to extrapyramidal symptoms than to sedation or orthostatic hypotension. However, the scientific evidence suggesting one or the other as first-line choice is limited. The clinician should choose either a high- or low-potency antipsychotic as first-line agent and observe for response and side effects. If patients do not respond or if they develop side effects, an alternative neuroleptic should be chosen, preferably with a different side effect profile. Rarely, psychotic symptoms respond to mood stabilizers or lithium carbonate.

In patients with Parkinson's disease or parkinsonism who are psychotic and who cannot tolerate neuroleptics, a trial of ondansetron 12 to 20 mg/day may be considered for the delusions (16). Also, there is some evidence that a cholinomimetic agent such as physostigmine, donepezil, or tacrine (17) may ameliorate the delusions of Alzheimer's disease.

Disturbances of the Drives

Clinical Features

All major drives, including feeding, sleep, and sexuality, may be disrupted in patients with dementia. Many lose weight slowly over a long time. This is unexplained. Weight loss is associated with early disease stages, when patients may forget to eat or are unable to prepare meals or feed themselves. However, weight loss occurs in dementia patients even when their food intake is supervised. Some speculate that patients with dementia are less active and therefore require

fewer calories. Clinical experience suggests that over time most patients equilibrate and stop losing weight. They may become thin although usually not cachectic.

Patients from time to time develop overeating and gain significant amounts of weight or stop eating almost completely and lose significant amounts of weight. Both of these circumstances should be dealt with immediately, particularly if patients are losing weight. Overeating is commonly associated with Klüver-Bucy syndrome. Undereating is typically associated with a general medical problem (possibly cancer), pain on swallowing, trouble swallowing, constipation, depression, paranoia, or delusions. When patients are losing weight and have stopped eating, they should carefully be assessed for these conditions.

Disturbances of sleep occur frequently in dementia patients. Most common are insomnias with patients staying up late, then falling asleep in the early morning and sleeping late into the day. Some patients develop complete reversal of the sleep-wake cycle. Few patients with dementia develop hypersomnia. Those who do are in the very advanced stages of disease, regressed and chair- or bed-bound.

Sexual disturbances also afflict dementia patients (18–19). These have been inadequately studied. Some patients, particularly men, may develop hypersexuality, manifested by inappropriate propositioning, inappropriate touching, or public displays of masturbation. In women with dementia, repeated touching and rubbing of the genital area may be the result of vaginal infection, uterine prolapse, or similar physical problems. Often, hypersexuality accompanies irritability or maniclike states. It may also occur in association with aggression and Klüver-Bucy syndrome. Isolated hypersexuality has also been reported.

Treatment

Treatment for hyperphagia is best accomplished through behavioral measures such as restricting the patient's access to food and providing supervision and structure. If the hyperphagia gets out of hand and leads to morbid obesity (this is quite rare) or if it is associated with the other elements of Klüver-Bucy syndrome, pharmacologic efforts to reduce appetite with an

SSRI, such as sertraline or fluoxetine, or one of the stimulants, typically methylphenidate, may be attempted.

Treatment of weight loss involves treatment of the underlying cause, whether it be a medical problem (such as carcinoma), depression, or paranoia. Concurrently, supportive care is provided, along with an aggressive effort to maintain nutrition. Treatments for depression, delusions, or paranoia should be attempted as discussed earlier. ECT should be a primary treatment consideration for a depressed patient who is losing weight. A nasogastric tube or intravenous nutrition may be used temporarily in a patient who is severely malnourished and who is undergoing ECT treatment.

Treatment of insomnia and sleep-wake cycle disturbance should begin with improvement of sleep hygiene. This consists of efforts to get the patient to go to sleep late every day, around 10 or 11 PM, while keeping him or her in a dark room for as long as possible into the next morning. Attempts should also be made to provide sufficient activity and to prevent patients from falling asleep during the day. Many sleep-wake cycle disturbances involve disruption of the body clock; these may respond to bright-light therapy in the morning for approximately an hour using 10,000 lux lights at 3 feet. If the sleep disturbance is associated with depression, suspiciousness, or delusions, that condition should be specifically treated.

For primary sleep disturbances with which bright-light therapy and good sleep hygiene are not successful, hypnotics such as trazodone 25 to 150 mg at bedtime, chloral hydrate 500 to 1500 mg a day, or zolpidem 5 to 10 mg a day may be used. Benzodiazepines are best avoided for treatment of sleep disturbances, since they have to be given chronically and carry a propensity for addiction or cognitive disturbance in dementia patients.

If hypersexuality occurs in association with another recognizable syndrome such as mania, treatment of the specific syndrome should be attempted. In men with dementia who are dangerously hypersexual or aggressive, a trial of an antiandrogen (20–21) may be attempted to reduce their sexual drive. Patients may be tried on pro-

gesterone 5 to 15 mg orally a day at first. If they respond well, they may be treated with 10 mg of depot intramuscular progesterone every 2 weeks to maintain a reduction of sexual drive. An alternative treatment to reduce sexual drive is leuprolide acetate 5 to 10 mg intramuscularly every month; this agent is also an antiandrogen.

Apathy
Clinical Features

Apathy is a state of reduced motivation and interest in the absence of sadness or lack of enjoyment (6). Patients are socially withdrawn and uninterested, and they may sit in a chair or lie in bed most of the day. They may agree to participate in activities but then make no effort to do so. Apathetic patients are not sad or anhedonic, do not report fatigue, do not worry or ruminate, and are not anxious or fearful of the future. Apathy is well studied and can be quantified reliably with the Apathy Evaluation Scale. It is likely to occur in any type of dementia, including Alzheimer's disease, vascular dementia, Huntington's disease, and Parkinson's disease. Apathy may be mistaken for depression and treated as depression. Also, apathy in the eyes of some caregivers is a state that should be corrected. These caregivers may attempt to get apathetic dementia patients to do things that do not interest them. This may provoke the patient to explosiveness, resistance, or aggression.

Treatment

Apathy does not always produce morbidity and mental suffering in and of itself. However, it may appear to independent observers that apathetic dementia patients are sad or unhappy. Additionally, there are concerns that apathy may lead to deconditioning if patients spend much of their time doing nothing. When patients are suffering from apathy or are becoming deconditioned, it is reasonable to attempt specific apathy treatments to see whether patients show more interest in day-to-day activities. However, if the primary problem of apathy is the demands that the environment or the caregiver is placing on the apathetic patient and the patient seems content, it is best to recommend modifications to the environment or to the caregiver's behavior so as to reduce the demands on the patient. If there are good reasons to reduce patients' apathy, a variety of pharmacologic measures may be tried. Apathy has been associated with reductions in dopamine, serotonin, and acetylcholine neurotransmission. Thus, rational pharmacologic treatments include the antidepressants, amantadine 50 to 200 mg a day, levodopa, methylphenidate, and other stimulants (all of the latter augment dopamine neurotransmission). The augmentation of acetylcholine neurotransmission through the use of cholinesterase inhibitors such as tacrine or donepezil may also be considered.

Aggression and Agitation
Clinical Features

Agitation and aggression (22) are nonspecific terms used to describe a variety of disturbances. When a patient is described as agitated or aggressive, it should first be clarified what is meant by the term. In many cases agitation refers to an activated state in which patients are driven, pacing, irritable, delusional, or hallucinating. It is preferred that the behavioral disturbance be classified along these more specific lines rather than be called agitation. The same is true for aggression, which may occur in the context of any of the other behavioral disturbances discussed. Agitation or aggression occurring in the context of any other behavioral disturbance should be thought of as secondary to another disturbance so that its treatment follows treatment of the primary disturbance.

At times, often in patients with severe dementia, aggression or agitation occurs in isolation and cannot be classified otherwise. The most common forms of such aggression are verbal (yelling, threatening) and physical (slapping, punching, biting, and hitting), often in the context of daily care or toileting. Verbal aggression is more common than physical aggression. Usually physical aggression does not carry sufficient force to damage property or seriously hurt others, although it can be quite damaging at times. Aggression may also occur after some other provocation from the environment, such as when other nursing home residents approach and invade the patient's personal space. Unprovoked aggression, in which a patient approaches and hits someone, throws things, or kicks at the wall, is much less common. Unprovoked aggression is seen most often in advanced or severe dementia patients. Any episode of aggression should be decoded, with interventions designed to target contributing causes. When decoding does not reveal any other obvious cause of the aggression, it is reasonable to believe that the aggression is intimately related to the dementing disease.

Treatment

Behavioral approaches to aggression, such as distraction, supervision, routine, and structure, are critical and should be tried first. Behavior modification approaches using token economies, rewards, and other contingencies have been reported to reduce some aggressive behaviors. Since unprovoked aggression is infrequent (events occurring once a week or less often), it is very difficult to develop and implement a consistent and sustained behavior modification plan. Many clinicians resort to pharmacologic interventions. Sequential trials of the following may be considered for unprovoked aggression: neuroleptics, antidepressants, mood stabilizers (divalproex sodium, carbamazepine, lithium, gabapentin), buspirone, β-blockers (which in animal studies have suggested the ability to block aggressive acts), antiandrogens, and benzodiazepines.

The success rate of treating unexplained and unprovoked aggression in dementia has not been established. With each medication trial there is probably no more than a 10 to 20% chance of benefit with the commensurate side effects that accompany the medicine. At times, patients with unprovoked aggression require restraint to prevent harm to others. Restraint may be in the form of sedation and/or physical restraint, such as a geriatric chair. If restraining measures are necessary, careful supportive care should be provided to the restrained patient. Over time, efforts should be made to reduce the amount of restraint and to determine whether the patient can tolerate independence without becoming aggressive. The ability to wean from restraint after episodes of unprovoked aggression, even in severe dementia, has repeatedly been observed in clinical practice.

Calling Out

Clinical Features

In moderate and severe dementia, particularly in institutions (probably because of selection bias), some patients call out intermittently in a disruptive way (23). The calling out may take the form of calling somebody's name, asking for help, requesting something specific (something to drink or eat), moaning, or unintelligible vocalizations. Many of these calling out behaviors (at times called clazomania) are secondary to a medical problem or another psychiatric syndrome. They may also occur independently, presumably as a consequence of brain damage from the dementing disease. Calling out is a particularly disruptive problem in institutions, as it can affect unit milieu and other residents. Also, patients who call out appear to be suffering, which makes treatment attempts compelling.

Treatment

Clinicians should first strive to identify what the patient is communicating by calling out and respond to the request. If this fails or if the request is clear but is repeated continuously after it has been addressed, nonspecific or environment-modifying approaches should be attempted. If these are not successful and the problem persists, it may be necessary to remove the patient from stimulating or noisy environments (dining room, activity area), when the calling out is worst. If the patient appears to be suffering while calling out or if the problem is severely disruptive to a unit milieu, pharmacologic treatments may be attempted. While the likelihood of the success is low, β-blockers, trazodone, buspirone, SSRIs, tricyclic antidepressants (21), neuroleptics, mood stabilizers, and antiandrogens, have been associated with reductions in calling out.

Disinhibition, Stimulus-Bound Behaviors, and Frontal Lobe Behaviors

Clinical Features

Behaviors that suggest disinhibition, such as wandering, intrusiveness, grabbing things, cursing, being distracted by stimuli, inattention, uri-nating in trash cans, and utilization behaviors, have all been described in patients with frontal lobe dysfunction. Similar behaviors have been described in dementia patients, particularly in those who are severely cognitively impaired. Many of these behaviors are harmless, and patients can be allowed to continue engaging in them so long as they are not suffering and there are no safety issues. However, from time to time these behaviors become problematic, particularly if they lead to aggression or adversely affect caregivers and other patients in institutions. Such behaviors also make patients vulnerable to elopement or victimization (theft, being hit by others).

Treatment

The preferred approach to these behaviors is to provide behavior management and to increase supervision, if possible with constant or one-to-one observation. This allows patients to continue with their disinhibited routines and provides someone to keep them out of trouble. This is a very labor- and time-intensive approach, although it typically bears fruit. Other approaches include attempts to distract patients. However, given the severity of dementia, by the time patients exhibit these behaviors, it is hard to engage them in new activities. These behaviors resemble the hyperactivity and inattention of children with attention deficit disorder and of adults who have suffered traumatic brain injury affecting the frontal lobes. For this reason, pharmacologic treatments using dopamine augmentors such as bupropion, levodopa, and psychostimulants have had success in treating them. Other treatment approaches may include β-blockers, DVS, and SSRI antidepressants.

Compulsive and Repetitive Behaviors

Clinical Features

Patients with severe dementia at times develop repetitive routinized behaviors. These include repetitive hoarding, tapping, pushing at doors, marching in place, picking in the air, pulling things out of closets, flushing the toilet, putting things in the mouth, and others. These resemble compulsions, although it is impossible to know whether patients are having true obsessions, given that their mental state is usually not accessible. Most of the time it is best to allow these behaviors to occur, if safe, because trying to stop them may be frustrating and lead to explosiveness and aggression. When patients are suffering or if the behaviors become seriously intrusive to others, attempts to stop them should be considered.

Treatment

Very little has been presented in the literature about how to approach these specific behaviors. However, their resemblance to compulsions suggests that medicines effective against obsessive compulsive disorders, such as clomipramine, and SSRIs (including fluvoxamine) may be attempted. Behavior modification has not been studied adequately, although our experience suggests that they are not effective for these types of disturbances.

Klüver-Bucy–like Behaviors

Clinical Features

Klüver-Bucy syndrome includes the triad of exploratory wandering, hyperphagia, and hypersexuality. Elements of this syndrome may develop in advanced dementia patients. They may walk around constantly testing doors, pulling at things, and looking into everything, although without a specific purpose. The presence of the entire triad is probably rare in dementia patients, although it definitely occurs, particularly in later stages of Alzheimer's disease.

Treatment

Providing nonspecific interventions and tolerating and compensating for these behaviors is probably the best treatment approach. A safe environment, free of hazardous substances that can be ingested and of vulnerable peers, is optimal for this approach to succeed. Pharmacologic treatment may also be used, although chances of success are uncertain. Possible treatments are amantadine, levodopa, stimulants, SSRIs, tricyclic antidepressants, and neuroleptics. Case history reports have noted benefits of these medicines in patients with brain injury, particularly the mentally retarded.

CONCLUSION

Behavioral disturbances are common in dementia and are an important focus of treatment in all settings with dementia patients. In approaching the demented patient with a behavioral disturbance, it is important to conduct a detailed, systematic evaluation followed by description and classification of the disturbance. This should be followed by decoding to determine contributing causes to the disturbances. Treatment planning is based on the results of the description and decoding of the behavioral disturbances. Effective treatments for behavioral disturbance in dementia include preventive interventions, caregiver education, behavior management, behavior modification, pharmacologic treatments, bright-light therapies, and environmental modifications to accommodate the patient's condition.

Acknowledgment. Supported in part by the Copper Ridge Institute. We are grateful to Betty Bourgeois for typing this manuscript and to Glenn Treisman and Diana Klein for their review and comments.

REFERENCES

1. Behavioral and Psychological Signs and Symptoms of Dementia: Implications for Research and Treatment. Proceedings of an international consensus conference. Lansdowne, Virginia, April 1996. Int Psychogeriatr 1996;8(suppl 3):215–552.
2. Practice guideline for the treatment of Alzheimer's disease and other dementias of late life. American Psychiatric Association. Am J Psychiatry 1997;154(suppl): 1–39.
3. Weiner MF, Edland SD, Luszczysnka H. Prevalence and incidence of major depression in Alzheimer's disease. Am J Psychiatry 1994;151:1006–1009.
4. Devanand DP, Jacobs DM, Tang MX, et al. The course of psychopathologic features in mild to moderate Alzheimer disease. Arch Gen Psychiatry 1997;54:257–263.
5. Lyketsos CG, Steele C. The care of patients with dementia. Rev Clin Gerontol 1995;5:179–197.
6. Marin RS, Fogel BS, Hawkins J, et al. Apathy: a treatable syndrome. J Neuropsychiatry Clin Neurosci 1995;7:23–30.
7. Carlson DL, Fleming KC, Smith GE, Evans JM. Management of dementia-related behavioral disturbances: a nonpharmacologic approach. Mayo Clinic Proc 1995;70:1108–1115 (review).
8. Rovner BW, Steele CD, Shmuely Y, Folstein MF. A ran-

domized trial of dementia care in nursing homes. J Am Geriatr Soc 1996;44:7–13.

9. Cummings JL, Mega M, Gray K, et al. The neuropsychiatric inventory: comprehensive assessment of psychopathology in dementia. Neurology 1994;44:2308–2314.

10. Loreck DJ, Bylsma FW, Folstein MF. The Dementia Signs and Symptoms Scale: a new scale for comprehensive assessment of psychopathology in Alzheimer's disease. Am J Geriatr Psychiatry 1994;2:60–74.

11. Alexopoulos GS, Abrams RC, Young RC, Shamoian CA. Cornell Scale for depression in dementia. Biol Psychiatry 1988;23:271–284.

12. Marin RS, Biedrzycki RC, Firinciogullari S. Reliability and validity of the Apathy Evaluation Scale. Psychiatry Res 1991;38:143–162.

13. Hyman SE, Arana GW, Rosenbaum JF. Handbook of Psychiatric Drug Therapy. Boston: Little, Brown, 1995.

14. Mishima K, Okawa M, Kishikawa Y, et al. Morning bright light therapy for sleep and behavior disorders in elderly patients with dementia. Acta Psychiatr Scand 1994;89:1–7.

15. Price TR, McAllister TW. Safety and efficacy of ECT in depressed patients with dementia: a review of clinical experience. Convuls Ther 1989;5:1–74.

16. Zoldan J, Friedberg G, Goldberg-Stern H, Melamed E. Ondansetron for hallucinosis in advanced Parkinson's disease. Lancet 1993;341 (letter).

17. Haddad PM, Benbow SM. Sexual problems associated with dementia: 2. Aetiology, assessment, and treatment. Int J Geriatr Psychiatry 1993;8:631–637.

18. Kaufer DI, Cummings JL, Christine D. Effect of tacrine on behavioral symptoms in Alzheimer's disease: an open-label study. J Geriatr Psychiatry Neurol 1996;9:1–6.

19. Haddad PM, Benbow SM. Sexual problems associated with dementia: 1. Problems and their consequences. Int J Geriatr Psychiatry 1993;8: 547–551.

20. Kyomen HH, Nobel KW, Wei JY. The use of estrogen to decrease aggressive physical behavior in elderly men with dementia. J Am Geriatr Soc 1991;39:1110–1112.

21. Ott BR. Leuprolide treatment of sexual aggression in a patient with dementia and the Klüver-Bucy syndrome. Clin Neuropharmacol 1995;18:443–447.

22. Patel V, Hope T. Aggressive behavior in elderly people with dementia: a review. Int J Geriatr Psychiatry 1993;8: 457–472.

23. Friedman R, Gryfe CI, Tal DT, Freedman M. The noisy elderly patient: prevalence, assessment, and response to the antidepressant doxepin. J Geriatr Psychiatry Neurol 1992;5: 187–191.

CHAPTER 17

LISA N. GELLER AND WILLIAM REICHEL

Alzheimer's Disease: Biologic Aspects

Alois Alzheimer's description of senile (amyloid) plaques and neurofibrillary tangles associated with dementia laid the groundwork for contemporary research in the disease that bears his name. The clinical presentation of Alzheimer's disease is consistent, and histopathologic analysis continues to be the standard used for definitive diagnosis of the disease. However, it is now clear that a number of different factors can play a role in the etiology of Alzheimer's disease for any person. Indeed, it has been suggested that Alzheimer's disease is not a disease as such, but a syndrome (1). Factors involved in Alzheimer's disease include neurotransmitters, cellular stress response, advancing age, and genetics. It is useful to think of the pathology of Alzheimer's disease as a disturbance or malfunction of a multistep biochemical pathway. Many different circumstances can disrupt the pathway leading to the same end point disease. Some of the better known factors contributing to the disease are considered below. However, in most cases, the extent to which each factor plays a role in causing Alzheimer's disease and the ways in which they interact are not yet clear.

EPIDEMIOLOGY

Much of our understanding of the etiology of Alzheimer's disease is based on epidemiologic information. Genetic theories and understanding of environmental risk factors, including the possible roles of head injury, trace elements such as aluminum, and other causal hypotheses demand a reliable epidemiologic database.

Although a wide range of prevalence rates has been reported for senile dementia of the Alzheimer type, all estimates emphasize the large number of people likely to show symptoms of the disorder. It has been estimated that about 10% of those 65 years old or older in the United States have Alzheimer's disease (Alzheimer's Association, 1996). Worldwide, approximately 4% of persons over 65 years of age have a severe form of senile dementia and about 10 to 20% have mild forms. Alzheimer's Disease International (ADI) estimates that by the year 2025, 34 million people will have dementia, a large proportion of them having Alzheimer's disease, and that 71% of those persons will be in developing countries. Prevalence rises sharply with age such that for persons over 85 years of age, 20% have a severe form of Alzheimer's disease (2–4). This means that in the future there are likely to be large increases in the number of persons with Alzheimer's disease. One estimate is that, at the present, 1% of the population has senile dementia at age 65 years, 10% at age 75 years, and 25–30% at age 85 years. These numbers are only estimates; a community-based study in East Boston, Massachusetts reported a prevalence of more than 47% in persons over 85 years (5). As life expectancy is increasing (principally because of the decrease in the death rate from heart disease and stroke) an increase can be expected in the number of elderly with Alzheimer's disease in each decade past 60 years (6).

Some studies, using data from hospitals and long-term care institutions, show a predominance of Alzheimer's disease among women and persons of low socioeconomic status. Others show equal prevalence among men and women and criticize the use of information largely gathered from institutional experience. Differences between cultural and racial groups have only begun to be studied. For example, one study of Cherokees suggests a protective gene in this population (7). At present very little is known about Alzheimer's disease according to race, rural versus urban populations, nationality except in western Europe and the United States, and other cross-cultural comparisons, although a few studies indicate that the importance of certain genetic factors cannot be generalized between races.

A number of studies show that the clinical diagnosis of Alzheimer's disease is confirmed pathologically approximately 90% of the time when strict criteria such as those proposed by the National Institute of Neurological and Communicative Disorders and Stroke (NINCDS)-Alzheimer's Disease and Related Disorders Association committee or in the fourth edition of *Diagnostic and Statistical Manual of Mental Disorders* (DSM-IV) are used. However, the clinical diagnosis of vascular dementia is much less accurate, and this type of dementia may be more common than previously thought (8). Furthermore, approximately 10% of demented persons do not meet pathologic criteria for either Alzheimer's disease or vascular dementia, the two most common causes of dementia. The meaning of such studies is sometimes difficult to evaluate. For example, studies done during the 1970s and 1980s suggest that vascular dementia was more common in Japan than in the United States or Western Europe (9). More recent epidemiologic studies in Japan report lower rates of the diagnosis of vascular dementia and higher rates of Alzheimer's disease (10). It is unclear whether this is a change in diagnostic practice or a change in the epidemiologic pattern of the disorder.

BIOLOGIC BASES OF ALZHEIMER'S DISEASE

The volume and complexity of information on the biology of Alzheimer's disease can seem overwhelming. Part of this difficulty is because multiple factors can contribute to the disease process. Studying these factors not only facilitates understanding of the pathologic processes of Alzheimer's disease but also helps to elucidate the normal multistep biochemical pathway that is disrupted in the disease. Researchers have identified many of the components that can disturb this biochemical pathway and lead to disease but do not yet have a complete picture of the normal or pathogenic pathways. Eventually, it should be possible to draw a coherent picture of the disease process.

The common thread between the different causes of Alzheimer's disease appears to be the formation of amyloid plaques through a two-part process. First, a protein termed Aβ, a major component of the amyloid plaque, is produced. In the second step, Aβ forms an insoluble aggregate that is deposited into amyloid plaques. This very simple view of the disease process provides a framework for analyzing information on Alzheimer's disease.

Neurotransmitter-Related Studies

Alzheimer's disease affects specific areas of the brain, particularly cholinergic neurons. In 1976, Davies and Maloney (11) reported significantly lower activity of choline acetyltransferase in the cerebral cortex of patients with "senile dementia of the Alzheimer type" than in age-matched normal persons. This finding has been confirmed by others. There is a correlation between the change in neurochemical activity and cognitive loss and brain pathology, particularly the number of neuritic plaques seen at autopsy. In contrast, reduction in the activity of choline acetyltransferase is not noted in multi-infarct dementia or depression (12). The decrease in choline acetyltransferase suggests a possible role for replacement therapy.

Whitehouse et al. (13, 14) found that the nucleus basalis of Meynert in the basal forebrain of patients with Alzheimer's disease demonstrated substantially fewer neurons than those of age- and sex-matched controls. Since the nucleus basalis provides diffuse cholinergic input to the neocortex, loss of this neuronal population may be an important anatomic correlate of the markedly reduced activity of choline acetyltransferase in Alzheimer's disease. This demonstration of selective degeneration of nucleus basalis of Meynert neurons may provide the first documentation of loss of a transmitter-specific neuronal population in a major disorder of higher cortical function. Whether nucleus basalis cell death leads to neocortical deficits remains unanswered. However, recent evidence favors other initial sites for the disease, including the cortex (15) and especially the hippocampus (16). Since cholinergic activity in Alzheimer's disease is diminished, many strategies of drug development for Alzheimer's disease focus on enhancing acetylcholine synthesis, preventing breakdown of acetylcholine, or both. In this regard, Alzheimer's disease can be compared with Parkinson's disease as to the hope of chemical manipulation.

Other neurotransmitter deficits identified in Alzheimer's disease include norepinephrine, serotonin, somatostatin, and corticotrophin-releasing factor (17). This suggests that replacement strategies may have to combine several drugs or that individual patients will require different treatment regimens based on their pattern of deficits.

Amyloid Plaques and Neurofibrillary Tangles

The two definitive neuropathologic findings of Alzheimer's disease, amyloid plaques and neurofibrillary tangles, have been the focus of an enormous research effort. Amyloid plaques are found in several areas of the brain in patients with Alzheimer's disease but are most prominent in areas associated with memory, such as the hippocampus and neocortex. The amyloid plaque is an extracellular structure composed primarily of Aβ and α_1-antichymotrypsin, a protease inhibitor. Aβ appears to be an abnormal product derived from the amyloid precursor protein (APP). APP is a membrane protein whose normal function is unknown. Several peptides are produced by cleavage of APP, most prominently a 40-amino acid fragment (Aβ 1–40) and a 42-amino acid fragment (Aβ 1–42). References to Aβ in the causation of Alzheimer's disease generally imply the 42-amino acid fragment. This fragment is produced in relatively large amounts in Alzheimer's disease brain and is thought to be a major factor in the pathologic process. Some studies have shown that Aβ is toxic to cells, leading to the suggestion that this protein is the causative agent in

Alzheimer's disease. Aβ can be soluble or form an insoluble β-pleated sheet structure. It is the latter that appears to be toxic to cells. The production of APP, its processing, and the production of toxic Aβ peptide appear to be key factors in the causation of Alzheimer's disease. These factors appear to be a common link between all cases of Alzheimer's disease, regardless of cause (18, 19).

Several hypotheses of the mechanism of deposition of Aβ in Alzheimer's disease have been presented. For example, it has been proposed that neuronal injury is an early step leading to the formation of dystrophic neurites that accumulate APP. This process would precede the formation of Aβ. In another prominent hypothesis, amorphous Aβ deposits, also known as diffuse plaques, are an early cause of the disease. The reason for the specificity to brain of amyloid plaque formation in Alzheimer's disease is interesting because Aβ appears to be produced and secreted in a variety of other tissues, including blood (20). α_1-Antichymotrypsin, a component of amyloid plaques, is specifically induced in β-amyloid peptide amyloidoses (21), although it is not clear whether it plays a role in plaque formation.

The other major neuropathologic feature of Alzheimer's disease, neurofibrillary tangles, is a feature shared with other neurodegenerative disorders. Studies have shown that neurofibrillary tangles are composed principally of tau, a normal component of neurons that binds to microtubules (22). In the neurofibrillary tangles of Alzheimer's disease, phosphates are attached to tau in an abnormal array, resulting in the pathologic tangle structure. Research continues to focus on the mechanisms that cause this hyperphosphorylation of tau and results in neurofibrillary tangles. Interestingly, the hyperphosphorylated tau appears to be a normal product during development. While many researchers believe that the formation of neurofibrillary tangles is not an initial event in Alzheimer's disease, these structures may play an important role in later stages of the disease.

Immune System Involvement

There is increasing evidence for the involvement of the immune system in Alzheimer's disease. Immunoglobulins and complement components have been reported to be associated with amyloid plaques (23). Reactive microglia, the macrophages of the brain, and reactive astrocytes have been found around amyloid plaques (24). As discussed later, the presence of these cells is consistent with the theory of acute-phase response involvement in the disease process. Using cell cultures, it was shown that microglia are activated by various forms of Aβ (25). Astroglia appear to produce transforming growth factor β (TGF-β₁) in response to brain injury but may also be involved in amyloidogenesis (26). Various humoral antibodies directed against Alzheimer's disease tissue and specifically against cholinergic neurons have been reported in Alzheimer's disease patients. It is not clear whether an immune response is a primary inducing factor in Alzheimer's disease or a response to preexisting damage.

Acute-Phase Response

The acute-phase response is an inflammatory response to physiologic stress that has been described primarily in the liver (27) and may involve the immune system. Accumulating evidence supports the hypothesis that the amyloidogenesis of Alzheimer's disease results from the acute-phase response elicited when certain areas of the brain are subjected to stress, whether biologic or environmental (28–30). A major component of the amyloid plaques, α_1-antichymotrypsin, is an acute-phase protein that appears to be specifically upregulated in β-amyloidoses (21). Based on the model for the acute-phase response in liver, this theory prescribes roles for interleukin-1 (IL-1), IL-6, tumor necrosis factor, and perhaps nerve growth factor in Alzheimer's disease (31). Indeed, IL-1 has been reported to increase the amount of APP mRNA in culture cells (32).

Oxidative Damage

Oxidative stress has been suggested to play a role in the etiology of Alzheimer's disease (33). Free radicals produced during such stress may act in Alzheimer's disease by damaging the membranes of neuronal cells or by altering proteins in harmful ways. Reactive oxygen metabolites have been observed to be generated by microglia in culture, and may play an important role in the acute-phase response (34). Clues indicating a role for oxidative damage in Alzheimer's disease include reports that cells from Alzheimer's patients may be particularly sensitive to damage by reactive oxygen metabolites (35) and may show increased levels of enzymes indicating oxidative stress. A number of treatments that reduce oxidative damage have been suggested, and some are being subjected to clinical trials. These include α-tocopherol (vitamin E) and selegiline (Deprenyl). The modest effects of a ginkgo biloba extract (EGb 761) on Alzheimer's disease patients with mild to moderate disease are hypothesized to be mediated by the free radical scavenging effects of components of the extract (36).

Mitochondrial Metabolism

Energy metabolism is abnormally low in the brains of Alzheimer's patients. This implies that these patients have altered mitochondrial metabolism. It was reported that cytochrome oxidase activity is low in the blood platelets and brains of Alzheimer's patients (37). A study demonstrating that many patients have a mutation in a cytochrome oxidase gene suggests a role for this mitochondrial factor in predisposing persons to Alzheimer's disease (38). A defect in cytochrome oxidase activity can result in increased free radical production, a condition associated with Alzheimer's disease. Although there is no clear proof that mitochondrial mutations can actually contribute to the development of Alzheimer's disease, these results suggest that mitochondria may play a role in the causation of the disease in some persons.

Estrogen

Considerable interest has been focused on a possible role for estrogen in Alzheimer's disease. Lack of estrogen has been postulated to account, at least in part, for the higher incidence of Alzheimer's disease in women than in men. Animal studies have shown that cholinergic neurons of the basal forebrain contain estrogen receptors (39). In addition, estrogen acts as an antioxidant without requiring the presence of its receptor. It may also act as an anti-inflammatory agent and decrease the levels of apolipoprotein E (ApoE) in plasma. This information coupled with primarily anecdotal accounts of reduced incidence of Alzheimer's disease in post-menopausal women undergoing estrogen therapy led to the suggestion that estrogen deficiency may constitute a risk factor for Alzheimer's disease. Recent studies have supported this observation (40, 41). However, some studies (42) report no consistent evidence of a positive effect of estrogen on cognitive function. Nevertheless, the use of estrogen for therapeutic or preventive interventions is intriguing, although the relative risks and benefits of estrogen treatment in postmenopausal women must be carefully weighed.

Cerebrovascular Disease

The brains of many aged people have significant numbers of senile plaques and neurofibrillary tangles at autopsy, even though the person demonstrated no behavioral signs of Alzheimer's disease. This prompted some investigators to look for conditions that coexist with the plaques and tangles that provide better indicators of behavioral disease. Snowdon et al. (43) have shown that one such factor may be cerebrovascular disease. In this study there was a significant relation between cognitive function and lacunar brain infarcts in the basal ganglia, thalamus, and deep white matter in elderly women who had Alzheimer's disease. While this result requires confirmation, it suggests that the prevention of cerebrovascular disease may also prove helpful in diminishing the clinical expression of Alzheimer's disease.

Genetics of Alzheimer's Disease

There is no question that there is a genetic component to some cases of Alzheimer's disease (44). The most striking genetic evidence is apparent in early-onset cases. Nearly all early-onset Alzheimer's disease has been linked to genetic causes with autosomal dominant transmission. A small number of the early-onset cases are caused by several mutations on chromosome 21 (45). These mutations lie in the APP gene that is responsible for the production of Aβ. This finding

is particularly interesting because nearly all persons with Down's syndrome (trisomy 21) who survive into their third or fourth decade develop the pathology of Alzheimer's disease, and many of those persons develop clinical dementia.

Even more striking, more than 70% of cases of early-onset familial Alzheimer's disease have been linked to chromosome 14 (46–49). The gene on chromosome 14 linked to these cases is generally called presenilin I (50). A related gene on chromosome 1 is associated with a small number of early-onset cases (51). Interesting as these studies are, the utility of testing for mutations in these genes for diagnosis of Alzheimer's disease is limited, since the three genes known to be associated with early-onset disease account for fewer than 2% of Alzheimer's disease cases (52).

Although the identification of specific genes involved in early-onset Alzheimer's disease is not directly useful to many patients (e.g., for diagnostic or predictive testing, if desired), these data reveal some of the steps involved in the biochemical pathway that can lead to Alzheimer's disease. Studies to determine how presenilins fit into the causation of Alzheimer's disease suggest that presenilins can be a substrate for an enzyme involved in apoptotic (as opposed to necrotic) cell death, namely, a caspase-3. In cultured neuronal cells, caspase-3 inhibitors block the novel cleavage of presenilins that occurs in Alzheimer's disease or apoptotic cell death (53).

Most Alzheimer's disease cases are of late onset, and there is evidence for a genetic component to at least some late-onset disease. Data from a study conducted in Sweden examining the concordance rate of Alzheimer's disease in twins suggest that even in late-onset disease there is a substantial genetic effect. However, the study also found that environmental factors were important in determining whether and when a person would get the disease (44). Some late-onset and early-onset cases of Alzheimer's disease have been linked to a locus on chromosome 19 encoding apolipoprotein E (ApoE). Specifically, the ApoE ε4 allele is associated with a predisposition to Alzheimer's disease. ApoE is a plasma protein involved in cholesterol transport. Persons who are homozygous for the ApoE ε4 allele are at greater risk for getting Alzheimer's disease and tend to have an earlier age of disease onset than heterozygotes. Estimates of the percentage of cases attributable to ApoE ε4 are quite variable. In one study those aged 65 and over with at least one copy of the ApoE ε4 allele were only about twice as likely to have Alzheimer's disease as persons who were ε3/ε3 (54).

However, not everyone with ApoE ε4 gets the disease. Approximately half of the people with two copies of the ApoE ε4 gene live into their 80s, and estimates are that about a third of those with Alzheimer's disease have no ApoE ε4 alleles. Furthermore, as with much other medical research, results on one population cannot always be generalized to another. For example, a study of Nigerians showed no association between ApoE ε4 and Alzheimer's disease (55). A study by Farrer et al. (56) shows that the ApoE ε4 allele is a significant risk factor for white and Japanese subjects but appears to be less of a risk factor in African-Americans and Hispanics and that the risk associated with ApoE ε4 decreases with age. Despite the interest in ApoE as a marker for a predisposition to Alzheimer's disease, experts do not recommend genetic testing for ApoE in asymptomatic persons, nor is it clear that it is a useful diagnostic test in patients presenting with dementia (57–59).

The mechanisms of ApoE action are not understood. Some have reported the presence of ApoE-like immunoreactivity in amyloid plaques. Different ApoE alleles have been observed to have different effects on activated microglia (27). Wisniewski et al. (60) reported that ApoE can interact with the amyloid protein and so suggest a role for ApoE in plaque formation (61), although there are mixed reports as to whether ApoE ε4 facilitates or slows the formation of Aβ aggregates.

A fifth genetic locus associated with Alzheimer's disease is on chromosome 12 (62). Other possible susceptibility loci have been identified on chromosomes 4, 6, and 20. Confirmation of these associations has not been made, nor is it known what genes may be involved.

The number of genetic loci implicated in Alzheimer's disease is evidence that it has multiple causes. Except for age of onset and rate of progression, the pathology and clinical presentation among these different genetic entities are indistinguishable (63). There is considerable vari-

ation in at least the age of onset in genetic cases of Alzheimer's disease and in the contribution of some genetic factors such as ApoE ε4. This underlines the importance of other (e.g., environmental) factors.

ENVIRONMENTAL FACTORS IN ALZHEIMER'S DISEASE
Viral Theories

Several slow virus diseases, kuru and Creutzfeldt-Jakob disease in man and scrapie in sheep, are interesting for the insights they may offer into the dementing process, and in the past they have been proposed as models for Alzheimer's disease. The report by Gajdusek et al. (64) reviews Creutzfeldt-Jakob disease, kuru, scrapie, and transmissible mink encephalopathy. There is no convincing evidence, however, that there is any relation between slow viruses and Alzheimer's disease.

Aluminum, Copper, and Other Trace Elements

Although studies since 1973 have reported increases in aluminum levels in the brains of Alzheimer's patients (65), the role of aluminum in Alzheimer's disease is still not established. Additional research is necessary to determine whether aluminum plays any role in this degenerative process. Copper can bind APP and may play a role in vesicular trafficking. It has been suggested that copper-mediated toxicity may occur in Alzheimer's disease, acting to cause free radical damage, which, in turn, causes aggregation of the toxic Aβ monomers (66). Zinc can also bind to APP and has been proposed to play a role in Alzheimer's disease.

A role for iron is suggested both by the association of iron with amyloid plaques and neurofibrillary tangles and by the appearance of the binding protein p97 (melanotransferrin) with reactive microglia associated with amyloid plaques in Alzheimer's disease brains (67). Iron, zinc, and aluminum all may increase the rate of Aβ precipitation into its insoluble form, thus playing a role in the proposed crucial second step of the Alzheimer's disease. Whether any of these metals are significant factors in the development of Alzheimer's disease requires further investigation.

Head Injury

Head injury resulting in punchdrunk syndrome, or dementia pugilistica, appears to be indistinguishable pathologically from Alzheimer's disease (68, 69). Similarly, a history of severe head trauma such as concussion has been reported to be a risk factor for Alzheimer's disease (70). While the mechanisms by which head injury contributes to Alzheimer's disease are not understood, it is likely that they are associated with cellular stress, as described earlier. ApoE ϵ4 deposition has also been associated with the deposition of Aβ after head injury (71). Elucidation of the mechanisms by which these processes contribute to Alzheimer's disease remains an important area of future research.

DIAGNOSTIC TESTS

A number of diagnostic tests, largely relying on genetic contributions, real and putative, are being developed, and some such tests are available. However, physicians should carefully consider what benefits, if any, will result from a test administered to any given patient. Guidelines published by a number of organizations caution that it is rarely, if ever, appropriate to test persons for a predisposition to Alzheimer's disease. Some groups advise against the use of tests even for diagnostic purposes. A draft report issued by Stanford University's Program in Genomics, Ethics, and Society (October 25, 1997) pointed out that the value of information obtained from a genetic test must be weighed against the possible negative consequences of these tests. These consequences may be financial (including the possible loss or increased cost of health insurance), psychologic, and social. The Statement on Use of Apolipoprotein E Testing for Alzheimer's Disease by the American College of Medical Genetics and the American Society of Human Genetics Working Group on ApoE and Alzheimer's Disease states, "At the present time it [ApoE testing] is not recommended for use in routine clinical diagnosis nor should it be used for predictive testing" (57).

Diagnostic tests based on biochemical markers have been proposed, and some are available. Most of these tests are of little if any use. This is primarily because there is considerable overlap between levels of the tested compound in normal persons and those with Alzheimer's disease. For example, knowledge of Aβ and APP have raised the hope of developing diagnostic tests for Alzheimer's disease that measure these entities. Although some investigators have reported a lower level of an APP derivative in the cerebrospinal fluid of persons with familial Alzheimer's disease than in their unaffected siblings, there is overlap between the levels detected in the two groups. In addition, many potential biochemical tests require analysis of cerebrospinal fluid, which is unacceptably invasive for many patients. Cerebrospinal fluid sampling is also unreliable because there is often a gradient of a given compound in the spinal column. Therefore, the measured concentration of a compound depends not only on the location of the tap but also on factors such as the height of the patient. These factors make it difficult to normalize samples unless there is a substantial difference between normal and Alzheimer's patients in the concentrations of the tested compound. Tests that entail measuring components in serum are less invasive, although overlapping test values between normal and disease populations remain a problem. Other test possibilities are extant. For example, it has been suggested that early detection of Alzheimer's disease could be accomplished by measuring serum levels of the iron binding protein p97.

POSSIBLE THERAPEUTIC AGENTS

As a result of the accumulated scientific knowledge, many therapeutic possibilities have been considered. Available drugs focus on the cholinergic deficit of Alzheimer's disease. One method of trying to correct this deficit is by administering drugs that inhibit cholinesterase, the enzyme that breaks down acetylcholine. One such drug is tacrine hydrochloride (Cognex), an acridinamine derivative, that has been approved for use in Alzheimer's disease. However, clinical reports suggest that tacrine has at best a low efficacy (72–76). Tacrine appears to improve cognition in a minority of Alzheimer's disease victims with mild to moderate dementia. Unfortunately, there is no conclusive evidence from controlled trials that tacrine use results in significant long-term improvement or in long-term prevention of decline. In addition, tacrine can cause hepatic changes, particularly elevations in serum alanine aminotransferase activity, focal necrosis, and granulomatous hepatitis. In the presence of liver toxicity, the dosage should be reduced or the drug stopped. Hepatic toxicity has been reversible with discontinuation of tacrine in virtually all cases thus far. In addition to the hepatic changes, other side effects of tacrine include nausea and drug interactions.

More recently, donepezil (Aricept) has been investigated for use in treatment of Alzheimer's disease (77). This cholinesterase inhibitor appears to help cognitive function without the serious hepatotoxicity produced by tacrine. From the limited evidence of early trials it appears that donepezil may be useful, but because it has not yet been extensively studied, its exact benefit and potential side effects are not fully known. The practicing physician will be faced with pressure from loving and distraught families to use any new drugs that emerge from this line of research. In each case, the risk-benefit ratio in light of the incomplete information available must be carefully considered for the individual patient.

Other drugs that may act as inhibitors of acetylcholinesterase are being identified and tested. For example, a component of a Chinese herbal medicine derived from the moss *Huperzia serrata* named huperzine A (HupA) is a reversible inhibitor of acetylcholinesterase activity with possible clinical potential (78). Because faulty proteolytic processing of APP is thought to be central to Alzheimer's disease, protease inhibitors are considered possible therapeutic agents. However, highly specific protease inhibitors must be found because administration of nonspecific proteases could cause tremendous damage. Effort is also being put into identification of substances that inhibit the aggregation of Aβ.

In keeping with the finding that inflammatory responses are involved in the causation of Alzheimer's disease, preliminary studies suggest that the use of anti-inflammatory drugs decreases the likelihood of Alzheimer's disease (79–82). The production of destructive oxygen radicals (possibly related to an immune response component to the disorder) may be another mechanism in the disease process amenable to therapy. Therefore, the efficacy of antioxidants such as α-tocopherol and nonsteroidal anti-inflammatory agents are being studied. In one published study, selegiline 10 mg/day and α-tocopherol 2000 IU/day were administered for 2 years to patients with moderate Alzheimer's disease (83). Both agents, separately and together, slowed the progression of the disease.

As mentioned earlier, the tantalizing but unsubstantiated role of estrogen deficiency in the degenerative process of Alzheimer's disease may someday lead to new treatment. In a prospective study of the effects of estrogen replacement therapy, Kawas et al. (84) found that postmenopausal women who took estrogen were about half as likely to be diagnosed with Alzheimer's disease as were women who did not take the hormone. Therefore, the therapeutic use of estrogen replacement therapy in postmenopausal women may provide hope for preventing or slowing the progress of Alzheimer's disease.

These are only a few of the interventions for Alzheimer's disease being investigated. Although they are promising, it is unclear which of these or any of the other proposed interventions will be most effective. Additional clinical studies will clarify the efficacy of these possible therapeutic agents. In the future, selection of the optimal treatment regimen for any person may require determining the cause of the disease for that person. Administration of preventive treatments may require evaluation of multiple Alzheimer's disease risk factors for a person.

ETHICAL CONSIDERATIONS

Although our understanding of Alzheimer's disease is far from complete, considerable progress has been made. As discoveries are made in understanding the full biologic picture of Alzheimer's disease, there will be increasing pressure to use new preventive or therapeutic agents, even for marginal benefit. At the same time, the physician must bear in mind his or her duty to help the patient while avoiding doing harm. The physician must be concerned if agents that are approved for use possess low efficacy and demonstrate significant side effects. The physician must also question the fast-emerging research findings that may be translated into new therapies before they are adequately understood. Therefore, the physician must work hard at monitoring developments in the field.

Another major area of ethical concern is the role of diagnostic tests that are becoming available, almost certainly before sound therapeutic modalities are available. It is easy to imagine the psychologic and social turmoil that will be engendered by the ability to determine that a fetus, a young adult, or a middle-aged adult may eventually develop Alzheimer's disease. It is therefore important to distinguish between testing asymptomatic persons who regardless of age may have positive tests for certain genetic or other biologic factors and testing persons who are in the early stages of dementia and who may therefore benefit from a differential diagnosis, for example, of vascular dementia. At least five professional groups have advised against presymptomatic testing for Alzheimer's disease. This is emphasized by current National Institutes of Health guidelines, which recommend professional counseling for patients before and after genetic testing and state flatly that "genetic testing in asymptomatic persons is unwarranted" except perhaps in cases of autosomal dominant early-onset families (85). Nearly the same ethical issues are concerns for both genetic and biochemical tests. Genetic tests have the added burden of providing information about family members who may not want the information and may be harmed by it.

CONCLUSION

Although we do not yet have a good understanding of the causal factors in Alzheimer's disease, rapid progress is being made. By virtue of the genetic information available, it is clear that Alzheimer's disease is the end stage of more than one basic cause. Many physiologic mechanisms and molecules have been implicated. The next decade should see enormous progress in understanding the causation of this devastating disease. With an improved understanding of causative factors, more specific preventive or therapeutic measures should become available.

Physicians will have to sort out various physiologic hypotheses and therapeutic interventions regarding Alzheimer's disease. In medical and scientific journals and in the lay press, physicians will read that Alzheimer's disease has its origin in a wide array of genetic and environmental factors. Physicians will be faced with many episodes in which family members and caregivers will demand drugs that are receiving attention in the public press as possible treatments for this illness. The dilemmas created by the availability of multiple pharmacologic interventions are only some of the issues that practicing physicians and other health professionals must consider during the emergence of the many discoveries and claims about the biology of Alzheimer's disease. Wurtman (86) has compared various pathophysiologic hypotheses to the tale of six blind men and the elephant. The original story (87) of the six blind men reads:

Once upon a time a king gathered some blind men about an elephant and asked them to tell him what an elephant was like. The first man felt a tusk and said an elephant was like a giant carrot; another happened to touch an ear and said it was like a big fan; another touched its trunk and said it was like a pestle; still another, who happened to feel its leg, said it was like a mortar; and another, who grasped its tail, said it was like a rope. Not one of them was able to tell the king the elephant's real form.

It is likely that with the convergence of major scientific discoveries, the true "elephantness" of Alzheimer's disease will soon be understood.

REFERENCES

1. Shua-Haim JR, Gross JS. Alzheimer's syndrome, not Alzheimer's disease. J Am Geriatr Soc 1996;44:96–97.
2. Brody JA. An epidemiologist views senile dementia—facts and fragments. Am J Epidemiol 1982;115:155–162.
3. Brody JA. An epidemiologist's view of the senile dementias: pieces of the puzzle. In: Wertheimer J, Marois M, eds. Senile Dementia: Outlook for the Future. New York: Alan R Liss, 1984:383.
4. Jorm AF, Korten AE, Henderson AS. The prevalence of dementia: a quantitative integration of the literature. Acta Psychiatr Scand 1987;76:465–479.
5. Evans DA, Funkenstein HH, Albert MS, et al. Prevalence of Alzheimer's disease in a community of older persons: higher than previously reported. JAMA 1989;262:2551–2556.

6. Jorm AF. The Epidemiology of Alzheimer's Disease and Related Disorders. London: Chapman and Hall, 1990.

7. Rosenberg R, Richter R, Risser T, et al. Genetic factors for the development of Alzheimer disease in the Cherokee Indian. Arch Neurol 1996;53:997–1000.

8. Skoog I, Nilsson L, Palmertz B, et al. A population-based study of dementia in 85-year-olds. N Engl J Med 1993; 328:153–158.

9. Endo H, Yamamoto T, Kuzuya F. Predispositions to arteriosclerotic dementia and senile dementia in Japan. In: Book of Abstracts of the XIIIth International Congress of Gerontology, New York, July 12–17, 1985. Washington: International Association of Gerontology, 1985:163.

10. Hasegawa K, Homma A, Imai Y. An epidemiological study of age-related dementia in the community. Int J Geriatr Psychiatry 1986;15:120–122.

11. Davies P, Maloney AJ. Selective loss of central cholinergic neurons in Alzheimer's disease [letter]. Lancet 1976; 2:1403.

12. Perry EK, Tomlinson BE, Blessed G, et al. Correlation of cholinergic abnormalities with senile plaques and mental test scores in senile dementia. BMJ 1978;2:1457–1459.

13. Whitehouse PJ, Price DL, Clark AW, et al. Alzheimer disease: evidence for selective loss of cholinergic neurons in the nucleus basalis. Ann Neurol 1981;10:122–126.

14. Whitehouse PJ, Price DL, Struble RG, et al. Alzheimer's disease and senile dementia: loss of neurons in the basal forebrain. Science 1982;215:1237–1239.

15. Perry RH. Recent advances in neuropathology. Br Med Bull 1986;42:34–41.

16. de Leon MJ, Golomb J, George AE, et al. The radiologic prediction of Alzheimer disease: the atrophic hippocampal formation. Am J Neuroradiol 1993;14:897–906.

17. Hardy JA, Higgins GA. Alzheimer's disease: the amyloid cascade hypothesis. Science 1992;256:184–185.

18. Rumble B, Rettallack R, Hilbich C, et al. Amyloid A4 protein and its precursor to Down's syndrome and Alzheimer's disease. N Engl J Med 1989;320:1446.

19. Epstein CJ, Avraham KB, Lovett M, et al. Transgenic mice with increased Cu/Zn-superoxide dismutase activity: animal model of dosage effects in Down syndrome. Proc Natl Acad Sci U S A 1987;84:8044.

20. Selkoe DJ. The molecular pathology of Alzheimer's disease. Neuron 1991;6:487–498.

21. Abraham CR, Shirahama T, Potter H. Alpha 1-antichymotrypsin is associated solely with amyloid deposits containing the beta-protein. Amyloid and cell localization of alpha 1-antichymotrypsin. Neurobiol Aging 1990;11:123–129.

22. Kosik K. Alzheimer's disease: a cell biological perspective. Science 1992;256:780–783.

23. McGeer PL, Akiyama H, Itagaki S, McGeer EG. Immune system response in Alzheimer's disease. Can J Neurosci 1989;16:516–527.

24. Rozemuller JM, Eikelenboom P, Stam FC, et al. A4 protein in Alzheimer's disease: primary and secondary events in extracellular amyloid deposition. J Neuropathol Exp Neurol 1989;48:674–691.

25. Barger SW, Harmon AD. Microglial activation by Alzheimer amyloid precursor protein and modulation by apolipoprotein E. Nature 1997;388:878–881.

26. Wyss-Corray T, Masliah E, Mallory M, et al. Amyloidogenic role for cytokine TGF-β1 in transgenic mice and in Alzheimer's disease. Nature 1997;389:603–606.

27. Heinrich PC, Castell JV, Andrus T. Interleukin-6 and the acute phase response. Biochem J 1990;265:621–636.

28. Vandenabeele P, Fiers W. Is amyloidogenesis during Alzheimer's disease due to an IL-1-/IL-6-mediated 'acute phase response' in the brain? Immunol Today 1991;12: 217–219.

29. Potter H, Nelson RB, Das S, et al. The involvement of proteases, protease inhibitors, and an acute phase response in Alzheimer's disease. Ann N Y Acad Sci 1992; 674:161–173.

30. McGeer PL, McGeer EG. The inflammatory response system of brain: implications for therapy of Alzheimer and other neurodegenerative diseases. Brain Res Rev 1995;21:195–218.

31. Mrak RE, Sheng JG, Griffin WS. Glial cytokines in Alzheimer's disease: review and pathogenic implications. Hum Pathol 1995;26:816–823.

32. Forloni G, Demicheli F, Giorgi S, et al. Expression of amyloid precursor protein mRNAs in endothelial, neuronal and glial cells: modulation by interleukin-1. Mol Brain Res 1992;16:128–134.

33. Harmon D. A hyothesis on the pathogenesis of Alzheimer's disease. Ann NY Acad Sci 1996;786:152–158.

34. Evans PH. Free radicals in brain metabolism and pathology. Br Med Bull 1993;49:577–587.

35. Piersanti P, Tesco G, Latorraca S, et al. Alzheimer skin fibroblasts susceptibility to oxygen radical damage. Neurobiol Aging 1992;13:81–111.

36. Le Bars PL, Katz MM, Berman N, et al. A placebo-controlled, double-blind, randomized trial of an extract of ginkgo biloba for dementia. JAMA 1997;278:1327–1332.

37. Parker WD Jr, Filley CM, Parks JK. Cytochrome oxidase deficiency in Alzheimer's disease. Neurology 1990;40: 1302–1303.

38. Davis RE, Miller S, Herrnstadt C, Ghosh SS. Mutations in mitochondrial cytochrome c oxidase genes segregate with late-onset Alzheimer disease. Proc Natl Acad Sci U S A 1997;94:4526–4531.

39. Toran-Allerand CD, Miranda RC, Bentham WD, et al. Estrogen receptors colocalize with low affinity nerve growth factor receptors in cholinergic neurons of the basal forebrain. Proc Natl Acad Sci U S A 1992;89: 4668–4672.

40. Wickelgren I. Estrogen stakes claim to cognition. Science 1997;276:675–678.

41. Tang MX, Jacobs D, Stern Y, et al. Effect of oestrogen

during menopause on risk and age at onset of Alzheimer's disease. Lancet 1996;348:429–432.

42. Barrett-Connor E, Kritz-Silverstein D. Estrogen replacement therapy and cognitive function in older women. JAMA 1992;269:2637–2641.

43. Snowdon DA, Greiner LH, Mortimer JA, et al. Brain infarction and the clinical expression of Alzheimer disease: the nun study. JAMA 1997;277:813–817.

44. Gatz M, Pederson NL, Berg S, et al. Heritability for Alzheimer's disease: the study of dementia in Swedish twins. J Gerontol 1997;52A:M117–M125.

45. Mullan M, Crawford F. Genetic and molecular advances in Alzheimer's disease. Trends Neurosci 1993;16:398–402.

46. Schellenberg G, Bird T, Wijsman E, et al. Genetic linkage evidence for a familial Alzheimer's disease locus on chromosome 14. Science 1992;258:668–671.

47. Mullan M, Houlden H, Windelspecht M, et al. A major locus for familial early onset Alzheimer's disease is on the long arm of chromosome 14, proximal to α-antichymotrypsin. Nat Genet 1992;2:340–343.

48. Van Broeckhoven C, Backhovens H, Cruts M, et al. Mapping of a gene predisposing to early-onset Alzheimer's disease to chromosome 14q24.3. Nat Genet 1992;2:335–339.

49. St George-Hyslop P, Haines J, Rogaev E, et al. Genetic evidence for a novel familial Alzheimer's disease locus on chromosome 14. Nat Genet 1992;2:330–334.

50. Sherrington R, Rogaev EI, Liang Y, et al. Cloning of a gene bearing missense mutations in early-onset familial Alzheimer's disease. Nature 1995;375:754–760.

51. Rogaev EI, Sherrington R, Rogaeva EA, et al. Familial Alzheimer's disease in kindreds with missense mutations in a gene on chromosome 1 related to the Alzheimer's disease type 3 gene. Nature 1995;376:775–778.

52. Farrer LA. Genetics and the dementia patient. Neurologist 1997;3:13–30.

53. Kim TW, Pettingell WH, Jung YK, et al. Alternative cleavage of Alzheimer-associated presenilins during apoptosis by a caspase-3 family protease. Science 1997; 277:373–376.

54. Evans DA, Beckett LA, Field TS, et al. Apolipoprotein E ε4 and incidence of Alzheimer disease in a community population of older persons. JAMA 1997;277:822–824.

55. Osuntokun BO, Sahota A, Ogunniyi AO, et al. Lack of an association between apolipoprotein E epsilon 4 and Alzheimer's disease in elderly Nigerians. Ann Neurol 1995;42:1097–1105.

56. Farrer LA, Cupples LA, Haines JL, et al. Effects of age, sex, and ethnicity on the association between apolipoprotein E genotype and Alzheimer disease. A meta-analysis. APOE and Alzheimer Disease Meta Analysis Consortium. JAMA 1997;278:1349–1356

57. American College of Medical Genetics/American Society of Human Genetics Working Group on APOE and Alzheimer's Disease. Statement on the use of apolipoprotein E testing for Alzheimer's disease. JAMA 1995;274:1627–1629.

58. Relkin NR, Tanzi R, Breitner J, et al. Apolipoprotein E genotyping in Alzheimer's disease: position statement of the National Institute on Aging/Alzheimer' Association Working Group. Lancet 1996;347:1091–1095.

59. Lehrman S. Genetic testing for Alzheimer's disease 'not appropriate.' Nature 1997;389:898.

60. Wisniewski T, Golabek A, Matsubara E, et al. Apolipoprotein E: binding to soluble Alzheimer's β-amyloid. Biochem Biophys Res Commun 1993;192:359–365.

61. Strittmatter C, Wisgraber KH, Huang DY, et al. Binding of human apolipoprotein E to synthetic amyloid β peptide: isoform-specific effects and implications for late-onset Alzheimer disease. Proc Natl Acad Sci U S A 1993;90:8098–8102.

62. Pericak-Vance MA, Bass MP, Yamaoka LH, et al. Complete genomic screen in late-onset familial Alzheimer disease: evidence for a new locus on chromosome 12. JAMA 1997;278:1237–1241.

63. Lopera F, Ardilla A, Martínez A, et al. Clinical features of early-onset Alzheimer disease in a large kindred with an E280A presenilin-1 mutation. JAMA 1997;277:793–799.

64. Gajdusek DC, Gibbs CJ Asher DM, et al. Precautions in medical care of and in handling materials from patients with transmissible virus dementia (Creutzfeldt-Jakob disease). N Engl J Med 1977;297:1253–1258.

65. Edwardson JA, Candy JM, Ince PG, et al. Aluminium accumulation, beta-amyloid deposition and neurofibrillary changes in the central nervous system. Ciba Found Symp 1992;169:165–185.

66. Multhaup G, Schlicksupp A, Hesse L, et al. The amyloid precursor protein of Alzheimer's disease in the reduction of copper (II) to copper (I). Science 1996; 271:1406–1409.

67. Kennard ML, Feldman H, Yamada T, Jefferies WA. Serum levels of the iron binding protein p97 are elevated in Alzheimer's disease. Nat Med 1996;2:1230–1235.

68. Roberts GW. Immunocytochemistry of neurofibrillary tangles in dementia pugilistica and Alzheimer's disease: evidence for common genesis. Lancet 1988;2:1456–1458.

69. Roberts GW, Allsop D, Bruton C. The occult aftermath of boxing. J Neurol Neurosurg Psychiatry 1990;53:373–378.

70. Mortimer JA, Van Duijn CM, Chandra V, et al. Head trauma as a risk factor for Alzheimer's disease: a collaborative re-analysis of case-control studies. Int J Epidemiol 1990;20(suppl 2):S28–S35.

71. Nicoll JAR, Roberts GW, Graham DI. Apolipoprotein E ε4 allele is associated with deposition of amyloid β-protein following head injury. Nat Med 1995;1:135–137.

72. Eagger SA, Levy R, Sahakian BJ. Tacrine in Alzheimer's disease. Lancet 1991;337:989–992.

73. Davis KL, Thal LJ, Gamzu ER, et al. A double-blind, placebo-controlled multicenter study of tacrine for Alzheimer's disease. N Engl J Med 1992;327:1253–1259.

74. Farlow M, Gracon SI, Hershey LA, et al. A controlled trial of tacrine in Alzheimer's disease. JAMA 1992;268:2523–2529.

75. Knapp MJ, Knopman DS, Solomon PR, et al. A 30-week randomized controlled trial of high-dose tacrine in patients with Alzheimer's disease. JAMA 1994;271:985–991.

76. Winker MA. Tacrine for Alzheimer's disease. JAMA 1994;271:1023–1024.

77. Rogers SL, Friedhoff LT. The efficacy and safety of donepezil in patients with Alzheimer's disease: results of a U.S. multicentre randomized double-blind, placebo-controlled trial. The Donepezil Study Group. Dementia 1996;7:293–303.

78. Raves ML, Harel M, Pang YP, et al. Structure of acetylcholinesterase complexed with the nootropic alkaloid, (−)−huperzine A. Nat Struct Biol 1997;4:57–63.

79. Breitner JC, Welsh KA, Helms MJ, et al. Delayed onset of Alzheimer's disease with nonsteroidal anti-inflammatory and histamine H2 blocking drugs. Neurobiol Aging 1995;16:523–530.

80. Rogers J, Kirby LC, Hempelman SR, et al. Clinical trial of indomethacin in Alzheimer's disease. Neurology 1993:43:1609–1611.

81. McGeer PL, Schulzer M, McGeer EG. Arthritis and anti-inflammatory agents as possible protective factors for Alzheimer's disease: a review of 17 epidemiologic studies. Neurology 1996;47:425–432.

82. Stewart WF, Kawas C, Corrada M, Metter EJ. Risk of Alzheimer's disease and duration of NSAID use. Neurology 1997;48:626–632.

83. Sano M, Ernesto C, Thomas RG, et al. A controlled trial of selegiline, alpha-tocopherol, or both as treatment for Alzheimer's disease. N Engl J Med 1997;336:1216–1222.

84. Kawas C, Resnick S, Morrison A, et al. A prospective study of estrogen replacement therapy and the risk of developing Alzheimer's disease: the Baltimore Longitudinal Study of Aging. Neurology 1997;48:626–632.

85. Post SG, Whitehouse PJ, Binstock RH, et al. The clinical introduction of genetic testing for Alzheimer disease: an ethical perspective. JAMA 1997;277:832–836.

86. Wurtman RJ. Alzheimer's disease. Sci Am 1985;252:62–71.

87. Bukkyo Dendo Kyokai. The Teaching of Buddha. 72nd rev ed. Tokyo: Kosaido, 1984:75.

CHAPTER 18

MARTY WYNGAARDEN KRAUSS, JAN S. GREENBERG, AND MARSHA MAILICK SELTZER

Aging in Adults With Developmental Disabilities and Severe and Persistent Mental Illness

This chapter examines the health and social status of older persons with developmental disabilities (DD) and older persons with severe and persistent mental illness (SPMI). Although distinct populations, they share a variety of characteristics that affect their clinical needs and, hence, their interactions with community-based health care practitioners. For example, for both groups, community-based living and services are now the norm. This is a sharp contrast to several decades ago, when residential, social, and health services were provided largely in isolated state-supported institutional settings. Their historic segregation from the general public has resulted in lack of knowledge about and limited exposure to these populations by health practitioners, particularly with respect to their health conditions and needs. Furthermore, the population of persons with DD and SPMI is particularly large because of the aging of the baby boom generation. The persons in this cohort are in midlife and will reach old age during the first decades of the next century, resulting in an increasingly large subgroup of older persons with these disabilities. Third, both groups rely heavily on the care and assistance provided by family members. Although the social stigma associated with SPMI and to a lesser extent DD has masked the prevalence of family-based care, greater awareness of and support for family caregivers has resulted in

increased demands for basic social and health services for impaired relatives. Furthermore, since few adults with DD or SPMI marry and most outlive their parents, their siblings often inherit some measure of responsibility during old age.

In this chapter we discuss the populations with DD and SPMI sequentially. We start each section with the definition of the population. We then present relevant information for practitioners regarding social and health situations, data on the settings in which they live, social issues that condition use of services, and specific health concerns associated with the aging process.

DEVELOPMENTAL DISABILITIES
Definition

Clinicians should be familiar with the controversies about the criteria used to diagnose a person as having DD. Each state has developed its own definition, and variation from state to state is common. Professional associations offer yet other definitions of DD (1). The central issue of the controversy is whether the definition is based on diagnostic categories (e.g., mental retardation, autism) or on functional limitations that result from these diagnostic conditions. The federal definition of DD has taken the latter approach. A developmental disability, as defined initially by PL 95–682 (the Developmental Disabilities Bill of Rights Act of 1978), is a severe chronic disability of a person that (*a*) is attributable to a mental or physical impairment or a combination of mental and physical impairments; (*b*) is manifested before the person attains age 22; (*c*) is likely to continue indefinitely; (*d*) results in substantial functional limitations in three or more of the following areas of major life activity: self-care, receptive and expressive language, learning, mobility, self-direction, capacity for independent living, economic self-sufficiency; and (*e*) reflects the person's need for a combination and sequence of special, interdisciplinary, or generic care, treatment, or other services that are lifelong or extended in duration and are individually planned and coordinated.

Although the federal definition of DD is based on the functional characteristics of the affected person, the most commonly included categories of DD are mental retardation (MR), cerebral palsy (CP), epilepsy, and autism. The largest subgroup of this population consists of persons with MR, from whom most of our knowledge about older persons with DD has been generated. According to the American Association on Mental Retardation, MR is defined as significantly subaverage general intellectual functioning (an IQ score of approximately 75 or below) existing concurrently with deficits in adaptive behavior and manifested before age 18 (1). The most prevalent known cause of MR is Down's syndrome (DS).

Population Characteristics and Demographic Trends
Population Size

The true size of the older population with DD is not known. First, there is ambiguity regarding when old age begins for persons with DD. Because some subgroups, such as those with DS, evidence premature aging (2), many have advocated the use of a lower age boundary to demarcate older from middle-aged DS populations. Second, there are no public registries listing persons with DD, and therefore those not known to the service system are not counted. Third, there is variation from state to state regarding who is counted among service recipients. Whereas virtually all states count those with MR, states are less consistent in the extent to which

those with epilepsy or CP are included in counts of service recipients.

Prevalence estimates suggest that about 1% of the adult population in the United States has MR. In 1985 it was estimated that there were 200,000 to 500,000 older adults with MR in the United States and that the numbers would double in the next 40 years (3). Furthermore, about 12% of the total population with MR is estimated to be aged 65 and older, a similar proportion as in the population without MR (4).

Life Expectancy and Mortality

There has been a marked increase in the life expectancy of persons with DD, primarily as a result of improved health care. For example, one third of babies born with DS have congenital heart defects (5). In the past these children died young, but corrective surgical procedures now extend their life well into the middle years.

Data have been assembled on mortality rates of persons with MR (6). Death rates are highest before age 5 and after age 55 and higher among those with severe or profound retardation than those with mild or moderate levels of disability (7). Among persons aged 40 or older, the greatest predictors of mortality are age, lack of mobility (which increases the risk of death from choking and pneumonia), and poor self-care skills (inability to feed one's self and lack of bowel and bladder control) (8). Persons with DS have an elevated risk of premature death, reflecting their general earlier onset of aging, including Alzheimer's disease (AD). Their rate of death increases sharply after age 50 (9). In subgroups other than those with DS or other organic causes of DD, life expectancy approaches that of the general population. As a result, the population of older persons with DD is considerably larger than in the past.

The Aging of Cohorts

As noted earlier, the population of adults with DD has grown because of the aging of the baby boom generation. Another cohort effect stems from the reduction in infant mortality in children with DD (10), so as these children grow up, the adult population will increase.

In summary, although the population of older persons with DD is difficult to estimate, this group is getting larger because of longer life expectancy and increases in the sizes of successive cohorts. Therefore, health care providers can reasonably expect to encounter more and more older persons with DD in need of medical care and health maintenance.

Age-Related Changes

The paucity of longitudinal studies of the development of persons with DD and the difficulty of disentangling cohort effects from the effects of aging make strong statements about age-related changes hazardous. Having acknowledged this, we describe what is known about changes in cognitive abilities, functional abilities, and health status in older adults with DD. Regarding cognitive abilities, studies have demonstrated maintenance of such abilities among adults with DD over time, and, indeed in some cases, evidence of intellectual gains (11). Those with DS have an increased risk of age-related declines in cognitive abilities after age 50 (2), a pattern distinct from those with other causes of DD, who show cognitive declines after age 60.

The pattern for age-related changes in functional abilities mirrors that of cognitive abilities. Studies show that declines in functional abilities are related to level of retardation; the less impaired, the slower the declines (12). However, the age-based rate of decline is faster than that of the nondisabled population, and those with DS decline fastest (9).

Many older persons with DD manifest behavioral problems, including stereotypies, withdrawn and resistant behaviors, aggression, and annoying behaviors. Such problems, which are prevalent in persons living in licensed settings and with their families (13), can complicate diagnosis and treatment regimens. Although reports indicate reduction of problematic behaviors with aging (14), they remain a significant contributor to stress among caretakers and may result in reduced social integration for persons with DD.

The DD population is notable for the prevalence of polypharmacy and for the frequent complications associated with long-term use of multiple medications (15). Long-term use of psychoactive and neuroleptic medications is common. As a result, tardive dyskinesia is widespread,

with estimates suggesting that up to 80% of the persons with MR who are withdrawn from neuroleptic medication display induced movement disorders, including stereotypic actions (16).

The most common health problems among older persons with DD include arthritis, heart disease, and high blood pressure (4). However, older persons with DD probably exhibit greater heterogeneity in age-related changes than does the general population. Health providers must evaluate each person in the context of the unique medical and social history and special concerns. A significant challenge is obtaining accurate histories. Communication difficulties among persons with DD are common, and they result in increased reliance on caregivers and family members as sources of medical histories. Clinical reports indicate that a major issue in the provision of health services is the extended time needed for obtaining relevant information, diagnostic testing, and explanation of treatments. Furthermore, some adults with DD have to be desensitized before invasive procedures.

Formal and Informal Supports

Almost by definition, older persons with a DD have high needs for formal and informal supports. Formal supports are most frequently provided by the network of community-based health, social, residential, and vocational services that now exist in every state. Informal supports are provided by family members, including parents, siblings, and extended family members. Furthermore, a variety of advocacy organizations, such as the national, state, and local chapters of the Association for Retarded Citizens of the United States, provide critical oversight and assistance to persons with DD. Despite the development of community-based systems of care and the active involvement of family members and advocacy groups, most persons with DD are lonely and do not participate in many of the traditional activities of adult life, including marriage, paid employment, civic involvement, diverse friendships, vacations, and so on. Given the well-documented importance of social support for health maintenance, the fragility of support that is characteristic of many older persons with DD has implications for the delivery of services and management of health needs.

There is considerable diversity of residential settings for older persons with DD. The family is the primary provider of informal support to persons with DD throughout their lives, as up to 85% of persons with DD live with or under the supervision of their families (17). The system of formal licensed residential care is extensive, however. As of 1996 there were approximately 325,000 persons with DD living in licensed residential settings (18), including large state-operated institutional facilities, psychiatric facilities, nursing homes, state-operated community residences, privately operated licensed community residences, and foster family care. In addition, more than 45,000 persons with DD live in homes they lease or own.

Other nonresidential supports that are critical to older persons with DD have proliferated in the past 10 years (19). Recognizing that the needs of older persons with DD are often similar to those of older persons in the general population, legislation has been passed to increase the access of the DD population to the generic system of aging services (Older Americans Act, PL 89–73; Developmental Disabilities Assistance and Bill of Rights Act, PL 100–142). Efforts to foster collaborative program planning between the aging and DD service sectors have resulted in increased presence of older persons with DD in senior center and senior companion programs, nutrition programs, and senior adult day programs. To a large extent, day programs for elders with DD focus on establishing and maintaining social connections, leisure activities, community inclusion opportunities, and health surveillance.

Special Populations

Down's Syndrome

Although the life expectancy of persons with DS has increased dramatically during this century and now approaches age 60, there is still a shorter life expectancy for this group than other adults with DD. Their primary causes of death in adulthood are dementia, stroke, and infection. Extensive evidence of premature aging within this population includes early menopause, hypothyroidism, presbycusis, cataracts, obstructive sleep apnea, immune senescence, osteoarthritis, and Alzheimer's disease (20–22).

Virtually all persons with DS over age 35 dis-play the neuropathologic changes associated with AD, although clinical manifestation of cognitive and functional decline is less common prior to age 50 than previously believed. The age-specific prevalence of dementia for adults with DS over age 50 is estimated at 40% (23). In some cases functional and cognitive losses may be the result of depression or other treatable illness rather than AD. Nevertheless, older persons with DS are less proficient in daily living skills than are either younger persons with DS or age-matched persons with other forms of MR (9).

Cerebral Palsy

There is great heterogeneity in the population of adults with CP regarding the extent of physical disability and any associated mental retardation. These factors affect health care needs throughout the life course. Although clinical information on aging among persons with CP is sparse, evidence suggests that these persons have considerable difficulty getting access to medical care (24). Problems associated with aging include urinary tract infections, incontinence, mobility difficulties, osteoporosis, and psychologic problems arising from the loss of expected functioning. Clinical evidence suggests an increase in stiffness, arthritis, and neck, back, and shoulder pain among older persons with CP, as well as seizures, hip fractures, and difficulty swallowing (22). Communication problems for people with CP result in an increased reliance on family and caretakers in clinical situations. Advances in medical care, including gastrostomy feeding, antibiotic treatment, and enhanced management of respiratory infections, have increased the life expectancy of persons with CP (24, 25).

Autism

Autism is considered both a developmental disability and a type of severe mental illness. No research about persons with autism in old age has been conducted. This diagnosis is relatively new (26), and hence the first persons to be diagnosed with autism are now in their 50s. The sparse data available suggest that two thirds of adults with autism do not live independent lives (27) and about half live in residential placements (28). The hallmark characteristics of autism, including difficulty forming close relationships (29) and abnormalities in communicative abilities, persist into adulthood (30). Several organic disorders occur frequently in persons with autism, including seizures (in about one third of such persons), tuberous sclerosis, hyperlactosemia, and neurofibromatosis (31).

SEVERE AND PERSISTENT MENTAL ILLNESS

Definition

SPMI, formerly known as chronic mental illness, has been described by the National Advisory Mental Health Council in terms of diagnosis, disability, and duration (32). SPMI in adults age 18 or older refers to disorders commonly accompanied by psychotic symptoms, including schizophrenia, schizoaffective disorder, bipolar disorder, and severe forms of major depression that are long-term or chronic conditions resulting in significant impairment in daily living activities and social, vocational, and educational functioning. Although technically organic brain disorders such as Alzheimer's could be included in the definition of SPMI, they traditionally have not been considered chronic mental illnesses and therefore are not discussed in this chapter.

Older adults with SPMI are a diverse and heterogenous group with respect to their level of social, occupational, and psychologic functioning. The largest subgroup of the population with SPMI consists of persons with schizophrenia. Longitudinal research suggests that the life course of schizophrenia is not necessarily progressive decline. Rather, many persons have long periods when they are relatively asymptomatic, and still others appear to recover (33). However, even elders who show few residual signs of having suffered a long-term mental illness face many challenges because of the secondary effects of the mental illness, such as chronic unemployment and long-term psychotropic medication use.

Population Characteristics and Demographic Trends

Population Size

Data from two major national studies, the National Comorbidity Survey (NCS) and the Epidemiologic Catchment Area (ECA) survey, are the major sources of data on the prevalence of SPMI in the adult population. The ECA, a general population survey of five local areas in the United States that was carried out between 1980 and 1985, assessed the prevalence of disorders listed in the third edition of *Diagnostic and Statistical Manual of Mental Disorders* (DSM-III), among persons aged 18 and older (34). The NCS was conducted in 1990–1991 to assess the prevalence of DSM-III-R (DSM-III revised) disorders in a nationally representative sample of adults aged 18 to 54. An analysis of NCS suggested that 2.6% of the adult population, representing approximately 4.8 million adults, meet the criteria for SPMI (35). However, the data suggest that there is a considerably lower rate of SPMI among those aged 55 and older, for reasons discussed later. Analysis of the Baltimore ECA indicates that the prevalence of SPMI among the population aged 55 and over living in the community is only 0.8% (35). In addition, a substantial number of older people living in the community have some of the symptoms associated with SPMI, although they may not meet all the criteria for a diagnosis of SPMI (36).

Life Expectancy and Mortality

It is generally recognized that persons with SPMI have a shorter life expectancy than the general population. The average life span of persons with schizophrenia is approximately 10 years shorter (37), in part because of an elevated risk of suicide, which typically occurs prior to age 40 (38). Older adults with affective disorders have a mortality rate 2.5 times that of the general population (39). This excess mortality is due to both higher rates of suicide and higher rates of death from medical problems (40).

Social Characteristics

There are a number of social characteristics that either increase the risk of SPMI or result from it. For example, the prevalence of SPMI is notably high among the poor and poorly educated persons in our society (41). These adults are less likely to marry and have children than the general population. Many older adults with SPMI reside in nursing homes, including almost half of the patients who have been deinstitutionalized (42). The 1985 National Nursing Home Survey (43) found that almost 200,000 nursing home residents, or 13.1% of such residents, had a diagnosis of schizophrenia or other psychotic disorder.

Demographic Trends

The composition of future cohorts of older adults with SPMI will be substantially different from that of today. They will enter old age with fewer health problems and more social supports, as they have not had the debilitating effects of long-term institutionalization. They will be better educated and more racially diverse, mirroring the larger demographic trend occurring in the general aging population. Health care professionals must take into account the changing nature of the aging cohort as they plan services for the next generation of older adults with SPMI.

Health Care Issues

Physical Health

The available research indicates that the relation between psychiatric disorders and medical illness is complex and poorly understood. A recent study addressed physical comorbidity among older adults with psychiatric disorders (44). Compared with patients with Alzheimer's disease and schizophrenia, older adults with major depression had significantly higher rates of degenerative joint disease, hypertension, and coronary artery disease. Several researchers have reported an association between depression and increased risk of medical illnesses (39, 45). A review of the literature on medical comorbidity and schizophrenia notes that the evidence is inconclusive as to whether schizophrenia is related to an increased risk of physical illnesses (37). Some health problems (e.g., cardiovascular disease) are particularly common in persons with schizophrenia, whereas others (e.g., rheumatoid arthritis) are less common than in the general population, and for still others (e.g., cancer) the findings have been inconsistent.

Additionally, older adults with SPMI appear to be at considerable risk for undiagnosed health problems. In a study examining the prevalence of physical disease in psychiatric patients in California, it was found that only 47% of the patients' physical illnesses were recognized by the mental health staff (46). Health care professionals may tend to overlook coexisting medical problems in patients with severe psychiatric symptoms (e.g., hallucinations and delusions), because of the prominence of the psychiatric symptoms (44). Also, because of the use of neuroleptics, which reduce pain sensitivity (47, 48), older persons with serious mental illness may fail to report mild pain or discomfort that is an early warning sign of disease. For these reasons, health care professionals should use screening instruments (e.g., the Cumulative Illness Rating Scale for Geriatrics) (49, 50) in primary care settings to aid in the detection of physical health problems in older adults with SPMI.

Cognitive Impairment

A large body of research indicates that schizophrenia is associated with moderate levels of cognitive impairment (51, 52), but that in general the cognitive impairment associated with schizophrenia is not progressive. It is less clear whether any subgroups of patients with schizophrenia are at particular risk for developing Alzheimer's disease. Researchers studied a cohort of long-term state hospital patients with schizophrenia (53). Brain autopsies revealed that 28% had cellular changes associated with Alzheimer's disease. Others have found increased cognitive decline with severe negative symptoms of schizophrenia (e.g., flat affect, withdrawal). These findings are consistent with the notion that schizophrenia may not be a unitary illness and that certain subtypes of schizophrenia may be associated with an increased risk of developing dementia.

If dementia is suspected in an elderly patient with SPMI, a comprehensive medical workup is indicated to seek out treatable causes (e.g., medication side effects, physical illnesses). Furthermore, as schizophrenia is associated with significant deficits in learning, health care providers should take into account these learning difficulties when working with these older persons. Helpful communication strategies include presenting new information linked to previously learned information and breaking down complex tasks into their component parts. Instructions may have to be repeated on several occasions before they are fully understood, and the use of more than one modality, such as both oral and written instructions, may facilitate the retention of new information.

Functional Status

Our knowledge about the functional status of older persons with SPMI is very limited. Cross-sectional surveys of persons with SPMI indicate, as expected, that older persons are likely to have more limitations in personal care and instrumental activities of daily living than younger adults (41). One study compared 55 outpatients with schizophrenia to 72 unaffected persons ranging in age from 45 to 86 years (54). The persons with schizophrenia had greater impairment than controls with respect to communication, transportation, finance, and shopping skills. There were no differences in more basic activities of daily living, such as eating and grooming.

Sensory Impairment

The research evidence as to whether older adults with SPMI are at greater risk for sensory impairments than their age peers is inconclusive. For example, no significant differences were found between persons aged 45 and over with psychiatric disorders and a comparison group of healthy similarly aged subjects in terms of their uncorrected hearing or visual abilities (55). However, psychiatric patients had significantly more problems with hearing and vision when using corrective devices such as hearing aids and eyeglasses than did the subjects without psychiatric disorders. This may indicate that older persons with SPMI are at greater risk for being improperly fitted with eyeglasses and hearing aids, possibly because they have difficulty clearly communicating their needs during an examination. Or it may result from the fact that older persons with SPMI face greater barriers in obtaining routine treatment for sensory impairments because of the lack of insurance coverage or expense of hearing and vision services (37). Teaching older adults with SPMI about vision and hearing losses and corrections may increase the likelihood that these persons receive proper care for their sensory deficits (55). Also, health care providers can assist older adults to use corrective aids correctly and periodically re-evaluate them to determine that such devices are properly fitted.

Formal and Informal Supports

Formal Mental Health Services

A study of the mental health needs of the chronically mentally ill elderly found that fewer than half had regular contact with a psychiatrist or psychiatric nurse (56). Similarly, among the ECA sites, only 42% to 55% of older persons with a current psychiatric diagnosis received some type of mental health services (57). Older adults with psychiatric disorders were more likely to seek outpatient treatment from a medical provider than a mental health professional.

Informal Supports

The social networks of persons with SPMI are smaller and include a higher proportion of family members than the social networks of those in the general population (58). Since women develop schizophrenia up to a decade later than men (59), they are more likely to marry and have children before they become mentally ill (60), and hence they have a different array of social supports than their male counterparts.

Little is known about family care of persons with SPMI after they reach old age, in part because in the past many older persons were transferred directly from state mental hospitals to nursing homes. Research on families of young and middle-aged adults with SPMI indicates that while families play a major role in caregiving, this care results in considerable emotional and social cost to the family (61, 62). Psychoeducational programs have reduced familial burden of families caring for a young or middle-aged adult with SPMI, and they may also be helpful for caregivers coping with the care of an elderly relative with SPMI.

Special Populations

Comorbidity: Substance Abuse and SPMI

Rates of substance abuse, which are particularly high among older adults with SPMI, are associated with medication noncompliance, medical illnesses, and risk of suicide. One study found that 31% of the older persons with schizophrenia met the DSM-III-R criteria for lifetime alcohol abuse or dependence as compared with 8% in the unaffected comparison group (37). Another study found that 32% of older adults with schizophrenia had a substance abuse problem, considerably higher than the 13 to 17% of older adults with major depressive disorders who were substance abusers (63). We know from general population studies that alcoholism is often undiagnosed in the elderly, and we suspect this similarly occurs with older adults with SPMI. The use of a screening tool, such as the Michigan Alcoholism Screening Test (MAST) (64) or the CAGE (65), may be a mechanism to encourage health care providers to evaluate their older patients with SPMI for problems with alcohol dependency.

Elders of Color

The ethnic elderly population in the United States is growing at least twice as rapidly as the elderly population as a whole. By 2030 elders of color are expected to constitute a quarter of the older population. A study of public housing residents in Baltimore who were 60 years and older (primarily poor African-American women), found prevalence rates 10 times as high for schizophrenia and 4 times as high for mood disorders as those found at the Baltimore ECA. Little is known, however, about the mental health needs of this population (66).

Homelessness

About 600,000 persons are homeless on any given night (67), of whom about 10% are age 60 and over. About one out of every three homeless people in the U.S. suffers from SPMI (68), and the prevalence of severe psychiatric disorders among the older homeless population has been found to be nearly equivalent to that among younger homeless persons (69). Many of these older persons are burdened by substance abuse, physical illness, and other adverse consequences of lifelong poverty. Although many homeless older adults with SPMI are eligible for federal and other targeted benefit programs, few are enrolled. Health care professionals have a important role in identifying such persons, who may need support and assistance to gain such entitlements.

FINAL CONSIDERATIONS

Several specific issues are often confronted by health care practitioners serving these populations. First, guardianship status may have to be clarified. Many persons with mental disabilities have legal guardians with either full or limited powers who therefore must participate in clinical and treatment decision making. Second, while most persons with MR and/or SPMI are poor and may be covered by Medicaid, state-based differences in covered benefits must be considered. Third, most states have specialists experienced in the provision of health services to people with MR and/or SPMI. Practitioners should locate such specialists for consultation and assistance. This is particularly important for the management of problematic behaviors (a condition characteristic of both populations), for which the propensity to overuse medication should be balanced with the activation of behavioral intervention programs and community supports.

The lack of knowledge about the aging process for these diverse groups is complicated by the common absence of detailed medical histories and the reliance on family caregivers as health surveillance reporters. With current projections for increases in the size of both populations, access to high-quality health care is critical. To this end, health care practitioners can be both active participants in increasing the quality of life of persons with DD and SPMI and contributors to a growing literature on their health care needs.

Acknowledgment. Support for the preparation of this chapter was provided, in part, by R01 AG08768 from the National Institute on Aging, R03 MH465644 from the National Institute on Mental Health, the Waisman Center at the University of Wisconsin-Madison, and the Starr Center for Mental Retardation of the Heller School at Brandeis University.

REFERENCES

1. Luckasson R, ed. Mental Retardation: Definition, Classification, and Systems of Support. 9th ed. Washington: American Association on Mental Retardation, 1992.
2. Zigman WB, Seltzer GB, Silverman WP. Behavioral and mental health changes associated with aging in adults

with mental retardation. In: Seltzer MM, Krauss MW, Janicki JP, eds. Life Course Perspectives on Adulthood and Old Age. Washington: American Association on Mental Retardation, 1994:67–92.

3. Jacobson JW, Sutton MS, Janicki MP. Demography and characteristics of aging and aged mentally retarded persons. In: Janicki MP, Wisniewski HM, eds. Aging and Developmental Disabilities. Baltimore: Brookes, 1985: 115–142.

4. Anderson DJ. Health issues. In: Sutton E, Factor A, Hawkins B, et al., eds. Older Adults With Developmental Disabilities. Baltimore: Brookes, 1993:29–48.

5. Pueschel SM. Health concerns in persons with Down syndrome. In: Pueschel SM, Tingey C, Rynders JE, et al., eds. New Perspectives on Down Syndrome. Baltimore: Brookes, 1987:113–134.

6. Eyman R, Grossman H, Tarjan G, Miller C. Life Expectancy and Mental Retardation (Monograph 7). Washington: American Association on Mental Retardation, 1987.

7. Eyman RK, Call TL, White JF. Mortality of elderly mentally retarded persons in California. J Appl Gerontol 1989;8:203–215.

8. Strauss D. The prediction of mortality for elderly people with mental retardation: a multivariable approach. Technical report 313. Riverside, CA: University of California, Department of Statistics, 1994.

9. Zigman WB, Schupf N, Sersen E, Silverman W. Prevalence of dementia in adults with and without Down syndrome. Am J Ment Retard 1995;100:403–412.

10. Lubin RA, Kiely M. Epidemiology of aging in developmental disabilities. In: Janicki MP, Wisniewski HM, eds. Aging and Developmental Disabilities. Baltimore: Brookes, 1985:95–114.

11. Eyman RK, Widaman KF. Life-span development of institutionalized and community-based mentally retarded persons, revisited. Am J Ment Defic 1987;91:559–569.

12. Janicki MP, Jacobson JW. Generational trends in sensory, physical, and behavioral abilities among older mentally retarded persons. Am J Ment Defic 1986;90: 490–500.

13. Seltzer MM, Hong J, Krauss MW. Behavior problems in adults with mental retardation and maternal well-being. Paper presented at the 30th Annual Gatlinburg Conference on Research and Theory in Mental Retardation, Riverside, CA, March 13, 1997.

14. Edgerton RB, Gaston MA. I've Seen It All! Lives of Older Persons With Mental Retardation in the Community. Baltimore: Brookes, 1991.

15. Adlin M. Health care issues. In: Sutton E, Factor A, Hawkins B, et al., eds. Older Adults With Developmental Disabilities. Baltimore: Brookes, 1993:49–60.

16. Sprague RL, van Emmerik RE, Slobounov SM, Newell KM. Facial stereotypic movements and tardive dyskinesia in a mentally retarded population. Am J Ment Retard 1995;100:345–358.

17. Seltzer MM, Krauss MW. Aging parents with coresident adult children: the impact of lifelong caregiving. In: Seltzer MM, Krauss MW, Janicki MP, eds. Life Course Perspectives on Adulthood and Old Age. Washington: American Association on Mental Retardation, 1994:3–18.

18. Prouty RW, Lakin KC, eds. Residential Services for Persons With Developmental Disabilities: Status and Trends Through 1996. Minneapolis: University of Minnesota Research and Training Center on Community Living, Institute on Community Integration, 1997.

19. Sutton E, Factor AR, Hawkins BA, et al., eds. Older Adults With Developmental Disabilities. Baltimore: Brookes, 1993.

20. Adlin M. Older adults with developmental disabilities and chronic mental illness. In: Reichel W, Gallo JJ, Busby-Whitehead J, et al., eds. Care of the Elderly: Clinical Aspects of Aging. 4th ed. Baltimore: Williams & Wilkins, 1995:161–167.

21. Schupf N, Zigman W, Kapell D, et al. Early menopause in women with Down syndrome. J Intellect Disabil Res 1997;41:264–267.

22. Seltzer GB, Luchterhand C. Health and well-being of older persons with developmental disabilities. In: Seltzer MM, Krauss MW, Janicki MP, eds. Life Course Perspectives on Adulthood and Old Age. Washington: American Association on Mental Retardation, 1994:109–142.

23. Schupf N, Silverman W, Sterling RC, Zigman W. Down syndrome, terminal illness, and risk for dementia of the Alzheimer-type. Brain Dysfunct 1989;2:181–188.

24. Baladin S, Morgan J. Adults with cerebral palsy: What's happening? J Intellect Devel Disabil 1997;22:109–124.

25. Janicki MP. Aging, cerebral palsy, and older persons with mental retardation. Aust N Z J Devel Disabil 1989; 15:311–320.

26. Kanner L. Autistic disturbances of affective contact. Nerv Child 1943;2:217–250.

27. Adams WV, Sheslow DV. A developmental perspective of adolescence. In: Schopler E, Mesibov GB, eds. Autism in Adolescents and Adults. New York: Plenum, 1983: 11–36.

28. Hitzing W. Community living alternatives for persons with autism and related severe behavioral problems. In: Cohen DL, Donnellan AM, Paul R, eds. Handbook of Autism and Pervasive Developmental Disorders. New York: Wiley, 1987:396–417.

29. Rumsey JM, Rappaport JL, Sceery WR. Autistic children as adults: psychiatric, social, and behavioral outcomes. J Am Acad Child Adolesc Psychiatry 1985;24:465–473.

30. Charlop MH, Haymes LK. Speech and language acquisition and intervention: behavioral approaches. In: Matson JL, ed. Autism in Children and Adults: Etiology, Assessment, and Intervention. Pacific Grove, CA: Brooks/Cole, 1994:213–240.

31. Sturmey P, Sevin JA. Defining and assessing autism. In: Matson JL, ed. Autism in Children and Adults: Etiology, Assessment, and Intervention. Pacific Grove, CA: Brooks/Cole, 1994:13–36.

32. Health care reform for Americans with severe mental illnesses: Report of the National Advisory Mental Health Council. Am J Psychiatry 1993;150:1447–1465.

33. Harding CM, Brooks GW, Ashikaga T, et al. The Ver-

mont longitudinal study of persons with severe mental illness: II. Long-term outcomes of subjects who retrospectively met DSM-III criteria for schizophrenia. Am J Psychiatry 1987;144:727–735.

34. Regier DA, Farmer ME, Rae DS, et al. One-month prevalence of mental disorders in the United States and sociodemographic characteristics: the Epidemiologic Catchment Area study. Acta Psychiatr Scand 1993;88:35–47.

35. Kessler RC, Berglund PA, Zhao S, et al. The 12-month prevalence and correlates of serious mental illness. In: Manderscheid RW, Sonnenschein MA, eds. Mental Health. United States Department of Health and Human Services publication (SMA)96–3098. Washington: Superintendent of Documents, US Government Printing Office, 1996:59–70.

36. Blazer DG, George LK, Hughes D. Schizophrenia symptoms in an elderly community population. In: Brody JA, Maddox GL, eds. Epidemiology and Aging. New York: Springer, 1988:134–149.

37. Jeste DV, Gladsjo JA, Lindamer LA, Lacro JP. Medical comorbidity in schizophrenia. Schizophr Bull 1996;2: 413–430.

38. Drake RE, Gates C, Whitaker A, Cotton PG. Suicide among schizophrenics: a review. Compr Psychiatry 1985;26:90–100.

39. Rabins PV, Harvis K, Koven S. High fatality rates of late-life depression associated with cardiovascular disease. J Affect Disord 1985;9:165–167.

40. Tsuang MT, Woolson RF, Fleming JA. Premature deaths in schizophrenia and affective disorders. Arch Gen Psychiatry 1980;37:979–983.

41. Barker PR, Manderscheid RW, Hendershot GE, et al. Serious Mental Illness and Disability in the Adult Household Population: United States, 1989. National Center for Health Statistics, Vital Health Statistics, 1992:218.

42. Talbott JA. The national plan for the chronically mentally ill: a programmatic analysis. Hosp Commun Psychiatry 1981;32:699–704.

43. Strahan GW. Prevalence of selected mental disorders in nursing and related care homes. In: Manderscheid RW, Sonnenschein MA, eds. Mental Health, United States, 1990. National Institute on Mental Health. Department of Health and Human Services Publication (ADM) 90–1708. Washington: US Government Printing Office, 1990:227–240.

44. Lacro JP, Jeste DV. Physical comorbidity and polypharmacy in older psychiatric patients. Biol Psychiatry 1994; 36:146–152.

45. Rodin G, Voshart K. Depression in the medically ill: an overview. Am J Psychiatry 1986;143:696–705.

46. Koran LM, Sox HC, Marton KI, et al. Medical evaluation of psychiatric patients. Arch Gen Psychiatry 1989;46: 733–740.

47. Dworkin RH. Pain insensitivity in schizophrenia: a neglected phenomenon and some implications. Schizophr Bull 1994;20:235–248.

48. Patt RB, Proper G, Reddy S. The neuroleptics as adjuvant analgesics. J Pain Symptom Manag 1994;9:446–453.

49. Miller MD, Paradis C, Houck PR, et al. Rating chronic medical illness burden in geropsychiatric practice and research: application of the Cumulative Illness Rating Scale (CIRS). Psychiatry Res 1992;41:237–248.

50. Parmelee PA, Thuras PD, Katz IR, Lawton MP. Validation of the Cumulative Illness Rating Scale in a geriatric residential population. J Am Geriatr Soc 1995;43:130–137.

51. Heaton RK, Drexler M. Clinical neuropsychological findings in schizophrenia and aging. In: Miller NE, Cohen GD, eds. Schizophrenia and Aging. New York: Guilford Press, 1987:145–161.

52. Davidson M, Haroutunian V. Cognitive impairment in geriatric schizophrenia patients. In: Bloom FE, Kupfer DJ, eds. Psychopharmacology: The Fourth Generation of Progress. New York: Raven Press, 1995:1447–1549.

53. Prohovnik I, Dwork A, Kaufman MA, Willson N. Alzheimer-type neuropathology in elderly schizophrenia patients. Schizophr Bull 1993;19:805–816.

54. Klapow JC, Evans J, Patterson TL, et al. Direct assessment of functional status in older patients with schizophrenia. Am J Psychiatry 1997;154:1022–1024.

55. Prager S, Jeste DV. Sensory impairment in late-life schizophrenia. Schizophr Bull 1993;19:755–772.

56. Meeks S, Carstensen LL, Stafford PB, et al. Mental health needs of the chronically mentally ill elderly. Psychol Aging 1990;5:163–171.

57. George LK, Blazer DG, Winfield-Laird I, et al. Psychiatric disorders and mental health service use in later life: evidence from the Epidemiologic Catchment Area Program. In: Brody JA, Maddox GL, eds. Epidemiology and Aging. New York: Springer, 1988:189–219.

58. Cohen CI, Sokolovsky J. Schizophrenia and social networks: Ex-patients in the inner city. Schizophr Bull 1978;4:546–560.

59. Lewine RRJ. Gender and schizophrenia. In: Tsuang MT, Simpson JC, eds. Handbook of Schizophrenia: Nosology, Epidemiology, and Genetics of Schizophrenia. 3rd ed. New York: Elsevier, 1988:379–398.

60. McGlashan TH, Bardenstein KK. Gender differences in affective, schizoaffective, and schizophrenic disorders. Schizophr Bull 1990;16:319–330.

61. Greenberg JS, Seltzer MM, Greenley JR. Aging parents of adults with disabilities: the gratifications and frustrations of later-life caregiving. Gerontologist 1993;33: 542–550.

62. Lefley HP. Family Caregiving in Mental Illness. Thousand Oaks, CA: Sage, 1996.

63. Mulsant BH, Stergiou A, Keshavan MS, et al. Schizophrenia in late life: elderly patients admitted to an acute care psychiatric hospital. Schizophr Bull 1993;19:709–721.

64. Selzer ML. The Michigan Alcoholism Screening Test: the quest of a new diagnostic instrument. Am J Psychiatry 1971;1:1653–1658.

65. Ewing JA. Detecting alcoholism: the CAGE questionnaire. JAMA 1984;252:1905–1907.

66. Rabins PV, Black B, German P, et al. The prevalence of psychiatric disorders in elderly residents of public hous-

ing. J Gerontol A Biol Sci Med Sci 1996;51:M319–M324.

67. National Institute on Mental Health. Outcasts on Main Street: Report of the Federal Task Force on Homelessness and Severe Mental Illness. Washington: US Department of Health and Human Services, Council on Homelessness, 1992.

68. Tessler RC, Dennis DL. A Synthesis of NIMH-Funded Research Concerning Persons Who Are Homeless and Mentally Ill. Rockville, MD: National Institute on Mental Health, 1989.

69. Cohen C, Onserud H, Monaco C. Outcomes for the mentally ill in a program for older homeless persons. Hosp Commun Psychiatry 1993;44:650–656.

CHAPTER 19

DOROTHY H. COONS AND NANCY L. MACE

Improving the Quality of Life in Long-Term Care

Our system of long-term care will face a tremendous challenge over the next several decades, with the predicted increase in the numbers of the old old in the population and of the elderly who will be afflicted with dementia. This chapter describes a number of the criteria that have been identified as essential to the establishment of therapeutic environments in long-term care settings and ways in which imaginative administrators and other personnel have created facilities that are positive and supportive and enable the elderly to live with dignity and satisfaction. It also suggests potential roadblocks to the implementation of such milieus and steps that can be taken to deal with or circumvent the barriers to change.

Fortunately, many positive changes in the care of older people have occurred since the era of the custodial county hospitals that housed the frail, indigent elderly in the 1930s and 1940s. Yet in traditional long-term facilities many of the practices still prevail, such as multiple occupancy sleeping areas, regimentation and rigid schedules, sterile environments, and limited opportunities for satisfying and enjoyable activities.

The decade ahead will be a crucial period in examining the methods and concepts that have shaped our system of long-term care. Some of the new approaches and ideas that have influenced a number of the better specialized dementia care units suggest ways long-term care in general can be improved. There is an urgent need for innovation, creativity, and openness to new ideas if facilities in long-term care are to enable the elderly to enjoy their final years (1).

QUALITY OF LIFE ISSUES

A number of criteria for providing a good quality of life for elderly residents of retirement homes and nursing facilities have emerged over the years as new and innovative programs were introduced (2).

Maintaining Identity

It is crucial that deliberate efforts be made to help each resident maintain a sense of person with history, feelings of worth, and a sense of achievement. For this to occur it is essential that staff become familiar with the history of each person and recognize his or her past in a number of ways. If residents themselves are unable to recall past events, family members can help staff by providing life histories or albums illustrating events in the person's life. Some facilities include residents' life histories in newsletters or display posters of their lives with pictures and stories.

Control Over One's Life

Most people prefer to have maximum control of their own lives, and yet the regimentation and rigid schedules in many long-term care facilities essentially strip residents of opportunities for decision making. This loss of control can be devastating and can lead to withdrawal, depression, anger, and/or resentment. Much of the regimentation becomes so much a pattern of operation that staff see no alternatives (3).

While alert older persons are usually able to make decisions about complex issues related to how they wish to live their lives, the person who is cognitively impaired also has preferences, although he or she may not be able to express them clearly. Even giving persons choices about what they will wear (perhaps a choice between two items) helps to give them a sense of having some control over their lives. Many of the difficult behaviors of persons with dementia occur when residents are forced to conform to schedules that are contradictory to their own lifestyles. For example, some people are early risers; others prefer to sleep late. If breakfast can be made available over several hours, the early morning hours become leisurely and relaxed instead of pressured and regimented. Bath schedules, too, should be made flexible to fit earlier life patterns of residents.

Many retirement homes have elected resident councils, but they have varying degrees of power and control over the life of a facility. The administrative staff members are the determining factor over how much influence the resident councils will have and how frequently their decisions will be accepted and implemented. In truly therapeutic milieus, staff members are strong advocates for residents, encouraging them to make decisions about life in the facility that often take precedence over those made by staff or governing boards (T Whyte, personal communication, 1992).

Continuation of Normal Social Roles

Role loss can be devastating for persons living in long-term care facilities. In younger life most persons assume a number of roles—family member, friend, social being, worker, learner, volunteer. Roles give meaning to each person's life and determine values and the way he or she will live. When meaningful roles are stripped from residents when they move to long-term care facilities and the only role that remains for them is that of sick old patient, life loses meaning and purpose.

The therapeutic and wellness-fostering facility makes every effort to provide access to normal social roles for residents. Opportunities are offered to create a welcoming and comfortable environment for families and friends from the community so as to enable the older person to continue relationships. Many social and educational events offer occasions to continue the roles of learner and social being. Many retirement homes and some nursing homes have a variety of volunteer activities and work tasks available for residents who are interested. The richness of such environments provides incentive for even frail elderly persons to function in normal and wholesome ways.

Right to Privacy

Few people question the need for privacy, and yet in some settings getting the job done on time takes priority over privacy. Having one's toileting needs announced in front of other residents can be very embarrassing to a sensitive person. One of the greatest indignities that elderly people face in some settings is being forced to share a room with a complete stranger. Because of the cost differential between single and double rooms, the trend is toward the latter. Pynoos and Regnier (4) cited this arrangement as the ultimate loss of privacy. Advocates for double or triple rooms claim that such arrangements help to prevent loneliness, yet they fail to recognize that forced relationships seldom result in friendships. Social spaces where activities and events occur enable residents to choose, as they would in the outside community, the friends with whom they feel compatible.

ROADBLOCKS TO GOOD QUALITY OF LIFE IN LONG-TERM CARE
Mixed Populations

One of the very serious problems that has plagued long-term care facilities for years is the wide mix in the degrees and types of impairment of residents. This presents a serious challenge to nursing homes and is a strong deterrent to the designing of a good quality of life for persons in need of care. In many facilities both the physically and the cognitively impaired are housed in the same unit. This presents many problems. The alert but physically impaired are often disturbed by the behaviors of those with dementia. The confused residents become more disoriented and agitated and often combative. The climate and ambiance of such a unit cannot accommodate the needs of either group.

Sterile Environments

Life in some long-term care settings consists almost solely of the absolute essentials of living— dressing, bathing, eating—and staff do not have the time or feel it is not essential to provide a more interesting life. In some of the more custodial settings staff make no effort to carry on conversations with residents while doing activities of daily living. Staff have been observed feeding residents, helping them dress, or bathing them without speaking to them during the entire activity except to give occasional instructions. Some nursing home chains actually discourage activities and social interactions between staff and residents through budget cutting. Because of limited staff, aides have so many people to care for that they can do nothing more than the bare essentials of caretaking. There are few or no diversions, entertaining events, or light-hearted exchange in some facilities. It is not surprising that residents in such settings withdraw, become depressed, or rebel against a life they find intolerable.

Staff Turnover

Nursing homes and especially dementia care units are increasing in staggering numbers in this country in an effort to meet the anticipated demand of the future. With this increase comes competition for staff. Even without this competition, however, staff turnover has been a serious problem in many facilities, sometimes because of the stress of the job and sometimes because of the lack of support, rewards, and job satisfaction employees receive. Because of this constant turnover staff are often inadequately trained in the principles of providing supportive care.

Physical Design

Physical design may have less effect on the quality of life in a facility than social relations, but it does have influence. Unfortunately, new facilities that resemble those of several decades ago are still being built. Designed after acute-care hospitals, they are stark and uninviting; long bare corridors are lined with rooms on either side; activity rooms are large and overwhelming;

walls have drab neutral colors; the blare of the intercom is confusing and disrupting; and the noise level is overwhelming. The message is of sickness. Many of the problems are a result of building codes that have gone unchanged for years (5). The regulations and the interpretation of regulations are interfering with the proper design and operation of many special care units.

Negative Management Methods

Few involved in long-term care would question that the quality of life in any facility is largely determined by the administrator. His or her attitudes and management methods influence not only the day-to-day operation but the general ambiance and quality of a setting. A number of methods, no longer considered productive and appropriate by management experts, can create an environment that is depressing and unwholesome for both staff and residents. For some administrators, fiscal issues take priority over quality of life even when the actions to improve quality of life do not create financial problems. Change does not occur without taking risks and trying new approaches. For traditional and conservative administrators, however, risk taking is unacceptable and unsafe (6). The hierarchical system in which orders are handed down from above and expected to be obeyed without question by direct service staff has unfortunately been in operation in many long-term care settings for years. This ignores the possibility that all staff may have knowledge and special skills that would benefit residents if they were allowed to use them. Some administrative personnel view evaluations as opportunities to criticize and reprimand staff with a total disregard of positive performances and skills they bring to the job. Management in some facilities fear change and much prefer that routines and practices remain consistent and unquestioned. Such a climate is an open opponent to innovation and creativity.

INNOVATIONS TO IMPROVE QUALITY OF LIFE
Dealing With the Problems of Mixed Populations

One of the innovations in specialized dementia care units that has led to the development of some really excellent facilities has been the establishment of graded units. Residents are carefully screened and placed in the unit that is designed for their level of impairment. Staff are well trained, and in some settings the physical environments are similar, so that as a resident becomes more impaired he or she can be transferred without trauma to an environment that is less active and more benign. If similar specialized units were implemented in nursing homes, it would resolve some of the very difficult and nontherapeutic situations that arise when populations range from the alert but physically impaired to the severely cognitively impaired.

Some retirement homes that have small populations of confused persons offer educational programs for alert persons to help them understand the changes that occur when residents become cognitively impaired and some of their difficulties. These homes also offer special small group activities specifically designed for those who are no longer able to cope with or enjoy large group activities.

Responding to Difficult Behaviors

One of the challenges that staff face in many settings is the difficult behaviors of residents. These behaviors may occur in persons with dementia, in those with physical or mental problems, or in alert and physically able persons who are angry or upset. Resident-to-staff violence is emotionally destructive to both residents and staff. It essentially reduces the staff's capacity to be affectionate and friendly. The violence, however, is inevitably caused by a negative environment and is therefore treatable. Many of the behaviors are normal reactions to situations that are blatantly disturbing. For a number of years physical restraints and excessive medication have been used to control behaviors. Fortunately, there is now a movement toward restraint-free environments and a careful monitoring of medications (7–9).

The management of problem behaviors is a topic that arises again and again in the operation of specialized units. The administration and staff of dementia units must accept the fact that tender loving care is not enough when working with cognitively impaired persons. The boredom and frustration in many such settings lead inevitably

to so-called difficult behaviors. All staff should be able to implement spontaneous activities that are distracting and diverting and that create a climate of fun and light-heartedness. For example, the period after the evening meal (the sundowning period) can be especially difficult. Residents may be searching for relatives or trying to escape to return home. If staff are prepared to improvise a simple exercise program or a sing-along, the attention of residents is quickly and easily drawn to the activity in progress.

Sharing snacks also creates feelings of warmth. For example, if a resident resists bathing, the staff person can suggest that they have juice and cookies together as soon as the bath is completed. This can be mentioned several times during the process of bathing to focus attention away from the activity that is causing the problem. As mentioned earlier, the elimination of rigid schedules in dementia units, such as breakfast times, bathing, and going to bed, can create a more relaxed environment that allows persons to continue habits and patterns of their earlier lives.

A Dynamic Program of Activities and a Full and Satisfying Life

If residents in long-term care are to continue in the normal social roles that gave meaning to their earlier lives, they need the opportunities and the options to become involved in a variety of activities and events as an ongoing part of the life of the facility. This in turn creates a sense of belonging and feelings of excitement and anticipation as new and interesting opportunities arise. The emphasis is on involvement and on being very much a part of the action rather than on sickness and losses. The following quotations of residents and a family member were taken from a weekly newsletter in one of the facilities that exemplifies a full life for residents (10).

"I don't think I will have my afternoon nap at all this week, I'm so busy with programs and meetings."

"One of these days I'll go to my daughter's for a rest. There is so much going on here."

A son said to his mother, "I should have looked at your appointment book to see if I could make an appointment with you, mom. You are busy all the time."

Such dynamic programs are not built on an occasional craft class. They offer opportunities for involvement throughout the day and are designed to enable residents to continue activities that provide continuity with their earlier lives. Good medical care is essential, but much more is needed if residents are to continue to live satisfying lives (11, 12).

Children in facilities add a delightful dimension to the lives of residents (13). In some retirement homes, residents are involved individually and with small groups of children, reading to them or sharing other activities. Some homes have established child care centers that enable the children and the elderly in retirement homes, nursing homes, and special dementia units to develop close relationships and spend time together almost daily (K Boling, personal communication, 1996). Teenage volunteers are now frequently trained to visit residents and share in activities.

Visiting pets have been a part of programs in a number of settings for years, but more often now live-in pets are accepted as a normal part of the life of a facility and a way to reduce loneliness and despair. One facility housing 80 residents has adopted, under the guidance of its physician, the Eden Alternative, a concept fostering the development of a habitat within the setting of a myriad of birds and animals and an abundance of plants and flowers (14). The program, which was initiated there, boasts a collection of 80 parakeets, 10 finches, 2 love-birds, 6 cockatiels, and 2 canaries in addition to 2 dogs, several cats, rabbits, and chickens. Children are also very much a part of the human habitat.

Clowning has been especially appealing in special Alzheimer's units that have children visiting frequently. Several staff and residents dress as clowns and do a variety of activities and performances with the small visitors.

Many older people who are cognitively impaired can still do or share tasks that were familiar to them when they lived in their own homes. Well-trained staff can involve residents by sharing such activities as bed making, dusting, working with food, or caring for plants. This not only gives residents feelings of usefulness but provides opportunities for them to have pleasant experiences with staff (15).

An innovative and risk taking director of an Alzheimer's unit in Michigan took nine residents from the facility to Florida on what a local newspaper labeled "a vacation from dementia." The success of the venture lay in the detailed planning and staffing. Eight staff members and volunteers accompanied the nine residents. The director's goal was that the residents experience "unbridled, abstract joy, however ethereal." The experience was so successful that other trips have followed (16; K Collins, personal communication, 1997).

In an effort to help residents of dementia units recall earlier events in their lives, their successes and achievements, and retain a sense of identity, some facilities hold self-esteem sessions, each with four or five residents. Personal memorabilia, scrapbooks, pictures, and newspaper articles can be used to help the group members recall incidents from their past. These meetings can also give residents an opportunity to discuss feelings about memory loss and other worries. The group sessions seem not only to relieve the concerns of residents but help them to continue to communicate and share thoughts and especially to maintain a sense of identity (A Robinson, G Gardner, personal communication, 1997).

Supportive Administrators

Because the administrator is usually the principal figure in determining the policies, structure, and organizational methods of a facility, it is crucial that he or she understand the role of an effective supervisory figure and the techniques for helping staff function effectively and get job satisfaction (17).

Hierarchical methods and punitive action are recognized as ineffective in helping staff to grow on the job and provide the best possible climate for older people. Even criticism can be given in ways that are positive, informative, and helpful. For example, if a staff person is having difficulty with a specific resident, he or she can be reprimanded; or the supervisor can suggest an approach that was successful with another resident.

The effective administrator shares information with staff members and involves them in decision making relative to their special responsibilities. In many situations the direct service staff are more knowledgeable about residents' interests, desires, and problems than are supervisory staff. The strong administrator sees joint planning and decision making as essential in helping staff to grow and commit to improving the quality of care.

Some change does occur without risks. Changes may be met with resistance from families or staff, or they may seem to conflict with state regulations. The wise administrator meets with potential resistors and gives the rationale for the changes. Some relatives, for example, may resist efforts to have restraints removed from a frail relative, fearing falls and injury. The new movement toward restraint-free facilities should be explained carefully to family members, and they should be reassured that special care and attention will be given to protect the person involved. Changes that seem to conflict with state regulations must be discussed with a state inspector before they are initiated. Frequently, when the inspector understands the purpose of the change, he or she can suggest ways in which it can be done in conformation with regulations.

The progressive and dynamic administrator is open to new ideas, methods, and innovations. The status quo is never viewed as satisfactory. He or she establishes a climate that enables staff members at all levels to feel comfortable in making suggestions for change. If the new idea is successful, it provides an occasion to give special recognition to the person who presented the idea and encourages others to be imaginative and creative. If the idea fails, it can provide an opportunity to consider alternatives. The failure should not lead to punitive action. Instead it should be made clear to staff that the administration values suggestions and is willing to take full responsibility if the ideas are unsuccessful.

Nurturing Staff

There are many reasons for nurturing staff. Personnel who are well treated and whose talents and abilities are recognized usually become more stable and less likely to leave a facility. Employees in long-term care facilities in large cities may have difficult personal lives and lack confidence, and yet they are often very good employees and deserve recognition. Direct service staff who are well treated and happy in their work usually create a positive and supportive relationship with residents (18).

In custodial and traditional settings, the only role available to direct service staff is that of caregiver. It is a limiting and frustrating role, and the job is often extremely demanding, with unrealistic time schedules imposed. In that situation the only goal is to get residents bathed, fed, or dressed or beds made. Good relations with residents are considered unimportant, in fact a waste of time.

In the therapeutic environment, staff members are encouraged to minimize the role of caregiver and instead become enablers, friends, and advocates. These roles require time. Helping older persons do as much as possible for themselves takes much more time that doing the task for them. Developing friendships also requires time to share experiences, ideas, information, and history (19, 20). In the more progressive facilities, all staff are encouraged to share activities with residents and to use their special talents. Direct service staff, housekeeping, and maintenance workers, for example, may have musical talents, craft skills, or other interests and abilities. If they are given time and training to work with small groups of residents, the lives of both residents and employees are enhanced.

The somber climate in many nursing home settings is symbolic of custodial care. Seldom is laughter heard, and there is little if any light-hearted repartee between residents and staff. Shared humor is an important element in facilities that provide a nurturing environment for both residents and staff.

There are many ways in which administrative staff can recognize abilities and successes of employees. Some give awards for jobs well done. Others give special recognition in stories about staff published in the units' regular newsletters. Some facilities videotape special events so that both residents and staff can see themselves and their achievements when the tapes are played.

Training Staff

Staff training methodology and content are extremely important for improving the quality of life in long-term care settings. The following topics are essential in an effective training series:

1. The aging process; potential changes as persons age; problems many elderly people face as a result of changes
2. An overview of dementia; the changes that occur over time and their possible effects on the person's ability to function
3. Criteria for designing therapeutic and health-fostering environments in long-term care settings
4. Communication skills and staff approaches
5. A discussion of possible causes of difficult behaviors; responding to the needs of the person to help reduce the frequency of difficult behaviors
6. Helping residents avoid dependency; enabling them to do as much as possible for themselves
7. The need for interesting and creative activities for elderly persons in all levels of care
8. Examining the physical environment for sensory cues, stimulation, and noninstitutional impact
9. Methods for designing a welcoming and involving program for families
10. Issues and methods essential for bringing about effective change
11. Problem-solving techniques
12. Methods for developing an effective and cohesive team of staff members that share information and are mutually supportive

Lectures are crucial for the dissemination of information and concepts, but other methods are needed to help staff understand new techniques and to change attitudes. For example:

1. A number of excellent videotapes demonstrate effective ways to help older people continue to function maximally, illustrate examples of interesting activities, and identify a variety of features of a therapeutic physical environment.
2. Exercises are especially useful in teaching skills and in changing attitudes and approaches. They can be designed to meet specific objectives. For example, an exercise

dealing with difficult behavior focuses first of all on a graphic description of the behaviors of a specific resident with whom staff are having problems. The second half of the exercise asks trainees to identify the strengths and needs of the same person and ways in which staff can build on the person's strengths and respond to his or her needs. The exercise is effective because of the changes in staff approaches in altering behaviors of alert persons as well as those with dementia.

A training series is most effective when all levels of staff are involved in the sessions. This enables persons to exchange ideas and experiences and develop a common understanding of the goals, methods, and concepts presented in the training sessions.

Noninstitutional Designs of Physical Environments

A number of new and attractive designs of facilities are replacing the traditional buildings that have dominated the field for years. Discarded are the long corridors, the huge, remote activity rooms, and the multiple-bed sleeping rooms.

One of the most creative designs for dementia facilities uses small cluster units surrounding an area for activities. The cluster contains six single bedrooms, a living and dining area, and a small kitchen (E Conard, personal communication, 1997). The homelike ambiance of each unit provides a relaxing, nonstressful environment. The small kitchen enables residents to work with food if they are able and interested.

Another design has single rooms surrounding an activities-dining-living area. Residents can leave their rooms and be drawn immediately to where activities are in progress. In therapeutic settings residents or their families are encouraged to furnish their rooms with personal furniture and memorabilia that give each person a sense of continuity and pride. Color cues and labels should be used throughout to help with orientation and area finding. To avoid the feeling of institution and sickness the stark whites and beiges, symbolic of acute care facilities, are discarded for tasteful homelike decorations, furniture, and accessories (21).

CONCLUSION

With the predicted increase in the number of elderly in need of care over the next several decades, we are faced with a formidable test of innovation in the United States and other countries to provide a life for mentally and physically impaired older persons that makes old age a reward and not an overwhelming burden. We will meet this challenge only with creativity and with a clearly defined focus that places a good quality of life as a primary objective in providing care for the elderly.

REFERENCES

1. Kosberg J, Garcia JL, Dulka IM. Ensuring the adequacy of long term care of AD patients: special challenges and advocacy mechanisms. Am J Alzheimer Dis 1997;12:3–9.
2. Coons DH, Mace NL. Quality of Life in Long-Term Care. New York: Haworth Press, 1996:3–16.
3. Lidz CW, Fischer L, Arnold RM. The Erosion of Autonomy in Long-Term Care. New York: Oxford University Press, 1992.
4. Pynoos J, Regnier V. Improving residential environments for the frail elderly: bridging the gaps between theory and application. In: Birren JE, Lubber JE, Rowe JC, Deutchman DE, eds. The Concept and Measurement of Quality of Life in the Frail Elderly. New York: Academy Press, 1991:91–117.
5. Hyde J. Special Care Units for People With Alzheimer's and Other Dementias: Consumer Education, Research, Regulatory, and Reimbursement Issues. Office of Technology Assessment OTA-H-543. Washington: US Government Printing Office, August 1992.
6. Rader J. Individualized Dementia Care. New York: Springer, 1995.
7. Mace NL The management of problem behaviors. In: Mace NL, ed. Dementia Care: Patient, Family, and Community. Baltimore: Johns Hopkins University Press, 1990:74–112.
8. Sloane PD, Rader J, Barrick AL, et al. Bathing persons with dementia. Gerontologist 1995;35:672–678.
9. Mace NL, Rabins PV. The 36-Hour Day. Baltimore: Johns Hopkins University Press, 1991.
10. Quotes. The Voice of the Village, Issue #813, January 24, 1997. Fir Park Village, Port Alberni, British Columbia, 1997 (weekly newsletter).
11. Hellen C. Alzheimer's Disease: Activity Focused Care. Boston: Andoner Medical, 1992.
12. Logsdon RG, Teri L. The pleasant events schedule—AD: psychometric properties and relationship to depression and cognition in Alzheimer's disease patients. Gerontologist 1997;37:40–45.
13. Friedman A, Robinson A. Wesley Hall: A Special Life. Innerimage Productions. Distributed by Terra Nova Films, Chicago, 1986 (film or videotape, 29 min).
14. Thomas WH. Life Worth Living: The Eden Alternative in Action. Acton, MA: Vander Wyk and Burnham, 1996.
15. Zgola JM. Therapeutic activity. In: Mace NL, ed. Dementia Care: Patient, Family, and Community. Baltimore: Johns Hopkins University Press, 1990;148–172.
16. Windsor S. A vacation from dementia. Ann Arbor (MI) News, June 4, 1995.
17. Coons DH. Improving the quality of care: the process of change. In: Coons DH, ed. Specialized Dementia Care Units. Baltimore: Johns Hopkins University Press, 1991; 25–35.
18. Walton M. The Deming Management Method. New York: Putnam, 1986.
19. Foner N. The Caregiving Dilemma: Work in an American Nursing Home. Berkeley, CA: University of California Press, 1994.
20. Pillemer KA. Solving the Frontline Crisis in Long-Term Care. Cambridge, MA: Frontline, 1996.
21. Cohen U, Weisman GD. Holding on to Home: Designing Environments for People With Dementia. Baltimore: Johns Hopkins University Press, 1991.

CHAPTER 20

REVA B. KLEIN AND JANICE E. KNOEFEL

Neurologic Problems in the Elderly

PARKINSON'S DISEASE

Movement disorders are a fascinating group of diseases and quite common among the elderly. Most practitioners have seen patients with Parkinson's disease and essential tremor and are quite familiar with the common symptoms they manifest. Treatment rationale has shifted as new medications became available. This section focuses on the principles of diagnosis, differential diagnosis, treatment approaches in early and late phases, and some theories of pathophysiology.

Idiopathic Parkinson's disease is one of the most prevalent neurodegenerative diseases encountered in the elderly. It can be very difficult to diagnose based solely on clinical grounds; therefore prevalence rates vary widely, from 10 to 405 per 100,000. The prevalence rate increases with age, also contributing to wide variations in estimates of prevalence (1).

The differential diagnosis of Parkinson's disease is extensive, and no confirmatory laboratory or radiologic tests are available. Among neurologists expert in movement disorders, the antemortem diagnosis is correct 75 to 85% of the time when confirmed by autopsy (2). In general, Parkinson's disease is an idiopathic, relentlessly progressive disorder with the hallmark findings of tremor, bradykinesia, rigidity, and postural instability. Other findings include dysautonomia, dementia, dysarthria, dysphagia, dystonia, sleep abnormalities, and an asymmetric presentation (3).

Briefly, parkinsonism can be classified as primary (idiopathic), secondary (acquired), here-dodegenerative, and multiple system degeneration (Parkinson's plus). Primary idiopathic Parkinson's disease is caused by loss of the pigmented dopamine-producing cells of the substantia nigra of the midbrain and confirmed at autopsy by the presence of Lewy bodies in the same distribution. The cause of cell loss is unknown (3).

Acquired Parkinson's can result from infections (postencephalitic, slow virus); medications, such as antipsychotics, antiemetics, reserpine, lithium (3), verapamil, diltiazem, valproate, and phenytoin; alcohol withdrawal (2); toxins (1-methyl-4-phenyl-1,2,3,6-tetrahydropyridine [MPTP], carbon monoxide, manganese, mercury, methanol, ethanol); vascular disease (multi-infarct state); trauma (pugilistic encephalopathy); tumors; normal pressure hydrocephalus; hepatocerebral degeneration; hypothyroidism; and parathyroid abnormalities (3).

Heredodegenerative disorders that can cause parkinsonian features include Huntington's disease, Wilson's disease, Hallervorden-Spatz disease, olivopontocerebellar and spinocerebellar degeneration (ataxia), and neuroacanthocytosis, among others. These are rare disorders accounting for 0.6% of the patients in this group (3).

The group classified as Parkinson's plus presents the greatest diagnostic challenge. There is much overlap and similarity among entities. Accurate diagnosis can take years, and even with autopsy, results may not be diagnostic. Detailed descriptions of each is beyond the scope of this discussion but Parkinson's plus should be considered in patients not responding to standard Parkinson's disease treatment and in patients presenting in an atypical clinical manner or deviating from the expected disease course. These include progressive supranuclear palsy (prominent ocular palsies), Shy-Drager syndrome (prominent autonomic dysfunction), striatonigral degeneration (prominent bulbar findings), parkinsonism-dementia-amyotrophic lateral sclerosis complex, corticobasal ganglionic degeneration (prominent apraxia and myoclonus), and diffuse Lewy body disease (thought to be an overlap between Parkinson's disease and Alzheimer's disease) (3).

There has been much written on the treatment of (idiopathic) Parkinson's disease and much controversy as to the best approach. Controversies being investigated include the concept of levodopa (the most effective symptomatic treatment available) as a neurotoxin adding to oxidative stress and cell death, then only contributing to the progression of disease; the antioxidant selegiline's ability to slow the progression of disease; long-acting levodopa carbidopa preparations or dopamine agonists delaying the onset of motor fluctuations and dyskinesias (consequences of long-term dopamine therapy); and dopamine receptor agonists differing in clinical effect because of specific target receptor properties (4). There has also been much work trying to identify patients with preclinical disease to improve outcome. So far there have not been established any criteria that are reliable before the onset of clinical signs, and often the diagnosis takes 5 years or more to confirm without autopsy. Biologic markers have not been defined (5).

Treatment can be divided into two main phases. First is the early stage with more subtle findings and perhaps an uncertain diagnosis. Second is the late phase, in which complications of therapy are evident, requiring a different treatment strategy.

Traditionally levodopa has been the mainstay treatment of choice for early Parkinson's symptoms. It is easy to start and monitor, and more important, there is a dramatic effect on symptoms. However, there is some evidence suggesting that levodopa may be neurotoxic to dener-

vated nigrostriatal dopamine pathways and may hasten long-term consequences of therapy. Dopamine receptor agonists (previously reserved for the onset of motor fluctuations) are now thought to bypass this problem. Agonists act on postsynaptic dopamine receptors and are therefore independent of dopamine synthesis in the degenerating presynaptic neurons in the substantia nigra. They were found to contribute only infrequently to complications of long-term therapy (motor fluctuations and dyskinesias). By initiating monotherapy early in the disease, it is possible to delay the use of levodopa, decreasing the overall total exposure to levodopa and reducing motor complications. Receptor agonists may not relieve symptoms as well as dopamine, and levodopa should be introduced once the level of impaired function or other symptoms become intolerable to the patient. There are many agents with differing receptor properties and thus differing side effect profiles and effectiveness. The three most widely used agents are bromocriptine (D1 antagonist, D2 agonist), pergolide (weak D1 agonist, D2 agonist), and pramipexole (D2 agonist only). Ropinirole is a newly released D2 agonist. The stimulation of D1 is thought to contribute to dyskinesias and the stimulation of D2 to reduce the symptoms of Parkinson's. Pramipexole and ropinirole, second-generation agonists, are not ergot derivatives, which limits the rare but serious adverse effects (edema, Raynaud's phenomenon, pleuropulmonary and retroperitoneal fibrosis) seen in the other agents. Other less worrisome side effects of all of these agents include nausea, dizziness, somnolence, orthostatic hypotension, hallucinations, and dyskinesias. In patients over 70 years of age, levodopa monotherapy can safely be initiated, keeping doses low to avoid the more common side effect of hallucinations (6).

Managing the late complications of Parkinson's disease remains one of the most challenging issues in neurologic disease. Almost all patients on chronic levodopa therapy eventually develop these complications. Motor responses include end-dose wearing-off, on-off, peak-dose dyskinesias, dystonias, and freezing. Behavioral and psychiatric disorders include dementia, depression, hallucinations, psychosis, and sleep disorders (7).

Motor fluctuations are thought to reflect the extent of degeneration in the dopamine systems. As the disease progresses, there are fewer and fewer neurons available to process exogenous levodopa and convert it to usable dopamine. In advanced disease the pattern of response to levodopa shifts to short duration. This is most readily seen in the wearing-off effect at the end of the dose and with dyskinesias and dystonias at the peak dose. Wearing off is predictable, occurring most often 2 to 4 hours after a dose. Treatment strategies include adding a dopamine agonist, lowering levodopa doses, shortening the interval dosing of levodopa, and using sustained-release preparations. Dyskinesias usually reflect too much dopamine activity and dystonias, too little. Dyskinesias often respond to lowering the levodopa dose, adding a dopamine agonist (which allows a lower levodopa dose), and using long-acting preparations. Dystonias are mostly an off phenomenon, especially in the early morning hours, when there is commonly a long dose interval following the bedtime dose or a sustained-release preparation. These respond readily to giving levodopa either as an additional dose or as an increased dose. On-off fluctuations are much more difficult to treat. They are sudden and unpredictable. The patient shifts abruptly from a state of adequate treatment or overtreatment to a state of undertreatment. Adding or increasing doses of levodopa may help the off state but also increases dyskinesias. The goal is to smooth out treatment response. Sometimes small doses with the same total daily dose at very frequent intervals (even as much as 60 to 90 minutes) can help. Liquid preparations may also help, but they must be prepared at home by crushing large numbers of tablets on a daily basis. As a practical matter both approaches become difficult (7). Sustained-release levodopa is also quite useful in smoothing out treatment response, although some patients miss the dramatic surge of motor response seen with the immediate-release formula.

Psychiatric complications may be even more debilitating. Often psychosis, confusion, agitation, hallucinations, and delusions respond to decreasing levodopa and/or dopamine agonists as well as decreasing or discontinuing anticholinergics, amantadine, or selegiline. Treatment with low doses of atypical neuroleptics is also helpful (8). Underlying precipitants of mental status changes should also be sought. These include acute infections, metabolic changes, new strokes, or tumors. Dementia occurs in 18 to 70% of patients and reflects both disease severity and advanced age. Psychiatric side effects occur most frequently in demented patients. Depression, which is found in about 40 to 60% of Parkinson's patients, correlates with duration of disease and with periods of being off. Treatment is standard antidepressant therapy and adjustment of Parkinson's disease treatment to minimize the off times (7).

There are surgical treatments for Parkinson's disease. Thalamotomy targets patients with debilitating tremor who fail to respond to pharmacologic therapy. Patients without gait abnormalities or bradykinesia respond best. Pallidotomy helps with bradykinesia, tremor, rigidity, and dyskinesias induced by levodopa. In this procedure the globus pallidus is stereotactically ablated unilaterally. Bilateral destruction, while very effective for dyskinesias, can induce cognitive deficits. Deep brain stimulation of the thalamus, subthalamic nuclei, or globus pallidus targets severe tremor. Most controversial is the transplantation of tissue from the adrenal medulla or mesencephalon (the dopamine-producing cells). These can be allografts (adult or fetal, adrenal or mesencephalic) or autografts from the adrenal. Clinical consensus regarding efficacy of this treatment is lacking (7).

Another approach with obvious benefit is to alter the natural course of the disease instead of just treating symptoms. This approach is under intense investigation, centering on theories of cause. Oxidative stress causing the release of cytotoxic free radicals leading to cell death is the focus. Stopping this reaction with antioxidants providing neuroprotection has been variably successful. One study looked at both tocopherol (a component of vitamin E that scavenges free radicals) and selegiline (a monoamine oxidase B inhibitor). In this initial study there was no effect from the tocopherol, but selegiline 10 mg per day delayed the onset of disability in Parkinson's disease (9). Subsequent studies did not find any effect on disease progression itself, and in fact there was no difference in levels of disability after several years between treated and untreated patients. However, the early symptomatic effects of the drug were confirmed, showing slowing in the progression of signs and symptoms. Another advantage in the early use of selegiline is the lowered requirement for levodopa. In this manner both the dopamine agonists and monoamine oxidase B inhibitors were found to delay progression of symptoms. Low doses of levodopa may actually be neuroprotective, while the higher doses may be neurotoxic. To summarize the neuroprotective approach: begin selegiline at the time of diagnosis, begin dopamine agonists once bothersome symptoms consistently occur, and add levodopa only when symptoms cause functional disability or great concern to the patient (10). Keep in mind that the late complications of therapy discussed earlier occur in almost all patients within approximately 5 years of starting levodopa therapy (8).

Questions regarding the use of amantadine in the treatment of Parkinson's disease often arise. The mechanism of action is unknown, and its benefits were discovered by chance. It seems to improve rigidity and bradykinesia. The side effects are similar to those of anticholinergics, causing impairment of memory, hallucinations, dry mouth, constipation, and urinary retention. In addition, amantadine can lead to ankle edema and livedo reticularis. Anticholinergics were used in the past in attempts to restore the balance between dopamine and acetylcholine and help raise the dopamine available in the synapse. They were somewhat helpful only for tremor. In general, the adverse effects of these medications outweigh the slight potential benefit, and they are rarely used to treat Parkinson's disease (11).

Essential tremor is thought by some to be the most common movement disorder. There is considerable controversy regarding its relation, if any, to Parkinson's disease. Patients with tremor are often told they have Parkinson's disease, even in the absence of the other cardinal motor signs needed for diagnosis. One large study (12) of 678 patients looked at the relation between essential tremor and other movement disorders, including Parkinson's disease. The researchers

defined essential tremor as "characterized by postural and kinetic tremor of the hands, head, and other body parts." They found a family history of tremor in 60% of patients. The body parts effected were the hands 90%, head 50%, voice 30%, legs 15%, and chin 15%. Of these patients 6.1% also had Parkinson's disease, which is a higher frequency than they found in the general population. It is controversial whether essential tremor is a risk factor for Parkinson's disease. Treatment of essential tremor with propranolol and primidone was found to be effective in only 40% of patients. Benzodiazepines are less effective (diazepam has not been studied; clonazepam was ineffective; and alprazolam was effective, thought to be from a sedating effect). Methazolamide, which inhibits carbonic anhydrase, was reported helpful by some patients but was not found to be effective in double-blind placebo trials (12). One study found the calcium channel blocker nimodipine to be effective in some patients (8 out of 15 showed improvement) (13). Deep-brain stimulation of the thalamus has been shown to control both essential tremor and the tremor of Parkinson's disease in 12-month follow-up (14).

HEADACHES

Headache is an extremely prevalent complaint among patients in general and among the elderly as well. Some studies show a prevalence of 55% in women and 45% in men aged 65 years and older. However, the demographics change as the population ages, with so-called benign headaches becoming less frequent and the likelihood of underlying disease increasing (15).

Headaches can be thought of as two broad categories of primary and secondary disorders. The primary disorders include migraine, cluster, tension, and hypnic headaches. Secondary headaches have causes such as mass lesions, temporal arteritis, medication, trigeminal neuralgia, postherpetic neuralgia, systemic disease, stroke, and Parkinson's disease. In general, the onset of headache is likely to be a primary disorder in the young patient and a secondary disorder in the elderly (16). One exception to this seems to be tension type headache, which increases in the elderly, perhaps related to the increased incidence of accompanying cervical osteoarthritis and/or depression (17). Headaches related to diseases of the eyes, ears, nose, sinuses, teeth, jaw, and face in general do not appear to be statistically different between younger and older patients (18).

Tension type headache is the more common complaint in the elderly and may also be described as muscle contraction headache. This often starts early in life but persists into old age, becoming chronic, more than the other primary headache disorders. New-onset tension headaches in the elderly are not common. Symptoms often include recurrent vague complaints of neck stiffness extending to the temples and forehead (15). These can be accompanied by photophobia, phonophobia, or nausea. Physical activity does not usually worsen symptoms. Treatment can be nonpharmacologic (relaxation, biofeedback) or pharmacologic. Drug therapy is usually effective with a tricyclic antidepressant (amitriptyline), β-blocker (propranolol), calcium channel blocker, or nonsteroidal anti-inflammatory (15, 16). These agents work best when used as prophylactic agents and can be used in much lower doses in the elderly patient, allowing several weeks for effect (15).

Hypnic (induced by sleep) headaches are rare, considered a primary disorder, and have the unique characteristic of having their onset in the older population (usually 65 to 84 years old). These are diffuse and throbbing and often awaken the patient at the same time every night. They resemble cluster headache in this respect but fail to exhibit the accompanying autonomic symptoms. They can last up to an hour and may be associated with REM (rapid eye movement) sleep. They often respond well to lithium 300 mg at bedtime, but a higher dose may be necessary if they recur (16). The mechanism of action may be related to enhanced serotonergic effect on the circadian rhythm in this cyclic disorder (19).

In contrast, cluster headaches are most often unilateral, periorbital or temporal, severe and with prominent autonomic features (16). They can last up to several hours and occur at any interval from every other day to 8 times in one day and can last weeks or months. Autonomic symptoms include conjunctival injection, lacrimation, nasal congestion, rhinorrhea, sweating, miosis, and ptosis. Most often these occur in men, having onset at age 20 to 40. Onset in the elderly is most common among women (15). Even with onset in the young, they tend to persist into old age or may recur after a long remission (16). For an acute attack, 100% oxygen 7 L per minute for 15 minutes can be an effective short-term therapy (15). Prophylactic agents include verapamil 80 mg 2 to 3 times a day, prednisone 20 mg twice a day, lithium 300 mg twice a day, methysergide 4 to 8 mg per day, and valproic acid (15, 16). A trial of at least 3 to 4 weeks should be given before switching agents (15). Other therapies include nerve blocks and ophthalmic nerve rhizotomy (16).

Migraine is usually found in the young and is quite rare in the elderly. Attacks tend to decrease in both frequency and severity with age. They resolve completely in some postmenopausal women. Menopause triggers their onset in about 10% of women. Symptoms are characterized by throbbing unilateral recurring attacks of pain lasting up to several days. Often they are accompanied by nausea, vomiting, photophobia, and phonophobia. They are made worse by physical activity. There may (classic) or may not (common) be an aura consisting of neurologic symptoms such as numbness, dizziness, blind spots, or scintillating scotomas (15). In patients who have an aura, the headache may eventually disappear altogether, leaving only the aura; this is termed aura without headache, migraine sine headache, or late-life migraine equivalent. Rarely, these present for the first time in the elderly and have to be differentiated from transient ischemic attacks, other vascular disorders, and seizures (16). In general, a transient ischemic attack lasts less than 15 minutes, while a migraine equivalent often persists beyond 20 minutes (15). Another pattern seen in the elderly is for migraine to evolve into chronic daily headache. Treatment can be aimed at aborting an acute attack with a nonsteroidal anti-inflammatory, vasoconstrictive (ergot alkaloids such as sumatriptan), or antiemetic (metoclopramide, chlorpromazine) medication. All of these must be used with extreme caution in the elderly because of their potential for severe side effects. If attacks are frequent and debilitating, prophylactic therapy should be initiated. The most efficacious agents include antidepressants (amitriptyline), β-blockers (propranolol), and calcium channel blockers (verapamil). Again, it is necessary to watch the side effect profiles in the elderly, especially with concomitant medical illness (15, 16).

Any elderly patient presenting with a headache for the first time or with a change in the character of the headache should be worked up for a secondary organic cause. Mass lesions, which form with increasing frequency, are most often subdural hematomas or tumors, either primary or metastatic. The most frequent primary tumors are gliomas, meningiomas, and pituitary adenomas. Metastatic lesions are most commonly from lung, breast, melanoma, or colon (16). Other symptoms that may predate the headache include vomiting, change in mental status (confusion, drowsiness, change in personality), and seizures (15). The pattern of pain is highly variable, depending on tumor size, location, and intracranial pressure. It may be worse on rising, awaken the patient from sleep, or worsen with cough or other Valsalva maneuvers. Subdural hematomas present in a similar manner but because of their extra-axial location are less likely to produce focal deficits. There may or may not be a history of trauma. Trauma is less likely in advanced age, during which there is more likely to be cerebral atrophy and thus a greater potential for spontaneously tearing bridging veins (16).

Giant cell or temporal arteritis is always a consideration in an older patient with a new headache. The headache is nonspecific, and often this is difficult to diagnose. Classically, there is temporal artery hardening, transient monocular blindness, jaw claudication, accompanying polymyalgia rheumatica, and elevated erythrocyte sedimentation rate. However, all of these are present in extreme variability, and all may even be absent. The diagnosis is made by a temporal artery biopsy. Skip lesions may be present, so a long segment of the temporal artery is needed, and even then, up to two thirds can be negative. Other blood vessels that can be affected include the aortic arch, the coronaries, the carotids, and the vertebrals, leading rarely to stroke, aortic rupture, or myocardial infarct. Intracranial arteries are typically spared and intraorbital branches most likely affected. The optic nerve is often involved as well, causing an acute ischemic optic neuropathy. Central retinal artery occlusion can cause a retrobulbar optic neuropathy. If untreated, bilateral blindness often ensues. The treatment consists of oral steroids, which can be started even before a biopsy is performed. In severe cases a dose of prednisone as high as 120 mg per day is needed. The dose is titrated and tapered according to the patient's response, as determined by the erythrocyte sedimentation rate. Side effects of the steroids include compression fractures, myopathy, psychosis, immunosuppression, and diabetes (20).

Other cerebrovascular disorders can cause headache. These include stroke, aneurysm, arteriovenous malformation, carotid dissection, intracranial hemorrhage, and sudden severe hypertension. Treatment of the underlying cause alleviates the headache (15).

Medications can induce headaches or exacerbate underlying headaches. The most common precipitants are alcohol, nitroglycerin, hormones (birth control pills, estrogen replacement), caffeine, and theophylline. Rebound headache can occur with opioids, aspirin, acetaminophen, barbiturates, ergot alkaloids, and caffeine. Nonsteroidal anti-inflammatories are thought not to be a cause of rebound headache (16).

Other neurologic conditions that can cause headache include trigeminal neuralgia, postherpetic neuralgia, and Parkinson's disease. Systemic disease contributing to secondary headaches in the elderly include Lyme disease, acute and chronic Epstein-Barr infection, hypoxia, hypercarbia, sleep apnea, severe anemia, hypercalcemia, and dialysis (16).

Type, pattern, cause, course, and prognosis of headache in the elderly are different from those in the younger population. A secondary cause must be pursued more vigorously in new-onset headaches and the side effect profiles of medications used for treatment watched vigilantly. There is at least one headache syndrome unique to the elderly, the hypnic headache.

SEIZURES

A seizure is an abnormal electrical discharge of neurons in the central nervous system. Epilepsy is recurrent seizures. There is generally a bimodal peak of incidence occurring first in infancy and childhood and again in the elderly. The incidence remains stable throughout adult life at approximately 15/100,000 per year, beginning to increase about age 50. By age 60 it reaches 50/100,000 and by 75 it is 75/100,000 per year (21). This is in large part due to a shift in causation from congenital anomalies and inborn errors of metabolism to structural and toxic causes. The most common cause in the elderly is cerebrovascular disease followed by tumor, trauma, and toxic or metabolic causes, including drugs and alcohol (22). Other causes include infections of the nervous system, dementia and degenerative disorders, anoxia, and cerebral amyloid angiopathy (21).

Seizures may be partial when they originate unilaterally or generalized when they originate bilaterally. Partial seizures are further subclassified as simple, with preservation of level of consciousness, or complex, with altered mental status. Either type of partial seizure can generalize (23). Partial seizures are more prevalent in the elderly, constituting 45 to 80% of seizure type compared with 9% to 50% for generalized seizures (22). Classification is important for determination of underlying causation, establishing prognosis, and choosing an appropriate treatment.

The differential diagnosis of seizures in the elderly includes transient ischemic attacks, syncope, drop attacks, transient global amnesia, psychiatric disorders, and sleep disorders. General guidelines may help differentiate these overlapping and similar events. Symptoms usually progress faster in an ischemic attack than in other conditions; syncope may precipitate an anoxic seizure; drop attacks often have an electroencephalogram (EEG) with a normal interictal pattern; transient global amnesia has a long duration of isolated memory deficit; new-onset psychiatric disorders in the elderly are exceedingly rare; and sleep disorders often can be confirmed with video polysomnography (23).

A thorough workup should include a thorough history to help classify the event, determine risk factors for stroke, and note any trauma. The medical history should include diabetes and other chronic diseases and the use of alcohol and drugs including prescription, over-the-counter, and illicit agents. A careful physical and neurologic examination helps to identify causative factors and look for focal deficits of the nervous system. Metabolic screen should include, at a minimum, electrolytes, blood urea nitrogen and creatinine, glucose, calcium, magnesium, and toxic screen.

The preferred neuroimaging is magnetic resonance imaging owing to its sensitivity, alleviating the need for iodinated contrast (which in rare instances can precipitate status epilepticus) and allowing detailed analysis of the temporal lobes, a frequent site of seizure (21).

EEG is more problematic in determining the diagnosis than one might imagine. There are some characteristic patterns, such as frontal intermittent rhythmic delta activity (FIRDA), seen in parasagittal meningiomas, and periodic lateralized epileptiform discharges (PLEDs), seen following a stroke; however, by and large specific patterns are more helpful in children. In addition, characteristic changes associated with aging can add to the confusion. Generalized slowing may be associated with normal aging as well as an increased number of focal abnormalities (21). Another age-associated change of uncertain significance is bursts of temporal slowing, often only on the left (22). EEGs are helpful in the evaluation of nonconvulsive status presenting as confusion, of possible metabolic encephalopathies, and of suspected psychogenic seizures when concurrent video monitoring can be used (23). Lumbar puncture to rule out meningitis or encephalitis is indicated in the presence of fever and no other discernible cause of seizures. Otherwise routine use of cerebrospinal fluid analysis is not recommended (23).

Approximately half of new-onset seizures in the elderly are thought to be related to cerebrovascular disease. Early single seizures do not appear to be a risk factor for later epilepsy but instead are related to the acute cerebral event. Later-onset seizures are most likely related to structural changes and are associated with a higher incidence of developing epilepsy (22). Strokes most likely to be associated with seizures include hemispheric cortical ischemic strokes, multilobar lesions, embolic strokes affecting the cerebral cortex, intracerebral hemorrhages, and subarachnoid hemorrhage. Small-vessel lacunar infarcts, subcortical infarcts, and posterior strokes are rarely associated with seizures (21).

Brain tumors are the next most common cause of seizures in the elderly. These include primary neoplasms as well as metastatic disease. Seizure may be the presenting manifestation in as many as 20% of cases. Metastases to the brain most often come from lung, breast, and melanoma. Pathophysiology includes necrosis, inflammation, mass effect, ischemia, and local membrane effects. Most often seizures are focal, with or without generalization. Occasionally, frontal-lobe tumors present as status epilepticus (21).

Toxic and metabolic disorders are an important consideration in the evaluation of new-onset seizures. Underlying factors to rule out are non-ketotic hyperglycemia, hypoglycemia, renal failure, hyponatremia, anoxia, and drug-induced causes. The latter is an especially important issue in the elderly because of age-associated changes in pharmacodynamics and increased sensitivity to epileptogenic properties of various drugs. Medications to beware of include penicillin, cephalosporins, imipenem, ciprofloxacin, theophylline, meperidine, intravenous iodinated contrast, lidocaine, antipsychotics, tricyclic antidepressants, bupropion, and lithium (21).

Many degenerative neurologic diseases are associated with seizures, the most common being dementia of the Alzheimer's type. These usually generalized tonic-clonic seizures occur in about 10% of patients. These may be associated with overall worsening of neurologic status and seem to be most common in the familial younger-onset forms of the disease. Myoclonus is frequently associated as well. Other forms of dementia can also exhibit epileptiform activity.

There are several general principles of treatment to keep in mind when initiating therapy in the elderly. There are age-related factors affecting drug absorption, volume of distribution, metabolism, and excretion. The best approach is to start with one agent, begin at a low dose, and titrate slowly with frequent clinical follow-up (22). Seizure control, not necessarily therapeutic ranges of drug levels, should be the end point of dosing. Sometimes control can be accomplished with a low drug level. Clinical response is far more important than the drug level (23).

There are many antiepileptic drugs available once the decision to treat has been made. Which agent to choose depends on the type of seizure and the side effect profile. Phenytoin (Dilantin) is indicated for partial and secondarily generalized tonic-clonic seizures. Side effects include nystagmus, drowsiness, ataxia, diplopia, and in very long term use, gingival hyperplasia, coarsening of facial features, and hirsutism. Dosing can be once daily, usually at bedtime. Carbamazepine (Tegretol) is also indicated for partial and secondarily generalized tonic-clonic seizures. Side effects include rash, drowsiness, blurred vision, diplopia, headache, ataxia, nausea and vomiting, and transient leukopenia. Occasionally severe agranulocytosis with severe neutropenia can persist, in which case the drug must be discontinued. Valproate (Depakote, Depakene) is approved for absence or multiple seizure types but has been found to be efficacious for partial and secondarily generalized tonic-clonic seizures. Side effects include drowsiness, nausea, vomiting, thrombocytopenia, liver failure, and hyperammonemia even with normal liver functions that can cause encephalopathy. Phenobarbital is useful also in partial and generalized tonic-clonic seizures, but cognitive side effects make it less tolerable. These include sedation, poor concentration, changes in behavior, and depression (24).

There are several newer agents on the market. Felbamate (Felbatol) was approved for monotherapy or add-on therapy in the treatment of partial and generalized tonic-clonic seizures but has been associated with serious or fatal aplastic anemia. It is in use for seizures refractory to all other first-line antiepileptic drugs. Gabapentin (Neurontin) is approved only for adjunctive therapy in refractory partial and secondarily generalized seizures but has had some use as monotherapy as well. There is no hepatic metabolism and no effect on hepatic enzymes, and therefore it does not affect other antiepileptic drugs. Side effects are drowsiness, ataxia, fatigue, and nystagmus. These are usually transient and mild, making this a very well tolerated medication (24). Lamotrigine (Lamictal) is another newly released drug approved for adjunctive therapy for partial seizures in adults. It is associated with potentially life-threatening dermatologic syndromes but is usually well tolerated and effective. Topiramate (Topamax) and tiagabine (Gabitnil) are two additional newly approved drugs for adjunctive treatment of partial seizures in adults with as yet little general experience in the treatment of seizures in the elderly.

There is a multicenter clinical trial now under way to determine the effectiveness and side effects of carbamazepine, gabapentin, and lamotrigine as monotherapy for seizures in adults aged 65 and over. Until the results of that trial are known, the best recommendation for antiepileptic drug selection is to consider the individual characteristics of the patient and seizure type. In general, carbamazepine, valproate, and phenytoin should be considered for monotherapy. Our preference is in that order.

GAIT DISORDERS

Gait disorders are critical to evaluate thoroughly (25–27). There are many neurologic causes of gait disturbance in general and many specific to the elderly. In fact, there are some changes in gait patterns due only to the aging process. Whether to deem these pathologic is the subject of a debate. The important issue is the effect on the patient's functional ability and quality of life. The first and perhaps the most significant is the issue of falling. This often makes the difference between living independently and the need for institutionalization. Up to 40% of nursing home admissions cite falls or instability as a contributing factor in placement (28). In persons over 65 years of age, about 30% fall in the space of a year (25). About 5% of these result in a fracture (26). Sequelae of unintentional injury are the sixth leading cause of death in people over age 65 (25). Even without injury, falls often lead to fear of falling, which in turn leads to restricting activities with loss of mobility and independence (26). The cost in mortality and morbidity is enormous, with the annual cost of acute care

alone for fall-related fractures estimated to be about $10 billion (25).

Nonneurologic causes of falls include syncope, arrhythmias, orthostatic hypotension, and a general decline in musculoskeletal function (26). The neurologic causes are even more prevalent. These include seizures, stroke, Parkinson's disease, Alzheimer's disease, myelopathy, cerebellar degeneration, tumors, hydrocephalus, and neuropathies. In one prospective study a potentially treatable cause was found in one third of the patients admitted consecutively to a neurology service with the chief complaint of difficulty walking (27).

Of course it seems prudent to try to identify certain risk factors for falling before the event occurs. These can be thought of in terms of intrinsic factors (the patient's physical condition and activity) and extrinsic (environmental factors). Intrinsic factors making a fall likely include visual problems, vestibular abnormalities, decreases in proprioception, cervical degeneration, peripheral neuropathy, dementia, musculoskeletal disorders, foot disorders, orthostatic hypotension, and medication. Environmental factors include lighting, floor surfaces and thresholds, stairs, kitchen setup, bathroom adaptations, entrances, clutter, and footwear. About half of the elderly who fall do so repeatedly. Once risk factors are identified, modifications can be made to reduce these hazards (28).

While the list of causative factors in gait disturbance is long, there seems to be a final common pathway leading to an actual fall. Studies indicate the most likely changes to contribute to a fall are decline in walking speed and stride length. This end point can occur both with pathologic states and with age-related physiologic changes. The effect of age seems to be most directly related to loss of muscle strength. In fact, regular exercise to increase strength may be able to stop the decrease in walking speed (29). Of the many neurologic diseases affecting gait, most affect the stride length. There is also a well-described pattern, known as the senile gait, common to many patients with neurologic impairments affecting gait. It is described as stooped posture, decreased stride and speed, reduced arm swing, increased double stance time (both feet on the floor at once), loss of normal heel-toe sequencing, and decreased hip and knee rotation (30). Gait disorders are not an inevitable result of aging, and the senile gait may indicate very subtle disease in the extrapyramidal, pyramidal, frontal, or peripheral nervous system (31).

Peripheral neuropathy is a general term for dysfunction of the peripheral nerve. There are many causes of such dysfunction, but in developed countries the most common is related to diabetes mellitus. About half of the diabetics over 60 have some peripheral neuropathy, while 10% of nondiabetics have neuropathy. The other neuropathies are most often due to alcohol, chronic lung disease, monoclonal gammopathy, neoplasm, medications (Dilantin, lithium, isoniazid, vincristine), renal disease, thyroid disease, and vitamin B_{12} deficiency (32). Overall, about 20% of elderly have some form of peripheral neuropathy (33, 34).

Peripheral neuropathy, an often overlooked cause of falls, is thought to be directly related to loss of somatosensory function. This system, along with the visual and vestibular systems, is instrumental in allowing people to remain upright. In one study more than 50% of patients with peripheral neuropathy fell each year (32).

Proprioception is critical to unipedal stance and walking on uneven surfaces, especially if vision is impaired. Normally a person should be able to balance on one foot for at least 10 seconds, but those with neuropathy were found to be able to do this for less than 4 seconds (32). Tests of unipedal balance appear to be even more sensitive than the Romberg in detecting peripheral neuropathy (34). In testing vibration, a 128-Hz tuning fork should be used, with the normal being able to detect the sensation at the metatarsophalangeal joint for at least 10 seconds (32). Some studies indicate that loss of proprioception is a part of normal aging and not a reliable indicator of neuropathy. Light touch and pain loss are thought to be more reliable indicators of pathology. Ankle jerks are absent in neuropathy but may also be absent in as many as 70% of normal aged individuals (35).

Intervention is aimed first at correcting the underlying cause of neuropathy, such as thyroid or vitamin deficiency. In diabetes it is adequate

glycemic control. This is not only to maximize nerve conduction velocities but to prevent the vascular compromise to nerves as well. It was found that with close monitoring, three or more daily injections of insulin lowered the incidence of neuropathy by 60%, compared with one or two injections in controls. Autonomic neuropathies from diabetes also contribute to falls with orthostatic hypotension, arrhythmias, and silent myocardial infarctions (33). Other interventions include physical and occupational therapy instruction in compensatory strategies with vision, adaptive equipment, environmental modifications, proper shoes and orthotics, and balance and strengthening exercises (32).

Cervical spondylosis is a significant cause of gait disturbance and falls in the elderly. Although it is not always clinically significant, radiologic evidence can be seen in more than 80% of those over 55 years (36). Caused by degenerative disc disease, it can lead to myelopathy and radiculopathy. It usually presents with intermittent neck pain that is very responsive to modification of activity, immobilization, exercise, and medications. If neurologic symptoms do occur, magnetic resonance imaging of the spine is indicated. Surgical intervention is reserved for those with severe intractable pain or progressive neurologic deterioration (37).

Myelopathy with upper motor neuron signs (spasticity, hyperreflexia, up-going toes, and occasionally bowel and bladder incontinence) is the more serious consequence, but this too is often responsive to conservative measures. Even with surgery and an initial improvement, functional outcome in myelopathy declines over time as the natural course progresses. The natural course is highly variable; some patients have a mild protracted course, while others have progressive disability. Overall, 30 to 50% improved with conservative therapy (37).

Radiculopathy is characterized by pain, sensory loss, motor loss, and/or reflex changes in a dermatomal distribution. This is most often due to a herniated disc with or without trauma causing irritation to a nerve root. Pain can be severe with a burning quality or there can be numbness and tingling. Pain may increase with Valsalva maneuvers. The most common level affected in the upper extremity is the C5 to C6 level with C6 radiculopathy. Pain radiates laterally to the thumb, index, and middle fingers; biceps and triceps are weak; and the brachioradialis reflex may be diminished. The next most common level is C6 to C7 with C7 radiculopathy. Here pain radiates posterolaterally down the arm, with numbness in the index, middle, and ring fingers, weakness of the triceps and pronator, and decreased triceps reflex. Again, most respond to conservative measures such as rest, immobilization, anti-inflammatories, exercise, steroid injections, or quick steroid pulses. Indications for surgery for a herniated disc include compression of the root or cord, instability of the spinal column (spondylolisthesis), and deformity (severe kyphosis with traction on other nerve roots) (38). Radiculopathies also occur in the lower extremity dermatomes in a similar pattern and respond to the same treatments. Gait impairment is related to pain, sensory loss, weakness, and limitation of range of motion.

Normal-pressure hydrocephalus (NPH) produces a characteristic gait abnormality and has an associated dementia thought to be reversible with treatment. The diagnosis is difficult and treatment efficacy difficult to predict. In one study as many as 80% of those shunted showed improved cognitive ability when examined carefully with neuropsychologic testing before and after surgery. Best results are found in those with duration of disease less than 12 months and with a known cause (39). Onset of gait abnormality before dementia also seems to predict a better outcome (40), although postoperative complications should be kept in mind. These include shunt failure, subdural hematomas, infections, and seizures (41). Causes of NPH include head trauma, intracranial hemorrhage, intracranial infection, carcinomatous meningitis, increased cerebrospinal fluid protein, and cerebellar hemangioblastoma. Often no underlying cause is found. Classically the patient presents with the triad of gait apraxia, dementia, and incontinence. The gait abnormality is described as magnetic, as though the feet were sticking to the floor and the patient has forgotten how to initiate swing. Once the patient is walking, the gait is slow and wide based, with small shuffling steps.

Pyramidal and extrapyramidal signs (weakness, spasticity, bradykinesia) are usually absent. Diagnosis is based on clinical examination and neuroimaging studies showing enlarged ventricles and periventricular hypodensities (42). Dynamic radioisotope studies of cerebrospinal fluid flow are not always definitive.

VERTIGO AND DIZZINESS

The nonspecific complaint of dizziness in the elderly is common, as much as 30% of patients over age 65 in some studies (43–46). It has a multitude of causes, and the diagnosis can be difficult. This is compounded by the fact that patients' histories are often vague and imprecise. In most cases, however, the diagnosis can be based on the history and office examination. An organized and systemic approach is critical to achieving this goal.

The first step is an accurate history. This is often the most difficult step, partly because of the imprecise use of the terms dizziness and vertigo. They are often ill defined in the mind of both the health care provider and the lay public, making it difficult to sort out the true nature of the problem. The patient must be allowed to use his or her own words to describe the symptoms. Questions must remain open ended, pressing for descriptive rather than definitive words. A sensation or feeling of movement, either of the patient in the environment or of the environment around the patient, is vertigo. This includes not only the classic, often-sought description of the room spinning but also of internal rotatory movement, a feeling of tilting, veering, or oscillating. There may also be a history of motion sickness or vague unsteadiness. True vertigo localizes to the vestibular system, either central or peripheral (43).

Another category of complaints is the impending faint. The patient may describe lightheadedness, unsteadiness, sweating, palpitations, and true loss of consciousness. The origin in this case is diffuse cerebral ischemia caused by a plethora of medical conditions, usually cardiovascular (43).

Another complaint may be pure dysequilibrium, i.e., a balance disorder causing an unsteady gait. This is caused by lesions of the vestibulospinal tract, proprioceptive systems, or somatosensory system or is related to cerebellar or other motor systems (43).

The last category to consider is psychogenic disorder, often related to severe anxiety, depression, or rarely, frank psychosis. These patients' complaints do not fit into any of the above categories and are often vague and bizarre (44).

Once the chief complaint determines the category of true vertigo, presyncope, dysequilibrium, or psychogenic disorientation, further history should begin to narrow down the possibilities. Main areas of concern should focus on time course, precipitating factors, and predisposing factors (43). The main vertiginous disorders are benign positional vertigo, Ménière's syndrome, central vascular events (vertebrobasilar insufficiency, cerebellar lesions, brainstem infarcts, labyrinthine infarcts), tumors (cerebellopontine angle, temporal bone, brain), infections (viral neurolabyrinthine, otomastoiditis, otitis externa), and demyelinating lesions of multiple sclerosis. Presyncope is most often related to cardiac disease, orthostatic hypotension, vasovagal attacks, and hyperventilation. Vestibulopathy, proprioceptive loss, somatosensory loss, motor lesions, or cerebellar lesions may cause dysequilibrium. Psychogenic dizziness is most often anxiety, panic, or depression.

Benign positional vertigo is a problem of the inner ear with many causes, although about half the time the exact cause cannot be elucidated. Most often the cause is head trauma or a postviral neurolabyrinthitis. The characteristic symptoms consist of brief episodic bouts of vertigo associated with changes in position. Usually they occur when the patient turns in bed, straightens up after bending, or extends the neck to look up. The pathophysiology is thought to be secondary to unilateral deposits in the posterior semicircular canal. The vertigo, which is associated with nystagmus, has the qualities of latency and fatigability. Most often this remits spontaneously (43). If there is no latency to onset and no adaptation to the vestibular stimulus, an alternative cause must be sought (44).

Ménière's disease involves hearing loss and tinnitus in addition to the vertigo (44). Usually the tinnitus and hearing loss associated with a sensation of fullness in the affected ear predates the vertigo. Onset of bouts of vertigo is rapid, with resolution over hours and residual unsteadiness sometimes for days. Early on the hearing loss is reversible, but it later becomes permanent. Pathology involves distension of the endolymphatic system with eventual rupture causing mixing of endolymph and perilymph. Again, most of the cases are idiopathic, but known causes include infections from bacteria, viruses, and syphilis. Treatment is with antivertiginous medications, salt restriction, and diuretics (43).

Vertigo related to ischemia in the vertebrobasilar system can affect the labyrinth, the vestibular nerve, or the vestibular nuclei in the brainstem. Onset is abrupt, lasts minutes, and is usually associated with acute nausea and vomiting. There are almost always accompanying signs, such as visual changes, diplopia, visual field cuts, weakness, and visceral sensations (43). Vertigo in isolation is rarely if ever due to posterior fossa ischemia. There are almost always associated neurologic deficits (3). One possible exception is an isolated small caudal cerebellar infarct. The underlying cause is most likely an infarct in the posterior inferior cerebellar artery territory or on occasion, the vertebral artery from either occlusion or emboli. If the anterior inferior artery distribution is the cause, there is usually hearing loss as well. Symptoms usually remit over several weeks (45). Other cerebellar signs should be sought if an infarct is suspected. These include ataxia, dysmetria, and symmetric gaze-evoked nystagmus (43).

Both benign and malignant tumors can invade the temporal bone causing vertigo. There are often accompanying signs, such as hearing loss, cranial neuropathies, or even brainstem findings, depending on the exact location and extent of the tumor growth. Tumors include meningiomas, gliomas, glomus body, acoustic neuromas, and metastatic disease (43).

Vertigo can be the presenting symptom in many infections. Direct erosion of the inner ear or labyrinth can occur with chronic bacterial otomastoiditis causing a cholesteatoma. Otitis externa can become virulent and spread to the adjacent temporal bone. Herpes zoster oticus causes a viral neuritis that can invade both the vestibular and facial nerves (43). Rarely, the sensory branch of the trigeminal nerve can also be affected.

A few patients with vertigo are found to have multiple sclerosis; however, a large proportion of patients with known multiple sclerosis also have vertigo. Most likely this is related to demyelination of the vestibular nuclei and its connections (44). Approximately 25% of patients have vertigo as the initial symptom, but 75% develop it at some point in the course of their disease.

The second main category, more frequently described as a light-headedness, usually is a precursor to syncope. Orthostatic hypotension is extremely common, and in fact most people have had it on at least one occasion. Recurrent episodes are more serious. This is mostly due to medications, severe anemia or volume contraction, or prolonged bed rest after a protracted illness. Many of the elderly take multiple medications, and this is a common problem with antihypertensives, antidepressants, and major tranquilizers (43). Occasionally autonomic dysfunction is a cause, as seen in diabetic neuropathy or the Shy-Drager syndrome, a variant of parkinsonism.

Vasovagal events, or common fainting, can be precipitated by extreme fear or anxiety. This in turn stimulates the medulla to decrease the heart rate and blood pressure, lowering cardiac output and decreasing cerebral blood flow (43). Hyperventilation can cause light-headedness along with perioral numbness and distal paresthesias (44). The mechanism is related to lowering of the carbon dioxide level, causing vasoconstriction of the cerebral blood vessels. Chronic hypocapnia can also occur in the absence of hyperventilation (43).

Presyncope in the elderly, which often has a cardiac or vascular origin, may be caused by an arrhythmia that lowers cardiac output. Underlying cardiac lesions include severe valvular disease, recurrent myocardial infarction, congestive heart failure, and severe hypertension. Dysequilibrium is more vague by history and more multifactorial than either true vertigo or lightheaded presyncope. Falls in the elderly are common and a very serious cause of morbidity and mortality. This is discussed further in the section on gait abnormalities. Psychogenic dizziness is a diagnosis of exclusion.

The elderly patient with a complaint of vertigo or dizziness remains a diagnostic challenge. The clear definition of the patient's symptoms is key to categorizing possible causes. Once the category is determined to be vertigo, presyncope, dysequilibrium, or psychogenesis, the localization becomes much easier. Once the problem can be localized, the workup and use of needed consultants can be targeted more efficiently.

REFERENCES

1. de Rijk MC, Breteler MM, Graveland GA. Prevalence of Parkinson's disease in the elderly: the Rotterdam Study. Neurology 1995;45:2143–2146.
2. Sage JI, Mark MH. Clinical review diagnosis and treatment of Parkinson's disease in the elderly. J Gen Intern Med 1994;9:583–589.
3. Stacy M, Jankovic J. Differential diagnosis of Parkinson's disease and the parkinsonism plus syndromes. Neurol Clin 1992;10:341–355.
4. Stern MB. The changing standard of care in Parkinson's disease: current concepts and controversies. Neurology 1997;49:S1.
5. Koller WC, Montgomery EB. Issues in the early diagnosis of Parkinson's disease. Neurology 1997;49:S10–S25.
6. Watts RL. The role of dopamine agonists in early Parkinson's disease. Neurology 1977;49:S34–S48.
7. Waters CH. Managing the late complications of Parkinson's disease. Neurology 1997;49:S49–S57.
8. Stern MB. Contemporary approaches to the pharmacotherapeutic management of Parkinson's disease: an overview. Neurology 1997;49:S2–S9.
9. Effects of tocopherol and deprenyl on the progression of disability in early Parkinson's disease. The Parkinson's Study Group. N Engl J Med 1993;328:176–183.
10. Olanow WC. Attempts to obtain neuroprotection in Parkinson's disease. Neurology 1997;49:S26–S33.
11. Calne DB. Treatment of Parkinson's disease. N Engl J Med 1993;329:1021–1027.
12. Koller WC, Busenbark K, Miner K, et al. The relationship of essential tremor to other movement disorders: report on 678 patients. Ann Neurol 1994;35:717–723.
13. Biary N, Bahou Y, Sofi MA, et al. The effect of nimodipine on essential tremor. Neurology 1995;45:1523–1525.
14. Busenbark KL, Wilkinson SB, Pahwa R, et al. Twelve month follow-up of deep brain stimulation (DBS) for essential tremor. Mov Disord 1996;11:254.
15. Ruioff GE. Headache in elderly patients: how to recognize and manage benign types. Postgrad Med 1993;94: 109–110, 113–116, 119–121.
16. Lipton RB, Pfeffer D, Newman LC, Solomon S.

Headaches in the elderly. J Pain Symptom Manage 1993;8:87–97.

17. Solomon GD, Kunkel RS, Frame J. Demographics of headache in elderly patients. Headache 1990;30:273–276.

18. Pascual J, Berciano J. Experience in the diagnosis of headaches that start in the elderly people. J Neurol Neurosurg Psychiatr 1994;57:1255–1257.

19. Raskin N. Short-lived head pains. Neurol Clin 1997; 15:143–152.

20. Caselli RJ, Hunder GG. Giant cell (temporal) arteritis. Neurol Clin 1997;15:893–902.

21. Thomas RJ. Seizures and epilepsy in the elderly. Arch Intern Med 1997;157:605–615.

22. Scheuer ML, Cohen J. Seizures and epilepsy in the elderly. Neurol Clin 1993;11:787–804.

23. Drury I, Beydoun A. Seizure disorders of aging: differential diagnosis and patient management. Geriatrics 1993;48:52–59.

24. Drugs for epilepsy. Med Lett 1995;37:37–40.

25. Tinetti ME, Baker DI, McAvay G, et al. A multifactorial intervention to reduce the risk of falling among elderly people living in the community. N Engl J Med 1994; 331:821–827.

26. Nevitt MC, Cummings SR, Kidd S, et al. Risk factors for recurrent nonsyncopal falls, a prospective study. JAMA 1989;261:2663–2668.

27. Fuh J, Lin K, Wang S, et al. Neurologic diseases presenting with gait impairment in the elderly. J Geriatr Psychiatr Neurol 1994;7:91–94.

28. Tinetti ME, Speechley M. Prevention of falls among the elderly. N Engl J Med 1989;320:1055–1059.

29. Woo J, Ho S, Lau J, et al. Age-associated gait changes in the elderly: pathological or physiological? Neuroepidemiol 1995;14:65–71.

30. Elble RJ, Hughes L, Higgins C. The syndrome of senile gait. J Neurol 1992;239:71–75.

31. Alexander NB. Gait disorders in older adults. J Am Geriatr Soc 1996;44:434–451.

32. Richardson JK, Ashton-Miller JA. Peripheral neuropathy, an often over-looked cause of falls in the elderly. Postgrad Med 1996;99:161–172.

33. Belmin J, Valensi P. Diabetic neuropathy in elderly patients. What can be done? Drugs Aging 1996;8:416–429.

34. Richardson JK, Ashton-Miller JA, Lee SG, Jacobs K. Moderate peripheral neuropathy impairs weight transfer and unipedal balance in the elderly. Arch Phys Med Rehabil 1996;77:1152–1156.

35. Thomson FJ, Masson EA, Boulton AJ. The clinical diagnosis of sensory neuropathy in elderly people. Diabet Med 1993;10:843–846.

36. Swagerty DL Jr. Cervical spondylotic myelopathy: a cause of gait disturbance and falls in the elderly. Kans Med 1994;95:226–227.

37. McCormack BM, Weinstein PR. Cervical spondylosis, an update. West J Med 1996;165:43–51.

38. Smith MD. Cervical radiculopathy: causes and surgical treatment. Minn Med 1995;78:28–45.

39. Thomsen AM, Borgesen SE, Bruhn P, et al. Prognosis of dementia in normal-pressure hydrocephalus after a shunt operation. Ann Neurol 1986;20:304–310.

40. Graff-Radford N, Godersky J. Normal-pressure hydrocephalus: onset of gait abnormality before dementia predicts good surgical outcome. Arch Neurol 1986;43: 940–942.

41. Jack C, Mokri B, Laws E, et al. MR findings in normal-pressure hydrocephalus: significance and comparison with other forms of dementia. J Comput Assist Tomogr 1987;6:923–931.

42. Friedland RP. Normal-pressure hydrocephalus and the saga of the treatable dementias. JAMA 1989;262:2577–2581.

43. Baloh RW. Dizziness in older people. J Am Geriatr Soc 1992;40:713–721.

44. Drachman DA, Hart CW. An approach to the dizzy patient. Neurology 1972;22:323–334.

45. Norrving B, Magnusson M, Holtas S. Isolated acute vertigo in the elderly: vestibular or vascular disease? Acta Neurol Scand 1995:91:43–48.

46. Colledge NR, Barr-Hamilton RM, Lewis SJ, et al. Evaluation of investigations to diagnose the cause of dizziness in elderly people: a community based controlled study. BMJ 1996;313:788–792.

Rehabilitation and the Aged

The philosophy, clinical approach, and therapeutic interventions of rehabilitation medicine can benefit many older adults. Those who are recovering from an acute illness and/or who have chronic illness are at risk for disabilities and functional loss. Some 86% of adults over age 65 have at least one chronic medical problem, and 53% of those over age 75 are limited in at least one activity of daily living (ADL) (1).

Rehabilitation is an approach to care provided by a team of professionals. Although physicians specializing in physical medicine and rehabilitation, physical therapists, and occupational therapists are most closely identified with rehabilitation practice, the rehabilitation approach is applicable to older patients being cared for by geriatricians, primary care physicians, orthopaedists, neurologists, nurses, psychologists, social workers, and most other health care professionals. Principles of successful rehabilitation include the following:

- A comprehensive approach that incorporates physical, emotional, and social factors in the care process
- A team effort that is multidisciplinary in membership and interdisciplinary in process
- A continuous and ongoing intervention that is not time limited
- A focus on function, whether it be lost function that may be restored (restorative therapy) or remaining function to be modified and strengthened to accommodate other disability (maintenance therapy) (2)

A useful model of disease progression and functional loss has been developed by the World Health Organization. When a disease becomes symptomatic at the organ level, the person is aware of an *impairment*. Examples of impairments include sensory loss, muscle weakness, and joint pain. *Disabilities* are the functional consequences of impairments. Examples of disabilities include difficulty walking and the inability to perform personal care. A disadvantage resulting from a disability is a *handicap*. A handicap limits or prevents the fulfillment of a role that is normal for the affected person. The nature and severity of a handicap are determined by the interaction of the adaptation of the person to the social and environmental surroundings and the adjustments made by society to accommodate the impaired person. Buildings and public transportation inaccessible to a person in a wheelchair may result in a handicap (1, 3). Whereas in the traditional medical model physicians are trained to interact at the level of disease, rehabilitation occurs at all levels, disease, impairment, disability, and handicap.

Although rehabilitation medicine offers hope of reducing disability and handicap among older adults, research in this area is limited (1). A few studies document the benefits of inpatient assessment and rehabilitation (4–6) and the application of geriatric and rehabilitation principles to specific clinical problems (7–11). These studies should be replicated in other settings and with a broader range of patients. Nonetheless, rehabilitation and geriatric medicine professional organizations strongly advocate that rehabilitation services be available in all settings in which older persons receive health care (12, 13).

This chapter reviews the rehabilitation process and the use of teams, the settings in which rehabilitation can occur, and the prescription of assistive devices. The role of the primary care physician in the rehabilitation process is discussed, as are specific approaches to stroke, hip fracture, Parkinson's disease, and arthritis.

ASSESSMENT

Rehabilitation focuses on restoring and maintaining functional ability; thus, assessment of the patient must be oriented to function. The optimal process is interdisciplinary, involving all disciplines relevant to a particular case; identifies not just disease but impairments, disabilities, and handicaps; involves physical, mental, and social spheres; and results in the establishment of objective goals. Assessment and goal setting must be individualized, capitalize on the patient's strengths and abilities, and restore or make adaptive changes to foster independence. The family and social network should be involved, and assessment should be ongoing, not static, with goals regularly reassessed.

In a given case, all disciplines involved have a discipline-specific focus to their portion of the comprehensive assessment. Table 21.1 lists and briefly describes the roles of various rehabilitation professionals. The physician's physical assessment should include the traditional medical history and physical as well as a functional assessment of ADLs, instrumental ADLs (IADLs), and mobility. Observing the patient perform functional tasks such as eating, dressing, putting on glasses, and combing hair helps identify diseases, impairments, disabilities, and handicaps not previously recognized. A patient's apraxia, hemineglect, or visual field cut, which may have been missed by a standard examination, becomes apparent in the functional assessment. The patient's problem list should include functional (e.g., incontinence, impaired mobility) as well as traditional medical problems, and the rehabilitation team should address each problem. Also, sexual function should not be overlooked as part of the rehabilitation assessment and program for the older patient.

Sensory impairments, very common among older persons, affect all aspects of the rehabilitation process. Unfortunately, even moderate and severe impairments can go unrecognized or untreated. Early identification of such impairments is particularly important because obtaining a hearing aid, low-vision aid, or glasses may take time, and the absence of such assistive devices may slow or preclude progress in a rehabilitation program.

Table 21.1

Rehabilitation Professionals

Professional	Role
Physiatry (physician trained in physical medicine)	Evaluates patient, integrates assessment data, determines potential, coordinates rehabilitation plan
Primary care physician	Manages acute and chronic medical care
Rehabilitation nurse	Integrates medical, nursing, rehabilitation plan
Physical therapist	Addresses mobility, strength, range of motion
Occupational therapist	Addresses activities of daily living and self-care
Speech pathologist	Addresses communication, swallowing
Psychologist and neuropsychologist	Diagnosis and treatment of mood, behavioral, and cognitive conditions
Social worker	Works with family, patient; financial counseling, discharge planning
Nutritionist	Assesses nutrition status, diet plan
Pharmacist	Reviews medication use
Audiologist	Provides hearing assessment and treatment
Vocational counselor	Evaluates work potential, provides training
Recreational therapist	Assists with hobbies, leisure activities, motivation
Orthotist, prosthetist	Makes and fits orthopaedic aids

The assessment of mental function should cover both psychologic and cognitive function. In assessing mood the clinician should have a high index of suspicion for depression, common and very treatable among rehabilitation populations. Cognitive function is particularly important with the older patient, as the prevalence of dementia rises dramatically with age (14, 15). Standard mental status tests, such as the Mini-Mental State Examination (MMSE) (16) and longer and more sensitive measures are essential components of the comprehensive rehabilitative assessment. A patient's cognitive ability influences all aspects of rehabilitation, including eligibility, choice of setting, assessment, goal setting, therapeutic interventions, and outcome. Although some persons with severe dementia are not candidates for rehabilitation, many cognitively impaired persons and their families benefit greatly from the rehabilitation process (17). Thus, cognitive impairment per se is not necessarily a reason to exclude a patient from rehabilitation.

An older person's family and social network are essential in the design and implementation of a rehabilitation program. It is important to make a realistic assessment of the strengths and weaknesses of the patient's social network. Financial resources must also be assessed because the availability of paid home health care workers, in addition to family and friends, will greatly influence the rehabilitation goals and outcomes.

The clinical assessment of rehabilitation patients can be facilitated by the use of the many standardized assessment instruments. Adequate test-retest and interobserver reliability of standardized instruments are valuable in monitoring a patient's progress during rehabilitation. Standardized instruments are available to assess specific disease states, global disability, ADLs and IADLs, mental status, motor function, balance, mobility, speech and language, and depression. A recent clinical practice guideline on stroke rehabilitation included a critical review of standardized instruments (18). Recommended instruments include the Barthel Index and the Functional Independence Measure (FIM) for the measurement of ADLs (19, 20). Both of these scales are widely used in rehabilitation settings.

REHABILITATION SETTINGS

Rehabilitation can occur in a variety of settings, and care can be provided by a single discipline or by many disciplines. When more than one discipline is involved, care can be provided in both multidisciplinary and interdisciplinary models. The site and number of disciplines depend on the needs and resources of the patient. An interdisciplinary model is preferred in all but the most straightforward cases. Table 21.2 outlines the range of settings in which rehabilitation is provided as well as general criteria for patients cared for in them.

Comprehensive inpatient medical rehabilitation is divided into three categories: acute and two subacute levels (21). The levels are not specific to the site of care but are defined by the medical stability of the patient and the intensity of rehabilitation. Acute hospital-based rehabilitation generally requires that a patient tolerate and need 3 or more hours of therapy per day and that the patient benefit from the involvement of two or more disciplines (e.g., physical therapy and occupational therapy). The acute hospital rehabilitation setting is the ideal and most intensive setting for the most medically complex patients. However, the older deconditioned patient may not tolerate such intensive therapy, and a subacute, skilled nursing facility (SNF) or home-care program may be more appropriate in many cases (22).

An example of a patient ideally suited for SNF-based rehabilitation is the person recovering from a hip fracture who needs skilled physical therapy on a daily basis but does not need any other rehabilitation. Patients with more complex needs requiring multiple rehabilitation disciplines and interdisciplinary care who cannot tolerate the intensity of an inpatient program can also be served in an SNF with a subacute rehabilitation program. Care provided in an SNF does not preclude return to a hospital when the patient can tolerate increased intensity of therapy.

Home care programs are best suited to those who have adequate social resources and are medically stable. The unavailability of cumbersome equipment (e.g., whirlpool, parallel bars) in the home can be a limiting factor, however. Reimbursement for home treatment also re-

Table 21.2

Rehabilitation Settings and Their Characteristics

Settings	Characteristics
Comprehensive Inpatient Medical Rehabilitation	
Category 1 (acute): Hospital	High risk for medical instability; requires two or more disciplines; generally 3 hours of therapy a day; Medicare coverage same as for other types of acute hospitalization
Category 2 (subacute): Hospital, hospital-based SNF, SNF	Moderate risk for medical instability; requires two or more disciplines; generally 3 hours of therapy a day; Medicare coverage varies
Category 3 (subacute): Hospital-based SNF, SNF	Low risk for medical instability; skilled therapy 5 times a week; less than 3 hours per day; one or more disciplines; Medicare covers 20 days in full, and days 21–100 partially
Home care program	Patient must be homebound; single or multiple therapies; limited Medicare coverage; adequate social supports required
Outpatient CORF	Complexity requires interdisciplinary process; multiple disciplines involved; adequate social resources required; limited Medicare coverage
Individual therapies	Limited number of disciplines; less complex cases; adequate social resources required; limited Medicare coverage

quires that the patient be homebound. In the outpatient setting, a comprehensive outpatient rehabilitation facility (CORF) is ideal for providing care to the patient who requires multiple disciplines and an interdisciplinary team process. Social support and transportation must allow daily travel to the CORF and provide a safe home environment. Individual therapies provided on an outpatient basis are appropriate when a single discipline is all that is required.

Medicare covers comprehensive medical inpatient rehabilitation in acute and subacute settings. Continued coverage requires documentation of functional improvement resulting from the therapy. However, many secondary private health insurance programs have significant limitations and require preauthorization for rehabilitation services. Medicare covers SNF care fully for 20 days and partially for days 21 to 100. Most supplemental insurance policies pick up a portion of the deductible but do not extend coverage beyond 100 days. Home care programs requiring skilled therapies are covered by Medicare for a limited time. CORF programs and individual therapies on an outpatient basis are also covered by Medicare, with a limit on the to-

tal dollar amount of therapy that can be provided per incident of illness.

Few data compare the effectiveness of various rehabilitation settings for restoring function and preventing long-term nursing home placement. A recent study compared the outcomes after hip fracture and stroke for patients receiving rehabilitation in hospital units, subacute units, or SNF units (23). Patients with stroke (but not with hip fracture) had better functional recovery in the hospital units. Subacute units were better at returning stroke patients to the community than were traditional nursing homes.

ASSISTIVE DEVICES

Assistive devices are used to relieve pain and maintain or restore function. Patients who need an assistive device also need help choosing appropriate equipment. Various assistive devices address problems with hearing, vision, mobility, and most ADLs and IADLs. Most require that the patient be trained in proper use. Physical and occupational therapists can assist the physician, patient, and family in the selection and proper use of products. Table 21.3 (24–27) is a brief summary of selected assistive devices.

Table 21.3

Selected Assistive Devices

Problem	Device	Comments
Bathing	Soap on a rope, long-handled back sponge, hand-held shower hose	Help when reaching is impaired; require adequate grip, range of motion
	Grab bars	Reduce risk of falls
	Tub seat or bench	Allows safe sitting in the bathtub
	Tub transfer bench	Bridges tub side with two legs in tub and two legs beside tub; reduces risk of falls while getting into and out of tub
Toileting	Raised toilet seat	Toilet seat 20″ from floor; handrails attached to wall or a freestanding frame; all reduce risk of falls
	Versa frames	
	Bedside commode	
Oral care	Toothbrush grip	
Dressing	Reaching device	Aids in picking things off floor
	Buttonhook	Helps with hand weakness, loss of agility
	Sock donner	Helps if hip flexion is limited
	Velcro closures	Substitute for buttons, shoelaces
	Elastic shoelaces	Aid in dressing
	Clothes hook	
	Long shoehorn	
Grooming	Electric razor	
	Tilt mirror	
	Built-up handle grips	
Eating	Built-up grips	Help with arthritis, decreased strength
	High-edged plates and nonskid pads	Keep food on plate and plate on table
	Rocker knife	Allows one-handed food cutting
	Cup with lid	Prevents spills with intention tremor
Mobility		
Orthoses	Foot	Modified shoes, lifts
	Ankle-foot	Plastic shell or metal brace for mild limb weakness (foot drop) after stroke; aids weight-bearing, alignment
	Knee-ankle-foot	Aids knee support, with or without hinge
Cane	Hemicane, hemiwalker	Four-point frame considerably supports hemiplegic patient; all canes held on side opposite involved leg
	Tri or quad cane	More support than single-point cane; wide or narrow base
	Standard cane	Pistol grip best; with tip on ground, elbow flexed 25°
Walker	Standard	Rubber tips; lift when moving; helps with weakness or imbalance if grip poor; can be fitted with platform grip attached to forearm if proximal strength adequate
	Roller	Front, 3-, or 4-wheel; can have brakes, cargo basket; help with balance but less support than

continued

Table 21.3 (*continued*)

Selected Assistive Devices

Problem	Device	Comments
		standard walker; helps patients with Parkinson's, unstable gait, or limited cardiorespiratory reserve who cannot tolerate lifting (e.g., COPD, CHF)
Wheelchair	Standard	For limited endurance or inability to walk; must carefully fit seat width, arm height, seat cushion, foot rests. Folding models available; expensive, requires physiatry input
Scooter	Powered	Three-wheeled electric scooter for mobility over long distances

Adapted from Brummel-Smith K. Rehabilitation. In: Ham R, Sloane P, eds. Primary Care Geriatrics. 2nd ed. St. Louis: Mosby-Year Book, 1992;137–161. Friedmann LW, Capulong ES. Specific assistive aids. In: Williams TF, ed. Rehabilitation in the Aging. New York: Raven Press, 1984;315–344. Wasson JH, Gall V, MacDonald R, Liang MH. The prescription of assistive devices for the elderly: practical considerations. J Gen Intern Med 1990;5:46–54. Wilson GB. Progressive mobilization. In: Sine RD, Liss SE, Roush RE, et al., eds. Basic Rehabilitation Techniques. 3rd ed. Rockville, MD: Aspen, 1988;132–136.

Deciding which is the most appropriate device and teaching the patient its appropriate use are probably beyond the scope of the average primary care physician. However, many older persons use canes for which they were never appropriately evaluated, and as many as 75% may use the wrong type of cane or one that is in ill repair, use it improperly, or have the wrong size. Thus, the primary care physician who sees a patient with a cane should ascertain that it is in good repair (rubber tip, no cracks, and so on), that it is the right size (height of greater trochanter) and that the patient uses it properly (e.g., for osteoarthritis, advances cane at the same time as the affected hip but holds the cane on the contralateral side).

STROKE

The rehabilitation of stroke patients is an enormous challenge because the condition is common and the functional consequences are often serious. Stroke mortality rates have been declining steadily since the early 1950s in the United States, but still, about 25% of stroke sufferers die within a month of the stroke, and up to 40% are dead within a year (28). Survivors with cerebral infarction show some improvement at 2 to 3 weeks, when the cerebral edema has resolved. In general, 50% of expected functional recovery occurs by 1 month, 75% at 3 months, 90% at 6 months, and nearly 100% at a year (29). Overall, 80% of survivors attain independent walking, and two thirds become independent in ADLs (30).

The rehabilitation approach to the older stroke patient may be supportive, preventing complications while spontaneous recovery occurs, or more active, involving intensive rehabilitation therapy. The effectiveness of aggressive stroke rehabilitation therapy and its relative contribution to recovery of function as compared with spontaneous recovery is controversial. It is also unclear whether intensive rehabilitation is most beneficial immediately after the stroke or 2 to 4 weeks after the initial event, when spontaneous recovery may allow for more intensive therapy.

The clinical approach to stroke is usually divided into three phases: acute (admission to 48 hours), subacute (48 hours to 3 months), and chronic (3 months and after). During the acute phase the patient is stabilized and a functional assessment is initiated. Measures to prevent deep vein thrombosis should be implemented until the patient is walking. Low-dose heparin or low-molecular-weight heparin is more effective than warfarin, pneumatic compression, or elastic stockings. Management of the acute phase of stroke is discussed in Chapter 10.

The subacute and rehabilitation phases of stroke care have recently been reviewed and a clinical practice guideline published (18). Though observation studies provide considerable information on the natural history of stroke, few well-controlled clinical studies document benefit from rehabilitation. A particularly challenging problem is the distinction of rehabilitation effects from spontaneous neurologic recovery after a stroke.

After stroke patients are stabilized, it is helpful to identify those with the best chance of benefiting from intensive rehabilitation. Although a number of negative prognostic indicators have been identified (Table 21.4), early prognostication is unreliable for the individual patient. Age has not been shown to be an independent predictor of outcome, although many older stroke patients also have comorbidities that can affect recovery.

Rehabilitation treatment for the stroke patient derives from an ongoing team assessment. The physical therapist's focus is on strength, endurance, and mobility. Motor recovery frequently follows a predictable sequence: initial flaccid paralysis, then flexor pattern synergy (flexion with movement), then extensor pattern synergy, then flexor selection, and lastly, extensor selection. Although this sequence varies from case to case, it is helpful to recognize that certain patterns can be capitalized on to assist with particular activities (e.g., extensor synergy and walking) (24). Treatment begins with bed mobility and progresses to balance training and sitting. Walking requires adequate strength and trunk stability. Patients with severe impairments may begin walking in parallel bars and then be advanced to a walker or cane. If the lower leg is weak, an ankle-foot orthosis (short leg brace) can promote more efficient walking by ensuring fixed dorsiflexion at the ankle and minimizing toe dragging in the swing phase of gait.

The occupational therapist addresses upper extremity function and the ability to perform ADLs, IADLs, and visual spatial perception deficits. Maintenance of range of motion in the affected upper extremity is essential to prevent a painful shoulder or contractures. Wrist splints are prescribed for distal upper extremity spasm. To avoid shoulder subluxation, transfers are managed without additional stress on the shoulder joint, and pillows and arm boards are used to support the affected arm. These positioning techniques maintain the humeral head in its proper position when the muscles usually responsible for this alignment are flaccid. Dressing aids, such as clothes reachers, button hooks, sock donners, and Velcro closures, may be prescribed. Feeding aids, such as rocker knives and plate guards, can be helpful.

Impairment of language function can be the most frustrating consequence of stroke. Dysarthria and aphasia require assessment by a speech pathologist. Communication boards can be provided to help the patient with expressive aphasia make his wishes known. The speech pathologist can also help rehabilitation team members communicate with the patient. The patient's ability to swallow should be assessed before oral fluids and food are started.

A number of complications may interfere with functional recovery from stroke (Table 21.5). Identification and aggressive treatment of these problems is important during both active rehabilitation and maintenance therapy. Clinical depression occurs in as many as 60% of stroke patients; and if unrecognized and untreated, it

Table 21.4

Predictors of Poor Functional Outcome After Stroke

Preexisting or new impairment in cognitive function
Previous stroke
Coexistent symptomatic cardiovascular disease
Large lesion on computed tomography
Initial coma
Perceptual-spatial deficit
Aphasia
Neglect or denial syndrome
Multiple neurologic deficits
Incontinence 2 weeks after stroke
No motor return 1 month after stroke

Adapted from Kelly J. Stroke rehabilitation for elderly patients. In: Kemp B, Brummel-Smith K, Ramsdel S. Geriatric Rehabilitation. Boston: College-Hill Press, 1990.

Table 21.5

Poststroke Complications That May Impair Functional Recovery

Medication toxicity	Sensory deprivation syndrome
Cognitive impairment	Depression
Aphasia	Dysphagia
Spasticity	Contractures
Shoulder problems	Pressure sores
Urinary incontinence	Constipation and fecal incontinence
Peripheral nerve palsies	Poor adjustment to disability
Caregiver withdrawal or burnout	

Adapted from Kelly J. Stroke rehabilitation for elderly patients. In: Kemp B, Brummel-Smith K, Ramsdel S. Geriatric Rehabilitation. Boston: College-Hill Press, 1990.

can interfere with rehabilitation. Shoulder-hand syndrome (reflex sympathetic dystrophy) can result in severe pain. Early therapy can reduce the risk or effect of this syndrome. Adequate range of motion of the shoulder joint, isometric muscle exercises, and elevation to reduce edema can help. If the syndrome progresses, oral steroids and stellate anesthetic blocks may help the pain (31).

HIP FRACTURE

About 250,000 hip fractures occur each year in the United States, and the incidence of femoral neck fractures is rising by about 40% per decade (32). During the year following the fracture, 20% of patients spend time in a nursing home, and 10 to 20% die. Although some data suggest better outcomes for patients who have operative repair within 24 hours of hospitalization, other findings support the importance of taking time to correct metabolic and hydration status and attending to other unstable medical conditions (33, 34). Postoperative care and rehabilitation can affect outcome (9). Mental status and the patient's functional status before the fracture are also important predictors of functional recovery. Rapid return to walking (by 2 weeks) is another good predictor of successful outcome. During the past decade reimbursement from Medicare and other payers has shifted hip fracture rehabilitation from the hospital to the outpatient, nursing home, and home settings (35).

Hip fractures are classified into three major categories according to anatomic location:

femoral neck (subcapital or intracapsular), intertrochanteric, and subtrochanteric. Femoral neck fractures, which account for a third of the hip fractures in the elderly, place the blood supply to the femoral head at risk, resulting in a high incidence of avascular necrosis. Intertrochanteric fractures, which constitute most of the other two thirds of hip fractures, usually unite, but they are associated with significant blood loss and more early complications than femoral neck fractures. Subtrochanteric fractures are uncommon in the older patient, result from very significant force, and are more difficult to repair.

The fracture site and the surgical technique greatly affect the course of rehabilitation. In older patients a stable repair that allows for early weight bearing is crucial to avoid postoperative complications and deconditioning. Occult or impacted femoral neck fractures can be treated with internal fixation with multiple pins, allowing early walking. In most older patients with displaced femoral neck fractures, prosthetic replacement is the best option, reducing the risks of nonunion and necrosis of the femoral head and allowing for immediate weight bearing. Patients with prosthetic hip repairs are instructed to follow precautions to prevent dislocation: no flexion of the hip greater than 90°, no internal rotation of the hip, and no adduction past the midline. Although intertrochanteric fractures can be treated with traction for 4 to 8 weeks, operative repair with a compression screw and plate allows for early weight bearing with a walker.

Avoidance of medical complications in the immediate postoperative period is imperative. Warfarin 10 mg prior to surgery and 5 mg the evening after surgery or low-molecular-weight heparin therapy reduces the occurrence of deep venous thrombosis. Removal of bladder catheters soon after surgery helps avoid urinary tract infections. Adequate skin care requires exemplary nursing. A 4-inch or thicker egg crate mattress is required, and heel protectors may be helpful. Sedative drugs should be avoided, and analgesics should be monitored closely.

Most orthopaedic surgeons recommend specific weight-bearing orders for hip fracture patients. These can include non-weight bearing, touchdown (10 to 15% body weight on limb), partial (30%), 50%, and full weight bearing (75 to 100%). There is considerable controversy in orthopaedic medicine concerning the rate of progression of the degree of weight bearing versus fracture healing (36). Many surgeons are quite cautious with older patients, which can result in unnecessary delay in postoperative mobilization. Also, partial weight bearing is very difficult for some older patients, leaving the physical therapist withholding treatment while awaiting more liberal orders from the attending surgeon. The older patient with a preexisting cognitive deficit may be unable to participate in any therapy that involves degrees of weight bearing. They may not be able to learn or remember to apply less than full weight. Thus, it is important to choose an operative repair that allows the earliest possible full weight bearing in this population.

PARKINSON'S DISEASE

Parkinson's disease (PD) is a chronic progressive disorder that is uncommon before age 50 and that has an increasing incidence through the eighth decade. Rehabilitation has not been shown to retard the progression of the illness. However, rehabilitation can lessen the influence of the illness by helping a person maximize functional abilities and maintain independent function for as long as possible (37–39). Therapy, which can usually be provided in the outpatient setting, should begin early in the course of the illness. Unfortunately, pharmacologic interventions are usually emphasized, and physical interventions are often overlooked. Physical and occupational therapists as well as speech pathologists should be consulted early in the course of the illness.

The physical therapist can focus on body alignment, gait, strength, and range-of-motion (ROM) exercises, as well as transferring. Patients are taught to look up and consciously lift their toes during the swing phase of gait. They should keep their feet wide apart (12 to 15 inches) and concentrate on lengthening their step. A program of regular exercises can improve or maintain strength and range-of-motion as well as prevent contractures. Group exercise programs can also help prevent the social isolation common in patients with Parkinson's disease. The patient should avoid rubber-soled shoes, which tend to stick when the patient walks, and canes, which are difficult for the person with a typical parkinsonian posture. When a Parkinson's patient needs a walker, it should have front wheels. A pickup walker is inappropriate for a person who has difficulty initiating motions (such as repeatedly picking up the walker) and the person with retropulsion, in which the motion of picking up a walker may cause backward falling.

The occupational therapist can enhance the patient's independence in performing ADLs. To simplify dressing, it can be helpful to use Velcro closures or zippers and over-the-head rather than buttoned clothing. Slip-on shoes with elastic shoelaces can also be helpful. Adaptive equipment can be used to assist with eating. If the patient is poorly coordinated, large-rimmed dishes or plate guards as well as weighted plates and cups can help minimize handicap. Environmental aids such as grab rails in the bathtub and near the toilet, a raised toilet seat, and raising the back legs of chairs by 1 to 3 inches to facilitate rising from a chair are also helpful.

The speech pathologist can help with communication and swallowing. Hypokinetic dysarthria is common in Parkinson's disease, and therapeutic efforts designed to improve respiration by teaching the patient diaphragmatic breathing exercises can improve the volume of sound and the number of words spoken per breath. The prevalence and type of swallowing disorders associated with Parkinson's disease varies. Nonetheless, individualized swallowing and stimulation techniques taught by a speech pathologist may be beneficial.

Hospitalization for intercurrent illnesses poses a particular risk for Parkinson's patients. It is important to avoid bed rest while continuing exercise programs during hospitalization. Should hospitalization or an intercurrent illness result in a significant decline in functional status, treatment in an acute hospital or SNF-level rehabilitation unit may be necessary.

ARTHRITIS

The goals of therapy for any arthritic condition are to improve or maintain functional ability and relieve or minimize pain. Physical therapies address both goals; they should begin early in the course of a symptomatic disease. Nonpharmacologic interventions should be individualized to the patient, the specific arthritic condition, and the stage of the disease. Rheumatologic diseases are dynamic, and thus periodic monitoring and reevaluation are necessary to adjust treatment as the condition progresses. Therapeutic interventions include rest, exercise, orthotics, assistive devices, and heat and cold as well as patient and family education.

Local rest of inflamed joints reduces pain and inflammation and may prevent contracture (40). Short rest periods to interrupt daily activities lasting more than 30 minutes (energy conservation program) have been shown to increase physical activity level in patients with rheumatoid arthritis (RA) (41). Systemic rest should be reserved for times when the patient with RA has multiple inflamed joints and fails to respond to conventional pharmacologic and nonpharmacologic interventions. It may also benefit patients with polymyalgia rheumatica (PMR) during the acute phase of the illness. However, systemic rest can lead to deconditioning and should be used cautiously.

Exercise for patients with arthritis can increase or maintain ROM, strengthen muscles, increase endurance, and improve the biomechanical function of joints (42). Exercise programs should take into account the degree of joint inflammation or effusion, the condition of surrounding muscle, the patient's overall endurance, mechanical derangement of the joint, and other comorbid illnesses. Therapeutic heat and cold have been used to provide relief of pain and promote increased range of joint motion. However, few controlled trials in the use of these modalities have been conducted (10, 43). The use of cold seems most appropriate for the acutely inflamed joint. Cold can decrease pain and relax surrounding spastic muscles. Later, in the subacute period, when inflammatory pain is subsiding and stiffness is present, either cold or superficial heat may be appropriate. Splints and orthotics are used to unweight joints, stabilize joints, decrease joint motion, or support joints in a position of maximal function and to increase joint motion (i.e., dynamic splint). Orthotics for the upper extremity, mainly confined to the wrist and hand, include resting splints, functional wrist splints, thumb post splints, ring splints, and dynamic splints. They are most commonly used in rheumatoid arthritis and carpal tunnel syndrome. Orthotics of the lower extremity are most useful for the foot and ankle and much less so for the knee. Shoes with a wide toe box can be used for the wide forefoot, cock toes, and hallux valgus deformity seen in RA and osteoarthritis (OA).

OA, the most common type of arthritis in older persons, can result in significant pain and disability. Involvement of the hip, knee, foot, and carpal carpometacarpal joints is common and can result in disability. Given the joints commonly affected and OA's primarily noninflammatory nature, rehabilitation of OA patients is somewhat different from that of RA patients. Hip OA rehabilitation management involves relieving weight-bearing stress by using an appropriate assistive device (e.g., cane) and stretching exercises to maintain ROM and strengthen hip musculature. Jogging can cause undue joint stress and should generally be avoided, whereas swimming is an optimal exercise. Bicycling is also acceptable. Unilateral hip disease has a high association with increased leg length on the affected side, and a lift for the opposite shoe is indicated if there is a disparity in length of more than 0.25 inch. OA of the knee can restrict range of motion and cause contractures of the joint capsule and hamstring, an unstable joint, and valgus or varus deformity. Patients should avoid using a pillow under the knee at night because this encourages knee and hip flexion contractures. A functionally important goal is to maintain knee extension, because more than a 10° flexion contracture results in less than optimal knee biomechanics and increases stress with weight bearing. For strengthening, non-weight bearing quadriceps isometric exercises should be done twice daily by patients with OA of the knee. This is particularly important for the patient with OA who is hospitalized with an intercurrent illness. Rising from a toilet or chair that is too low can increase joint stress and should be avoided by using chairs of the appropriate height and high toilet seats. Therapeutic exercise can improve physical capacity, relieve symptoms, and improve functional ability in short-term studies of persons with knee OA (11). OA commonly results in hallux valgus with or without bunions, hallux rigidus with cocked toes, metatarsal head calluses, and abrasions on the dorsum of the toes. Thus, a properly fitting wide-toe box shoe is essential. The carpometacarpal joint is frequently affected by OA. Using a thumb post splint to immobilize the thumb in a functionally abducted position relieves pain and allows for performance of functional activities.

Strengthening exercises are also important in the rehabilitation management of RA, but care must be taken to avoid aggravating the inflamed joint. Brief isometric exercises performed with joints in the least painful posture (usually mid-joint range) can allow for strengthening with the least harm. A 6-second maximal contraction twice daily for each muscle group is adequate to maintain strength (41). Progressive ROM exercises can be used to maintain or regain ROM in the patient with RA. However, it is important to avoid aggravating inflamed joints, and it must be recognized that once subluxation or dislocation has occurred, no exercises will restore alignment.

When pharmacologic and nonpharmacologic interventions fail to relieve pain or restore function, surgery should be considered for OA of the hip and knee and to a lesser extent, for RA. Rehabilitation can enhance the outcome of surgery in many situations, and the involvement of the appropriate rehabilitation professionals should occur early, preferably before the surgery.

THE PRIMARY CARE PHYSICIAN

The primary care physician plays a key role in the rehabilitative care of the older patient. The nature of the role varies with the specific condition, the phase of the illness, the setting, and regional variations in resources and standard practices. Regardless, the primary care physician should function to some extent as a team leader. This role may be explicit in some situations, e.g., when the primary care physician is the designated team leader on an inpatient rehabilitation unit. However, more often the role is implicit, such as in the SNF, home care, or outpatient setting. As the team leader, no matter how explicit the role, the primary care physician must coordinate services, facilitate an interdisciplinary process, and use function as the bench mark for establishing goals, monitoring progress, and assessing outcomes. When teams are well established, the role is relatively straightforward. However, when this is not the case, the task can be cumbersome, time consuming, and unreimbursed. Nonetheless, it is essential for good outcomes. Furthermore, when done well, it is extremely gratifying for the patient, the family, the rehabilitation professionals, and the primary care physician.

REFERENCES

1. Cole TM, Edgerton VR, eds. Medical Rehabilitation Research: Report of the Task Force. Bethesda, MD: National Institutes of Health, 1990:29.
2. Erickson RV. Principles of rehabilitation. In: Beck JC, ed. Geriatrics Review Syllabus. 2nd ed. New York: American Geriatrics Society, 1991:73–88.
3. World Health Organization. International Classification of Impairments, Disabilities and Handicaps. Geneva: World Health Organization, 1980:184.
4. Applegate WB, Miller ST, Graney MJ, et al. A randomized, controlled trial of a geriatric assessment unit in a community rehabilitation hospital. N Engl J Med 1990: 322:1572–1578.
5. Rubenstein LZ, Josephson KR, Wieland GD, et al. Effectiveness of a geriatric evaluation unit: a randomized clinical trial. N Engl J Med 1984;311:1664–1670.
6. Landfeld CS, Palmer RM, Kresevic DM, et al. Randomized trial of care in a hospital medical unit especially designed to improve the functional outcomes of

acutely ill older patients. N Engl J Med 1995;332:
1338–1344.

7. Granger CV, Hamilton B, Gresham G. The stroke rehabilitation outcome study. Part I. General description.
Arch Phys Med Rehabil 1988;59:506–509.

8. Granger CV, Hamilton B, Gresham G. The stroke rehabilitation outcome study. Part II. Relative merits of the
total Barthel index score and a four-item subscore in
predicting patient outcomes. Arch Phys Med Rehabil
1989;70:100–103.

9. Kennie DC, Reid J, Richardson IR, et al. Effectiveness of
geriatric rehabilitative care after fractures of the proximal femur in elderly women: a randomised clinical trial.
BMJ 1988;297:1083–1086.

10. Puett DW, Griffin MR. Published trials of nonmedical
and noninvasive therapies for hip and knee osteoarthritis. Ann Intern Med 1994;121:133–140.

11. Ettinger WH, Afable RF. Physical disability from knee osteoarthritis: the role of exercise as an intervention. Med
Sci Sports Exerc 1994;26:1435–1440.

12. American Geriatrics Society Public Policy Committee.
Geriatric rehabilitation. J Am Geriatr Soc 1990;38:
1049–1050.

13. Dixon TP. Rehabilitation across the continuum: managing the challenges. Arch Phys Med Rehab 1997;78:115–
119.

14. Evans DA, Harris F, Albert MS, et al. Prevalence of
Alzheimer's disease in the community population of
older persons. JAMA 1989;262:2551–2556.

15. Skoog I, Nilsson L, Palmertz B, et al. A population based
study of dementia in 85-year-olds. N Engl J Med 1993;
328:153–158.

16. Folstein MF, Folstein SE, McHugh PR. "Mini-mental
state". A practical method for grading the cognitive state
of patients for the clinician. J Psychiatr Res 1975;12:
189–198.

17. Goldstein FC, Strasser DC, Woodard JL, Roberts VJ.
Functional outcome of cognitively impaired hip fracture
patients on a geriatric rehabilitation unit. J Am Geriatr Soc
1997;45:35–42.

18. Gresham GE, Duncan PW, Stason WB, et al. Post-Stroke
Rehabilitation. Clinical Practice Guideline 16 (AHCPR
95-0662). Rockville, MD: US Department of Health and
Human Services, Public Health Service, Agency for
Health Care Policy and Research, 1995.

19. Mahoney FI, Barthel DW. Functional evaluation: the
Barthel Index. Md State Med J 1965;14:61–65.

20. Keith RA, Granger CV, Hamilton BB, Sherwin FS. The
functional independence measure: a new tool for rehabilitation. In: Eisenberg MG, Grzesiak RC, editors. Advances in Clinical Rehabilitation. Vol 1. New York:
Springer-Verlag, 1987:6–18.

21. Commission on Accreditation of Rehabilitation Facilities.
Section 2.IIA. Medical rehabilitation programs; comprehensive inpatient, categories one through three. In: Supplement to the 1994 Standards Manual and Interpretive
Guidelines, Organizations Serving People With Disabili-

ties. Tucson, AZ: Commission on Accreditation of Rehabilitation Facilities, 1994:1–14.

22. Weber DC, Fleming KC, Evans JM. Rehabilitation of
geriatric patients. Mayo Clin Proc 1995;70:1198–1204.

23. Kramer AM, Steiner JF, Schlenker RE, et al. Outcomes
and costs after hip fracture and stroke: a comparison of
rehabilitation settings. JAMA 1997;277:396–404.

24. Brummel-Smith K. Rehabilitation. In: Ham R, Sloane P,
eds. Primary Care Geriatrics. 2nd ed. St. Louis: Mosby-
Year Book, 1992:137–161.

25. Friedmann LW, Capulong ES. Specific assistive aids. In:
Williams TF, ed. Rehabilitation in the Aging. New York:
Raven Press, 1984:315–344.

26. Wasson JH, Gall V, MacDonald R, Liang MH. The prescription of assistive devices for the elderly: practical
considerations. J Gen Intern Med 1990;5:46–54.

27. Wilson GB. Progressive mobilization. In: Sine RD, Liss
SE, Roush RE, et al., eds. Basic Rehabilitation Techniques. 3rd ed. Rockville, MD: Aspen, 1988:132–136.

28. Bonita R. Epidemiology of stroke. Lancet 1992;339:
342–344.

29. Caronna JJ. Cerebrovascular diseases. In: Kelley WN,
ed. Textbook of Internal Medicine. 2nd ed. Philadelphia: Lippincott, 1992:2166.

30. Kelly J. Stroke rehabilitation for elderly patients. In:
Kemp B, Brummel-Smith K, Ramsdel S, eds. Geriatric
Rehabilitation. Boston: College-Hill, 1990.

31. Fishburn MJ, deLateur BJ. Rehabilitation. In: Reuben
DB, Yoshikawa TT, Besdine RW, eds. Geriatrics Review
Syllabus. 3rd ed. Dubuque, IA: Kendall/Hunt for Amer-
ican Geriatrics Society, 1996:101.

32. Bonar S, Tinetti M, Speechly M, Cooney L. Factors associated with short- versus long-term skilled nursing facility placement among community-living hip fracture
patients. J Am Geriatr Soc 1990;38:1139–1144.

33. Hoenig H, Rubenstein LV, Sloane R, et al. What is the
role of timing in the surgical and rehabilitative care of
community-dwelling older persons with acute hip fracture? Arch Intern Med 1997;157:513–520.

34. Cooney LM. Hip fracture outcomes. Arch Intern Med
1997;157:485–486.

35. Pryor GA, Williams DR. Rehabilitation after hip fractures: home and hospital management compared. J
Bone Joint Surg 1989;71:471–474.

36. Goldstein TS. Geriatric Orthopaedics: Rehabilitative
Management of Common Problems. Gaithersburg, MD:
Aspen, 1991:39–55.

37. Gauthier L, Dalziel S, Gauthier S. The benefits of group
occupational therapy for patients with Parkinson's disease. Am J Occup Ther 1987;41:360–364.

38. Palmer SS, Mortimer JA, Webster DD, et al. Exercise
therapy for Parkinson's disease. Arch Phys Med Rehabil
1986;67:741–747.

39. Comella CL, Stebbins GT, Brown-Toms N, Goetz CG.
Physical therapy and Parkinson's disease: a controlled
clinical trial. Neurology 1994;44:376–378.

40. Hicks J, Gerber L. Rehabilitation of the patient with

arthritic and connective tissue disease. In: Delisa JA, et al., eds. Rehabilitation Medicine: Principles and Practice. 2nd ed. Philadelphia: Lippincott, 1993:1047–1081.

41. Gerber L, Furst G, Shulman B, et al. Patient education program to teach energy conservation behaviors to patients with rheumatoid arthritis. Arch Phys Med Rehabil 1987;68:442–45.

42. Hicks J, Gerber L. Rehabilitation of the patient with arthritic and connective tissue disease. In: Delisa JA, et al., eds. Rehabilitation Medicine: Principles and Practice. 2nd ed. Philadelphia: Lippincott, 1993:1047–1081.

43. Swezey RL. Rehabilitation in arthritis and allied conditions. In: Kottke FJ, Lehmann JF, eds. Krusen's Handbook of Physical Medicine and Rehabilitation. 4th ed. Philadelphia: Saunders, 1990:679–716.

CHAPTER 22

JONATHAN TAYLOR AND RICHARD A. NORTON

Gastrointestinal Disease in the Aged

In the few years since the previous edition of this book was published, some of the digestive problems besetting the elderly population, such as peptic ulcer disease of the stomach and duodenum, have come under greater control. Other problems, including malignancies of the tubular gut, the pancreas, and the liver, are still very prevalent and difficult to treat effectively, although the diagnosis is easier to make in many patients.

ESOPHAGEAL PROBLEMS

Gastroesophageal reflux, or heartburn, is one of the most common complaints in the older patient. About 40% of adults have heartburn at least once a month (1). These patients may develop reflux or heartburn because of transient lower esophageal sphincter relaxations or a weak lower esophageal sphincter with or without a hiatus hernia. Esophageal injury occurs when caustic gastric contents come into contact with the esophageal mucosa. The degree of mucosal injury is related to the duration of contact. Patients with heartburn typically complain of a burning sensation in the epigastric region that radiates to the neck. The pain of acid reflux, however, may mimic angina pectoris or the pain of an acute myocardial infarction. Other patients with severe esophagitis may be asymptomatic. On endoscopy there may be evidence of esophagitis, and if the inflammation is severe, ulcerations, esophageal stricture, or Barrett's esophagus may develop. Other causes of esophagitis include irradiation, infections (*Candida,* herpes, cytomegalovirus), medications (tetracycline, KCl, aspirin, quinine), and ingestion of caustic substances.

Patients with persistent reflux symptoms, odynophagia, or dysphagia should be evaluated with upper gastrointestinal endoscopy. Complications of gastroesophageal reflux disease (GERD) can be identified at that time and any areas of esophageal mucosa that appear to be abnormal can be sampled for biopsy. An alternative study is an upper gastrointestinal radiology study, but the sensitivity of this test for detecting reflux is low (2). If an upper endoscopy is normal, esophageal manometry with continuous 24-hour pH monitoring helps identify patients with reflux. The sensitivity and specificity of 24-hour pH monitoring are greater than 90% when the intraesophageal pH is lower than 4 for more than 10.5% of time when the patient is upright and 6% when supine (3).

Treatment for heartburn includes lifestyle modifications and pharmacologic therapy. Initial management with lifestyle modifications may reduce reflux. Patients are advised to elevate the head of the bed on 6-inch blocks, lose weight if obese, eat small meals, avoid bedtime snacks, stop drinking alcohol and smoking, avoid caffeinated beverages, coffee, carminatives such as garlic, onions, peppermint, fatty foods, chocolate, tomato, and citrus fruit juices. H_2 receptor blockers help heal the majority of patients with mild esophagitis who do not respond to lifestyle modifications. In patients with severe esophagitis, the proton pump inhibitors (PPIs) are potent inhibitors of gastric acid secretion, and almost all esophagitis is healed after 8 weeks of therapy (4, 5). PPIs are also more effective than H_2 blockers in maintaining GERD remission (6).

Persistent gastroesophageal reflux may cause esophageal stricture or Barrett's esophagus.

Some 13% of patients who have endoscopic examinations for evaluation of reflux have Barrett's esophagus (7, 8), in which the normal stratified squamous epithelium that lines the distal esophagus is replaced by columnar epithelium. Barrett's esophagus is clinically important because esophageal carcinoma may arise from dysplastic Barrett's epithelium.

The annual incidence of adenocarcinoma in patients with Barrett's esophagus has been estimated at 0.8% (9). Of patients with Barrett's esophagus and high-grade dysplasia, 25% developed carcinoma within 1.5 years (10). Treatment of Barrett's esophagus focuses on the control and healing of reflux esophagitis along with regular endoscopic surveillance for dysplasia. For patients with persistent, confirmed high-grade dysplasia, surgery is advised to resect all of the esophagus lined with columnar epithelium. If surgery is contraindicated by other medical problems, Barrett's esophagus may be ablated with electrocoagulation or photodynamic therapy. Most clinicians perform surveillance endoscopy every other year in patients with Barrett's esophagus without dysplasia. If patients have low-grade dysplasia, intensive antireflux therapy for 2 to 3 months is followed by more frequent endoscopic surveillance.

Patients with symptomatic esophageal strictures due to reflux esophagitis can be treated with the PPI. After endoscopy is performed to rule out malignancy, a symptomatic stricture with a lumen diameter of less than 13 mm can be dilated with bougies. Dilators (bougies) with diameters of 5 to 20 mm are used to stretch the narrowed esophagus at monthly or longer intervals. If a stricture cannot be successfully dilated, surgery may be performed. When an elderly patient has dysphagia and marked dilation of the proximal or middle esophagus, two diagnoses, achalasia and esophageal dilation due to an infiltrating carcinoma of the gastric cardia, should be considered. Although an upper gastrointestinal radiograph is helpful, the diagnosis is confirmed by endoscopy with multiple biopsies and esophageal motility study.

Achalasia presents only infrequently in patients over age 50 (11). All patients with achalasia have dysphagia to solids, and most also have dysphagia to liquids. Patients may complain of regurgitation of undigested food, chest pain, heartburn, and weight loss. Esophageal manometry studies typically show an increased basal pressure of the lower esophageal sphincter, incomplete lower esophageal sphincter (LES) relaxation after swallowing, and aperistalsis of the distal esophagus. Once malignancy has been excluded, the patient may treated with pneumatic dilation or endoscopic botulinum toxin injection into the LES. Approximately two thirds of patients have relief of dysphagia after botulinum toxin injection 6 months after therapy (12). Botulinum toxin treatment also has fewer side effects than balloon dilation.

Esophageal adenocarcinoma usually arises from Barrett's epithelium in the distal esophagus. In patients who have esophageal adenocarcinoma, up to 86% have a columnar lined esophagus (13). The mean age at diagnosis is 64 years. Most patients have advanced disease at the time of diagnosis, and there is a disappointingly low 5-year survival rate. Surgical excision of the tumor in selected patients with limited disease may improve survival. For palliation of dysphagia, a stent can be placed through the tumor. Radiotherapy, laser therapy, photodynamic therapy, and cauterization with diathermy equipment also may improve swallowing.

Squamous cell carcinoma of the esophagus is more common than adenocarcinoma in the United States. Predisposing conditions include smoking, excessive alcohol consumption, corrosive injury of the esophagus, achalasia, and tylosis. Incidence of squamous carcinoma is higher for men than for women and higher for blacks than for whites. Barium radiography or endoscopy is the initial diagnostic study, and endoscopic biopsy confirms the diagnosis. Surgical treatment by esophagogastrectomy has a 7.1% mortality rate but a 5-year survival rate of only 6% (14). Similar survival rates have been reported in patients treated with radiotherapy.

Some patients complain of a lump in the back of the throat or a globus sensation, which often follows emotional stress. This symptom is constant and usually does not cause difficulty swallowing. Once organic disease has been ruled out, the diagnosis can be made using a provocative test. The patients should be coached to swallow several times over a few minutes, and as the supply of saliva is depleted, the back of the tongue is lubricated less and less adequately. Friction of the back of the tongue produces the feeling of an obstructing lump. The treatment is to advise the patient to swallow less frequently and to drink water or juice when the globus sensation develops. For most patients, reassurance, retraining, and drinking fluids is fully effective in relieving the symptoms.

Zenker's diverticulum occurs most commonly in the elderly. Also known as a pharyngoesophageal diverticulum, it is a pouch of mucosa that is directed posteriorly just above the upper esophageal sphincter. Some are tiny and asymptomatic. Others are large and may cause dysphagia, regurgitation of undigested food, and halitosis. When the patient is horizontal, reflux of contents of the Zenker's diverticulum into the airway can lead to aspiration pneumonia and lung abscess. Diagnosis is made with a barium swallow. Since the condition results from a hypertensive or poorly coordinated relaxation of the upper sphincter, surgical weakening of the sphincter is usually an effective treatment. If the diverticulum is large, removal or inversion of it can also relieve symptoms.

Several conditions in the elderly population may result in severe dysphagia with aspiration pneumonia and an inability to maintain hydration and nutrition. These conditions include esophageal cancer, head and neck cancer, cerebrovascular accident, and muscular dystrophy. To manage the immediate problem of feeding and hydration, insertion of a percutaneous endoscopic gastrostomy (PEG) tube is recommended. The PEG is more comfortable for the patient and is much less likely to be dislodged than a nasogastric or Dobbhoff tube. It is usually placed through the patient's left upper abdominal wall under light intravenous sedation as an outpatient procedure. If the patient's underlying condition improves, as may occur after a brainstem stroke, the PEG may be removed.

GASTRIC PROBLEMS

Drugs that regularly cause gastritis include alcohol, aspirin and other nonsteroidal anti-inflammatory drugs, iron, potassium chloride, and chemotherapeutic agents. Because of the widespread use of nonsteroidal anti-inflammatory drugs for joint pain, the incidence of gastritis and ulcer disease in the aging population is increasing (15).

The incidence of type B or antral gastritis caused by *Helicobacter pylori* infection increases as a population ages. The prevalence increases progressively from 10% at 20 years of age to 50% at 60 years of age (16). There is also a strong association between *H. pylori* infection and duodenal and gastric ulcers. Eradication of *H. pylori* infection in these patients significantly reduces recurrence of duodenal and gastric ulcers (17, 18). A number of antibiotic regimens have been used to treat *H. pylori* infection. One common regimen consists of a 2-week course of Pepto-Bismol 2 tablets 4 times a day, metronidazole 250 mg 3 times a day, and tetracycline 500 mg 4 times a day. This regimen produces cure rates above 90% (19). To help heal ulcers, an H_2-blocker or a PPI should be continued for 4 to 8 weeks. A repeat endoscopy or upper gastrointestinal radiograph should be performed to document gastric ulcer healing and rule out gastric carcinoma.

The incidence of gastric cancer has been falling dramatically in all industrialized countries since about 1950. The reasons for this decline are not clear. Patients usually do not present until the disease is advanced. The symptoms include weight loss, abdominal pain, anorexia, vomiting, and bleeding. Screening with radiography or upper endoscopy locates the lesion, and biopsy confirms the diagnosis. The most important prognostic factors are depth of invasion and regional lymph node status. The overall 5-year survival rate is 20% in patients who are candidates for complete surgical resection (20). Chemotherapy unfortunately does not generally seem to improve survival.

Gastric outlet obstruction usually arises from either a pyloric channel ulcer that has scarred the pylorus or from infiltration by a gastric carcinoma. Diagnosis of a carcinoma, even with endoscopic biopsy, may be difficult, since biopsies may miss the malignant cells buried deeply in the tissue. Therapy for gastric outlet obstruction requires surgical bypass (gastrojejunostomy) unless the obstruction is relieved by treatment with nasogastric suction and aggressive therapy with a PPI.

Failure of the stomach to empty may also result from a failure of normal motility, known as gastroparesis. Causes include bowel surgery (immediate postoperative period), diabetic neuropathy, infiltrating carcinoma, and idiopathic causes. Various prokinetic agents have been used to treat gastroparesis. Cisapride given before meals significantly accelerates gastric emptying of both liquids and solids, and side effects are rare.

PROBLEMS OF THE SMALL AND LARGE BOWEL

One of the most common causes of diarrhea in elderly patients is lactose intolerance. Up to a third of American whites and two thirds of persons of Asian, African, and Latin-American groups are lactase deficient. Symptoms of lactose intolerance include abdominal distension, bloating, pain, flatulence, and diarrhea. The diagnosis can be confirmed with a lactose tolerance test or a lactose breath test. Alternatively, the patient can test himself or herself at home by drinking a glass of room temperature milk on an empty stomach. If significant flatulence, pain, or diarrhea occurs within 2 hours, the test is considered positive. Nutritional counseling can focus on elimination of lactose from the diet. Most patients markedly improve their symptoms by eating a low lactose diet and taking lactase before each meal.

Inflammatory bowel disease, including Crohn's ileitis, colitis, and ulcerative colitis, may occur in older patients, although initial presentation is not common after age 60. Blood, stool studies, radiography, and colonoscopy with biopsy are therefore important to confirm the diagnosis and define the extent of the disease. Controlling the inflammation is the goal of treatment. Acutely, prednisone can suppress disease activity. Other agents, such as sulfasalazine and other 5-aminosalicylates, 6-mercaptopurine, and antibiotics can be used chronically to keep patients in remission. Surgical resection is curative for patients with ulcerative colitis, and it eliminates the risk of colorectal cancer. Conversely, for patients with Crohn's disease surgery is not curative, and there is a recurrence rate of approximately 50% within 10 years after surgery (21).

Elderly patients with diarrhea offer a diagnostic challenge. This is a useful approach for evaluating diarrhea:

1. Is there microbial infection of the small or large bowel? Stool studies for parasitic and bacterial pathogens occasionally identify the specific agent. If there is an infection, antibiotic therapy helps eliminate the infection.
2. Is there local disease of the rectum and colon? Rectal examination, flexible sigmoidoscopy and barium enema, and colonoscopy are useful procedures to identify patients with ischemic colitis, antibiotic-associated colitis, inflammatory bowel disease, or infectious colitis.
3. Is there significant steatorrhea? A 72-hour stool collection with laboratory estimation of fat content gives the most dependable answer to the question. Steatorrhea is defined as more than 7 g of fat per 24 hours of stool output. Qualitative study of a single stool specimen may be used as a screening test, but this tends to be inaccurate.
4. If steatorrhea is present, is the small bowel capable of absorbing nutrients, especially fats? This can be evaluated by a d-xylose test, since the carbohydrate xylose is absorbed in approximately the same portion of the small bowel as fat. If the small intestine is diseased, further study should lead to appropriate treatment. Examples of small bowel disease include celiac sprue, extensive involvement by scleroderma, and advanced Crohn's ileocolitis.
5. If steatorrhea is present and small bowel absorption is normal, pancreatic insufficiency may be the cause of the diarrhea. The pancreas may fail to produce adequate enzymes for lipolysis within the lumen of the small bowel. A hydrogen breath test following ingestion of 100 g of rice carbohydrate may differentiate between pancreatic and small bowel disease. The rise in breath hydrogen is early with small bowel disorders and late with pancreatic insufficiency (22). Treatment is discussed later under pancreatic disease.
6. Is there bacterial overgrowth in the upper small intestine? This may be determined by radiography of the small bowel, to identify

any diverticula in this area. The intestinal juice can be sampled by a fluoroscopically placed tube to determine the flora. Treatment with courses of antibiotics for a week every month should give good results.

ISCHEMIC COLITIS

In patients with ischemic colitis, 60% are over age 70 (23). Causative factors include atherosclerosis, aortic surgery, hypotension, and embolic events. Patients present with abdominal pain and bloody diarrhea, but the pain frequently is mild or absent. Chronic ischemic changes in the colon may lead to fibrosis and colonic strictures. Acute transmural ischemia can progress to gangrene with perforation or peritonitis. Most patients, however, have a more limited benign course with transient and reversible ischemia and symptoms that last a day or two. The endoscopic changes can mimic inflammatory bowel disease. Flexible sigmoidoscopy or colonoscopy is the procedure of choice to diagnose ischemic colitis. Surgical intervention is indicated for patients with peritonitis, perforation of the colon, or symptomatic stricture.

COLONIC DIVERTICULAR DISEASE

Colonic diverticular disease is another diagnostic challenge. Diverticulosis is defined as the herniation of the mucosa and submucosa of the colon through the muscular layer of the colonic wall. These pouches or pockets are common, and approximately 50% of the elderly population have colonic diverticula (24). This condition is thought to be caused by increased intraluminal pressures causing herniation of the colonic mucosa through the colonic wall. Diverticula most commonly occur in the sigmoid colon but may be found in any part of the colon. Diverticulitis, or inflammation of the peridiverticular tissues, occurs in a minority of patients with diverticulosis and is characterized by abdominal pain, usually in the left lower quadrant, tenderness with or without a palpable mass, and fever. During an acute attack computed tomography (CT) of the abdomen and pelvis can be performed to rule out other causes of abdominal pain and fever, including appendicitis and abdominal abscesses.

After antibiotic treatment has resolved the infection and inflammation, a barium enema or colonoscopy can be carried out. If patients have repeated attacks, resection of the involved segment of the colon is effective treatment.

CANCER OF THE COLON

A major health problem for elderly patients is colorectal adenocarcinoma. At present there is no consensus as to the most cost-effective screening for this disease. The American Cancer Society, World Health Organization, National Cancer Institute, and American College of Surgeons recommend that asymptomatic patients over age 50 have fecal occult blood testing annually and flexible sigmoidoscopy every 3 to 5 years (25, 26). Patients with colon cancer in a first-degree relative should begin screening at age 40 with a colonoscopy or flexible sigmoidoscopy and barium enema. In the future, genetic testing may help identify patients at particular risk for colon cancer.

When an elderly patient reports rectal bleeding or when there occult blood in the stool, a complete study of the colon and rectum, either by colonoscopy or by sigmoidoscopy and barium enema radiography, is indicated. Hemorrhoids are the most frequent source of rectal blood loss. When other potential sites of bleeding have been excluded, the hemorrhoids should be treated initially with dietary counseling and conservative measures, such as high-fiber diet, adequate fluid intake, sitz baths, suppositories, and ointments. If the problem persists, the hemorrhoids may be coagulated by infrared light, which is safe and highly effective (27). If polyps are present, they should be removed endoscopically and examined histopathologically. Patients with an adenomatous polyp should have a follow-up colonoscopy 3 years after the baseline examination (28). Of these patients, 30 to 40% have another adenoma detected during the follow-up examination (29). Another cause of rectal bleeding in the elderly patient is fragile superficial blood vessels in the colon, known as arteriovenous malformations, or angiodysplasias. For patients in whom these lesions are prominent or actively bleeding, electrocautery through the endoscope often eliminates bleeding. Diverticulosis of the colon may be a site of bleeding, but this occurs rarely and is difficult to prove.

Constipation is a common problem in the elderly population (see section on constipation in Chapter 6). If there is an abrupt change in bowel habits, the colon should be studied to exclude an anatomic lesion such as colon cancer. There are many causes of constipation, such as diabetes; hypothyroidism; electrolyte abnormalities, including hypercalcemia and hypokalemia; and drugs, including anticholinergics, antiparkinsonians, antidepressants, antipsychotics,, opioids, calcium channel blockers, and anticonvulsant medications. Treatment of idiopathic constipation consists of increased physical activity and fluid intake, a high-fiber diet, and an agent such as psyllium or methylcellulose, which increases the bulk of the stool. Hyperosmolar laxatives, such as lactulose and sorbitol, or magnesium citrate can also be used to treat this problem.

Rectal prolapse, more common in women than men, is related to poor pelvic muscle tone and multiple episodes of severe constipation and straining. It is associated with fecal incontinence. Medical management consists of keeping the stool soft and manually reducing the prolapse when it occurs to prevent complications such as ulceration, bleeding, and perforation. If rectal prolapse persists, surgical repair should be considered.

Fecal incontinence, which plagues many older patients, is particularly common in bedridden institutionalized patients. Evaluation can help determine whether there is diarrhea, fecal impaction, an anorectal lesion, or a neurologic cause. If fecal impaction is noted on rectal examination, disimpaction should help relieve the incontinence. A high-fiber diet and increased fluid intake should help correct this problem. Exercises several times a day to strengthen the anal sphincter muscle may be successful. It is also useful to regulate the diet to produce a firmer stool. Antidiarrheal medication such as loperamide may also be effective.

IRRITABLE BOWEL SYNDROME

Irritable bowel syndrome is almost as common in the elderly as in middle-aged persons (30). It is defined as at least 3 months of continuous or recurrent abdominal pain relieved by passage of a bowel movement. In addition, these patients complain of frequent bowel movements and looser stool, with the onset of abdominal pain, constipation alternating with diarrhea, abdominal bloating, passage of mucus, and straining or incomplete evacuation (31, 32). The pathogenesis is not known, but it probably is a disease of disordered intestinal motility or visceral sensation. There is no identifiable organic disorder. The challenge for the physician is to differentiate functional symptoms from specific organic symptoms. What are the clues that a patient has irritable bowel syndrome? (*a*) It arises soon after the most stressful events of the patient's life and disappears soon afterward. (*b*) The abdominal pain does not awaken the patient during the night. (*c*) The patient has at least moderate psychologic stress. (*d*) The symptoms are not typical of any organic disease.

Although the diagnosis of irritable bowel syndrome is usually based on the clinical symptoms, most patients have a complete blood count, erythrocyte sedimentation rate, thyroid function tests, and stool examination for enteric pathogens, ova and parasites, and fecal leukocytes to exclude organic diseases. Flexible sigmoidoscopy rules out a distal obstructing cancer, ischemic colitis, and inflammatory bowel disease. If there are upper gastrointestinal complaints, radiography, endoscopy, or ultrasound studies may be indicated.

When treating the patient with irritable bowel syndrome, a nonjudgmental, confident approach is helpful. Discussion of the results of the laboratory test and evaluation, the cause of pain, and other symptoms is important. In addition, the absence of long-term health risks and other serious diseases such as cancer should be emphasized. Most patients are relieved when they hear this information. This is a list of practical recommendations for treatment of irritable bowel syndrome:

1. Some patients note that certain foods exacerbate their symptoms. Foods to avoid include fried, fatty, and ice-cold foods. Foods that cause bloating include milk and milk products, onions, broccoli, Brussels sprouts, celery, carrots, and beans. Baked or broiled meat, fish, poultry, and any cooked fruits and vegetables are better tolerated. When the pa-

tient's symptoms have improved for 2 weeks, one food per day may be reintroduced.

2. Drinking a cup of comfortably hot water upon arising and every 2 hours may relieve some patients' symptoms.
3. For severe abdominal cramping, it is recommended that local heat be applied to the abdomen with a hot water bottle or a heating pad 1 to 3 times per day.
4. Regular physical exercise for 30 to 60 minutes at least twice a week helps relieve stress, which may exacerbate irritable bowel syndrome.
5. Many patients with irritable bowel syndrome respond to fiber supplements. Fiber increases gut transit, reduces constipation, and may slightly reduce abdominal discomfort.
6. Although no medication has been shown to have a therapeutic effect in treating irritable bowel syndrome, a number of drugs have provided some symptomatic relief to specific subgroups of patients. Antispasmodic medications, tricyclic antidepressants, and antidiarrheal medications should be avoided if possible unless the patient's symptoms do not respond to the other measures outlined here.

JAUNDICE

The differential diagnosis of jaundice is very important to the elder patient. Fortunately diagnostic and laboratory tests help the physician make a rapid diagnosis. Liver function tests, including a fractionated bilirubin level, alkaline phosphatase, and aminotransferases help differentiate whether there is evidence of hepatitis or obstruction of the biliary tree. Patients with hepatocellular disease have at least fivefold elevations of the aminotransferases, and hepatitis serologies occasionally identify the specific virologic agent. Obstruction leads to a threefold to fivefold elevation of the alkaline phosphatase. It is not possible, however, to determine the site of the obstruction from the blood tests alone. When jaundice is present, the clinician makes use of noninvasive tests initially and then orders invasive studies if indicated. The history, physical examination, initial blood studies, and virologic serologies usually establish or exclude hepatocellular disease. Fine-needle liver biopsy confirms the diagnosis.

If cholestasis is the problem, the next step is to determine the site of obstruction. In the majority of patients with dilated bile ducts an ultrasound study of the liver and pancreas can show whether the biliary tree is dilated. Occasionally a tumor mass is identified. Computed tomography is more sensitive than ultrasound examination to rule out pancreatic, biliary, and hepatic masses. Invasive studies, such as endoscopic retrograde cholangiopancreatography (ERCP) and percutaneous transhepatic cholangiography (PTC), may be required to locate the obstruction. With both ERCP and PTC it is possible to relieve the obstruction by removal of stones or placement of stents to allow drainage of bile. Hepatitis is no more frequent in the elderly population than in the young, and the clinical course may be milder (33). As with other disorders, when the course of hepatitis becomes complicated, the morbidity and mortality may rise steeply in the older patient.

BILIARY OBSTRUCTION

Older patients are at particular risk for tumors of the biliary tract and for cancers of the pancreas that invade and obstruct the bile ducts. ERCP may allow removal of stones or stenting of obstructing neoplasms. Biliary stones are moderately common in North America and Western countries. Approximately 20 million Americans have gallstones; at least 20% of women and 10% of men over age 40 have gallstones. The majority of patients with gallstones never have symptoms. In one prospective study, only 18% of a cohort of patients developed biliary colic after 20 years (34). Since only a minority of patients have pain or other symptoms due to gallstones, it is not necessary to treat patients with asymptomatic gallstones.

Biliary colic typically is episodic and severe. It lasts for hours and is located in the epigastrium. The pain is steady, not waxing and waning. When this characteristic pain occurs and when the patient and the physician agree that removal is indicated, laparoscopic surgery is the treatment of choice. Laparoscopic cholecystectomy (LC) is contraindicated in patients with empyema of the gallbladder, adhesions or inflammation that prevents the surgeon from identifying the anatomy of the gallbladder, cirrhosis with portal hypertension, gallbladder cancer, or cholangitis with septic shock. LC generally is well tolerated. Approximately 5% of patients who undergo LC have complications, including bleeding, infection, or injury to the bile duct or bowel. This compares favorably with a 21% rate of complications for patients having open cholecystectomy (35). The incidence of bile duct injury is related to the number of laparoscopic procedures performed by the surgeon. The bile duct injury rate drops from 2.2% to 0.1% after the 13th case (36). LC-related mortality is rare, ranging from 0 to 0.13% (37). Open cholecystectomy mortality rates are also low, varying according to the patient's age. For patients over age 60 mortality is 1.3% versus 0.15% for those less than 60 years of age (38). Postoperatively patients recover more quickly after LC and have less pain. The mean hospital stay in the United States is 1 day, and most patients return to work after 10 days. After open cholecystectomy the mean length of hospital stay is 5 days, and patients returned to work 31 days after patients who underwent LC. There are also significant cost savings, more than $1000, for the patient who has LC versus open cholecystectomy (39).

Acute pancreatitis in an otherwise healthy elderly person often is due impacted gallstones causing obstruction of the papilla and pancreatic duct. It is controversial whether endoscopic treatment within the first 72 hours of admission reduces complications and mortality. ERCP enables gastroenterologists to make a diagnosis of gallstone pancreatitis. During the procedure the stones can be extracted from the ampulla of Vater, and subsequently the pancreatic duct can drain normally. The endoscopic sphincterotomy is carried out with a knife that consists of a wire on one side of the tip of a slender plastic catheter. When the tube has been properly placed under endoscopic vision in the orifice of the ampulla, an electric current is passed through the wire so that the local tissue is cut and cauterized. Bleeding is usually minor, although aberrant arteries in the duodenal wall occasionally bleed when cut. Common bile duct stones can be extracted with a variety of instruments, including tiny rubber balloons, wire baskets, and heavy wire snares that can crush the stones.

Chronic pancreatitis resulting from overuse of alcohol or from unknown causes may produce little or no pain, and the resulting scarring may leave the gland incapable of secreting adequate amounts of proteolytic and lipolytic enzymes into the pancreatic juice. Weight loss is moderate to severe, as is weakness and fatigue, due to the nutritional deficiency. Diagnosis may be made according to the algorithm in the discussion of diarrhea, and treatment consists of adding pancreatic extract to the patient's program. It may be difficult for the patient to ingest enough extract to overcome the steatorrhea, so some regimens call for taking two to three tablets before, during, and again after each meal. Once the treatment plan is in place and working, however, there is usually gratifying weight gain and return of the patient's baseline energy and sense of well-being.

Pancreatic cancer usually affects patients between 60 and 80 years of age. The presenting symptoms, which are nonspecific, include abdominal pain, weight loss, and jaundice. The pain is vague, poorly localized, and made worse by eating. Lying curled up on one's side may give relief. Anorexia and weight loss follow, and later there is jaundice from biliary obstruction. No immunologic tests or tumor markers are specific enough to diagnose pancreatic cancer. Pancreatic masses are routinely identified using ERCP, ultrasound, or CT. Subsequent needle biopsy under CT or ultrasound guidance confirms the diagnosis. A double duct sign during ERCP signifies that the biliary and pancreatic ducts are invaded by the same malignant process. Surgical resection offers the only hope for cure, but unfortunately only a minority of patients are candidates for curative resection. Combination chemotherapy and radiation therapy results in only a very modest improvement in survival. The prognosis remains poor.

REFERENCES

1. Nebel O, Fornes M, Castell D. Symptomatic gastroesophageal reflux: incidence and precipitating factors. Digest Dis 1976;21:953–956.
2. Ott D, Gelfand D, Wu W. Reflux esophagitis: radiographic and endoscopic correlation. Radiology 1979; 130:583–588.
3. Schindlbeck N, Heinrich C, Konig A, et al. Optimal thresholds, sensitivity, and specificity of long-term pH-metry for the detection of gastroesophageal reflux disease. Gastroenterology 1987;93:85–90.

4. Sontag S. The medical management of reflux esophagitis. Gastroenterol Clin North Am 1990;19:683–712.
5. Hetzel D, Dent J, Reed W, et al. Healing and relapse of severe peptic esophagitis after treatment with omeprazole. Gastroenterology 1988;95:903–912.
6. Klinkenberg-Knol E, Jansen J, Lamers C, et al. Use of omeprazole in the management of reflux oesophagitis resistant to H2-receptor antagonists. Scand J Gastroenterol Suppl 1989;166:88–93.
7. Schnell T, Sontag S, Wanner J, et al. Endoscopic screening for Barrett's esophagus, esophageal adenocarcinoma and other mucosal changes in ambulatory subjects with symptomatic gastroesophageal reflux. Gastroenterology 1985;88:1576.
8. Winters C, Spurling T, Chobanian S, et al. Barrett's esophagus: a prevalent, occult complication of gastroesophageal reflux disease. Gastroenterology 1987;92:118–124.
9. Spechler S, Goyal R. The columnar-lined esophagus, intestinal metaplasia, and Norman Barrett. Gastroenterology 1996;110:614–621.
10. Levine D, Haggitt R, Blount P, et al. An endoscopic biopsy protocol can differentiate high-grade dysplasia from early adenocarcinoma in Barrett's esophagus. Gastroenterology 1993;105:40–50.
11. Barrett N. Achalasia of the cardia: reflections upon a clinical study of over 100 cases. BMJ 1964;1:1135–1140.
12. Pasricha P, Ravich W, Hendrix T, et al. Intrasphincteric botulinum toxin for the treatment of achalasia. N Engl J Med 1995;332:774–778.
13. Haggitt R, Tryzelaar J, Ellis F, et al. Adenocarcinoma complicating columnar epithelium-lined (Barrett's) esophagus. Am J Clin Pathol 1978;70:1–5.
14. Galandiuk S, Hermann RE, Cosgrove DM, Gassman JJ. Cancer of the esophagus. The Cleveland Clinic experience. Ann Surgery 1986;203:101–108.
15. Gilinsky N. Peptic ulcer disease in the elderly. Gastroenterol Clin North Am 1990;19:255–271.
16. Dooley C, Cohen H, Fitzgibbons P, et al. Prevalence of *Helicobacter pylori* infection and histologic gastritis in asymptomatic persons. N Engl J Med 1989;321:1562–1566.
17. Graham D, Lew G, Klein P, et al. Effect of treatment of *Helicobacter pylori* infection on the long-term recurrence of gastric or duodenal ulcer. Ann Intern Med 1992;116:705–708.
18. Hentschel E, Brandstatter G, Dragosics B, et al. Effect of ranitidine and amoxicillin plus metronidazole on the eradication of *Helicobacter pylori* and the recurrence of duodenal ulcer. N Engl J Med 1993;328:308–312.
19. Walsh J, Peterson W. The treatment of *Helicobacter pylori* infection in the management of peptic ulcer disease. N Engl J Med 1995;333:984–991.
20. Parker S, Tong T, Bolden S, Wingo P. Cancer statistics, 1996. CA Cancer J Clin 1996;46:5–27.
21. Trnka Y, Glotzer D, Kasdon E, et al. The long-term outcome of restorative operation in Crohn's disease. Ann Surg 1982;196:345–355.
22. Kerlin P, Wong L, Harris B, et al. Rice flour, breath hydrogen, and malabsorption. Gastroenterology 1984;87:578–585.
23. Abel M, Russell T. Ischemic colitis: comparison of surgical and nonoperative management. Dis Colon Rectum 1983;26:113–115.
24. Parks T. Natural history of diverticular disease of the colon. Clin Gastroenterol 1975;4:53–69.
25. Levin B, Murphy G. Revision in American Cancer Society recommendations for the early detection of colorectal cancer. CA Cancer J Clin 1992;42:296–299.
26. Winawer S, St. John D, Bond J, et al. Prevention of colorectal cancer: guidelines based on new data. WHO Collaborating Center for the Prevention of Colorectal Cancer. Bull World Health Organ 1995;73:7–10.
27. Johanson JF, Rimm A. Optimal nonsurgical treatment of hemorrhoids: a comparative analysis of infrared coagulation, rubber band ligation, and injection sclerotherapy. Am J Gastroenterol 1992;87:1601–1606.
28. Bond J. Polyp guideline: diagnosis, treatment and surveillance for patients with nonfamilial colorectal polyps. Ann Intern Med 1993;119:836–843.
29. Winawer S, Zauber A, O'Brien M, et al. Randomized comparison of surveillance intervals after colonoscopic removal of newly diagnosed adenomatous polyps. N Engl J Med 1993;328:901–906.
30. Thompson W, Heaton K. Functional bowel disorders in apparently healthy people. Gastroenterology 1980;79:283–288.
31. Talley N, Phillips S, Melton L, et al. Diagnostic value of the Manning criteria in irritable bowel syndrome. Gut 1990;31:77–81.
32. Manning A, Thompson W, Heaton K, et al. Towards positive diagnosis of the irritable bowel. BMJ 1978;2:653–654.
33. Zauli D, Crespi C, Fusconi M, et al. Different course of acute hepatitis B in elderly adults. J Gerontol 1985;40:415–418.
34. Gracie W, Ransohoff D. The natural history of silent gallstones. N Engl J Med 1982;307:798–800.
35. Scher K, Scott-Conner C. Complications of biliary surgery. Am Surg 1987;53:16–21.
36. Meyers W et al. A prospective analysis of 1518 laparoscopic cholecystectomies. N Engl J Med 1991;324:1073–1078.
37. Lee V, Chari R, Cucchiaro G, et al. Complications of laparoscopic cholecystectomy. Am J Surg 1993;165:527–532.
38. Berci G, Sackier J, The Los Angeles experience with laparoscopic cholecystectomy. Am J Surg 1991;161:382–384.
39. Stoker M, Vose J, O'Mara P, et al. Laparoscopic cholecystectomy: a clinical and financial analysis of 280 operations. Arch Surg 1992;127:589–595.

Infections of the Elderly

The physician caring for an elderly patient with a possible infectious disease undertakes a study of complexity mired in ambiguity. The elderly patient may have multiple diagnoses with the passage of years, alterations in physiologic response due to chronic diseases, numerous medications with potential adverse effects, subtle or misleading presentations of both common and unusual infectious diseases, and challenging ethical choices about appropriate therapy. In his book, *On the Affected Parts,* Galen wrote, "There are very few essential symptoms of disease which do not point to the affected part. In fact, the alterations of function point directly to the affected part" (1). However, in this era of medicine, finding a single infectious disease that can account for all presenting signs and symptoms may be difficult, and Galen's dictum often may not hold when older persons are considered.

COMMON COMPLAINTS AND SYMPTOMS

Mental status changes are frequently the primary complaint reported for elderly persons with infectious disease. The clinician may wish to assess the patient in two levels of risk for infectious disease. The highest immediate infectious disease risk in a patient with mental status changes or confusion is for a disease such as meningitis or sepsis. The probability of such high-mortality diseases generally warrants immediate intravenous antibiotic therapy, aggressive evaluation, and support. At somewhat lower risk but greater frequency are common illnesses such as viral, respiratory tract, and urinary tract infections (UTIs). In these cases mental status changes indicate se-

vere disease, and a very careful effort at specific diagnosis and treatment is required. Decreased intake of food and fluid is an insidious presentation of most infections in the elderly. In these cases rectal or tympanic temperature measurements are important to document fever possibly missed with oral thermometers.

Cough is a final common pathway for the expression of abnormal conditions that arise anatomically anywhere from the nose to the terminal alveoli. The high morbidity and mortality associated with pneumonia in the elderly is emphasized by recognizing that pneumonia may be the most frequently missed diagnosis found at autopsy. Less common pathophysiologic mechanisms for cough, including drugs (e.g., ACE inhibitors, amiodarone), bronchospastic reflex cough from esophageal reflux, and cardiac conditions (e.g., cardiomyopathy with congestive heart failure), must be differentiated from infectious disease.

Urinary incontinence often complicates the care of demented patients and embarrasses those who are not demented. The new onset of incontinence with lower tract symptoms of dysuria or frequency generally indicate an active infection that requires treatment. Fever, chills, and back pain usually indicate upper tract disease, such as pyelonephritis, for which the initial antibiotic therapy should usually be delivered by the intravenous route. Skin irritation from incontinence contributes to the development of skin ulcers and complicates healing. Although both condom and indwelling urinary catheters may assist in control of incontinence, they are frequently associated with the development of UTIs and potentially life-threatening bacteremias. Perineal, rectal, or low back pain in elderly men often indicates prostatitis, which may present with or without a fever.

The elderly are susceptible to enteric pathogens because of antacid therapy and decreased gastric acid production, decreased motility, and decreased mucosal immunity. Diarrhea is often complicated by issues of self-care and hygiene in institutional settings. Antibiotic usage in the elderly increases the frequency of *Clostridium difficile* colitis, as well as occasional colitis from toxins of *Staphylococcus aureus* and other species of *Clostridium*. The *C. difficile* toxin assay is valuable, and symptomatic patients should be treated with metronidazole 250 mg 3 times a day orally for 7 to 14 days or, if the patient is unable to take it orally, 500 mg every 8 hours intravenously, with vancomycin 125 mg 4 times a day orally reserved for those who fail to respond (2). Rapid fluid loss and profound dehydration are possible with diarrheal infections in the elderly, especially if intake is limited by vomiting or by access to fluids.

RELEVANT COMORBIDITIES FROM THE HISTORY

Experienced clinicians often begin the evaluation of a patient by reviewing the problem list with a search for possible diagnoses based on pattern recognition. The patterns are combinations of diagnoses commonly accepted as increasing the probability of comorbidities. For example, the nursing home patient with late-stage Parkinson's disease and a cough may be anticipated to have aspiration pneumonia causing a fever. Similarly, a patient being treated with broad-spectrum antibiotics and having loss of appetite with difficulty chewing and swallowing may be expected to have candidal stomatitis or esophagitis. In diabetic women a finding of candidal stomatitis or thrush should prompt consideration of yeast dermatitis or vaginitis. Identifying such patterns, whether based on experience or didactic learning, allows the physician to expand differential diagnoses as well as anticipate other problems.

Each identified problem requires a review for the expected physiologic changes associated with the disease process, for the possible routes of access for infectious pathogens, and for the ef-

fects on the patient if such an infectious disease process occurs. For example, the physiologic changes found with immobility and bedridden states such as advanced dementia are associated with pneumonia, decubiti, and UTIs. Indwelling urinary catheters and vascular sites of access are commonly the routes of nosocomial infection, often with resistant organisms. Other more unusual routes and organisms may be considered, such as electronic thermometers, which have been implicated in vancomycin-resistant enterococci transmission (3) and shower heads with contaminated water supplies, which are believed to provide an aerosol route for *Legionella*. The only measures that can be easily applied to prevent such transmission of *Legionella* are hyperchlorination and high water temperature (4).

Knowledge of past disease conditions is important in anticipating recurrent problems, especially when risk factors persist or the effects on the patient cannot be abated. For example, erysipelas caused by a β-hemolytic streptococcus frequently recurs at the same site, and prompt antibiotic therapy may avoid hospitalization. In these cases the possibility of staphylococcal cellulitis or resistant or unusual organisms must also be considered. Physicians and health systems should track patients with methicillin-resistant *S. aureus* (MRSA) or vancomycin-resistant enterococci (VRE). MRSA can be detected by culture of the anterior nares, wounds, or sputum (5). Mupirocin applied to the nares or wound may clear the MRSA, but recurrences have been noted in 40%, and resistance to mupirocin develops (6). The majority of readmitted MRSA carriers remain colonized for more than 3 years. Vancomycin is the mainstay of treatment for deep MRSA infections, but resistance is emerging. VRE are also increasingly common, especially in patients who are taking cephalosporins or vancomycin or who have *C. difficile* diarrhea. The Centers for Disease Control and Prevention (CDC) have advised infection control measures for limiting the spread of MRSA and VRE and can assist in obtaining investigational drug treatment (7).

UTIs warrant emphasis because of their frequency, potential severity, and recurrence rate in the elderly. One common mistake is to diagnose a UTI based on findings in a clean-caught urine sample when the presence of many squamous epithelial cells or growth of mixed bacterial skin organisms indicates contamination of the specimen. In elderly women with fever, flank pain, mental status changes, or any other signs of systemic infection, it is important to obtain a catheterized specimen for accurate culture and urinalysis. The use of minicatheters or female catheterization kits is technically easier and perhaps psychologically less invasive than the standard straight or Foley catheter.

Cultures from patients with chronic indwelling urinary catheters should be interpreted with great caution, as colonization occurs promptly and progressively resistant organisms develop under the pressure of antibiotic therapy. Symptomatic patients with infections originating from chronic indwelling urinary catheters usually require catheter change to assess for urinary obstruction and to obtain adequate cultures. Discussions of catheter-associated "urinary fever" date to at least 1884, and yet it remains a common and difficult task to determine whether a fever is a result of catheter-associated bacteriuria that has become invasive or whether something else is causing the fever (8). Infections associated with chronic urinary catheters should generally be treated initially with intravenous antibiotics to cover Enterobacteriaceae (most likely *Escherichia coli*) and enterococci. Prior cultures are often helpful in selecting from the several appropriate antibiotic choices. Urinary catheter changes may also cause recurrent symptomatic urine infections. If such a pattern emerges, it is reasonable to consider antibiotic prophylaxis (sulfamethoxazole 800 mg plus trimethoprim 160 mg, two tablets orally prior to catheter change) (9).

Asymptomatic bacteriuria in the very elderly person does not require antibiotic treatment. Uncomplicated cystitis may be diagnosed only in the absence of the many factors that increase the risk to the patient, including prior exposure to antibiotics or surgical instruments, anatomic abnormalities, or signs of systemic involvement such as fever, chills, and flank pain. Uncomplicated cystitis may be successfully treated with any of several oral antibiotics, with treatment limited to

only a few days. Almost all other UTIs carry a risk of gram-negative sepsis and other significant morbidity and mortality. In potentially septic patients antibiotic selection must cover Enterobacteriaceae, *Pseudomonas,* and enterococci, with consideration of the patient's prior cultures and probability of resistant organisms. Attention to potential renal toxicity is especially important with use of aminoglycosides. A calculation of the creatinine clearance based on the Cockroft formula is essential in adjusting antibiotic dosages (see Chapter 27). After cultures have returned, it is often possible and cost effective to change patients to oral administration of quinolones or sulfamethoxazole with trimethoprim.

SURGICAL HISTORY: HUNTER'S JUDGMENT

John Hunter (1736–1793) believed, as do all good surgeons, that the healer's greatest skill is his judgment, especially the judgment that restricts surgical operations to situations in which more conservative measures are to no avail (10). Prior surgery changes the differential diagnosis considerations and modifies approaches to surgical intervention in elderly patients with infectious disease. This principle is most evident in abdominal disease, in which prior abdominal surgery may be associated with adhesions leading to intestinal obstruction, and adhesions may complicate the use of laparoscopic surgical approaches. In the extremely frail elderly and those for whom use of anesthetics carries an unacceptably high risk, a surgeon may decide to treat intestinal obstruction or cholecystitis conservatively with a relatively long course of nasogastric suction and antibiotics.

Prior surgical interventions may also contribute to infectious disease. For example, bacterial colonization of the bile ducts with organisms such as *E. coli* and *Klebsiella* commonly follows choledochojejunostomy. This is well tolerated unless bile duct strictures develop, in which case the decrease in bile flow may result in bacteremia and sepsis. Recognition of this unusual source of abdominal sepsis can be difficult. While pancreatitis is usually easily diagnosed, it may be difficult to decide about surgical intervention for pseudocysts or bacterial infections. In all such situations the patient's prior response to surgery is an important consideration.

Surgical interventions may be considered as possible underlying causes of endocarditis, which may have an unusual presentation and delay of diagnosis in the elderly. The most common operations contributing to endocarditis are tooth extractions, urologic procedures, and cardiac surgery. Patients who are undergoing surgery and who are at risk for developing endocarditis should receive prophylaxis according to published standards (11). Even though prophylaxis is frequently not given, relatively few cases of endocarditis develop compared with the vast numbers of situations in which prophylaxis should be considered. Only 29% of cases of infective endocarditis have been found to be nosocomial, but the excess nosocomial mortality (40% compared with 18% mortality for community-acquired infective endocarditis) argues for additional attention to prophylaxis for invasive procedures, especially intravascular and genitourinary surgery. In the hospital or nursing home setting the diagnosis may be especially difficult to establish because of coexisting infections. Recent advances in transesophageal echocardiography have contributed to the assessment of patients with small vegetations and periannular complications (12–14).

PREVENTIVE HEALTH MEASURES

The fourth leading cause of death for all ages in 1993 in the United States was chronic obstructive pulmonary disease (COPD) and allied conditions; the sixth was pneumonia and influenza (15). Few interventions can match the benefits of an annual influenza vaccination, since 95% of influenza deaths occur among patients who are 60 years of age or older. While vaccination reduces the risk of influenza by about 50% in the elderly, influenza vaccinations have also been shown to reduce mortality and hospital admissions by 60 to 70%. The reduction in admissions is also demonstrated for pneumonia, acute and chronic respiratory disease, and congestive heart failure. Amantadine 100 mg or less daily by mouth or rimantadine 100 mg orally once or twice a day should be considered if influenza A is epidemic, especially in nursing homes, where viral spread may be rapid (16, 17). Lower doses

may be considered to avoid central nervous system side effects.

There is still controversy regarding the efficacy and duration of protection afforded by the pneumococcal polysaccharide vaccine, but the paucity of significant side effects and low cost argue for its use, especially in high-risk patients, among whom there is increasing evidence of efficacy. Universal revaccination is not indicated. However, revaccination is recommended for the elderly who were given the vaccine prior to age 65 and more than 5 years previously and for patients at high risk (such as patients with nephrotic syndrome, renal failure, splenectomy, immunosuppression for transplants, and possibly human immunodeficiency virus-infected patients who received pneumococcal vaccine more than 6 years ago) (18).

Although only about 50 cases of tetanus are reported annually in the United States, the elderly are disproportionately affected, and vaccination should be given every 10 years after completion of the primary series. For clean minor wounds tetanus adsorbed toxoid (Td) should be given if it has been more than 10 years since the last dose or if the primary series of three doses is not known to have been completed; tetanus immune globulin (TIG) is not required. For all other wounds, including but not limited to punctures, burns, avulsions, crush injuries, and those contaminated with dirt, feces, soil, or saliva, Td is given unless the primary series is completed and the most recent dose was less than 5 years ago; TIG is also given if the primary series is not known to have been completed (19).

The tuberculosis (TB) case rate among the elderly living in nursing homes is almost 4 times that of the elderly living elsewhere. Purified protein derivative (PPD) testing is advised for all residents on entering institutional care and annually thereafter, for high-risk groups, and for those who have signs of disease or close contact with persons with documented cases. Persons who test positive should have chest radiographic evaluation. Persons who test negative should be retested in a week. Although tuberculin cannot sensitize an uninfected person, retesting may enhance the hypersensitivity reaction from a remote tuberculous infection. Tuberculin test positivity only after boosting is common in the elderly, in persons with nontuberculous mycobacteria, and in bacille Calmette-Guérin-vaccinated persons. Each of these groups is considered at low risk in the absence of pulmonary findings. Since this booster effect can persist for up to a year, it is important to perform the booster test promptly rather than interpret a test a year later as a recent converter (20).

Dental care in the elderly should be provided because of the association of dental disease with discomfort, malnutrition, endocarditis, and aspiration pneumonia. Podiatric care is advised annually, more frequently for diabetics and patients with peripheral vascular disease.

The use of home intravenous antibiotic therapy with long-term indwelling catheters also presents difficulties in determining sources of bacteremia and sepsis. Strict adherence to infection control practices, dedicated medical record keeping with data shared among all sites of medical care, and the improvement of outpatient protocols for catheter care may assist in reducing morbidity and mortality.

To prevent puerperal fever, in 1848 Semmelweis argued for the simple measure of washing the hands in a chlorine solution until the cadaver smell was gone (21). Today, hand washing remains the single most important and effective method for preventing the spread of infectious disease.

SOCIAL AND COMMUNITY INFORMATION: ON EPIDEMICS

Ideally, clinicians should know the infectious disease patterns in their community, whether that is the hospital, nursing home, or community. Hospitals publish their bacterial resistance profile annually and are required to report significant infectious diseases. Many of the risks associated with hospitals may also be ascribed to chronic care facilities, especially for nosocomial pneumonia. There was a 46.6% increase in the age-adjusted COPD death rate from 1976 to 1993, so the growing population of the elderly will undoubtedly continue to suffer from the associated pulmonary and cardiovascular diseases (22).

Influenza, parainfluenza, or respiratory syncytial virus may cause epidemics in institutions or close living quarters. In contrast to bacterial infections in debilitated persons, viral epidemics may spread to all exposed persons and therefore require restrictive isolation. Elderly persons living in the community appear to have the same rate of pneumonia as younger persons, but once pneumonia has developed, older adults respond less well to treatment.

In 1883, Gustav Neuber of Kiel built a private hospital with a dust-free ventilating system, and he was the first to operate in surgical cap and gown. William Stewart Halsted of Baltimore started using rubber gloves in 1889. Ernst von Bergmann of Berlin introduced steam sterilization in 1886 and established the basic aseptic ritual in 1891 (23). Now we are again facing increasing numbers of patients with contagious diseases, perhaps with resistant organisms or active TB. Our modern approach includes negative-pressure air-filtered rooms, gowns and gloves, and sterilization techniques. Debate continues about the effectiveness and cost of high-efficiency particulate air filters (HEPA respirators) (24).

Hospitals are developing protocols for the care of patients who may have TB, since the diagnosis is often delayed and costly preventive measures of isolation must be applied early to protect health care providers and other patients. Primary TB infection typically produces only a transient, mild febrile illness with malaise. However, a primary infection may progress to produce chronic cavitary TB or even death, which may be mistakenly ascribed to antibiotic-unresponsive pneumonia. Elderly persons who are known to be tuberculin reactive are at a greater risk for developing active TB than are younger reactors. Physical signs are not very helpful in diagnosing pulmonary TB. The chest radiograph is essential to document the infiltrative process; any distribution of infiltrates may be consistent with TB. In reactivation of TB the most common abnormality is reticulonodular infiltration in the apicoposterior segments of the upper lobes, with or without cavitation. Miliary TB is more common in the aged than any other age group and generally follows the rupture of a caseous site into the bloodstream. Interestingly, relapse rates for TB are not increased in appropriately treated patients with extensive disease, cavitation, or surgery. Likewise, there is no requirement for additional drugs or increasing the duration of therapy when there are coexisting diseases such as diabetes, malignancy, or corticosteroid therapy (25). Consideration should be given to the expansion of programs for directly observed therapy to reduce noncompliance-associated relapse rates and the development of multidrug-resistant organisms (26).

MEDICATION REVIEW: READING THE TEA LEAVES

One challenging technique used to teach the principles of geriatric physiology and pharmacology is to have students develop their own list of the patient's diagnoses based exclusively on a lengthy current medication list. Recurrently hospitalized or institutionalized patients may be taking more than 20 medications, while the average drug use in patients more than 65 years of age is 5 to 12 drugs per day. Such exercises develop an appreciation for the common definition of a well-trained physician caring for the elderly as a physician who stops medications. Physicians should learn the variety of mechanisms by which drugs can affect the care of patients with infectious disease, and for difficult or high-risk patients the physician should readily consult with clinical pharmacologists and infectious disease specialists (27).

PHYSICAL EXAMINATION: GERHARDT'S DICTUM

Examination comes first, then judgment, and then one can give help [28].
                              —Carl Gerhardt (1833–1902)

The laboratory principles of sensitivity and specificity are difficult to apply to the physical examination of a patient with infectious disease. However, the concepts are useful to the practitioner, given the variations encountered in the diverse geriatric population. For example, in patients with documented COPD a finding of crackles at the base of a lung may be nonspecific, indicating chronic hypoventilatory changes, exacerbation of COPD, onset of heart failure, or pneumonia. In the presence of fever, however, crackles may be relatively sensitive and very specific for pneumonia if it was known that the lungs were clear on a prior examination. In the absence of fever, the crackles are considered less specific,

since congestive heart failure is a common consideration.

VITAL SIGNS

Since early detection of infectious disease allows a greater opportunity for effective intervention, professionals who care for the elderly must be alert to subtle changes in vital signs. The elderly often have disorders of homeostasis associated with chronic and debilitating diseases, so the vital signs must be assessed for changes from the baseline status as well as altered from "normal" standards.

A characteristic of infection is fever, but fever may be absent in elderly patients with a serious infection such as pneumonia or cholecystitis (29, 30). The assessment of fever must take into consideration the use of medications with antipyretic properties, such as nonsteroidal anti-inflammatories, steroids, and over-the-counter preparations. Chronic diseases, such as renal failure, also may alter the febrile response. However, fever in the elderly cannot be dismissed lightly, since it is relatively unlikely to be a benign viral infection (only 17% in one study) (31). The concept equating 98.6°F (37°C) with normal body temperature dates from the axillary temperature measurements of Wunderlich in the 1860s. A modern study found a mean temperature in healthy persons of 98.2°F (36.8°C) (32). Tympanic thermometers can measure core temperatures fast and accurately (33). Tachycardia may serve as a valuable guide for severity when fever is absent. β-Blockers and cardiac disorders also alter the expected heart rate response. Respiratory rates increase in a variety of infectious diseases in response to many stimuli, including fever, hypoxia, and acidosis. Respirations in excess of 25 breaths per minute constitute a relative risk factor indicating the need for hospital treatment of pneumonia or other disease.

NUTRITION AND FLUID ASSESSMENT

Nursing home patients with recurrent infections may lose weight out of proportion to their decrease of intake. Some degree of inadequate nutrition may be found in significant proportions of the institutionalized elderly (34, 35). Protein-calorie malnutrition in the elderly may contribute to immune deficiency, increased infections, and bedsores. A diet deficient in zinc may contribute to immune deficiency, poor wound healing, and poor antibody response to influenza vaccine (36). Diets high in fiber are advocated for persons who have had diverticulitis. On the other hand, high dietary fiber in bedfast persons may be constipating and can lead to megacolon or volvulus with presenting signs of an acute abdomen. Many elderly patients eat in a semirecumbent position, which may increase the risk of aspiration and pneumonia. Such considerations are important, since some immune deficiencies can be reversed and the risk of major septic complications can be significantly decreased by appropriate nutritional replacement therapy.

An assessment of the recent fluid intake and output for elderly patients is important because of the role of hypodipsia leading to dehydration and electrolyte disorders, which often accompany infections. Decreased urine flow may contribute to the development of UTIs. Urosepsis and other infections predisposing to shock require fluid support, but intravenous fluid administration and other osmotic loading must be monitored closely because of the reduced cardiac reserve in many elderly.

THE FOCUS OF THE EXAMINATION

All bedridden patients are at risk for skin breakdown and decubiti. Immobility and incontinence of bowel and bladder often contribute to the loss of skin integrity. Assessment of tissue oxygenation and perfusion is important, and findings of deficiency should lead to institution of measures to improve cardiac and pulmonary function. The single most important factor for improving the care of the skin and preventing decubiti is the regular observation of the skin for changes and the progression of any erythema, ischemia, or wounds. Only by turning the patient and inspecting decubiti can the clinician make appropriate and timely choices about therapy. Local care and debridement of decubiti without antibiotic therapy is adequate treatment unless there is sepsis or widespread cellulitis. In many cases the possibility of underlying osteomyelitis must be evaluated with radiographs or nuclear bone scans. Patients septic from decubiti require initial polymicrobial antibiotic coverage and subsequent therapy directed by culture results. A variety of regimens are available, and the choice should be guided by local hospital or nursing home antibiotic resistance patterns.

Infectious disease with associated skin changes may not present in a typical fashion in the elderly, which contributes to delay or failure to diagnose and treat properly. For example, pyogenic infections such as *Staphylococcus* and β-hemolytic streptococci may not develop the characteristic heat, redness, and pain. Cellulitis may present as an indolent swelling and a furuncle, as a cold abscess. In patients who are immunosuppressed or on high-dose steroids, the depth and extent of fasciitis is often underestimated. In cases of fasciitis it is often necessary to obtain surgical tissue for accurate cultures early in the course of the disease.

Early recognition of herpes zoster, which most commonly affects persons aged 50 to 70, is important because prompt therapy decreases the risk of postherpetic neuralgia. Famciclovir 750 mg 3 times a day for 7 days or valacyclovir 1 g 3 times a day for 7 days, if started within 72 hours of symptom onset, may be more effective than acyclovir 800 mg 5 times a day for 7 days in shortening the duration of the rash and in decreasing postherpetic neuralgia (37).

Skin cultures yielding exotic organisms such as unusual anaerobes, gram-negative bacteria, or yeastlike fungi should not be dismissed lightly as contaminants. In the elderly, tinea pedis often extends beyond the fifth digital interspace and is accompanied by onychomycosis. Patients with tinea often develop secondary staphylococcal infections requiring antibiotic treatment. A high index of suspicion is warranted for scabies when there is a widespread pruritic eruption.

Staphylococci, streptococci, and gram-negative bacteria are frequent causes of conjunctivitis, but fungi, toxins, irritating chemicals, and drug allergies should also be considered. Viral conjunctivitis is typically bilateral, with red eyes, but is less exudative than bacterial conjunctivitis. Pharyngitis is sometimes associated with viral conjunctivitis. Viruses may cause infection of the cornea and conjunctiva simultaneously and may warrant ophthalmologic consultation, especially if herpes is suspected. Blepharitis is a common and chronic disorder in the elderly and may require antibiotic treatment for acute forms.

External otitis frequently accompanies cerumen impactions, the most easily treated cause of hearing loss. Polymyxin B-neomycin-cortisone drops are very effective against the usual organisms, *Pseudomonas, Proteus,* and Enterobacteriaceae. Treatment failures may result from difficulty in delivering the drops deep into the canal or from infection with fungi. Malignant otitis externa is recognized when external otitis progresses to *Pseudomonas* cellulitis in poorly controlled diabetics. Mild cases may respond to outpatient therapy with ciprofloxacin 500 to 750 mg orally twice a day, but intravenous antipseudomonal antibiotics are commonly required for more severe cases, perhaps with surgical debridement.

Examination of dentition is important, as the teeth are a potential site of abscesses and a source of organisms in infective endocarditis and aspiration pneumonia. Oral candidiasis may present with minimal signs and yet lead to inadequate oral intake, especially when esophageal candidiasis is present. Treatment with nystatin 500,000 U oral swish and swallow 4 times a day for 14 days or with clotrimazole 10-mg troches 5 times a day for 14 days is usually well tolerated, producing a response within 4 days. HIV-infected patients with thrush have been found to be more responsive to fluconazole 200 mg single dose orally or 100 mg a day for 5 days than to clotrimazole (38). Patients with poor response, resistant organisms, or immunosuppression such as with acquired immunodeficiency syndrome may require amphotericin B, for which infectious disease consultation is advisable.

Neck stiffness is difficult to interpret as a sign of meningitis when there is associated Parkinson's disease or cervical arthritis. A high index of suspicion for meningitis is warranted, since mortality may be reduced from 41 to 19% with adequate early therapy for community-acquired meningitis. The most common pathogen associated with meningitis in older persons, *Streptococcus pneumoniae*, has demonstrated increasing resistance to penicillin as well as cefotaxime and ceftriaxone. Coliforms, *Haemophilus influenzae, Listeria monocytogenes, Pseudomonas aeruginosa,* and *Neisseria meningitidis* constitute less likely organisms. Gram-negative bacilli are more frequent in nosocomial infections. Initial therapy in areas with higher pneumococcal resistance should include vancomycin and cefotaxime or ceftriaxone. There are limited data on the effectiveness of dexamethasone, which may be considered for patients with meningitis when the spinal fluid Gram stain indicates many bacteria or the patient is in coma with evidence of increased intracranial pressure or cranial nerve paralysis (39). There are no significant differences in mortality related to common pathogens, but a higher mortality may be expected for patients aged 60 years or older who have an obtunded mental status upon admission or who have seizures within 24 hours of admission. Empiric therapy should be given within 30 minutes of presentation. When neurologic deficits are present, prompt antibiotic therapy may necessitate administration of antibiotics prior to a cranial computed tomography and lumbar puncture (40). Infectious disease consultation is appropriate for patients with bacterial meningitis.

The ability accurately to assess and record pulmonary findings remains the essential first step in initiating timely and cost-effective therapy for pulmonary disorders. Diagnostic and therapeutic decisions often require specific knowledge of the premorbid status of the patient. Elderly patients often present with pulmonary findings that may have both infectious and cardiovascular causes.

The cardiac examination is especially important in the setting of infective endocarditis; attention must be directed toward finding any new or changing murmurs, which may indicate valvular destruction or the extension of a periannular abscess. Auscultation for pericardial rubs is often the key to establishing the diagnosis of tuberculous, bacterial, or viral pericardial disease. Repeated examinations in multiple positions are essential because of the intermittent presentation of pericardial rubs.

In caring for the elderly patient, a high index of suspicion and an awareness of the insidious symptoms of acute abdominal disease are mandatory. The elderly suffer the most from wound dehiscence and have higher complication rates than younger persons. For example, appendicitis is less common in the elderly than in the young, but symptoms are more likely to be ignored by the patient, and the mortality is higher, up to 10%. The classical sequence of symptoms is uncommon. The elderly are more likely to have a period of abdominal discomfort with nausea and anorexia but without vomiting. Rebound tenderness and guarding are present only half the time. Nearly all of the mortality with appendicitis in the elderly is associated with delay in diagnosis and perforation or gangrenous bowel at surgery (41).

Biliary tract disease is the most common indication for abdominal surgery in the elderly, accounting for 26 to 40% of acute abdominal disease. In patients with suppurative cholecystitis, one fourth may not have abdominal tenderness, one third may have no temperature elevation, one third may have no white blood cell count (WBC) elevation, and one third may have no peritoneal signs. Because the elderly so often have minimal findings with florid peritonitis, acute cholecystitis must be considered an indication for emergency surgery.

Clinicians should be mindful of effective antibiotic therapy for recurrent gastric ulcers from *Helicobacter pylori*. Recent trials have shown effectiveness for a variety of well-tolerated and shorter-term antibiotic regimens (42).

Volvulus may present with massive abdominal distension but only a mild degree of discomfort. Sepsis, shock, and severe pain occur late in the course along with increasing bowel wall tension. The twisting of a redundant portion of colon on a narrowed mesentery occurs most commonly in the sigmoid colon and is less likely in the cecum. Patients with volvulus typically have comorbidities of severe pulmonary, cardiac, neurologic, or psychiatric disorders with inactivity and chronic constipation. Although sigmoid volvulus constitutes only about 5% of large bowel obstruction, the subtleties of presentation require special consideration in the elderly with any signs or symptoms of an acute abdomen.

Diverticulitis is common and often recurrent in the elderly. The usual organisms are Enterobacteriaceae, bacteroides, and enterococci. Primary treatment consists of oral antibiotics such as sulfamethoxazole 800 mg plus trimethoprim 160 mg orally twice a day or ciprofloxacin 500 to 750 mg orally twice a day with metronidazole 500 mg orally 4 times a day until a clinical response is obtained. Assessment of severe forms of this extraluminal disease may require evaluation with computed tomography in addition to contrast studies or endoscopy. Treatment may require intravenous antibiotics and surgical resection. Patients taking steroids often have very misleading symptoms and examination even in the presence of colonic perforation (43).

Examination of the lower extremities with a finding of ulcers or poor wound healing should prompt consideration of underlying venous insufficiency or diabetes. Venous insufficiency ulcers usually have *S. aureus* and various gram-negative bacilli. Diabetic ulcers commonly have complex isolates of aerobes and anaerobes. Decubitus cultures also reflect this complex flora, and blood cultures may yield more than one organism. Arterial insufficiency also must be assessed in lower extremity ulcers that fail to heal, especially in diabetics and other persons known to have arteriosclerosis.

LABORATORY AND IMAGING STUDIES

And therefore before a man sets forward he should ask himself this question: Am I not upon the verge of something unnecessary [44]?

—Marcus Aurelius (121–180 AD)

In the well elderly there is no evidence in laboratory reference ranges for a loss of general metabolic homeostasis. The elderly, however, do demonstrate a higher probability of metabolic disturbances when they are ill. As with the assessment of vital signs, it is important to focus on changes in laboratory values in addition to comparison with established reference ranges.

Laboratory and imaging studies not only establish diagnoses but also assist in the recognition of host factors that influence the prognosis. An albumin of less than 3 g/dL or total protein of less than 5.5 g/dL constitutes a poor prognostic sign in the elderly. Low cholesterol levels also are an indicator of protein-calorie malnutrition and have been correlated with mortality in the long-term health care setting (45). A total lymphocyte count of less than 1500/mL has been used as a sign of malnutrition. Loss of cell-mediated immunity may be suspected in patients with lymphocyte counts less than one third of normal. Such readily available data may indicate the need for nutritional support early in the course of an infectious or surgical disease.

The WBC must be interpreted carefully, since some healthy persons maintain baseline counts of 10,000 to 12,000/mL, while other equally healthy persons have counts in the range of 3,000 to 4,000/mL (46). It is generally accepted that granulocytes have to be decreased to less than 10% of normal before an increased susceptibility to infection is manifested. In the particular case of bacterial pneumonia, a WBC of less than 10,000/mL is not unusual, but early forms (left shift) are usually increased. The absence of leukocytosis and fever in elderly patients with pneumonia correlates with increased mortality (47).

Sputum specimens are often difficult to obtain in the elderly because of their inability to cooperate, ineffective cough with decreased ciliary transport, and disease states such as dehydration, congestive heart failure, and chronic pulmonary disease. Studies in patients with pneumonia suggest that no likely organism may be found in up to half of the cases, and the organisms to which the pneumonia is ascribed may have been selected largely by judgment of the treating physician. Interpretation of sputum specimens must take into consideration that patients from long-term care facilities may have colonization of the oropharynx with gram-negative organisms without pneumonia. Changes in the antibiotic regimen for pneumonia should not be based on each new resistant organism recovered from repeated sputum specimens. Such specimens obtained during antibiotic therapy are expected to yield resistant organisms. Sputum cultures should be limited to use as an indication of the probable cause of pneumonia rather than as a method to assess the response to therapy.

Reliable interpretation of chest radiographs requires not only the wisdom of experience but also knowledge of the current symptoms and prior films for comparison. In patients with pneumonia it is common to find that chest radiographs may progressively worsen in spite of appropriate initial treatment, so reliance should be placed on other parameters of response to therapy. Hydration may also accentuate infiltrates of patients with pneumonia. If a patient fails to respond, the clinician should review the possibility of a wrong diagnosis, inappropriate or inadequate levels of antimicrobial therapy, superinfection, adverse drug reaction such as a fever, and an inadequate host response. Follow-up radiographs several weeks after apparent recovery are important to determine that pulmonary infiltrates have cleared and to exclude pulmonary lesions such as bronchogenic neoplasms. Bronchoscopy and percutaneous needle biopsy under computed tomography are used increasingly to obtain specimens for culture and cytology.

ASSESSMENT: VIRCHOW'S EMPHASIS

The basis of understanding disease is the study of the way in which it distorts not only normal structure, but normal function as well [48].
—Rudolf Virchow (1821–1902)

In geriatrics, assessment must extend beyond the diagnosis and treatment to include the probability of complications, the expected functional level, and ethical concerns. The most characteristic measure of aging may be the reduced ability to respond adaptively to environmental challenges such as infectious disease. *Frailty* is a useful concept for indicating an inherent vulnerability to diseases and other challenges. Frailty is often applied to patients of extreme age and to younger elderly who have chronic diseases or limitations that decrease their ability to respond to the stress of illness or treatment in a hospital. Optimal outcomes in the frail elderly require identifying multiple-organ disease states to avoid unexpected adverse results from diagnostic or therapeutic efforts. Translated from Hippocrates' *Epidemics,* this emphasis becomes "to help, or at least do no harm" (49).

Prognosis is correlated with functional level in the recovery from infectious disease. Patients with infectious diseases in nursing homes have some of the same high risk factors for morbidity and mortality as hospitalized patients, again principally because of their age, functional level, and comorbidities. Very often when nursing home residents become acutely ill, they simply need a few days of close observation with intravenous antimicrobials and hydration, as might be the case for a lower respiratory infection or UTI. Decisions about hospitalization in these situations depend on the abilities of the physician and nursing home staff to provide services, the preferences of the resident and the family, and the availability of acute hospital care. Many cases of nursing home–associated pneumonia can be treated successfully with oral antibiotics, but nursing home treatment failed 31% of patients in one study. As with so many diseases of the elderly, failure of treatment for pneumonia in the nursing home setting is associated with the functional losses of feeding dependency, the need for mechanically altered diets, and abnormal vital signs (50).

MEDICATION: THE SILVER BULLETS

Remember how much you do not know. Do not pour strange medicines into your patients [51].
— Sir William Osler (1849–1919)

Given the wide variation in drug absorption and metabolism in the elderly, it is essential to individualize the treatment program carefully. In the hospital, the number of drugs prescribed increases with age and length of stay, so ongoing assessment of the possibility of interactions with antibiotics and other agents is required. Age alone affects drug absorption less than disease conditions, concurrent drug therapy, and meals. Coadministration of food may reduce the absorption of drugs such as penicillin and cephalosporins. Cholestyramine binds penicillin. Antacids may reduce the absorption or bioavailability of tetracycline, quinolones, and isoniazid. Drugs with anticholinergic effects may reduce the absorption of tetracycline and other drugs.

In the elderly, the daily production of creatinine decreases with the age-associated decrease in lean body mass. Thus, the loss of glomerular filtration may not be revealed by the serum creatinine alone. An assessment of renal function, as measured with creatinine clearance or estimated with the Cockroft formula, is the most important consideration in antibiotic prescribing for the elderly (52). Special consideration must be given to patients with hypertension, diabetes, vascular disease, prior renal disease, obstructive uropathy, or recent insults to renal function such as shock or contrast agents. Considerable caution must be exercised with aminoglycoside agents because of their high potential for nephrotoxicity. Serum peak and trough levels of the aminoglycosides are required, since underdosing is also a frequent problem.

Antibiotic therapy in the elderly is complicated for many reasons in this population at risk. Treatment is too often delayed because the disease presentation may not have the typical signs and symptoms. Patients in long-term care facilities may present with unusual and resistant bacterial flora. The elderly have more polymicrobial infections than younger patients, especially more mixed aerobic-anaerobic bacterial infections. Finally, treatment duration in the elderly is generally longer because of functional or disease-related changes that predispose to treatment failure.

Because of the high incidence of complications during the care of the elderly there is increasing emphasis on research in prophylactic treatments. For example, studies have indicated that the risk of nosocomial pneumonia in mechanically ventilated patients receiving stress ulcer prophylaxis appears to be less with sucralfate than with antacid or ranitidine (53).

The principles of antibiotic prophylaxis for surgery are increasingly well defined. Hospitals now publish guidelines and monitor both procedure and individual physician infection rates with a focus on appropriate antibiotic selection, timely intravenous administration (infusion completed prior to skin incision), and duration of postoperative antibiotic therapy. Evidence supporting a single preoperative dose is mounting, with most advocates recommending another dose if the operation lasts more than 2 or 3 hours (54).

PROGNOSIS

A conservative approach in caring for the elderly with infectious disease is to assume that a patient may have defective host defenses. In the elderly, the outcome of any acute illness often depends more on the various attributes of the host than on the virulence of the infecting organism.

When confronted with a poor outcome, physicians may say, "But the patient looked so good!" Since the presentation of infectious disease in the elderly is so variable, the general appearance of a patient should not be used to exclude a diagnosis. A corollary to this principle relates to decisions about appropriate disposition or level of care after a patient has been diagnosed with an infectious disease. Such decisions about care settings should be based on the initial diagnosis and the presenting condition of the patient rather than on the condition shortly after treatment has begun. As an example, the elderly patient with a fever spike, shaking chills, and leukocytosis should be evaluated and treated for probable bacteremia rather than assuming a relatively benign prognosis based on an afebrile state following response to acetaminophen and fluids. Indeed, some patients with infectious diseases succumb in spite of an initial response to timely and appropriate treatment with all available supportive therapy. "Sometimes the bugs win" (D Thomas Crawford, personal communication, 1997).

REFERENCES

1. Nuland SB. Doctors: The Biography of Medicine. New York: Random House, 1989:153.
2. Bartlett JG. The 10 most common questions about *Clostridium difficile*-associated colitis. Infect Dis Clin Pract 1992;1:256–259.
3. Livornese LL Jr, Dias S, Samel C, et al. Hospital acquired infection with vancomycin-resistant *Enterococcus faecium* transmitted by electronic thermometers. Ann Intern Med 1992;117:112–116.
4. Alary M, Joly JR. Factors contributing to the contamination of hospital water distribution systems by legionellae. J Infect Dis 1992;165:565–569.
5. Sanford MD, Widmer AF, Bale MJ, et al. Efficient detection and long-term persistence of the carriage of methicillin-resistant *Staphylococcus aureus*. Clin Infect Dis 1994;19:1123–1128.
6. Kauffman CA, Terpenning MS, He X, et al. Attempts to eradicate methicillin-resistant *Staphylococcus aureus* from a long-term-care facility with the use of mupirocin ointment. Am J Med 1993;94:371–378.
7. Interim guidelines for prevention and control of staphylococcal infection associated with reduced susceptibility to vancomycin. MMWR Morb Mortal Wkly Rep 1997; 46:626–635.
8. Clark A. The discussion on catheter or urinary fever. Lancet 1884;1:137.
9. Harding GK, Nicolle LE, Ronald AR, et al. How long should catheter-acquired urinary tract infections in women be treated? A randomized controlled study. Ann Intern Med 1991;114:713–719.
10. Nuland SB. Doctors: The Biography of Medicine. New York: Random House, 1989:194.
11. Deajani AS, Taubert KA, Wilson W, et al. Prevention of bacterial endocarditis: recommendations by the American Heart Association. Circulation 1997;96:358–366.
12. van der Meer JT, van Wijk W, Thompson J, et al. Awareness of need and actual use of prophylaxis: lack of patient compliance in the prevention of bacterial endocarditis. J Antimicrob Chemother 1992;29:187–194.
13. Chen SC, Dwyer DE, Sorrell TC. A comparison of hospital and community-acquired infective endocarditis. Am J Cardiol 1992;70:1449–1452.
14. Shapiro SM, Young E, De Guzman S, et al. Transesophageal echocardiography in diagnosis of infective endocarditis. Chest 1994;105:377–382.
15. Mortality patterns—United States, 1993. MMWR Morb Mortal Wkly Rep 1996;45:161–164.
16. Govaert TM, Thijs CT, Masurel N, et al. The efficacy of influenza vaccination in elderly individuals. A randomized double-blind placebo-controlled trial. JAMA 1994; 272:1661–1665.
17. Prevention and control of influenza: recommendations of the Advisory Committee on Immunization Practices (ACIP). MMWR Morb Mortal Wkly Rep 1997;46(Rr-9):1–25.
18. Prevention of pneumococcal disease: recommendations of the Advisory Committee on Immunization Practices. MMWR Morb Mortal Wkly Rep 1997;46(Rr-8):1–24.
19. Tetanus surveillance—United States, 1991–1994. MMWR Morb Mortal Wkly Rep 1997;46(Ss-2):15–25.
20. Menzies R, Vissandjee B, Rocher I, St Germain Y. The booster effect in two-step tuberculin testing among young adults in Montreal. Ann Intern Med 1994; 120:190–198.
21. Nuland SB. Doctors: The Biography of Medicine. New York: Random House, 1989:247.
22. Mortality patterns—United States, 1993. MMWR Morb Mortal Wkly Rep 1996;45:161–164.
23. Nuland SB. Doctors: The Biography of Medicine. New York: Random House, 1989:382.
24. Adal KA, Anglim AM, Palumbo CL, et al. The use of high-efficiency particulate air-filter respirators to protect hospital workers from tuberculosis: a cost effectiveness analysis. N Engl J Med 1994;331:169–173.
25. Initial therapy for tuberculosis in the era of multidrug resistance. MMWR Morb Mortal Wkly Rep 1993;42(Rr-7):1–8.
26. Weis SE, Slocum PC, Blais FX, et al. The effect of directly observed therapy on the rates of drug resistance and relapse in tuberculosis. N Engl J Med 1994;330:1179–1184.

27. Stein BE. Avoiding drug reactions: seven steps to writing safe prescriptions. Geriatrics 1994;49:28–30.

28. Nuland SB. Doctors: The Biography of Medicine. New York: Random House, 1989:200.

29. Metlay JP, Schultz R, Li Y, et al. Influence of age on symptoms at presentation in patients with community-acquired pneumonia. Arch Intern Med 1997;157:1453–1459.

30. Norman DC, Toledo SD. Infections in elderly persons: an altered clinical presentation. Clin Geriatr Med 1992; 8:713–719.

31. Keating HJ III, Klimek JJ, Levine DS, Kiernan FJ. Effect of aging on the clinical significance of fever in ambulatory adult patients. J Am Geriatr Soc 1984;32:282–287.

32. Mackowiak PA, Wasserman SS, Levine MM. A critical appraisal of 98.6° F, the upper limit of the normal body temperature, and other legacies of Carl Reinhold August Wunderlich. JAMA 1992;268:1578–1580.

33. Edge G, Morgan M. The Genius infrared tympanic thermometer: an evaluation for clinical use. Anaesthesia 1993;48:604–607.

34. Pinchofsky-Devin GD, Kaminski MV. Correlation of pressure sores and nutritional status. J Am Geriatr Soc 1986;34:435–440.

35. Silver AJ, Morley JE, Strome LS, et al. Nutritional status in an academic nursing home. J Am Geriatr Soc 1988; 36:487–491.

36. Prasad AS. Zinc: the biology and therapeutics of an ion. Ann Intern Med 1996;125:142–144.

37. Kost RG, Straus SE. Drug therapy: postherpetic neuralgia: pathogenesis, treatment, and prevention. N Engl J Med 1996;335:32–42.

38. Koletar SL, Russell JA, Fass RJ, Plouffe JF. Comparison of oral fluconazole and clotrimazole troches as treatment for oral candidiasis in patients infected with human immunodeficiency virus. Antimicrob Agents Chemother 1990;34:2267–2268.

39. Townsend GC, Scheld WM. The use of corticosteroids in the management of bacterial meningitis in adults. J Antimicrob Chemother 1996;37:1051–1061.

40. Durrand ML, Calderwood SB, Weber DJ, et al. Acute bacterial meningitis in adults: a review of 493 episodes. N Engl J Med 1993;328:21–28.

41. Burns RP, Cochran JL, Russell WL, Bard RM. Appendicitis in mature patients. Ann Surg 1985;201:695–704.

42. Sung JJ, Chung SC, Ling TK, et al. Antibacterial treatment of gastric ulcers associated with *Helicobacter pylori*. N Engl J Med 1995;332:139–142.

43. Chappuis CW, Chon I Jr. Acute colonic diverticulitis. Surg Clin North Am 1988;68:301–313.

44. Gibbons R, ed. In Their Own Words. New York: Random House Gramercy Press, 1995:112.

45. Rudman D, Mattson DE, Nagraj HS, et al. Antecedents of death in the men of a Veterans Administration nursing home. J Am Geriatr Soc 1987;35:496–502.

46. Bender BS, Nagel JE, Adler WH, Andres R. Absolute peripheral blood lymphocyte count and subsequent mortality in elderly men: the Baltimore Longitudinal Study of Aging. J Am Geriatr Soc 1986;34:649–654.

47. Ahkee S, Srinath L, Ramirez J. Community-acquired pneumonia in the elderly: association of mortality with lack of fever and leukocytosis. South Med J 1997;90: 296–298.

48. Virchow R. The archive of pathological anatomy and physiology and clinical medicine. In: Nuland SB. Doctors: The Biography of Medicine. New York: Random House, 1989:312.

49. Nuland SB. Doctors: The Biography of Medicine. New York: Random House, 1989:16.

50. Degelau J, Guay D, Straub K, et al. Effectiveness of oral antibiotic treatment in nursing home-acquired pneumonia. J Am Geriatr Soc 1995;43:245–251.

51. Thayer WS. Osler the teacher. In: Thayer WS, ed. Osler and Other Papers. Baltimore: Johns Hopkins University Press, 1931:3.

52. Cockroft DW, Gault MH. Formula for calculating creatinine clearance from serum creatinine. Nephron 1976;16:31.

53. Prod'hom G, Leuenberger P, Koerfer J, et al. Nosocomial pneumonia in mechanically ventilated patients receiving antacid, ranitidine, or sucralfate as prophylaxis for stress ulcer: a randomized controlled trial. Ann Intern Med 1994;120:653–662.

54. Nichols RL. Update: antibiotic prophylaxis in surgery. Infect Dis Clin Pract 1996;5:S77–S84.

CHAPTER 24

TOM J. WACHTEL, MICHAEL D. STEIN, AND DAVID L. RABIN

HIV Infection in Older People

EPIDEMIOLOGY

The acquired immunodeficiency syndrome (AIDS) epidemic in the United States has affected primarily young adults because the prevalence of behaviors that result in infection with human immunodeficiency virus (HIV) is highest in that age group. Indeed, industrial nations are still in the epidemiologic pattern in which 80 to 90% of HIV transmission is attributable to male homosexual contact or intravenous drug usage (IDU) (1). However, the proportion of cases attributed to heterosexual transmission increased from 3% during the 1980s to 10% during the 1990s. Furthermore, the drug-using community is aging (2), and persons past age 50 are less likely to use condoms or undergo HIV testing than are younger ones (3). According to data from states with confidential reporting, about 5% of new HIV infections occur in persons aged 50 or more, both in men and in women (4). Women constitute a larger percentage of AIDS cases with increasing age: 13.2% for those aged 60 to 69 and 28.7% for those aged 65 or more. With 10.4% of cases in persons aged 50 or more (5), 573,800 cumulative cases in the United States in 1981 through 1996 (6), and an increasing proportion of AIDS deaths in the elderly, geriatricians cannot ignore the epidemic (7).

Blood transfusion is the mode of transmission in only 1% of cases in those aged 13 to 49, but it causes 6% of cases among those aged 50 to 59, 28% in persons aged 60 to 69, and 64% in those aged 70 or above (8). The rate of transfusion-associated AIDS peaked at age 55 to 64 for men and age 65 to 74 for women (9). Blood transfu-

sion is a very efficient mode of inoculation, with each contaminated unit associated with a 90% probability of infection (1). Most of the transfusion-acquired HIV infections in one study occurred during coronary bypass surgery (10). Since the introduction in 1985 of routine screening of blood products for antibodies to HIV, it is estimated that the risk of contracting HIV by transfusion is now lower than 1/150,000 units transfused (11).

PRIMARY CARE OF HIV-INFECTED OLDER PERSONS
History

Up to age 70, homosexual contact is the most common mode of transmission, but heterosexual transmission is an increasing risk, and most elderly remain sexually active (5). As HIV infection continues to occur in the elderly, both women and men, questions about sexual activity are important for those aged 50 and above of both sexes. In our experience older people are willing to discuss these sensitive areas. Questions specifying high-risk sexual activities should be asked directly and nonjudgmentally. A history of sexually transmitted disease should be considered a marker for HIV infection. Inquiry should be made about condom use. Unless the relationships are monogamous and HIV status is known, condoms should be recommended to prevent sexually transmitted diseases and HIV infection. As women are postmenopausal and not at risk of pregnancy, they may not appreciate their need for protection. Indeed, those aged 50 and above with sexual risk were only one sixth as likely to use condoms during sex as those in their 20s (3). The injection of illicit drugs should be discussed openly, but the yield of this area of inquiry generally is lower than in younger persons.

Equally important is a history of transfusions between 1978 and 1984. An estimated 20,300 persons over age 50 received transfusions contaminated with HIV (12). Since the incubation period between inoculation and a diagnosis of AIDS is estimated to average 8 to 10 years (13), the crest of this mode of transmission is behind us, so we can expect over the next few years a shift from transfusion-associated AIDS to sex- or drug-associated infection among older people. This shift emphasizes the need for attention to prevention of HIV for the elderly. While condom use has increased for younger people, in part owing to education about HIV prevention, most educational campaigns emphasize young people, impeding use or awareness of the need for condoms by the elderly (14). The elderly have much less awareness and knowledge about HIV and AIDS than younger people (15).

The review of systems should focus on constitutional symptoms (weight loss, fever, night sweats, fatigue), decreased physical or mental function, pain, and specific symptoms such as lymphadenopathy, rashes, oral lesions, headaches, decreased vision, cough, dyspnea, recurrent pneumonias, abdominal pain, diarrhea, recurrent vaginal discharge, and abnormal bleeding (16).

Physical Examination

The patient's weight should be recorded at each visit. The oral cavity is often the site of early manifestations of HIV infection. These include herpetic lesions, thrush, bacterial periodontitis, hairy leukoplakia (plaques on the side of the tongue), and nodules that may indicate Kaposi's sarcoma or lymphoma. The skin can also be involved early in the course of HIV infection; common skin disorders include viral infections (herpes simplex, herpes zoster, molluscum contagiosum, human papillomavirus), fungal infections (candidiasis, cryptococcosis), bacterial infections (*Staphylococcus,* syphilis), and noninfective disorders (seborrheic dermatitis, psoriasis, pruritic papules, Ka-

posi's sarcoma, and drug reactions). The lymph node groups should be examined; general lymphadenopathy may be the only manifestation of HIV disease. Lymph node biopsy should not be routine but should be considered if a single lymph node is rapidly enlarging, if the patient has the B type of symptoms of lymphoma, or if confirmation of a diagnosis of fungal or mycobacterial disease is needed. The pulmonary and cardiovascular examination should be documented for baseline purposes, together with liver and spleen size. The genitalia and rectum should be examined for any sexually transmitted disease. In women, recurrent *Candida* vaginitis is considered a marker of HIV disease, and the increased risk of cervical cancer in HIV-infected women calls for Pap smears every 6 months. The nervous system is involved in as many as 80% of patients with HIV disease, because the AIDS virus itself and many of the complicating opportunistic infections (e.g., *Cryptococcus*) and malignancies (e.g., lymphoma) have an affinity for it. Therefore, a careful baseline neurologic examination is important. It should include cranial nerve, motor, sensory, cerebellar, and reflex testing. HIV infection has been recognized as an important cause of dementia in older persons (16). In one study, HIV encephalopathy was diagnosed in 24% of patients above age 55, compared with only 9% of patients under age 40 (8). Therefore, a formal mental status examination (see Chapters 2 and 13) should be performed in all elderly persons with HIV infection every 3 to 6 months.

Diagnostic Studies

Testing for HIV is clearly the first step in the diagnosis of HIV infection (Table 24.1). The actual ordering of an HIV test should always be preceded by pretest counseling. Test recipients should be advised that testing can be performed anonymously at various testing sites or that it can be performed confidentially in the doctor's office. People have many misconceptions about the test. They should be told that a positive test does not imply AIDS but rather infection with the virus that causes AIDS and while they may remain asymptomatic for many years, they are contagious and must be taught how the virus is transmitted. Test recipients also should be told that while it is very accurate, the predictive value

Table 24.1

Management of Older Persons With HIV Disease

	CD4 Count		
	750 Cells/mm^3	350 Cells/mm^3	50 Cells/mm^3
Routine physical examination	Q 3–6 mo	Q 3 mo	Q mo
HIV test	Once	Once	Once
Pelvic examination, Pap smear	Q 6 mo	Q 6 mo	Q 6mo
Cognitive testing	Q 6 mo	Q 3 mo	Q mo
CBC	Q 3–6 mo	Q mo	Q mo
BUN and/or creatinine	Yearly	Q 3–6 mo	Q 3–6 mo
Transaminase, alkaline phosphatase	Yearly	Q 3–6 mo	Q 3–6 mo
Syphilis serology	Once	Once	Once
CD4 count	Q 6 mo till < 600; then q 3 mo	Q 3 mo	Q 3 mo
HIV RNA	Q 3–6 mo	Q 3 mo	Q 3 mo
PPD	Yearly	Yearly	Yearly
Chest radiography	Baseline	Pulmonary symptoms or as otherwise needed	Pulmonary symptoms or as otherwise needed
Pneumococcal vaccine	Once, perhaps q 5–10 years	Once, perhaps q 5–10 years	Once, perhaps q 5–10 years
Influenza vaccine	Yearly	Yearly	Yearly
Antiretroviral therapy	For high viral load	Yes	Yes
PCP prophylaxis	No	No	Yes
MAI prophylaxis	No	No	Yes

CBC, complete blood count; BUN, blood urea nitrogen; PPD, purified protein derivative (tuberculosis test); PCP, *Pneumocystis carinii* pneumonia.

of a positive test can be low if the pretest probability is low (i.e., in low-risk persons). The physician must be aware of state laws regarding the reporting of test results, the notification of partners, and the limits of confidentiality. False-negative tests may occur early in the course of infection during the window of seroconversion. Therefore, persons participating in HIV-risk activities may need to be retested. Causes of false-positive test results include chronic liver disease, autoimmune diseases, multiple myeloma, and infection with other retroviruses. Test results should always be given in person, which allows patients to ask questions and express feelings, as well as permits the development of a management plan.

Most laboratories perform both enzyme-linked immunosorbent assay (ELISA) and Western blot tests on a specimen submitted for HIV testing. ELISA is extraordinarily sensitive (99.5%) but less specific (98%). The Western blot test, used for confirmation of a positive ELISA, is less sensitive (98%) than the ELISA test but very specific (99.7%). Other tests for HIV infection include radiofluorescent antibody (RFA) and polymerase chain reaction (PCR).

The CD4 helper lymphocyte is a direct target of HIV, and its count is the most widely used indicator of a patient's level of immunodeficiency. The CD4 count is used to guide decisions regarding antiretroviral therapy and prophylaxis against opportunistic infections. Because there is variation in CD4 results depending on laboratory expertise, intercurrent infection, and time of day the blood is drawn, treatment decisions should be based on several values. Many staging systems have been suggested, the most widely used being the Centers for Disease Control and Prevention (CDC) classification system for HIV infection (17). In the clinical setting we find it more useful to sort patients into groups according to the CD4 count and the plasma HIV RNA quantification (viral load). This stratification allows predictions of prognosis and vulnerability to specific HIV-related disorders. Having more than 500 CD4 cells per cubic millimeter indicates a robust immune system; most persons have low levels of HIV RNA (fewer than 30,000 copies per milliliter), and patients are almost always asymptomatic. Between 200 and 500 cells per cubic millimeter most patients are asymptomatic but susceptible to bacterial and minor fungal infections; most begin antiretroviral therapy aimed at postponing the onset of symptomatic disease during this time. Below 200 cells per cubic millimeter antiretroviral therapy is continued and prophylaxis against opportunistic infections is suggested. Patients with fewer than 200 cells per cubic millimeter should be protected against *Pneumocystis carinii* pneumonia (PCP). Most patients with counts below 50 cells per cubic millimeter have advanced disease and are most susceptible to opportunistic infections (discussed later).

It is now clear that at least 10 billion HIV particles are produced and destroyed daily and that this viral turnover drives HIV pathogenesis. The level of HIV RNA in plasma has been shown to be the strongest predictor of long-term outcomes. While CD4 count and HIV RNA are in general inversely proportional, both are needed for optimal prognostic staging. The CD4 count should direct prophylaxis of opportunistic infections, and HIV RNA should direct initiation of antiretroviral therapy; changes in the HIV RNA and CD4 cell count determine the degree of clinical benefit conferred by specific antiretroviral drugs.

Other important diagnostic studies include complete blood counts, renal function tests, liver function tests, baseline hepatitis and syphilis serology, skin testing for anergy and tuberculosis, and a baseline chest radiograph. There is substantial consensus for planning the follow-up care and laboratory testing of persons according to CD4 count (18). Cancer screening should be offered as recommended by the American Cancer Society except for Pap smears, which should be obtained every 6 months.

Treatment

Specific textbooks in AIDS recommend appropriate management of opportunistic infections and malignancies (19). This section deals principally with the management of HIV disease in the primary care setting.

Antiretroviral Therapy

As of September 1997, 11 antiretroviral medications have been approved by the U.S. Food and Drug Administration (FDA). Each has a specific in vivo potency, side effect profile, and drug interaction concerns. The central goal of HIV therapy is to suppress viral replication to keep the viral load below the level of detection provided by current HIV RNA assays and to maintain this level of suppression as long as possible. In most cases this translates to the use of combination antiretroviral drug therapy. Studies over the past decade demonstrate that monotherapy (using nucleoside analog reverse transcriptase inhibitors (RTIs, such as zidovudine, ddI, ddC, 3TC, D4T) often only partially suppresses viral replication or suppresses it for short periods. Two-drug therapy may suppress replication for persons with low viral load levels (fewer than 30,000 copies per milliliter), but the duration of effect is usually found to be limited to 6 to 12 months. Higher initial viral load levels often require three-drug therapy for effective and durable suppression.

Because such regimens (usually including two RTIs and a protease inhibitor, such as indinavir, nelfinavir, ritonavir, or saquinavir) are complex and potentially toxic, maintaining long-term patient adherence is a challenge (20). Detailed discussion about the number of pills required, their timing, and medications to avoid is a particular concern for asymptomatic persons and those with other medical problems who are beginning lifelong HIV treatment. The financial cost of triple drug therapy is substantial, and some elderly do not have insurance that covers the cost of therapy. Some 40% of those with AIDS have Medicaid, but not all Medicaid programs cover triple drug therapy (21). Those on Medicare do not have drug coverage unless they have supplementary coverage. Furthermore, eligibility for Medicaid usually occurs late in disease, when institutional care expenses are great and the patient is impoverished; unfortunately, triple drug therapy should begin long before this time. Indeed, those with HIV infection and not AIDS are more likely not to be insured. Those with public insurance have broader coverage than those with private coverage. Elderly and disabled persons who have Medicare have broad home health care, hospice, and skilled nursing facility coverage, all desirable in caring for the late stages of disease.

It is likely that short-term nonadherence can result in the emergence of drug-resistant HIV strains, which can limit future options. Thus, making regular contact with the patient (often weekly at first) is critical to success. For patients who are unwilling to start triple-drug therapy, double-drug therapy may be recommended rather than deferral of therapy.

Successful continuation therapy should reduce HIV RNA levels to undetectable values within 1 month of initiation. The most likely cause of incomplete viral suppression early in three-drug therapy is noncompliance with the regimen by the patient, although resistance is also possible very late in disease. The likelihood of noncompliance is particularly great for those without drug insurance; even those on AIDS drug assistance programs may have difficulty, as the increasing costs of drug therapy have outpaced the ability of many states' programs to remain solvent throughout a year (22). Beyond 2 years, the durability of effect of triple-drug regimens remains unknown.

Prophylaxis of Pneumocystis carinii Pneumonia

When the CD4 count falls below 200 cells per cubic millimeter, oral trimethoprim-sulfamethoxazole (Bactrim, Septra) is recommended at one double-strength tablet daily or every other day. This regimen is more effective than aerosol pentamidine (23), which should be reserved for patients who develop toxic reactions (usually a rash) to trimethoprim-sulfamethoxazole. Aerosol pentamidine 300 mg is administered monthly. Oral dapsone 100 mg per day is as effective as aerosol

pentamidine in the primary prevention of PCP, and like trimethoprim-sulfamethoxazole, it may have the additional benefit of preventing toxoplasmosis.

Prophylaxis for Other Opportunistic Infections

At CD4 cell counts below 100 per cubic millimeter, patients are most susceptible to opportunistic infections. At this time, many clinicians offer clarithromycin 500 to 1000 mg per day, azithromycin (1200 mg once a week) or rifabutin (300 mg per day) to prevent *Mycobacterium avium* intracellulare (MAI), a progressive systemic infection characterized by fevers, diarrhea, and weight loss (24). Similarly, oral ganciclovir may lower the incidence of cytomegalovirus disease (most often retinitis), and fluconazole (50 to 100 mg per day) has been used to prevent cryptococcosis and candidiasis. Recurrent herpes simplex can be prevented with valacyclovir.

Vaccination

All patients with HIV infection should be given pneumococcal vaccination once, as early in the course of illness as possible to increase the likelihood that the patient will develop protective antibodies. Indeed, bacterial infections, while not AIDS-defining illnesses, play an important role in the morbidity and mortality of patients with HIV disease.

Influenza vaccination should be given yearly for the same reason. Hepatitis B vaccination should be reserved for patients whose personal behavior places them at risk for infection, and who show no laboratory signs of previous immunity. Of course, tetanus vaccination should be up to date (every 10 years) as in all adults.

Table 24.1 displays the routine diagnostic and therapeutic measures that the authors use as guidelines for the management of all elderly persons with HIV infection.

COURSE OF ILLNESS
Prognosis

The prognosis of HIV disease is considerably worse in persons over age 50 than in younger persons (25, 26). Many studies of prognosis are flawed by inaccurate information on the date of seroconversion and the finding that older people with HIV infection are diagnosed later in the course of infection (6, 9). Nevertheless, the information available from numerous cohorts of HIV-infected patients indicates rather convincingly that survival time after an AIDS diagnosis is inversely related to age (27, 28), that the period between inoculation and an AIDS diagnosis is inversely related to age (27), and that survival time from inoculation is shorter in older than in younger adults (29, 30). Causes of death in older patients with AIDS are similar to those described in younger patients (7, 31), with opportunistic infections and bacterial infection leading the list in all age groups.

However, recent findings indicate that progression of AIDS is particularly fast in the elderly because their HIV infection is likely to go unrecognized (32) and because of the coinfection and comorbidity that accompany the late diagnosis (33). It is likely that geriatricians have had less experience with HIV and AIDS, an unexpected diagnosis in the elderly. Physicians' experience with AIDS affects survival (34), which may account in part for the worse prognosis of AIDS in the elderly.

Finally, it is important to consider quality of life of patients with HIV disease, as it is in any terminal illness. Quality of life can be reliably measured with the Medical Outcomes Study Instrument (35), which explores six dimensions of well-being: physical function, role functions, social function, mental health, health perception, and pain. All other known parameters being equal, old age is associated with lower quality of life scores in all of the dimensions measured by the instrument. Equally important was the finding that symptoms are the strongest correlates of well-being, suggesting that aggressive management of patients' complaints in HIV disease can considerably improve their quality of life.

REFERENCES

1. Holmes KK. The changing epidemiology of HIV transmission. Hosp Pract 1991;26:153–178.
2. Zellweger U, Wang J, Heusser R, Somaini B. Trends in age at AIDS diagnosis in Europe and the United States: evidence of pronounced "ageing" among injecting drug users. AIDS 1996;10:1001–1007.
3. Stall R, Catania J. AIDS risk behaviors among late middle-age and elderly Americans: the National AIDS Behavioral Surveys. Arch Intern Med 1994;154:57–63.
4. Catania JJ, Truman H, Kegiles JM, et al. Older Americans and AIDS: transmission risks and primary prevention research. N Engl J Med 1989;29:372–381.
5. First 500,00 AIDS cases—United States, 1995. MMWR Morb Mortal Wkly Rep 1995;44:849–853.
6. Update: trends in AIDS incidence, deaths, and prevalence—United States, 1996. MMWR Morb Mortal Wkly Rep 1997;46:165–173.
7. US Centers for Disease Control and Prevention. HIV/AIDS surveillance report. MMWR Morb Mortal Wkly Rep 1996;8:1–40.
8. Ship JA, Wolff A, Selik RM. Epidemiology of acquired immune deficiency syndrome in persons aged 50 or older. J Acquir Immune Defic Syndr 1991;4:84–88.
9. Selik RM, Ward JW, Buehler JW. Demographic differences in cumulative incidence rates of transfusion-associated acquired immunodeficiency syndrome. Am J Epidemiol 1994;140:105–112.
10. Ferro S, Salit IE. HIV infection in patients over 55 years of age. J Acquir Immune Defic Syndr 1992;5:348–353.
11. Cumming PD, Wallace EL, Schorr JB, Dodd RY. Exposure of patients to human immunodeficiency virus through the transfusion of blood components that test antibody negative. N Engl J Med 1989;321:941–946.
12. Peterman TA, Lui KJ, Lawrence DN, Allen JR. Estimating the risks of transfusion-associated acquired immunodeficiency syndrome and human immunodeficiency virus infection. Transfusion 1987;27:371–374.
13. Medley GF, Anderson RM, Cos DR, Billard L. Incubation period of AIDS in patients infected via blood transfusion. Nature 1987;328:719–721.
14. Feldman MD. Sex, AIDS and the elderly. Arch Intern Med 1994;154:19–20.
15. LeBlanc AJ. Examining HIV-related knowledge among adults in the U.S. J Health Soc Behav 1993;34:23–26.
16. Lynn LA. Primary care for HIV infection. Hosp Pract 1992;27:48–64.
17. Karon JM, Buehler JW, Byers RH, et al. Projections of the number of persons diagnosed with AIDS and the number of immunosuppressed HIV-infected persons—United States, 1992–1994. MMWR Morb Mortal Wkly Rep 1992;41(Rr-18):1–29.
18. Stein MD, O'Sullivan P, Rubenstein L, et al. The ambulatory care of HIV-infected persons: a survey of physician practice patterns. J Gen Intern Med 1992;7:180–186.
19. Sande MA, Volberding PA. The Medical Management of AIDS. 5th ed. Philadelphia: Saunders, 1996.
20. Deeks SG, Smith M, Holodniy M, Kahn JO. HIV-1 protease inhibitors. A review for clinicians. JAMA 1997;277:145–153.
21. Diaz T, Chu SY, Conti L, et al. Health insurance coverage among persons with AIDS: results from a multi-state surveillance project. Am J Public Health 1991;84:1015–1018.
22. State AIDS Drug Assistance Programs: A National States Report on Access. Washington: National Alliance of State and Territorial AIDS Directors, 1997.

23. Bozzette SA, Finkelstein DM, Spector SA, et al. A randomized trial of 3 antipneumocystis agents in patients with advanced human immunodeficiency virus infection. N Engl J Med 1995;332:693–699.

24. Ostroff SM, Spiegel RA, Feinberg J, et al. *Mycobacterium avium* complex disease in patient infected with human immunodeficiency virus. Clin Infect Dis 1995;21:572–576.

25. Piette JD, Mor V, Fleishman JA. Patterns of survival with AIDS in the United States. Health Serv Res 1991;26:75–95.

26. Sutin DG, Rose DN, Mulvihill M, Taylor B. Survival of elderly patients with transfusion-related acquired immunodeficiency syndrome. J Am Geriatr Soc 1993;41:214–216.

27. Stehr-Green JK, Holman RC, Mahoney MA. Survival analysis of hemophilia-associated AIDS cases in the United States. Am J Publ Health 1989;79:832–835.

28. Goedert JJ, Kessler M, Aledort LM, et al. A prospective study of human immunodeficiency virus type 1 infection and the development of AIDS in subjects with hemophilia. N Engl J Med 1989;321:114–118.

29. Santagostino E, Gringeri A, Cultraro D, et al. Factors associated with progression to AIDS and mortality in a cohort of HIV-infected patients with hemophilia followed up since seroconversion. Cell Mol Biol 1995;41:371–380.

30. Darby SC, Ewart DW, Giangrande PL, et al. Importance of age at infection with HIV-1 for survival and development of AIDS in UK hemophilia population. Lancet 1996;347:1573–1579.

31. Stein M, O'Sullivan P, Wachtel T, et al. Causes of death in persons with human immunodeficiency virus infection. Am J Med 1992;93:387–390.

32. Alpert PL, Shuter J, DeShaw MG, et al. Factors associated with unrecognized HIV-1 infection in an inner-city emergency department. Ann Emerg Med 1996;28:159–164.

33. Shast DJ, Rubenstein E, Carley H, et al. The importance of co-morbidity in HIV-infected patients over 55: a retrospective case control study. Am J Med 1996;101:605–611.

34. Kitahata MM, Koepsell TD, Deyo RA, et al. Physicians' experience with the acquired immunodeficiency syndrome as a factor in patients' survival. N Engl J Med 1996;334:701–706.

35. Wachtel T, Piette J, Mor V, et al. Quality of life in persons with human immunodeficiency virus infection: measurement by the medical outcomes study instrument. Ann Intern Med 1992;116:129–137.

CHAPTER 25

B. LYNN BEATTIE AND VICTORIA Y. LOUIE

Nutrition and Aging

Mark Twain said, "The only way to keep your health is to eat what you don't want, drink what you don't like, and do what you'd druther not." Nutrition, health, and aging are related, and in recent decades choices of food and drink have made healthful eating easier. The objective of this chapter is to provide some understanding of the role of nutrition in aging, health, and disease, along with some practical guidelines for assessment and thoughtful intervention. It is hoped that these comments are more useful than Mark Twain indicated, since "nutrition is the environmental factor most subject to human control in contributing to the health of the aging and aged" (1).

Fries (2) speculated that the goal of a long and vigorous life may be attainable as a result of the compression of morbidity from chronic disease into very late life. However, it appears that increasing longevity is usually accompanied by only fair or poor health and limited activity, especially in the ninth and tenth decades of life (3). There is evidence in North America today that mortality from "lifestyle diseases," such as heart disease and stroke, is declining (4–6). Is personal responsibility for health producing the change? How much of this responsibility is related to nutrition?

Exton-Smith (7) observed that individual dietary patterns in most old people remain similar to those that have been acquired by habit established at a younger age. Nutritional health education is, therefore, a responsibility to the young. There is a great need for longitudinal studies and standardized surveys that measure dietary intake and incorporate clinical examination and laboratory investigation to develop meaningful descriptions of the specific nutritional needs of the elderly population. The American Dietetic Association (8) position statement emphasizes the relations among nutrition, aging, and health. The association supports "comprehensive nutrition services for the elderly as an integral component of the continuum of health care." Good health with increased physical activity stimulates appetite and thereby promotes better intake of nutrients.

Aging brings progressive loss of tissue function along with possible accumulation of diseases, including osteoporosis, atherosclerosis, cancer, obesity, diabetes mellitus, and hypertension. Application of knowledge of nutritional risk factors may influence the effects of these diseases on our society. Hazzard (9) commented in legal prose:

Whereas all age-related diseases are (by definition) time-dependent; and
Whereas all such processes are multifactorial in origin;
therefore:
Single modality intervention late in life is unlikely to yield appreciable benefit;
Intervention should be multifactorial and begin at an early age.

NUTRITION AND LONGEVITY

Knowledge of the relations between nutrient intake and duration of life span is expanding. Dietary restriction in laboratory animals can be brought about by reducing daily intake of a nutritionally adequate diet (one that supports maximal growth), intermittently feeding a nutritionally adequate diet (e.g., feeding every second, third, or fourth day) and feeding ad libitum a diet containing insufficient amounts of protein to support maximal growth (10).

McCay et al. (11, 12) showed that although growth was retarded, the life span of rats was increased with dietary restriction. Masaro (13) notes from animal studies that food restriction retards aging, extending the life and altering the rate of increase in age-specific mortality. This is apparently due to energy restriction, not restriction of a specific nutrient or nutrients. The mechanism may include a reduced rate of production of reactive oxygen molecules, an increased ability to scavenge them, increased ability to repair molecular damage, or a combination thereof. Whether these findings apply to human aging is debated. A cohort of persons from Germany who follow vegetarian diets and health-conscious lifestyles have been followed longitudinally (11 years), and mortality from all causes was half that of the general population (14). Factors other than diet, such as abstinence from smoking and selection bias, no doubt played a role.

There is an urgent need for research into levels of specific nutrients and eating patterns that optimize physical and mental development in youth, physiologic performance during adulthood, and retention of health and vigor in senescence. This research should be extended from laboratory animals to persons.

NUTRITION AND AGING

With aging, physiologic changes may affect ingestion and enjoyment of food. The sense of taste changes with aging. The number of taste buds on the lateral surfaces of the tongue that detect sweet and salty tastes decrease, leaving the central taste buds, which identify sour and bitter tastes, to predominate. The sense of smell tends to decline also, and the combined loss of gustatory and olfactory senses may lead to less interest in food. Decreased salivary flow, poor dentition, and decreased power of mastication that accompany the aging process may limit the amount and variety of foods eaten. The superimposition of various pathologic conditions may emphasize these physiologic changes. Ingestion may be hampered by the toothlessness, gingival lesions, mucous membrane erosions, or difficulty swallowing. Appetite may decrease because of physiologic or psychologic factors. Effects of intercurrent illness, surgery, or excessive alcohol ingestion may decrease intake.

Digestion tends to be slower with aging. There is a reduced capacity to regulate metabolism, hormonal induction of enzymes requires more time, and reduced numbers of hormone receptors are evident on cell surfaces. These factors may be increasingly significant in the face of pathologic changes such as hiatus hernia, reflux, and/or atrophic gastritis. Absorption appears to be little affected by aging, but many factors, including quality of nutrients, medications, and various disease states, may affect this function.

Some general effects of aging on body systems may be modified through attention to nutrition. Morley (15) reviewed nutritional modulation of behavior and immunocompetence suggesting that there are parallels with aging changes and protein-energy undernutrition (PEU). Some work shows that caloric supplementation restores immunocompetence, mitigating the aging decline.

Taylor et al. (16) described decreased lens and retinal function with increasing age, more so in smokers, and suggested that nutrient intake can delay cataract development, a common problem with increasing age. Snodderly (17) suggested that carotenoids and antioxidant vitamins may help to retard some of the destructive processes in the retina and retinal pigment epithelium that lead to age-related degeneration of the macula. The macula is rich in the carotenoid lutein found in spinach and other greens, broccoli, green beans, peas, and corn.

The cumulative effects of the changes of aging become more prominent as the years go on. Pathology may be superimposed. Awareness of the changes is necessary when assessing nutritional vulnerability and evaluating nutritional interventions to modulate phenomena that may not be inevitable.

NUTRITION SCREENING

It is cost effective to screen and identify for further assessment and intervention the elderly who are at high nutritional risk. The principles of the Canadian Task Force on Periodic Health Examination include screening for risk factors associated with malnutrition, including tobacco use, alcohol use, physical inactivity, and loneliness (18). The American Academy of Family Physicians, the American Dietetic Association, and the National Council on Aging, Inc., completed a 5-year multifaceted Nutrition Screening Initiative (NSI) to promote routine screening and better nutrition care of older Americans consistent with the report *Healthy People 2000* (19). The NSI developed a simple self-administered questionnaire for the elderly, the "Determine Your Nutritional Heath Checklist," based on known risk factors and indicators of poor nutrition (20). These include factors affecting diet quality and quantity, such as not eating for one or more days, eating fewer than two meals a day, regularly eating less than the recommended servings from the Food Guide Pyramid, difficulties eating or swallowing, extensive food avoidances, therapeutic diets used inappropriately or not provided, refusal to eat, eating fewer than 70% of meals provided in a long-term care facility, partial or total feeder dependency, and inability to make choices or express food preferences. Other factors relating to food insecurity and conditions that increase nutritional risk include alcohol use; polypharmacy; weight loss; dependency for food, feeding, and activities of daily living; oral health problems; recent hospitalization, surgery, or traumatic life events; altered mental states; nursing home admission; dehydration; dysphagia; and diarrhea, especially with fever and vomiting.

The checklist, or level I, screen permits identification of the elderly at high nutritional risk. The level II screen completed by health and medical professionals provides more specific diagnostic information on nutritional status and level of interventions. The interdisciplinary approach to delivering nutritional intervention incorporates social services, oral health, mental health, medication use, nutrition education and counseling, and nutrition support.

ASSESSMENT OF NUTRITIONAL STATUS

Nutritional status is the health condition of a person as influenced by his or her intake and use of nutrients. Nutritional assessment and intervention are essential components of nutrition services

and integral to the continuum of health care. In the elderly, the assessment of nutritional status is complicated by age-related changes in routinely measured parameters and by lack of appropriate standards for their interpretation. Its assessment requires the corroboration of data from clinical, dietary, anthropometric, and biochemical evaluations. Simultaneous use of these techniques substantiates findings and increases the sensitivity by which persons at risk for nutrient deficiencies or overnutrition may be identified.

Clinical History

When addressing nutritional assessment, it is important to assess attitude and interest in life and the activities of daily living. The role of physical disabilities in either procurement or preparation of foods is significant. Problems in ingestion and digestion must be addressed. Food avoidances and preferences are noteworthy. A history of bone fracture or abdominal surgery may be relevant. A complete drug history, including prescribed medications, over-the-counter medications, and laxatives, is necessary. Bowel and urinary habits may influence eating habits. The health of nails, hair, and skin and the predisposition to infection and ability to heal are important indicators of nutritional and general health.

The physician may assess nutritional risk through review of clinical status by history, physical examination, and assessment of the general intake of the major food groups. Baker et al. (21) studied the effectiveness of clinical evaluation of nutritional status, and examiners agreed in 81% of cases. This clinical evaluation correlated well with objective measures, although the oldest patient was only 76 years. Referral to a dietitian for a more extensive dietetic history is indicated when risk is evident and when intervention is recommended.

Dietary Assessment

The assessment of dietary status is important as an indicator of nutritional status. It predicts nutritional risk and substantiates the presumptive diagnosis from biochemical, anthropometric, and other observations. It entails estimation of the person's habitual intakes of food, conversion of food into nutrients using a food composition table, and comparison of nutrient intakes with dietary standards to determine their adequacy (22).

Methods for collecting data on dietary intake vary in their validity, reliability, and precision, and they depend on the food being recorded and the subject's characteristics. The elderly as a group may have limited ability to recall, impaired hearing and/or vision, and intakes that vary because of chronic diseases. There are two categories of methods for data collection, based on the time at which data are collected.

Retrospective methods estimate the amount and type of food and fluids consumed over the past 24 hours, several days, weeks, months, or years. These include the 24-hour recall, food frequency recall, semiquantitative food frequency recall, and Burke type of dietary histories. All are subject to considerable errors of recall. While the 24-hour recall is objective and convenient to administer, longer retrospective recalls provide data more representative of foods consumed by season, region, and ethnicity. The 24-hour recall, which is frequently used among free-living and institutionalized or hospitalized elderly, may be validated by repeated multiple recalls, direct observation, and other methods.

Prospective methods to assess current intakes include food diary, weighed food records, and direct observation. The foods consumed are recorded as estimated or weighed. Although a 7-day record is most representative of the usual intake, a 3-day record produces better record keeping by motivated older subjects who are able to read and write. Dietary assessment often depends on recall and good interview techniques. The presence of a relative or significant other and use of a checklist may be helpful. Data are compared against the nutritional standards, i.e., the Recommended Dietary Allowances (RDAs) and the Recommended Nutrient Intakes (RNIs).

Clinical Assessment

Clinical evaluation entails assessment of the mouth, skin, hair, eyes, nails, lower extremities, and various organs and systems. Angular stomatitis or cheilosis may be associated with niacin, riboflavin, or pyridoxine deficiency, but both are seen with ill-fitting dentures. Poor oral hygiene and periodontal disease produce changes that are indistinguishable from deficiency glossitis and gingivitis. The raw appearance of the tongue with filiform papillary atrophy is associated with niacin deficiency, and a magenta color reflects riboflavin deficiency, although irritants, systemic antibiotics, and uremia also may cause the discoloration. Soft and spongy bleeding gums indicate ascorbic acid deficiency or poor oral hygiene. The condition of the skin may reflect a person's nutritional status. Dry, inelastic skin may be associated with aging alone, dehydration, or follicular hyperkeratosis of vitamin A deficiency; nasolabial seborrhea, with lack of pyridoxine; and skin lesions of the exposed parts of the body, with niacin deficiency. Dryness, thickening, and opaqueness of the conjunctivae are observed with progressive vitamin A deficiency. Pale mucous membranes and cupping of the nails suggest inadequate iron. Lack of luster, depigmentation, and easy pluckability of the hair may accompany protein deficiency. Edema of the extremities may be associated with thiamin lack or protein deficiency from many causes. Enlargement of the liver or the thyroid, petechiae, ecchymoses, and other nonspecific findings should be considered in the overall assessment. Clinical assessment is highly subjective, and physical signs may indicate multiple nutrient deficiencies, nonnutritional influences, or combinations.

ANTHROPOMETRIC MEASUREMENT

Anthropometry measures changes in the body's composition of fat and fat-free mass as a reflection of how well the diet supplies the nutritional needs of the body. It is noninvasive, inexpensive, and easy to perform. However, it is subject to errors of measurement and interpretation. It is also nonspecific and usually imprecise unless the newer, more costly techniques for estimating body composition are employed. The most common measures are stature, body weight, triceps skin fold thickness, and upper arm circumference.

Stature and Body Weight

Accurate measurement of height is important because of its use in computing other indices of nutritional status. Baseline standing height should be measured annually because of age-related progressive bone loss and shortening of the spinal column. Where there is spinal curvature, flexion contraction of the legs, severe arthritis, paralysis, or amputations, the knee height distance between the sole of the foot and the apex of the knee with each joint flexed at a 90° angle may be used to predict adult height. Alternatively, stature may be estimated as twice the distance of the arm span from the sternal notch to the longest finger of the dominant hand.

Body weight is an estimate of total body energy stores. It is measured under standard conditions to minimize errors introduced by diurnal variation, clothing, different scales, and other factors, such as artificial limbs, casts, and orthopaedic shoes. Serial weights should be taken using the same scale, preferably a balance or wheelchair scale that is calibrated annually. The weight is monitored for changes in energy, protein, and water balance and is interpreted with caution in the presence of edema, ascites, and tumor.

Body weight is evaluated against the person's usual or previous weight. It is also compared with a reference standard for height and age of a healthy elderly population. The 1983 Metropolitan Height and Weight Tables show average weights for different body frame sizes associated with the lowest mortality for men and women up to age 59 only. Frisancho (23) has also compiled average weights as percentile distributions for up to age 74, based on data from the National Health and Nutrition Examination Survey (NHANES) I. The best, most comprehensive data on average weight for height up to 94 years are from Master et al. (24). Actual body weight that is 20% below or above the desirable weight is consistent with undernutrition and obesity respectively. Weight loss of more than 0.5 kg per day indicates a negative balance in either energy or water compartment or both (25). Loss of more than 10 pounds or 5% of the previous body weight in a month, or 10% or more in 6 months, is clinically significant. In chronic weight losses in which the absolute body weight is less than 55 to 60% of desirable, the energy reserve is near the survival limits of starvation. The minimum for survival is 48 to 55% of desirable body weight, corresponding to less than 5% fat or a body mass index (BMI) of 13 to 15. Weight loss also carries a prognostic value for outcome of treatment and disease. According to Windsor and Hill (26), loss of 10 to 20% of body weight before illness is accompanied by functional abnormalities in some patients, while loss of more than 20% of body weight before illness is associated with protein-energy malnutrition (PEM) and multiple functional abnormalities in almost all patients.

Another index of nutritional status based on height and weight for the estimation of body fat is BMI. Desirable BMI for persons over age 65 is 24 to 29; the lower and higher values suggest poor nutritional status and obesity respectively. BMI may be increased by high muscle mass or large body frame.

Skin Folds and Circumferences

Skin fold and circumferential measurements provide estimates of body fatness and energy stores, as well as estimates of lean tissue indices, total protein, and functional compartments (25). Serial measurements may be used to evaluate outcomes of nutrition intervention. These measurements include the following: triceps, biceps, subscapular, and suprailiac skin folds and mid upper arm, midthigh, and midcalf circumferences. Generally the more measurements at multiple sites, the more reliable the estimates. In practice, triceps skin fold and mid-upper arm circumference are most frequently taken. All measurements are subject to interobserver variation, individual variation in fat distribution, and changes in fat distribution with nutritional status. Since prediction equations were developed in healthy subjects, they are inaccurate when used in obese or undernourished seriously ill patients. In the elderly, they are made imprecise by hydration status, reduced skin elasticity and compressibility, and internalization of subcutaneous fat with aging (27).

After total body fat is computed, determinations are made for fat-free mass (FFM), total body energy, total body protein, and skeletal muscle protein. These values are compared with standards. Because of the nonspecificity of anthropometric measurements, the assessment for PEM requires correlation with laboratory analysis.

Other Methods

The creatinine height index (CHI) provides an estimate of muscle protein from the 24-hour creatinine excretion of a person compared with the standard healthy person of the same height. This tool is most practical in a research setting and may lack validity in older adults.

Bioelectrical impedance is a relatively new, economical, inexpensive, and simple but as yet insufficiently standardized technique for assessing lean body mass and fatness. Attention has been drawn to skeletal muscle function. Jeejeebhoy (28) has demonstrated that the force-frequency curve of the adductor pollicis muscle, obtained by stimulating the ulnar nerve at the wrist, is a sensitive and specific measure of nutrient intake or withdrawal. This technique is seen not to be affected by age and disease and has the advantage of being useful for ill or sedentary persons.

Recording of serial weight measurements remains the most practical means of assessing significant fluctuations in nutritional status or change in chronic disease states. Age- and gender-specific values must be applied when using standards.

LABORATORY ANALYSIS

Biochemical analysis provides an objective and noninvasive evaluation of nutritional status from determinations of essential nutrient and metabolite concentrations in bodily fluids. Biochemical indices are precise, sometimes providing early indicators of malnutrition, and they substantiate clinical, dietary, and anthropometric findings.

The initial laboratory evaluation should include albumin and a complete blood count with red cell indices and white cell differential (29). If anemia is a possibility, further investigations are warranted to differentiate deficiencies of iron, folate, and vitamin B_{12} from anemia of chronic disease. These include serum ferritin, which indicates early stages of iron deficiency; plasma iron, transferrin, and total iron-binding capacity, which assess the ability of transferrin to bind iron and free erythrocyte protoporphyrin; and red blood cell folate and serum vitamin B_{12} levels. The level of lymphocytes recalculated as to-tal lymphocyte count is a simple estimate of immunocompetence that is suppressed in PEM. In the absence of physiologic stress such as infection or injury and catabolic illness, serum albumin is a valid indicator of likely nutritional risk and likely benefit from nutritional interventions (25). Serum albumin responds slowly to protein repletion and is modified by other factors, such as congestive heart failure, bed rest, hydration, renal or hepatic failure, trauma, and surgery. Other plasma transport proteins with shorter half-lives responding more quickly to depletion and repletion are thyroxine-binding prealbumin, transferrin, and retinol-binding protein. Although they are also nonspecific, these indices reflect recent dietary protein-energy status and are good tools to monitor response to nutrition interventions.

Among other commonly used tests are fasting blood glucose to measure carbohydrate metabolism; thyroid-stimulating hormone (TSH) level to detect changes in thyroid function as consideration in malnutrition; blood urea nitrogen and creatinine, not as indicators of poor nutrition but to detect changes in hydration; and plasma sodium and potassium to analyze disturbances in fluid, electrolyte, and acid-base homeostasis.

Among all of the biochemical indices available, serum albumin carries the highest prognostic value for morbidity and mortality in the elderly. Recent studies by Sahyoun et al. (30) demonstrate serum albumin below 40 g/L as a predictor of 3-year mortality in institutionalized elderly and 9- to 12-year mortality in free-living elderly. Among hospitalized elderly, hypoalbuminemia is recognized as a marker of risk for complications in hospital, long hospital stays, frequent readmissions, and increased mortality in hospital and after discharge (31, 32).

DIETARY STANDARDS

The recommended daily intakes of energy and nutrients set out in the U.S. RDAs, last updated in 1989, are under revision after many years of consultation with the food and nutrition community (33). The new approach applies the concept of a safe intake range in which four reference points for a given nutrient are identified according to available scientific evidence. The comprehensive and complex guidelines called Dietary Reference Intakes (DRIs) comprise four categories: Recommended Dietary Allowances, Adequate Intakes, Estimated Average Requirements, and Tolerable Upper Intake Levels. In a paradigm shift, DRIs now establish levels of intake of nutrients for heath maintenance in meeting the requirements of almost all healthy persons in the population, for prevention of diet-related chronic disease, and for multiple uses by health professionals and nutrition policy makers. Given the heterogeneity of the elderly, age groupings to reflect age-associated physiologic and metabolic changes in nutrient requirements are 51 to 70 years, 71 to 80 years, and over 81 years (34).

The first group of recommendations released recently are for calcium, phosphorus, magnesium, vitamin D, and fluoride, nutrients related to bone health and other body functions. All other recommendations will be developed by the year 2000 and released sequentially, starting with folate and B vitamins (1998); then antioxidants (e.g., selenium, vitamins C and E); macronutrients (e.g., protein, fat, carbohydrates); trace elements (e.g., iron, zinc); electrolytes and water; and other nonnutrient food components (e.g., fiber, phytoestrogens).

The 1995 "Dietary Guidelines for Americans" (Table 25.1) support the seven key food-based recommendations of the previous guidelines (35). It is different from the nutrient-based recommendations of the DRIs. The new emphasis is on activity and exercise in achieving energy balance for weight control and health. The Food Guide Pyramid of 1990 replaces the Basic Four Food Groups as an educational tool to explain and interpret the dietary guidelines. It describes five major food categories depicted as a pyramid corresponding to the ideal relative proportion of each in the diet starting from the base to its apex: bread, cereal, rice, and pasta group; fruit group; vegetable group; meat, poultry, fish, dry beans, eggs, and nuts group; milk, yogurt, and cheese group. The greater emphasis on fruit and vegetables at present is reflected in a nationwide campaign, the "5 a Day for Better Health," to pro-

Table 25.1

Dietary Guidelines for Americans

1. Eat a variety of foods.
2. Balance the food you eat with physical activity. Maintain or improve your weight.
3. Choose a diet low in fat, saturated fat, and cholesterol.
4. Choose a diet with plenty of grain products, vegetables, and fruits.
5. Choose a diet moderate in sugars.
6. Choose a diet moderate in salt and sodium.
7. If you drink alcoholic beverages, do so in moderation.

Reprinted from Dietary Guidelines for Americans. 4th ed. Washington: US Departments of Agriculture and Health and Human Services, 1995.

mote the consumption of at least five servings a day of fruit and vegetables.

Nutrition Recommendations for Canadians

In Canada the Recommended Nutrient Intakes (RNIs) published in 1990 are the standard (36). Since Canada and the United States are collaborating in the development of the DRIs, it is likely that the same reference intakes will be applied in the revision of the RNIs. Similar nutrition messages are conveyed in Canada's *Guidelines for Healthy Eating,* amended in 1991, based on the *Nutrition Recommendations for Canadians* released in 1990 on healthful eating for disease prevention. The companion *Canada's Food Guide to Healthy Eating* provides guidance in food selection (37).

Energy

The RDA for people aged 51 and older is 2300 kcal for a 77-kg reference man and 1900 kcal for a 56-kg reference woman. The Canadian RNI for energy is comparable for ages 50 to 74 years at 2300 kcal for men and 1800 kcal for women. These are correspondingly reduced for 75 years and older to 2000 kcal and 1700 kcal respectively. Although there is a decrease in energy requirement with advancing age, there is no parallel decrease in the need for most other nutrients.

Estimated energy requirements are based on predictions of total energy expenditure (TEE). Its measurement is subject to inherent errors associated with attempts to categorize the typically varied activities usually performed by the elderly over 24 hours. It is compounded by interlaboratory variation in analytic procedures and computations, small sample size, heterogeneity of study group, study design, and scarcity of data (38). Roberts (38) reviewed six studies on TEE in elderly men and women. When published values are adjusted, the revised estimated energy needs are above the RDA. The percent body fat was the most significant predictor of TEE, which falls with age as the proportion of body fat increases. Alternatively, physical activity is the major determinant of variation in TEE.

While upward revision of the RDA may be warranted, recommendations to maintain regular physical activity into the later years are in keeping with the *Surgeon General's Report on Physical Activity and Health* (39). Physical activity prevents sarcopenia and preserves muscle strength and functional capacity while affording the elderly greater energy consumption and the likelihood of obtaining the recommended nutrients.

Protein

The RDA for protein is 0.8 g/kg per day based on extrapolations from nitrogen-balance studies conducted in younger people. This corresponds to 63 g/day for the reference man consuming 2300 kcal and 50 g/day for the reference woman on intake of 1900 kcal daily. There is not much information from the very few studies completed over the past 20 years on protein requirements in the elderly. Campbell and Evans (40) identified inherent errors in nitrogen balance studies to explain the conflicting results. Short-term studies tend to overestimate requirements because of inadequate equilibration periods to lower protein intakes. Long-term studies underestimate requirements when protein equilibrium is achieved at the expense of reduced body cell mass and muscle mass. The extent of contribution to nitrogen disequilibrium from inevitable age-related loss of lean body mass over the study period is also not known. In other studies reporting weight loss, the resulting negative energy balance contributed to negative nitrogen balance. Moreover, nonstandardized formulas for calculating nitrogen balance and safe level of protein intake were used.

Campbell and Evans applied standard procedures to data from several earlier studies and recalculated the mean protein requirement for the study group. When data from all studies were combined and adjusted to cover the needs of the majority of the elderly, findings were that the safe protein intake for both men and women exceeds the RDA at 1 g/kg per day or more. Although protein synthesis is decreased with aging, there is a corresponding decrease in protein degradation, so that protein balance in the healthy elderly is not altered. However, the elderly appear to show diminished efficiency in protein use (41). Gersovitz et al. (42) also noted that protein requirement was higher in the presence of acute and chronic diseases and in response to physiologic stresses such as wound healing and decubitus ulcer.

On the other hand, Millward et al. (43) argued for no revision in the 1985 Food and Agriculture Organization of the United Nations, World Health Organization, and United Nations University recommendation for protein from which the RDA was derived. Their studies using leucine balance studies found lower metabolic demand and lower apparent protein requirement with age without impairment in efficiency of protein use. Although there is no age-related change in whole-body protein turnover rates, there is a fall in skeletal muscle protein turnover. While it presumably contributes to loss of skeletal muscle mass and muscle strength, resistance training in elderly subjects restored the protein synthesis rates to those seen in younger adults. Similarly, the isotope balance technique used in determining protein requirement is not without its problems.

Carbohydrates and Fiber

There is no RDA for carbohydrates. The guideline places greater emphasis on intake of complex carbohydrates, up to 55 to 60% of total calories, which provides 20 to 35 g of dietary fiber daily. Complex carbohydrates comprise both starch and nonstarch nonnutrient polysaccharides. The proportion of dietary starch that becomes resistant starch is determined by numerous physical factors, including degree of processing, and physiologic factors, such as extent of chewing and rate of passage through the small intestine. Resistant starch resists digestion and is preferentially fermented to butyric acid, which improves colonic health and may protect against colon cancer (44).

Nonnutrient dietary fiber comprises insoluble and soluble fibers. Insoluble fiber containing cellulose, hemicellulose, and lignin is characterized by water-binding capacity. It is found in wheat bran, whole-grain breads and cereals, and skins of fruits and vegetables. Soluble fiber containing pectin, mucilages, and gums, forms gel matrices that slow down intestinal absorption and are metabolized almost completely in the large intestine by bacteria, giving rise to short-chain fatty acids as fermentation products. Sources of soluble fiber are oat bran, gums, fruits, vegetables, and legumes.

The role of dietary fiber in the treatment of constipation, hemorrhoids, and diverticular disease is well recognized. By its water retention capacity, a high fiber diet contributes to a softer, larger fecal mass that naturally stimulates peristalsis and reduces fecal transit time. Soluble fiber is also recommended for its viscosity and resultant delayed absorption of glucose and cholesterol in the control of diabetes and hypercholesterolemia respectively.

Fat

The risk of CHD (coronary heart disease) increases with elevated total cholesterol and other factors including smoking, hypertension, and diabetes. Decreasing the risk of CHD must address all risk factors, not just total cholesterol alone. It is reasonable to recommend modification of lifestyle and treatment for known risk factors including obesity, hypertension, and diabetes. The availability of highly effective drugs such as reductase inhibitors, which decrease cholesterol production, and the interest of the pharmaceutical companies in these products, which may be presented to 15 to 20% of the population estimated to have hypercholesterolemia, provide a major challenge to the medical community. The availability of these drugs must not preclude appropriate dietary and lifestyle management. Dietary prudence and lifestyle modifications in middle age may well reduce the burden of atherosclerosis in older age.

The recommendation is to limit dietary fat to 30% or less of total energy, of which essential fatty acids constitute 2 to 3%, and to reduce total cholesterol intake to no more than 300 mg per day. The recommendation is consistent with other guidelines offered by the National Institutes of Health Consensus Development Panel, the American Heart Association, and the National Heart, Lung and Blood Institute and is the goal of the National Cholesterol Education Program.

Over the 18 years between 1972 and 1990, the NHANES (45) reported on changes in the consumption of dietary fat and cholesterol that are consistent with nutrition education and health promotion initiatives to improve the cardiovascular health of the population. There were reductions in dietary fat, saturated fat, dietary cholesterol, and serum cholesterol. The percentages of energy derived from total, saturated, and polyunsaturated fats were 34%, 11.7%, and 7.1%. Mean cholesterol intake declined from 355 to 291 mg, with a corresponding decrease in average age-adjusted serum cholesterol concentration from 213 to 205 mg/dL. This is reflected in improved cardiovascular lipid profile, with declines in low-density lipoprotein (LDL) cholesterol from 213 to 205 mg/dL. This is in line with the *Healthy People 2000* goal of mean serum cholesterol concentration of 200 mg/dL by the year 2000. The reductions in serum cholesterol coincide with a reported decline in combined death rate from all cardiovascular disease by 45% between 1973 and 1993. Chapter 26 reviews lipid abnormalities in the elderly.

Vitamin Requirements

The RDAs for most vitamins are the same for younger and older adults. The exceptions are thiamin, niacin, and riboflavin, which are lower as a reflection of the lower energy needs of the elderly. In the face of lower energy needs, the nutrient density of the diet is important for meeting the recommended vitamin requirements. Energy intake of less than 1000 kcal per day is unlikely to furnish the needed vitamins and minerals.

There is evidence that aging changes requirements for some vitamins.

B Vitamins

FOLATE. The RDA for folate is 200 μg for men and 150 mg for women. There is a suggestion for revising it upward. Folate deficiency anemia occurs most frequently in the elderly (46). Low dietary folate intake is coupled with drug-induced folate deficiency from use of certain anticonvulsant and antibacterial agents, antifolate cancer therapeutics, anti-inflammatory drugs, and sulfasalazine. Folate absorption is also reduced by factors that alter intestinal pH, such as gastric atrophy and antacid use. In addition, cigarette smoking, alcohol use, and disease are also contributory. Yet the recent Boston Nutritional Status Survey reported mean plasma levels of less than 7 nmol/L in 2.5% of the 686 free-living and 266 institutionalized elderly (47). On the other hand, the Survey in Europe on Nutrition and the Elderly found no indications of biochemical deficiencies among persons 70 to 75 years old in towns of 10,000 to 20,000 population across 12 countries (48). It is possible that food folate is generally underestimated, as food composition tables are incomplete for folate. The extent of its bioavailability is altered by food processing and is variable from a mixed diet.

Low folate levels are associated with an elevated plasma homocysteine level, now considered an independent risk factor for CHD based on epidemiologic studies (46). It has a prevalence rate of 28 to 42% in various populations with CHD and carries a high risk of premature occlusive vascular disease. Previously considered normal folate levels in the elderly are also associated with high levels of homocysteine (49). High-dose folic acid (typically 5 mg/day) has a homocysteine-lowering effect in both healthy and affected subjects. It is possible that the level of food folate needed to prevent anemia is different from that which suppresses homocysteine. Supplementation either with folate or vitamin B_{12} is effective only if the elevation in total homocysteine is secondary to the vitamin deficiency.

There is evidence to support a role for folate in the regulation of mood and mediation of antidepressant drug effect (50). Folate deficiency resulting in megaloblastic anemia is commonly associated with depressive symptoms, followed by dementia and peripheral neuropathy. Conversely, marginal or deficient folate levels have been detected among patients with depressive disorders. Low levels of folate and its derivatives are correlated with the degree of severity and duration of these symptoms. The recent initial finding that low folate levels were related to poor treatment outcome with the selective serotonin reuptake inhibitor fluoxetine suggests a role of folate as an adjunct to antidepressant therapy.

Sources of dietary folate include leafy green vegetables, orange juice, fortified breakfast cereals, and grain products. It is most concentrated in spinach, liver, and yeast extract. However, the major contributors in the U.S. diet are orange juice, white bread, rolls and crackers, and dried beans. Food folate is degraded by heat, air, and ultraviolet light, resulting in losses during food preparation and cooking, and it is leached and lost in cooking water.

VITAMIN B_{12}. The 1989 RDA for vitamin B_{12} is 2 μg in elderly men and 1.6 μg in elderly women. It may be prudent to revise it upward, given the irreversible neurologic damage of vitamin B_{12} deficiency and given that increasing folate in the food supply through recent folate fortification of bread and grains can mask and delay diagnosis of vitamin B_{12} deficiency.

The metabolism of folate and vitamin B_{12} is intimately connected (51). Both are required in the methylation of homocysteine to methionine and other methylation reactions involving neurotransmitter metabolism. It is postulated that a defect in methylation processes is central to the biochemical basis of the neuropsychiatry disturbances of these vitamin deficiencies. While folate deficiency commonly causes depression, vitamin B_{12} deficiency is associated with peripheral neuropathy. Both cause dementia and cognitive impairment.

Vitamin B_{12} deficiency is present in up to 15% of the elderly, based on elevated methylmalonic acid (MMA) with or without elevated total homocysteine concentrations in combination with low or marginal vitamin B_{12} levels (52). Both folate and vitamin B_{12} deficiencies result in elevated total homocysteine levels, while only vitamin B_{12} deficiency raises MMA levels. In the elderly serum vitamin B_{12} concentrations lack sensitivity and specificity. Metz et al. (53) correlated evidence of tissue vitamin B_{12} deficiency at relatively high serum concentrations of the vitamin, more than 150 pmol/L. It is therefore imperative that vitamin B_{12} deficiency be actively screened and treated to prevent permanent neurologic damage. The elderly are at risk for developing preclinical vitamin B_{12} deficiency with age because of loss of intrinsic factor and to a larger extent food-cobalamin malabsorption due to achlorhydria, gastric atrophy, bacterial overgrowth, and *Helicobacter pylori* infection of the stomach (54).

The Normative Aging Study (55) showed lower cognitive performance in spatial copying skills in men aged 54 to 81 whose elevated total homocysteine levels were significantly correlated with low concentrations of folate and vitamin B_{12}. Higher levels of plasma vitamin B_6 among younger subjects was associated with better performance only on two tests of memory.

VITAMIN B_6. The 1989 RDA for vitamin B_6 defined in relation to protein intake is 2 mg/day in men and 1.6 mg/day in women. Vitamin B_6 is a cofactor in the synthesis of several essential neurotransmitters. Vitamin B_6 deficiency is associated with peripheral neuropathy and convulsions. Some data support a higher requirement for the elderly. In the SENECA study median dietary intakes of vitamin B_6 for all of the towns studied were below the RDA, with overall prevalence of biochemical deficiency at 23.3% (56). In the Boston survey 56% of the elderly men and women had dietary intakes below two thirds of the RDA, while only 5% had biochemical evidence of poor vitamin B_6 status. From a depletion-repletion study of people aged 61 to 71 years, Ribaya-Mercado et al. (57) estimated levels that normalized plasma and urine indices of B_6 status at 1.96 mg/day and 1.9 mg/day for men and women respectively. Vitamin B_6 depletion is associated with depressed lymphocyte proliferation and response and impaired interleukin-2 production (58). Low levels of B_6 are also related to high levels of homocysteine, though that relation is weaker than the one between folate and homocysteine.

Antioxidant Vitamins

There is as yet no conclusive evidence for protective effects of antioxidant vitamin C, vitamin E, β-carotene and the carotenoids in prevention of cancer or cardiovascular disease (CVD). The current RDA is 60 mg for vitamin C; 10 and 8 mg α-tocopherol equivalent for adult men and women respectively; and 1000 and 800 mg retinol equivalents for men and women respectively. Buring and Hennekens (59) reviewed the results of four large-scale randomized trials. In the Chinese Cancer Prevention Study, the use of combination regimens of nine supplements, including retinol, β-carotene, vitamin E, vitamin C, and selenium preclude differentiating the effect of any one supplement. There was a significant reduction in total mortality for groups assigned the combination of selenium, vitamin E, and carotene.

Similarly the Alpha-Tocopherol, Beta-Carotene Cancer Prevention Study (ATBC) found that over 6 years neither 50 mg vitamin E nor 20 mg β-carotene daily supplements protected Finnish male smokers aged 50 to 69 years against CVD. However, there were statistically significant increases in mortality from ischemic heart disease and in incidence of lung cancer in the β-carotene group. There was also a significant increase in deaths from cerebral hemorrhage in the vitamin E group. Another study, the Beta-Carotene and Retinol Efficacy Trial, was terminated early when similar findings in the direction of the ATBC became evident with a treatment combination of β-carotene and vitamin A.

The Physicians' Health Study over 12 years showed no effect of supplementation with β-carotene on cancer, total CVD, or mortality among 22,071 U.S. male physicians aged 40 to 84 who were current or past smokers. However, in a subgroup analysis of 333 doctors with a history of chronic stable angina or coronary revascularization procedure, there was a possible reduction in vascular disease events on 50 mg β-carotene taken every other day.

In another study of a subset of 747 community-dwelling elderly in Massachusetts, there was a significant finding that those in the quintiles taking the most vitamin C had the lowest overall mortality from heart disease (60). The inverse relation was evident with intakes starting at 400 mg of vitamin C, corresponding to the middle-intake quintiles. However, there were no associations between vitamin E or β-carotene with overall mortality from heart disease and cancer.

The outcome of ongoing randomized trials may provide definitive evidence of the roles of β-carotene, vitamin E, and vitamin C. These include the Women's Antioxidant Cardiovascular Study, the Canadian Heart Outcomes Prevention Evaluation Study, the U.K. Heart Protection Study, and the Italian GISSI Prevention Trial. Supplementation with antioxidant vitamins is unwarranted. The consumption of a diet rich in fruits, vegetables, and whole grains consistent with the Food Guide Pyramid supplies all known micronutrients and fiber and possibly a myriad of other naturally occurring phytochemicals with health protective benefits, such as flavonoids, and phenolic compounds (61). The plant foods offering the highest anticancer activity include ginger, soybeans, cabbage, licorice, and the umbelliferous vegetables, including carrots, celery, cilantro, parsley, and parsnips. The phytochemicals in whole-grain products and soy also reduce the risk of cardiovascular disease.

ANTIOXIDANT VITAMINS AND IMMUNOCOMPETENCE. Nutrition is a critical determinant of immunocompetence (62). Conversely, malnutrition and specific nutrient deficiency as a common cause of immunodeficiency may involve vitamins A, C, E, and B_6; folic acid; zinc; selenium; iron; and copper. Aging induces changes in immune responses, placing the elderly at risk for infections, cancer, and autoimmune and inflammatory diseases. Myelin et al. (63) reviewed the few clinical trials completed to date in both institutionalized and community-dwelling elderly supplemented with vitamin E, β-carotene, or glutathione. There is a suggestion of enhanced immune response with prolonged supplementation of high-dose vitamin E.

Chandra (62) reported on age-related changes in immune responses, including repressed stem cell kinetics and reserve, cutaneous delayed hypersensitivity to ubiquitous recall antigens reduced in frequency and size, slightly reduced number of circulating T lymphocytes, decreased thymulin activity, depressed natural killer cell activity, and decreased primary antibody production. These findings support the use of immunologic tests as prognostic indices of surgical outcomes and in assessment of nutritional status and nutritional support. Nutritional support in the form of extra energy or single or multiple micronutrients can enhance impaired immunity in the elderly.

Salt

Carruthers (64) expressed concern that physicians and their patients have accepted too readily the option of long-term medication for hypertension rather than the review and revision of nutritional habits. He maintained that there is unequivocal evidence of a clear correlation between obesity and hypertension and focused on the association between high sodium intake and excessive caloric intake. The control of dietary salt intake may be offset by sodium in many foodstuffs and in medications. Fast foods and processed foods such as canned soups are notorious for salt content. Medications also may add substantial salt intake.

Awareness of the potential preventive aspects of limiting salt in the diet should be maintained. Restaurants and fast food outlets should use less salt; customers should be allowed to determine their own salt preference. Not salting food discourages the expectation of saltiness, and because the taste preference for sodium diminishes after a few months of restriction, good adherence is achievable. Hypertensive patients should use less salt. The effectiveness of thiazide therapy in hypertension is enhanced by reduced salt intake.

Bone Health

Calcium, phosphorus, magnesium, vitamin D, and fluoride are important to the development and maintenance of bone and other calcified tissues (65). Adequate Intake (AI) is proposed for vitamin D and fluoride, while RDAs are given for phosphorus and magnesium. The daily AI for calcium is 1200 mg for adults aged 51 or more. Osteoporosis leading to fractures affects 25 million mostly American women, and its incidence increases with age (66). It is preventable and treatable. Bone health is influenced by diet, exercise, and estrogen. Preventive strategies focus on reducing age-related bone loss through increasing intake of calcium-rich foods, engaging in regular weight-bearing or strength training exercises, smoking cessation, moderation in drinking, and, for postmenopausal women, estrogen replacement therapy or its alternative if not contraindicated. Osteoporosis as a heterogeneous multifactorial disorder is discussed in Chapter 33.

Calcium intake above the previous RDA for the elderly is needed to slow age-related bone loss and compensate for a decrease in efficiency of intestinal calcium absorption. Supplementation with vitamin D where exposure to sunlight is limited may enhance calcium and phosphorus homeostasis and bone retention. Sun exposure to hands, arms, and face for 5 to 15 minutes may provide sufficient amounts of vitamin D, but longer exposure is required with use of sunscreen, by people with dark skin, in cloudy, smoggy areas, and in northern latitudes (67). High intakes of protein, sodium, and caffeine and high-phosphorus foods, including meat, all increase the urinary excretion of calcium. For every gram of protein consumed and every 2300 mg of sodium added to the diet, urinary calcium loss is increased by 1 mg and 40 to 80 mg respectively. Caffeine in equivalent amounts of two to three servings of brewed coffee consumed daily may accelerate bone loss in healthy postmenopausal women when calcium intake is below 800 mg (68).

Iron

The 1989 RDA for iron is 10 mg per day for both men and women. Wood et al. (69) reviewed iron nutriture and recommended no revision of the RDA. There is no evidence that aging affects iron absorption or homeostasis. Although there are no data on the very old, results from NHANES II, the Boston Nutritional Status Survey, and the Baltimore Longitudinal Study of Aging showed that median iron intakes in the elderly either meet or exceed the RDA. Iron deficiency anemia among the elderly is estimated at 1 to 6%, higher in Hispanic women and

the poor. There is a question whether serum ferritin concentration is still a good measure of iron stores, since inflammation associated with chronic diseases tends to elevate it falsely.

Zinc

The 1989 RDA for zinc is 15 mg/day for men and 12 mg/day for women. The limited studies support no age-associated reduction in zinc absorption efficiency (69). There is no consensus on whether plasma, serum, or polymorphonuclear leukocyte zinc concentration is the most reliable indicator of zinc status. Although there is no evidence of zinc deficiency in the elderly, numerous surveys have shown that dietary intake of zinc at less than the RDA parallels the decline in energy consumption with age. Preliminary results suggest that zinc therapy improves night vision, prevents macular degeneration, enhances T-cell function, and improves wound healing (70).

Water Metabolism

The elderly are at risk for both water intoxication and dehydration from age-related decline in renal capacity to excrete water and impaired thirst response. Total body water is reduced with age, from about 80% at birth to 60 to 70% in old age (71), i.e., 17% in women and 11% in men from the third to the eighth decade. It is a reflection of the decline in intracellular water concomitant with age-related loss in lean body mass or total body cell mass (72). Water homeostasis is also altered by disease processes and pharmacologic agents that induce changes in solute concentration and water volume in either the extracellular or intracellular compartments.

The Baltimore Longitudinal Study of Aging demonstrated a mean decrease in glomerular filtration rate (GFR) of 0.75 mL per minute per year in a sample of 254 normal healthy subjects (73). However, only a third of the group was so affected. It is suggested that this decline in GFR is not immutable and may reflect secondary aging. In the presence of reduced GFR, the capacity to excrete free water and thereby concentrate or dilute urine is diminished. Free water loading may result in a systematically hypo-osmolar state. Other studies show age-related declines in renal mass and renal blood flow (74). All are implicated in the physiologic derangement of osmoregulation and volume regulation commonly observed in the elderly.

Balance between water intake and output is maintained through thirst, arginine vasopressin (AVP) or antidiuretic hormone (ADH), and renal function. When water intake is increased and blood osmolality reduced, AVP release is suppressed and the excess water is excreted as dilute urine. Conversely, reduced water intake and increased plasma tonicity stimulate thirst and ADH secretion. Water is then reabsorbed in the renal collecting tubules, and urine concentration increases until normal blood osmolarity is restored.

Dehydration, a common problem among nursing home residents, often leads to hospitalization. Diseases such as stroke and cognitive impairment can further decrease the thirst response, and limited access to water in the elderly confined to bed or restrained in wheelchair or gerichair is common. The loss of the circadian rhythm of AVP that occurs with aging leads to nocturia and increased fluid loss. Dehydration can result in postural hypotension, constipation, and delirium.

Hyponatremia is not rare. Both low-salt diets and inadequate salt in tube-feeding solutions are important causes, as is the frequent use of diuretics. The syndrome of inappropriate antidiuretic hormone is associated with many of the diseases that result in institutionalization. Several drugs result in decreased free water clearance and hyponatremia; beside thiazides, these include chlorpropamide, carbamazepine, morphine, tricyclic antidepressants, haloperidol, and phenothiazines. Water retention can also lead to hyponatremia and may complicate the ability to manage diuretic-induced hyponatremia.

Water Intoxication

The recommended fluid intake is 1.5 to 2 L per day. The formula that best adjusts for extremes in body weight is 100 mL/kg for first 10 kg of body weight, 50 mL/kg for the next 10 kg, and 15 mL per remaining kilogram. Other standards frequently used are 30 mL/kg body weight or 1 mL/kcal energy consumed. The majority of fluids are usually taken at mealtimes. The most reliable nonmeal sources are fluids given with medications, which increase with the number and frequency of medications.

Protein-Energy Malnutrition and Undernutrition

Good nutrition is essential to the elderly in maintaining their health, functional abilities, and independent living. Malnutrition, whether undernutrition or obesity, detracts from the quality of life, as it exacerbates chronic disease; increases disability; lowers resistance to infection, extending hospital stays; and accelerates admission to a nursing home.

The prevalence of PEM is estimated at 15% in community-dwelling seniors, 5 to 12% of homebound older persons, 20 to 65% of hospitalized patients, and 5 to 85% of institutionalized elderly (75). In PEM there is depletion of lean body mass and adipose tissue, with weight loss and its attendant deficiencies in one or more nutrients. Loss of more than 20% of body weight before illness and hypoalbuminemia at less than 35 g/L indicate PEM.

PEM is associated with hospital complications, long hospital stays, frequent readmissions, and increased mortality in hospital and after discharge. Serum albumin below 40 g/L is a predictor of 3-year mortality in institutionalized elderly and 9- to 12-year mortality in free-living elderly. In the elderly PEM induces severe immunodeficiency affecting cell-mediated immunity, phagocyte function, complement system, secretory immunoglobulin A antibody concentrations, and cytokine production (62) and therefore is associated with high risk of infection. Hypoalbuminemia is also a significant risk factor for development of decubitus ulcers and a major determinant in wound healing (76).

Morley (77) hypothesized that chronic weight losses with advancing age may be attributed to dysregulation of food intake, described as physiologic anorexia of aging. The elderly person fails to maintain food intake because of loss of hedonistic qualities of food, increased circulation of the satiating hormone cholecystokinin, and possible decline in the opioid feeding drive and neuropeptide Y. The anorexia of aging may place the elderly at greater risk for reducing food intake and development of PEU.

There are social, psychologic, and medical causes of PEU (77). Social factors include poverty; social isolation; elder abuse; functional dependency in activities of daily living, such as feeding, food procurement, and meal preparation; and poor knowledge of nutrition. In the institutional setting other factors that may contribute to weight loss are ethnic food preferences, monotony of institutionalized food, and socially unacceptable dining behaviors.

A number of psychologic factors that influence the well-being of the elderly are associated with weight loss (77). Depression is one of the most important treatable causes of apathy, weakness, stomach pains, nausea, anorexia, and diarrhea resulting in weight loss. Bereavement, alcoholism, late-life mania, late-life paranoia, anorexia, tardive dyskinesia associated with excessive oral control, and sociopathy wherein the locus of control interferes with the intake of food all contribute to weight loss. Dementia is also associated with slow progressive weight loss from failure to eat due to cumulative losses of cognition and sensory and motor control, high energy expenditure related to continuous pacing, and apraxia of swallowing (78).

Weight loss may be due to a medical condition that alters appetite, increases metabolism, and causes malabsorption (77). Dyspepsia due to *H. pylori* is associated with anorexia and weight loss. Intestinal bacterial overgrowth causes malabsorption, anorexia, and weight loss. Increased metabolism contributing to weight loss is associated with hyperthyroidism, pheochromocytoma, and movement disorders such as parkinsonism, Huntington's chorea, and tardive dyskinesia. Chronic obstructive pulmonary disease contributes to weight loss through increased energy expenditure from use of accessory muscles for breathing and anorexia due to severe dyspnea associated with eating. In cardiac cachexia, anorexia and weight loss are associated with depletion of lean body mass because of elevated circulating levels of tumor necrosis factor and interleukin-1, which cause hypermetabolism and hypercatabolism (79). On the other hand, anorexia, excessive muscle wast-

ing, and weight loss in rheumatoid arthritis are associated with increased concentrations of tumor necrosis factor and interleukin-1β (77). Other factors contributing to weight loss include oral disease, dysphagia, malignant disease, gallstones, chronic and recurrent infections, and late-onset gluten enteropathy, particularly in association with diabetes mellitus.

Prevention of PEM involves assessment for risk factors and timely intervention of progressive PEU. Hypoalbuminemia in community-dwelling elderly (80) is correlated with older age; receiving welfare; vomiting at least 3 days per month; surgery for gastrointestinal tumor; self-reported heart failure; recurring cough attacks; feeling tired or worn out; little or no exercise; a condition interfering with eating; toothlessness or fair or poor condition of teeth; trouble chewing meat; a low-salt diet; self-reported protein albumin, blood, or sugar in urine; and current cigarette smoking. These sociodemographic, lifestyle, and disease-related factors, which are independent predictors of serum albumin 38 g/L or less or progressively lower albumin concentrations less than 40 g/L, identify risk of death.

Weight loss and concomitant PEU are common nutritional concerns in institutionalized elderly (81). Depression and adverse drug-nutrient interaction are the most common causes of weight loss. Abbasi and Rudman (82) identified 15 causes of PEU that are modifiable. These include prolonged use of restricted diets; use of drugs impairing desire or ability to eat; need for assistance or devices for eating; ineffective technique of eating assistance; dining environment not conducive to eating and socialization; provision of maintenance instead of repletion diets; inadequate nutritional support during illness; unrecognized febrile illness; need for modified diet; management of complications in tube feeding; poor dentition; need for assessment of dysphagia; and treatment of dysphagia.

Protein-Energy Overnutrition

Solomon and Manson (83) recently reviewed epidemiologic data on obesity and its association with all-cause mortality. Obesity remains a major health issue that is increasing in magnitude.

Between 1988 and 1991 at least one third of adults were estimated to be obese as defined by BMI at or above 27.3 in women and 27.8 in men, corresponding to body weight *at or above* 120% of ideal body weight. Women and nonwhites in particular have high prevalence rates. Obesity is both a risk factor for and cause of mortality from coronary artery disease, stroke, diabetes mellitus, hypertension, dyslipidemia, and some cancers.

Body weight commonly increases with age, and in the elderly, modest obesity thought to be protective used to be recommended. However, the results of earlier studies were biased by overexclusion of high-risk groups and confounding of leanness from previous smoking and unrecognized illness associated with weight loss. Therefore, the adjusted optimal weights associated with the least mortality are somewhat controversial. These are below average weights in both men and women, and they apply throughout adult life. Weight gain in adulthood is associated with increased mortality, and the central type of fat accumulation estimated by waist-to-hip measurement appears detrimental.

Health care workers and other professionals as well as families should be aware of risk factors that may lead to malnutrition and should be alert to the need for preventive intervention. The NSI material noted earlier in this chapter is a tool for awareness and education. Housebound persons are often already known to health and social service agencies. Help with shopping, assistance in preparing meals, Meals on Wheels, luncheon clubs, and day centers can help. "Health foods" and dietary supplement use should be monitored, because such products tend to erode purchasing power needlessly and do not guarantee a balanced diet.

Identification of persons at risk for malnutrition is important whether they are at home or in acute or long-term institutions. The frail elderly are especially vulnerable. Prevention requires attention to nutritional status. Treatment of acute medical or surgical illness requires early intervention, possibly with enteral nutritional supplements, to modify or prevent the downhill course of nitrogen depletion.

NUTRITION AND ACTIVITY

As noted earlier in this chapter, nutrition and physical activity are inextricably bound. Decrease in muscle mass and strength with increasing age has been linked to frailty, falls, functional decline, and impaired mobility. Factors include chronic illness, sedentary lifestyle, nutritional deficiencies, and aging. Fiatarone et al. (84) undertook a randomized controlled trial comparing progressive resistance exercises, multinutrient supplementation, both, and neither in a 10-week trial in institutionalized persons with an average age of 87 years. They found that multinutrient supplementation without concomitant exercise did not decrease muscle weakness or reduce physical frailty. Evans (85) examined a population of healthy men, one group with protein calorie supplement and one without. The ones with supplement had greater gains in muscle mass. He also applied the programs to persons over age 90 in an institution and showed increase in muscle strength by 174% and muscle size by 9%. Persons who received the supplement and did not exercise decreased their ad lib intake. In those who exercised, weight and intake increased.

Encouraging older persons to remain active, be it in the community or even performing basic activities of daily living in an institutional setting, leads to improved self-esteem, muscle tone, and interest in and intake of nutrients.

NUTRITION AND DEMENTIA

Several aspects of dementia and nutrition should be considered: (*a*) the role of nutrient deficiencies in the development of dementia, particularly Alzheimer's disease and other syndromes of impaired cognition; (*b*) the role of nutrients in the treatment of dementia, particularly Alzheimer's disease and reversible cognitive impairment (B_{12}, thiamin); (*c*) the potential for malnutrition due to self-neglect in some cases of dementia; (*d*) the potential for malnutrition due to high energy use in some persons with dementia.

Many amino acids, including tyrosine, tryptophan, threonine, histidine, and choline, are precursors for neurotransmitters. Vitamin precursors include A, B_6, B_{12}, thiamin, niacin, riboflavin, C, D, E, and folic acid. The role of amino acid and vitamin deficiencies in dementing disorders has been evaluated (86), but their effects in the pathogenesis of Alzheimer's disease are uncertain. The role of minerals, including aluminum, in the development of Alzheimer's disease remains controversial. The use of supplements such as choline and lecithin has not been shown to be effective in treating the dementia or slowing the disease. In multi-infarct dementia, diet may play a role through effects on blood pressure and related risk factors, and nutritional control may alter progress of this type of dementia. Studies to date suggest that persons with multi-infarct dementia tend to have less weight loss than those with Alzheimer's disease (86).

Another common dementia is due to alcohol excess. Abstinence and good nutrition, including thiamin replacement, may improve this form of dementia. In clinical situations, however, there is a group of patients who may well have complex pathogenesis with an early history of alcohol excess; despite withdrawal from alcohol, they may develop a progressive dementing disorder of the Alzheimer type.

Loney et al. (87) suggested that in dementia the disease itself does not affect nutrition, but secondary effects such as neglect, forgetting mealtimes, decreased motor skills, depression, paranoid reactions, and eating nonfoods or spoiled food may be more relevant. Malnutrition is most likely to be found in newly institutionalized demented persons and is reversible, although unfortunately the dementia remains. The effects of Vitamin E, ginkgo biloba, and other nutrients are being explored as modulators of development or progress of dementia.

Monitoring weights is crucial among demented persons (86, 88). Rheaume et al. (89) used a pedometer to measure daily miles (despite some difficulties encouraging demented persons to keep these in place) and presumed walking at 3 miles per hour. They found the pacing group walked 3.9 plus or minus 0.4 miles per day, and the sedentary group of demented persons walked 2.4 plus or minus 0.9 miles per day. From their calculations, they determined that pacers required an additional 1600 kcal per day. Appetites may increase, but energy intake is seldom adequate, and ongoing weight loss is frequent.

Gray (86) suggested a number of strategies for providing adequate nutrition to demented persons, including understanding behavioral and functional changes associated with the disorder (attention to energy requirements, olfactory and gustatory changes, difficulties with chewing and swallowing, and the often time-consuming and emotionally draining task of assisting with feeding). Dietary supplements may be in order.

NUTRITION AND THE INSTITUTIONAL MILIEU

The need for institutionalization is often precipitated by a deterioration in the capacity for self-care or the loss of caretakers. Very few elderly view placement in an institution as an ideal living arrangement. The loss of independence and privacy and the inability to maintain lifestyles make the adjustment more difficult. Adaptive capacities may be diminished by illness. The food service in an institution has the monumental task of providing attractive and nutritious meals that are pleasing to the palate. The quality of food service in any institution is constrained by budgetary restrictions necessitated by spiraling food and labor costs. Nevertheless, a dietitian's skills can translate the resident's nutritional needs into an individualized plan. Retraining residents to feed themselves should be encouraged whenever possible. Follow-up is critical to any plan to do this. In this case, observation of meal service allows the dietitian, nurse, or other staff to evaluate actual intake and alter the diet if necessary. Table 25.2 identifies some nutrient intake problems and possible solutions.

Food acceptance itself is a complex reaction determined by the physiologic, psychologic, biochemical, social, educational, and sensory reactions of persons moving in a framework of race, religion, tradition, economic status, and environmental conditions. Some degree of dissatisfaction is inevitable. Food preferences fall into distinct patterns, and knowledge of these patterns for an institutionalized group may minimize dissatisfaction and increase consumption. Barr et al. (90) studied nutrient intakes of a group of women over 80 in a care facility. They found that only 75% of the food provided was consumed, with mean intake of vitamin C, iron, niacin, and ri-

Table 25.2

Problems of Nutrient Intake and Solutions

Problem	Solution
Poor appetite and poor intake	Reassess eating capabilities and diet consistency
	Provide small portions, more frequent meals
	Tailor diet to personal preferences and food intolerances
	Offer selective menu
	Capitalize on breakfast, usually the best-eaten meal
	Consider use of high-calorie supplements or complete meal replacement formulas
	Schedule aperitifs
	Allow sufficient time for meals
	Maintain oral hygiene and personal grooming
	Plan seating arrangements for compatibility
	Appeal to the senses by describing the aroma, taste, and visual appeal of a meal
	Remove from other residents with highly objectionable eating habits
	Establish rapport
	Maximize comfort and tolerance by proper positioning and management of pain and energy level
	Encourage use of dining room to increase socialization
	Encourage families to bring in favorite home-cooked or ethnic foods
	Use outings and catering to encourage participation
Low energy level	Keep food warm by using heat-retaining dishes
	Use high-calorie supplements
	Offer smaller portions, more frequent feeding
	Place liquids and beverages in paper or plastic foam cups
	Make foods easily accessible on tray, e.g., removing lids and opening packaged items; spreading butter and jam
	Allow sufficient time for meals by providing early trays
	Assist with feeding as necessary
Impaired vision	Ensure adequate lighting
	Orient to tray or table setting
	Help set up tray
	Place food in reach
	Place tray in field of vision
Mastication	Assess need for dentures
	Ensure properly fitting dentures
	Modify food consistency, avoiding purees whenever possible
	Offer purees as a last resort
Hemiparesis	Offer bite-size portions, finger foods
Poor hand-to-mouth coordination	Help set up tray; place beverage to resident's functional side
	Use mechanical aids or adapted eating utensils
Dysphagia	Suction excess saliva before meals
	Allow sight and smell of food to stimulate salivation and prepare swallowing reflex
	Seat upright with the head flexed slightly forward
	Encourage thorough chewing of food
	Offer solid foods—soft, moist, full-bodied, and held together well, e.g., fish, souffle, canned pears, ripe bananas

continued

Table 25.2 (*continued*)

Problems of Nutrient Intake and Solutions

Problem	Solution
	Exclude pureed, sticky, stringy, grainy, acidic, or dry foods
	Provide thick fluids, e.g., tomato juice, fruit nectar, eggnog
	Serve jello, sherbet, frozen juice, etc., if imbibing fluids is a problem
	Serve cold foods cold and hot foods hot to stimulate the senses
	Suggest exercise to improve swallowing, e.g., sucking on ice chips, frozen fruit juices
Objectionable behavior	Permit staff to role model desirable behaviors
	Seat according to compatibility and level of function
	Allow ample time to eat and provide flexible times of meal service
	Maintain calm, relaxed atmosphere; reduce background noise; minimize distraction by serving one food at a time
	Provide special plates and adapted utensils to maintain independence
	Encourage peer interaction and support
	Offer praise and encouragement for improvements

The authors acknowledge the contribution of members of the Gerontological Practice Group of the British Columbia Dieticians' & Nutritionists' Association, Canada.

boflavin adequate compared with the RDAs and RNIs, but average intakes of protein, calcium, vitamin A, thiamin, and zinc were lower than the standards. Advanced age was negatively correlated with overall dietary adequacy.

Mealtime is a reference time of day for some persons and the highlight of the day for others. Intake of food produces a psychologic need for social interchange. Many times, the feeding situations in early life have a strong influence. The first sustained human contact and socially important transaction is feeding. It makes the world dependable, comforting, satisfying, and nonthreatening (91). For the institutionalized aged, food may again become a symbol of security. The patient may reject food to manipulate the staff or family. Staff attitudes may inadvertently promote dependency. Staff must be encouraged to patient accommodation of individual needs. If food on trays is attractively presented and judiciously chosen, monitoring of returns on trays may indicate a spectrum of problems from quality of food preparation to failure to address mental and physical handicaps of consumers. Table 25.3 describes considerations for planning institutional food services.

Asplund et al. (92) assessed psychogeriatric institutionalized patients. They found energy and protein undernutrition in 30% and obesity in 4% of the patients. Undernutrition did not correlate with duration of stay and was less frequent in subjects with their own teeth than in toothless persons. Because food intake was similar in patients with and without undernutrition, possible interactions between malnutrition and chronic psychiatric disorders in the elderly were considered, such as general dysmetabolism in handling of substrates. Morgan et al. (93) observed that women with severe dementia in a psychiatric hospital weighed 15 kg less as a group than a comparison group of active elderly women living in the community and consuming a similar calorie intake. The role of occult disease in the institutionalized group is uncertain.

Anderson (94) compared a group of institutionalized veterans with a group of clinic patients. The greatest dietary difference between the clinic and domiciliary patients was not related to the use of dentures. Findings suggested that regardless of earlier diet, older persons in institutions eat nutritionally important foods if given the opportunity. Staff attitudes are important for institutional food services. If staff expect old people to be dependent and conforming

Table 25.3

Components of Institutional Food Service and Considerations for Planning

Component	Consideration for Planning
Menu design	Provide attractive meals based on the four food groups to meet the nutritional needs of residents
	Consider day-to-day variations in color and visual appeal, texture, consistency, size, shape, and flavor combination in each meal
	Survey ethnic, religious, and regional preferences
	Note and update personal preferences on residents' menus when a selective daily menu is not available
	Plan for long menu cycle; 4 or more weeks is desirable
	Consider the type of meal pattern, the number of food items offered, and the times meals are served, e.g., a choice of three-meal-a-day plan; four-meal plan consisting of a continental breakfast, late morning brunch, main meal in the late afternoon, and a substantial snack in the evening; or five-meal plan
	Choose a meal pattern compatible with the sleeping habits of residents (i.e., early risers, early retirers)
	Ensure that no more than 15 hours elapse between the last meal of one day and the first meal of the following day
	Adjust menu to reflect holiday items, special occasions, and social activities
	Offer alternatives compatible with therapeutic dietary modifications
	Semiannually review menu for quality review standards, production efficiency, and cost factor
	Revise menu to incorporate seasonal fruits and economical food items
	Establish daily feedback for updating preferences, assessing acceptability of menu selection, and monitoring residents' nutritional intake
	Select china for stability and ease of eating; consider use of plate guards and rimmed plates
Type of meal service and staffing	Family-style dining, i.e., delivery of bulk food to be distributed
	Buffet—smorgasbord service, self-served selection
	Encourage socialization of dietary staff with residents during mealtimes to provide individual attention and maintain rapport
	Adopt a policy for dietary and nondietary staff to help with serving, tray returns, etc.
Atmosphere of dining room	Create a comfortable homelike environment with subdued painted walls and good lighting
	Partition room with mobile dividers for intimacy
	Provide soft, unobtrusive background music
	Arrange for attractive table setting that highlights the season and special events or themes
	Group no more than six residents around small tables
	Make tables available for singles or couples
	Position tables for ease of movement
	Offer choice of seating companion to stimulate socialization
	Base seating arrangements on the need for supervision, assistance, and level of orientation

continued

Table 25.3 (*continued*)

Components of Institutional Food Service and Considerations for Planning

Component	Consideration for Planning
	Encourage use of dining room for group cooking activities
	Minimize background noise from television, trolley, clatter of cutlery and plates, and staff talk; consider use of thick wall hangings, baffles, and padded placemats
	Separate noisy and difficult residents and those with objectionable table manners
Food-related activities	Meal preparation, baking session
	Men's group; ladies' friendship tea
	Reminiscence group (to discuss favorite, traditional, bygone foods)
	Pub and family nights
	Outings to restaurants
	Outdoor picnics, barbecue
	Champagne breakfast
Cooking facility for residents' use	Small kitchenette with storage facilities
	Sink, stove, oven, refregerator
	Electric kettle, toaster, pots, and pans
	Plates, bowls, teacups, and saucers
	Supply of tea, coffee, sugar, cream, bread, butter, cheese, cookies, milk, juice

Modified from Beck C. Dining experiences of the institutionalized aged. J Gerontol Nurs 1981;7:104–107. Davies L, Holdsworth MD. An at-risk concept used in homes for the elderly in the United Kingdom. J Am Diet Assoc 1980;76:264–267. Mahaffey MJ, Mennes ME, Miller BB. Food Service Manual for Health Care Institutions. Chicago: American Hospital Association, 1981.

(91), they may inadvertently extinguish independence. There is a nutritional bill of rights (American Dietetic Association 1976) in which the resident has a right to be as independent as possible in eating.

Institutional food is simply not everyone's home-cooked meal. The residents can participate in menu revision. They may be solicited for menu suggestions and feedback once these are implemented. A representative of the dietary department should be identified so that the resident may direct criticism and communicate changing food preferences. The dietitian or delegate must maintain a high profile to establish, observe, direct, encourage, and teach residents, families, and staff. Training dietetic and food service staff to monitor and note tray returns as part of their cleanup procedure is an asset.

NUTRIENT–DRUG INTERACTIONS

Lamy (95, 96) suggested that food–drug interactions are probably more common than indicated in the literature. Some associations between nutritional status and drugs include reduced albumin with consequences for highly protein-bound drugs (antimicrobials, cardiac drugs), changes in microsomal liver enzymes with alterations in effects of drugs metabolized in the liver (digitoxin, tricyclics), effects on urinary pH with change in the excretion patterns of drugs (urinary antimicrobials), and altered absorption (chelation of iron, calcium) (97).

Many commonly used drugs affect vitamin and mineral status (98, 99). The elderly, particularly those with chronic illness, may be vulnerable to subclinical deficiencies. Drugs may stimulate (tricyclic antidepressants) or depress (digoxin) appetite and thereby induce overnutrition or undernutrition. Ethanol has many effects. It can stimulate appetite as an aperitif. Excessive ethanol ingestion may impair pyridoxine or folate metabolism or promote zinc and magnesium losses. Pharmacotherapy in the elderly is common. Awareness of potential drug–food interactions may allow interventions that will preclude undesirable side effects.

DIET AND CANCER

Farber (100) reviewed some aspects of nutrients and cancer. Diet may influence the incidence of cancer in some sites, such as the colon, breast, and endometrium. Carcinogens may occur in food as natural substances, as contaminants, or as products of food preparation. Balducci et al. (101) suggested that dietary prevention of cancer may be effective in advanced age and that the dietary guidelines of the National Academy of Sciences should be implemented in this population. The American Cancer Society has suggested reducing fat intake to 20% to prevent breast and colon cancer.

Micronutrients have a role in the endogenous formation of carcinogens. Dietary amines and drugs such as oxytetracycline and chlorpromazine, for example, can react with nitrous acid generated in the stomach to form nitroso compounds. These compounds are carcinogenic to laboratory animals. They may be inhibited by dietary ascorbic acid and vitamin E. Fiber content plus vitamins C and E are being considered as modulators of carcinogens generated in the feces.

Plumlee et al. (102) reviewed the harmful effects of cooking methods that produce carcinogens (e.g., benzo[a]pyrene). They described their process for setting priorities for food items to be tested for possible mutagen information when cooked. Weisburger (103) addressed the role of the food type, quality, and mode of cooking in the causation of carcinoma in the gastrointestinal tract and endocrine-sensitive organs. If current concepts are correct, risk of gastric cancer can be reduced by ensuring that appropriate amounts of food containing vitamin C are eaten with each meal and by reducing salt,

which acts as an adjuvant. Reduced intake of fried foods and fat reduces risk of colon, breast, and prostate cancer. These and other observations have led to dietary recommendations by the American Cancer Society.

Nutritional strategies are now incorporated into management plans for cancer patients. The effects of the disease on appetite, digestion, and other factors, such as nausea, vomiting, and anorexia, which frequently accompany radiotherapy and chemotherapy, require ongoing monitoring, prevention, and intervention (104).

The promotion and prevention of carcinogenesis by micronutrients is an intriguing field ripe for study. Cancer patients require attention to specific strategies to promote adequate nutrition in treatment programs. The relations among genetic background, disease risks, and lifestyle factors, including diet, are worthy of further evaluation.

SUMMARY

Consumption of a nutritionally adequate, balanced, and tasty diet is recommended for optimal health. This must be individualized to each person's needs and preferences. Intakes of calorie-rich foods low in nutrients is discouraged. Dietary standards must be continually monitored, and the relations among nutrition, environment, and lifestyle must be researched more thoroughly.

Education and personal responsibility for health are lifetime pursuits. Knowledge and application of the principles of good nutrition may go a long way toward enhancing prospects for successful aging. We should not be misled by extremists, lay or professional, who would consign us to a life of Spartan diets and galley-slave exertion as a recipe for long life. Moderation has been touted for generations as a prescription for good health. There is no evidence that this advice is out of date.

REFERENCES

1. Justice CL, Howe JM, Clark HE. Dietary intakes and nutritional status of elderly patients: study in a private nursing home. J Am Diet Assoc 1974;65:639–646.
2. Fries JF. Aging, natural death, and the compression of morbidity. N Engl J Med 1980;303:130–135.

3. Disability and health: characteristics of persons by limitation of activity and assessed health status, United States, 1984–1988. In: Advance Data From Vital Health and Statistics of the National Center for Health Statistics. No. 197, May 21, 1991.

4. Garraway WM, Whisnant JP, Furlan AJ, et al. The declining incidence of stroke. N Engl J Med 1979;300: 449–452.

5. Morgan PP, Wigle DT. Medical care and the declining rates of death due to heart disease and stroke. Can Med Assoc J 1981;125:953–954.

6. Walker WJ. Changing United States life-style and declining vascular mortality: cause or coincidence? N Engl J Med 1980;297:163–165.

7. Exton-Smith AN. Malnutrition in the elderly. Proc R Soc Med 1977;70:615–619.

8. American Dietetic Association. Position of the American Dietetic Association: Nutrition, aging and the continuum of health care. J Am Diet Assoc 1993;93:80–81.

9. Hazzard WR. Aging and atherosclerosis: interactions with diet, heredity and associated risk factors. In: Nutrition, Longevity and Aging: Proceedings of the Symposium on Nutrition, Longevity and Aging, Miami. New York: Academic Press, 1976:143.

10. Barrows CH, Kokkonen GC. Relationship between nutrition and aging. Adv Nutr Res 1977;1:253.

11. McCay CM, Crowell MF, Maynard LA. The effect of retarded growth upon the length of life span and upon the ultimate body size. Nutrition 1989;5:155–171.

12. McCay CM, Sperling G, Barnes LL. Growth, ageing, chronic diseases and life span in rats. Arch Biochem 1943;2:469–479.

13. Masoro EJ. Retardation of aging processes by food restriction: an experimental tool. Am J Clin Nutr 1992; 55:1250S–1252S.

14. Chang-Claude J, Frentzel-Beyme R, Eilber U. Mortality pattern of German vegetarians after 11 years of follow-up. Epidemiology 1992;3:395–401.

15. Morley JE. Nutritional modulation of behavior and immunocompetence. Nutr Rev 1994;52:S6–S8.

16. Taylor A, Jacques PF, Epstein EM. Relations among aging, antioxidant status, and cataract. Am J Clin Nutr 1995;62(suppl):1439S–1447S.

17. Snodderly DM. Evidence for protection against age-related macular degeneration by carotenoids and antioxidant vitamins. Am J Clin Nutr 1995;62(suppl):1448S–1461S.

18. The periodic (vs. annual) health examination. Canadian Task Force on Periodic Health Examination. Can Med Assoc J 1979;121:1193–1254. 1984;130:4–16. 1986; 134:724–727. 1988;138:618–626.

19. White JV, Dwyer JT, Posner BM, et al. Nutrition screening initiative: development and implementation of the public awareness checklist and screening tools. J Am Diet Assoc 1992;92:163–166.

20. Dwyer JT. Screening older Americans' nutritional health: current practices and future possibilities. Washington: Nutrition Screening Initiatives, 1991.

21. Baker JP, Detsky AS, Wesson DE, et al. Nutritional assessment: a comparison of clinical judgment and objective measurements. N Engl J Med 1982;306:969–972.

22. Dwyer JT. Dietary assessment. In: Shils ME, Olson JA, Shike M, eds. Modern Nutrition in Health and Disease. 8th ed. Philadelphia: Lea & Febiger, 1994:842–860.

23. Frisancho AR. New standards of weight and body composition by frame size and height for assessment of nutritional status of adults and the elderly. Am J Clin Nutr 1984;40:808–819.

24. Master AM, Lasser RP, Beckman G. Tables of average weight and height of Americans age 65 to 94 years. JAMA 1960;114:658–662.

25. Heymsfield SB, Tighe A, Wang Z-M. Nutritional assessment by anthropometric and biochemical methods. In: Shils ME, Olson JA, Shike M, eds. Modern Nutrition in Health and Disease. 8th ed. Philadelphia: Lea & Febiger, 1994:812–841.

26. Windsor JA, Hill GL. Weight loss with physiologic impairment. Ann Surg 1988;207:290–296.

27. Kubena KS, McIntosh WA, Georghiades MB, Landmann WA. Anthropometry and health in the elderly. J Am Diet Assoc 1991;91:1402–1407.

28. Jeejeebhoy KN. Common modes of assessment of nutritional status. Front Clin Nutr 1992;1:1–6.

29. Ham RJ. Indicators of poor nutritional status in older Americans. Am Fam Physician 1992;45:219–228.

30. Sahyoun NR, Jacques PF, Dallal G, Russell RM. Use of albumin as a predictor of mortality in community-dwelling and institutionalized elderly populations. J Clin Epidemiol 1996;49:981–988.

31. Herrmann FR, Safran C, Levkoff SE, Minaker KL. Serum albumin level on admission as a predictor of death, length of stay, and readmission. Arch Intern Med 1992; 152:125–130.

32. Ferguson RP, O'Connor P, Crabtree B, et al. Serum albumin and prealbumin as predictors of clinical outcomes of hospitalized elderly nursing home residents. J Am Geriatr Soc 1993;41:545–549.

33. Food and Nutrition Board. Recommended Dietary Allowances. 9th ed. Washington: Food and Nutrition Board, National Academy of Sciences, National Research Council, 1989.

34. Food and Nutrition Board. How should the recommended dietary allowances be revised? A concept paper from the Food and Nutrition Board. Nutr Rev 1994;52: 216–219.

35. Report of the Dietary Guidelines Advisory Committee. Dietary Guidelines for Americans. Nutr Rev 1995;53: 376–379.

36. Scientific Review Committee. Nutrition Recommendations: The Report of the Scientific Review Committee. Ottawa: Canadian Government Publishing Center, 1990.

37. Health and Welfare Canada. Action towards healthy eating: Canada's guidelines for healthy eating and recommended strategies for implementation. Ottawa: Supply and Services Canada, 1990.

38. Roberts SB. Energy requirements of older individuals. Eur J Clin Nutr 1996;50(suppl 1):S112–S117.

39. Summary of the Surgeon General's report addressing physical activity and health. Nutr Rev 1996;54:280–284.

40. Campbell WW, Evans WJ. Protein requirements of elderly people. Eur J Clin Nutr 1996;50(suppl 1):S180–S185.

41. Uauy R, Scrimshaw NS, Young VR. Human protein requirements: nitrogen balance response to graded levels of egg protein in elderly men and women. Am J Clin Nutr 1978;31:779–785.

42. Gersovitz M, Motil K, Munro HN, et al. Human protein requirements: assessment of the adequacy of the current recommended dietary allowance for the dietary protein in elderly men and women. Am J Clin Nutr 1982; 35:6–14.

43. Millward DJ, Fereday A, Gibson N, Pacy PJ. Aging, protein requirements and protein turnover. Am J Clin Nutr 1997;66:774–786.

44. Schneeman BO, Tietyen J. Dietary fiber. In: Shils ME, Olson JA, Shike M, eds. Modern Nutrition in Health and Disease. 8th ed. Philadelphia: Lea & Febiger, 1994:89–100.

45. Ernst ND, Sempos CT, Briefel RR, Clark MB. Consistency between US dietary fat intake and serum total cholesterol concentrations: the National Health and Nutrition Examination Surveys. Am J Clin Nutr 1997;66 (suppl 4):965S–972S.

46. McNulty H. Folate requirements for health in different population groups. Br J Biomed Sci 1995;52:110–119.

47. Russell RM, Suter PM. Vitamin requirements of elderly people: an update. Am J Clin Nutr 1993;58:4–14.

48. Haller J, Lowik MR, Ferry M, Ferro-Luzzi A. Nutritional status: blood vitamins A, E, B6, B12, folic acid and carotene. Euronut SENECA investigators. Eur J Clin Nutr 1991;45(suppl 3):63–82.

49. Selhub J, Jacques PF, Wilson PW, et al. Vitamin status and intake as primary determinants of homocystinemia in an elderly population. JAMA 1993;270:2693–2698.

50. Alpert JE, Fava M. Nutrition and depression: the role of folate. Nutr Rev 1997;55:145–149.

51. Bottiglieri T. Folate, vitamin B12, and neuropsychiatric disorders. Nutr Rev 1996;54:382–390.

52. Stabler SP, Lindenbaum J, Allen RH. Vitamin B12 deficiency in the elderly: current dilemmas. Am J Clin Nutr 1997;66:741–749.

53. Metz J, Bell AH, Flicker L, et al. The significance of subnormal serum vitamin B12 concentration in older people: a case control study. J Am Geriatr Soc 1996;44: 1355–1361.

54. Carmel R. Cobalamin, the stomach and aging. Am J Clin Nutr 1997;66:750–759.

55. Riggs KM, Spiro A III, Tucker K, Rush D. Relations of vitamin B12, vitamin B6, folate, and homocysteine to cognitive performance in Normative Aging Study. Am J Clin Nutr 1996;63:306–314.

56. Cruz JA, Moreiras-Varela O, van Staveren WA, et al. Intake of vitamins and minerals. Euronut SENECA investigators. Eur J Clin Nutr 1991;45(suppl 3):121–138.

57. Ribaya-Mercado JD, Russell RM, Sahyoun N, et al. Vitamin B6 requirements of elderly men and women. J Nutr 1991;121:1062–1074.

58. Myelin SN, Ribaya-Mercado JD, Russell RM, et al. Vitamin B6 deficiency impairs interleukin 2 production and lymphocyte proliferation in elderly adults. Am J Clin Nutr 1991;53:1275–1280.

59. Buring JE, Hennekens CH. Antioxidant vitamins and cardiovascular disease. Nutr Rev 1997;55:S53–S58.

60. Sahyoun NR, Jacques PF, Russell RM. Carotenoids, vitamins C and E, and mortality in an elderly population. Am J Epidemiol 1996;144:501–511.

61. Craig WJ. Phytochemicals. J Am Diet Assoc 1997;97 (suppl 2):S199–S204.

62. Chandra RK. Nutrition and the immune system: an introduction. Am J Clin Nutr 1997;66:460S–463S.

63. Myelin SN, Wu D, Santos MS, Hayek MG. Antioxidants and immune response in aged persons: overview of present evidence. Am J Clin Nutr 1995;62(suppl): 1462S–1476S.

64. Carruthers SG. Nutrition and hypertension. J Can Diet Assoc 1980;41:274–281.

65. Food and Nutrition Board. Calcium and related nutrients: overview and methods. Nutr Rev 1997;55:335–341.

66. McBean LD, Forgac T, Finn SC. Osteoporosis: visions for care and prevention: a conference report. J Am Diet Assoc 1994;94:668–671.

67. Holick MF. Vitamin D and bone health. J Nutr 1996;126(suppl):1159S–1164S.

68. Harris SS, Dawson-Hughes B. Caffeine and bone loss in healthy postmenopausal women. Am J Clin Nutr 1994; 60:573–578.

69. Wood RJ, Suter PM, Russell RM. Mineral requirements of elderly people. Am J Clin Nutr 1995;62:493–505.

70. Boosalis M, Stuart MA, McClain CJ. Zinc metabolism in the elderly. In: Morley JE, Glick Z, Rubenstein LZ, eds. Geriatric Nutrition: A Comprehensive Review. 2nd ed. New York: Raven Press, 1995:115–121.

71. Chidester JC, Spangler AA. Fluid intake in the institutionalized elderly. J Am Diet Assoc 1997;97:23–28.

72. Pfeil LA, Katz PR, Davis PJ. Water metabolism. In: Morely JE, Glick Z, Rubenstein LZ, eds. Geriatric Nutrition: A Comprehensive Review. 2nd ed. New York: Raven Press, 1995:145–151.

73. Chernoff R. Thirst and fluid requirements. Nutr Rev 1994;52(8 Pt 2):S3–S5.

74. Morley JE, Silver AJ. Nutritional issues in nursing home care. Ann Intern Med 1995;123:850–859.

75. Mion LC, McDowell JA, Heaney LK. Nutritional assessment of the elderly in the ambulatory care setting. Nurse Pract Forum 1994;5:46–51.

76. Osterweil D, Wendt PF, Ferrell BA. Pressure ulcers and nutrition. In: Morley JE, Glick Z, Rubenstein LZ, eds. Geriatric Nutrition: A Comprehensive Review. 2nd ed. New York: Raven Press, 1995:335–342.

77. Morley JE. Anorexia of aging: physiologic and pathologic. Am J Clin Nutr 1997;66:760–773.

78. Finley B. Nutritional needs of the person with Alzheimer's disease: practical approaches to quality care. J Am Diet Assoc 1997;97(suppl 2):S177–S180.

79. Freeman LM, Roubenoff R. The nutrition implications of cardiac cachexia. Nutr Rev 1994;52:340–347.

80. Reuben DB, Moore AA, Damesyn M, et al. Correlates of hypoalbuminemia in community-dwelling older persons. Am J Clin Nutr 1997;66:38–45.

81. Morley JE, Silver AJ. Nutritional issues in nursing home care. Ann Intern Med 1995;123:850–859.

82. Abbasi AA, Rudman D. Undernutrition in nursing home: prevalence, consequences, causes and prevention. Nutr Rev 1994;52:113–122.

83. Solomon CG, Manson J. Obesity and mortality: a review of the epidemiologic data. Am J Clin Nutr 1997;22 (suppl):1044S–1050S.

84. Fiatarone MA, O'Neill EF, Ryan ND, et al. Exercise training and nutritional supplementation for physical frailty in very elderly people. N Engl J Med 1994;330:1769–1775.

85. Evans WJ. Effects of aging and exercise on nutrition needs of the elderly. Nutr Rev 1996;54:S335–S339.

86. Gray GE. Nutrition and dementia. J Am Diet Assoc 1989;89:1795–1802.

87. Loney LA, Hutton JT, Stewart JR, Spallholz JE. Nutritional concerns for patients with Alzheimer's disease. Tex Med 1987;83:40–43.

88. Litchford MD, Wakefield LM. Nutrient intakes and energy expenditures of residents with senile dementia of the Alzheimer's type. J Am Diet Assoc 1987;87:211–213.

89. Rheaume Y, Riley ME, Ladislav V. Meeting nutritional needs of Alzheimer patients who pace constantly. J Nutr Elderly 1987;7:43–52.

90. Barr SI, Chrysomilides SA, Willis EJ, Beattie BL. Nutrient intakes of the old elderly: a study of female residents of a long-term care facility. Nutr Res 1983;3:417–431.

91. Beck C. Dining experiences of the institutionalized aged. J Gerontol Nurs 1981;7:104–107.

92. Asplund K, Normark M, Pettersson V. Nutritional assessment of psychogeriatric patients. Age Ageing 1981;10:87–94.

93. Morgan DB, Newton HM, Schorah CJ, et al. Abnormal indices of nutrition in the elderly: a study of different clinical groups. Age Ageing 1986;15:65–76.

94. Anderson EL. Eating patterns before and after dentures. J Am Diet Assoc 1971;58:421–426.

95. Lamy PP. Drug interactions and the elderly: a new perspective. Drug Intell Clin Pharm 1980;14:513–515.

96. Lamy PP. Nutrition and the elderly. Drug Intell Clin Pharm 1981;15:887–891.

97. Thomas JA. Drug-nutrient interactions. Nutr Rev 1995;53:271–282.

98. Roe DA. Therapeutic significance of drug-nutrient interactions in the elderly. Pharmacol Rev 1984;36(suppl 2):109S–1022S.

99. Roe DA. Therapeutic effects of drug-nutrient interactions in the elderly. J Am Diet Assoc 1985;85:174–181.

100. Farber E. Chemical carcinogenesis. N Engl J Med 1981;305:1379–1389.

101. Balducci L, Wallace C, Khansur T, et al. Nutrition, cancer, and aging: an annotated review: I. Diet, carcinogenesis, and aging. J Am Geriatr Soc 1986;34:127–136.

102. Plumlee C, Bjelanes LF, Hatch FT. Priorities assessment for studies of mutagen production in cooked foods. J Am Diet Assoc 1981;79:446–449.

103. Weisburger JH. Mechanism of action of diet as a carcinogen. Cancer 1979;43:1987–1995.

104. Dwyer J. The spectrum of dietary and nutritional approaches to cancer. Nutrition 1989;5:197–199.

Lipid Abnormalities in Older People

This chapter is an introduction to lipid and lipoprotein metabolism and its abnormalities in older people. Since the mechanisms that regulate lipid and lipoprotein levels in older people are the same as those found in younger people, effects of genetics, environment, diseases, and drugs on lipid and lipoprotein levels are described with particular emphasis on aspects that are different in older persons. Clinical evaluation and treatment of dyslipoproteinemias in older people to modify risk of atherosclerosis are outlined.

LIPIDS AND LIPOPROTEINS

Lipoproteins contain nonpolar lipids (mostly triglycerides and cholesteryl esters), polar lipids (mostly phospholipids and unesterified cholesterol), and specific apolipoproteins. Chylomicrons, synthesized in the intestine, and very low density lipoproteins (VLDL), synthesized in the liver, are the carriers of triglycerides synthesized from dietary fat and carbohydrates. Both are metabolized in peripheral tissues by the action of lipoprotein lipase (LPL). Clinically, chylomicrons and VLDL are most important as carriers of dietary energy. By themselves they are not risk factors for atherosclerosis. However, high levels of chylomicrons appear to cause acute pancreatitis, and high levels of VLDL are associated with poor glucose control in diabetics.

The products of chylomicron and VLDL metabolism include chylomicron remnants, intermediate-density lipoproteins (IDL), low-density lipoproteins (LDL), and the lipoprotein Lp(a). These products of chylomicron and VLDL metabolism are associated with increased risk of atherosclerosis. Thus the chylomicron remnants IDL, LDL, and Lp(a) are the "bad" lipoproteins, and elevated levels lead to accumulation of cholesterol in fatty streaks in arterial walls. They also play a role in the progression of fatty streaks to complex calcified plaques. Several factors influence this process: (a) direct infiltration of LDL into the arterial wall where they are taken up by cells, stimulating pathologic changes in the arterial wall, (b) increased transport and atherogenicity of certain LDL subfractions, and (c) oxidation of LDL-forming LDL, which are especially atherogenic.

High-density lipoproteins (HDL) are intermediaries in lipoprotein metabolism. In population studies, high levels of HDL are associated with reduced risk for atherosclerosis. The association of high HDL levels with low atherosclerosis rates, the role of HDL and lecithin-cholesterol acyl transferase (LCAT) in removal of cholesterol in LCAT deficiency, and experimental evidence for a role of HDL in cholesterol transport from cells to lipoproteins in vitro has led to the hypothesis that HDL in some way is responsible for removal of cholesterol from peripheral tissue and prevention of the accumulation of cholesterol in arteries, which eventually leads to atherosclerosis. This so-called reverse cholesterol transport is the prevailing hypothesis regarding the mechanism of HDL in protecting against atherosclerosis (1).

GENETIC REGULATION OF LIPID AND LIPOPROTEIN LEVELS

Genetic abnormalities in the apolipoproteins, cell receptors that bind apolipoproteins, and enzymes that regulate lipoprotein metabolism affect the levels of all lipoproteins (2, 3). Genetically high levels of chylomicrons caused by LPL deficiency are associated with increased risk of pancreatitis. Genetically high levels of VLDL, IDL, and Lp(a) caused by low levels of LPL, isoforms of apolipoprotein E, and genetic differences in apolipoprotein Lp(a) are associated with increased risk of atherosclerosis (4). Genetically low levels of chylomicrons, VLDL, chylomicron remnants, IDL, LDL, and Lp(a) found in people with abetalipoproteinemia are associated with deficiencies in fat-soluble vitamins, particularly vitamin E. Genetically high levels of HDL caused by either increased rates of synthesis of HDL apolipoproteins or decreased levels of cholesterol ester transfer protein (CETP) are associated with low rates of atherosclerosis. About half of genetically low levels of HDL are associated with high rates of atherosclerosis; the rest are associated with low or normal rates of atherosclerosis.

Homozygous familial hypercholesterolemia, one of the best-studied genetic diseases affecting LDL levels, is associated with premature atherosclerosis and early mortality. There are relatively few elderly people who are even heterozygous for familial hypercholesterolemia, which suggests that this gene is also associated with short life (5). Similar studies show a relatively low prevalence of the apolipoprotein E2 phenotype in older people. Apolipoprotein E2 in the homozygote state is associated with markedly high risk of atherosclerosis, and it appears to shorten life even in the heterozygote state. Small family studies of people who are extremely long lived suggest that genetically increased HDL levels may be associated with particularly long life.

EXERCISE, BODY COMPOSITION, AND DIET

Exercise, diet, and body fat affect lipid and lipoprotein levels. In general, exercise increases HDL levels and decreases levels of chylomicrons and VLDL. To a lesser extent, exercise decreases LDL levels. People with a high percent of body fat, particularly those with concomitant glucose intolerance, have relatively high levels of VLDL and LDL. LPL is higher in people who exercise, those with low body fat, and those with high muscle mass. Reducing the percent of body fat by exercise and diet and increasing the relative amount of

muscle decrease triglyceride levels and increase HDL levels by modulating LPL activity.

The major dietary effects on lipid and lipoprotein levels are due to total calories, total cholesterol, relative amounts of saturated and transunsaturated fatty acids, and relative amounts of omega-3 fatty acids in the diet. Decreasing the total calories and total fat in the diet decreases chylomicron, VLDL, chylomicron remnant, IDL, and LDL levels. Similarly, decreasing the amounts of cholesterol, saturated fatty acids, and transunsaturated fatty acids also decreases the levels of atherogenic lipoproteins. Under certain circumstances, however, decreasing total cholesterol intake also decreases total HDL levels, especially when saturated fatty acids are replaced by complex carbohydrates and polyunsaturated fats in the diet. Increasing intake of omega-3 fatty acids appears to decrease serum clotting rates and may decrease acute cardiac and cerebrovascular disease. However, ingesting large amounts of fish oil increases triglyceride levels and decreases HDL levels in some people.

DISEASES AFFECTING LIPOPROTEIN LEVELS

Hypothyroidism is well known to raise cholesterol levels. LDL levels in particular are elevated, and thyroid replacement normalizes cholesterol levels. Reverse T3, an analog of the active thyroid hormone triiodothyronine, lowers LDL levels, though its use as a lipid-lowering drug is limited because of its side effect profile.

Diabetes causes increased triglyceride levels along with increased cholesterol levels. In poorly controlled diabetics, the principal elevated lipoprotein is VLDL. Good diabetic control normalizes triglyceride levels and reduces cholesterol levels proportionally. The relation of triglyceride levels to diabetic control is so close that diabetics with elevated triglycerides must be evaluated for poor control.

Usually, inflammatory diseases decrease levels of triglyceride, cholesterol, and all lipoprotein classes, VLDL, LDL, and HDL. Occasionally triglyceride and VLDL levels are increased because of deficiencies in LPL. The reduction in LDL and HDL appears to be due to direct effects cytokine mediators of inflammation, which inhibit hepatic lipoprotein production. In severe inflammatory disease, acquired LCAT deficiency leads to relative elevations of unesterified cholesterol. Recovery from the cause of inflammation, such as acute arthritis, pneumonia, or myocardial infarction, leads to normalization of lipoprotein levels within a few months. These effects of inflammation on lipoprotein levels are so marked that lipoprotein levels measured immediately after myocardial infarction are not reliable. Evaluation of patients with myocardial infarction for secondary prevention strategies must be delayed until 2 to 3 months after the infarction.

EFFECTS OF DRUGS ON LIPID AND LIPOPROTEIN LEVELS

Several drugs, particularly hormones and antihypertensive agents, affect lipid and lipoprotein levels. As mentioned, thyroid replacement decreases cholesterol, primarily by decreasing LDL levels. Estrogens in general reduce LDL levels and raise HDL levels. The beneficial effect of estrogens on LDL and HDL makes estrogen treatment one of the first considerations in treating dyslipoproteinemias in older women because of its beneficial effects on both bone and lipid metabolism. In contrast to estrogen, testosterone and other androgens increase LDL and decrease HDL levels; and people taking anabolic steroids often have profoundly low HDL levels. Recent reports suggest that growth hormone treatment increases HDL levels. Among antihypertensive agents, thiazide diuretics increase LDL levels, and population studies have shown that people taking β-blockers also have increased LDL levels.

AGE-ASSOCIATED CHANGES IN LIPIDS AND LIPOPROTEINS

Age-associated changes in lipid and lipoprotein levels have been studied both longitudinally and cross-sectionally (6, 7). In general, total and LDL cholesterol levels increase with age until approximately ages 55 to 65 in men, after which they show a slight decrease. In women the increase in cholesterol and LDL occurs primarily after the menopause, and the peak occurs about 10 years later than in men, between ages 65 and 75. HDL levels decrease significantly at male pu-

berty. After this decrease HDL levels in men remain relatively low compared with those of women until late in life. In men the HDL levels increase slightly after age 65 or 75 in association with decreasing levels of testosterone. HDL levels in women are fairly constant throughout life, although there is a slight decrease after menopause.

PREVENTION OF ATHEROSCLEROSIS BY MODIFYING LIPOPROTEIN RISK FACTORS

Elevated levels of atherogenic lipoproteins are associated with increased risk of cardiovascular and cerebrovascular disease, and the major clinical reason to measure cholesterol, triglyceride, and lipoprotein levels is to evaluate and modify risk of heart disease and stroke (8). The goal of the National Cholesterol Educational Program (NCEP) is to reduce LDL levels in all people who have elevated cholesterol levels (9).

There are three major prevention strategies: primary prevention, secondary prevention, and atherosclerosis regression. Primary prevention, which is accomplished by modifying risk factors before disease develops, is addressed mostly to people below age 65 (9,10). Secondary prevention is accomplished by reducing risk factors after an event caused by atherosclerosis, such as myocardial infarction or stroke. Regression of atherosclerosis has been demonstrated with noninvasive techniques to image arteries and determine degrees of atherosclerosis before myocardial infarction or stroke. Regression appears to be accomplished by aggressively lowering levels of atherogenic lipoproteins and eliminating other risk factors. Vigorous treatment in this fashion may reduce atherosclerosis long before effects on incidence of myocardial infarction and stroke can be demonstrated (11).

Other risk factors may be more important than lipid and lipoproteins (12, 13). The most significant reversible risk factor is smoking; and smoking cessation reduces the risk of cardiovascular and cerebrovascular disease much sooner than lowering levels of atherogenic lipoproteins. Similarly, uncontrolled hypertension causes greater short-term risk for cardiovascular and cerebrovascular disease than elevated lipid and lipoprotein levels. Finally, certain diseases, such as uncontrolled diabetes, should be addressed along with elevated lipid levels.

The premise for modifying lipid and lipoprotein risk factors for coronary and cerebrovascular disease is that data from primary prevention, secondary prevention, and regression trials carried out primarily in younger people apply in general to older people. There are no data suggesting that the mechanisms regulating lipid and lipoprotein levels that operate in younger people are at all different in older people. The few clinical trials of older people have shown no difference in the effect of modifying lipid and lipoprotein levels on reducing risk for development of atherosclerosis and subsequent coronary and cerebroarterial disease (14–17). The primary results of these intervention trials suggest that reducing cholesterol levels, particularly LDL cholesterol levels, reduces the incidence of new coronary artery disease, symptoms (e.g., angina), and events (e.g., myocardial infarction) (18–20). The same holds true for reducing triglyceride levels, although this effect is less pronounced for reasons that are still unknown. The primary lipoprotein decreased in these trials is LDL. However, reduced levels of LDL also are accompanied by reduced levels of chylomicron remnants, IDL, and Lp(a). Reducing LDL cholesterol levels does not actually reduce the death rate; rather it decreases the incidence of new cardiac and cerebrovascular events. Thus, while life is not necessarily prolonged, active life expectancy is prolonged because of the reduced rate of disabling heart attacks and strokes.

Secondary prevention and reversal of atherosclerosis can be accomplished by decreasing the same atherogenic lipoprotein levels that are lowered in primary prevention (11, 21). In secondary prevention, people who have already had a myocardial infarction are vigorously treated for all of their risk factors, including elevated levels of lipids and atherogenic lipoproteins. People who have had heart attacks and whose lipid and lipoprotein levels are vigorously treated have a lower incidence of second heart attacks, and this reduced incidence can be seen within 5 years of beginning the secondary prevention.

Recently it has been shown, with noninvasive techniques to image arteries and measure the de-

gree of atherosclerosis, that very vigorous treatment of hyperlipidemias along with modifying other risk factors can reduce the amount of atherosclerosis in large vessels. Reversal of atherosclerosis is accomplished in part by lowering the cholesterol level to less than 160 mg/dL with a combination of strict diet, often a vegetarian diet, and lipid-lowering drugs. Reversal can be seen in less than 5 years, which suggests that a rapid beneficial effect on clinical end points such as new symptoms and coronary or cerebrovascular events will eventually be described.

The observation in population studies that high HDL levels are associated with lower risk for coronary and cerebrovascular disease leads to the expectation that raising HDL levels would also reduce the risk of heart attack or stroke. However, there are no interventions that specifically raise HDL levels, and this idea has not been tested. Modalities that raise HDL levels include those that lower triglyceride, cholesterol, and atherogenic lipoprotein levels. Moreover, elevated HDL levels are associated with relative leanness and increased exercise tolerance. (Reducing body fat and increasing exercise tolerance has benefits to most people's feeling of well being, and therefore, things that raise HDL levels are generally beneficial.) An exception to this is alcohol. Although it has been reported that modest intake of alcohol raises HDL levels, excessive alcohol intake is deleterious and can be life threatening.

ROLE OF AGE IN TREATMENT DECISIONS

Treatment of dyslipoproteinemias in older people has to be placed in the context of other diseases they may have. Primary prevention of coronary and cerebroarterial disease does not show beneficial effects in fewer than 5 to 10 years. Therefore a rule of thumb is that patients with less than 10 years' life expectancy do not benefit from primary prevention of atherosclerosis by reduction of cholesterol levels. People in this category include those with cancer or end-stage heart, lung, or other organ disease and the very old. The average life expectancy of someone 65 years old is about 17 years, and therefore, a person of this age should be considered a candidate for primary prevention. However, the life expectancy of men in the United States decreases to 10 years by about age 73; and in women the life expectancy decreases to 10 years by about age 78. Therefore, men over age 75 and women over age 85 are probably not candidates for primary prevention of atherosclerosis by reduction of cholesterol levels unless they are in exceptionally robust good health. Although an 85-year-old man or woman in perfect health may live to be 100 and may benefit from primary prevention of atherosclerosis even after age 85, such persons are rare and difficult to identify. Similar consideration must be given to secondary prevention.

Given the effect of vigorous treatment of hypercholesterolemia on quality of life and the possibility that unregulated dietary modifications to lower cholesterol levels can cause dietary deficiencies of calcium, for example, which would shorten both active and total life, vigorous treatment of people over age 85 must be considered the exception rather than the rule. Additionally, all of these arguments about the advisability of treating hyperlipidemia in very old people are modulated by any chronic life-shortening diseases such as Alzheimer's disease. Since the average patient with Alzheimer's disease does not live much more than 10 years beyond initial diagnosis, patients with Alzheimer's disease should usually not be treated for hyperlipidemia. Since similar shortened life spans are seen in other dementing diseases (e.g., multi-infarct dementia), a clinical rule of thumb is that demented people, regardless of age, should not be treated for hyperlipidemias.

CLINICAL EVALUATION OF LIPID AND LIPOPROTEIN LEVELS

When considering modification of lipid and lipoprotein levels to reduce risk for cardiovascular and cerebrovascular disease, cholesterol level is the most important (22). In general, cholesterol levels over 220 mg/dL should be further studied. The more the cholesterol level exceeds 200 mg/dL, the more important it is to perform further evaluation and consider intervention, since the risk of cardiovascular and cerebrovascular disease increases directly with the cholesterol level above that. People with levels sub-

stantially over 350 mg/dL are at very high risk for early death.

In actuality, however, the relation of risk of death to cholesterol level is a U-shaped curve (23). The U shape appears to be more pronounced in older than in younger people. While elevated cholesterol levels are associated with increased risk of coronary and cerebrovascular disease, very low cholesterol levels (less than 150 mg/dL) are commonly associated with other life-threatening problems, including cancer, acute infection, other inflammatory disease, starvation, and other causes of malnutrition. Hence, a clinician observing an older person with a very low cholesterol level must consider that the low cholesterol level may indicate another disease requiring further evaluation. There is no evidence to suggest that lowering previously high cholesterol levels below 160 mg/dL causes these diseases. It has been speculated, however, that very low cholesterol levels may be associated with depression (24). Whether this is a cause of depression or an effect of poor food intake during depression or whether both low cholesterol levels and depression are caused by the same condition (e.g., cancer) remains to be established.

Triglyceride is often measured at the same time as cholesterol in an initial screening. Utility of this without HDL cholesterol levels is limited. Nonetheless, very high triglyceride levels (over 1 g/dL) must be immediately evaluated and treated, because they are associated with the development of acute pancreatitis. In addition, as mentioned earlier, very high triglyceride levels should alert the clinician to the possibility of uncontrolled diabetes. Very high triglyceride levels also occur in nephrotic syndrome, although by the time triglyceride elevation is seen, the edema of nephrotic syndrome is usually pronounced.

After observation that the cholesterol level is high, systemic disease must be ruled out. The two most important diseases affecting older people that are associated with high cholesterol levels are hypothyroidism and diabetes. Hypothyroidism is associated with markedly high cholesterol levels, sometimes as high as 350 mg/dL. Most of the elevated cholesterol is in the form of LDL. Both the total cholesterol and LDL levels are rapidly normalized with appropriate thyroid replacement. Uncontrolled diabetes is primarily associated with elevated triglyceride levels. However, since triglyceride-rich lipoproteins also contain cholesterol and since most screening programs measure cholesterol but not triglyceride, it is necessary to consider that a person with newly recognized cholesterol elevation may have previously undiagnosed diabetes or diabetes that is not properly controlled. As in the case of hypothyroidism, proper diabetic control promptly normalizes triglyceride levels and reduces cholesterol levels proportionately.

After ruling out systemic diseases that may be responsible for high cholesterol levels, it is necessary to repeat the cholesterol measurement, measure triglycerides, and measure HDL cholesterol levels. LDL can be calculated from these measurements. The calculation usually used is LDL cholesterol equals total cholesterol minus HDL cholesterol minus the quantity triglyceride level divided by 5. This formula is based on the assumption that in most people the amount of cholesterol in the triglyceride-rich lipoproteins is equal to one fifth of the triglyceride level when measured in milliliters per deciliter. Two methods are used to assess the LDL level calculated in this way. The method proposed by the National Cholesterol Education Program is to recognize that people with LDL cholesterol levels over 160 mg/dL are at increased risk for developing cardiovascular and cerebrovascular disease. An alternative approach is to calculate the LDL-HDL ratio. Such a calculation takes into account the fact that higher HDL levels are associated with lower risk of cardiac and cerebrovascular disease. Thus, an LDL-HDL ratio greater than 5 suggests increased risk of these cholesterol-associated diseases.

TREATMENT OF HIGH CHOLESTEROL AND TRIGLYCERIDE LEVELS

Treatment of elevated lipid and lipoprotein levels must begin by establishing purposes and goals of treatment. Age- and disease-dependent life expectancy modifies the goals, since all of the treatments, including dietary modification, have potential adverse side effects and may adversely affect quality of life. The goals and likelihood of accomplishing them must be carefully discussed. Second, the goals must address which specific lipids and lipoproteins are going to be modified. Triglyceride-lowering uses somewhat different diets and drugs from those of cholesterol lowering. In many cases both cholesterol and triglyceride levels are high, and certain LDL-lowering diets and drugs can reduce triglyceride levels as well as LDL cholesterol levels. Finally, many people would be well advised to raise HDL cholesterol levels. Drugs and diets that increase HDL levels are not well developed, and it is quite common that reducing cholesterol levels also drops HDL cholesterol levels. While low cholesterol levels, especially below 160 mg/dL, found in populations at screening are associated with bad outcome, there is no evidence that reducing cholesterol levels causes increased morbidity and mortality.

The first means to modify cholesterol and triglyceride levels is to modify behavior (25). Initially, all risk factors for cardiovascular and cerebrovascular diseases must be addressed, since many are affected directly by behavior. Moreover, risk factors for other problems causing morbidity and mortality must also be addressed. It is important to counsel patients about use of seat belts while driving, prevention of accidents and falls, smoking cessation, control of hypertension, and regulation of diabetes if present (26).

Diet is the first behavior to modify. Generally, trained dietitians should be used whenever possible to help set goals and procedures. The first step is to reduce total caloric intake. The American Heart Association (AHA) Step 1 Diet calls for a 30% reduction in calories. In addition to reducing calories, it is important to reduce intake of cholesterol and saturated fats. It is especially important in older people to prevent deficiencies, particularly in fat-soluble vitamins (vitamins A and D) and minerals (e.g., iron and calcium). Iron and calcium deficiency must be prevented, especially when meat intake is specifically reduced. An important motivational factor in getting people to adhere to diets is that weight reduction due to improved diet causes other benefits: it improves glucose control, it improves self-image, and it increases physical energy.

The second behavior to modify is exercise. Increased exercise reduces percent of body fat and increases the percent of lean mass. Concomitant with this, exercise decreases triglyceride levels. Exercise can increase HDL levels somewhat, an effect that is most marked in competitive male athletes. Increased exercise carries benefits similar to those of weight reduction due to diet: improved glucose control, improved self-image, and increased energy to do important activities.

It is reasonable to consider addition of pharmaceuticals after 3 to 6 months' trial of diet and exercise. It is critical, if pharmaceutical treatment is contemplated, to compare the goals in terms of reducing specific lipids and lipoproteins with the drugs that will be used. Costs and side effects must also be considered. First-line treatment of hypercholesterolemia can be niacin (27), a fibric acid derivative, a bile salt-binding resin, or an β-hydroxy-β-methyglutaryl and coenzyme A (HMG-CoA) reductase inhibitor (28). First-line pharmaceutical treatment of hypertriglyceridemia includes niacin or a fibric acid derivative. In women who are trying to reduce cholesterol levels, strong consideration should be given to beginning cyclic estrogen therapy, since estrogens in women both lower cholesterol and raise HDL levels.

All of the cholesterol-lowering drugs are associated with side effects. Niacin (nicotinic acid) causes flushing even at low doses, although this can be ameliorated if an aspirin is taken prior to the nicotinic acid. Fibric acid derivatives cause nausea and other gastrointestinal symptoms. Bile salt-binding resins cause constipation. HMG-CoA reductase inhibitors cause many gastrointestinal side effects. In vigorous attempts to reduce cholesterol levels, which are necessary to cause regression of atherosclerosis, the major side effect is elevated liver function tests, especially if several drugs are used. The use of the drug combination lovastatin and gemfibrozil has been discouraged because of reports of associated severe myopathy, rhabdomyolysis, and renal failure.

FOLLOW-UP

Once treatment has been initiated for a patient, annual (or more frequent) follow-up is critical to determine its effectiveness and to monitor side effects. Therapeutic goals must be periodically reviewed. As with all medications used in older patients, both initial and maintenance treatment should be the lowest possible dose necessary to achieve satisfactory results. Particular attention should be paid to possible drug interactions, as polypharmacy is a major cause of morbidity in the older population.

CONCLUSION

Although some changes in lipid and lipoprotein levels are associated with aging, metabolism in older people is similar to that in younger people. Thus, high LDL cholesterol levels are "bad" and high HDL cholesterol levels are "good" in older people, as they are in younger ones. When treating older people for lipid abnormalities, however, the presence of other diseases may modify decisions to treat or not to treat; in addition, there is less time remaining in the lives of older people for treatment to be effective. Since improvement in morbidity or mortality may not be as great in older people, careful attention must be paid to adverse side effects and other factors affecting quality of life, even extensive changes in diet. In conclusion, abnormalities in lipoproteins in older people should be carefully evaluated. Treatment decisions, however, must be carefully considered in the light of other medical problems, chronic disorders and diseases, and life expectancy.

REFERENCES

1. Gordon DJ, Rifkind BM. High-density lipoprotein: the clinical implications of recent studies. N Engl J Med 1989;321:1311–1316.
2. Thieszen SL, Hixson JE, Nagengast DJ, et al. Lipid phenotypes, apolipoprotein genotypes and cardiovascular risk in nonagenarians. Atherosclerosis 1990;83:137–146.
3. Rader DJ, Brewer HB Jr. Lipoprotein(a). Clinical approach to a unique atherogenic lipoprotein. JAMA 1992;267:1109–1112 (clinical conference) (erratum, JAMA 1992;267:1922).
4. Scanu AM, Lawn RM, Berg K. Lipoprotein(a) and atherosclerosis. Ann Intern Med 1991;115:209–218.
5. Murano S, Shinomiya M, Shirai K, et al. Characteristic features of long-living patients with familial hypercholesterolemia in Japan. J Am Geriatr Soc 1993; 41:253–257.
6. Gofman JW, Young W, Tandy R. Ischemic heart disease, atherosclerosis, and longevity. Circulation 1966;34: 679–697.
7. Kronmal RA, Cain KC, Ye Z, Omenn GS. Total choles-

terol levels and mortality risk as function of age. Arch Intern Med 1993;153:1065–1073.

8. Grundy SM. Cholesterol and coronary heart disease. Scand J Clin Lab Invest Suppl 1990;199:17–24.

9. Goodman DS. The National Cholesterol Education Program: guidelines, status, and issues. Am J Med 1991;90 (suppl 2A):32S–55S.

10. Muldoon MF, Manuck SB, Matthews KA. Lowering cholesterol concentrations and mortality: a quantitative review of primary prevention trials. BMJ 1990;301: 309–314.

11. Barth JD, Arntzenius AC. Progression and regression of atherosclerosis, what roles for LDL-cholesterol and HDL-cholesterol: a perspective. Eur Heart 1991;12: 952–957.

12. Grundy SM. Multifactorial etiology of hypercholesterolemia: implications for prevention of coronary heart disease. Arterioscler Thromb 1990;11:1619–1635.

13. Harris T, Cook EF, Kannel WB, Goldman L. Proportional hazards analysis of risk factors for coronary heart disease in individuals aged 65 or older. J Am Geriatr Soc 1988;36:1023–1028.

14. Hazzard WR. Dyslipoproteinemia in the elderly. Clin Geriatr Med 1992;8:89–102.

15. Karvonen MJ. Determinants of cardiovascular diseases in the elderly. Ann Med 1989;21:3–12.

16. Aronow WS, Starling L, Etienne F, et al. Risk factors for coronary artery disease in persons older than 62 years in long-term health care facility. Am J Cardiol 1986; 57:518–520.

17. Denke MA, Grundy SM. Hypercholesterolemia in elderly persons: resolving the treatment dilemma. Ann Intern Med 1990;112:780–792.

18. The Lipid Research Clinics Coronary Primary Prevention Trial results. I. Reduction in incidence of coronary heart disease. JAMA 1984;251:351–364.

19. The Lipid Research Clinics Coronary Primary Prevention Trial results. II. The relationship of reduction in incidence of coronary heart disease to cholesterol lowering. JAMA 1984;251:365–374.

20. Shepherd J, Cobbe SM, Ford I, et al. Prevention of coronary artery heart disease with pravastatin in men with hypercholesterolemia. N Engl J Med 1995;333:1301–1307.

21. Sacks FM, Pfeffer MA, Moye LA, et al. The effect of pravastatin on coronary artery events after myocardial infarction in patients with average cholesterol levels. N Engl J Med 1996;335:1001–1009.

22. Kannel WB, Doyle JJ, Shephard JF, et al. Prevention of cardiovascular disease in the elderly. J Am Coll Cardiol 1987;10:25A–28A.

23. Verdery RB, Goldberg AP. Hypocholesterolemia as a predictor of death: a prospective study of 224 nursing home residents. J Gerontol 1991;46:M84–90.

24. Oliver MF. Serum cholesterol: the knave of hearts and the joker. Lancet 1981;2:1090–1095.

25. Stamler J. Risk factor modification trials: implications for the elderly. Eur Heart 1988;9(suppl D):9–53.

26. Hermanson B, Omenn GS, Kronmal RA, et al. Beneficial six-year outcome of smoking cessation in older men and women with coronary artery disease. N Engl J Med 1988;319:1365–1369.

27. Canner PL, Berge KG, Wenger NK, et al. Fifteen year mortality in coronary drug project patients: long-term benefit with niacin. J Am Coll Cardiol 1986;8:1245–1255.

28. Grundy SM. HMG-CoA reductase inhibitors for treatment of hypercholesterolemia. N Engl J Med 1988; 319:24–31.

CHAPTER 27

SUMANT S. CHUGH, BARBARA A. CLARK, AND HENRY M. YAGER

Principles of Fluid and Electrolyte Balance and Renal Disorders in the Older Patient

THE AGING KIDNEY

As with all of the body's organ systems, the human kidney gradually develops anatomic and physiologic changes with aging. These changes are well compensated and generally not perceptible unless superimposed illness upsets the homeostasis. Elderly persons have increased susceptibility to disorders of fluid and electrolytes as well as renal failure when physiologically challenged. The first section of this chapter focuses on the anatomic and physiologic basis of these susceptibilities that may contribute to morbidity in the elderly.

Anatomic Changes

Significant changes occur in the vasculature of the kidney. The arteries develop medial hypertrophy, intimal proliferation with reduplication of elastic tissue (1). An increasing number of cortical arterioles end blindly because of the loss of cortical glomeruli. In the juxtamedullary region a number of afferent and efferent arterioles are connected via obsolescent glomerular tufts rather than ending blindly, forming a sort of afferent-efferent arteriovenous fistula (2–4). The blood supply to the medulla is better preserved than that to the cortex (2, 5). The anatomy of the tubules also changes, with decreased tubule length and development of tubular diverticula of the distal convoluted tubules (1). Some investigators believe these changes may be the predecessors of ac-

quired renal cysts, which are commonly seen after the fifth decade of life (6). The renal interstitium gradually becomes mildly fibrotic, especially in the renal pyramids (5–8). The overall mass and size of the kidney decrease with advancing age. Intravenous pyelographic studies demonstrate a loss in length of about 0.5 cm per decade after age 50 (9). Other studies report a 20 to 40% decrease in size from the third to the eighth decade (8–11). Most of the tissue loss occurs in the cortex, with a 30 to 40% decrease in number of glomeruli and an increase in the number of sclerotic, nonfunctioning glomeruli (12–14). The glomeruli undergo microscopic changes that include a decrease in surface area, expansion of the mesangial area, and an increase in basement membrane thickness (2, 12–14).

Glomerular Filtration Rate and Renal Blood Flow

Several investigative groups have sought to determine the effects of these changes in the renal parenchyma on measurable physiologic functions (15–19). Results of the National Institute on Aging longitudinal study in Baltimore, which were first published in 1976, included creatinine clearance results from 584 men in their third to eighth decade of life studied at 12- to 18-month intervals (15). They noted an average creatinine clearance value of 140 mL per minute per 1.73 m^2 at ages 25 to 30, with a significant progressive decline in creatinine clearance, approximately 8 mL per minute per 1.73 m² per decade, beginning in the mid 30s. Interestingly, the presence of hypertension or prostatic enlargement did not significantly alter creatinine clearance in this sample, presumably because of good medical management and follow-up. They also reported a small rise in serum creatinine with advancing age from 0.813 mg/dL from ages 25 to 34 to 0.843 mg/dL by ages 75 to 84. Therefore serum creatinine progressively overestimates glomerular filtration rate (GFR) with advancing age. This can be explained by the decrease in muscle mass associated with decrease in creatinine production and excretion (15). In a follow-up of the Baltimore Longitudinal Study of Aging published in 1985, Lindeman et al. (20) again noted a mean decline in creatinine clearance of 0.75 mL per minute per year with a normal distribution of values around the mean. Some 30% of the population showed no deterioration of renal function over time. This finding emphasizes the fact that individual variation must be taken into account when considering the effect of aging on kidney function and that a measurable decrease in GFR with age is far from universal.

Several authors have developed nomograms to estimate creatinine clearance (CrCl) based on the serum creatinine and expected fall in GFR with age (15, 21). The most widely used of these was published by Cockcroft and Gault in 1976 (21):

$$CrCl \text{ (milliliters per minute) in men} = \frac{(140 - age) \times Weight \text{ in kilograms}}{72 \times Serum \text{ creatinine (milligrams per deciliter)}}$$

For women, multiply the result by 0.85.

This method provides an estimate, as individual variability makes it imprecise. The estimation is valid only in the steady state and not useful when renal function is changing daily, as in acute renal failure. Furthermore, 24-hour creatinine clearance itself is an overestimate of GFR (as compared with inulin or iothalamate clearance) because of the small contribution of tubular creatinine secretion to urinary creatinine concentration. This difference is exaggerated with advancing age, as the percentage of urinary creatinine concentra-

tion attributable to tubular secretion increases with age (16).

The mechanism of glomerular atrophy and the decline in GFR with aging is unknown, and a variety of theories have been proposed. Some of the decline may be secondary to vascular changes of aging (3–5, 16). An alternative theory suggests the possibility of injury due to excessive intraglomerular pressure, or hyperfiltration, although the mechanisms and mediators are not fully defined (22–24). Diets consistently high in protein induce excessive filtration and accelerate the development of sclerotic glomeruli at a younger age than expected in the rat kidney (22, 24). Methods that reduce intraglomerular capillary pressure, such as chronic angiotensin-converting enzyme (ACE) inhibition are capable of attenuating age-related glomerulosclerosis in the rat (25, 26). However, inhibition of advanced glycation end products, which have been implicated in diabetes related glomerular injury, is also capable of ameliorating the glomerulosclerosis seen in aging rats (27), suggesting that events other than hemodynamically mediated injury are also involved in the age-associated decline in GFR. The relevance of these studies to human aging remains unclear.

Tubular Functions

Proximal tubular functions, such as transport of glucose and amino acids, decline progressively with age (28). These changes parallel the fall in GFR, suggesting that the decline is related to a decreased number of functioning nephrons with age rather than a specific defect in transport. However, studies in animals suggest that aging may be associated with some decrease in tubular enzyme concentrations, lower concentrations of sodium-potassium adenosine triphosphatase (ATPase), decreased sodium-hydrogen exchange, and sodium-dependent phosphate transport (29–31).

Acid-Base Homeostasis

Renal acid excretion and acid-base balance in aging are well maintained under basal conditions. However, the ability to respond to an acid load is somewhat impaired (32, 33). The decrease in renal acid excretion is due to a decrease in both urinary ammonium and phosphorus and parallels the decline in GFR. One meta-analysis reports a slight age-related reduction in serum bicarbonate levels and increase in hydrogen ion in the circulation (34). The slight defects in renal acid handling have been attributed to the decrease in nephron mass with age.

Sodium Homeostasis

Renal sodium handling is determined by the interaction of a variety of factors. Advancing age has been associated with declines in the renin-aldosterone system (35), increases in atrial natriuretic hormone (ANH) (36–38), declines in urinary prostaglandin E_2 and dopamine (39–41), increases in circulating β-adrenergic catecholamines (42, 43), and decreased β-adrenergic receptor activity (43, 44).

The elderly appear to have some defects in responding to both increases and decreases in sodium intake. The response to decreases in dietary sodium intake was demonstrated in classic studies by Epstein and Hollenberg in which healthy young (less than 30 years old) and healthy old (over 60 years) subjects were placed on very low sodium diets (less than 10 mEq/day) (45). The half-time to achieve sodium balance (i.e., when daily sodium output equals intake) was 18 hours in the young compared with 31 hours in the old. This suggests a relative sodium wasting in the elderly, a paradoxic finding in view of the well-recognized age-related reduction in plasma renin and aldosterone levels. However, the clinical implications of this are unclear. One study reports an increased susceptibility to orthostatic hypotension in the elderly following sodium deprivation (46). However, in other studies the elderly do not appear especially susceptible to salt depletion during sodium deprivation (35). Weidmann et al. (35), comparing responses to a sodium intake of 10 mEq per day, did not find any difference in body weight (a reflection of total body sodium loss) after 6 days in young versus old; both groups lost approximately 2.5% of body weight. This suggests that the defects in sodium conservation may not universally represent serious problems with excess sodium wasting, at least in the healthy elderly.

The data on the renal response to increases in sodium intake are also conflicting. Virtually all studies report that the elderly are more likely than the young to develop increases in blood pressure in response to increases in sodium intake (47–49). Elderly exhibit more weight gain than the young and take longer to excrete the sodium, with a higher proportion excreted at night (50). In addition, the elderly are more susceptible to the sodium-retaining effects of antinatriuretic pharmacologic agents such as nonsteroidal anti-inflammatory drugs (NSAIDs) (48). Conversely, other studies report exaggerated blood pressure and natriuretic responses to acute intravenous sodium loading (as compared with oral sodium loading) in healthy elderly, a response reminiscent of that seen in younger patients with hypertension, especially those with low plasma renin levels or salt sensitivity (51, 52).

The natriuretic response to exogenous infusions of ANH or dopamine are well maintained in the healthy elderly human kidney, even in the absence of increases in GFR (53–55). Conversely, aging may impair the renal vasodilatory and natriuretic response to the nitric oxide precursor l-arginine, although this has been documented only in hypertensive humans (56). The elderly have less diuretic and natriuretic response to loop diuretics, attributed to the age-related decrease in functioning nephrons rather than tubular insensitivity to these agents (57).

Atrial Natriuretic Hormone

ANH is a 28-amino acid peptide hormone secreted primarily by atrial myocytes in response to atrial stretch usually induced by volume expansion (36–38). Plasma ANH levels rise with age (36–38). The reasons for the elevated levels and the relevance to aging physiology remain to be elucidated. Some elderly patients with the syndrome of acquired hypoaldosteronism have higher ANH levels than age-matched healthy controls (58), implicating excessive ANH as a possible factor in the pathophysiology of this disorder.

While ANH levels are higher in the healthy elderly than in the young, they are even further elevated in cardiovascular disease states in the elderly (59). In one nursing home study ANH levels were high even before overt manifestations of congestive heart failure and were proposed as a noninvasive marker for early detection of congestive heart failure (CHF) (59).

Renin-Angiotensin System

Evidence suggests that alterations in the renin-aldosterone system have a significant effect on the hemodynamics and volume homeostasis in aging. Not only do basal renin and aldosterone levels decline with age, but stimulation of renin or aldosterone release in response to upright posture, salt depletion, or potassium infusion is also blunted (35, 60, 61). Weidmann et al. (35) found that the aldosterone response to adrenocorticotropic hormone (ACTH) stimulation was similar in young and old, suggesting that the main defect lies in renin secretion and/or the aldosterone release in response to renin. Both a decrease in renin synthesis and impairment in renin release are seen with aging (62, 63). However, the elderly have been reported to have an increased density of angiotensin II receptors which may somewhat compensate the age-related decline in renin levels (64). While the renal vasoconstrictive response to angiotensin infusion is similar in young and elderly humans (5), the hypotensive effects of ACE inhibitors may be more pronounced, at least in hypertensive elderly (64).

Water Homeostasis

Numerous systems affect the regulation of water balance, and each of these may be influenced to some degree by aging. Renal concentrating and diluting abilities are impaired with age (65–67). The maximal concentrating ability and minimum urine volume are impaired in the elderly in response to water deprivation (66). In one study the mean maximum urine osmolality following a 24-hour water deprivation in elderly (aged 60 to 79) was 882 plus or minus 49 mosm/kg versus 1109 plus or minus 22 in young (aged 20 to 39) (66). The factors responsible for the decreased concentrating ability in the elderly kidney are not completely clear. Likely contributing factors are age-related decline in GFR and the relative increase in medullary, as compared with juxtaglomerular, flow, with a resultant washout of the medullary countercurrent

concentrating gradient. A number of studies have investigated whether aging is associated with defects in pituitary release of or renal response to antidiuretic hormone (ADH) (67–69). Although the elderly may have exaggerated ADH responses to hypertonicity, they appear to have diminished responses to posture- or diuretic-induced volume depletion (i.e., volume pressure sensitivity) (69). Elderly persons have greater ADH responses to nicotine (a potent stimulus for ADH release) but not to insulin-induced hypoglycemia (70).

Elderly persons also have a reduced ability to excrete a water load (65, 67, 71). There may be a slight impairment in the maximal diluting capacity in the elderly kidney, but it is not enough to account for all of the impairment in free water excretion that has been observed (67, 71). This suggests that age-related changes in GFR, anatomic changes in renal vasculature, or differences in neurohumoral mediators that affect distal tubular flow may be important. Healthy elderly subjects appear to have defects in renal prostaglandins, which are known to be important in water diuresis (37, 72). Studies in healthy elderly women reveal diminished urinary excretion of prostaglandin E_2 in response to water loading (39).

Hypernatremia

Defects in water conservation, diminished thirst, illness-induced water loss, and lack of access to water because of immobility or neurologic disease make the elderly especially susceptible to dehydration and hypernatremia. Hypernatremia has been used as a marker for poor prognosis and for evidence of neglect in nursing homes (73–75). The symptoms of hypernatremia are lethargy, obtundation, or coma due to neuronal cell dehydration and shrinkage. Hypernatremia may result from loss of water and sodium, either renal or extrarenal, with greater water than sodium loss; predominant water loss, as with central or nephrogenic diabetes insipidus or water deprivation; or exogenous excessive sodium administration. History, physical examination, and evaluation of urinary osmolality and sodium distinguish among these. Therapy consists of hypotonic fluids in the first scenario, water alone in the second scenario, and diuretics plus water in the third. If severe dehydration with hypotension is present, initial fluid should consist of isotonic fluids until cardiovascular stability is established. (These will still be hypotonic relative to the patient's osmolality). The water deficit can be calculated by the following formula:

$$Water\ deficit = Normal\ total\ body\ water - \\ Observed\ total\ body\ water$$

$$Observed\ total\ body\ water = Weight\ in\ kilograms \times 0.6$$

$$Normal\ total\ body\ water \times Normal\ serum\ sodium = \\ Observed\ total\ body\ water \times Observed\ serum\ sodium$$

Use either observed present body weight or known prior body weight in the equation. For example, an elderly man goes the emergency room with confusion and a serum sodium of 163. He cannot be weighed, but a weight of 70 kg was recorded 3 weeks earlier, when he was alert and well:

$$Normal\ total\ body\ water = 70 \times 0.6 = 42\ L \\ 42\ L \times 140 = 5880 = X \times 163 \\ X = 36\ L \\ Water\ deficit = 42\ L - 36\ L = 6\ L$$

Half of this amount should be replaced in the first 24 hours and the remainder, over the next 24 to 48 hours. The brain can generate idiogenic osmoles to defend against excessive intracellular water loss to the extracellular space. Overly rapid correction does not allow dissipation of these idiogenic osmoles and may lead to intracerebral cellular swelling with worsening mental status or seizures.

Hyponatremia

Just as with hypernatremia, the prevalence of hyponatremia increases with age (65, 76–80). In one study 11.3% of patients in an inpatient geriatric unit had serum sodium concentration less than 130 mEq/L, and 4.5% had less than 125 mEq/L (77). Another study reported a 22% prevalence of hyponatremia in a chronic disease facility (79), and yet another reported an 8% prevalence in a group of geriatric outpatients (78). Several prospective studies of hyponatremia in hospitalized patients demonstrate that as many as 60 to 70% of cases occur in the el-

derly (76–80). In one retrospective study of 405 ambulatory geriatric outpatients, 46 were found to have hyponatremia, with the syndrome of inappropriate antidiuretic hormone secretion (SIADH) the apparent cause in 27 (81). Of these SIADH cases 7 were in the very old and had no apparent underlying cause. The authors suggested that aging itself may be a risk factor for development of an SIADH-like hyponatremia in a subset of very old patients.

Hyponatremia, like hypernatremia, also appears to be a marker for more serious illness. In one study, the likelihood of death was 8.7% in hyponatremic patients as compared with 1% in normonatremic patients (82). Mild hyponatremia is usually asymptomatic, but severe hyponatremia (sodium less than 125 mEq/L) is often accompanied by lethargy, somnolence, seizures, or coma, probably related to neuronal cell swelling and increased intracranial pressure. Hyponatremia can occur in the setting of sodium and volume depletion (as in diuretic use, adrenal insufficiency, or gastrointestinal (GI) losses), sodium and volume overload (as in CHF, cirrhosis, and nephrotic syndrome), or with euvolemia (as in SIADH). The latter can be induced by drugs, respiratory disorders, central nervous system (CNS) disorders, or cancer. Although the cause of hyponatremia is often multifactorial, diuretic-induced hyponatremia is particularly common in the elderly. Diuretics may be implicated in up to 20 to 30% of cases in some series (76, 77, 79, 80, 83). Thiazide diuretics are particularly likely to predispose to hyponatremia via any of a number of mechanisms, including increased renal sodium losses, volume-mediated nonosmotic stimulation of ADH, potassium depletion, and interference with formation of a maximally dilute urine in the distal tubule (83, 84). Under these circumstances the intake of hypotonic fluid by patients depleted of salt and water may lead to hyponatremia. Even healthy elderly appear susceptible to hyponatremia with thiazide diuretic use if excessive water is ingested concomitantly. Therefore, it seems reasonable to caution elderly patients taking thiazide diuretics (which may a good drug of choice for hypertension in the elderly) to avoid habitual drinking of large volumes of water and to avoid the simultaneous use of NSAIDs without close medical supervision.

Hypovolemic hyponatremia should be treated with isotonic saline. After rapid correction of hypotension, the infusion should be slowed to replace ongoing losses plus enough to raise serum sodium concentration approximately 0.5 mEq/L per hour. Patients with hyponatremia resulting from edema should have salt and water restrictions. If serum sodium is below 115 mEq/L or if seizures occur, loop diuretics and 3% saline are given to raise serum sodium at 2 mEq/L per hour until seizures are controlled or at 0.5 mEq/L per hour until serum sodium concentration reaches 125 mEq/L. In SIADH water intake should be restricted to 700 to 1000 mL per day. Administration of 3% saline plus a loop diuretic should be reserved for severe hyponatremia or seizures, as in patients with edema-associated hyponatremia (85). Overly rapid correction or overcorrection, particularly if the hyponatremia developed over a long period, can lead to delayed worsening of the neurologic status, with delirium, seizures, or coma. This clinical scenario has been associated with pathologic defects in the brainstem, a condition known as central pontine myelinolysis (85).

Potassium Metabolism

Because aging is associated with declines in aldosterone levels, GFR, and some distal tubular functions, the elderly are at risk for hyperkalemia (86). Hyporeninemic aldosteronism with associated hyperkalemia is predominately a syndrome of the elderly (86, 87). The distal tubule constitutes the major site for excretion of potassium. At this site sodium is reabsorbed from the tubular lumen in exchange for potassium secreted from the tubular interstitium. This exchange is enhanced in the presence of aldosterone. Elderly humans have diminished aldosterone responses to stimulation by upright posture (i.e., mediation via renin and angiotensin) (35, 60) or intravenous potassium infusion (61). The diminished aldosterone response to hyperkalemia may be explained at least in part by the reduction in plasma renin and the rise in plasma levels of ANH that are characteristic of aging.

Handling of acute potassium loads entails both renal and extrarenal mechanisms. The main effect of aldosterone is on the renal excretion of potassium rather than on extrarenal uptake. Extrarenal uptake of potassium (i.e., shifting potassium intracellularly) is the primary defense against acute potassium loads. This process is mediated predominantly by insulin and sympathetic β-adrenergic activity (88). β-Adrenergic activity declines with age in many tissues (43, 44). However, there are few studies on the extrarenal handling of potassium in the elderly. In potassium infusion studies, serum potassium levels rise to the same degree in elderly as young persons, despite the blunted aldosterone response in the elderly (61), suggesting intact mechanisms of extrarenal potassium metabolism. A study using strenuous exercise with associated release of potassium from exercising muscle revealed a faster rise in serum potassium levels in the elderly (89), suggesting either a defect in extrarenal potassium uptake or faster muscle potassium loss. Elderly subjects also display a delayed decrease in serum potassium levels toward normal after potassium infusion, consistent with delayed renal excretion (62).

Many medications commonly prescribed to older patients are inhibitors of the renin-angiotensin-aldosterone system. ACE inhibitors suppress aldosterone release by inhibiting the conversion of angiotensin I to angiotensin II. β-Blockers and NSAIDs also suppress renin release (88). β-Blockers additionally interfere with intracellular potassium uptake (88). Spironolactone, an aldosterone antagonist, and other potassium-sparing diuretics interfere with potassium excretion. Heparin may suppress aldosterone by directly inhibiting its adrenal synthesis (88). Trimethoprim interferes with secretion of potassium in the distal tubule. Careful monitoring of potassium levels is therefore indicated when prescribing agents that may interfere with potassium regulation to the elderly patient.

ACUTE RENAL FAILURE

The incidence of acute renal failure increases with age (90, 91). The incidence of acute renal failure in the elderly hospitalized has been reported to be at least 5 times that of a younger population (91). As in any age group, the causes of acute renal failure fall into one of three categories: prerenal, renal, and postrenal. All three categories are common in the elderly. Defects in renal sodium handling, frequent use of diuretics and drugs that can interfere with autoregulation of glomerular hemodynamics (such as ACE inhibitors and NSAIDs), lead to a higher frequency of prerenal azotemia in the elderly. This is particularly relevant when superimposed illness, such as CHF, GI fluid loss, or sepsis, threatens the circulation. Postrenal azotemia is also more common in the elderly than in the young, largely because of the increased occurrence of prostatic enlargement, although other causes of bladder or ureteric dysfunction may also be implicated. The aged kidney is also more susceptible to ischemic and nephrotoxic acute renal failure (90). Additional causes of intrinsic acute renal failure in the elderly include atheroembolic disease, multiple myeloma, cortical necrosis, urate obstruction, glomerulonephritis, interstitial nephritis, and vasculitis. Advanced age is considered to be a risk factor for radiocontrast nephropathy (92). The reasons for the increased susceptibility of the older kidney to ischemic and nephrotoxic acute renal failure are not fully delineated. Mechanisms important in the defense against acute renal failure include factors that preserve renal blood flow, particularly to the renal medulla, which exists at low oxygen tensions at all times (93). These intrinsic mechanisms include renal autocrine systems such as prostaglandins, dopamine, nitric oxide, and endothelin. Recent magnetic resonance imaging (MRI) techniques that can visualize differences in renal parenchymal oxygen tension reveal less ability to modulate medullary oxygenation in the kidneys of healthy elderly volunteers than in healthy young subjects (94). Fixed structural vascular changes and/or alterations in renal autocoids may contribute to this relative medullary hypoxia in the elderly.

The diagnosis and management of acute renal failure in the elderly population does not differ from that of a younger population. A decrease in either urinary sodium or fractional excretion of sodium remains a good indicator of prerenal azotemia. Measures that can be useful in preventing nephrotoxic renal failure include adequate hydration and discontinuation of NSAIDs,

particularly prior to radiocontrast studies (93). Studies examining outcomes of acute renal failure in the elderly suggest that the elderly may have the same rates of recovery as younger patients without any additional adverse consequences of dialysis (91, 95, 96). Therefore, age alone is not necessarily a poor prognostic indicator in cases of acute renal failure and should not be used as a reason to withhold acute dialysis if other organ systems are intact.

RENOVASCULAR DISEASE

The two common forms of renovascular disease in the elderly are renal artery stenosis (RAS) and atheroembolic renal disease. Approximately 15% of cases of end-stage renal disease (ESRD) result from renovascular disease (97).

Renal Artery Stenosis

Narrowing of the renal artery is fairly common in the elderly patient. In an autopsy series of 295 patients, narrowing of the intraluminal diameter by more than 50% was noted in 17% of normotensive patients and 56% of hypertensive patients (98). It may also be an incidental finding during angiograms done for unrelated reasons. For example, in one study 59% of patients undergoing arteriography to evaluate peripheral vascular disease had stenosis of at least one renal artery (99). The most prevalent cause of renal artery stenosis in this age group is atherosclerosis. Atheromatous plaques commonly involve the proximal third of the renal artery. In some cases ostial lesions are formed by encroachment of plaques in the wall of the aorta on the ostium of the renal artery. Other causes of renal artery stenosis, such as fibromuscular dysplasia and arteritis, are much less common.

There are several clinical presentations of RAS. First, it may be new-onset hypertension in the elderly or difficulty in controlling previously stable hypertension. Renin secretion is generally increased in renovascular hypertension (RVH) in the setting of both unilateral and bilateral (or unilateral in a solitary kidney) RAS. There is evidence to suggest that volume expansion (i.e., salt and water retention) plays a greater role in hypertension due to bilateral RAS than unilateral RAS (100–102). On physical examination, abdominal bruits, present in up to 40% of patients, usually signify RAS, although they may originate from other vessels (103). Retinopathy is more pronounced in patients with RVH than in those with primary hypertension because of its briefer and stormier course (103). It is important to stress that demonstration of RAS in a hypertensive patient does not necessarily establish a diagnosis of RVH, because essential hypertension also accelerates the development of atheromatous plaques, which may occur in the renal arteries and elsewhere (103).

Second, some elderly patients have progressive azotemia in the presence of other evidence of atherosclerotic disease. This condition, called ischemic nephropathy, which is being increasingly recognized, may contribute to the increased frequency of ESRD attributed to hypertension in the past decade (104, 105). Typical features include hypertension, peripheral vascular disease, inactive urinary sediment, and urinary protein excretion less than 1 g per day (106). However, the sensitivity of these signs for identifying patients with ischemic nephropathy is relatively low.

Third, RAS should be suspected in patients who develop acute renal failure after treatment with ACE inhibitors. This phenomenon also occurs with other classes of antihypertensive drugs (107), though less commonly, and in patients with essential hypertension without evidence of RAS.

Fourth, recurrent pulmonary edema in patients with poorly controlled hypertension and renal insufficiency is now recognized as a marker of bilateral renal artery stenosis (108). The occurrence of pulmonary edema is not related to the severity of hypertension or renal failure. Although it is more common in patients who have associated coronary artery disease, it also occurs in patients with normal coronaries (109).

The gold standard for the diagnosis of RAS is selective renal arteriography. However, since it is invasive and carries the risk of contrast nephropathy, atheroembolism, and vascular trauma, arteriography is not recommended as a screening test. More recently the use of intra-arterial digital subtraction angiography has replaced conventional angiography because high-quality images may be obtained with low dye loads and smaller-lumen catheters may diminish the incidence of atheroembolism and arterial tears. Of several noninvasive tests, captopril renography has become popular in view of its high sensitivity (92%) and specificity (93%) (110, 111). It is also useful in predicting the likelihood of improvement in blood pressure after revascularization (112). Proponents of Doppler ultrasonography have noted similar sensitivity (95%) and specificity (90%) (113). However, Doppler ultrasonography is operator dependent and may have limited value in the presence of extreme obesity or poor bowel preparation (114). Other rapidly evolving techniques, including magnetic resonance angiography and spiral CT angiography, have comparable sensitivity and specificity and the advantage of delineating the arterial anatomy, but use of them is limited by high cost.

RVH in the elderly can be treated medically, surgically, or by angioplasty. Since severe RAS may impair renal function as well as cause hypertension, some form of revascularization is preferred. Surgical revascularization is the traditional treatment of choice. The 10-year survival is 70% in surgically treated patients with isolated atherosclerosis and 30% in patients with diffuse atherosclerosis (115). The leading cause of mortality in these patients is atheromatous disease elsewhere in the body. Neither age nor impaired renal function should exclude patients from revascularization, since in a study of patients older than 60 years surgical mortality was 2.8% and not significantly higher in patients with serum creatinine above 1.4 mg/dL (116). Angioplasty produces results similar to those of surgical revascularization and is becoming increasingly popular, especially for patients with nonostial stenosis. It is particularly beneficial for patients turned down for surgery because of severe comorbid conditions. Recently patients with ostial stenosis have had nonsurgical placement of intravascular stents with good results (117). The main concerns with medical management in patients deemed unsuitable for surgery or angioplasty are progression of RAS and the hemodynamic effects of blood pressure reduction on renal function. ACE inhibitors should be used with great caution in patients with bilateral

RAS, since they often precipitate a dramatic decline in renal function. In patients with unilateral RAS and renovascular hypertension, one retrospective analysis (118) noted a significant association between ACE inhibitors and the development of progressive renal artery occlusion, whereas another (119) found no adverse effect on renal function or kidney size after a year of therapy. Dihydropyridine calcium channel blockers have been shown to reduce blood pressure in patients with bilateral RAS with less impairment of function of the ischemic kidney than ACE inhibitors in short-term studies (120), but comparative long-term data are lacking (121).

Treatment of ischemic nephropathy follows the same general principles as treatment of RAS. Revascularization in some form is preferred, since conservative management with antihypertensive medications is often unsuccessful, and reduction of blood pressure with ACE inhibitors and other antihypertensive agents in patients with bilateral RAS may cause a significant decline in GFR. The combination of diuretics and ACE inhibitors should be avoided, since it increases the risk of acute renal failure (103).

Atheroembolic Renal Disease

Atheroembolic renal disease is progressive renal insufficiency due to embolic obstruction of small and medium sized renal arteries by atheromatous material. Other organs and tissues often involved include the retina, brain, pancreas, skin, and muscles. Predisposing conditions include aortic surgery; angiography of the aorta or coronary or carotid circulation, especially via the femoral route; cardiopulmonary resuscitation; use of intra-aortic balloon pumps; anticoagulation; and thrombolytic therapy for acute myocardial infarction. Occasionally, atheroembolic renal disease occurs spontaneously. The clinical spectrum of disease varies from episodic and labile hypertension to the insidious onset of progressive renal insufficiency 1 to 4 weeks after the after the initial insult to a more explosive syndrome of acute renal failure associated with purple discoloration of toes, livido reticularis of the lower extremities and/or abdominal wall, GI bleeding, pancreatitis, myocardial infarction, retinal ischemia, cerebral infarc-

tion, and severe hypertension. Other clinical and laboratory features include fever, elevated erythrocyte sedimentation rate, eosinophilia, eosinophiluria, transient hypocomplementemia, rise in serum glutamic-oxaloacetic transaminase (SGOT) and lactate dehydrogenase (LDH), hematuria without casts, and proteinuria, occasionally in the nephrotic range. Although ophthalmic examination and skin and muscle biopsies are often helpful, definitive diagnosis may require renal biopsy. Differential diagnosis includes contrast-induced acute renal failure, polyarteritis nodosa, cryoglobulinemia, allergic vasculitis, atrial myxoma, and endocarditis. The time course usually differentiates it from contrast-induced acute renal failure, which generally occurs within 1 to 4 days after the angiographic procedure. Atheroembolic renal failure is most commonly irreversible and progressive, though stabilization and improvement have been documented in some instances. Since no definitive treatment is available, careful risk-benefit assessment should be carried out before performing invasive angiographic procedures in patients with widespread atherosclerotic disease. Once renal failure progresses to ESRD, supportive therapy, including dialysis, should be offered. Peritoneal dialysis has the theoretic advantage of avoiding transient heparinization commonly used with hemodialysis.

Thromboembolic Renal Disease

Renal artery thromboembolic disease is total or partial occlusion of the renal arteries from clot emboli that arise outside the kidney or from thrombosis arising within the renal arteries (122). Emboli most commonly originate from the heart in patients with atrial arrhythmias or mural thrombi (123). In situ renal artery thrombosis is less common and is generally superimposed on an atheromatous plaque but may also complicate traumatic intimal tears. The clinical presentation is that of renal infarction, including abdominal or flank pain, nausea, vomiting, fever, and sudden onset of hypertension or exacerbation of previously controlled hypertension (122). The diagnosis is often missed, since this presentation may mimic that of nephrolithiasis, pyelonephritis, bowel infarction, or acute cholecystitis. Urinalysis reveals nonnephrotic proteinuria and microscopic hematuria. Serum enzymes, including SGOT, LDH, and alkaline phosphatase, rise in proportion to the extent of tissue damage and follow a predictable time course. SGOT rises within 24 hours and decreases in 4 to 7 days. LDH increases within the first 2 days and remains elevated for up to 2 weeks. Alkaline phosphatase starts rising by day 3 to 5 and may remain elevated for up to 4 weeks. Elevated urinary LDH and alkaline phosphatase may allow differentiation from infarction of other organs. The diagnosis is suggested by nonvisualization or absence of function on intravenous pyelography, isotope renography, or computed tomography (CT), but definitive evidence may require arteriography. In addition, transesophageal echocardiography is useful in evaluating for a cardiac source of embolism.

Management of thromboembolic renal disease includes control of hypertension, restoration of renal blood flow, and prevention of further episodes. Both systemic anticoagulation with heparin or warfarin and systemic or intraarterial thrombolytic therapy have been successful in restoring renal blood flow. Surgical thrombectomy or embolectomy is reserved for cases in which anticoagulation and thrombolysis are contraindicated, i.e., in the setting of bilateral renal artery occlusion, severe uncontrolled hypertension, or bleeding from renal infarction. Anticoagulation with warfarin should be continued as long as the risk of recurrent thromboembolism persists. Hypertension is usually well controlled with standard antihypertensives, including ACE inhibitors.

GLOMERULAR DISEASE IN THE ELDERLY

The true incidence of glomerular disease in the elderly is difficult to establish (124). Data from renal biopsy series (Table 27.1) do not give an accurate estimate of the incidence of various forms of glomerular disease, since most patients with an established systemic disease such as diabetes or cancer presenting with a glomerular syndrome do not have biopsies and are therefore underrepresented.

The clinical presentation of glomerular disease

Table 27.1

Renal Biopsy Results in Patients 65 Years of Age and Older

Proliferative or necrotizing glomerulonephritis	147
Membranous glomerulopathy	114
Focal segmental glomerulosclerosis	52
Crescentic glomerulonephritis[a]	41
Arterionephrosclerosis[b]	39
Minimal change glomerulopathy	38
Diabetic glomerulosclerosis	29
Chronic glomerulopathy with advanced sclerosis	27
Membranoproliferative glomerulonephritis[c]	24
Atheroembolic disease	23
Amyloid	18
Interstitial nephritis	16
Acute tubular necrosis	13
Thrombotic microangiopathy	10
Myeloma cast nephropathy	7
Light-chain deposition disease	5
Neoplasm	4
Fibrillary glomerulonephritis	4
Cortical necrosis	2
Thin basement membrane nephropathy	2
Miscellaneous (nonglomerular)	6
Miscellaneous other glomerular lesions	15
No pathologic diagnosis (normal)	2
Nonspecific abnormalitites	33
Inadequate tissue for diagnosis	69
End-stage kidney	5
Total	745

Reprinted with permission from Falk RJ, Jennette JC. Glomerular disease in the elderly. In: Jacobson HR, Striker GE, Klahr S, eds. The Principles and Practice of Nephrology. St. Louis: Mosby, 1995:518–524.
[a]>80% crescents.
[b]Primary diagnosis.
[c]Including types I, II, and III.

can be divided into five syndromes: (*a*) acute glomerulonephritis (acute GN), (*b*) rapidly progressive glomerulonephritis (RPGN), (*c*) chronic glomerulonephritis (CGN), (*d*) nephrotic syndrome (NS), and (*e*) persistent urinary abnormalities with few or no symptoms.

Acute GN is characterized by a relatively abrupt onset of hematuria, proteinuria, hypertension, salt and water retention, diminished GFR, and occasionally oliguria. Frequently accompanying microbial infection, acute GN commonly recovers spontaneously. The classic example is postinfectious GN, a type of diffuse proliferative GN more commonly associated in the elderly with subclinical than clinically obvious infection. Therefore, in addition to evaluating the throat and skin for evidence of streptococcal infection, the workup should include evaluation for low-grade endovascular infections. Circulatory congestion and renal insufficiency are more common in the elderly than in the young, possibly as a result of impaired cardiopulmonary and renal reserve.

RPGN is characterized by a relatively insidious onset and progressive loss of renal function, often accompanied by oliguria. Spontaneous recovery is rare, and the temporal association with microbial infection is not a constant feature. The classic example is pauci-immune crescentic GN, the most common cause of aggressive GN in patients older than 65. Crescentic GN is discussed in more detail later.

CGN is a general term referring to progressive renal function impairment of insidious onset accompanied by varying degrees of hematuria, proteinuria, and hypertension. The course extends over decades, and toward the end it becomes difficult to say whether the cause of renal failure was glomerular, tubular, interstitial, or vascular.

NS is characterized by proteinuria exceeding 3.5 g per day accompanied by hypoalbuminemia and associated with varying degrees of hypertension, edema, hyperlipidemia, and lipiduria. Common causes of NS in the elderly include diabetes mellitus, membranous nephropathy, and minimal change disease (MCD). Some of the other less common causes include focal sclerosis, membranoproliferative GN, and paraproteinemias. Serologic studies for the evaluation of NS include antinuclear antibodies (ANA), C3, C4, hepatitis B and C blood studies, blood cultures, urine and serum protein electrophoresis, human immunodeficiency virus (HIV) serology (if applicable), and an initial search for malignancy. The most common types of NS in the elderly are likely to have a negative serologic profile. Therefore, renal biopsy plays an important role in diagnosis and treatment. In the hands of an experienced operator, the complication rate of renal biopsy under real-time ultrasound guidance is similar in old and young patients.

Asymptomatic hematuria and/or proteinuria (less than 3 g per day) occurs in the absence of any systemic abnormality such as hypertension, reduced renal function, hypoproteinemia, or edema. Hematuria, either gross or microscopic, may be recurrent or persistent and may occur in the absence of proteinuria. Hematuria may occur in up to 10% of asymptomatic men above age 50. Hematuria of glomerular origin is characterized by small, dysmorphic red blood cells accompanying proteinuria and red blood cell casts. Common nonglomerular causes of hematuria include stones, prostatitis, tumors of the urinary tract (kidney, prostate, bladder), and chronic or intermittent bladder catheterization. If lower urinary tract bleeding is suspected, a triple voided urine specimen may be helpful. Initial hematuria indicates a urethral source; terminal hematuria indicates a bladder source; and hematuria through the entire sequence indicates bleeding from the upper urinary tract. An important cause of isolated proteinuria in the elderly is multiple myeloma, in which light-chain proteinuria is often negative by dipstick, which detects albumin, but positive by the sulfosalicylic acid method.

Rapidly Progressive Glomerulonephritis

Based on immunohistologic and serologic criteria, RPGN or crescentic GN is divided into 3 groups, pauci-immune GN (described later), immune complex GN (e.g., systemic lupus erythematosus, infective endocarditis), and antiglomerular basement membrane antibody disease. Pauci-immune necrotizing GN is the predominant cause of RPGN in the elderly. More than 80% of these patients have antineutrophil cytoplasmic antibodies (ANCA) positive in the serum and evidence of small-vessel vasculitis (e.g., Wegener's granulomatosis or microscopic polyarteritis). In a retrospective study of patients diagnosed with Wegener's granulomatosis and stratified above or below age 60, the prevalence of upper respiratory tract involvement and hemoptysis at initial presentation was less common in elderly patients, although pulmonary infiltrates were commonly seen during the course of the disease in both groups (125). In the same series, renal insufficiency at the time of diagnosis was more common in the elderly, and the incidence of CNS involvement was 4.5 times as high in this group. Treatment of most forms of pauci-immune GN with corticosteroids and cyclophosphamide has been shown to reduce mortality. Since the elderly are especially prone to complications of these agents, frequent clinical and laboratory follow-up is essential. In a recent placebo-controlled trial, cotrimoxazole significantly reduced the incidence of relapses in patients with Wegener's granulomatosis (126).

Membranous Nephropathy

Membranous nephropathy is the most common cause of NS in the elderly. A unique feature of this condition is its association with malignancy in up to 20% of cases (127). The incidence of cancer in the elderly patient with membranous nephropathy is 5 times as high as in the general population (128). Lung, colon, and other cancers of the GI tract have been most commonly associated with this condition. Lymphomas and leukemias have also been associated, though less commonly. There are scattered reports of remission of NS after surgical removal of the cancer or treatment of lymphoma or leukemia. Proteinuria occurs simultaneously with or precedes malignancy in 80% of cases, and malignancy precedes proteinuria in about 20% of patients. Thus, a negative screen for malignancy at the time of presentation with NS does not exclude the possibility of detecting malignancy on follow-up. In general, an exhaustive search for an occult malignancy is not required. A good history and physical examination and basic hematology and chemistry profiles, recommended screening tests such as chest radiograph, mammography, flexible sigmoidoscopy, and stool evaluation for occult blood should be done. Any abnormalities in these screening tests should prompt a more aggressive search for an occult malignancy. These patients should be followed closely for 12 to 18 months to determine whether a malignancy becomes manifest.

Untreated idiopathic membranous GN is usually a slowly progressive disease, with intermittent clinical remissions and exacerbations of NS

(129). Poor prognostic factors associated with development of progressive renal failure include male sex, old age at onset, severe proteinuria (less than 10 g per day), poorly controlled hypertension, severe hypercholesterolemia, reduced GFR at onset, and renal biopsy showing advanced disease (130). Adults with non-nephrotic-range proteinuria have a favorable prognosis, with a 10-year renal survival rate of 85 to 95%. Therefore, specific treatment in this group of patients is not recommended (131). ACE inhibitors are useful for control of hypertension as well as reduction of proteinuria. Adults with NS, normal renal function, and proteinuria less than 10 g per day should be managed conservatively with ACE inhibitors and observed for either spontaneous remission or progression (130). Patients with persistent, severe proteinuria (more than 10 g per day), symptomatic NS, or progressive renal failure are best treated with a combination of oral cyclophosphamide and glucocorticoids or sequential chlorambucil and glucocorticoids (130). Patients with advanced chronic renal failure (serum creatinine less than 3 to 4 mg/dL) are best managed by conservative means and optimal control of hypertension with ACE inhibitors.

Minimal Change Disease

MCD, a frequent cause of NS in elderly patients, is characterized by abrupt onset of heavy proteinuria, hypoalbuminemia, and hyperlipidemia. Unlike children with MCD, the elderly frequently have systolic hypertension probably unrelated to the underlying glomerular disease. Distinctive features of MCD in adults include occasional presentation with acute renal failure and an association with lymphoproliferative disorders. Some authors (124) propose that acute renal failure results from a sudden decrease in vascular filling pressures as a consequence of massive proteinuria and hypoalbuminemia. This process overwhelms the kidney's ability to autoregulate, especially when it is already compromised by arteriosclerosis. Patients treated with corticosteroids and diuretics usually recover function, but some require several weeks of dialysis before recovery. The most commonly associated neoplasm is Hodgkin's disease. Other neoplastic processes identified with MCD are non-Hodgkin's lymphoma; tumors of the uroepithelium, pancreas, prostate, colon, lung, and kidney; oncocytomas; and mesotheliomas.

Corticosteroids are the treatment of choice for MCD in all age groups, with remission of NS achieved in approximately 80% of adults. In general, it takes longer to achieve remission in adults than in children. In a study of the treatment of MCD in adults, 60% achieved remission within 8 weeks and 73% within 16 weeks of corticosteroid therapy (132). Relapses are common and should be treated with corticosteroids. In some studies alternate-day steroid therapy has been shown to be as effective as daily dosing (133) while reducing steroid toxicity. Once remission is achieved, corticosteroids should be tapered over 2 to 3 months. If a relapse occurs during tapering, the dose should be immediately increased to the level at which the remission occurred. For patients who are resistant to steroids, relapse frequently, or are steroid dependent, cyclophosphamide for 8 to 12 weeks is a reasonable alternative, and elderly patients may tolerate it better. Cyclosporin has also been used in cyclophosphamide-resistant patients.

Multiple Myeloma

Multiple myeloma typically occurs in the elderly, with a mean age of onset of 68 years. Patients frequently present with back and rib pain aggravated by movement; increased susceptibility to infections, including pneumonia and pyelonephritis; renal failure; anemia; hypercalcemia; and occasionally manifestations of the hyperviscosity syndrome.

The renal presentation may be acute renal failure or chronic progressive renal insufficiency. Evidence of tubular damage due to light-chain excretion is almost always present. The earliest manifestation of tubular damage is the adult Fanconi syndrome (type 2, proximal renal tubular acidosis) with loss of glucose and amino acids in the urine and defects in the ability of the kidney to acidify urine. Renal failure is often multifactorial, including cast nephropathy, volume depletion, hypercalcemia, nephrocalcinosis, and uric acid nephropathy. The majority of patients have large amounts of Bence Jones proteinuria,

which tests negative for protein by dipstick but positive by the sulfosalicylic acid test. Less commonly the glomerulus is involved by AL amyloid deposition, monoclonal immunoglobulin deposition, or immune complex disease, which manifests as heavy nonselective proteinuria, including light chains and albumin. The serum anion gap is often reduced because the circulating light chains are cationic. Serum and urine protein electrophoresis are useful diagnostic tests.

Treatment includes management of hypercalcemia, maintenance of euvolemia, chemotherapy, and treatment of infection. Parenteral radiocontrast agents should be avoided in view of an increased risk of contrast-induced acute renal failure.

Primary Amyloidosis

Primary amyloidosis, another disease predominantly affecting the adult and elderly population, involves tissue infiltration by the amino terminal portion of the variable region of the immunoglobulin light chains (AL) produced by abnormal plasma cells. Major clinical manifestations include nephrotic syndrome, restrictive cardiomyopathy, orthostatic hypotension due to autonomic neuropathy, peripheral neuropathy, chronic liver disease, and purpuric skin lesions. Differentiation from multiple myeloma, a more common plasma cell disorder, may be difficult, but less than 25% plasma cells in bone marrow, smaller amounts of monoclonal protein in serum or urine, and absence of associated anemia, hypercalcemia, or lytic bone lesions suggest amyloidosis rather than myeloma.

The kidney is affected in 50% of patients with NS as the predominant presentation. Most patients have nonselective proteinuria, including plasma proteins and lambda light chains. Hypercholesterolemia is less frequent than in other forms of NS. Median survival in patients with symptomatic cardiac involvement is 6 months, whereas predominant renal involvement is associated with a median survival of 21 months (134). Survival in patients with urinary kappa light chains is superior to that in patients with lambda light chains (135). Therapeutic modalities include melphalan, prednisone, and colchicine, but response to therapy in most cases is less than desirable. Preliminary results from treatment of selected patients with high-dose melphalan and prednisone in conjunction with stem cell rescue are somewhat more encouraging (134). Only 18% of patients with primary amyloidosis undergo dialysis for chronic renal failure, with a median survival on dialysis of 8.2 months (136).

Diabetic Nephropathy

Diabetic nephropathy is a clinical syndrome characterized by persistent proteinuria (more than 150 mg in 24 hours), progressive decline in GFR, and hypertension. In the United States diabetic nephropathy is the leading cause of ESRD. The various risk factors for development of diabetic nephropathy in patients with non-insulin-dependent diabetes mellitus (NIDDM) include microalbuminuria (urinary albumin excretion 30 to 300 mg in 24 hours) (137), male sex (138), family history (139), ethnicity (Native Americans more than African Americans; African Americans more than Mexican Americans; Mexican Americans more than Asian Indians; Asian Indians more than European white patients) (140) and poor glycemic control (141). When compared with diabetic patients without microalbuminuria, the risk ratio of developing diabetic nephropathy ranges from 4.4 to 21 (median 8.5) in patients with NIDDM and microalbuminuria (142). Urinary albumin excretion increases by approximately 20% annually in NIDDM patients with persistent microalbuminuria (143). The prevalence of microalbuminuria and macroalbuminuria in NIDDM is about 30% and 35% respectively (142). Once overt nephropathy is established, the mean rate of decline in GFR is approximately 5.7 mL per minute per year, though some patients decline at as much as 22 mL per minute per year (144).

While there is a definite role of tight metabolic control in slowing the progression from normoalbuminuria to microalbuminuria in patients with insulin-dependent diabetes mellitus (IDDM), no similar data are available for NIDDM. Similarly, large-scale trials studying the effect of tight glycemic control on progression from microalbuminuria to overt nephropathy in patients with NIDDM are ongoing. However, ACE inhibitors have been shown to slow the pro-

gression from the stage of microalbuminuria to overt nephropathy in patients with NIDDM (143). Treatment of overt nephropathy should focus on the control of hypertension and reduction of proteinuria with ACE inhibitors, with the addition of other antihypertensive agents if necessary to keep blood pressure in the normal range.

About 60% of NIDDM patients with proteinuria have a diabetic retinopathy (145). Blindness resulting from proliferative diabetic retinopathy or maculopathy is 5 times as common in diabetic patients with proteinuria as in their normoalbuminuric counterparts (145). Peripheral neuropathy is present in most patients with advanced nephropathy. Macrovascular disease, including stroke, carotid artery stenosis, coronary artery disease, and peripheral vascular disease, is 2 to 5 times as common in nephropathic patients as in normoalbuminuric patients (145). There is a notably increased frequency of nondiabetic glomerular disease in NIDDM patients, including acute endocapillary proliferative GN, membranous GN, crescentic GN, MCD, amyloidosis, and ischemic nephropathy (146). Therefore, the appearance in NIDDM patients of impaired renal function and an abnormal urine sediment in the absence of a diabetic retinopathy should raise suspicion of nondiabetic glomerular disease.

As renal insufficiency progresses, the insulin dose required to maintain optimal glycemic control usually falls. Hyperkalemia at relatively low serum creatinine levels, which is usually related to hyporeninemic hypoaldosteronism in these patients, may be exacerbated by medication such as ACE inhibitors, potassium-sparing diuretics, and β-blockers. In most cases it is controlled with a loop diuretic such as furosemide. Management of ESRD with dialysis or transplantation is discussed in a subsequent section.

INTERSTITIAL NEPHRITIS

Aging is associated with histologic and physiologic changes in the renal interstitium, collectively labeled tubulointerstitial nephropathy of the elderly. However, beyond these changes, elderly people are susceptible to a number of types of interstitial injury broadly classified as either acute interstitial nephritis (AIN) or chronic interstitial nephritis (CIN).

Acute Interstitial Nephritis

AIN is described in 1 to 15% of renal biopsies in different centers (147, 148). The hallmark of this condition is inflammatory cells (mainly T cells and monocytes) in the interstitium, sparing the glomeruli. While lesions associated with renal dysfunction are usually diffuse, drug-induced interstitial nephritis is often patchy, involving the deeper cortical layers. The infiltrate and the interstitial edema separate the tubules from their usual contiguous configuration. In severe cases the tubular basement membrane may be disrupted.

AIN is classified as drug related, infection related, or idiopathic. Drugs commonly implicated include penicillins, sulfonamides, NSAIDs, cephalosporins, rifampicin, Dilantin, furosemide, and thiazide diuretics. Clinical features of drug-induced AIN, including rash, fever, and eosinophilia, are typically seen with penicillinlike drugs but are uncommon with NSAIDs. Urinalysis reveals subnephrotic-range proteinuria, hematuria (sometimes gross), eosinophiluria, and white blood cell casts. However, none of these features is specific for drug-induced AIN. NSAIDs may cause minimal-change nephrotic syndrome in association with AIN (149). Renal failure occurs variably after days or weeks of taking the drug. In most patients it follows the course of a typical immune response, peaking at 2 weeks or so. A common clinical occurrence is a febrile patient who defervesces in response to antibiotic treatment and whose fever recurs several days later. However, renal failure may occur over months, as in diuretic-induced AIN (150). A history of allergy to the drug is only rarely obtained. Infection-related AIN is most commonly seen in the setting of acute pyelonephritis. However, AIN and renal failure may also accompany systemic infections as a response to the infection rather than to seeding of the kidney by the infection. Idiopathic AIN is less common than the other two categories and is frequently associated with antitubular basement membrane antibodies. Fever is common, but rash and eosinophilia are rare.

In general, the first step in the treatment of drug-induced AIN is identification and removal of the offending agent. Unless this is done, progression to ESRD is likely. In some patients removal of the offending agent is followed by improvement of renal function within days. The likelihood of complete recovery is inversely proportional to the duration of renal failure. In patients with idiopathic AIN, spontaneous resolution may occur, but more than 50% of patients have residual renal dysfunction. The second step in the treatment of AIN is undertaken if no spontaneous recovery of renal function occurs within days of removal of the offending agent. Although well-randomized and controlled trials documenting the efficacy of steroids in AIN are lacking, some nephrologists recommend using 1 mg/kg per day of prednisone in the absence of infection (151). If renal function improves within 2 weeks, the drug should be continued at lower doses for another 2 to 4 weeks. If no improvement occurs, cyclophosphamide 2 mg/kg per day may be added, and if it is effective, continued for 1 year. If neither steroids nor cyclophosphamide is effective within 6 weeks, both should be withdrawn. As with steroids, well-controlled trials establishing the efficacy of cyclophosphamide in this clinical setting are lacking.

Chronic Interstitial Nephritis

The pathologic hallmark of CIN is dilated, atrophic tubules, interstitial fibrosis, and cellular infiltrates, primarily lymphocytes, in the interstitium. While the glomeruli may be normal in the initial stages, segmental sclerosis, periglomerular fibrosis, and ultimately global sclerosis may develop as CIN progresses. The causes of CIN include drugs (analgesics, lithium, cyclosporin, cisplatin), metabolic disorders (diabetes mellitus, hypercalcemia, hyperuricemia), immunologic disorders (vasculitis, transplant rejection, Wegener's granulomatosis), hematologic disorders (multiple myeloma, lymphoma), urinary tract obstruction, hereditary diseases (autosomal dominant polycystic kidney disease), and infections. Most patients have symptoms of the primary disease. The rest have nonspecific symptoms of renal failure, including weakness, malaise, nausea, nocturia, and altered sleep pattern, or are incidentally noted to have an abnormal urinalysis or serum creatinine. Other laboratory features include the presence of nonnephrotic-range proteinuria, microscopic hematuria, pyuria, glycosuria, acidifying defects (proximal or distal renal tubular acidosis), and concentrating defects. Serum uric acid levels are usually low for the degree of renal failure because of defects in the reabsorption of uric acid. More than 50% of patients have hypertension. Anemia occurs early in the course of renal failure, since erythropoietin is produced in the interstitium. Treatment of CIN generally entails treatment of the underlying cause. If the patient presents with advanced renal insufficiency or has a systemic disorder with no specific treatment, renal biopsy may not be indicated, since it does not influence therapy.

Of the causes listed here, the ones of major interest in the elderly include multiple myeloma, hypercalcemic nephropathy, and obstructive uropathy. Hypercalcemia, which is often related to malignancy in this age group, causes renal dysfunction due to renal vasoconstriction, decrease in glomerular ultrafiltration coefficient, and volume contraction due to nephrogenic diabetes insipidus. In prolonged hypercalcemia, nephrocalcinosis may arise from deposition of calcium around the tubular basement membranes, initially in the medullary tubules, then in the cortical proximal and distal tubules, and finally in the interstitial space.

Obstructive uropathy is a common cause of CIN and renal failure in the elderly. Benign prostatic hypertrophy is the most frequent cause in elderly men. Symptoms of bladder outlet obstruction occur in 75% of men over age 50. Malignant neoplasms such as prostate and bladder cancers and metastatic involvement of the ureters or pelvic nodes also cause urinary tract obstruction in this age group. Other nonmalignant causes include uterine prolapse, large-bowel diverticulitis involving the left ureter, abdominal aortic aneurysm causing retroperitoneal fibrosis, and direct pressure from an aneurysm. Diagnosis of bladder outlet obstruction is suggested if the bladder is palpable or percussible above the symphysis pubis. Renal and bladder ultrasound examination establishes the diagnosis by demonstrating hydronephrosis and determines the bladder residual volume after voiding. Complete or partial obstruction results in a decline in GFR,

decreased reabsorption of solutes, impaired tubular secretion of H^+ and K^+, and nephrogenic diabetes insipidus. Treatment of obstructive uropathy includes treatment of the underlying condition and relief of the obstruction.

RENAL REPLACEMENT THERAPY IN THE ELDERLY

According to the United States Renal Data System, the overall prevalence of ESRD is increasing by approximately 7 to 8% every year (152). The increase is greatest among the elderly, and by the year 2000, 50 to 60% of patients with ESRD are predicted to be above age 65. The two most common causes of ESRD among the elderly are diabetes mellitus and hypertensive nephrosclerosis; each accounts for 34% (152). Among elderly patients on renal replacement therapy in the United States, 82.4% are on in-center hemodialysis, 0.7% are on home hemodialysis, 9.7% are on chronic peritoneal dialysis, and 5.8% have a functioning transplant. In 1.3% of patients, modality of treatment was not available (152).

Hemodialysis

Hemodialysis is the primary treatment modality of ESRD patients in the United States. The overall 1- and 5-year survival of ESRD patients aged 65 or older in the United States is 73.2% and 26.5% respectively. The most common complications in elderly patients with ESRD on chronic hemodialysis include hypotension, GI bleeding, malnutrition, infections, and dialysis-related amyloidosis (153). Hypotension during dialysis is most commonly caused by major fluid shifts from the intravascular space. Other major contributing factors include diminished cardiac reserve due to concomitant heart disease and the use of antihypertensives with vasodilatory or negative inotropic effects that reduce the ability of the patient to compensate for changes in the intravascular volume. GI bleeding in these patients is frequently due to gastritis, diverticular disease, angiodysplasia, or malignancy, and the risk is increased by the concomitant use of NSAIDs. If the bleeding time is prolonged and bleeding does not subside upon use of specific measures for each condition (e.g., H_2-blockers, stopping NSAIDs), desmopressin (DDAVP) 0.3 µg/kg intravenously or conjugated estrogens 0.6 mg/kg intravenously daily for 4 to 5 days may be used.

Malnutrition is common in elderly ESRD patients. The mortality rate of patients with serum albumin concentrations between 3.5 and 4 mg/dL is twice that of patients with serum albumen above 4 mg/dL. A diet providing at least 35 kcal/kg per day and 1 g/kg per day protein is recommended for patients on hemodialysis. After myocardial infarction, septicemia is the second most common cause of death in this patient population. Common portals of entry include the lungs, vascular access, and GI and genitourinary tracts. Sepsis from vascular access is commonly staphylococcal, whereas gram-negative organisms predominate in the genitourinary tract. β_2-Microglobulin amyloidosis develops in patients on long-term hemodialysis and manifests as bony cysts, carpal tunnel syndrome, and less commonly, GI hemorrhage. β_2-Microglobulin is a normal component of the major histocompatibility complex that is normally degraded by the kidneys but is inadequately cleared by hemodialysis. No specific treatment is available for this condition. Some studies suggest a lower incidence of this condition with synthetic dialysis membranes than with conventional cellulose membranes (154).

Chronic Peritoneal Dialysis

Chronic peritoneal dialysis (CPD) uses the peritoneal membrane for diffusion of uremic waste products and excess water. Dialysis fluid is instilled and drained cyclically. In continuous ambulatory peritoneal dialysis (CAPD), the exchanges are done manually throughout the day, usually 4 to 6 times, whereas in continuous cyclic peritoneal dialysis (CCPD), an automated device is used to cycle the exchanges over 6 to 12 hours overnight. The most frequent cause of hospitalization is peritonitis. Other common complications include catheter blockage, inguinal hernia, fluid leakage, vascular ischemia, hypotension, and congestive heart failure.

The main advantage of CPD over hemodialysis is that the patient retains independence by performing dialysis at home. Patients with reduced cardiovascular reserve tolerate CPD better than hemodialysis because of its reduced tendency to cause hypotension. Disequilibrium syndrome is avoided, since urea is removed more gradually, and loss of residual renal function is slower than with hemodialysis. As a result of losing up to 25 g of protein in the dialysate per day, CPD patients must eat about 100 g of dietary protein per day to avoid malnutrition. These patients also tend to maintain a higher hematocrit. The major advantages of hemodialysis over CPD is in patients who are unable to perform their own dialysis. In general, patients with inadequate social support and cognitive impairment are not appropriate candidates for CPD. This form of therapy is ideal when a family member or friend can be actively involved in the therapy of the elderly patient. The major disadvantage of CPD is a high dropout rate after episodes of peritonitis. Neither dialysis modality has a clearly demonstrated superior survival rate. An Italian multicenter study (155) suggested better survival on CAPD for patients older than 53.5 years, but data from the United States (156) indicate worse survival among older diabetics on CAPD. The Canadian Renal Failure Registry (157) showed no difference in the survival of elderly patients on hemodialysis versus CPD, although CPD had a higher rate of technique failure. For unclear reasons, the survival of elderly patients (age over 65 years) on CPD at 18 months in Canada is greater than in the United States (82% versus 61.1%) (158).

Renal Transplantation

As mentioned earlier, only 5.8% of the elderly ESRD patient population has a functioning renal allograft. The lower prevalence of transplantation in the elderly is largely because of a general preference of younger people for this form of therapy and the perception of increased risks of transplantation in the elderly. This view is gradually changing, since allograft and survival have improved with the introduction of cyclosporin. In the precyclosporin era, patient and graft survival in the elderly population 1 year post transplant (70% and 58% respectively) was clearly inferior to the results in the cyclosporin era (81% and 72% respectively) (153). The two most common causes of graft failure among elderly patients in the cyclosporin era are death with a functional graft and graft rejection. The major causes of mortality within the first 3 months of transplantation are cardiovascular disease and pulmonary infection. Older transplant patients require less immunosuppression, and there is a tendency in the cyclosporin era in some centers to reduce the dose of steroids significantly and even progressively eliminate them from the immunosuppressive regimen, thereby reducing the adverse effects of steroid therapy. Elderly patients are less likely to develop acute allograft rejection than younger patients.

The critical question often posed to the clinician is whether or not to consider an elderly patient for transplantation. A recent study (159) did not find any significant difference in 5-year patient and allograft survival between 24 cadaveric renal transplant recipients aged 65 to 74 years and 404 concurrent first cadaver kidney transplant recipients aged 20 to 44 years (86% versus 92% and 77% versus 63% respectively). To obtain comparable results, it is important to be careful in choosing elderly patients for renal transplantation. In general, primary cadaveric transplantation can be performed in patients older than age 65 if they pass through a selection algorithm that excludes active infection, active malignancy, unsuitable anatomy for technical success, high probability of operative mortality, and noncompliance. However, as transplantation in the elderly becomes more prevalent, it raises an ethical issue, as it exacerbates the shortage of cadaveric kidneys. To offset this, some centers have begun using cadaveric kidneys from elderly donors. While some studies show that survival of old-donor kidneys is inferior to that of young-adult-donor kidneys (153), one recent study (160) concluded that long-term patient and graft survival may be achieved by transplanting these organs. Other authors have transplanted both kidneys from elderly donors into a single recipient with excellent 1-year survival (161). This approach should have further evaluation.

In summary, renal transplantation is a viable option for therapy in a select subset of the elderly ESRD population, and the percentage of elderly patients with a functional renal transplant is likely to increase in the future.

REFERENCES

1. Darmady EM, Offer J, Woodhouse MA. The parameters of the aging kidney. J Pathol 1973;109:195–207.
2. Ljungqvist A, Lagergren C. Normal intra-renal arterial patterns in adult and aging human kidney. J Anat 1962; 26:285.
3. Reynes M, Coulet T, Diebold J Jr. Microvascularization of normal and aging kidney. Pathol Biol 1968;16:1081.
4. Takazakura E, Wasabu N, Handa A, et al. Intrarenal vascular changes with age and disease. Kidney Int 1972; 2:224–236.
5. Hollenberg NK, Adams DF, Solomon HS, et al. Senescence and the renal vasculature in normal men. Circ Res 1974;34:309–316.
6. Baert L, Steg A. Is the diverticulum of the distal and collecting tubules a preliminary stage of the simple cyst in the adult? J Urol 1977;118:707–710.
7. Kappel B, Olsen S. Cortical interstitial tissue and sclerosed glomeruli in the normal human kidney, related to age and sex. A quantitative study. Virchows Arch [Pathol Anat] 1980;387:271–277.
8. Aschinberg LC, Koskimies O, Bernstein J, et al. The influence of age on the response to renal parenchymal loss. Yale J Biol Med 1978;51:341–345.
9. McLachlan M, Wasserman P. Changes in size and distensibility of the aging kidney. Br J Radiol 1981;54:488–491.
10. Dunnill MS, Halley W. Some observations on the quantitative anatomy of the kidney. J Pathol 1973;110:113–121.
11. Gourtsoyiannis N, Prassopoulos P, Cavouras D, Pantelidis N. The thickness of the renal parenchyma decreases with age: a CT study of 360 patients. AJR Am J Roentgenol 1990;155:541–544.
12. Steffes MW, Barbosa J, Basgen JM, et al. Quantitative glomerular morphology of the human kidney. Lab Invest 1983;49:82–86.
13. Goyal VK. Changes with age in the human kidney. Exp Gerontol 1982;17:321–331.
14. Kaplan C, Pasternack B, Shah H, Gallo G. Age related incidence of sclerotic glomeruli in human kidneys. Am J Pathol 1975;80:227–234.
15. Rowe JW, Andres R, Tobin JD, et al. The effect of age on creatinine clearance in man: a cross sectional and longitudinal study. J Gerontol 1976;31:155–163.
16. Davies DF, Shock NW. Age changes in the glomerular filtration rate, effective renal plasma flow and tubular excreting capacity in adult males. J Clin Invest 1950;29: 496.
17. Olbrich O, Ferguson MH, Robson JS, Stewart CP. Renal function in aged subjects. Edinburgh Med J 1950;57: 117.
18. Papper S. The effects of age in reducing renal function. Geriatrics 1973;28:83–87.
19. Hosoya T, Tushima R, Icida K, et al. Changes in renal function with aging among Japanese. Intern Med 1995;34:520–527.
20. Lindeman RD, Tobin J, Shock NW. Longitudinal stud-

ies on the rate of decline in renal function with age. J Am Geriatr Soc 1985;33:278–285.

21. Cockcroft DW, Gault MH. Prediction of creatinine clearance from serum creatinine. Nephron 1976;16:31–41.

22. Anderson S, Brenner BM. Effects of aging on the renal glomerulus. Am J Med 1986;80:435–442.

23. Brenner BM, Meyer TW, Hostetter TH. Dietary protein intake and the progressive nature of kidney disease. N Engl J Med 1982;307:652–660.

24. Neuringer JR, Brenner BM. Hemodynamic theory of progressive renal disease: a 10 year update in brief review. Am J Kidney Dis 1993;22:98–104.

25. Anderson S, Rennke HG, Zatz R. Glomerular adaptations with normal aging and with long-term converting enzyme inhibition in rats. Am J Physiol 1994;267: F35–F43.

26. Heudes D, Michel O, Chevalier J, et al. Effect of chronic ANG I-converting enzyme inhibition on aging processes. I. Kidney structure and function. Am J Physiol 1994;266:R1038–R1059.

27. Li YM, Steffes M, Donnelly T, et al. Prevention of cardiovascular and renal pathology of aging by advanced glycation inhibitor aminoguanidine. Proc Nat Acad Sci U S A 1996;93:3902–3907.

28. Miller JH, MacDonald RK, Shock NW. Age changes in the maximal rate of renal tubular reabsorption of glucose. J Gerontol 1952;7:196–200.

29. Kinsella JL, Sacktor B. Renal brush-border NA$^+$-H$^+$ exchange activity in the aging rat. Am J Physiol 1987; 252:R681–R686.

30. Beuchene RE, Fanestil DD, Barrows CH Jr. The effect of age on active transport and Na-K activated ATPase activity in renal tissue of rats. J Gerontol 1965;20:306–310.

31. Burich RJ. Effects of age on renal function and enzyme activity in male C57 B46 mice. J Gerontol 1975;30:539–545.

32. Adler, Lindeman RD, Yiengst MJ, et al. Effect of acute acid loading on urinary acid excretion by the aging human kidney. J Lab Clin Med 1968;72:278–289.

33. Agarwal BN, Cabebe RG. Renal acidification in elderly subjects. Nephron 1980;26:291–295.

34. Frassetto Z, Sebastian A. Age and systemic acid-base equilibrium: analysis of published data. J Gerontol 1996;51:B91–B99.

35. Weidmann P, De Myttenaere-Bursztein S, Maxwell MH, de Lima J. Effects of aging on plasma renin and aldosterone in normal man. Kidney Int 1975;8:325–333.

36. Ohashi M, Fujio N, Nawata H, et al. High plasma concentration of human atrial natriuretic polypeptide in aged men. J Clin Endocrinol Metab 1987;64:81–85.

37. Haller BG, Zust H, Shaw S, et al. Effects of posture and aging on circulating atrial natriuretic peptide levels in man. Hypertension 1987;5:551–556.

38. Clark BA, Elahi D, Epstein FH. The influence of gender, age and the menstrual cycle on atrial natriuretic peptide levels in man. J Clin Endocrinol Metab 1990;70:349–352.

39. Kuhlik A, Elahi D, Epstein FH, Clark BA. Decline in urinary excretion of dopamine and PGE2 with age. Geriatr Nephrol Urol 1995;5:79–83.

40. Armando I, Nowicki S, Aguirre J, Barontini M. A decreased tubular uptake of dopa results in defective renal dopamine production in aged rats. Am J Physiol 1995;268:F1087–F1092.

41. Rathaus M, Greenfeld Z, Podjarny E, et al. Altered prostaglandin synthesis and impaired sodium conservation in the kidneys of old rats. Clin Sci 1992;83: 301–306.

42. Zeigler MJ, Lake CR, Kopin JJ. Plasma noradrenaline increases with age. Nature 1976;261:333–336.

43. Bursztyn M, Bresnahan M, Gavras I, Gavras H. Effect of aging on vasopressor, catecholamines and alpha2-adrenergic receptors. J Am Geriatr Soc 1990;38:628–632.

44. Galbusera M, Garattini S, Remuzzi G, Mennini T. Catecholamine receptor binding in rat kidney: effect of aging. Kidney Int 1988;33:1073–1077.

45. Epstein M, Hollenberg NK. Age as a determinant of renal sodium conservation in normal man. J Lab Clin Med 1976;87:411–417.

46. Shannon RP, Wei JY, Rosa RM, et al. The effect of age and sodium depletion on cardiovascular response to orthostasis. Hypertension 1986;8:438–443.

47. Elliott P, Stamler J, Nichols R, et al. Intersalt revisited: further analysis of 24 hour sodium excretion and blood pressure within and across populations. BMJ 1996;312: 1248–1253.

48. Mulkerrin EC, Clark BA, Epstein FH. Increased salt retention and hypertension from non-steroidal agents in the elderly. Q J Med 1997;90:411–415.

49. Finnerty FA Jr. Hypertension in the elderly. Postgrad Med 1979;65:119–125.

50. Luft FC, Weinberger MH, Fineberg NS, et al. Effects of age on renal sodium homeostasis and its relevance to sodium sensitivity. Am J Med 1987;82:9–15.

51. Luft FC, Fineberg NS, Weinberger MH. The influence of age on renal function and renin and aldosterone responses to sodium-volume expansion and contraction in normotensive and mildly hypertensive humans. Am J Hypertens 1992;5:520–528.

52. Krakoff LR, Goodwin FJ, Baer L, et al. The role of renin in the exaggerated natriuresis of hypertension. Circulation 1970;42:335–345.

53. Mulkerrin E, Epstein FH, Clark BA. Reduced renal response to low dose dopamine infusion in the elderly. J Gerontol 1995;50:M271–M275.

54. Clark BA, Elahi D, Shannon RP, et al. Influence of age and dose on the end-organ responses to atrial natriuretic peptide in humans. Am J Hypertens 1991;4:500–507.

55. Mulkerrin EC, Brain A, Hampton D, et al. Reduced renal hemodynamic response to atrial natriuretic peptide in elderly volunteers. Am J Kidney Dis 1993;22:538–544.

56. Campo C, Lahera V, Garcia-Robles R, et al. Aging abolishes the renal response to L-arginine in essential hypertension. Kidney Int 1996;55:S126–S128.

57. Oberbauer R, Krivanek P, Turnheim K. Pharmacokinetics and pharmaco-dynamics of the diuretic bumetanide in the elderly. Clin Pharmacol Ther 1995;57:42–51.

58. Clark BA, Brown RS, Epstein FH. Effect of atrial natriuretic peptide on potassium-stimulated aldosterone secretion: potential relevance to hypoaldosteronism in man. J Clin Endocrinol Metab 1992;75:399–403.

59. Davis KM, Fish LC, Elahi D, et al. Atrial natriuretic peptide levels in the prediction of congestive failure risk in frail elderly. JAMA 1992;267:2625–2629.

60. Noth RH, Lassman N, Tan SY, et al. Age and the renin-aldosterone system. Arch Intern Med 1977;137:1414–1417.

61. Mulkerrin E, Epstein FH, Clark BA. Aldosterone responses to hyperkalemia in healthy elderly humans. J Am Soc Nephrol 1995;6:1459–1466.

62. Jung FF, Kennefick TM, Ingelfinger JR, et al. Down-regulation of the intrarenal renin-angiotensin system in the aging rat. J Am Soc Nephrol 1995;5:1573–1580.

63. Corman B, Barrault MB, Klinger C, et al. Renin gene expression in the aging kidney: effect of sodium restriction. Mech Ageing Dev 1995;84:1–13.

64. Belmin J, Levy BI, Michel JB. Changes in the renin-angiotensin-aldosterone axis in later life. Drugs Aging 1994;5:391–400.

65. Shannon RP, Minaker KL, Rowe JW. Aging and water balance in humans. Semin Nephrol 1984;4:346–353.

66. Rowe JW, Shock NW, DeFronzo RA. The influence of age on the renal response to water deprivation in man. Nephron 1976;17:270–278.

67. Miller JH, Shock NW. Age difference in the renal response to antidiuretic hormone. J Gerontol 1953;8:446–448.

68. Hilderman JH, Vestal RE, Rowe JW, et al. The response of arginine vasopressin to intravenous ethanol and hypertonic saline in man: the impact of aging. J Gerontol 1978;33:39–47.

69. Rowe JW, Minaker KL, Sparrow D, Robertson GL. Age-related failure of volume-pressure-mediated vasopressin release. J Clin Endocrinol Metab 1982;54:661–664.

70. Chiodera P, Capretti L, Marchesi M, et al. Abnormal arginine vasopressin response to cigarette smoking and metoclopramide (but not to insulin induced hypoglycemia) in elderly subjects. J Gerontol 1991;46:M6–M10.

71. Clark BA, Shannon RP, Rosa RM, Epstein FH. Increased susceptibility to thiazide induced hyponatremia in the elderly. J Am Soc Nephrol 1994;5:1106–1111.

72. Anderson RJ, Berl T, McDonald KM, Schrier RW. Prostaglandins: effects on blood pressure, renal blood flow, sodium and water excretion. Kidney Int 1976;10:205–215.

73. Phillips PA, Rolls BY, Ledingham JG, et al. Reduced thirst after water deprivation in healthy elderly men. N Engl J Med 1984;311:753–759.

74. Mahowald JM, Himmelstein DW. Hypernatremia in the elderly: relation to infection and mortality. J Am Geriatr Soc 1980;24:177.

75. Himmelstein DW. Hypernatremia in nursing home patients: an indication of neglect. J Am Geriatr Soc 1983;31:466.

76. Lye M. Electrolyte disorders in the elderly. Clin Endocrinol Metab 1984;13:377.

77. Sunderam SG, Mankikar GD. Hypernatremia in the elderly. Age Aging 1983;12:77–80.

78. Miller M. Fluid and electrolyte balance in the elderly. Geriatrics 1987;42:65.

79. Kleinfield M, Casimir M, Bora S. Hyponatremia as observed in a chronic disease facility. J Am Geriatr Soc 1979;27:156–161.

80. Hachman I, Cabili S, Peer G. Hyponatremia in internal medicine ward patients: causes, treatment and prognosis. Isr J Med Sci 1989;25:73–76.

81. Miller M, Hecker MS, Friedlander DA, Carter JM. Apparent idiopathic hyponatremia in an ambulatory geriatric population. J Am Geriatr Soc 1996;44:404–408.

82. Tierney WM, Martin DK, Greenlee MC, et al. The prognosis of hyponatremia at hospital admission. J Gen Intern Med 1986;1:380–385.

83. Booker JA. Severe symptomatic hyponatremia in elderly outpatients: the role of thiazide therapy and stress. J Am Geriatr Soc 1984;32:108–113.

84. Fichman MP, Vorherr H, Kleeman CR, Telfer N. Diuretic induced hyponatremia. Adv Nephrol 1984;13:1–28.

85. Sterns RH, Capuccio JD, Silver SM, Cohen ED. Neurologic sequelae after treatment of severe hyponatremia: a multicentric perspective. J Am Soc Nephrol 1994;4:1522–1530.

86. DeFronzo RA. Hyperkalemia and hyporeninemic hypoaldosteronism. Kidney Int 1980;17:118–134.

87. Kokko JP. Primary acquired hypoaldosteronism. Kidney Int 1985;27:690–702.

88. Clark BA, Brown RS. Potassium homeostasis and hyperkalemic syndromes. Endocrinol Metab Clin North Am 1995;24:573–591.

89. Ford GA, Blaschke TF, Wiswell R, Hoffman BB. Effect of aging in changes in plasma potassium during exercise. J Gerontol 1993;48:M140–M145.

90. Fillit H, Rowe JW. The aging kidney. In: Brocklehurst JC, Tallis RC, Fillit HM, eds. Textbook of Geriatrics and Gerontology. London: Churchill Livingstone, 1992:612–628.

91. Pascual J, Liano F, Ortuno J. The elderly patient with acute renal failure. J Am Soc Nephrol 1995;6:144–153.

92. Brezis M, Epstein FH. A closer look at radiocontrast-induced nephropathy. N Engl J Med 1979;320:179–181.

93. Brezis M, Rosen S, Epstein FH. The pathophysiological implications of medullary hypoxia. Am J Kidney Dis 1989;13:253–258.

94. Prasad PV, Edelman RR, Clark BA, Epstein FH. Age related differences in medullary PO2 during water diuresis as determined by Bold MRI. J Am Soc Nephrol 1996;7:1832 (abstract).

95. Kumar R, Hill CM, McGeown MG. Acute renal failure in the elderly. Lancet 1973;1:90–91.

96. Rodgers H, Staniland JR, Lipkin GW, Turney JH. Acute renal failure: a study of elderly patients. Age Aging 1990;19:36–42.

97. Rimmer JM, Gennari FJ. Atherosclerotic renovascular disease and progressive renal failure. Ann Intern Med 1993;118:712–719.

98. Holley KE, Hunt JC, Brown AL, et al. Renal artery stenosis: a clinical-pathologic study in normotensive and hypertensive patients. Am J Med 1964;37:14–22.

99. Choudhri AH, Cleland JG, Rowlands PC, et al. Unsuspected renal artery stenosis in peripheral vascular disease. BMJ 1990;301:1197–1198.

100. Vensel LA, Devereux RB, Pickering TG, et al. Cardiac structure and function in renovascular hypertension produced by unilateral and bilateral renal artery stenosis. Am J Cardiol 1986;58:575–582.

101. Pickering TG, Herman L, Devereux RB, et al. Recurrent pulmonary edema in hypertension due to bilateral renal artery stenosis: treatment by angioplasty or surgical revascularization. Lancet 1988;2:551–552.

102. Sutters M, Al-Kutoubi MA, Mathias CJ, Peart S. Diuresis and syncope after renal angioplasty in a patient with one functioning kidney. BMJ 1987;295:527–528.

103. Pickering TG, Blumenfeld JD, Laragh JH. Renovascular hypertension and ischemic nephropathy. In: Brenner BM, ed. The Kidney. Philadelphia: Saunders, 1996: 2106–2125.

104. Corradi B, Malberti F, Farina M, et al. Chronic renal failure due to atheromatous renovascular disease in the elderly. Contrib Nephrol 1993;105:167–171.

105. Zucchelli P, Zucchala A. Ischemic nephropathy in the elderly. Contrib Nephrol 1993;105:13–24.

106. Jacobson H. Ischemic renal disease. Kidney Int 1988; 34:729–743.

107. Textor SC, Novick AG, Tarazi RC, et al. Critical perfusion pressure for renal function in patients with bilateral atherosclerotic renal vascular disease. Ann Intern Med 1985;102:308–314.

108. Messina LM, Zelenock GB, Yao KA, Stanley JC. Renal revascularization for recurrent pulmonary edema in patients with poorly controlled hypertension and renal insufficiency: a distinct subgroup of patients with atherosclerotic renal artery occlusive disease. J Vasc Surg 1992;15:73–82.

109. Harding MB, Smith LR, Himmelstein SI, et al. Renal artery stenosis: prevalence and associated risk factors in patients undergoing routine cardiac catheterization. J Am Soc Nephrol 1992;2:1608–1616.

110. Elliott WJ, Martin WB, Murphy MB. Comparison of two noninvasive screening tests for renovascular hypertension. Arch Intern Med 1993;153:755–764.

111. Fommei E, Ghione S, Palla L, et al. Renal scintigraphic captopril test in the diagnosis of renovascular hypertension. Hypertension 1987;10:212–220.

112. Setaro JF, Chen CC, Hoffer PB, Black HR. Captopril renography in the diagnosis of renal artery stenosis and prediction of improvement with revascularization: the Yale Vascular Center experience. Am J Hypertens 1991; 4:698S–705S.

113. Hoffman U, Edwards JM, Carter S, et al. Role of duplex scanning for the detection of atherosclerotic renal artery disease. Kidney Int 1991;39:1232–1239.

114. Canzanello VJ, Textor SC. Noninvasive diagnosis of renovascular disease. Mayo Clin Proc 1994;69:1172–1181.

115. Lawrie GM, Morris GC, Glaeser DH, DeBakey ME. Renovascular reconstruction: factors affecting long-term prognosis in 919 patients followed up to 31 years. Am J Cardiol 1989;63:1085–1092.

116. Bedoya L, Ziegelbaum M, Vidt DG, et al. Baseline renal function and surgical revascularization in atherosclerotic renal arterial disease in the elderly. Cleve Clin J Med 1989;56:415–421.

117. Blum U, Krumme B, Flugel P, et al. Treatment of ostial renal artery stenosis with vascular endoprostheses after unsuccessful balloon angioplasty. N Engl J Med 1997; 336:459–465.

118. Postma CT, Hoefnagels WH, Barentsz JO, et al. Occlusion of unilateral stenosed renal arteries: relation to medical treatment. J Hum Hypertens 1989;3:185–190.

119. Arzilli F, Giovannetti R, Meola M, et al. ACE-inhibition vs surgical treatment in the outcome of ischemic kidney of renovascular patients: a one year follow-up. High Blood Press 1992;1:47–50.

120. Ribstein J, Mourad G, Mimran A. Contrasting acute effects of captopril and nifedipine on renal function in renovascular hypertension. Am J Hypertens 1988;1: 239–244.

121. Epstein M. Calcium antagonists and renal protection: current status and future perspectives. Arch Intern Med 1992;152:1572–1584.

122. Yager HM, Harrington JT. Renal artery embolism and thrombosis. In: Hurst JW, ed. Medicine for the Practicing Physician. Stamford, CT: Appleton & Lange, 1996: 1400–1402.

123. Hoxie HJ, Coggins CB. Renal infarction: statistical study of two hundred and five cases and detailed report of an unusual case. Arch Intern Med 1940;65:587.

124. Falk RJ, Jennette JC. Glomerular disease in the elderly. In: Jacobson HR, Striker GE, Klahr S, eds. The Principles and Practice of Nephrology. St. Louis: Mosby, 1996;518–524.

125. Krafcik SS, Covin RB, Lynch JP, Sitrin RG. Wegener's granulomatosis in the elderly. Chest 1996;109:430–437.

126. Stegeman CA, Cohen Tervaert JW, de Jong PE, Kallenberg CG. Trimethoprim-sulfamethoxazole (co-trimoxazole) for the prevention of relapses of Wegener's granulomatosis. N Engl J Med 1996;335:16–20.

127. Eagen J, Lewis EJ. Glomerulopathies of neoplasia. Kidney Int 1977;11:297–303.

128. Brueggemeyer CD, Ramirez G. Membranous nephropathy: a concern for malignancy. Am J Kidney Dis 1987; 9:23–26.

129. Donadio JV, Torres VE, Velosa J, et al. Idiopathic membranous nephropathy: the natural history of untreated patients. Kidney Int 1988;33:708–715.

130. Glassock RJ, Cohen AH, Adler SG. Primary glomerular diseases. In: Brenner BM, ed. The Kidney. Philadelphia: Saunders, 1996:1392–1497.

131. Schieppati A, Mosconi L, Perna A, et al. Prognosis of un-

treated patients with idiopathic membranous nephropathy. N Engl J Med 1993;329:85–89.

132. Nolasco F, Cameron JS, Heywood EF, et al. Adult-onset minimal-change nephrotic syndrome: a long-term follow-up. Kidney Int 1986;29:1215–1223.

133. Nair RB, Date A, Kirubakaran MG, Shastry JC. Minimal-change nephrotic syndrome in adults treated with alternate-day steroids. Nephron 1987;47:209–210.

134. Falk RH, Comenzo RL, Skinner M. The systemic amyloidoses. N Engl J Med 1997;337:898–909.

135. Gertz MA, Kyle RA. Prognostic value of urinary protein in primary systemic amyloidosis. Am J Clin Pathol 1990;94:313–317.

136. Gertz MA, Kyle RA, O'Fallon WM. Dialysis support of patients with primary systemic amyloidosis: a study of 211 patients. Arch Intern Med 1992;152:2245–2250.

137. Viberti GC, Hill RD, Jarrett RJ, et al. Microalbuminuria as a predictor of clinical nephropathy in insulin-dependent diabetes mellitus. Lancet 1982;1:1430–1432.

138. Ballard DJ, Humphrey LL, Melton LJ III, et al. Epidemiology of persistent proteinuria in type II diabetes mellitus: population-based study in Rochester, Minnesota. Diabetes 1988;37:405–412.

139. Seaquist ER, Goetz FC, Rich S, Barbosa J. Familial clustering of diabetic kidney disease: evidence of genetic susceptibility to diabetic nephropathy. N Engl J Med 1989;320:1161–1165.

140. Cowie CC, Port FK, Wolfe RA, et al. Disparities in incidence of diabetic end-stage renal disease according to race and type of diabetes. N Engl J Med 1989;321:1074–1079.

141. Hanssen KF, Dahl-Jørgensen K, Lauritzen T, et al. Diabetic control and microvascular complications. Diabetologia 1986;29:677.

142. Parving HH, Osterby R, Anderson PW, Hsueh WA. Diabetic nephropathy. In: Brenner BM, ed. The Kidney. Philadelphia: Saunders, 1996:1864–1892.

143. Ravid M, Savin H, Jutrin I, et al. Long-term stabilizing effect of angiotensin-converting enzyme inhibition on plasma creatinine and on proteinuria normotensive type II diabetic patients. Ann Intern Med 1993;118:577–581.

144. Gall MA, Nielsen FS, Smidt UM, Parving HH. The course of kidney function in type 2 (non-insulin dependent) diabetic patients with diabetic nephropathy. Diabetologia 1993;36:1071–1078.

145. Gall MA, Rossing P, Skøtt P, et al. Prevalence of micro- and macroalbuminuria, arterial hypertension, retinopathy and large vessel disease in European type 2 (non-insulin-dependent) diabetic patients. Diabetologia 1991;34:655–661.

146. Gambara V, Mecca G, Remuzzi G, Bertaini T. Heterogenous nature of renal lesions in type II diabetes. J Am Soc Nephrol 1993;3:1458–1466.

147. Wilson DM, Turner DR, Cameron JS, et al. Value of renal biopsy in acute intrinsic renal failure. BMJ 1976;2:459–461.

148. Laberke HG, Bohle A. Acute interstitial nephritis: correlations between clinical and morphological findings. Clin Nephrol 1980;14:263–273.

149. Pirani CL, Valeri A, D'Agati V, Appel GB. Renal toxicity of nonsteroidal anti-inflammatory drugs. Contrib Nephrol 1987;55:159–175.

150. Lyons H, Pinn VW, Cortell S, et al. Allergic interstitial nephritis causing reversible renal failure in four patients with idiopathic nephrotic syndrome. N Engl J Med 1973;288:124–128.

151. Kelly CJ, Neilson EG. Tubulointerstitial diseases. In: Brenner BM, ed. The Kidney. Philadelphia: Saunders, 1996:1655–1679.

152. United States Renal Data System: USRDS 1997 Annual Data Report. Bethesda, MD: National Institutes of Health, National Institute of Diabetes and Digestive and Kidney Diseases, Division of Kidney, Urologic, and Hematologic Diseases, 1997.

153. Shapiro WB. Renal replacement therapy in the elderly. In: Jacobson HR, Striker GE, Klahr S, eds. The Principles and Practice of Nephrology. St. Louis: Mosby, 1996:533–541.

154. van Ypersele de Strihou C, Jadoul M, Malghem J, et al. Effect of dialysis membrane and patient's age on signs of dialysis-related amyloidosis. Kidney Int 1991;39:1012–1019.

155. Maiorca R, Vonesh EF, Cavalli PL, et al. A multicenter selection adjusted comparison of patient and technique survivals on CAPD and hemodialysis. Perit Dial Int 1991;11:118–127.

156. Held PJ, Port FK, Turenne MN, et al. Continuous ambulatory peritoneal dialysis and hemodialysis: a comparison of patient mortality with adjustment for comorbid conditions. Kidney Int 1994;45:1163–1169.

157. Posen GA, Jeffery JR, Fenton SS, Arbus GS. Results from the Canadian renal failure registry. Am J Kidney Dis 1990;15:397–401.

158. Churchill DN, Thorpe KE, Vonesh EF, Keshaviah PR. Lower probability of patient survival with continuous peritoneal dialysis in the United States compared with Canada. J Am Soc Nephrol 1997;8:965–971.

159. Barry JM, Lemmers MJ, Meyer MM, et al. Cadaveric kidney transplantation in patients more than 65 years old. World J Urol 1996;14:243–248.

160. Wyner LM, Novick AC, Hodge EE, et al. Long-term follow-up of kidneys transplanted from elderly cadaveric donors. World J Urol 1996;14:265–267.

161. Johnson LB, Kuo PC, Schweitzer EJ, et al. Double renal allografts successfully increase utilization of kidneys from older donors within a single organ procurement organization. Transplantation 1996;62:1581–1583.

Urologic Problems of the Elderly

As people age, changes in body functions increase with distressing regularity. Bowel and urinary tract decompensation are very common complaints of the geriatric patient. With few exceptions, men's voiding habits change and their sexual ability decreases. In addition, few men lack information concerning prostate cancer. Women, often beginning in the middle years, are troubled by increasing bladder incontinence. Almost half of women over 65 have some type of urinary tract infection. This chapter addresses common alterations of the lower urinary system of older men and women. Urinary incontinence is discussed in Chapter 29.

BENIGN PROSTATIC HYPERPLASIA

By far the most common urologic concern of older men is various conditions that affect the prostate. Though men are certainly susceptible to infection and irritation at any age, enlargement of the prostate, or benign prostatic hyperplasia (BPH), usually begins about 40 to 45 years of age. The prostate is stimulated to grow and is maintained in size and secretory function by the continued presence of serum testosterone. BPH is a proliferative process that involves both the stromal and epithelial elements of the prostate.

Until recently prostatectomy and watchful waiting were the usual treatment options. However, the past 10 years have seen the introduction of a number of medical therapies as a successful alternative to prostatectomy or tolerance of minimal or moderate symptoms. Not only has medical treatment of BPH seen an expansion of alternatives, but new invasive procedures and minimally invasive techniques have been developed.

Medical Treatment

There are two principal categories of medical treatment of minimal to moderate symptoms of prostatic hyperplasia. In this context, it is important to emphasize symptomatic disease, as there is no evidence that treating asymptomatic BPH is beneficial. The two drug categories are 5α-reductase inhibitor (finasteride, or Proscar) and the α-adrenergic antagonist drugs terazosin (Hytrin), doxazosin (Cardura), and tamsulosin (Flomax). As more experience and careful studies have accumulated since 1991, when these medications were introduced, their role in the treatment of BPH has been debated (1–4).

Finasteride has been shown to have beneficial effects only on prostates of significant volume (5). Its effects on prostates of small volume are no different from those of placebo (1). Again it is important to state that not all large-volume prostate glands are symptomatic. The use of this drug and other medical treatments of BPH should be limited to patients who have symptoms. Most men with symptomatic BPH have a low-volume prostate gland. In this group, one of the α-adrenergic antagonist drugs give the best results. The development of α-adrenergic drugs followed findings that two factors lead to symptoms in BPH, a static and a dynamic component (6). The static component consists of the enlargement of the adenoma; the dynamic component is the tone or degree of contraction of prostatic smooth muscle. The dynamic function of the prostate was determined to be mediated primarily by α receptors in the capsule and adenoma (7). Therefore it is not surprising that medication with an α-adrenergic blocking activity relieves symptoms of BPH.

There is no doubt that the introduction and successful use of both finasteride and the α-adrenergic blockers has had a dramatic effect on the frequency of standard prostatectomy (transurethral resection, or TUR). No urologist in practice even 10 years has seen similar declines in the numbers of TURs performed after 1991. There still remain patients who present in urinary retention or very late in the progression of BPH, for whom medical therapy is not effective. In addition, some patients are intolerant of the side effects of medical therapy and must turn to invasive procedures to obtain relief from symptoms. Before discussing invasive management of BPH, it is appropriate to address medical therapy.

More and more, men are presenting to urologists asking about or actually taking some form of plant extract (so called phytotherapy). Such treatment is common in Europe, especially England, and Canada. It is very likely that primary care physicians are also being asked for information about these extracts, partly because of the extensive marketing campaigns of the companies that sell these products. The most commonly used plant extract is saw palmetto (*Serenoa repens*). It is difficult as yet to advise patients of the benefits of these forms of treatment for several reasons. Few studies have been done, and the studies that are available are not randomized or controlled. Most of the products contain several ingredients (such as vitamin E, vitamin C, and zinc) along with saw palmetto, so that it is not clear that any beneficial effects derive from the saw palmetto. An appropriate response to questions about these products appears to be that they are probably safe but may not be effective.

Invasive Management

Despite the preference of most patients, many physicians, and some insurance agencies to remedy obstructive symptoms due to BPH with noninvasive measures, such as medical therapy, failure of medical therapy is common. Invasive therapy becomes necessary when patients are in advanced stages of obstruction or cannot tolerate medical therapy. A variety of invasive therapies

for treatment of obstructive BPH are available, and additional techniques continue to evolve. Given the variety of therapeutic modalities, it is understandable that there should be confusion and uncertainty even among practicing urologists. "Minimally invasive" is a new catchphrase that has taken hold in public information as well as in the urology literature. Here is an overview of invasive and minimally invasive methods.

In the first part of the 20th century, obstructive BPH was managed by open surgical enucleation of the enlarged gland. Today this method is used infrequently, only for very specific indications. Transurethral surgical removal of the prostate was developed and used as early as the 1930s, but several decades went by before the procedure was generally accepted. TUR is now considered the standard approach to obstructive BPH. In older men with concomitant illness, even TUR is associated with some morbidity and mortality. For this reason newer procedures have been developed. In addition, new procedures that are minimally invasive also may be less costly.

A slight modification of TUR is transurethral electrovaporization of the prostate (TUEVP). It is essentially the same as TUR but does not entail cutting prostate tissue; instead the prostate tissue is vaporized. TUEVP requires general or spinal anesthesia, but the advantage over TUR is the reduction in overall risk. In particular, hemostasis in TUEVP is significantly better, and therefore the patient is less likely to require a transfusion. Patients who are hematologically compromised or whose religious convictions preclude the use of transfusions are especially suited for TUEVP over TUR.

In older men with a small prostate and in younger men in whom minimal chance of changing ejaculatory function is desired, a limited operative procedure called transurethral incision of the prostate (TUIP) is sometimes used. TUIP entails deep incisions through the bladder neck and along the length of the prostatic urethra to the level of the verumontanum. In addition to the maintenance of ejaculatory ability, other advantages of TUIP are the brevity of the procedure and greatly diminished blood loss.

The therapies discussed so far use equipment common to all operating rooms. The next group of minimally invasive treatment modalities require specialized equipment. In addition, the urologic surgeon needs additional expertise unless he or she has recently completed a residency program in which these procedures were part of the training. Laser therapy has been available for treatment of the prostate for more than 10 years. At least six types of laser therapy are employed (8) with varying degrees of success, but none is widely accepted as yet. Other forms of treatment for prostatic obstruction include cryotherapy (not in common use), microwave thermotherapy, interstitial placement of needle electrodes in the adenoma (TUNA, or transurethral needle ablation). TUNA has promise as an outpatient procedure done under local anesthesia or with light sedation (9).

Two additional therapies that do not entail surgery of the prostate are recommended by some physicians. Balloon dilation of the prostate became popular in the late 1980s but is done less often today. More interest is now given to the use of an intraurethral stent. Because stenting can be done under local anesthesia, it is especially appealing for patients too ill for other procedures.

CANCER OF THE PROSTATE

Prostate cancer is the most common cancer diagnosed in men in the United States and the second most common cause of cancer deaths. The news media frequently report the latest diagnostic or therapeutic advances to an anxious public. What remains unanswered is the ability to predict the longevity of a given patient with prostate cancer. A further dilemma arises in trying to craft the optimal treatment for a given patient. The protracted course of the disease makes these questions difficult to answer.

Early prostate cancer is asymptomatic. If urologic symptoms, such as hematuria, back pain, or obstruction, do occur with prostatic carcinoma, the cancer is at least locally extensive and possibly metastatic. The American Urologic Association recommendations for screening men consists of annual digital rectal examination (DRE) and assay for prostate-specific antigen (PSA) for men between 50 and 70 years of age. If the patient has a history of carcinoma of the prostate in a relative, it is recommended that annual evaluations begin at age 40. African-American men should begin annual surveillance at age 40 because they have a higher incidence of prostate cancer than do whites. On the other hand, there is little advantage to more screening than annual digital examination in men in their 80s or 90s. Even the value of routine screening of men in their 70s is debatable.

It is important to discuss not only the philosophy of screening in various age groups but also the limitation of the serum PSA. PSA is a protease produced by prostatic epithelium secreted into the seminal fluid. Therefore, obtaining a PSA level within 48 hours of ejaculation may result in a temporary elevation. Because prostatic disease alters the normal cellular barriers that keep PSA within the ductal system of the prostate, most prostatic disorders can raise the PSA. Prostatitis, urinary retention, BPH, and prostatic infarction as well as cancer can elevate the PSA. If the rectal examination strongly suggests a nodule or diffuse hardness, the PSA may be reliable even in the presence of prostatitis or another disorder. Obtaining a PSA should probably be deferred in men with a urinary tract infection or indwelling Foley catheter.

When evaluating a patient whose has had a PSA test, one must consider what is a "normal" level. When originally developed, a standard range for PSA of 0 to 4 ng/mL was established. As thousands of men were tested, factors besides concurrent disease of the prostate were found to change the PSA level. The volume of the prostate gland tends to alter PSA (10). Adjustment of the acceptable range according to age has been strongly argued (11). Studies recommend the following norms for PSA based on age: ages 40 to 50 years, 0 to 2.5 mg/mL PSA; ages 50 to 60 years, 0 to 3.5 mg/mL PSA; ages 60 to 70 years, 0 to 4.5 mg/mL PSA. Nevertheless, most PSA elevations occur between 4 and 10 mg/mL. Because BPH is so common, the most likely reason for the PSA elevation is prostate enlargement. A PSA level between 4 and 10 mg/mL in a man with a normal DRE is probably false-positive (12).

Verification of carcinoma of the prostate requires tissue sampling. Rectal ultrasonic guided biopsy sampling of the prostate performed on an outpatient basis is the accepted method of detection. Though rectal sonography alone adds little to the evaluation of most patients, sonography permits the needle to be guided in obtaining tissue samples. Usually three samples from each lobe of the prostate (a total of six biopsies) are taken.

PROSTATITIS

About 20% of men seen in urology clinics have evidence of prostatic inflammation. Several forms of prostatitis are recognized: bacterial and nonbacterial prostatitis and prostatodynia. Acute and chronic bacterial prostatitis can be confirmed with cultures. Mycobacterial prostatitis results in symptoms of inflammation as well as excessive inflammatory cells in the prostatic secretions with negative culture. Prostatodynia is diagnosed in patients who have symptoms consistent with prostatitis but who have negative culture and no sign of inflammation in prostatic secretions.

Bacterial prostatitis is most commonly associated with gram-negative organisms. The usual route of infection is the distal urethra. Younger men may develop prostatitis as a result of sexual activity, while in older men it usually results from instrumentation of the urinary tract (e.g., Foley catheter) or as a result of poor genital hygiene in an uncircumcised man. Acute bacterial prostatitis is characterized by sudden onset of fever, chills, perineal pain, urinary frequency, myalgias, and varying degrees of bladder outlet obstruction. Rectal examination reveals a tender, swollen prostate. An acutely inflamed prostate should *not* be massaged. If acute urinary retention accompanies the prostatitis, hospitalization and treatment with intravenous antibiotics is warranted. Usual therapy for acute prostatitis consists of 4 weeks of oral antibiotics.

Chronic prostatitis is most commonly encountered in the older man. Symptoms may include any of the following: burning on urination, urinary frequency, suprapubic discomfort, testicular or perineal discomfort, low back pain, nocturia, urgency, feeling of incomplete emptying of the bladder, and arthralgias. The rectal examination may show varying degrees of softness or swelling with or without tenderness. Massaged prostatic secretions are a helpful guide in evaluating inflammation. For a culture of prostatic secretions, a urine specimen is obtained after prostatic massage. The treatment of chronic prostatitis, whether bacterial or not, is associated with varying success. Patients with chronic prostatitis should be warned of the likelihood of recurrences. Antibiotics that are the most useful for treating men with chronic prostatitis include trimethoprim-sulfamethoxazole, doxycycline, carbenicillin, and the quinolones. For an initial episode, treatment for 10 to 14 days usually is successful. Longer courses of therapy, which should be individualized, are required when a recurrence is being treated. Treatment may be daily, every other day, 1 week each month, or as needed. In addition to antibiotics, dietary restrictions are often helpful. Eliminating colas, beer, and coffee should be recommended. Occasionally spicy foods and chocolates cause ongoing irritation and prostatitis. The role of prostatic massage in the treatment of chronic prostatitis remains controversial. Before the development of more effective antibiotics, prostatic massage was widely used. Even now, when the patient gives a history of significant allergies to many antibiotics, massage therapy may be a less troublesome method of treatment. Articles encouraging the use of prostatic massage for chronic prostatitis continue to appear (13).

Prostatodynia is a syndrome in which patients have symptoms similar to those of bacterial or nonbacterial prostatitis but no objective findings. Occasionally the prostatic examination is painful to the patient but there is no softness and the prostatic secretions are normal. Often these patients receive antibiotics without any improvement. In these cases urethral stricture or some other less common bladder condition must be ruled out by cystoscopy. Many patients with prostatodynia have some type of emotional distress. Regardless of the cause, symptoms suggest spasm of the internal urinary sphincter and nonrelaxation of the pelvic floor striated muscles. Relaxation of the urethral sphincter may be helped by use of α-adrenergic blockers, doxazosin, or terazosin. Sitz baths and addressing psychologic distress may also help.

DISEASES OF THE PENIS

Phimosis, paraphimosis, and balanoposthitis are penile problems frequently encountered in elderly men. Phimosis is a tightening of the foreskin around the glans, causing difficulty in retracting the foreskin and possibly inability to retract the foreskin at all. In paraphimosis, the retracted foreskin becomes trapped and swollen proximal to the corona of the glans (Fig. 28.1). Left untreated, paraphimosis results in necrosis and infection of the foreskin. Early treatment consists of manual reduction as illustrated in Figure 28.1. Advanced cases require surgical reduction and should be considered a urologic emergency. Balanoposthitis is an inflammatory condition of the glans and overlying foreskin. The most common underlying cause of this condition is diabetes. So often is this the case that diabetes should be sought in any patient not known to be diabetic who has balanoposthitis. Management consists of thorough cleansing of the glans and foreskin with mild soap followed by the application of an antifungal steroid ointment twice daily. If the balanoposthi-

tis recurs or fails to clear, a circumcision should be performed.

A patient complaining of a lump in the penis, curvature of the penis with erection, or painful erections most likely has Peyronie's disease. This is not really a disease but fibrous plaques that partially surround the cavernous sheath of the penis. Though it was described over a century ago, the cause remains unknown. Attention has focused on trauma, usually during vigorous sexual intercourse, as a significant causative factor. Treatment of Peyronie's disease remains uncertain and very limited. Some benefit is obtained by the use of vitamin E 400 U twice daily. p-Aminobenzoate (Potaba), probably the most widely used medical treatment, has its greatest benefit in men with painful plaques or painful erections. Other treatments that have been tried include ultrasonic treatments, steroid injections, and surgical excision of the plaques.

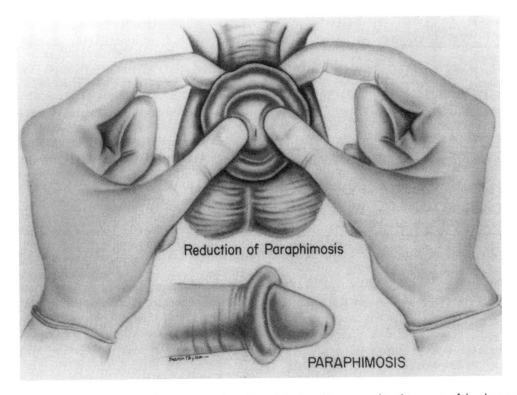

Figure 28.1.   Paraphimosis is the trapping and swelling of the foreskin proximal to the corona of the glans penis. Correction of the paraphimosis is usually done by firm constant pressure on the glans by thumbs, with the forefingers under the paraphimosis.

Carcinoma of the penis constitutes fewer than 1% of all malignancies that occur annually in men in the United States (14). The uncircumcised man is by far the most likely to develop carcinoma of the penis. In fact, neonatal circumcision essentially eliminates the risk of this malignancy. Poor hygiene and genital warts are contributing factors in the development of carcinoma of the penis. Most of these malignancies can be successfully managed by partial amputation or by laser surgery.

DISEASES OF THE SCROTUM AND SCROTAL CONTENTS
Epididymitis

The most frequently encountered acute problem of the scrotum is epididymitis. In the elderly man, epididymitis may follow instrumentation of the urinary tract, including the use of a Foley catheter. Cystitis or prostatitis may precede the onset of epididymitis. Symptoms include painful hemiscrotum with enlargement and tenderness of the epididymis, often with fever and malaise. Treatment of epididymitis includes bed rest, scrotal support, ice packs until the testis and epididymis are no longer tender, and appropriate oral antibiotics. In diabetic patients very close attention is necessary because progression to abscess formation, though not common, is possible.

Hydrocele

A diffuse cystic enlargement of the scrotum that transilluminates is diagnostic of a hydrocele. Hydroceles are usually unilateral and frequently are well tolerated and asymptomatic. Large hydroceles preclude satisfactory palpation of the surrounded testis. If there is concern about the testis, scrotal ultrasound can confirm the status of the testis. There are good techniques to perform hydrocelectomy safely and comfortably, with local anesthesia on an outpatient basis, on men requiring relief of significant symptoms. Careful aspiration of a symptomatic hydrocele may also be tried, but the results are often only temporary.

Spermatocele

Spermatocele is another cystic structure of the scrotum. The spermatocele also transillumi-nates but is usually above the upper pole of a clearly palpable testis. Most spermatoceles are asymptomatic, and their main importance lies in clarification to the patient of the nature of the lump in the scrotum. Occasionally an enlarging, painful spermatocele justifies surgical removal. Surgery can be done with local anesthesia on an outpatient; however, a spermatocele should not be aspirated.

Cancer of the Testis

Malignancy of the testis is normally a disease of younger men. In elderly men with testicular tumors, the most common types are lymphomas and metastatic carcinomas, including metastatic carcinoma of the prostate.

MALE SEXUAL DYSFUNCTION

Sexual dysfunction in men is mostly related to erectile dysfunction. The past decade has seen a marked increase in awareness and the willingness of older men to bring their difficulty performing sexually to the attention of their physician. A progressively larger cohort of healthy men are reaching their 70s and 80s. The sexual partners of older men have in great measure been more frank about their interests in sexual relations. Most people now expect to be sexually active when older than perhaps has been the norm in the past. Primary care physicians should be ready to assist older men with advice about sexual dysfunction.

A study of 1300 men showed that the prevalence of impotence tripled from ages 40 to 70 (15), so that age is the most important risk factor. The second most important factor was cigarette smoking: impotence occurred in 56% of smokers and 21% of nonsmokers. Other risk factors include diabetes mellitus, heart disease, and treated hypertension.

In evaluating a man with sexual dysfunction, a thorough history is mandatory. Special attention should be directed at the medication list (16). Table 28.1 lists the major antihypertensive medications that may contribute to erectile dysfunction. Table 28.2 lists other drugs often implicated in erectile dysfunction. The physical examination should include an assessment of the patient's general health. The abdomen should be

Table 28.1

Antihypertensive Medications Associated With Sexual Dysfunction in Men

Diuretics
  Thiazides
  Spironolactone
  Chlorthalidone
Antihypertensives
  α-Adrenergic blockers
    Phenoxybenzamine
    Phentolamine
    Prazosin
  β-Adrenergic blockers
    Propranolol
    Metoprolol
  Central sympatholytics
    Methyldopa
    Clonidine
    Reserpine
  Neurotransmitter depleter
    Guanethidine
  Vasodilators
    Hydralazine
    Minoxidil

examined for aneurysm. The status of the femoral and peripheral pulses should be determined. Examine the genitalia to rule out the penile plaques of Peyronie's disease and other structural abnormalities and examine the testes to rule out hypogonadism. A rectal examination to evaluate the prostate and to assess sphincter tone as an indicator of altered sacral neurologic status is recommended. Sometimes a more complete neurologic examination is warranted. Basic laboratory tests that complement the physical examination in evaluation of male sexual dysfunction include routine urinalysis, blood glucose, serum testosterone, and thyroid function tests.

Treatment of erectile dysfunction is an evolving area. While a number of men have psychologic causes that underlie sexual dysfunction, studies of impotence suggest that physical causes are more common. Invasive treatment for erectile dysfunction began with penile implants using rigid, semirigid, and inflatable prostheses. Occasionally men were found to have a correctable vasogenic cause and were treated with penile revascularization procedures. Revascular-

ization meets with mixed acceptance. Penile implants are established therapy for male erectile dysfunction, but their cost and invasive nature are limiting factors.

External erectile devices have become commonplace in the past 10 years. Men have to be sufficiently motivated to use the external vacuum devices effectively, but these methods do have the advantage of being noninvasive. Two minimally invasive modalities that have recently been developed appear to be acceptable and effective. Intracavernous injection of a mixture of papaverine-phentolamine and prostaglandin E_1 is successful in 60 to 70% of patients but has a high dropout rate. Another minimally invasive method of delivering medication for erectile dysfunction is alprostadil urethral suppository (MUSE). Most patients find insertion of a small suppository into the distal urethra more acceptable than an injection. Early claims are for 70% effectiveness, but only long-term studies will substantiate the value of MUSE. Oral preparations, aside from oral testosterone, have not been particularly numerous or effective. Yohimbine has been available for more than 15 years and is effective in a limited number of patients, mostly men with psychogenic erectile dysfunction. The release of the first in a series of oral medications, alprostadil (Viagra), has been enthusiastically received. An oral drug with few

Table 28.2

Other Drug Categories Associated With Sexual Dysfunction in Men

Psychoactive agents
  Phenothiazines
  Antidepressants
  Antianxiety agents
  Lithium carbonate
  Barbiturates
Anticholinergics
Miscellaneous drugs
  Cimetidine
  Clofibrate
  Digoxin
  Indomethacin
Addictive drugs
  Alcohol
  Nicotine
Opioids

side effects would be highly valued by patients. Oral alprostadil is contraindicated in men who are taking nitrates. In addition, use of Viagra in men who have significant cardiac disease, even if not on nitrates, should be deferred until safety parameters have been delineated. Some deaths have occurred in this group of men also. The long-term effectiveness of these new medications for male sexual dysfunction is not yet known.

LOWER UROLOGIC DISEASES IN WOMEN

Urethral Diseases in Women

The female urethra is normally 3 to 5 cm long. In the postmenopausal woman the urethra is subject to various inflammatory and anatomic changes. One common finding in the older woman is the hypospadiac urethra. In this condition the urethral meatus has retracted inside the vaginal vault. The more proximal location of the urethral meatus often makes catheterization difficult. The position of the meatus also predisposes to trauma and ascending urethritis. The re-

cessed urethra may also irritate the distal vagina by emptying urine into the vaginal vault (Figs. 28.2 and 28.3).

A frequent postmenopausal finding is urethral prolapse. The prolapsed appearance indicates eversion of the urethral mucosa. Treatment with either periodic urethral dilation or application of estrogen cream twice daily for about 2 weeks is often effective. A localized area of prolapse at the 6 o'clock position of the urethral meatus is called a urethral caruncle. Application of estrogen cream and sitz baths may reduce the local swelling, but if reasonably prompt resolution does not occur, excision of the lesion should be considered because of the occasional development of urethral carcinoma.

Two other frequent anatomic abnormalities of the older female urinary tract are urethroceles and urethral diverticula. A urethrocele is a protrusion into the vaginal vault of the anterior vaginal wall containing the urethra. Though usually associated with the loss or weakening of support of the anterior vaginal mucosa, it occasionally is due to dis-

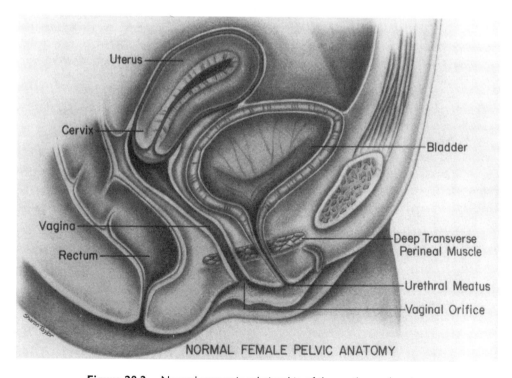

Figure 28.2. Normal anatomic relationship of the urethra and vagina.

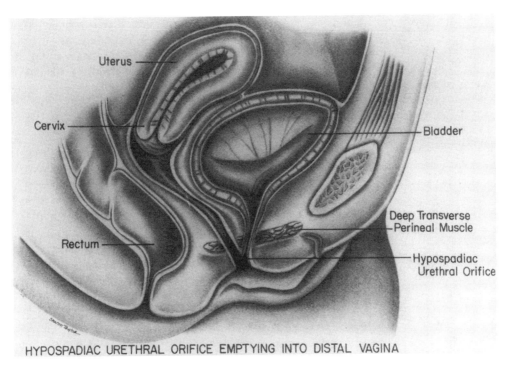

HYPOSPADIAC URETHRAL ORIFICE EMPTYING INTO DISTAL VAGINA

Figure 28.3.   Hypospadiac urethra often found in postmenopausal women.

tal urethral stenosis. A urethral diverticulum is a local outpouching of the urethra, most often the result of an infection of a periurethral gland. A urethral diverticulum should be considered in one of several situations: the expression of purulent discharge from the urethral meatus during a vaginal examination; a history of urethral discharge between urinations; and occasionally as a cause of recurrent cystitis. Urethral stenosis is yet another anatomic abnormality found in elderly women that may be due to postmenopausal estrogen deprivation with secondary tightening of the periurethral tissue, recurring urethritis, or trauma from urethral instrumentation. In other cases urethral stenosis is a lifelong condition. Symptoms that suggest urethral stenosis include hesitancy of the urinary stream, straining to void, and a small stream with a long time to complete urination. Senile urethritis is an inflammatory condition of the urethra that occurs often but is only occasionally symptomatic. When symptoms do occur, they are usually irritative, such as burning on urination, or frequency. Usually, the urine culture is sterile. Urinary analgesics alone or in combination with antispasmodics are helpful in clearing the symptoms. Topical or systemic estrogen replacement therapy has been found useful in reducing recurrent lower tract infections in postmenopausal women.

Hematuria

Hematuria is a cause for serious concern for primary care physicians and is a source of frequent referral to urologists. The level of concern varies according to whether the hematuria is gross or microscopic, and if microscopic, whether intermittent or persistent. In the elderly population gross painless hematuria, whether associated with anticoagulant therapy or not, should prompt a complete urologic workup. The workup should consist of either intravenous pyelography or renal ultrasound, urine for cytology, and in most cases, cystoscopy. If hematuria is associated with urinary symptoms such as dysuria, burning, or flank pain, the suspected condition, such as cystitis, prostatitis, or renal calculus, should be treated. If the suspected primary condition has cleared but the microscopic hematuria persists, the patient should be referred for urologic evaluation.

In a discussion of microscopic hematuria, one must first define what is normal and then determine whether any abnormality is intermittent or persistent. The most commonly accepted upper limit of normal for urinary red blood cells is three per high-powered field (17). The screening for microscopic hematuria by dipstick testing alone is not recommended (18). If the patient has only one episode of microscopic hematuria, a complete urologic workup is not indicated. Several episodes of microscopic hematuria, however, should warrant an ultrasound study of the upper urinary tract as well as urine cytology. Because the incidence of epithelial cancer increases with age, cystoscopy is also usually indicated for the older patient.

LOWER URINARY TRACT INFECTIONS

Comprehensive studies of urinary tract infections in the elderly have shown a marked increase with advancing age (19, 20) and a 3:1 ratio of women to men. Contributing to this rise in the rate of infections with age include menopause and consequent hormonal changes, prostatism, increased hypotonia of the bladder musculature, perineal soilage, impaired mental status, and the higher incidence of immobile or bedbound patients (21, 22).

Symptomatic urinary tract infections in patients of any age should be treated. Typical symptoms of lower urinary tract infections include dysuria, burning on urination, urgency, frequency, hematuria, nocturia, and suprapubic discomfort. Urinalysis shows pyuria and at times hematuria. Symptomatic relief can be provided by prescription of urinary analgesics (Pyridium) or a combination of analgesics and antispasmodics (Urised). The empiric use of an appropriate antibiotic often renders the patient asymptomatic by the time the results of a urine culture are available.

For the older woman with a first episode or only infrequent episodes of lower urinary tract infection, the first choice of medication is generally from a cost-effective group of antibiotics that includes synthetic penicillins (amoxicillin or ampicillin), sulfamethoxazole-trimethoprim, nitrofurantoins, and doxycycline or tetracycline. In men, however, the synthetic penicillins are often not very useful. In both men and women with known previous urinary tract infections, the use of second-line, albeit more expensive drugs, such as the cephalosporins and the quinolones, should be considered.

Occasionally success with a single megadose or a 3-day regimen of antibiotics has been reported for acute lower urinary tract infections in women (23, 24). Drugs used in these regimens include amoxicillin, sulfamethoxazole-trimethoprim, and the quinolones (25). Another study suggests that none of these short regimens is effective in elderly women (26).

Catheter-associated urinary tract infections warrant special mention. For many reasons, catheter drainage is common in the elderly and the presence of bacteriuria with chronic indwelling Foley catheters is unquestioned. In addition, the likelihood of urosepsis in older patients with Foley catheters is significant. Hence there are two important questions to be answered in the care of the patient with a chronic Foley catheter: What practical methods should be used in daily care of the patient with an indwelling catheter? What is the role, if any, of antibiotic therapy?

An essential factor in minimizing the likelihood of symptomatic infection is good fluid intake. A minimum of 1.5 L of fluid per day is recommended. Bladder irrigation with any substance has no value in preventing infection. Urinary acidification is difficult because of the chronic pyuria created by the foreign body presence of the catheter. There is disagreement about how often to change an indwelling Foley catheter. Some authors change the catheter only if drainage stops (27). But in other than an institutional setting, this is impractical and dangerous. Rather, most recommend changing the catheter at 4- to 6-week intervals.

The other question is the role of antibiotics in the patient with an indwelling Foley catheter. Ideally, if a patient can be successfully managed by the previous steps, it is not necessary to consider antibiotics. But the frequent occurrence of urosepsis and need for hospitalization raises the question of the value of antibiotic suppressive therapy, especially in patients who have demonstrated recurrent urosepsis. Unfortunately the medical literature does not provide clear guidance. My personal opinion is that the use of trimethoprim-sulfamethoxazole, nitrofurantoin, or occasionally a quinolone in a low daily dose prevents urosepsis for these patients. This observation has been borne out in nursing home, acute hospital, and community settings. A debilitated and deteriorating patient may well frustrate any management course.

The management of asymptomatic bacteriuria is another controversial topic. Some studies plead the importance of bacteriuria and shortened survival (28), while other studies support the view that asymptomatic bacteriuria is a benign condition (19, 20). Management of asymptomatic bacteriuria should include regular follow-up visits, encouraging good fluid intake (1.5 L per day), and urinary acidification if gram-negative organisms are present.

REFERENCES

1. Lepor H, Williford WO, Barry MJ, et al. The efficacy of terazosin, finasteride, or both in benign prostatic hyperplasia. N Engl J Med 1996;335:533–539.
2. Walsh PA. Treatment of benign prostatic hyperplasia. N Engl J Med 1996;335:586–587.
3. McConnell JD, Fitzpatrick JM, Hickel JC, Roehrburm CG. BPH therapy: an expanding number of alternatives. Contemp Urol 1998;10:55–62.
4. Osterling JE, Munda JM. A new reality for urology: drugs that alleviate BPH symptoms. Contemp Urol 1994;6:46–58.
5. Tammela TL, Kuntturi MJ. Urodynamic effects of finasteride in the treatment of bladder outlet obstruction due to benign prostatic hyperplasia. J Urol 1993;149:342–344.
6. Caine M. The present role of alpha-adrenergic blockers in the treatment of benign prostatic hypertrophy. J Urol 1986;136:1–4.
7. Caine M, Raz S, Zeigler M. Adrenergic and cholinergic receptors in the lumen prostate, prostatic capsule, and bladder neck. Br J Urol 1975;47:193–202.
8. Kabalin JN. Invasive therapies for benign prostatic hyperplasia. Monogr Urol 1997;18:19–47.
9. Schulman CC, Zlotta AR. TUMA: a promising new therapy for BPH. Contemp Urol 1995;7:59–69.
10. Dalkin BL, Almann FR, Kupp JB. Prostatic specific antigen levels in men older than 50 years without clinical evidence of prostatic carcinoma. J Urol 1993;150:1837–1839.
11. Osterling JE, Jacobsen SJ, Chute CG, et al. Serum prostate specific antigen in a community-based population of healthy men: establishment of age specific reference ranges. JAMA 1993;270:860–864.
12. Partin AW, Carter HB. Prostatic-specific antigen: use in clinical practice. Campbelli Urol Update 1994;10:1–12.
13. Loughlin KR, Whitmore WF. Managing prostate disorders in middle age and beyond. Geriatrics 1987;42:45–56.
14. Schellhammer PF. A concise plan for managing carcinoma of the penis. Contemp Urol 1992;4:13–25.
15. Feldman HA, Goldstein I. Matzicharistou DG, et al. Impotence and its medical and psychosocial correlates: results of the Massachusetts Male Aging Study. J Urol 1994;151:54–61.
16. Van Arsdaley KN, Wein AJ. Drug-induced sexual dysfunction in older men. Geriatrics 1984;39:63–70.
17. Classock RJ. Hematuria and pigmenturia. In: Massry SG, Classock RJ, eds. Textbook of Nephrology. Baltimore: Williams & Wilkins, 1989:491–495.
18. Sutton JM. Evaluation of hematuria in adults. JAMA 1990;263:2475–2480.
19. Yoshikawa TT. Chronic urinary tract infections in elderly patients. Hosp Pract 1993;28:103–118.
20. Smith IM. Infections in the elderly. Hosp Pract 1982;17:69–85.
21. Nicolle LE, Muir P, Harding GK, Norris M. Localization of urinary tract infection in elderly, institutionalized women with asymptomatic bacteriuria. J Infect Dis 1988;157:65–70.
22. Kaye D. Problems concerning bacteriuria in the elderly. J Infect Dis 1982;12:4–20.
23. Dontas AS. Management of urinary tract infections in the geriatric patient. Geriatr Med Today 1987;6:41–53.
24. Rubin RH, Fong LST, Jones SR, et al. Single dose amoxicillin therapy for urinary tract infection. JAMA 1980;244:561–564.
25. Hooton TM, Johnson C, Winter C. Single dose and three day treatment regimens of ofloxacin versus trimethoprim-sulfamethoxazole for acute cystitis in women. Antimicrob Agents Chemother 1991;35:1479–1483.
26. Ford S. New considerations in treatment of urinary tract infections in adults. Urology 1992;39:1–11.
27. Seiler WD, Stalelie HB. Practical management of catheter associated UTIs. Geriatrics 1988;43:43–50.
28. Dontas S. The effect of bacteriuria on survival in old age. Geriatr Urol 1983;2:74–79.

CHAPTER 29

JAN BUSBY-WHITEHEAD AND THEODORE M. JOHNSON II

Urinary Incontinence

Urinary incontinence, defined as the involuntary loss of urine, affects more than 10 million adults, including approximately 30% of community-dwelling older adults (1), 35 to 40% of older patients in acute care hospitals, and 50% of elderly nursing home residents. The loss of continence is not a natural consequence of aging, although specific age-related changes, such as functional impairment and reduction in bladder capacity, may contribute to urinary incontinence. Advanced age, female gender, upper and lower extremity weakness, dementia, affective disorder, and a history of gynecologic or urologic surgery are factors associated with an increased risk of incontinence (2–5). Urinary incontinence is an underreported condition. Most patients do not report it to health care providers (6), perhaps because they are embarrassed or believe nothing can be done to help (7). Because urinary incontinence is curable in many and can be managed in most cases (8), health care providers should ask about incontinence and evaluate the situation thoroughly. Interventions directed at treating the underlying causes of incontinence are frequently effective.

PATHOPHYSIOLOGY

Central nervous system control of bladder and sphincter function is mostly inhibitory through neural linkages from the sensorimotor cortex of the frontal lobes to the brainstem, cerebellum, thalamus, and spinal cord. Unless central inhibition occurs, the following sequence of events results in normal urination: Bladder emptying is mediated by cholinergic (parasympathetic) activity. Normal bladder filling increases cholinergic tone, stimulating the urge to void. The reflex controlling urination occurs through the cholinergic S2–S4 sacral nerve roots. With the urge to void, adrenergic (sympathetic) and somatic inhibition simultaneously occurs, allowing relaxation of the internal and external sphincters. Bladder contraction is enhanced while the urethral sphincters and pelvic floor muscles relax via input from the pudendal nerve. When the bladder is full, higher cortical inhibitory inputs eventually can be exceeded, resulting in the involuntary contraction of the bladder via the reflex arc.

Innervation of the lower urinary system is under cholinergic, adrenergic, and somatic control systems. Normal voiding requires storage of urine until the time of bladder emptying. Urine storage is mediated by adrenergic neural activity. β-Adrenergic receptors in the bladder dome are activated during filling and cause bladder relaxation, resulting in low intravesicular pressures despite increasing bladder volumes. Normal bladder capacity is 300 to 600 mL. Stimulation of α-adrenergic receptors in the bladder neck, bladder base, and proximal urethra results in constriction of the bladder neck and internal sphincter. The urethra has internal and external sphincters. The smooth muscle layers of the urethra form the internal sphincter. In postmenopausal women, lower levels of estrogen may affect urethral mucosal integrity. In older men the internal sphincter is vulnerable to damage during prostatic resection. The external sphincter is composed of urethral striated muscle that is under voluntary control and can interrupt voiding. Somatic innervation through the pudendal nerve allows voluntary contraction of the external sphincter and pelvic floor musculature that protects against urine loss from sudden increases in abdominal pressure.

Normal bladder emptying occurs when intravesicular pressure exceeds bladder outlet and sphincter resistance. This process requires the input of stimuli from the lower urinary tract and the coordination of central and peripheral neurologic responses and musculoskeletal activity. Disturbance of any component of this delicately balanced system may result in urinary incontinence.

CLASSIFICATION

Transient incontinence is defined as new incontinence that occurs suddenly, is generally associated with an acute medical or surgical illness or drug therapy, and is usually reversible with resolution of the underlying problem. Causes of transient incontinence are diverse (Table 29.1). Transient incontinence may arise from factors causing impaired cognition, including delirium and use of central nervous system (CNS) depressants such as opioids and sedative hypnotics. Causes of increased urine production, such as loop diuretics, hyperglycemia, and hypercalcemia, and volume overload states can also promote transient incontinence. Fecal impaction results in incontinence via unclear mechanisms, yet after relief of the impaction, continence is often restored. Bladder irritation from urinary tract infection, atrophic urethritis, or vaginitis can be addressed with improvement in continence. Restricted mobility may also cause transient incontinence.

Established incontinence is usually chronic, is not related to acute illness, requires investigation, and may be amenable to treatment with proper diagnosis. Established urinary incontinence that acutely becomes worse should also be approached initially as transient incontinence. Some patients with established causes of urinary incontinence have developed strategies for staying dry, such as staying near toilet facilities or reducing fluid intake. However, the problem may become acute if a patient becomes immobile, develops an acute infection, or begins a new medication. If incontinence persists despite correction of obviously contributing factors, a thorough evaluation

is requisite. Several types of incontinence may be present concurrently.

Table 29.1
Identification of Reversible Conditions That May Cause or Contribute to Urinary Incontinence

Conditions affecting the lower urinary tract
    Urinary tract infection (symptomatic with frequency, urgency, dysuria)
    Atrophic vaginitis or urethritis
    Prostatectomy
    Stool impaction
Drug side effects
    Diuretics: polyuria, frequency, urgency
    Caffeine: aggravation or precipitation of urinary incontinence
    Anticholinergic agents: urinary retention, overflow incontinence, stool impaction
    Psychotropic medications
        Antidepressants: anticholinergic actions, sedation
        Antipsychotics: anticholinergic actions, sedation, immobility, rigidity
        Sedatives, hypnotics, CNS depressants: sedation, delirium, immobility, muscle relaxation
    Opioid analgesics: urinary retention, fecal impaction, sedation, delirium
    α-Adrenergic blockers: urethral relaxation
    α-Adrenergic agonists: urinary retention (found in many cold and diet over-the-counter preparations
    β-Adrenergic agonists: urinary retention
    Calcium channel blockers: urinary retention
    Alcohol: polyuria, frequency, urgency, sedation, delirium, immobility
Increased urine production
    Metabolic disorders (hyperglycemia, hypercalcemia)
    Excess fluid intake
    Volume overload
        Venous insufficiency with edema
        Congestive heart failure
Impaired ability or willingness to reach the toilet
    Delirium
    Chronic illness, injury; restraint that interferes with mobility
    Psychologic disorders

Modified from Fantl JA, Newman DK, Colling J, et al. Urinary Incontinence in Adults: Acute and Chronic Management. Clinical Practice Guideline 2 (1996 Update) (AHCPR 96–0682). Rockville, MD: US Department of Health and Human Services, Public Health Service, Agency for Health Care Policy and Research, March 1996.

Functional Incontinence

Most functional incontinence results from the inability of an otherwise continent person to reach the toilet in time because of physical, pharmacologic, psychogenic, or environmental factors. Severe joint pain, muscle weakness, immobility, decreased visual acuity, and an inability to articulate the need to void are the primary physical causes of functional incontinence. Common medication classes that can precipitate urinary incontinence include diuretics, sedative-hypnotics, and anticholinergics. Theoretically, β-adrenergic agonists and calcium channel blockers may also impair proper bladder function, although this is infrequently observed. Functional incontinence may also result from lack of motivation (dementia, depression, or psychosis) or a history of frequent failure to reach the toilet in time (giving up). Environmental contributors include inconveniently located toilets, obstacles in the path to the toilet, and physical restraints.

Detrusor Instability (Urge Incontinence)

Detrusor instability, or urge incontinence, results from unsuppressed bladder contractions that are strong enough to overcome bladder outlet resistance and that generally result in involuntary bladder emptying. Transient causes of urge incontinence include local irritating processes such as urinary tract infection, inflammation from radiotherapy or chemotherapy, fecal impaction, and an enlarged prostate. Patients with detrusor instability usually present with frequent urination and nocturia associated with a loss of large urine volumes (more than 100 mL), although the history of urge incontinence is neither sensitive nor specific (9). An irresistible urge to void is a common complaint, but up to 20% of persons with detrusor instability do not have this symptom (10). Furthermore, patients with stress or overflow incontinence may also have urgency. Detrusor instability that causes frequent low-volume voiding may prompt patients to void on a schedule to avoid an accident. However, this maneuver may result in reduced bladder capacity and increased bladder tone. Detru-

sor instability may coexist with other types of incontinence.

Special categories of detrusor overactivity merit comment. Detrusor motor instability associated with a neurologic disorder is called detrusor hyperreflexia. Any insult to the structural integrity of the cholinergic inhibitory center of the CNS or the afferent innervation from the lower spinal cord where the reflex arc is located can cause detrusor hyperreflexia. Processes such as Alzheimer's disease, cerebrovascular atherosclerosis, multiple sclerosis, Parkinson's disease, spinal cord tumors or transection, and cervical spondylosis (among others) may result in incontinence by this mechanism (11). It still remains unclear whether these CNS disorders damage the central inhibitory pathways or impair the patient's overall functional capacity and ability to maintain normal urination (12). A subset of patients with a history suggesting urge incontinence may actually have detrusor hyperreflexia with impaired contractility (DHIC) associated with a bladder that empties about one third of its volume (13).

Outlet Obstruction and Atonic Bladder (Overflow Incontinence)

Anatomic obstruction to bladder emptying in men occurs primarily because of prostatic hypertrophy, prostatic neoplasm, or urethral stricture. Less commonly, urethral stricture or severe bladder prolapse impedes urine flow in women. Partial obstruction may become complete with the use of anticholinergic or α-agonist pharmacologic agents or with constipation. Low spinal cord lesions, diabetic or alcoholic neuropathy, and prescription of muscle relaxants, opioids, or antidepressants that block the cholinergic-induced contraction of the detrusor muscle may result in urinary retention.

The clinical presentation of outlet obstruction or atonic bladder can be urine loss due to overflow incontinence. Symptoms of frequent dribbling after urination or urgency to urinate may predominate. Patients may be found to have an enlarged, palpable bladder. This specific finding is not very sensitive for establishing the diagnosis of outlet obstruction. Patients may strain to urinate, and voluntarily and involuntarily voided urine volumes are frequently small.

Sphincter Insufficiency and Pelvic Floor Weakness (Stress Incontinence)

Stress incontinence occurs most commonly in women due to a hypermobile urethra, sphincter insufficiency, or reduced support by the pelvic floor musculature in the bladder outlet. Multiple childbirth, gynecologic surgery, and decreased effects of estrogen on pelvic tissues, vasculature, and urethral mucosa are probable contributory causes. Sphincter weakness may also be the result of urethral inflammation, neurologic disease, radiation therapy, or α-blocking drugs such as prazosin or methyldopa. In men, stress incontinence occurs less often, usually in those who have sustained sphincter or nerve trauma during prostatectomy.

Patients are likely to complain of losing small amounts of urine with coughing, straining, lifting, or changing posture. While this history is highly sensitive, it is only moderately specific, and many patients with these symptoms do not have stress incontinence (9). Nocturia is an uncommon complaint in the person with stress incontinence, but urgency may occur.

EVALUATION

The evaluation of the elderly incontinent patient should begin with a careful history directed at understanding the nature, severity, and burden of the problem and identifying the most easily remedied contributing causes of incontinence. Focus should be placed on urinary symptoms, noting onset and duration of incontinence, frequency, amount of urine lost per episode, and any contributing factors. An incontinence chart or diary that can be filled out before the patient's visit is an important means of documenting each episode.

A history of leakage occurring immediately following coughing, laughing, or posture change may have good positive predictive value in diagnosing stress incontinence (14). Classic symptoms of urge incontinence, such as urine loss with hand washing, hearing running water, or while rushing to the bathroom, are insensitive and nonspecific (14). Dysuria and frequency may indicate infection. A decrease in force of the urine stream and straining with urination suggest obstruction. An inability to stop urine flow voluntarily suggests pelvic muscle weakness. A low score on a mental status screening examination suggests dementia, which may be associated with detrusor instability, indifference to the symptoms, or both.

Important items of the medical history include data about childbirth, pelvic surgery, cancer, neurologic disease, diabetes mellitus, congestive heart failure, and previous treatment of urinary incontinence. Specific questions should be asked about mobility, prescription and over-the-counter medication use, alcohol use, and excessive fluid intake. Inquiries should be made about the physical layout of the patient's residence and whether impaired mobility limits access to toilet facilities. The patient should bring a bag containing all prescription and nonprescription drugs to the clinic so that medications that may contribute to incontinence can be identified.

The physical examination of patients with urinary incontinence should focus on the abdomen and urogenital, central, and peripheral nervous systems. The finding of a palpable bladder suggests outlet obstruction or an atonic bladder, yet this sign may be absent when the patient has significant postvoid residual volume (PVR). The rectal examination may reveal fecal impaction, a pelvic mass, or an enlarged prostate gland. The size of the prostate does not correlate well with obstruction (15). An important component of the physical examination of the patient with urinary incontinence is the assessment of perianal sensation and the patient's ability to contract and relax the anal sphincter voluntarily. An abnormal clinical sign such as sacral anesthesia or reduced anal sphincter tone can suggest potentially serious, even emergency lumbosacral disease. In women, a pelvic examination is indicated to assess urethral, uterine, or bladder prolapse and to evaluate the patient for any pelvic mass. A gray, dry vaginal mucosa may indicate lack of estrogen.

In women, a major diagnostic dilemma is to differentiate between urge incontinence and stress incontinence. In men, the primary distinction is between overflow incontinence and urge incontinence. Most studies show a poor correlation between the underlying cause and the patient's symptoms. Incontinence from several causes (mixed incontinence) in many older people limits the usefulness of evaluation algorithms based on symptoms and signs alone (16).

DIAGNOSTIC TESTS

Selected tests have generally been recommended for the evaluation of most incontinent patients. Obtaining a urinalysis and/or a urine culture is a standard part of the evaluation of the patient with incontinence. Properly collected clean-catch urine is adequate for culture even in the nursing home (17). While an unlikely yet serious cause of new incontinence is bladder carcinoma causing irritation, urine cytology is not recommended in the routine evaluation of the incontinent patient (8) as a screening test. Cystoscopy for bladder carcinoma should be used for patients with persistent hematuria and no indication of infection or renal disease. Blood testing (blood urea nitrogen, creatinine, glucose, and calcium) is recommended if compromised renal function or polyuria is suspected in patients not taking diuretics (8).

The PVR should be measured in all patients with symptoms of incontinence. This can be done by inserting a 14-Fr straight catheter into the bladder in sterile fashion or with the use of a bladder ultrasound scan 5 to 10 minutes after the patient has voided. Caution is indicated for patients with outflow obstruction, as a single catheterization may cause infection. Portable ultrasound has been shown to be highly reliable, especially at low and very high bladder volumes, and it may be considered for PVR determination (18). Although the definition of high PVR is controversial, a return of 200 mL or more suggests either obstruction or atonic bladder and is an indication for further urologic evaluation (8).

Clinical tests for stress incontinence in women are useful and highly specific (19). With a full bladder and wearing a preweighed pad, the patient should cough, laugh, or strain to induce urine leakage. The patient then voids, the urine volume is measured, and the pad is weighed. This test should be repeated if the urine volume in the pad and pan is less than 200 mL.

A bedside bladder-filling test has been proposed by several investigators to evaluate bladder capacity and to detect detrusor instability (20,

21). This test is usually performed after catheterization for PVR. Resistance to passage of the catheter provides information suggesting stricture or low obstruction. A 50-mL syringe without plunger attached to the catheter is held 15 cm above the pubic symphysis and filled gravitationally in 50-mL increments until the urge to void is noted by the patient. Filling is continued in 25-mL increments until involuntary contractions cause a rise in fluid level in the syringe or the patient notes feeling completely full. In one study of 171 older patients, mostly women, bedside cystometry had 75% sensitivity and 79% specificity for detrusor instability, compared with multichannel cystometry (21). The limitations of bedside cystometry include (*a*) inability to exclude detrusor hyperactivity completely; and (*b*) inability to diagnose impaired detrusor contractility and delayed emptying, which is thought to be an important cause of incontinence in nursing home populations. Also, stress and urge incontinence may not need to be fully characterized prior to prescribing treatment such as pelvic muscle exercises or scheduled voiding (13).

Formal Urodynamic Testing

After the basic evaluation, treatment for the presumed type of incontinence should be initiated unless there is an indication for further evaluation (8). Further evaluation is indicated for the following reasons: if the initial treatment fails, a history of surgery or radiotherapy, frequent urinary tract infections, marked prolapse on physical examination, severe hesitancy, PVR greater than 200 mL, inability to pass a catheter; or persistent hematuria (22). Common urodynamic tests that provide more detailed diagnostic information include urine flowmetry, voiding cystourethrography, multichannel cystometrogram, pressure flow study, urethral pressure profile measurement, and sphincter electromyography (8). A urologist or gynecologist generally performs these tests.

TREATMENT

Accurate diagnosis of urinary incontinence is essential for appropriate treatment. Any cause of transient incontinence identified during evaluation should be addressed specifically. Behavioral, pharmacologic, and surgical therapies are all effective in older people. It is generally advisable to begin a treatment regimen with the least risk and burden to the patient and caregiver. In all types of incontinence except those characterized by overflow (obstructed or atonic bladder), behavioral technique should be considered as first-line therapy unless the patient has a specific preference for another type of therapy (8).

Functional Treatment

Successful treatment of functional incontinence relies on recognition that physical, pharmacologic, psychologic, or environmental problems exist and can cause or worsen urinary incontinence. Providing the patient with assistive devices such as a urinal or bedside commode; reassessing drug indications, doses, and schedules; treating depression; addressing hostility; eliminating barriers in the path to the toilet; and removing restraints may improve incontinence dramatically. Timed voiding schedules are particularly useful in the cognitively impaired or physically disabled patient.

Detrusor Instability

The treatment of detrusor instability entails designing interventions to decrease or block uninhibited bladder contractions, improve bladder capacity, and prolong the time from symptoms of urgency to voiding. Behavioral and pharmacologic therapies are the mainstays of treatment. Behavioral techniques include bladder training or retraining, habit training, and pelvic muscle exercises with and without biofeedback. Bladder training comprises an educational program, scheduled voiding, and positive reinforcement to train the patient to resist sensations of urgency, postpone voiding, and urinate on a fixed timetable. A randomized, controlled study of bladder training in women diagnosed with urinary incontinence reported that 75% of the subjects reduced incontinent episodes by half and 12% became continent (23).

Habit training (timed voiding) also requires that the patient void according to a timetable. Using this method, the patient is taught to resist symptoms of urgency. In one controlled nursing home-based trial, 86% of subjects had significantly decreased frequency of incontinent episodes over 3 months (24). Prompted voiding is a technique requiring a caregiver to check for wetness at rou-

tine intervals and to prompt the patient to void. This is effective in dependent and cognitively impaired nursing home or home care patients, provided they can recognize some degree of bladder fullness or the need to void or can ask for assistance and respond when prompted to toilet (25).

Pelvic muscle exercises, or Kegel exercises, can reduce symptoms of urgency and prevent urge incontinence through feedback inhibition from the pelvic floor to the detrusor muscle (26). These techniques may be used with or without biofeedback with good results in reducing incontinence (27), yet many patients require repeated guidance in performing these exercises properly to obtain the maximal benefit. Only 50% of patients who had a single, simple verbal instruction in Kegel exercises were able to perform the technique properly (28). Bladder-sphincter biofeedback techniques record bladder, vaginal, and rectal pressures or electrical activity and display the information for the patient, who learns techniques to relax the bladder and contract pelvic floor muscles as reflected in changes measured by pressures or electrical activity. These procedures require insertion of sensors and the service of a trained technician. Biofeedback in conjunction with bladder retraining has been shown to be effective in teaching voluntary inhibition of detrusor contractions to selected patients, achieving 50% or greater improvement in incontinence. This approach is most useful for patients who are mobile and who have minimal cognitive impairment. Electrical stimulation via the sacral reflex arc has also been used to inhibit detrusor hyperactivity in selected patients (8).

Pharmacologic therapy has proved useful for many patients with detrusor instability. Anticholinergic agents are first-line drug therapy for these patients, and oxybutynin is the agent of choice. The dosage demonstrated to be effective in clinical trials is 2.5 to 5 mg 3 times a day, although some elderly patients benefit at a much lower dosage. Tolterodine, a muscarinic receptor antagonist, was found to be as effective as oxybutynin in double-blind studies but had a lower incidence and decreased severity of dry mouth. As with oxybutynin, tolterodine should not be used in patients with narrow-angle glaucoma or urinary retention. Other drugs observed in clinical trials to be beneficial include dicyclomine hydrochloride, propantheline, and tricyclic antidepressants, such as imipramine, doxepin, desipramine, and nortriptyline. Treatments recommended in the Agency for Health Care Policy and Research (AHCPR) 1996 clinical practice guideline *Urinary Incontinence in Adults* for treatment of detrusor instability are listed in Table 29.2. Only oxybutynin and flavoxate have been approved officially by the FDA for this use, and flavoxate is no longer a recommended treatment (8).

Sphincter Insufficiency and Pelvic Muscle Weakness

Behavioral, drug, and surgical therapies are all useful in treating stress incontinence. Kegel exercises are beneficial for strengthening the pelvic floor muscles and are recommended as first-line therapy for treatment of stress incontinence because of their effectiveness and lack of side effects. Patients must be properly taught the exercise in order to avoid performing a Valsalva maneuver, as the increased abdominal pressure might make the urine loss worse. A series of muscle contractions held for 3 to 10 seconds with 10-second rest periods in between are repeated 20 to 30 times, 3 times a day for at least 8 weeks (8). One study reported improvement in incontinence symptoms in 54% and cure in 16% of elderly women subjects (29). The use of conical vaginal weights that are squeezed by the patient may improve the effectiveness of Kegel exercises in selected patients (30). Electrical stimulation may also be useful for some patients, especially those who have difficulty in properly identifying their pelvic floor muscles or patients with very weak pelvic muscles.

Since sphincter contraction is mediated by α-adrenergic activity, drugs that stimulate α-receptors are the mainstays of treatment for stress incontinence. The most widely used α-adrenergic agonist is phenylpropanolamine, and the main contraindication to its use is hypertension. The recommended dose is 25 to 100 mg of the sustained-release preparation twice daily by mouth. Use of phenylpropanolamine has been shown to improve 30 to 60% versus placebo response in patients with stress incontinence. Estrogen has direct effects on urethral mucosa and periurethral tissues in women. While meta-analysis has shown estrogen therapy to reduce stress incontinence in women (31), estrogen given in hormonal replacement doses was not shown to be effective in reducing frequency or volume of urine loss in one recent trial (32). Estrogen may be a useful adjunct given orally or vaginally when single-drug therapy with an α-adrenergic agonist has proved inadequate (8). If long-term therapy with estrogen is planned, continuous daily dosing or cycling medroxyprogesterone (Provera) 2.5 to 10 mg daily should be given simultaneously to women with an intact uterus (Table 29.2).

When conservative therapy has failed, surgery may be appropriate. In patients with urethral hypermobility, retropubic or needle suspension of the urethrovesical junction is the procedure of choice, and cure rates of 78 to 84% have been reported (8). For intrinsic sphincter deficiency, periurethral bulking injections with collagen (less frequently with Teflon) that cause an increase in outlet resistance are recommended as first-line surgical treatment for women with stress incontinence who do not have coexisting urethral hypermobility. Urethral insufficiency is rare in men. Periurethral bulking injections and artificial sphincter implantation, which allows the patient to use a pump in the scrotal sac to inflate and deflate a balloon around the urethra, may be appropriate in severe cases (8).

Outflow Obstruction

For men with moderate to severe obstruction due to prostate enlargement, surgery is the treatment of choice. Terazosin (Hytrin), an α-adrenergic antagonist, minimizes symptoms related to prostatism (33), and possibly finasteride (Proscar) has a role, but neither is the treatment of choice where there is urinary retention. Transurethral prostatectomy has a high cure rate for patients with properly functioning bladders. Women with a significant cystocele may require surgical repair. In these patients, full evaluation, including urodynamic testing, prior to surgery is essential to rule out coexisting causes of incontinence.

Atonic Bladder

Smooth muscle contractions may occur in patients with atonic bladder in response to cholinergic agonists such as bethanechol. Patients respond to doses of 10 to 30 mg 3 or 4 times a day.

Table 29.2

Therapeutic Modalities in Urinary Incontinence

Type of Incontinence	Strongly Recommended Therapies	Potentially Useful Therapies
Urge		
Behavior therapy	Diet, fluid management Bladder training PME	Pelvic floor electrical stimulation PME with biofeedback

Drug therapy	First line
	  Oxybutynin; starting dose,
	    2.5 mg bid; target dose, up
	    to 5 mg tid
	  Tolterodine; starting dose,
	    1 mg bid; target dose,
	    up to 2 mg bid
	Second line
	  Propantheline; starting dose,
	    15 mg tid; target dose, up to
	    30 mg tid
		Imipramine; starting dose 10 mg hs;
		  target dose, up to 25–50 mg hs
		Dicyclomine; starting dose, 10 mg tid;
		  target dose, up to 20 mg tid

Stress		
Behavior therapy	PME, bladder training	

Drug therapy	First line (should not use in
	  patients with hypertension)
	Phenylpropanolamine; starting
	  dose, 25 mg SR bid; target
	  dose, 75 mg SR bid
		Adjunctive therapy
		
		Conjugated estrogen[a] (women); oral
		  starting dose, 0.3 mg–0.625 mg qd;
		  target dose up to 0.625 mg qd;
		  intravaginal starting dose, 0.5 g qd;
		  target dose, up to 1 g qd
		Imipramine; starting dose, 10 mg
		  hs; target dose, up to 25–50 mg hs
		Hypermobility
		  Anterior vaginal repair
		Intrinsic sphincter deficiency
		  Artificial sphincter

Surgery	Hypermobility
	  Retropubic suspension
	  Needle bladder neck suspension
	Intrinsic sphincter deficiency
	  Sling procedure
	  Periurethral bulking agents	

Overflow	Correction of cause of overflow
	  Surgical procedure to relieve
	  obstruction
		Intermittent catheterization
		Indwelling catheter

Functional	Address underlying cause	Timed voiding schedules

Modified from Fantl JA, Newman DK, Colling J, et al. Urinary Incontinence in Adults: Acute and Chronic Management. Clinical Practice Guideline 2 (1996 Update) (AHCPR 96–0682). Rockville, MD: US Department of Health and Human Services, Public Health Service, Agency for Health Care Policy and Research, March 1996.

PME, pelvic muscle exercises; SR, sustained release.

[a]Progestin (medroxyprogesterone 2.5 to 10 mg/day) continuously or intermittently for women with intact uterus.

Literature does not support the use of bethanechol longer than a month (34). In patients with milder dysfunction, scheduled voiding may be useful. In patients with severe neurologic deficits, intermittent clean catheterization every 2 to 4 hours by the patient or caregiver is often the best management. If this is not possible or practical, an indwelling catheter may be necessary. To reduce the frequency of complications, including urolithiasis, symptomatic bacteriuria, periurethral abscess, and acute pyelonephritis, the use of chronic indwelling catheters is generally not encouraged. Appropriate management of an indwelling catheter depends on proper insertion using sterile technique and maintaining a closed sterile system. Urethral cleansing, routine bladder irrigation, and prophylactic antibiotic therapy should be avoided (35), as these procedures do not prevent bladder colonization and are likely to result in the selection of resistant organisms. Overflow incontinence due to a hyporeflexic bladder is generally poorly responsive to behavioral or pharmacologic therapy. Surgery is not indicated.

SUMMARY

Urinary incontinence remains a common, underreported, and costly problem in elderly patients. However, new therapeutic options using behavioral, pharmacologic, and surgical approaches can lead to symptomatic improvements or cure of this important clinical problem and increased comfort for the patient.

REFERENCES

1. Herzog AR, Fultz NH. Prevalence and incidence of urinary incontinence in community-dwelling populations. J Am Geriatr Soc 1990;38:273–281.
2. Brown JS, Seeley DG, Fong J, et al. Urinary incontinence in older women: who is at risk? Study of Osteoporotic Fractures Research Group. Obstet Gynecol 1996;87:715–721.
3. Palmer MH, German PS, Ouslander JG. Risk factors for urinary incontinence one year after nursing home admission. Res Nurs Health 1991;14:405–412.
4. Tinetti ME, Inouye SK, Gill TM, Doucette JT. Shared risk factors for falls, incontinence, and functional dependence: unifying the approach to geriatric syndromes. JAMA 1995;273:1348–1353.
5. Wetle T, Scherr P, Branch LG, et al. Difficulty with holding urine among older persons in a geographically de-

fined community: prevalence and correlates. J Am Geriatr Soc 1995;43:349–355.
6. Burgio KL, Ives DG, Locher JL, et al. Treatment seeking for urinary incontinence in older adults. J Am Geriatr Soc 1994;42:208–212.
7. UmLauf MG, Goode S, Burgio KL. Psychosocial issues in geriatric urology: problems in treatment and treatment seeking. Urol Clin North Am 1996;23:127–136.
8. Fantl JA, Newman DK, Colling J, et al. Urinary Incontinence in Adults: Acute and Chronic Management. Clinical Practice Guideline 2 (1996 Update) (AHCPR 96–0682). Rockville, MD: US Department of Health and Human Services, Public Health Service, Agency for Health Care Policy and Research, March 1996.
9. Summitt RL Jr, Stovall TG, Bent AE, Ostergard DR. Urinary incontinence: correlation of history and brief office evaluation with multichannel urodynamic testing. Am J Obstet Gynecol 1992;166:1835–1840 (discussion 1840–1844).
10. Resnick NM, Yalla SV, Laurino E. The pathophysiology of urinary incontinence among institutionalized elderly persons. N Engl J Med 1989;320:1–7 (see comments).
11. Brocklehurst J, Dillane J. Studies of the female bladder in old age: 2. Cystometrograms in 100 incontinent women. Gerontol Clin 1966;8:306–319.
12. DuBeau CE, Resnick NM. Urinary incontinence and dementia: the perils of guilt by association. J Am Geriatr Soc 1995;43:310–311 (editorial; comment).
13. Resnick NM, Yalla SV. Detrusor hyperactivity with impaired contractile function: an unrecognized but common cause of incontinence in elderly patients. JAMA 1987;257:3076–3081.
14. Bergman A, Bader K. Reliability of the patient's history in the diagnosis of urinary incontinence. Int J Gynaecol Obstet 1990;32:255–259.
15. Frimodt Moller PC, Jensen KM, Iversen P, et al. Analysis of presenting symptoms in prostatism. J Urol 1984;132:272–276.
16. DuBeau CE, Resnick NM. Evaluation of the causes and severity of geriatric incontinence: a critical appraisal. Urol Clin North Am 1991;18:243–256.
17. Ouslander JG, Schapira M, Schnelle JF. Urine specimen collection from incontinent female nursing home residents. J Am Geriatr Soc 1995;43:279–281.
18. Ouslander JG, Simmons S, Tuico E, et al. Use of a portable ultrasound device to measure post-void residual volume among incontinent nursing home residents. J Am Geriatr Soc 1994;42:1189–1192.
19. Diokno AC, Normolle DP, Brown MB, Herzog AR. Urodynamic tests for female geriatric urinary incontinence. Urology 1990;36:431–439.
20. Sutherst JR, Brown MC. Comparison of single and multichannel cystometry in diagnosing bladder instability. BMJ (Clin Res Ed) 1984;288:1720–1722.
21. Ouslander J, Leach G, Abelson S, et al. Simple versus multichannel cystometry in the evaluation of bladder function in an incontinent geriatric population. J Urol 1988;140:1482–1486.

22. Kane RL, Ouslander JG, Abrass IB. Essentials of Clinical Geriatrics. New York: McGraw-Hill, 1989.

23. Fantl JA, Wyman JF, McClish DK, et al. Efficacy of bladder training in older women with urinary incontinence. JAMA 1991;265:609–613.

24. Jarvis GJ. A controlled trial of bladder drill and drug therapy in the management of detrusor instability. Br J Urol 1981;53:565–566.

25. Schnelle JF. Treatment of urinary incontinence in nursing home patients by prompted voiding. J Am Geriatr Soc 1990;38:356–360.

26. Nygaard IE, Kreder KJ, Lepic MM, et al. Efficacy of pelvic floor muscle exercises in women with stress, urge, and mixed urinary incontinence. Am J Obstet Gynecol 1996;174:120–125.

27. Burgio KL, Robinson JC, Engel BT. The role of biofeedback in Kegel exercise training for stress urinary incontinence. Am J Obstet Gynecol 1986;154:58–64.

28. Bump RC, Hurt WG, Fantl JA, Wyman JF. Assessment of Kegel pelvic muscle exercise performance after brief verbal instruction. Am J Obstet Gynecol 1991;165:322–327 (discussion 327–329).

29. Burns PA, Pranikoff K, Nochajski T, et al. Treatment of stress incontinence with pelvic floor exercises and biofeedback. J Am Geriatr Soc 1990;38:341–344.

30. Olah KS, Bridges N, Denning J, Farrar DJ. The conservative management of patients with symptoms of stress incontinence: a randomized, prospective study comparing weighted vaginal cones and interferential therapy. Am J Obstet Gynecol 1990;162:87–92.

31. Fantl JA, Cardozo L, McClish DK. Estrogen therapy in the management of urinary incontinence in postmenopausal women: a meta-analysis. First report of the Hormones and Urogenital Therapy Committee. Obstet Gynecol 1994;83:12–18.

32. Fantl JA, Bump RC, Robinson D, et al. Efficacy of estrogen supplementation in the treatment of urinary incontinence. The Continence Program for Women Research Group. Obstet Gynecol 1996;88:745–749.

33. Lepor H, Williford WO, Barry MJ, et al. The efficacy of terazosin, finasteride, or both in benign prostatic hyperplasia. Veterans Affairs Cooperative Studies Benign Prostatic Hyperplasia Study Group. N Engl J Med 1996;335:533–539 (see comments).

34. Ouslander J. Urinary incontinence. In: Hazzard W, Andres R, Bierman E, Blass J, eds. Principles of Geriatric Medicine and Gerontology. 3rd ed. New York: McGraw-Hill, 1990;1123–1142.

35. Wong E. Guidelines for Prevention of Catheter-Associated Urinary Tract Infections. Philadelphia: Saunders, 1974.

Geriatric Gynecology

As American women live longer and maintain health and vitality into advanced age, it is important for both patients and physicians to remain vigilant regarding detection of early disease and promotion of optimum health. Gynecologic care can be an area overlooked because of focus on a patient's other chronic disease states. Attitudes of both patients and physicians regarding sexuality, incontinence, and genital problems may also be barriers to appropriate gynecologic care. Conflicting recommendations from authoritative groups regarding intervals for cervical and breast cancer screening can leave patients and physicians confused about when to perform and when to discontinue regular Pap smears and mammograms. If routine Pap screening is discontinued, there may be a tendency to discontinue genital examinations entirely, resulting in missed diagnoses of vulvar, vaginal, cervical, uterine, ovarian, bladder, urethral, rectal, and colon disorders.

The average life expectancy at birth for an American woman in the 1990s is 77 years, 5 years longer than for men. But if a woman reaches menopause, it is probable she will live an additional 30 years (1). Issues related to menopausal changes can become a major concern for women and their physicians, especially during the perimenopausal period. Whether to prescribe hormone replacement and how to manage therapy are major issues. Managing premenopausal, perimenopausal, and postmenopausal symptoms and nontraditional approaches to menopause are becoming more interesting to patients and therefore to physicians who provide information, advice, and care.

If an older woman has gynecologic symptoms (e.g., postmenopausal vaginal bleeding, uterine prolapse, urinary incontinence, vulvar itching) the physician must be prepared to obtain a complete gynecologic history and perform an adequate genital, pelvic, and rectal examination. Certain special techniques may be required, as may a healthy index of suspicion for gynecologic problems.

HISTORY AND PHYSICAL EXAMINATION
Gynecologic History

Every woman should be queried regarding age of menarche, menstrual history (e.g., regularity, duration, flow, dysmenorrhea), age of menopause, menopausal symptoms (vasomotor, psychologic, and atrophic changes, cardiovascular disease, osteoporosis, disturbances of menstrual pattern), any history of postmenopausal bleeding, and hormone or other treatments for menopausal symptoms (e.g., over-the-counter hormones, herbs, nutritional supplements, and acupuncture). Any history of endometriosis, infertility, gynecologic cancer, and fibroids is also important. Asking about previous gynecologic surgery, especially hysterectomy and oophorectomy, is vital. Women who had hysterectomies prior to 1960 may have had a supracervical procedure and therefore should be examined for a remaining cervix. The reason for hysterectomy is important, as surgery for benign causes requires different Pap smear surveillance than surgery for uterine or cervical malignancy. Results of previous Pap smears are important, as is the date of the last Pap smear and frequency of prior screening.

A complete obstetric history is also necessary to assess risk of breast, ovarian, and uterine cancer and pelvic relaxation. Gravidity, parity, mode of delivery, and postpartum complications all are important information to the clinician. Sexual history should also be obtained. If the patient is sexually active, level of satisfaction and any specific concerns should be ascertained. Dyspareunia, bleeding after coitus, vaginal discharge, lack of lubrication, and genital pruritus can all be important symptoms requiring further evaluation and treatment. If the patient is not sexually active, questions about availability of relationships, partner issues regarding sexuality, masturbation, or lack of sexual interest may be important areas to explore with the patient.

It is important to discuss bowel and urinary symptoms, especially urinary incontinence, with older women. Because of social taboos, incontinence may not be an issue patients are comfortable in revealing without specific questioning, yet many types of urinary incontinence are treatable.

Physical Examination

Positioning a patient for a genital and pelvic examination is sometimes a challenge. Many elderly patients have musculoskeletal problems that limit external rotation of the hips, making the lithotomy position uncomfortable or impossible. Alternative positions include the left lateral decubitus position, in which the patient lies on her left side with both knees bent. An assistant holds the top leg up while the examiner inserts the speculum with the handle positioned posteriorly to the patient. The frog-leg position, in which the patient lies on her back with her feet together at the foot of the table, with her knees as far to the sides as possible, is another option. The speculum is inserted with the handle up. Placing an inverted bedpan covered by a towel under the sacrum may offer additional visualization by elevating the pelvis. The patient should empty her bladder prior to the pelvic examination.

Whatever position is used, the examiner begins with inspection of the external genitalia. Pubic hair becomes sparse postmenopausally, and atrophic skin changes of the vulva may be evident. Inspection for skin lesions, ulcerations, leukoplakia, bleeding, and infection precede the speculum examination. Most women with inadequate estrogen exhibit thinned and pale vaginal mucosa, and often urethral ectasia, in which internal urethral tissue has everted externally, giving the appearance of a hyperemic mass around the urethral opening. Palpation of the introitus for masses or tenderness is also important. Visual inspection and palpation for bladder or rectal prolapse and uterine descensus also take place prior to speculum or bimanual examination. Asking the patient to bear down or cough may accentuate these conditions.

Using the proper speculum for the patient's anatomy is critical. Many postmenopausal women have a stenotic introitus with a shortened vaginal vault, requiring the use of a narrow-blade Pederson speculum. A virginal speculum is sometimes necessary. If there is a great deal of tissue relaxation, a wide-blade Graves speculum may be needed. In any case, the speculum should be warmed, preferably with warm water, as lubricants introduced into the vagina may interfere with Pap smear interpretation. The introitus should be gently stretched with the examiner's gloved fingers and the speculum inserted gently. Often it is helpful to have the woman first tighten and then relax the pubococcygeus muscles, so that she can sense the amount of control she has over muscle tone (and therefore muscle relaxation) in this area. Often the patient relaxes when she can voluntarily control these muscles, and the examination is more comfortable for the patient. Once the speculum is in place, specimens from the ectocervix and endocervical canal can be obtained for Pap testing. In women with prolonged lack of estrogen, the cervix may be quite difficult to identify, as it thins out and flattens and can even become flush with the posterior vaginal wall. The vaginal mucosa is inspected as the speculum is withdrawn. Most frequently one finds pallor and thinning of the mucosa, with loss of the rugal folds normally found in younger women.

Finally, a bimanual vaginal and rectovaginal examination is performed. If palpation is especially difficult, a single finger in the vagina can be used. Any palpable ovarian tissue in a woman who is more than 3 years post menopause is abnormal and requires further investigation. Uterine size, position, and mobility are assessed. Masses or tenderness on rectal examination must be evaluated. Stool is tested for occult blood.

MENOPAUSE AND HORMONE REPLACEMENT THERAPY

A sentinel event for many women is the transition from the reproductive stage to the nonreproductive stage of life. Not only do major physiologic changes occur, but emotional, social and psychologic transitions take place as well. Some women have few if any physical or emotional symptoms during menopause, while others report major psychologic and organic changes. Strictly speaking, menopause is the total cessation of spontaneous menstrual periods, with complete failure of ovarian follicular development in the presence of adequate gonadotropin stimulation. It is determined in retrospect (for natural, not surgical menopause) after menses have ceased for 12 months. Climacteric is the perimenopausal period when the ovary progressively decreases estrogen production.

Symptoms of Menopause

There may be long or short ovulatory cycles during the climacteric, with unpredictable menstrual flow. Numerous vasomotor symptoms may begin during the climacteric phase and continue into menopause: hot flashes, a sudden feeling of warmth lasting 2.5 minutes, often followed by hot flushes, consisting of redness of the upper body, profuse sweating in some areas, surface temperature increased by 2.5°C, occurring within 1 minute and lasting up to 30 minutes. These symptoms often occur at night, causing insomnia. Other symptoms that frequently accompany menopause include fatigue, nervousness, depression, sweating, headaches, insomnia, irritability, dizziness, joint and muscle pain, and palpitations. The mean age of menopause in the United States is 51.4 years (2). Later symptoms of these hormonally mediated physiologic changes include atrophy (vaginal pain, itching, dryness, bleeding, dyspareunia, dysuria), osteoporosis, and cardiovascular disease.

Vasomotor symptoms occur in 80% of climacteric women, and up to 25% of women may have symptoms as long as 5 years after menopause.

Women with vasomotor symptoms have overall lower estrogen levels than those without symptoms. Those with lower body fat seem to have more symptoms, as do smokers (3). Vasomotor symptoms correspond to a surge in luteinizing hormone (LH) levels.

Hormonal Changes

In premenopausal women, the monthly surge of follicle-stimulating hormone (FSH) stimulates the development of 100 to 200 ovarian follicles. Only 1 follicle reaches maturity; the rest undergo atresia. But as they develop, the oocyte within each follicle enlarges, and the surrounding granulosa cells increase in number. As the follicles further enlarge, they accumulate a surrounding layer of interstitial theca cells. Under the influence of LH, the theca cells secrete steroid hormones, mainly the androgenic steroids testosterone and androstenedione. The follicular granulosa cells, under stimulation from FSH, convert these androgenic precursors to estrogen; estradiol, the principal human estrogen; and estrone, by aromatization. Thus the ovarian follicle has two major functions: production of mature germ cells and the secretion of active sex steroids.

The days of the menstrual cycle are numbered beginning with the first day of menstrual flow. During the follicular phase (the first 12 to 15 days of the cycle), the follicle destined for ovulation matures. In the latter half of the follicular phase, this follicle is the main source of estrogen, which provides a feedback loop to the pituitary and hypothalamus, where LH and FSH are stimulated. On about day 14 of the cycle, LH secretion peaks and ovulation is stimulated. The mature follicle transforms into a corpus luteum, which secretes large quantities of progesterone and estradiol, again under the influence of LH. Progesterone dominates the second half of the menstrual cycle, the luteal phase. The endometrium builds up a thick multilayered lining of straight glands during the follicular phase, and during the luteal phase it becomes secretory. Without implantation of a fertilized egg, the negative feedback effect of estrogen and progesterone inhibits the secretion of LH and the corpus luteum involutes. The endometrial lining is shed, and day 1 of the menstrual cycle begins again. Absent high levels of estrogen, FSH and LH levels rise and a new group of follicles begins to grow.

Estrogen acts not only on the genital tract and pituitary-hypothalamic axis but on many other tissues and organs. Peripheral actions of estrogen affect the development of breast tissue, subcutaneous fatty tissues, positive effect on lipoproteins, and positive calcium balance. Ovarian androgens are important in libido, mature body hair pattern, and maintaining sebaceous glands that keep skin and hair soft. While the adrenal glands also secrete estrogens and androgens, their primary estrogen is estrone, which is only about a third as potent as ovarian estradiol. Half of the biologically active circulating androgen in women comes from the adrenals (4).

As women reach their mid 40s, the number of follicles recruited to develop in each cycle decreases, and the plasma levels characteristic of the follicular phase begin to decline. Menstrual patterns begin to change, with variations in cycle length and bleeding volume. Incomplete luteinization following ovulation due to reduced follicular function earlier in the cycle can occur. This reduction in follicular function results in a short or inadequate luteal phase, low progesterone levels, and decreased fertility. Feedback to the pituitary at this stage results in gradually increasing FSH levels, resulting in failed ovulation, missed periods, and irregular bleeding. Finally, the number of available follicles drops, cyclic bleeding stops completely, FSH and LH levels remain elevated throughout the cycle, and estrogen, progesterone, and androgen levels fall. The transition from regular menstrual cycles to complete cessation of menses usually takes 1 to 2 years. This climacteric period is typically when hot flashes and other menopausal symptoms occur. By a year or so after menopause, the ovaries become fibrotic and contain no more follicles. Most of the physical and psychologic symptoms women undergo begin to dissipate. However, genital atrophy and adverse effects upon bones, lipid profile, hair, skin, and other body tissues and organs continue.

Diagnosing menopause is largely a clinical skill. The conventional diagnosis is 12 months without menstruation. Routine laboratory testing is usually not indicated. FSH and LH levels rise, FSH 10 to 20 times over premenopausal levels, and LH about 3 times premenopausal levels. In the perimenopausal period varying levels of FSH may be found, including high levels approximating those found in menopause. Nearly all of the sex steroids (estradiol, estriol, progesterone, testosterone, dehydroepiandrosterone, androstenedione) decline. Estrone, which is the steroid converted in adipose tissue by aromatization from androstenedione, declines less dramatically than the other sex hormones (5).

Hormone Replacement

When, how, and whether to replace female hormones continues to be an area of considerable controversy. Hormone replacement therapy (HRT) clearly resolves many of the vasomotor and psychologic symptoms encountered in the climacteric period for most women. There is very good evidence that HRT (especially estrogen replacement) prevents the acceleration of osteoporosis in aging women (6) and protects postmenopausal women from cardiovascular disease by elevating high-density lipoproteins (HDL), lowering low-density lipoproteins (LDL) (7), causing some degree of vasodilation, and activating antithrombotic factors in the blood. HRT also prevents genital tract atrophy and eliminates many of the symptoms and diseases that accompany these atrophic changes. There is new evidence to suggest that HRT can help delay the onset of Alzheimer's disease (8) and decrease the overall incidence of the disease.

Yet despite these major benefits, many women remain skeptical about using HRT (9) and worry about the risks of breast and endometrial cancer, hypertension, thromboembolic disease, cholelithiasis, and other as yet unknown side effects. Some patients and physicians wonder whether a natural condition of aging requires medical intervention, and many seek nonpharmacologic remedies for climacteric symptoms and pursue nondrug regimens for preventing osteoporosis and heart disease.

However, it has become standard to recommend HRT to women without contraindications to hormone therapy (Table 30.1). The U.S. Preventive Services Task Force recommends that

Table 30.1

Contraindications and Precautions to Estrogen Replacement Therapy

Absolute contraindications
  History of breast cancer
  Endometrial cancer
  Acute vascular thrombosis, or history of recurrent thrombosis
  Neuro-ophthalmologic vascular disease
  Acute liver disease
  Chronic impaired liver function
  Undiagnosed vaginal bleeding
Precautions; individualization required
  Posttreatment breast or endometrial cancer
  Difficult-to-control hypertension
  History of single thrombotic event
  Uterine leiomyomata
  Gallbladder disease
  Seizure disorders
  Hormone-sensitive migraine headaches
  Familial hyperlipidemia

physicians discuss the risks and benefits of HRT with all menopausal women so that the patient can make an informed decision (10).

A variety of estrogen and progestin compounds are available for prescription in the United States. It is now clear that all women with an intact uterus who take estrogen should take progestins too. The potential for endometrial overstimulation and development of endometrial hyperplasia and cancer are too great. Conversely, women treated with both an estrogen and a progestin actually have a lower incidence of endometrial cancer than those who are not treated with HRT (11). The questions for the patient and physician should be which hormone compounds, by what route, in what dose, with what timing, and for how long.

Patients who decide on hormonal therapy and do not have a uterus should use estrogen alone. For those with a uterus, however, combination therapy with estrogen and a progestin is required. Any of variety of regimens and combinations can be used. The most popular at this writing include daily continuous use of equine-derived conjugated estrogens 0.625 mg daily or 1 mg of oral micronized estradiol plus synthetic

medroxyprogesterone acetate (MPA) 2.5 mg daily. MPA is less androgenic than the other widely available oral progestin, norethindrone acetate. Norethindrone acetate, a component of many birth control pills, is rarely recommended for HRT regimens. The main goal of continuous therapy is amenorrhea, as irregular bleeding or the reinitiation of menses is a major reason for noncompliance. Withdrawal bleeding may occur during the first 6 months of continuous HRT, but endometrial sampling may be unnecessary during this initiation period.

Sequential therapy with conjugated estrogens or estradiol daily and at least 10 mg MPA for a minimum of 10 days monthly can also be used. Recommended sequential regimens usually include estrogen during days 1 through 25 of the month plus MPA on days 16 through 25. No hormone is taken day 25 through 30 or 31. Sequential regimens result in relatively predictable bleeding and can be used in the perimenopausal period, while a woman may still be menstruating. Vaginal bleeding during calendar days when the patient is on hormone therapy is an indication for endometrial biopsy. The patient may also have estrogen withdrawal symptoms during the days off estrogen. A combination of these approaches or continuous sequential HRT entails estrogen given daily throughout the month, with 5 mg MPA added during the first 2 weeks of the month. Most women have withdrawal bleeding on this regimen, and an endometrial sample should be taken if bleeding occurs prior to day 10 of the cycle.

Conjugated equine estrogens are sulfates of estrone, equilin, and equilenin. Native estrogens in the human woman, which are produced by aromatization of androgen precursors, are estrone (E_1), estradiol (E_2), and estriol (E_3). The physiologic potency of E_2 is the greatest, followed by E_1 (approximately one third the potency of E_2), with E_3 having the least hormonal activity. Estradiol is metabolized to estrone in the gastrointestinal tract. First-pass metabolism of estrogen in the liver also stimulates hepatocyte function, alters protein synthesis, and changes bile composition. These factors have implications for blood pressure control, risk of cholelithiasis, synthesis of clotting factors, and lipoprotein patterns. For these reasons some patients may find nonoral routes of estrogen administration preferable.

Available nonoral routes of administration include transdermal patches, vaginal creams, oral troches, and injection. Injections are rarely used today, and the popularity of transmucosal and transdermal delivery systems seem to be increasing. Transdermal delivery systems cause skin rash in about 15% of patients and are more expensive than oral preparations. Progestins can be given continuously via transmucosal (vaginal or oral troche) or oral routes.

Duration of treatment remains an unanswered question. Whenever HRT is discontinued, calcium loss proceeds rapidly. There is theoretically no objection to indefinite therapy as long as the patient remains free of side effects. The earlier HRT is started, the better for bone mineral density (12). There is little available information on the upper limit of age for starting HRT, although it appears that benefit occurs regardless of the starting age.

Although this is controversial, a small increase in the incidence of breast cancer may occur in patients using HRT, approximating a 10% additional risk over those not receiving HRT. It appears unlikely that HRT contributes significantly to hypertension, although nonoral routes may be preferable for those with preexisting hypertension, because stimulation of angiotensinogen estrogen may contribute to blood pressure elevation.

Alternative Therapies

Some women find relief from vasomotor symptoms and decreased libido from androgens (methyltestosterone 1.25 to 2.5 mg daily by mouth) or estrogen-testosterone combinations; however, androgens may have deleterious effects on the lipid profile and can cause masculinization with long-term use. Bellergal (phenobarbital, ergotamine, belladonna alkaloids) 1 tablet in the morning and at noon and two at bedtime has been useful for some women's hot flashes (13). Clonidine 0.1 mg by mouth 3 times daily or a clonidine patch has been used for the hot flashes associated with treatment for breast and prostate cancer and for climacteric vasomotor symptoms (14). Progesterone-only therapy may be useful for some women, especially those with contraindications to estrogen (Table 30.1). While this regimen may have deleterious effects on the lipid profile (15), it may inhibit bone resorption and promote bone formation, and thus reduce the risk of osteoporosis (16). Vasomotor headaches associated with menopause may be treated with a variety of approaches similar to those for vascular migraines, including verapamil hydrochloride, starting at 80 mg per day. There is reasonable evidence that physical exercise may reduce the frequency of hot flashes postmenopausally (17) and that relaxation training can be efficacious in the treatment of hot flashes and psychologic symptoms of menopause (18).

The popular literature is replete with books recommending a variety of "natural" approaches to managing menopausal symptoms, preventing and reversing osteoporosis, and maximizing cardiac health. Herbal remedies such as evening primrose oil (containing gamolenic acid) are marketed for hot flashes (19), as well as black cohosh, touted for its estrogenic activity (20). Dong quai, which contains numerous coumarin derivatives having mild antispasmodic activity as well as phytoestrogens, is consumed by thousands if not millions of women worldwide to treat a variety of gynecologic problems, including menopausal symptoms. Unfortunately, there is minimal scientific evidence that these herbs have any significant therapeutic effect (20, 21). Ayurvedic and homeopathic (22) remedies for menopause have been used by many patients for years, apparently without ill effects. While many of these modalities may hold promise, they have been underevaluated, and much more study is needed.

Natural progesterone creams, transmucosal troches, and plant sources of edible natural estrogens and progesterone for all the benefits of HRT without the risks of synthetic estrogen and progesterone are recommended by several popular authors (23–26). Such literature reflects a prevailing philosophy that plant-derived estrogens and progestins ("phytohormones") are more physiologic and can be obtained through proper diet and nutritional supplementation with foods high in estrogen (such as soybeans and their byproducts). Such plant products are high in estriol, which mimics human estriol activity, and contain other compounds that block access to procarcinogenic receptors, thus decreasing the risk of breast and endometrial cancer. Dehydroepiandrosterone (DHEA) is another hormone touted for many purposes, including being a precursor to both estrogens and androgens and therefore valuable for the management of menopausal states (27). While positive anecdotal testimonials abound, to date there have been only a few small studies of natural hormones and DHEA. It is hoped that we will soon see rigorous studies of these promising modalities.

POSTMENOPAUSAL VAGINAL BLEEDING AND UTERINE CANCER

Endometrial cancer is the most common gynecologic cancer, the incidence rising significantly after age 45 and peaking between ages 55 and 69 (28). Fortunately, endometrial cancer is often discovered at an earlier stage than many other gynecologic cancers, and is often cured with surgery, sometimes combined with irradiation. Approximately 75% of women with endometrial cancer present with vaginal bleeding, which is generally the only symptom of the disease. Table 30.2 lists risk factors for endometrial cancer.

Bleeding from the genital tract after menopause is a worrisome symptom, since approximately 10 to 20% of postmenopausal bleeding is due to malignancy, the likelihood increasing with age (29). Women should be instructed to report incidents of such bleeding to their health care provider, whether it is slight spotting or frank bleeding, since there is no correlation between amount of bleeding and stage of disease. With more women being prescribed hormone replacement therapy during and after menopause, there

Table 30.2

Risk Factors for Endometrial Cancer

Nulliparity
Age > 50 years
Age at menopause > 52 years
Unopposed estrogen therapy
Obesity
History of endometrial hyperplasia or adenomatous
  hyperplasia
Pelvic irradiation

is an increase in the incidence of postmenopausal vaginal bleeding. It is important to remember that there are many causes for a complaint of "vaginal" bleeding, some of which are not even genital. Table 30.3 lists a variety of causes of bleeding after menopause.

Evaluation of Postmenopausal Bleeding

Obviously, a thorough history and physical examination are needed for complaints of bleeding. The pattern, amount, and frequency of bleeding are important. It is important to ascertain any previous evaluation for postmenopausal bleeding and history of abnormal bleeding before menopause. Any history of vulvar or vaginal trauma is needed, as well as solicitation of other associated symptoms: dryness, pruritus, discharge, or vulvar lesions. An overall gynecologic and sexual history is in order, as well as any previous surgery, radiation exposure, prior Pap smear results, systemic diseases, and family history of gynecologic cancers. Of course, knowledge about medications the patient is taking, especially hormones, is vital.

Physical examination should include evaluation of the abdomen, back, and flank and rectal examination in addition to a complete genital and pelvic examination. The genital examination should pay particular attention to any obvious site of bleeding; skin lesions; vaginal atrophy and discharge; cervical friability and lesions; uterine size, mobility, tenderness, and surface contour; and ovarian size and tenderness.

Laboratory evaluation should include hemoglobin assessment, urinalysis, stool for occult blood, Pap smear, and evaluation of cervical and vaginal specimens for infection as indicated. Any suspicious lesions of the vulva, vagina, or cervix should be biopsied. If the bleeding is obviously uterine and the patient is *not* on HRT, endometrial biopsy should be undertaken. Newer techniques for evaluating vaginal bleeding, such as endometrial biopsy using a flexible plastic sampling device, have become safe, effective first-line office procedures for evaluating postmenopausal bleeding (30) and have essentially replaced dilation and curettage as a first-line diagnostic test for most patients.

Table 30.3
Causes of Postmenopausal Bleeding

Vulvar
    Angioma
    Ulceration, inflammation
    Vulvar dystrophy
    Condyloma
    Vulvar intraepithelial neoplasia
    Vulvar cancer
    Trauma
Urinary tract
    Urethra: ectasia, inflammation, tumor
    Bladder infection, malignancy, stone, polyp
    Ureter stone, malignancy
    Kidney stone, malignancy
Vaginal
    Atrophic vaginitis
    Angioma
    Ulceration, infection (vaginitis)
    Malignancy
    Vaginal intraepithelial neoplasia
    Trauma
    Condyloma
Cervical
    Irritation, infection
    Malignancy (squamous cell or adenocarcinoma)
    Dysplasia
    Polyp
    Condyloma
    Trauma
Uterine
    Endometrial hyperplasia
    Endometrial adenomyosis, polyp
    Endometrial malignancy
    Endometrial atrophy
    Endometritis
    Estrogen excess (exogenous, or adrenal or ovarian
        tumor)
    Other (e.g., sarcoma, fibroids)
Rectal
    Hemorrhoids
    Fissure
    Vascular lesion
    Malignancy
Other
    Tubal or ovarian malignancy
    Bleeding diathesis

The native postmenopausal endometrium is generally 1 mm or less. It is estimated that approximately half of women taking hormone replacement have an endometrial thickness of 4 to 5 mm. The most important finding in evaluating endometrial tissue is the degree of cellularity. More cellular tissue, which correlates with hyperplasia and cancer, is diagnosed by the gross amount of tissue found during sampling, ultrasound, and microscopic evaluation of endometrial tissue. If the endometrial sample is abnormal, further diagnosis and treatment are needed. If the sample is adequate and no disease is found, the workup is completed. Repeat endometrial biopsy should be undertaken for additional episodes of bleeding. If the sample is inadequate for diagnosis and was obtained correctly, minimal tissue is incompatible with cancer; the biopsy should be repeated if bleeding recurs. If the physician is unable to obtain a sample because of cervical stenosis, consideration for pelvic ultrasound, dilation and curettage, and/or referral to a gynecologist may be indicated.

Screening for endometrial cancer is not recommended by any authorities, although the American Cancer Society does recommend endometrial sampling for high-risk patients (obese, infertile, anovulatory, family history of endometrial or colon cancer, personal history of colon or breast cancer) and those who have abnormal bleeding. Ultrasound as a screening test has a very low sensitivity and is not recommended for asymptomatic women. Pap smears are not thought to be reliable screening tests for endometrial cancer. The presence of endometrial cells on Pap, however, should be further evaluated in postmenopausal women who are not on HRT or who have abnormal endometrial cells while on HRT.

CERVIX

Contrary to popular wisdom, cervical cancer continues to be a problem into old age. Nearly half of all cervical cancer deaths occur in women over age 65 (31). This startling statistic is due to the fact that many elderly women have not been routinely screened throughout their reproductive years, and the cancer is found at a more advanced, and hence less treatable stage. Approximately 16,000 new cases of cervical cancer are detected annually. Obtaining an adequate endocervical specimen in the elderly may be difficult, due to cervical stenosis and atrophy.

Pap Smear Screening

The U.S. Preventive Services Task Force made updated recommendations in 1996 for the frequency of Pap smear testing in the elderly population. Their most recent recommendations are that women who have been regularly screened with normal Pap results may be considered for discontinuation of testing at age 65. Those who have not had regular screening should have at least two normal Pap smears a year apart and then every 3 years thereafter (32). Medicare began covering triennial Pap smears in 1990. Evidence suggests that women who have had a hysterectomy for a benign cause do not need vaginal cuff Pap smears (33). However, those who had hysterectomies for cervical or uterine cancer should continue regular Pap smear testing of the vaginal cuff, as they are at increased risk for recurrence. Prior to the early 1960s, about a third of hysterectomies were performed supracervically. These women require Pap testing as if they had not had a hysterectomy.

For an adequate Pap smear, the cervix must be fully visualized. Sampling the transformation zone, the most important part of the screening test, is performed most effectively with a cytobrush. It is fairly common to have difficulty obtaining an adequate specimen because the patient is uncomfortable or there is difficulty locating the cervix in an atrophic vagina or inserting the cytobrush into a stenotic cervical os. A thinner endocervical brush inserted more deeply into the os may be a valuable adjunct in such cases.

Pap smear results are reported according to the standardized Bethesda reporting system developed by the National Cancer Institute in 1988. Because this system is always undergoing revision and refinement, terminology should be confirmed with local experts in the field or other current resources.

Further Testing

Further evaluation for high-risk patients and those with persistent abnormalities on follow-up Pap testing should be referred for colposcopy with directed biopsies, endocervical curettage, and definitive therapy, as indicated. Treatments may ultimately include cryotherapy, laser therapy, cervical conization, hysteroscopy or hysterectomy, depending upon the situation.

OVARIAN DISORDERS

Ovarian cancer accounts for approximately 12% of gynecologic cancers in women over age 75. Unfortunately, it tends to be diagnosed at a later stage in older women and carries a worse prognosis (34). Any palpable ovary in a postmenopausal woman requires further evaluation, including ultrasonography and probably laparoscopy or laparotomy, depending on the situation.

Symptoms of ovarian cancer are vague, often centering on ill-defined yet common gastrointestinal symptoms such as bloating and abdominal discomfort. The diagnosis of ovarian cancer should be at least entertained in any woman over 40 who complains of persistent gastrointestinal symptoms. Family history of ovarian cancer is one major risk factor. Other risk factors include family history of breast or colon cancer and personal history of breast, colon, or endometrial cancer. Early menarche and late menopause are also risk factors for ovarian cancer.

Screening for Ovarian Cancer

Pelvic examination is a poorly sensitive and specific screening test for ovarian cancer. By the time an ovarian cancer is palpable, it is likely to be metastatic. If an ovarian mass is appreciated, however, further evaluation must be undertaken. Such evaluation includes a pelvic ultrasound with vaginal probe and a CA-125 determination, although this test also lacks specificity. Laparoscopy may be necessary if the foregoing are abnormal or equivocal.

Screening asymptomatic women or even those at high risk (such as having one first-degree relative with ovarian cancer) with CA-125 testing or screening ultrasound are as yet unproven to be cost effective in detecting early ovarian cancer (35, 36). Work to develop an effective tumor marker for patients at highest risk is being done so that this relatively small group of women may have a better chance at early detection and improved survival.

DISORDERS OF THE VULVA

With loss of the protective effect of estrogen on urogenital tissue, the vulva undergoes significant change. The skin loses elasticity with loss of collagen and thinning of the epithelium. Any vulvar complaint should have immediate evaluation, and the skin should be thoroughly evaluated on a regular basis. Any lesion that does not respond promptly to treatment must be sampled for biopsy to exclude malignancy and to direct proper therapy.

Infection and Inflammation

Dermatologic irritants such as soaps, deodorants, and especially urine can cause significant inflammation and skin breakdown. Eliminating the irritant is, of course, the main objective. Topical steroids may be useful for a short time to reduce inflammation and pain but are not a substitute for definitive therapy for incontinence or chronic irritation from other sources.

Candidal infections are fairly common in postmenopausal women, especially diabetics, obese women with intertriginous maceration and fungal superinfection, and those undergoing antibiotic therapy. Treatment with topical antifungal creams with concomitant treatment of vaginal candidiasis is recommended. Newer oral antifungal agents (such as the one-dose fluconazole treatment) may be effective as well.

Older women, especially those who are sexually active, can be exposed to sexually transmitted diseases, such as chlamydia, gonorrhea, trichomoniasis, or herpes. An appropriate index of concern for these causes should be maintained despite a patient's chronologic age, and proper diagnostic testing and therapy should be undertaken. Bacterial vaginosis may appear in the face of sexual transmission or when the pH of the vagina becomes more alkaline, as occurs frequently in the postmenopausal state.

Atrophic vaginitis, or disuse vaginitis, is seen commonly in the menopausal woman, with a loss of rugation, thinning of the vaginal mucosa, and susceptibility to bleeding and irritation even from minor trauma. Bacterial superinfection can lead to malodorous discharge and irritation. In addition to treating any distinct infection, local treatment with vaginal estrogens or systemic estrogen treatment may be indicated. The clinician should remember that vaginal estrogens are absorbed systemically, so that any contraindication for estrogen therapy eliminates topical therapy as well. For some women, restoring the normally acidic pH of the vagina with acidic intravaginal gels may be helpful.

Dystrophic Changes

All vulvar abnormalities should be biopsied to determine proper therapy as well as to exclude malignancy, which often presents as irritation and pruritus. Vulvar dystrophy is the term used widely to describe a variety of nonneoplastic squamous changes of the vulva. The Nomenclature Committee of the International Society of Gynecological Pathologists has defined three categories of vulvar lesions: lichen sclerosis, squamous hyperplasia, and all other dermatoses. Vulvar dystrophy appears to be a precursor to vulvar carcinoma, as are history of human papilloma virus infection, advanced age, history of cervical neoplasia, smoking, and compromised immunity (37).

Lichen sclerosis (also lichen sclerosis et atrophicus, or LSA), which causes more than a third of vulvar dystrophies, may extend beyond the vulva to the thigh, groin, and perirectal areas. The skin appears dry and atrophic in leukoplakic patches, which are painful and may even bleed when the patient scratches to relieve the constant itching. Treatment remains somewhat controversial. For some time the most widely recommended therapy was topical testosterone cream. However, topical corticosteroids are the current treatment of choice (38), along with use of cotton underwear and avoidance of local irritants.

Squamous hyperplasia has a raised and thickened appearance and is extremely pruritic. Topical steroid creams and antihistamines to break the itch-scratch cycle may be useful.

Vulvar intraepithelial neoplasia (VIN) is a preinvasive neoplastic process that is often multifocal. The appearance of VIN lesions is variable, and any suspicious lesion must be sampled for biopsy. Pathologists classify the severity of cellular atypia as VIN I, II, or III. Patients with VIN of any grade should be referred for colposcopy.

Treatment can include laser ablation, local excision, or chemical destruction, depending on individual variables and extent of disease. Definitive treatment is required for VIN III.

Malignancies

Malignant melanoma and invasive vulvar carcinoma are seen with increasing frequency with advancing age. Some 5% of melanomas in women occur in the vulva. Any suspicious pigmented lesion should be excised completely and pathologically examined. Invasive neoplasms are likely to require radical surgical excision, with or without lymph node dissection.

Other Vulvar Conditions

Condylomata acuminata, a viral disease caused by the human papilloma virus, can affect women of all ages. Lesions can appear as small, flat, confluent plaques or as papillomatous cauliflowerlike lesions. Verrucous carcinoma and VIN can be indistinguishable from condyloma, so that biopsy and colposcopy are indicated for these lesions as well. For biopsy-proven condylomata acuminata, treatment can be accomplished with topical 5-fluorouracil, trichloroacetic acid, cryotherapy, or laser ablation.

DISORDERS OF THE VAGINA AND PELVIC SUPPORT

Vaginitis in the older woman is caused by the same bacteria and fungi as in younger women. However, the frequency of infections increases with age because of the higher vaginal pH after menopause. Evaluation with cultures, saline, and potassium hydroxide is the same as for younger women, as is treatment of causative organisms. (See discussion under Infection and Inflammation.)

Vaginal cancer is the rarest gynecologic cancer in women (1 to 2% of gynecologic malignancies). It usually presents with vaginal bleeding as the main complaint, although dysuria, dyspareunia, hematuria, and pelvic pain may be the presenting symptoms. Adenocarcinoma of the vagina is a higher risk in women exposed to diethylstilbestrol in utero, but squamous cell carcinoma is actually more common overall. Treatment usually is surgery and radiotherapy (39).

Atrophic Symptoms

Without estrogen, the vaginal tissues become friable and pale and lose elasticity. Dyspareunia, pruritus, burning, and leukorrhea are complaints commonly associated with atrophic vaginitis. The atrophic vaginal mucosa is also more susceptible to secondary infection. Systemic or topical estrogen nearly always resolves symptoms of vaginal atrophy. However, vaginal estrogen is absorbed systemically at approximately 50% of oral routes, so contraindications to systemic estrogens apply to the vaginal route of administration as well. Doses as low as 0.3 mg of conjugated estrogens intravaginally every 3 days have been reported to alleviate symptoms of atrophic vaginitis.

Pelvic Relaxation

Pelvic relaxation is a common condition in older women. A combination of childbirth trauma to the perineal tissues and loss of estrogen causing atrophy of pelvic connective tissue contributes to pelvic relaxation. However, nulliparous women may also have pelvic relaxation, which is a broad term that applies to uterine prolapse, cystocele, and rectocele, all of which may occur alone but are more common in combination. Grading of relaxation assists in classification and discussion of treatment options, and apply to degree of cystocele, rectocele, and uterine prolapse. First-degree prolapse is defined as descent of the structure into the upper two-thirds of the vagina. Second-degree prolapse occurs when the structure is near the vaginal introitus. Third-degree prolapse occurs when the structure is outside the introitus, and total procidentia is complete prolapse of the pelvic organs outside the vagina.

A cystocele is protrusion of the bladder into the anterior vaginal wall; the patient may have varying severity of stress urinary incontinence symptoms. A urethrocele is protrusion of the urethra into the vagina, and indicates that support of the urethrovesical junction has been lost. Both cystocele and urethrocele are easily demonstrated on pelvic examination, when pushing down the posterior vagina with the fingers and observing the anterior vaginal wall as the patient bears down, as in a Valsalva maneuver. With significant cystocele the bladder bulges into the vagina. If a sterile cotton swab is placed into the urethra and the patient asked to cough, it angles toward the ceiling in cases of significant stress incontinence, rather than toward the floor (with the patient in the lithotomy position), as found in a normal urethrovesical angle. Urodynamic testing is usually required to determine the cause of urinary incontinence in the older woman.

Similarly, a rectocele is protrusion of the rectum into the posterior vaginal wall, signifying relaxation of the rectovaginal fascia. In severe cases the patient is unable to defecate without placing her fingers in the vagina and pushing posteriorly to overcome the rectal bulge into the vagina. Uterine prolapse, or descensus, refers to the descent of the uterus from its normal position high in the vagina to varying degrees of descent toward the introitus and beyond. Patients usually complain of vaginal heaviness and the sensation that something is falling out of the vagina.

Treatment Options

Mild pelvic relaxation with minimal urinary stress incontinence can be treated nicely with Kegel exercises. The woman is taught how to tighten and relax the pelvic floor muscles at least 100 times daily. Most women with mild symptoms find significant relief within a few weeks. For advanced cases, surgical correction is likely to be needed, but surgery is a major undertaking, especially in a frail older woman. A variety of surgical procedures are available, including anterior colporrhaphy and Burch colposuspension, usually with hysterectomy.

For many patients, a pessary is a reasonable alternative (40). They do not work well with marked outlet relaxation, as some degree of muscle tone is needed to keep the pessary in place. Pessaries are available in various shapes (ring, cube, Gellhorn, Hodge, doughnut), sizes, and materials (rubber, plastic, silicone) and can be solid or inflatable. The ring pessaries and inflatable doughnut pessaries are relatively easy to use. They are placed similarly to a diaphragm, fitting between the symphysis pubis and posterior fornix of the vagina. Cube pessaries are relatively easy for the patient to insert and remove. Hodge pessaries, which may be indicated for more advanced uterine descensus, may require

visits to the physician every 6 weeks for removal and cleaning. Pessaries should be removed and cleaned weekly. Complications include ulceration, infection, and difficulty with use. Vaginal estrogen creams can strengthen the vaginal tissue and help prevent ulceration and irritation from the pessary.

GENITOURINARY SYSTEM
Urinary Incontinence

Involuntary loss of urine is a major problem, affecting 8 million to 12 million people, mainly older women, in the United States annually. Unfortunately, fewer than half of women suffering from this condition seek medical attention for it. Psychosocial dysfunction, including limitation of social contact, embarrassment, depression, decrease in activities of daily living, and decreased sexual activity are important consequences of untreated urinary incontinence. Physical complications include perineal skin maceration and increased urinary tract infections.

Understanding the anatomy and neurophysiology of the lower urinary tract can help determine the type of incontinence and guide treatment. The bladder is composed of three layers of smooth muscle called the detrusor muscle. It is innervated by parasympathetic and sympathetic nerve fibers and is under the control of the brainstem unless inhibited by the cerebral cortex. The detrusor muscle contracts in response to parasympathetic stimuli and relaxes with sympathetic and β-adrenergic stimulation. The bladder neck and proximal urethra contract in response to α-adrenergic stimulation.

Genuine stress incontinence results from the loss of structural support for the proximal urethra and bladder neck, resulting in loss of urine with any increase in intra-abdominal pressure, as the proximal urethra is no longer pressed against the pubic symphysis and urine is allowed to escape. Stress incontinence is the most common type of urinary incontinence, accounting for more than 80% of incontinence in women under age 60. The treatment of stress incontinence involves Kegel or pelvic floor strengthening exercises combined with local estrogen therapy. Biofeedback and bladder retraining programs can be useful adjuncts to muscle strengthening programs. Pessaries may be helpful, and surgical repair may be needed in advanced cases that do not respond to conservative measures.

Detrusor instability (also called detrusor hyperactivity or urge incontinence) is less common overall than stress incontinence, but it accounts for nearly 70% of urinary incontinence in the elderly. Urge incontinence can be caused by central nervous system (CNS) lesions that remove normal cortical ability to inhibit bladder contractions (e.g., stroke, demyelinating disorders, CNS infections, CNS tumors) or by bladder infections or tumors. Unfortunately, many cases of detrusor instability appear to be idiopathic. Diagnosis of urge incontinence can be made by urodynamic testing. On bedside urodynamic testing (introduction of sterile water or saline into the bladder in 50-mL increments) the patient feels the urge to void at low volumes (50 to 100 mL) if detrusor instability is the problem. Treatment for urge incontinence is bladder-retraining regimens and pharmacologic therapy with an anticholinergic agent (propantheline, oxybutynin, dicyclomine, tricyclic antidepressant) to suppress bladder contractility. Acupuncture is showing some promise in the treatment of urge incontinence. Surgery to denervate the bladder is an extreme last resort (41).

Overflow incontinence is less common than urge or stress incontinence. It occurs when the bladder is unable to empty normally because of obstruction of urinary outflow (urethral stricture, tumor, abnormal urethral sphincter contraction, medications, especially anticholinergics) or neurologic problems that inhibit detrusor activity (e.g., diabetes mellitus, vitamin B_{12} deficiency, herniated disc). In these cases the postvoid residue is high (greater than 100 mL), total bladder capacity is increased, the urinary stream may be weak and slow, and passage of a urethral catheter may be difficult if obstruction exists. Treatment is removal of any offending drug, optimal diabetic management, vitamin B_{12} if deficient, and removal of any anatomic obstruction. Pharmacologic therapy is aimed at increasing detrusor tone in the absence of outflow obstruction with an α-adrenergic agent such as bethanechol chloride.

Urinary Tract Infection

Because of postmenopausal atrophy, the urethra is shortened, the pelvic musculature is relaxed, and the vaginal pH changes. All of these factors make the older woman susceptible to urinary tract infections (UTIs). Different from their younger counterparts, older women may have more frequent UTIs, may become incontinent during the infection, and are more prone to pyelonephritis and sepsis from UTIs due to altered lymphocyte function. Therefore, bladder infections in older women should be treated vigorously with antibiotic therapy, directed by urine culture and sensitivity results. Generally, a long course of antibiotic therapy (10 to 14 days) is appropriate in the geriatric population. Follow-up cultures should always be performed to assure sterilization of the urine. Bacteria most commonly found in UTIs in older women include *Proteus, Klebsiella,* and enterococci.

Recurrent infections and chronic bacteriuria can be difficult to manage. Evaluation for cause of recurrence, such as renal calculi, abnormal urinary tract anatomy, enterovesical fistula, or other connection to the gastrointestinal tract should be evaluated with intravenous pyelography (IVP) or sonogram. If no structural abnormality is discovered, suppression with a urinary acidifying agent such as ascorbic acid may be a consideration. Long-term suppression with antibiotics is a more difficult decision, as selection of resistant strains of bacteria may make future therapy more difficult. For patients who seem to have intercourse-related UTIs, a postcoital regimen of single-dose antibiotic (e.g., nitrofurantoin 100 mg or trimethoprim-sulfamethoxazole one double-strength tablet) may serve well as a preventive measure. For the same anatomic reason that diaphragms may contribute to UTIs, so may pessaries, by pushing bacteria into the urethra from the vaginal introitus.

Treatment of asymptomatic bacteriuria (ASB) is more difficult. Some evidence suggests improved long-term prevention of pyelonephritis and sepsis with treatment of ASB, while other studies do not. Clinical judgment is required in such cases. Intravaginal use of estrogen cream may decrease susceptibility to UTIs and is worth using unless there are contraindications to estrogen use.

REFERENCES

1. McKinlay SM, Brambilla DJ, Posner JG. The normal menopause transition. Maturitas 1992;14:103–115.
2. McKinley SM, Brambilla DJ, Posner JG. The normal menopause transition. Maturitas 1992;14:103–115.
3. Scwingl PJ, Hulka BS, Harlow SD. Risk factors for menopausal hot flashes. Obstet Gynecol 1994;84: 29–34.
4. Harman M, Blackman MR. The postmenopausal state. In: Evans JG, Williams TF, eds. Oxford Textbook of Geriatric Medicine. Oxford: Oxford University Press, 1992:149–155.
5. Johnson CA. Menopausal symptoms. In: Johnson CA, Johnson BE, Murray JL, Apgar BS, eds. Women's Health Care Handbook. Philadelphia: Hanley & Belfus, 1996: 359–362.
6. Effects of hormone therapy on bone mineral density: results from the postmenopausal estrogen/progestin interventions (PEPI) trial. The Writing Group for the PEPI. JAMA 1996;276:1389–1396.
7. Effects of estrogen or estrogen/progestin regimens on heart disease risk factors in postmenopausal women. The Postmenopausal Estrogen/Progestin Interventions (PEPI) Trial. The Writing Group for the PEPI Trial. JAMA 1995;273:199–208.
8. Tang MX, Jacobs D, Stern Y, et al. Effect of oestrogen during menopause on risk and age at onset of Alzheimer's disease. Lancet 1996;348:429–432.
9. Salamone LM, Pressman AR, Seeley DG, Cauley JA. Estrogen replacement therapy: older women's attitudes. Arch Intern Med 1996;156:1293–1297.
10. Postmenopausal hormone prophylaxis: In: Guide to Clinical Preventive Services. Report of the U.S. Preventive Services Task Force. 2nd ed. Baltimore: Williams & Wilkins, 1996:829–844.
11. Persson I, Adami HO, Bergkvist L, et al. Risk of endometrial cancer after treatment with oestrogens alone or in conjunction with progestogens: results of a prospective study. BMJ 1989;298:147–151.
12. Schneider DL, Barrett-Connor EL, Morton DJ. Timing of postmenopausal estrogen for optimal bone mineral density. JAMA 1997;277:543–547.
13. Clayden JR, Bell JW, Pollard P. Menopausal flushing: double-blind trial of a non-hormonal medication. BMJ 1974;1:409–412.
14. Ylikorkala O. Clonidine in the treatment of menopausal symptoms. Ann Chir Gynaecol Fen 1975;64:242–245.
15. Lobo RA. The role of progestins in hormone replacement therapy. Am J Obstet Gynecol 1992;166:1997–2004.
16. Prior JC. Progesterone as a bone-trophic hormone. Endocrinol Rev 1990;11:386–398.
17. Hammar M, Berg G, Lindgren R. Does physical exercise influence the frequency of postmenopausal hot flushes? Acta Obstet Gynecol Scand 1990;69:409–412.
18. Irvin JH, Domar AD, Clark C, et al. The effects of relaxation response training for the treatment of menopausal symptoms. J Psychosom Obstet Gynecol 1996;17:202–207.
19. Chenoy R, Hussain S, Tayob Y, et al. Effect of oral gamolenic acid from evening primrose oil on menopausal flushing. BMJ 1994;308:501–503.
20. Tyler V. The Honest Herbal: A Sensible Guide to the Use of Herbs and Related Remedies. 3rd ed. New York: Pharmaceutical Products Press, 1993:45–46.
21. Tyler V. The Honest Herbal: A Sensible Guide to the Use of Herbs and Related Remedies. 3rd ed. New York: Pharmaceutical Products Press, 1993:113–114.
22. MacEoin B. Homeopathy for Menopause. Rochester, VT: Healing Arts Press, 1997.
23. Lee JR. What Your Doctor May Not Tell You About Menopause. New York: Warner Books, 1996.
24. Lee JR. Natural Progesterone: The Multiple Roles of a Remarkable Hormone. Sebastopol, CA: BLL Publishing, 1993.
25. Northrup C. Women's Bodies, Women's Wisdom. New York: Bantam, 1994.
26. Martin R. The Estrogen Alternative: Natural Hormone Therapy With Botanical Progesterone. Rochester, VT: Healing Arts Press, 1997.
27. Sahelian R. DHEA, A Practical Guide. Garden City Park, NY: Avery, 1996.
28. Feldman S, Berkowitz RS, Tosteson AN. Cost-effectiveness of strategies to evaluate postmenopausal bleeding. Obstet Gynecol 1993;81:968–975.
29. Boring CC, Squires TS, Tong T. Cancer statistics, 1993. CA Cancer J Clin 1993;43:7–26.
30. Stovall TG, Photopulos GJ, Poston WM, et al. Pipelle endometrial sampling in patients with known endometrial carcinoma. Obstet Gynecol 1991;77:954–956.
31. US Department of Health and Human Services. Vital Statistics of the United States. Washington: US Government Printing Office, 1984;2(Part A):PHS–88–1102.
32. Screening for cervical cancer. In: Guide to Clinical Preventive Services. Report of the U.S. Preventive Services Task Force. 2nd ed. Baltimore: Williams & Wilkins, 1996:105–118.
33. Fetters MD, Fischer G, Reed BD. Effectiveness of vaginal Papanicolaou smear screening after total hysterectomy for benign disease. JAMA 1996;275:940–947.
34. Grover SA, Cook EF, Adam J, et al. Delayed diagnosis of gynecologic tumors in elderly women: relation to national medical practice patterns. Am J Med 1989; 86:151–156.
35. Bombard AT, Fields AL, Aufox S, Ben-Yishay M. The genetics of ovarian cancer: an assessment of current screening protocols and recommendations for counseling families at risk. Clin Obstet Gynecol 1996;39:860–872.
36. Schwartz PE, Chambers JT, Taylor KJ. Early detection

and screening for ovarian cancer. J Cell Biochem Suppl 1995;23:233–237.

37. Ansink AC, Heintz AP. Epidemiology and etiology of squamous cell carcinoma of the vulva. Eur J Obstet Gynecol Reprod Biol 1993;48:111–115.

38. Bracco GL, Carli P, Sonni L, et al. Clinical and histological treatments of vulval lichen sclerosis. J Reprod Med 1193;38:37–40.

39. Manetta A, Pinto JL, Larson JE, et al. Primary invasive carcinoma of the vagina. Obstet Gynecol 1988;72:77–81.

40. Sulak PJ, Kuehl TJ, Shull BL. Vaginal pessaries and their use in pelvic relaxation. J Reprod Med 1993;38:919–923.

41. Urinary Incontinence Guideline Panel. Urinary Incontinence in Adults. Clinical Practice Guideline 2 (AHCPR 92–0038). Rockville, MD: US Department of Health and Human Services, Public Health Service, Agency for Health Care Policy and Research, 1992.

CHAPTER 31

REBECCA A. SILLIMAN AND LODOVICO BALDUCCI

Breast Cancer

Breast cancer is common in older women. If it is diagnosed in its early stages, survival rates comparable with those of women in most younger age groups can be attained (1). As is the case with many other conditions, an incomplete scientific knowledge base, combined with the complicating factors of comorbidity, impaired functional status, and diminished social support, create challenges for clinicians who care for older women with this disease. This chapter focuses primarily on issues related to the management of invasive early-stage disease but briefly discusses screening issues (see also Chapter 3), carcinoma in situ, and the approach to the patient with advanced disease.

EPIDEMIOLOGY AND PROGNOSIS

Breast cancer has become increasingly important in older women for three major reasons. First, the incidence of breast cancer increases dramatically with age, such that fully 60% of incident cases are diagnosed in women aged 60 or older (2). Second, the numbers of women aged 65 or older and, in particular, the numbers of women aged 85 or older are increasing rapidly (3). Third, the age-adjusted incidence of breast cancer is also increasing, in part because of the increased use of screening mammography (4, 5). Taken together, these factors have three important consequences: (*a*) the number of older women with newly diagnosed breast cancer will continue to increase; (*b*) the average age of women with newly diagnosed breast cancer will continue to rise; and (*c*) the number of older women who are survivors of breast cancer will grow.

Breast cancer is a serious disease in older women. For example, although the 10-year risk of recurrence for women aged 70 or older who are node negative with 1- to 5-cm tumors is 20 to 30%, the risk for women with one to three positive nodes and tumors of any size is 50%, and the risk for women with four or more positive nodes and tumors of any size is 80% (6). Furthermore, the most recent breast cancer mortality figures demonstrate a marked decline in mortality in all age groups except those aged 80 or older (7).

SCREENING

Although screening mammography has proven efficacy in women up to age 70 years, there is no good scientific evidence to support or refute its efficacy in women aged 70 or older (8). Nonetheless, there are several reasons screening older women makes good clinical sense. First, the positive predictive value of mammography and physical examination is higher in older women than in younger women (8). Second, the incidence of breast cancer continues to rise until the ninth decade of life (1). Third, life expectancy at age 85 is more than 6 years (9).

Yet it is older women who are least likely to be screened. Physicians less often recommend that older women receive mammography screening, and older women are more likely not to believe that such screening is necessary (10). Although rates of screening mammography have increased in recent years, according to 1992 National Health Interview Survey data, only 63.5% of women aged 70 to 79 years and 48.5% of women 80 or older reported ever having a mammogram. When asked about having had a mammogram in the past year, these numbers decreased to 39.8% and 21.6%, respectively (7). Although information from available clinical studies does not provide guidance about when to stop screening, the recommendations of the Forum on Breast Cancer Screening in Older Women are reasonable (11):

1. Clinical breast examination should be performed annually, and mammography should be performed approximately every 2 years for women aged 65 to 74.
2. Clinical breast examination should be performed annually, and mammography should be performed at regular intervals of approximately every 2 years for women aged 75 and over whose general health and life expectancy are good.
3. It is prudent for women aged 65 and over to perform monthly breast self-examination (BSE) to identify clinical lesions and seek professional care.

These guidelines emphasize the importance of general health and life expectancy in clinical decision making about screening for women aged 75 and older. They also emphasize that no one screening modality should be relied on. Neither negative self-examination nor a negative clinical examination should give one a sense of security; mammography is still indicated, and vice versa. Finally, these guidelines suggest that the interval between mammograms should be "approximately" every 2 years. Although Medicare now pays for annual mammography screening, the available data do not indicate that a 12-month interval is more effective than a 24-month interval (8).

CARCINOMA IN SITU

One of the consequences of increased mammography screening is the increasing incidence of carcinoma in situ. For example, the most common form, *ductal carcinoma in situ* (DCIS), increased 235% between 1979 and 1986 among women aged 50 or older (12). DCIS is a spectrum of diseases that carry with them differing propensities for recurrence. Because the tumor is commonly multicentric, the recommended treatment is either simple mastectomy or breast-conserving surgery and radiotherapy. Recent re-

finements in prognostic classification suggest that there may be some low-risk patients for whom breast-conserving surgery alone may be appropriate (13).

The much less common *lobular carcinoma in situ* (LCIS) is a risk factor for the development of bilateral breast cancer. The risk of developing invasive carcinoma, which is approximately 1% per year, persists indefinitely. Management is therefore either careful and close follow-up or bilateral prophylactic mastectomy (14).

A new and special problem is mixed tumors, i.e., ones that have an in situ component as well as an invasive component. The prognosis of these tumors is related to the size of the invasive component, which also guides the approach to therapy, as described next.

NEWLY DIAGNOSED INVASIVE BREAST CANCER

The new diagnosis of cancer at any age is frightening. When coupled with the prospect of having to see three or more new physicians (one or more surgeons and medical and radiation oncologists), it may be overwhelming. The primary care physician can play a critical role in cancer care for older patients by answering questions and reviewing the recommendations of specialists; clarifying the patient's values regarding the risks and benefits of various treatment options; and spending additional time with patients who may be inclined to choose the quickest treatment "just to get it over with." In addition to the older patients themselves, family members are likely to be involved in decision making, and they should be included in discussions about treatments. Their questions and fears need attention as well. Meeting needs of both the patient and the family requires a thorough understanding of the best available scientific evidence regarding treatment efficacy, including the gaps in knowledge and the areas of uncertainty.

EARLY-STAGE DISEASE: MANAGEMENT OF THE PRIMARY TUMOR

The 1990 NIH Consensus Development Conference on the treatment of early-stage breast cancer concluded that "breast conservation treatment is an appropriate method of primary therapy for the majority of women with stage I and II breast cancer and is preferable because it provides survival rates *equivalent* to those of total mastectomy and axillary dissection while preserving the breast." Here, breast conservation treatment refers to breast-conserving surgery (e.g., lumpectomy), level I or II axillary node dissection, and postoperative irradiation of the breast. In the view of the Consensus Development Conference, total mastectomy should be considered only when the cancer is multicentric or when the cancer and/or breast size would make the cosmetic results unacceptable to patients (15).

Note that these recommendations have been made for all women, regardless of age. While most would agree that basing treatment recommendations on age alone is inappropriate, generalizing treatment recommendations from studies of younger women may be equally problematic. Patients with major comorbidities have been excluded from clinical trials. Furthermore, it is probable that those with functional disabilities have been excluded as well, although no clinical trials have gathered data, either baseline or follow-up, regarding functional impairments (16–20).

Although breast-conserving surgery with axillary dissection followed by radiotherapy is recommended for the majority of women regardless of age and should be offered as a treatment option, other factors are likely to play a role in older women's decisions. First, for many, a mastectomy may be viewed as a more definitive procedure, particularly when risk of recurrence is considered to be important. Second, most women who choose mastectomy do not require radiotherapy. Although radiotherapy to the breast is well tolerated by most older women, the need for daily radiation treatments can be daunting. Arranging transportation, coping with long distances to radiotherapy facilities, and/or managing emotional and physical fatigue may not seem worth it. These barriers may sway women into deciding against breast-conserving surgery. Third, body image considerations are less important to many (but not all) older women. For those to whom these considerations are important, mastectomy with breast reconstruction may be an attractive alternative. Fourth, and perhaps

most important, physicians' recommendations have a powerful influence on older women's decisions. Silliman et al. (21) found that the two most important factors influencing older women's treatment decisions are physicians' recommendations and the desire to minimize the risk of recurrence (21). Regardless of the type of surgical procedure chosen, careful attention should be paid to preserving upper body, shoulder, and arm strength and mobility. During the early postoperative period, physical therapy and the judicious use of analgesics facilitate the preservation of function.

The problem for physicians trying to use an evidence-based approach to guide the care of older women is that these women have generally been excluded from clinical trials addressing treatment efficacy. As a result, there remain two very important unresolved controversies regarding primary tumor therapy: (*a*) the need for radiotherapy following breast-conserving surgery; and (*b*) the need for axillary dissection, regardless of the surgical management of the breast. Radiotherapy has not been shown to be effective either in preventing systemic disease or in prolonging survival (15). Second, it is not clear whether it prevents disease recurrence in older women, since older women appear to have lower recurrence rates than younger women (19, 22–25). Breast-conserving surgery without irradiation may be reasonable in older women for whom a course of radiation would be especially burdensome and in those who are at high risk for operative and/or postoperative complications. For these women, adjuvant tamoxifen may be a prudent addition to therapy, recognizing that clinical progression is likely even with this approach (26).

Axillary dissection has been advocated as a therapeutic intervention that both eliminates residual disease and stages patients. The goal of eliminating residual tumor has not been well studied in older women, although a recent report from Rhode Island suggests that women 65 and older who do not receive an axillary dissection do not live as long as those who receive definitive therapy (27). With respect to staging, a promising new diagnostic technique called lymphatic mapping and sentinel node biopsy has been pioneered at the University of South Florida and is now being used in many centers around the United States. Lymphatic node mapping uses a radioactive tracer to identify the sentinel node, the first node to receive lymphatic drainage from the breast. Initial results from a series of 57 patients indicate that it is 100% sensitive. No cases of skip metastases (metastases to level II or level III axillary nodes without involvement of level I nodes) were found (28). If these results hold in larger series, women with negative sentinel nodes will be spared from the morbidity as well as the costs of axillary dissection.

A final issue related to primary tumor management is the consideration of medical rather than surgical treatment. In studies comparing the survival of women initially treated with tamoxifen with those surgically treated, survival has been comparable. However, patients treated with tamoxifen alone have had more local progression than those treated surgically (29–31). These findings suggest that tamoxifen alone should be reserved as a treatment option only for women who are too frail to undergo surgery or who simply do not want to have it. One hopes that this applies to a very small number of patients, since the risks of breast-conserving surgery, in particular, are small.

EARLY-STAGE DISEASE: ADJUVANT TREATMENT
Tamoxifen

Unlike the case of primary tumor management, the benefits of tamoxifen in older women are fairly well understood. Adjuvant tamoxifen therapy has been shown to decrease rates of recurrence and mortality in older women with early-stage breast cancer. A meta-analysis of clinical trials worldwide that included 2656 women 70 years or older documented decreases in both recurrence (28%) and overall mortality (21%) rates among patients with node-positive disease treated with tamoxifen. Similar proportional risk reductions were found for node-negative and hormone receptor-poor patients, although the absolute risk reduction was less. Finally, treatment with tamoxifen prevents contralateral breast cancer (32). There are non-breast cancer benefits of therapy for postmenopausal women

as well. Tamoxifen may prevent osteoporosis (33) and reduce cholesterol levels (34). Recent reports suggest that tamoxifen reduces the risk of hospitalization for cardiovascular disease and for fatal myocardial infarction (35, 36).

Although there are proven health benefits, the costs and risks of tamoxifen therapy are not trivial. First, generic tamoxifen, at the recommended dose of 20 mg/day, costs most patients $85 a month or more. Second, menopausal symptoms caused or exacerbated by tamoxifen are common, particularly in the young old. Although side effects may be treated with transdermal clonidine or oral progesterone derivatives, their own side effects may limit their use. Third, treatment with tamoxifen increases the risk of conditions for which older women are already at risk. For example, deep vein thrombosis can complicate the use of tamoxifen, and this risk appears to be particularly high in women 65 years and older (37). In addition, there is a small but definite increase in the risk of endometrial cancer among tamoxifen users (38, 39). Finally, ocular toxicities, although uncommon at the usual doses, have been reported; they range from crystalline retinal deposits to corneal changes (40). On balance, treatment with tamoxifen is prudent for most older women with early-stage disease except those with an excellent prognosis (those with tumors smaller than 1 cm). Findings from clinical trials support 5 years of tamoxifen treatment (41).

Chemotherapy

The value of adjuvant chemotherapy alone or in conjunction with tamoxifen has not been well studied in women over age 70. Indeed, the meta-analysis of studies worldwide mentioned earlier included only 366 women in this age group who received adjuvant chemotherapy. Adjuvant chemotherapy did not appear to benefit these women (42). Chemotherapy may be efficacious in patients with aggressive disease, but this is not known. What is known is that older women are able to tolerate combination chemotherapy when renally excreted drugs are adjusted to creatinine clearance (43, 44). Furthermore, chemotherapy has become safer in older women since the introduction of safer drugs (e.g., gemcitabine and vinorelbine [Navelbine]) and of new antidotes to drug toxicity (e.g., hemopoietic growth factors and dexrazoxane for anthracycline cardiotoxicity) (45).

METASTATIC DISEASE

Survival rates in older women diagnosed with metastatic disease decrease with age. While the 1-year survival rate for women aged 65 to 74 is similar to that in the first postmenopausal age decade (55 to 64 years, 61%: 65 to 74 years, 58%), rates decline thereafter to 54% in those 75 to 84 years and 44% in those aged 85 and older (1). The 5-year survival rates across all age groups are uniformly dismal, ranging from 16 to 20%. These rates provide a compelling argument for a more systematic approach to screening and early diagnosis.

While hormonal treatment in these women has only a modest effect on survival, symptom palliation can be achieved in most patients (46, 47). Because it is well tolerated, tamoxifen is recommended as the first line of treatment, regardless of hormone receptor status. The average response rate is about 30%, with the highest response rates being among women who have positive hormone receptors, who have had a long disease-free survival, and who have soft tissue or bony metastases. Calcium levels should be monitored initially, since transient hypercalcemia can occur if bony metastases are present. Megestrol acetate or the aromatase inhibitor anastrazole may be useful when patients relapse. Anastrazole is more powerful than its predecessor aminoglutethimide and has fewer side effects (48).

Although the use of chemotherapy in older women with metastatic disease has not been well studied, recent reports suggest no age-related differences in response rates, time to progression, survival, or toxic side effects (42, 43). Older women whose disease has become refractory to hormonal therapy may be candidates for combination chemotherapy. Complete responses are rare, but partial responses lasting up to 6 to 12 months can be expected in about 40% of patients (2).

As is the case with all older patients with life threatening disease, treatment of women with metastatic disease must take into account risk and benefits, especially quality-of-life issues, and the patient's preferences. End-of-life care, including preferences for site of death and the use of hospice, also should be discussed. Decision making should be iterative; patients and families need to understand that the therapeutic plan can be flexible and change as the patient's needs change. (See Chapters 51, 63, and 67 for more thorough discussions of these issues.)

CARE OF SURVIVORS

As more women with treated breast cancer survive into old age, new questions arise for clinicians caring for them. One question that has received considerable attention in recent years is what kind and duration of follow-up care breast cancer survivors should receive. Although the question has not been answered for older women per se, studies of the value of routine follow-up testing demonstrate that such testing does not affect health outcomes (49–51). It is doubtful that studies specifically designed to address the question in older women would reach different conclusions.

Another question is whether hormone replacement therapy is safe for these women. The accumulated evidence does not support the continued prohibition of hormone replacement therapy in breast cancer survivors. Pending the results of definitive studies, hormone replacement therapy can be recommended, at least for breast cancer survivors receiving adjuvant tamoxifen therapy (52). Such therapy does not appear to increase the risk of recurrence or the development of contralateral disease; it may decrease the duration and severity of menopausal symptoms; and it may complement the cardiovascular and bone benefits of tamoxifen.

Additional questions that are especially germane to older women should addressed by well-designed follow-up studies of long-term survivors. These include the following: How long should surveillance mammography be continued? What are the long-term musculoskeletal complications of mastectomy, radiotherapy, and axillary dissection? What are the long-term pulmonary complications of postoperative radiotherapy? Are there long-term psychosocial issues that influence older women's quality of life?

SUMMARY AND CONCLUSIONS

The care of older women with breast cancer is complicated by the lack of a complete body of evidence supporting the efficacy of recommended screening and treatments. Physicians can best serve their older women patients by emphasizing the importance of screening and early detection. When breast cancer is diagnosed, the patient's preferences, comorbidity, functional status, life expectancy, risks and benefits of treatment, and family support all should be taken into account when developing a treatment plan. Given the need for better information on which to base treatment decisions, older patients should be encouraged to participate in studies that will expand our knowledge.

REFERENCES

1. Yancik R, Ries LB, Yates JW. Breast cancer in aging women: a population-based study of contrasts in stage, surgery, and survival. Cancer 1989;63:164–169.
2. Breast Cancer Factors and Figures 1996. Atlanta: American Cancer Society, 1995.
3. Schneider EL, Guralnick JM. The aging of American: impact on health care costs. JAMA 1990;263:2335–2340.
4. Lantz PM, Remington PL, Newcomb PA. Mammography screening and increased incidence of breast cancer in Wisconsin. J Natl Cancer Inst 1991;83:1540–1546.
5. Feuer EJ, Wun LM. How much of the recent rise in breast cancer incidence can be explained by increase in mammography utilization? A dynamic population model approach. Am J Epidemiol 1992;136:1423–1436.
6. Muss HB. The role of chemotherapy and adjuvant therapy in the management of breast cancer in older women. Cancer 1994;74:2165–2171.
7. Chu KC, Tarone RE, Kessler LG, et al. Recent trends in US breast cancer incidence, survival, and mortality rates. J Natl Cancer Inst 1996;88:1571–1579.
8. Costanza ME. Issues in breast cancer screening in older women. Cancer 1994;74:2009–2015.
9. Manton K. Cross-sectional estimates of active life expectancy for the US elderly and oldest-old populations. J Gerontol 1991;46:S170–S182.
10. Breen N, Kessler L. Changes in the use of screening mammography: evidence from the 1987 and 1990 National Health Interview Surveys. Am J Public Health 1994;84:62–67.
11. Breast cancer screening in older women: Screening recommendations of the forum panel. J Gerontol 1992;47: 5(special issue).
12. Morrow M, Schnitt SJ, Harris JR. Ductal carcinoma in situ. In: Harris JR, Lippman ME, Morrow M, Hellman S, eds. Diseases of the Breast. Philadelphia: Lippincott-Raven, 1996:355–368.
13. Silverstein MJ, Poller DN, Waisman JR, et al. Prognostic classification of breast ductal carcinoma "in situ." Lancet 1995;345:1154–1157.
14. Morrow M, Schnitt SJ. Lobular carcinoma in situ. In: Harris JR, Lippman ME, Morrow M, Hellman S, eds. Diseases of the Breast. Philadelphia: Lippincott-Raven, 1996:369–373.
15. NIH consensus conference. Treatment of early stage breast cancer. JAMA 1991;265:391–395.
16. Veronesi U, Saccozzi R, Del Vecchio M, et al. Comparing radical mastectomy with quadrantectomy, axillary dissection, and radiotherapy in patients with small cancers of the breast. N Engl J Med 1981;305:6–11.
17. Sarrazin D, Le M, Rouesse J, et al. Conservative treatment versus mastectomy in breast cancer tumors with macroscopic diameter of 20 millimeters or less. The experience of the Institut Gustave-Roussy. Cancer 1984;53:1209–1213.
18. Fisher B, Anderson S, Redmond CK, et al. Reanalysis and results after 12 years of follow-up in a randomized clinical trial comparing total mastectomy with lumpectomy with or without irradiation in the treatment of breast cancer. N Engl J Med 1995;333:1456–1461.
19. Veronesi U, Banfi A, Del Vecchio M, et al. Comparison of Halsted mastectomy with quadrantectomy, axillary dissection and radiotherapy in early breast cancer: long-term results. Eur J Cancer Clin Oncol 1986;22:1085–1089.
20. Habibollahi F, Fentiman IS. Breast conservation techniques for early breast cancer. Cancer Treat Rev 1989; 16:177–191.
21. Silliman RA, Troyan SL, Guadagnoli E, et al. The impact of age, marital status, and physician-patient interactions on the care of older women with breast carcinoma. Cancer 1997;80:1326–1334.
22. Nemoto T, Patel JK, Rosner D, et al. Factors affecting recurrence in lumpectomy without irradiation for breast cancer. Cancer 1991;67:2079–2082.
23. Clark RM, Whelan T, Levine M, et al. Randomized clinical trial of breast irradiation following lumpectomy and axillary dissection for node-negative breast cancer: an update. J Natl Cancer Inst 1996;88:1659–1664.
24. Kantorowitz DA, Poulter CA, Sischy B, et el. Treatment of breast cancer among elderly women with segmental mastectomy plus postoperative radiotherapy. Int J Radiat Oncol Biol Phys 1988;15:263–270.
25. Veronesi U, Luini A, Del Vecchio M, et al. Radiotherapy after breast-preserving surgery in women with localized cancer of the breast. N Engl J Med 1993;328:1587–1591.
26. Dunser M, Haussler B, Fuchs H, Martgreiter R. Lumpectomy plus tamoxifen for the treatment of breast cancer in the elderly. Eur J Surg Oncol 1993;19:529–531.
27. Wanebo HJ, Cole B, Chung M, et al. Is surgical management compromised in elderly patients with breast cancer? Ann Surg 1997;225:579–589.
28. Albertini JJ, Lyman GH, Cox C, et al. Lymphatic mapping and sentinel node biopsy in the patient with breast cancer. JAMA 1996;276:1818–1822.
29. Ciatto S, Cirillo A, Confortini M, Cardillo CD. Tamoxifen as primary treatment of breast cancer in elderly patients. Neoplasia 1996;43:43–45.

30. Gazet JC, Markopoulos C, Ford HT, et al. Prospective randomized trial of tamoxifen versus surgery in elderly patients with breast cancer. Lancet 1988;1:679–681.

31. Bates T, Riley DL, Houghton J, Fallowfield L, Baum M. Breast cancer in elderly women: a Cancer Research Campaign trial comparing treatment with tamoxifen and optimal surgery with tamoxifen alone. The Elderly Breast Cancer Working Party. Br J Surg 1991;78:591–594.

32. Systemic treatment of early breast cancer by hormonal, cytotoxic, or immune therapy: 133 randomised trials involving 31,000 recurrences and 24,000 deaths among 75,000 women. Early Breast Cancer Trialists' Collaborative Group. Lancet 1992;339:1–15.

33. Love RR, Mazess RB, Barden HS, et al. Effects of tamoxifen on bone mineral density in postmenopausal women with breast cancer. N Engl J Med 1992;326:852–856.

34. Love RR, Wiebe DA, Newcomb PA, et al. Effects of tamoxifen on cardiovascular risk factors in postmenopausal women. Ann Intern Med 1991;115:860–864.

35. McDonald CC, Stewart HJ. Fatal myocardial infarction in the Scottish adjuvant tamoxifen trial. BMJ 1991;303:435–437.

36. Rutqvist LE, Mattsson A. Cardiac and thromboembolic morbidity among postmenopausal women with early-stage breast cancer in a randomized trial of adjuvant tamoxifen. J Natl Cancer Inst 1993;85:1398–1406.

37. Fisher B, Brown A, Wolmark N, et al. Prolonging tamoxifen therapy for primary breast cancer: findings from the National Surgical Adjuvant Breast and Bowel Project clinical trial. Ann Intern Med 1987;106:649–654.

38. Fornander T, Rutqvist LE, Cedermark B, et al. Adjuvant tamoxifen in early breast cancer: occurrence of new primary cancers. Lancet 1989;1:117–120.

39. Fisher B, Costantino JP, Redmond CK, et al. Endometrial cancer in tamoxifen-treated breast cancer patients: findings from the National Surgical Adjuvant Breast and Bowel Project (NSABP) B-14. J Natl Cancer Inst 1994; 86:527–537.

40. Nayfield SG, Gorin MB. Tamoxifen-associated eye disease: a review. J Clin Oncol 1996;14:1018–1026.

41. Swain SM. Tamoxifen: the long and short of it. J Natl Cancer Inst 1996;88:1510–1512.

42. Early Breast Cancer Trialists' Collaborative Group. Systemic treatment of early breast cancer by hormonal, cytotoxic, or immune therapy: 133 randomized trials involving 31,000 recurrences and 24,000 deaths among 75,000 women. Part 2. Lancet 1992;339:71–85.

43. Gelman RS, Taylor SG. Cyclophosphamide, methotrexate and 5 fluorouracil chemotherapy in women more than 65 years old with advanced breast cancer: the elimination of age trends in toxicity by using doses based on creatinine clearance. J Clin Oncol 1984;2:1404–1413.

44. Christman K, Muss HB, Case LD, Stanley V. Chemotherapy of metastatic breast cancer in the elderly: the Piedmont Oncology Association experience. JAMA 1992; 268:57–62.

45. Balducci L, Extermann M. Cancer chemotherapy in the older patient: what the medical oncologist needs to know. Cancer 1997;80:1317–1322.

46. Pritchard RI, Sutherland DJA. The use of endocrine therapy. Hematol Oncol Clin 1989;3:765–806.

47. Ziegler LD, Buzdar AU. Recent advances in the treatment of breast cancer. Am J Med Sci 1991;301:337–349.

48. Hoffken K, Jonat W, Possinger JR, et al. Aromatase inhibition with 4-hydroxy-androstenedione in the treatment of postmenopausal patients with advanced breast cancer: a phase II study. J Clin Oncol 1990;8:875–880.

49. Marrazza A, Solina G, Puccia V, et al. Evaluation of routine follow-up after surgery for breast carcinoma. J Surg Oncol 1986;32:179–181.

50. Zwaveling A, Albers GH, Felthuis W, Hermans J. An evaluation of routine follow-up for detection of breast cancer recurrences. J Surg Oncol 1987;34:194–197.

51. Impact of follow-up testing on survival and health-related quality of life in breast cancer patients. A multicenter randomized controlled trial. The GIVIO Investigators. JAMA 1994;271:1587–1592.

52. Cobleigh MA, Berris RF, Bush T, et al. Estrogen replacement therapy in breast cancer survivors: a time for change. JAMA 1994;272:540–545.

CHAPTER 32

SHARI M. LING, JOHN A. FLYNN, AND FREDRICK M. WIGLEY

Musculoskeletal Disorders in the Elderly

Musculoskeletal pain and discomfort are common complaints for older adults (1). Recent studies suggest that arthritis is the leading chronic disease in the United States that increases in prevalence and incidence with age (2). Arthritis frequently results in painful symptoms that can result in compromised function, loss of mobility, and disability (3). The care of older adults with rheumatic conditions challenges practitioners at several levels. Symptom reporting and clinical presentation may differ in older adults. Patients may mistakenly attribute their painful and other symptoms to "old age" and dismiss them without reporting them to a physician (4). Patients may also inaccurately attribute their musculoskeletal pain to arthritis without the necessary medical confirmation. Clinicians are also challenged by atypical, nonclassical, and even vague presentations of rheumatic diseases in older adults (5).

GENERAL APPROACH TO THE ELDERLY PATIENT WITH MUSCULOSKELETAL DISORDERS

The list of diseases and disorders that can cause painful musculoskeletal symptoms is extensive (6). One should first ascertain that painful symptoms are due to arthritis or some periarticular or other process. Painful symptoms reproducible on active and passive joint range-of-motion and joint line tenderness characterize arthritis, and they are accompanied by crepitance and bony prominence in osteoarthritis. If arthri-

tis is present, one should next establish the number of joints involved. For example, arthritis of a single joint may be due to infection, crystalline disease, or trauma but cannot be explained by uncomplicated osteoarthritis except in the first carpal joint of the hand or knee. Painful active but normal passive range of motion suggests a periarticular process (tendinitis, bursitis) that may accompany arthritis and also may result in painful movement independent of arthritis. Systemic symptoms, including prolonged morning stiffness, weight loss, and fatigue should be elicited to determine whether the arthritis is inflammatory and whether systemic or metabolic illness should be aggressively sought.

The radiographic studies that clinicians frequently rely on in young adults may not be as reliable in the evaluation of older adults. Although radiographic studies can help to confirm arthritis, clinicians may be misled by the high prevalence of asymptomatic radiographic osteoarthritis and prematurely cease in their search for a diagnosis. Similarly, magnetic resonance imaging (MRI) can be helpful to confirm a clinical diagnosis of spine disease but can also reveal incidental disc disease. Therefore, the most appropriate use of radiographic studies is to confirm rheumatic diseases suspected because of history and physical examination, not to use them as screening tests for rheumatic diseases in the elderly.

The erythrocyte sedimentation rate (ESR), rheumatoid factor, and antinuclear antibodies

(ANA) are used to evaluate rheumatic disease and are reviewed extensively elsewhere (6). Their utility depends on the prevalence of a given rheumatic disease in the population under study; they are useful in confirming a suspected diagnosis such as rheumatoid arthritis or late-onset lupus. However, they should not be used as a screening test for "rheumatic disease," since healthy older adults may also have abnormal laboratory values.

The Westergren sedimentation rate can be elevated in older adults even in the absence of identifiable illness. The Westergren sedimentation rate is useful for evaluating the patient with headache, fever of unknown origin, or unintentional weight loss if temporal or giant cell arteritis is suspected but does not independently secure the diagnosis. High ESR can also accompany nonrheumatic systemic illness and therefore does not distinguish giant cell arteritis from systemic infection, myeloma, or other advanced malignancy.

Rheumatoid factor is an antibody (usually immunoglobulin-τ, or IgG) that reacts with the Fc fragment of IgG. These are detectable in 70 to 80% of patients with rheumatoid arthritis but are not specific to it (7). Rheumatoid factors are detectable in other rheumatic and nonrheumatic conditions that are characterized by chronic antigenic stimulation (e.g., granulomatous diseases, syphilis, endocarditis). Rheumatoid factors may also be detected in up to 30% of apparently healthy older adults, usually at a titer of 1:80 or less. This test may be most useful in the evaluation of the older adult with the symmetric inflammatory polyarthritis that is characteristic of rheumatoid arthritis. However, an isolated elevated rheumatoid factor does not establish a diagnosis of rheumatoid arthritis in an elderly patient with diffuse and vague musculoskeletal complaints in absence of inflammatory joint findings on examination.

ANAs are immunoglobulins that are directed against deoxyribonucleic acid (DNA), ribonucleic acid (RNA), and nuclear or cytoplasmic proteins. Although a variety of cell substrates have been used, rat kidney and liver substrates provide great sensitivity but little specificity. In comparison, the human monoclonal line (Hep2) offers greater specificity for rheumatic disease.

Both the pattern of immunofluorescence (rim, speckled, nucleolar, or diffuse) and titer provide useful clinical information. ANAs can be found in healthy older adults but in the absence of rheumatic disease are usually seen in a diffuse pattern at a low titer. High-titer ANAs may occur in older adults with systemic or drug-induced lupus, inflammatory muscle disease, and scleroderma. In summary, the aforementioned laboratory studies remain useful to confirm the presence of specific rheumatic conditions in older patients. However, these studies may be misleading when used inappropriately as tools to screen for the presence of rheumatic illnesses or when used alone to diagnose them.

MANAGEMENT OF RHEUMATIC CONDITIONS IN OLDER ADULTS

Effective management of arthritis in the elderly should include concurrent medicinal and nonmedicinal interventions for pain relief and preservation of functional independence, mobility, and quality of life. While acetaminophen is the recommended initial analgesic of choice for symptomatic osteoarthritis, this therapy alone is ineffective and inadequate to manage inflammatory arthritis. The glucocorticoid and non-steroidal anti-inflammatory medications that are important to the management of inflammatory rheumatic conditions are associated with toxicities that must be closely monitored in elderly patients who have little physiologic reserve.

The principles of "start low and go slow" apply to the management of older adults with rheumatic conditions. Other modes of therapy are often effective at relieving pain and can improve or help to maximize function. These include topical agents, local heat or ice, ultrasound, and stimulation with electrical devices (TENS). Physical therapy is mandatory for patients with lower extremity weakness and gait abnormalities, but may also benefit older adults prior to the development of these and other functional end points. The use of proper orthotic devices and shock absorbing shoes may also be joint protective and compensate for permanent functional deficits. Energy conservation and the implementation of proper joint mechanics are important concepts to convey to older adults with rheumatic illnesses and musculoskeletal diseases. Disease specific therapies are discussed in the following sections.

Avoiding Late Complications

Early assessment of function is crucial to detecting subtle but important changes during the course of management. Older adults are at high risk for developing gait impairment, for falls, and for functional decline, as defined by the need for assistance with mobility and/or self care (8–11). Difficulties with mobility, upper extremity function, household management, and self-care activities have been associated with arthritis and joint pain in several studies of the community-residing elderly (10–14). It has also been clearly shown that arthritis accompanied by other co-morbid conditions results in greater impairment of mobility than arthritis alone (11–13).

Because ambulation can be painful in patients with knee and/or hip osteoarthritis, disturbances of gait, such as an adductor lurch or antalgic gait, are common and may themselves predispose to falls (9, 14). In a recent review King and Tinetti highlight four prospective studies of risk factors for falls in older adults (15–18). Indeed, a self-reported history of "arthritis" and physical findings of painful or limited range of motion were predictive of recurrent nonsyncopal falls among community-residing elderly. Furthermore, these and other studies clearly demonstrate that a number of intrinsic and environmental factors other than arthritis contribute to risk of falling. These include lower extremity muscle weakness, deficits in balance, impaired visual, proprioceptive, and cognitive function, sedative medications, and comorbid medical conditions. This problem also applies to residents of nursing homes and assisted living facilities, 50% of whom experience difficulty with ambulation or recurrent falls, but in whom the prevalence of symptomatic arthritis is unknown.

In brief, all older adults with arthritis and other rheumatic disorders should be screened by interview for functional deficits including those of complex tasks (shopping, driving, finance management), self-care (bathing, dressing, toileting, etc.) (19, 20). In addition, objective task performance measures including the timed walk and sequential chair stands may be a worthy time investment since these measures detect and predict functional deficits before they are clinically apparent to either the physician or patient (21–24). Functional assessment is indicated at the time of the initial patient evaluation and every 1 to 3 years thereafter. Occupational therapy services provide valuable information regarding in-home function and can be particularly useful in the assessment of general home safety and risk of falls.

OSTEOARTHRITIS

Osteoarthritis (25) is the most common articular disease in the United States (26). Of the identified demographic risk factors for it, age is the most influential one for all sites (27, 28). Prevalence rates for both radiographic and, to a lesser extent, symptomatic osteoarthritis (moderate or severe) increase with a steep rise after age 50 in men and age 40 in women (28–31). The prevalence and incidence of radiographic and symptomatic osteoarthritis are also influenced by gender. Hand osteoarthritis is particularly prevalent among elderly women (29, 32, 33). In addition, polyarticular osteoarthritis and isolated knee osteoarthritis are slightly more common in women than men. Although hip osteoarthritis is more common in elderly men, women were more likely to report pain in all affected joints, including the hip (29, 32–35).

Clinical Presentation

Osteoarthritis is diagnosed by a triad of typical symptoms, physical findings, and radiographic changes (36). The American College of Rheumatology has set forth criteria that have excellent precision for identification of patients with symptomatic osteoarthritis and that do not rely solely on radiographic findings (Table 32.1) (37–39). The distal and proximal interphalangeal and first carpal-metacarpal joints of the hand, knees, hips, metatarsal phalangeal joints of the foot, and the lumbar and sacral spine are sites of osteoarthritis in the elderly.

Symptoms

Patients with early disease have pain in one or more joints that is aggravated by activity and is

Table 32.1

Does the Clinical Presentation Meet ACR Criteria for the Diagnosis of Osteoarthritis?

Hand[a]	Knee	Hip
Hand pain, aching, or stiffness *and* Hard tissue enlargement of 2 or more select joints *and* Fewer than 3 swollen metacarpophalangeal joints *and* 2 or more DIP hard tissue enlargement *or* deformity in 2 or more select joints	Knee pain *and* Radiographic osteophytes *and* 1 or more of the following: age 50 years or more, morning stiffness < 30 minutes, crepitus on motion	Hip pain *and* 2 or more of the following: ESR < 10 mm/hr, radiographic femoral or acetabular osteophytes, radiographic joint space narrowing

Modified from Cooke TD, Dwosh IL. Clinical features of osteoarthritis in the elderly. Clin Rheum Dis 1986;12:155–174. Hochberg MC, Altman RD, Brandt KD, et al. Guidelines for the medical management of osteoarthritis. Part I. Osteoarthritis of the hip. American College of Rheumatology. Arthritis Rheum 1995;38:1535–1540. Hochberg MC, Altman RD, Brandt KD, et al. Guidelines for the medical management of osteoarthritis. Part II. Osteoarthritis of the knee. American College of Rheumatology. Arthritis Rheum 1995;38:1541–1546. Altman R, Alarcon G, Appelrouth D, et al. The American College of Rheumatology criteria of the classification and reporting of osteoarthritis of the hand. Arthritis Rheum 1990;33:1601–1610.
[a]Select joints are DIP, proximal interphalangeal, first CMC.

relieved by rest. Morning stiffness and stiffness following inactivity, also known as gel phenomena, may be present but are limited to several minutes and must be distinguished from the prolonged stiffness that accompanies inflammatory joint diseases. The onset of symptoms is insidious, and they progress gradually. Patients with advanced disease may have pain at rest and may sense that their weight-bearing joints lock or give way because of internal derangement (36).

Physical Signs

Bony joint enlargement, the most common physical finding in osteoarthritis, may be accompanied by crepitus and limited range of motion. Heberden's and Bouchard's nodes of the distal and proximal interphalangeal joints of the hand are examples of joint enlargement in primary osteoarthritis. Tenderness on palpation at the joint line, painful motion, and limited range of motion are also common although not unique to osteoarthritis. Progressive cartilage destruction, malalignment, joint effusions, and subchondral bone collapse contribute to irreversible deformity. Periarticular muscle atrophy develops

quickly. Inflammatory signs such as soft tissue swelling and joint warmth rarely accompany osteoarthritis. Intense inflammatory signs should alert the clinician to another process, such as infection or crystal-induced arthritis (36).

Radiographic Signs

Standard radiographs augment the history and examination to confirm a diagnosis of osteoarthritis. The radiographic features of osteoarthritis, which include osteophyte formation, joint space narrowing, subchondral sclerosis, and cysts, are shown in Figure 32.1 (40, 41). Radiographs also assist in evaluating the patient whose symptoms fail to respond to conventional therapy or whose symptoms are suspicious for fracture or malignancy. MRI may be useful when there is a need to evaluate patients for spinal stenosis, internal knee derangements, or avascular necrosis. Bone scans have limited utility in the diagnosis and management of osteoarthritis.

When defined by radiographs, the distal and proximal interphalangeal joints of the hand are the most prevalent location of osteoarthritis. The knee and hip are the second and third most common locations of radiographic osteoarthritis, re-

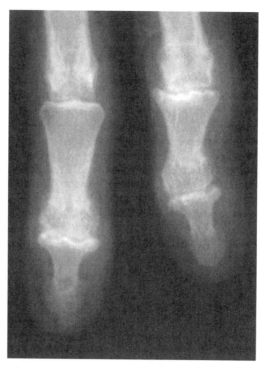

Figure 32.1. Radiographic abnormalities of osteoarthritis, including osteophytes, sclerosis, and joint space narrowing.

spectively, and, in contrast to the hand, are frequently symptomatic. The first metatarsal phalangeal and carpometacarpal joints are also frequent sites of radiographic osteoarthritis (42).

Subsets of Disease

Erosive inflammatory osteoarthritis is a subset of osteoarthritis that is characterized by relatively intense inflammatory changes in the small joints of the hands. Mild to moderate synovitis is present in the early stages, followed often by joint instability and later still ankylosis. Radiographic erosions are visible. Osteoarthritis in other peripheral joints, such as the shoulder, elbow, wrist, and metacarpophalangeal joints, usually is due to some secondary process, such as traumatic injury or neuropathy. Osteoarthritis can be the result of joint destruction due to inflammatory joint disease, injury, metabolic disorder, infection, neuropathic processes, or hypermobility. In elderly patients, calcium pyrophosphate dehydrate deposition disease is

likely the most common cause of secondary osteoarthritis.

When to Suspect Another Condition

Musculoskeletal complaints, which are common in the elderly, may arise from an expansive list of disorders ranging from benign to malignant (43–45). Although the diagnosis of osteoarthritis is straightforward, one should ascertain that painful symptoms are indeed attributable to osteoarthritis. Nerve entrapment and infectious and vascular disorders may be mistakenly attributed to osteoarthritis when typical radiographic abnormalities are present. In addition, periarticular syndromes and inflammatory diseases, such as calcium pyrophosphate disease, may be superimposed on osteoarthritis. We suggest the algorithm outlined in Table 32.2. The acute onset of joint pain accompanied by inflammatory findings should warrant prompt investigation, including arthrocentesis, to exclude infectious and/or crystalline disease.

Table 32.2

An Algorithmic Approach to Osteoarthritis

Are systemic symptoms present?	Yes →	Rheumatoid arthritis
Generalized morning sickness		Polymyalgia rheumatica
Fever		Gout, CPPD, hydroxyapatite
Anorexia		Systemic lupus
Weight loss		Sjögren's syndrome
Fatigue	No ↓	Carcinoma polyarthritis

Are painful symptoms due to disorders other than or superimposed on osteoarthritis?

Periarticular	Articular	Systemic
Bursitis	Infectious arthritis	Malignancy
Tendinitis	Crystalline diseases	Neuropathy
Fibromyalgia	Internal derangement	Thyroid disease
Primary bone	Hemarthrosis	Acromegaly
Primary muscle	Ochronosis	Hemochromatosis

Pathogenesis

Osteoarthritis can be thought of as a process of cartilage matrix degradation to which an ineffectual attempt at repair is made (46, 47). A progressive decrease in the number of chondrocytes with advancing age probably limits the ability of aging cartilage to maintain and repair itself. Thus, progressive depletion of proteoglycan and an alteration in the integrity of the collagen ultrastructure (i.e., type II collagen) are observed in osteoarthritic cartilage. Presumably in response to this degradative process, chondrocytes initially undergo increased proliferation and secrete enhanced amounts of proteoglycan molecules. As the disease progresses, however, the reparative process is outmatched by the degradative process, and a net loss of cartilage occurs. The superficial layer of cartilage initially shows fissuring, cracking, and erosion that progresses over time to the deeper layers.

A number of soluble proteins have been implicated in the pathogenesis of osteoarthritis by virtue of their abilities to degrade or inhibit repair of cartilage. A relative excess of destructive metalloproteinase (MMP) enzymes or proinflammatory cytokines, such as interleukin-1 (IL-1), favor cartilage destruction and development of osteoarthritis. A relative deficiency of protective mediators such as the IL-1 receptor antagonist or tissue metalloproteinase inhibitors can also result in the cartilage destruction that is characteristic of osteoarthritis. Although growth factors and oncogenic proteins have been identified in osteoarthritic cartilage, their roles in the development of osteoarthritis remain unclear.

Management

Effective management of osteoarthritis in the elderly includes concurrent pharmacologic and nonpharmacologic interventions with goals of pain relief and preservation of functional independence, mobility, and quality of life (48).

Nonpharmacologic Management

Recent guidelines set forth by the American College of Rheumatology for the management of hip and knee osteoarthritis highlight the importance of nonpharmacologic modes of therapy, including local heat or ice, ultrasound, and electrical stimulation to relieve pain (37, 38). Weight reduction, as little as 10 pounds, in obese patients and proper use of assistive devices and shock absorbing footwear can help protect the joint from further damage and improve joint biomechanics and overall function. Myths that patients with arthritis should avoid exercise have been dispelled by recent evidence indicating that joint loading and mobilization are essential for articular integrity (49). Others have shown that even moderately disabled persons with knee osteoarthritis benefit from low-impact aerobic or resistive exercise, with improvement in measures of disability, physical performance, pain, and gait without injury to joints (50–54). Studies of nursing home and community-dwelling elderly clearly demonstrate that a reduction in the number of falls is an additional benefit of exercise (55).

Current Medical Therapy

Until medications that modify or stop the progression of osteoarthritis become available, relief of painful symptoms will remain the goal of medicinal intervention. Acetaminophen up to 4 g daily is the initial analgesic of choice for symptomatic osteoarthritis, but it must be used cautiously by patients who consume alcohol or have hepatic impairment (37, 38, 56, 57). Some patients require nonsteroidal anti-inflammatory agents (NSAIDs) at anti-inflammatory doses to achieve adequate analgesia (58). However, all NSAIDs are to be used with great caution by elderly patients, since NSAID-induced gastrointestinal and renal toxicities occur with increased frequency. Consequently, concurrent use of the prostaglandin E_1 analog misoprostol or an H_2 blocker should be considered for patients at risk for gastrointestinal bleeding (59). In addition, renal function should be monitored at regular intervals. The cyclooxygenase-2 (COX-2) specific NSAIDs offer a theoretic advantage over nonselective cyclooxygenase inhibitors, as they may minimize NSAID-induced gastrointestinal and renal toxicity (60, 61).

Local therapies may include topical capsaicin and methyl salicylate creams as adjunctive agents in the management of knee and hand osteoarthritis (62, 63). Judicious use of intra-articular glucocorticoid injections is appropriate for elderly osteoarthritis patients with effusions or local inflammatory signs. Periarticular injections may effectively treat the bursitis or tendinitis that may accompany osteoarthritis. The need for frequent intra-articular injections suggests that orthopaedic intervention may be prudent.

Surgical Management

Severe pain that is unresponsive to maximal medical therapy and compromised function indicate the need for surgical intervention (46). Arthroscopic lavage may relieve pain for patients with significant crepitus or radiographically visible loose bodies of a large joint, although benefits are rarely permanent. The location and extent of articular damage, age of the patient, and integrity of the surrounding ligamentous structures determine whether an osteotomy or total joint replacement is indicated. Careful selection of patients for surgery is warranted, given the high incidence of perioperative and postoperative risks in elderly patients. Perioperative management should also anticipate the cardiovascular deconditioning that accompanies advanced lower-extremity osteoarthritis. Prolonged postoperative rehabilitation is often required, and it may be complicated by other medical problems. The long-term efficacy of intra-articular glycosaminoglycan injections remains to be proved.

REGIONAL MUSCULOSKELETAL DISORDERS
The Painful Spine

Low back pain is the most common local musculoskeletal complaint that confronts the physician (Table 32.3) (64–66). Although much of the medical literature on back pain pertains to young adults, it is helpful to distinguish an acute condition (7 days or less) from one that persists

Table 32.3

Common Causes of Low Back Pain in the Elderly Patient

Mechanical
  Osteoarthritis
  Degenerative disc disease
  Spinal stenosis
  Muscular strain
  Inflammatory spondyloarthropathy
Metabolic bone disease
  Osteoporosis
  Osteomalacia
Neoplastic
  Myeloma
  Leukemia
  Metastatic disease
Paget's disease
  Diffuse idiopathic skeletal hyperostosis (DISH)

or is chronic (3 months or more). The clinician should also be careful to consider malignant and other systemic processes in elderly patients with back pain because of their prevalence in this population.

Although acute low back strain occurs in the elderly, it is a much less common cause of back pain than in young adults. The first step in evaluating acute back pain is to exclude life- or function-threatening conditions. Complaints of writhing pain or back pain that is accompanied by claudicatory symptoms or syncope may be due to an abdominal aortic aneurysm. Urgent computed tomography (CT) and surgical evaluation are warranted to exclude this life-threatening condition. Claudicatory symptoms accompanied by bilateral sciatica and saddle anesthesia suggest compression or compromise of the cauda equina (cauda equina syndrome). Neurologic deficits should be sought and MRI and neurosurgical evaluation urgently obtained. Aneurysms and cauda equina syndrome are both more commonly encountered in elderly patients than with young adults.

Back pain may be a presentation of a majority of systemic disorders, including malignancy. The issue of axial malignancy is discussed later in this chapter. The following warning signs warrant further diagnostic evaluation: fever, antecedent weight loss, anorexia, pain that awakens the patient at night or that is more prominent with recumbency. Such pain may suggest a malignancy or occult infection of the spine or surrounding area. Early morning stiffness that persists beyond 1 hour raises the possibility of inflammatory spondyloarthropathy. Recent evidence suggests that inflammatory back disease can develop in the elderly.

The causes of persistent low back discomfort in the elderly differ significantly from those seen in younger age groups. Adults over age 55, especially those who have a history of malignancy, steroid use, or recent trauma or symptoms in the thoracic spine, should undergo radiographic evaluation of the symptomatic area to rule out a bony lesion.

Many diagnostic procedures are available. Plain radiographs of the spine are helpful in evaluating patients in whom malignancy or fracture is suspected. Lateral, anteroposterior, and oblique views should be obtained. Sacroiliac views must be requested specifically if inflammatory back disease is suspected. CT provides the best resolution of cortical bone and should be requested if cortical erosions are suspected but not visualized on plain radiographs of the spine or sacroiliac joints. MRI is the best available test when neurologic impairment or encroachment is a concern. MRI also provides the best resolution of intraosseous processes such as tumor and infection. Myelography provides information valuable in planning the surgical approach and excluding other lesions that are not clinically apparent prior to surgery.

Common Conditions in Elderly Patients With Back Pain

OSTEOARTHRITIS OF THE AXIAL SKELETON. Probably the most common cause of back pain and limitation of motion are osteoarthritis and degenerative disc disease. Complaints are usually about the lumbar and/or cervical areas. The pain is generally insidious in onset, often present since younger years (30 to 40 years of age), dull most of the time but sharp on extreme range of motion, and in the low back, aggravated by forward flexion. Pain in the neck that is aggravated by extension and relieved by flexion suggests osteoarthritis of the facet joints of the cervical vertebral bodies. Stiffness lasting several minutes after periods of inactivity is typical of osteoarthritis and/or degenerative disc disease. If the pain radiates into the legs or arms, a radiculopathy secondary to nerve root compression may be present. Sciatica secondary to impingement of L4-L5 or L5-S1 is the most common type of nerve root entrapment syndrome. In contrast, thoracic back discomfort is distinctly unusual and should not be attributed to axial osteoarthritis or degenerative disc disease. Approximately 70% of patients over age 70 have radiographic evidence of cervical degenerative disc disease, most frequently in C5-C6 or C6-C7. Radiographic evidence of structural problems of the axial lumbar apophyseal (facet) joints and/or degenerative disc disease are also highly prevalent in this population, affecting approximately 60% of women and 80% of all elderly patients. It is necessary for the clinician to question whether each patient's clinical presentation may account for the radiographic findings or is due to another process. Conservative medical management is appropriate unless the pain is not reasonably controlled or a progressive neurologic syndrome emerges. Medical management follows the same principles and precautions that are detailed in the section on osteoarthritis.

SPINAL STENOSIS. Spinal stenosis is an important cause of low back pain and dysfunction in the elderly (67, 68). It can be caused by compression of the spinal canal through extensive bony enlargement of the vertebral body facets and by soft tissue changes secondary to degenerative disc disease. It may also be a result of another acquired bony disease, such as Paget's disease, acromegaly, renal osteodystrophy, or late-stage ankylosing spondylitis, or secondary to malignant mass or bony collapse from tumor invasion. It may also occur in the cervical area. Spinal stenosis may also develop after laminectomy, attempted spinal fusion, or chemonucleolysis.

Typically the discomfort of spinal stenosis is dull and moderate, aggravated by moving into extension (lying down, stretching backward, standing up straight, walking down an incline or stairs), and improved with stooping forward by flexing the hips and knees. The pain may radiate into the posterior legs or buttock, causing discomfort that is often aggravated by walking (pseudoclaudication). Leg numbness or muscle weakness as well as other neurologic impairment can occur, including an upper motor lesion and/or bowel or bladder dysfunction. In lumbar spinal stenosis there are relatively few physical findings. Specifically, demonstrable sensory or muscular deficits are seen in the minority of patients. The straight-leg test is usually negative.

The neurogenic claudication of spinal stenosis must be differentiated from vascular claudication. Patients with vascular claudication are relieved by standing and lying flat and have diminished peripheral pulses; patients with spinal stenosis have worsened pain when standing upright in the extended position and may have normal distal lower extremity pulses. Bicycle exercise testing can occasionally distinguish neurogenic from vascular claudication by reproducing vascular claudication and not reproducing neurogenic claudication.

Plain radiographs offer little value in making the diagnosis of lumbar spinal stenosis. Electromyelography studies, however, are abnormal in about 80% of patients. The abnormalities are frequently seen in multiple levels in a bilateral distribution. MRI is being used most commonly for the diagnosis of spinal stenosis. However, if clinical suspicion for spinal stenosis is high and the MRI does not support this, CT myelography can be performed to allow further evaluation of the bony and soft tissue structures of the spine.

Conservative treatment is appropriate in the absence of significant pain or neurologic deficit. There is, however, no evidence to suggest that this offers any improvement in symptoms. Surgical decompressive laminectomy is the treatment of choice for relief of pain and functional improvement or when there is a neurologic deficit. It is important to appreciate the entire extent of spinal cord compression before surgery and carefully evaluate the patient as a candidate for surgery before considering this intervention. Pamidronate and calcitonin are under investigation as management options for this condition.

DIFFUSE IDIOPATHIC SKELETAL HYPEROSTOSIS. By age 50, approximately 60% of women and 80% of men form anterior and lateral osteophytes of the vertebral column (spondylosis deformans). Diffuse idiopathic skeletal hyperostosis (DISH) (69) is a disorder characterized by calcification and ossification of the anterior longitudinal ligament in the absence of degenerative disc disease or inflammatory back disease (68). Adult-onset diabetes mellitus can be found in up to 50% of patients with DISH. The ossification, which may extend over several vertebral bodies, is associated with moderate to marked limitations of movement of the thorax and low back. DISH is often an asymptomatic radiologic finding. However, it may be an important cause of complaints of decreased range of motion and stiffness with discomfort. Bony spurs may occur at other sites, including the tip of the elbow or the heel. This process rarely causes nerve root entrapment and generally can be managed with conservative measures of education and physical therapy. Axial manifestations of malignancy are discussed later.

Management

Relatively uncommon in elderly patients, simple muscular strain can be treated conservatively with rest (3 days is probably as effective as longer without risk of deconditioning), local measures such as gentle massage and heat, and the use of an analgesic such as acetaminophen, low doses of NSAIDs, or opioid analgesics if necessary. Patients should be taught about proper back mechanics to avoid further injury. Recovery should occur in 2 to 4 weeks. Because of this excellent prognosis, glucocorticoid injection therapies are rarely necessary, nor are they more effective than placebo in management of acute back pain due to disc herniation in young adults. Muscle relaxants have not been studied in the management of back pain in older adults, and they carry a risk of anticholinergic side effects, including drowsiness and urinary retention (70, 71).

Persistent back pain is more of a challenge. Standard strategies are based on data from young adult patients and may not be appropriate for older adults, whose back symptoms have vastly different origins. In contrast to acute back pain, in persistent back pain bed rest should be avoided, since deconditioning contributes further to disability without any proven benefit for these patients. Muscle relaxants, NSAIDs, and local glucocorticoid injections have not been systematically studied. Recent evidence suggests that tricyclic antidepressants provide some benefit for those who are also depressed but offer little to patients who are not depressed. Neuromuscular and/or transcutaneous electrical nerve stimulation (TENS) when used together are probably more effective than when either is used alone, but this also has not been studied in older adults (72–74). Experimental therapies, including epidural steroids and acupuncture, are under investigation.

The Painful Shoulder

The painful shoulder (75) is a common musculoskeletal complaint in the elderly, usually presenting as either unilateral or bilateral pain that radiates into the upper arm or deltoid muscle groups on elevation of the arm or arms laterally or over the head. Abduction of the arm to 45° involves the muscles of the rotator cuff. These muscles insert to the humeral head and lie beneath the acromion to the scapula. The insertion of these muscles has a limited blood supply and because of its location is subject to chronic impingement, injury, and microtears. Consequently, inflammation and deposition of calcium-containing crystals (hydroxyapatite) take place in these tissues. Patients present with a painful arch of motion of the arm from 0 to 45° of abduction, or they may have decreased motion of the arm (the frozen shoulder syndrome). They may also have an acutely painful shoulder girdle with signs of inflammation. The acute inflammatory events are secondary to bursitis or tendinitis as a reaction to the local release of calcium-containing crystals from the soft tissue into the bursae, tendons, or joints. The acute inflammatory event is best treated with rest and an NSAID. Alternatively, corticosteroids can be instilled into the subdeltoid region of the shoulder girdle. In the indolent phase of this process, protection of the shoulder and regular physical therapy to recover range of motion constitute the preferred treatment.

Acromioclavicular (AC) joint osteoarthritis can also cause shoulder pain. Patients have pain at the AC joint as they elevate the arm beyond 45° of abduction, such as raising the arm over the head. Biceps tendinitis can present as anterior shoulder girdle pain and swelling. This condition is aggravated by pronation of the forearm, flexion and extension of the forearm, or compression over the biceps tendon. Rest and short-term use of an NSAID almost always results in successful treatment.

In the absence of a neuropathy, true glenohumeral joint arthritis (the true shoulder joint) is not common in the elderly patient. Limitation of shoulder movement is almost always secondary to bursitis, rotator cuff disease, or the restriction from the chronic impingement syndrome.

Bursitis

Bursitis is inflammation in a bursal sac that normally lines and lubricates movement between bones, tendons, ligaments, and/or muscles. The bursae may become inflamed because of trauma (microbleeding or tears), overuse, infection, systemic inflammation (e.g., rheumatoid arthritis), microcrystalline deposition, or for no well-defined reason. Polymyalgia rheumatica can also cause bursitis of the subacromial area. The patient has pain that is local and aggravated with motion. If the bursa is superficial (e.g., the olecranon bursae), swelling, heat, or redness may be present. Fever is usually absent.

Sites of daily trauma, such as the olecranon bursa over the elbow and the prepatellar bursa of the knee, are the areas where bursitis is more likely to occur. Other sites include the trochanteric bursa (lateral upper thigh), anserine bursa (tibia at the anterior medial knee), ischial bursa (over the ischial tuberosity), and semimembranosus-gastrocnemius bursa behind the knee (Baker's cyst).

Baker's cyst has special importance because it can rupture and result in severe pain and swelling in the involved knee and leg. This typically occurs in those with some underlying arthritic knee condition. The patients typically complain of acute onset of calf pain and calf swelling that occurs when the popliteal cyst dissects down into the calf muscle. This may mimic thrombophlebitis and so has been called the pseudothrombophlebitis syndrome (76). In anyone with acute leg pain and swelling, Baker's cyst should be considered and should not mistaken for deep venous thrombosis. Traditionally, diagnosis was established with an arthrogram; however, now ultrasonography can detect a ruptured cyst. Therapy requires rest for the joint and intra-articular injection of corticosteroids. This should provide relief within a matter of hours.

Whenever possible an acutely inflamed bursae should be aspirated to obtain bursal fluid for examination (including polarization microscopy for crystals) and culture. Crystal-induced bursitis and infection have high leukocyte counts (25,000 to 50,000 cell per cubic millimeter), while in other causes the white count is usually low. The olecranon is a common site of septic bursitis, usually *Staphylococcus aureus* infection. Infectious bursitis requires both appropriate antibiotics and drainage. In the elderly patient, it is recommended that the patient be hospitalized initially for management of septic bursitis (77). Noninfectious bursitis can best be treated with rest and a short course of an NSAID. If this fails to resolve the situation, a local injection of corticosteroids may be helpful.

Tenosynovitis

Tenosynovitis, or tendinitis, can occur at any age, either secondary to overuse (exercise) or trauma or associated with generalized inflammatory arthritis (e.g., rheumatoid arthritis). Although any tendon can be involved, common sites include the flexor tendons of the fingers (the trigger finger), the abductor or extensor tendons of the thumb (de Quervain's syndrome), dorsal extensor tendons of the wrist, and insertion of muscles at the elbow (tennis and golfer's elbow). Tenosynovitis is best managed by splinting the involved area (rest) and using an NSAID for several days. Corticosteroid injections can be helpful when NSAIDs are contraindicated or ineffective. Tendinitis can be distinguished from ganglion cysts (cystic swelling of the synovial sheath) and Dupuytren's contracture (hyperplasia of the palmar fascia) because tendinitis tends to have an acute onset and a short course compared with the chronic noninflammatory nature of ganglion cysts and contracture. Diffuse palmar fascia thickening has been associated with ovarian carcinoma and long-standing diabetes.

MICROCRYSTALLINE DISEASE

The most common acute monarticular arthritis in the elderly patient is crystal induced. The main forms of microcrystalline arthritis are triggered by monosodium urate crystals (gout) and calcium pyrophosphate dihydrate crystals (pseudogout) (78, 79). Pseudogout clinically mimics gout, but the treatments are different (discussed later). It is therefore important to perform arthrocentesis to identify the exact crystal and distinguish crystal-induced arthritis from other causes of acute monarthritis, particularly septic arthritis.

Gout

In gout (80, 81) hyperuricemia leads to the deposition of monosodium urate crystals in soft tissue (the tophi) and in the structures of the joint. In the absence of defined secondary factors (e.g., renal insufficiency, diuretic use) young and middle-aged men are more likely to have an elevated serum uric acid level and gout than are premenopausal women. In fact, in men over age 30, gout is the most common cause of inflammatory arthritis. In the elderly population, hyperuricemia becomes equally prevalent in men and women and is seen more commonly in those with renal insufficiency and those using thiazide diuretics for hypertension. In this condition urate crystals are proinflammatory and provoke an acute arthritis that is usually monarticular and intense.

Symptoms

Gout classically presents as an acute severe monarticular arthritis, a soft tissue infection (cellulitis), or thrombophlebitis. The most frequently involved joints are those of the lower extremity, including the metatarsal phalangeal joint of the great toe (podagra), the ankle, and the knee. Typically, an attack begins abruptly for no apparent reason; the joint rapidly swells and becomes warm to touch, erythematous, and so exquisitely painful that the patient will not move the joint or allow it to be touched. Gouty arthritis is episodic and spontaneously resolves in 3 to 10 days without treatment. Occasionally the attacks occur in the upper extremity, particularly in the olecranon bursae. A polyarticular presentation is uncommon as an initial presentation in young adults but can occur in the elderly population. Also, multiple joint involvement may be a complication of untreated chronic tophaceous gout. Tophaceous deposits around the joints of the fingers can be mistaken for the nodules of osteoarthritis or even rheumatoid arthritis in the elderly patient (Fig. 32.2). Recurrent untreated gout attacks and local deposition of urate destroy bone and joints, leading to joint deformities and remarkable disability. The other major sequela of hyperuricemia is nephrolithiasis from uric acid stones. In a partially treated state, patients may also have attacks that are less intense and are difficult to diagnose.

Laboratory Diagnosis

During an acute gout attack the patient may have a remarkable leukocytosis associated with fever, causing a major concern for infection. The serum uric acid level is influenced by several factors and therefore has limited value during an acute attack. Specifically, up to a third of patients can have a normal serum uric acid level at the time of an acute attack. Arthrocentesis of the involved

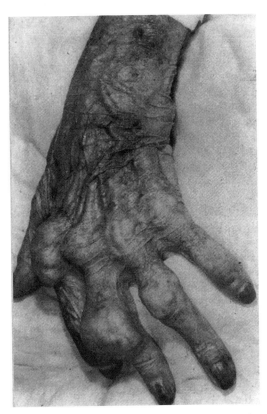

Figure 32.2.   Gouty arthritis with tophaceous deposits.

joint and synovial fluid analysis are important procedures to establish the diagnosis of gout. In gout, the joint fluid is inflammatory, with decreased viscosity, high protein level, and elevated polymorphonuclear leukocytes. The synovial fluid leukocyte count is generally above 50,000 cells per cubic millimeter, levels also seen in septic arthritis. Gram staining of the fluid sample and culture should be negative for bacteria. Monosodium urate crystals are easily identified in the joint fluid with a polarizing microscope; they are needle-shaped crystals, bright yellow when the crystal's long axis is parallel to the axis of light from the polarizer (negatively birefringent).

Management (80–82)

Patients who have asymptomatic elevations of the serum uric acid (no history of renal stones, tophi, or gouty arthritis) should not be treated unless levels exceed 13 mg/dL. Treatment of the acute gout attack and prevention of recurrent attacks are the main and separate issues to be addressed in the patient with gout. After diagnosis of acute gouty arthritis, the principal aim of therapy is to relieve pain and suppress inflammation. In the elderly it is important to do a careful review of other medical problems and the physiologic condition of the patient before starting any drug treatment for the acute inflammatory condition. Given the high prevalence of concurrent chronic illnesses, including renal insufficiency, coronary artery disease, congestive heart failure, and ulcer disease, it is important to keep in mind that gout is not a life-threatening condition. Gouty arthritis may be managed with analgesics alone; the risks of other therapies are significant.

NSAIDs rapidly reduce inflammation and pain in gouty arthritis and are as effective in older adults as they are in young adults. No one NSAID has been shown to be more efficacious than another in the treatment of gout. The NSAID should be started at full dose and continued until the attack resolves (usually within 24 to 48 hours). Contraindications to NSAIDs are evidence of renal or hepatic insufficiency and peptic ulcer disease. Elderly patients are at a high risk for NSAID-related gastritis, peptic ulceration, and gastrointestinal bleeding. NSAID-induced renal failure is common in elderly patients. If NSAIDs are to be used, caution should be exercised: first document normal renal function, and use a short-acting NSAID at a low dose for the briefest period necessary to control the attack.

Colchicine has been used successfully for more than 100 years for the treatment of acute gouty arthritis. It is thought to work by suppressing leukocytes from ingesting the urate crystal and by reducing the production of locally produced chemoattractants. It can be given orally in small, frequent doses; however, oral colchicine usually causes significant gastrointestinal distress, including abnormal cramps, diarrhea, or nausea and vomiting. These side effects can be avoided by giving colchicine by a slow intravenous infusion. This route of administration, however, has been complicated by a significant risk of severe toxic reactions. Patients with renal and hepatic insufficiency and/or elderly patients have a high risk of these toxicities.

Because of these risks, colchicine should be avoided in elderly patients as the initial drug treatment of acute gouty arthritis.

Corticosteroids are also very effective for suppressing the inflammation of acute gout. A corticosteroid should be considered as the medication of choice when an NSAID and colchicine are considered too risky. This can be administered either orally or intravenously in moderate doses to suppress inflammation (20 to 30 mg orally daily for several days). Intramuscular injections of adrenocorticotropic hormone (ACTH) or corticosteroids are not recommended. Preferably, intra-articular injection of corticosteroids follows joint aspiration; this is extremely effective when acute gout affects one joint.

Treatment of hyperuricemia should be delayed until the acute attack is suppressed and fully resolved for several weeks. After the acute attack has subsided, the physician should address any risk factors for hyperuricemia that can be corrected. For example, a myelodysplastic disorder (e.g., polycythemia vera) can cause excess uric acid production and hyperuricemia; excessive alcohol intake can both increase urate production and decrease its renal excretion; thiazide diuretics decrease renal uric acid secretion and increase serum uric acid. If hyperuricemia persists after potentially reversible causes of hyperuricemia are addressed, a drug that lowers serum uric acid should be considered. If the patient has had only one gout episode and if there is a low or normal excretion of urate (low risk for renal stone), colchicine alone can be used in low doses (0.6 mg orally once or twice daily) for prophylaxis against new attacks. Patients with renal insufficiency are at risk for developing colchicine-induced myopathy.

Recurrent acute gout can also be prevented by normalizing the serum uric acid level, decreasing the total body urate content. In the elderly, urate underexcretion is the most common cause of hyperuricemia. Thiazide use should be discontinued if possible, since thiazides favor uric acid reabsorption and impair clearance. Therapy to lower serum uric acid should be reserved for patients who have recurrent gouty attacks, a renal stone, or tophaceous gout. Uricosuric medication (probenecid) can be used in patients with low or normal uric acid excretion, no renal insufficiency, and no history of uric acid nephrolithiasis. The xanthine oxidase inhibitor allopurinol lowers the production of urate and is the more practical drug for the elderly patient to normalize the serum uric acid. It is recommended that allopurinol be started at 100 mg orally daily and increased by 100 mg every 2 weeks in the setting of normal renal function until the serum uric acid is normalized. The maximum dose usually required is 300 mg daily. Oral colchicine 0.6 mg orally once or twice a day should be started before allopurinol treatment to prevent a new gout attack, which may occur because tissue uric acid shifts rapidly during decreases in serum uric acid.

Pseudogout

The acute inflammatory monarthritis that is secondary to calcium pyrophosphate dihydrate (CPPD) crystals mimics gout and therefore is called pseudogout (78, 83). Deposition of CPPD crystals in the cartilage (chondrocalcinosis) is very common in the elderly. Chondrocalcinosis, usually an asymptomatic finding that is more common in men than in women, can be seen radiographically in the medial and lateral compartments of the knee and within the radiocarpal joint of the wrist.

Symptoms

Like gouty arthritis, pseudogout presents as an episodic acute, intense arthritis that can involve one or several joints. The attacks are typically self-limited and most usually affect the knee or the radiocarpal joint in the wrist. A minority of patients have a symmetric polyarthritis that mimics rheumatoid arthritis, including the constitutional symptoms of fatigue, morning stiffness, and low-grade fever. Pseudogout may also present as mini attacks or pseudo-osteoarthritis. It may also cause profound inflammation, fever, and a sepsislike picture. Arthrocentesis of the involved joint should be done when possible so that the crystal can be identified and joint fluid can be sent for culture. The CPPD crystals are rod-shaped and blue when viewed with parallel light on the polarizing microscope (positively birefringent).

Management

Chondrocalcinosis and attacks of pseudogout have been associated with a number of diseases, including hypothyroidism, hyperparathyroidism, and hemochromatosis. Treatment of pseudogout requires suppression of the acute inflammation with an NSAID or if necessary, corticosteroids. Colchicine may be used on an ongoing basis to prevent recurrent inflammation. There are no drugs to alter the tissue level CPPD crystals. Fortunately, unlike gout, pseudogout is only infrequently recurrent.

DIFFUSE SOFT TISSUE PAIN SYNDROMES

Diffuse pain syndromes (Table 32.4) may be either inflammatory or noninflammatory (80). The clinician should diligently exclude inflammatory causes of diffuse pain, often accompanied by morning stiffness, dry mouth and eyes, Raynaud's phenomena, and constitutional symptoms. Giant cell arteritis, polymyalgia rheumatica (PMR), malignancy including myeloma, and rheumatoid arthritis, which reach their peak prevalence rates after age 60, can cause diffuse pain. Less common

Table 32.4

Differential Diagnosis of Diffuse Pain in the Elderly

Noninflammatory
  Depression
  Chronic pain syndrome
  Metabolic disorder
  Hyperthyroidism
  Hypothyroidism
  Hyperparathyroidism
  Vitamin D deficiency
  Fibromyalgia (fibrositis)
  Malingering
Inflammatory
  Rheumatic diseases with late-set onset
    Polymyositis
    Rheumatoid arthritis
    Sjögren's syndrome
  Systemic lupus erythematosus
  Chronic infections
  Systemic vasculitis
    Giant cell arteritis
  Malignant neoplasms

inflammatory causes of diffuse musculoskeletal pain in the elderly include polymyositis, systemic lupus, and Sjögren's syndrome. These entities are discussed in detail later in this chapter.

Noninflammatory causes of diffuse musculoskeletal pain include metabolic and endocrine disorders and the fibromyalgia syndrome. The prevalence of hypothyroidism appears to be as high as 17% in adults older than 60 years. Hypothyroidism can result in a painful myopathy and gait abnormalities. The incidence of hyperthyroidism, which may lead to thyroid acropathy, periostitis, and digital clubbing, also increases considerably in older adults. Since Graves' disease and toxic multinodular goiter are most common in older adults, these conditions should be sought out with ultrasound and nuclear thyroid scans. Hyperparathyroidism can also result in accelerated osteoporosis and diffuse pain and may be accompanied by other features in the setting of renal disease.

Clinicians should be aware of the musculoskeletal manifestations of osteomalacia (85, 86), which may be associated with polyarthralgias and/or proximal muscle weakness. Symptoms include bone pain involving the spine, rib cage, pelvis, and shoulder girdle. Radiographic findings include diffuse osteoporosis, coarse trabeculation, and pseudofractures. Subnormal serum 25-hydroxyvitamin D levels provide the best measure of vitamin D stores. Despite average intakes of vitamin D in excess of twice the recommended dietary allowance of 200 IU per day, up to 50% of home-bound older adults living in the community have low vitamin D. Vitamin D replacement produces symptomatic and functional improvement.

Fibromyalgia syndrome is a disorder characterized by diffuse musculoskeletal pain accompanied by nonrestorative sleep, fatigue, and physical tender points. It is common in the elderly (87). Community-based studies have shown that the prevalence of fibromyalgia syndrome peaks in the 60s. Although early studies were careful to exclude patients with radiographic osteoarthritis, recent observations suggest that patients with rheumatic disorders and osteoarthritis may also develop fibromyalgia syndrome. It may respond to management with tricyclic antidepressants or cyclobenzaprine at low doses, but the anticholinergic side effects of these two agents limit their usefulness for older adults. As discussed earlier, NSAIDs may assist with pain management but should be prescribed cautiously. Opioid analgesics may also be used sparingly. Psychiatric illness including depression should also be sought out, as it may cause diffuse musculoskeletal complaints.

POLYMYALGIA RHEUMATICA

Polymyalgia rheumatica (PMR) (88–91) is a clinical syndrome that is seen almost exclusively in patients over age 50 (mean age of onset 70; range 50 to 90). It is most common in women and whites, particularly those of Scandinavian descent. The incidence of PMR increases with each decade over age 50 but varies with the ethnic background of the population. It has been estimated that in Olmstead County, Minnesota, the incidence is 19.8 per 100,000 in persons aged 50 to 59 and 112 per 100,000 in persons aged 70 to 79.

Symptoms

PMR is manifested by a symmetric aching discomfort and stiffness of the neck, shoulders, and hips. It commonly begins acutely over 2 weeks but may also have an insidious onset and course. Pain and stiffness are usually most prominent in the morning and after periods of rest (gelling). The pain generally improves as the patient moves the involved muscles and joints, but it can be progressive over time if untreated. In fact, the pain can be debilitating and compromise the patient's ability to provide self-care. Other clinical symptoms suggesting an inflammatory illness are usually prominent. These include a low-grade fever, weight loss, fatigue, mood changes, and lethargy. The symptoms of PMR may cause patients to withdraw from their usual social activity or produce profound depression. Although muscle weakness is uncommon, the patient may be unstable and subject to falls due to pain and stiffness.

Signs and Laboratory Findings

On physical examination the patient may appear chronically ill and may have a depressed affect. There is usually no objective evidence of muscle weakness. Range of motion of the shoulders and hips is frequently limited by pain and stiffness. PMR often involves the joints of the fingers and the wrist in a pattern similar to that of rheumatoid arthritis. Less commonly, the patient has swelling of the one or both sternoclavicular joints. Joint effusion, especially within the fingers, wrists, and knees, is not uncommon. Carpal tunnel entrapment may occur secondary to wrist synovitis. Laboratory studies will often show evidence of a systemic inflammatory reaction: a remarkably elevated ESR, mild leukocytosis, and a normochromic, normocytic anemia of "chronic disease." An elevated serum alkaline phosphatase is found in 20 to 60% of patients because of a nonspecific granulomatous process in the liver. The analysis of synovial fluid, when present, shows only moderate inflammation with typically fewer that 15,000 synovial white blood cells per cubic millimeter. Muscle enzyme levels and electromyelograms are normal.

PMR is a clinical syndrome that requires the exclusion of other specific diseases. Several disorders may mimic PMR. The arthritis of PMR is similar to rheumatoid arthritis. In fact, rheumatoid arthritis in the elderly patient may begin with months of muscular aches and stiffness before the onset of inflammatory joint changes. Some have suggested that late onset of seronegative rheumatoid arthritis in fact is the articular manifestation of PMR. Polymyositis has been confused with PMR, but patients with polymyositis usually have proximal muscle weakness and less muscular pain. Endocrine disorders such as hypothyroidism may have muscular pains and/or a myopathy with weakness. Malignancy and chronic infection may also resemble PMR (90). One must consider soft tissue pain syndromes as discussed earlier. Finally, giant cell arteritis, as discussed later, may present as a PMR syndrome.

Management

PMR has no known cause. Treatment is directed at the inflammatory process. It is reasonable to use an NSAID as an initial mode of treatment in patients without signs or symptoms of associated giant cell arteritis. However, an NSAID generally provides only mild to moderate relief of symptoms. PMR is dramatically responsive to relatively low doses of oral corticosteroids. In fact, the resolution of symptoms within 24 hours following an oral dose of up to 20 mg of prednisone is so characteristic and unique to PMR that this dramatic response to corticosteroids is helpful in confirming the diagnosis. Nonetheless, the toxicity of corticosteroid usage in the elderly patient must always be given careful consideration. The signs and symptoms of active disease resolve rapidly, so in most patients the prednisone dosage can be tapered to 5 mg daily within a few weeks. Patients who are resistant to corticosteroid therapy are so uncommon that the diagnosis of PMR should be questioned. If the patient is intolerant of or not responsive to corticosteroids, consideration can be given to immunosuppressive therapy.

GIANT CELL ARTERITIS

Giant cell arteritis (GCA) (92–94) is also called cranial or temporal arteritis because the signs and symptoms are a result of inflammatory lesions of the vessels extending off the aortic arch into the temporal and cranial arteries (sparing intracerebral blood vessels). Like PMR, GCA almost exclusively affects white patients over age 50. Approximately 10 to 20% of patients who have PMR have occult GCA detected by biopsy of an asymptomatic temporal artery, but this association varies with ethnic background.

GCA may manifest in a variety of ways, the most common being new and persistent headache. While temporal headache is characteristic, any location of headache may occur. In addition, even in the absence of headache, some patients with GCA may be profoundly ill with constitutional symptoms including fatigue, mood changes, weight loss, anorexia, and myalgia. Fever is usually low grade, but occasionally GCA causes fever of unknown origin. Visual disturbances, including diplopia, blurred vision, and unilateral or bilateral transient loss of vision, are common symptoms of GCA. These symptoms signal impending ophthalmic artery ischemia that may result in blindness. Other symptoms that affect the head and neck include the sensation of nodules over the scalp, pain in the jaws on chewing (jaw claudication), tongue pain, throat pain, and unexplained cough. GCA is a generalized process, so that ischemic injury can occur in the distribution of any major muscular artery, including the coronary circulation.

Laboratory studies typically show a markedly elevated ESR, leukocytosis, and a normocytic, normochromic anemia. Frequently the serum alkaline phosphatase level is mildly elevated. A definitive diagnosis requires a temporal artery biopsy with pathology demonstrating arterial wall necrosis and multinucleated giant cells within the medial portion of the vessel. Investigations suggest that a unilateral temporal artery biopsy misses the diagnosis in up to 15% of cases, while bilateral biopsies that are negative for arteritis exclude GCA 95% of the time.

Management

When there is a high clinical suspicion of active GCA, the patient should be started promptly on prednisone 1 mg/kg per day (prednisone 60 to 80 mg orally daily). Prompt treatment with corticosteroids may prevent blindness and other vascular events. Within several days after initiating corticosteroids the patient should undergo a diagnostic temporal artery biopsy in all suspected cases to confirm the clinical diagnosis. Whenever possible, the biopsy specimen should first be obtained from a symptomatic location. Because the inflammatory changes are not uniformly present in the temporal artery, the biopsy specimen should be at least 3 cm long to allow for careful pathologic sectioning and thorough evaluation of the vessel wall. Biopsy of the other temporal artery should be considered if the first biopsy specimen is negative and the diagnosis is unclear. Prednisone taper can begin slowly and cautiously a month after clinical signs and symptoms have resolved. The ESR and other laboratory findings should have dramatically improved. The corticosteroids can be tapered by lowering the dose by 5 mg every 5 to 7 days. Disease activity occasionally recurs as the dosage reaches approximately 5 to 15 mg. It has been reported that most patients can have corticosteroids stopped after 2 years, but in our experience a maintenance dose of 5 mg daily is needed in some cases. Methotrexate or azathioprine may allow steroid dose reduction.

MUSCLE WEAKNESS IN THE ELDERLY PATIENT

Age-associated reductions in muscle mass translate to overall reduced muscle strength for many older adults (95). These changes may be perceived as weakness or the need to exert greater effort to achieve a given amount of physical work. However, complaints of weakness should be met with careful scrutiny and an earnest effort to identify a potentially reversible cause. As with the evaluation of musculoskeletal pain, the clinician should follow a methodical approach to the elderly patient with weakness. Proximal muscle weakness should be clearly distinguished from distal weakness, since this distinction narrows the diagnostic possibilities and guides the evaluation. Impaired proximal muscle strength, as is seen with inflammatory myositis and myopathies, results in difficulty with activities such as rising from a chair and climbing stairs and in sustained self-care activities that necessitate raising the arms above the head. Complaints of choking, dysphonia, and visual alterations accompany weakness of the oropharyngeal and ocular muscles. In contrast, weakness of the distal extremities that is often accompanied by neurosensory abnormalities suggests a peripheral neuropathy.

Muscle

Metabolic causes of weakness include hypokalemia, hypocalcemia, hypomagnesemia, and hypophosphatemia. These reversible derangements can follow medical therapy but also occur sporadically in the older patient. Adrenal, parathyroid, and thyroid hyperfunction or hypofunction can result in proximal weakness that is reversible with proper treatment. Diabetic amyotrophy is also characterized by proximal weakness but usually accompanies long-standing diabetes with concurrent neuropathy. This condition may persist or worsen in spite of aggressive glycemic control. Clinicians must be careful to exclude toxic myopathy, which can complicate chronic alcohol use and also treatment with glucocorticoids, antimalarial medications, colchicine, zidovudine, and lipid-lowering agents (HMG coenzyme A reductase inhibitors). Older adults are at greater risk for drug-induced myopathy when renal or hepatic dysfunction is present. In addition to the aforementioned conditions that may be more common in older adults, infectious causes of weakness include viral (including human immunodeficiency virus [HIV]) and parasitic illnesses.

Polymyositis and Dermatomyositis

Polymyositis and dermatomyositis (96–100), systemic inflammatory muscle diseases that result in proximal weakness, usually affect adults 40 to 50 years old. Accompanying features may include nonerosive but deforming arthritis, interstitial lung disease, cardiac systolic dysfunction, and intestinal and rarely renal disease. Although skin abnormalities distinguish these two conditions, they are distinct clinical conditions for which distinct immune-mediated factors have been implicated. Serum creatinine kinase and aldolase enzymes are released from injured skeletal muscle during periods of disease exacerbations and fall during remission. Electromyographic testing reveals myofibril insertional irritability in most patients with active muscle inflammation but does not demonstrate these findings in muscle that has already atrophied. MRI of the proximal muscles using a fat suppression technique may be helpful in identifying an ideal biopsy site by detecting the edema that accompanies inflammation. Muscle biopsy remains the gold standard, both confirming the presence of inflammatory muscle disease and distinguishing polymyositis from dermatomyositis and the rare inclusion body myositis.

Inclusion body myositis (98, 101) (IBM) is an inflammatory myopathy characterized by proximal and distal weakness that is most commonly encountered in men over age 50. Its insidious onset, concurrent distal muscle and nerve involvement, and inexorable course distinguish this disease clinically from polymyositis and dermatomyositis, but this distinction is often subtle. Serum muscle enzymes may be marginally elevated if not normal. Unlike polymyositis and dermatomyositis, it may show neuropathic features on electrodiagnostic testing,. Although the recommended management is similar to that of polymyositis and dermatomyositis, IBM is less responsive to immunosuppressive therapy. Inflammatory myositis can accompany other systemic rheumatic illnesses including vasculitis, systemic lupus, rheumatoid arthritis, and systemic sclerosis. In these instances, other aspects of the disease should be sought. Tumor-associated myositis may occur without a rash typical of dermato-myositis and should be considered when there is a poor response to therapy (91–100).

Neuromuscular Junction

Although myasthenia gravis can occur at any age, its predilection is for women in their 20s and men in their 60s. This disease may complicate treatment with penicillamine. Myasthenia gravis is characterized by weakness with rapid muscle fatigability and partial recovery following periods of rest. The muscles innervated by cranial nerves are most commonly involved, resulting in ptosis or diplopia in most cases. Weakness of the pharyngeal and laryngeal muscles may result in regurgitation or aspiration. Confirmatory tests include objective improvement on administration of edrophonium (Tensilon), a short-acting cholinesterase inhibitor; progressive decrement in voltage on repetitive electrical stimulation, particularly in proximal muscles; and circulating anticholinesterase receptor antibodies. Treatment with pyridostigmine and prednisone can be initiated. Plasmapheresis is required for patients in acute crisis.

Eaton-Lambert syndrome is a paraneoplastic syndrome that results in fatigable weakness of proximal muscles. The incremental response of action potential on repetitive stimulation observed on electromyographic (EMG) testing is occasionally accompanied by clinical improvement as the day wears on. Although most commonly a correlate of lung carcinoma, it is also seen in association with other malignancies. It can improve following successful surgical removal or chemotherapy of the malignancy.

Peripheral Nerve

Cervical spondylosis with nerve root impingement may complicate the cervical spine osteoarthritis that is common in older adults (102). Radiculopathy can develop insidiously with neck pain. Myelopathy with sensory impairment, weakness, and blunted upper extremity reflexes with or without fasciculations may develop. Later, neck pain may resolve as lower extremity motor and sensory impairment become apparent. Surgical intervention may arrest progressive neurologic impairment.

Peripheral neuropathy is a common feature of

many rheumatic diseases. Clinical features include a burning, dysesthetic pain and weakness in the distribution of the involved nerves. Orthostatic hypotension may be an accompanying feature. EMG studies help to exclude neuropathy as a cause of the observed weakness and can differentiate mononeuropathy (e.g., carpal tunnel syndrome), distal symmetric polyneuropathy (e.g. diabetic neuropathy), and mononeuritis multiplex. Electrodiagnostic studies also distinguish demyelinating from axonal processes, further narrowing the diagnostic possibilities.

Central Nervous System Disease

Amyotrophic lateral sclerosis (ALS) is a neurodegenerative disease that afflicts older adults. It is characterized by corticospinal tract brainstem motor nuclei and spinal cord anterior horn dysfunction. Progressive muscle weakness with fasciculations result. Absence of sensory loss distinguishes ALS from cervical and lumbar spondylitic myelopathy that complicate spinal arthritis. Subacute combined degeneration of the spinal cord complicates B_{12} deficiency. Neurologic manifestations include cognitive impairment, gait imbalance, and recurrent falls due to posterior column dysfunction. Symmetric weakness and spasticity develop later. These and other neurologic conditions are discussed in detail elsewhere.

LATE-ONSET SYSTEMIC LUPUS ERYTHEMATOSUS

Although systemic lupus erythematosus (SLE, lupus) (103, 104) is predominantly a disease of women in the second to fifth decade of life, an estimated 6 to 20% of patients with SLE are over age 50. The female predominance noted in young adults is not prominent in late-onset lupus.

Clinical Presentation

Constitutional symptoms often dominate the clinical picture of late-onset lupus. Older adults with lupus are more likely to develop arthritis, pleuritis, or pericarditis than young adults with this disease and less likely to have central nervous system disease, lymphadenopathy, and Raynaud's phenomenon. Renal disease, a rare manifestation of late-onset lupus, is less likely to progress to renal failure than in early-onset lupus.

Laboratory Studies

ANAs, which uniformly accompany the aforementioned symptoms in late-onset lupus, present in a rim pattern in 57% of cases. Anti-Ro antibodies are also common. Recent evidence suggests that for elderly patients, the specificity of the ANA test and positive predictive value are modest (73% and 4% respectively), since an abnormal ANA can be found in older adults without rheumatic diseases. Antibodies to double-stranded (native) DNA, although less common in late-onset lupus, is fairly specific for this disease. For older adults, ANA testing has little value without other clinical features to suggest lupus or other rheumatic disease (105).

Management

Since the clinical presentation of late-onset lupus is quite similar to that of drug-induced lupus erythematosus (DILE), clinicians must be careful to exclude DILE. DILE may complicate the use of a variety of medications (e.g., procainamide, hydralazine) that older adults are commonly prescribed. DILE is also accompanied by ANAs, particularly antibodies to histone cellular components. Resolution of symptoms and laboratory abnormalities follows promptly after discontinuing the offending agent. Although hormonal influences have clearly been implicated in the pathogenesis of lupus in young adults, few have addressed this question in the elderly. One large prospective cohort study recently discovered that postmenopausal women taking hormonal replacement for 5 or more years had a 2.5 times greater risk of lupus than controls (106). However, the cardiovascular and bone protective effects of estrogens likely outweigh the risk of lupus.

Avoidance of the sun and use of topical agents that block ultraviolet light are indicated for all patients with lupus. Specific clinical subsets determine the appropriateness of various therapies. Serositis often responds to NSAIDs, but use of these agents can result in the gastrointestinal and renal toxicities described elsewhere. Antimalarial agents are effective management of cutaneous and arthritic manifestations, but their use requires regular ophthalmologic monitoring because of the prevalence of macular degeneration in elderly patients. Those with severe arthritis or serositis unresponsive to these therapies may require corticosteroids to establish control of the disease. The overall prognosis of late-onset lupus is better than that of early-onset disease by virtue of the low prevalence of life-threatening complications and central nervous system involvement.

RHEUMATOID ARTHRITIS IN THE ELDERLY

Clinical Presentation

Although it is significantly less prevalent than osteoarthritis, it has recently become apparent that rheumatoid arthritis (RA) is an important disease of the elderly. Up to 40% of patients with rheumatoid arthritis are over age 60; many have aged with their disease. Clinicians caring for these patients are challenged by the consequences of long-standing disease and complications arising from RA and its treatment. Cases of late-onset RA (LORA) develop after age 60 and account for 20 to 55% of elderly patients with RA. Patients with LORA may present similarly to young adults with acute inflammatory polyarthritis involving the small joints of the hands and feet (Fig. 32.3) accompanied by a positive rheumatoid factor. Other seronegative presentations that are unique to the elderly include an inflammatory arthritis of the shoulder and hips similar to PMR and remitting symmetric

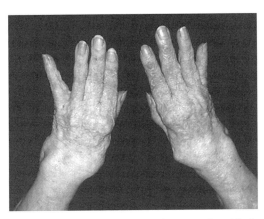

Figure 32.3. Rheumatoid arthritis in the elderly symmetric with inflammatory disease of the metacarpophalangeal, proximal interphalangeal, and wrist joints.

seronegative synovitis with peripheral edema (RS3PE syndrome). In fact, descriptive studies suggest that late-onset RA should be considered in the differential diagnosis of PMR and vice versa (6, 107). In contrast to young adults with RA, older patients with RA are more likely to have a high initial ESR. ANAs are detectable in up to 30% of patients. The utility of these laboratory studies is often tempered by the observation of these same laboratory abnormalities in the absence of identifiable rheumatic disease in the elderly.

Management

Descriptive studies suggest that patients with seropositive RA, even if late onset, should be managed aggressively, including use of disease-modifying agents (108, 109). It has been shown that some of these agents can be safely used in elderly patients with appropriate monitoring (Table 32.5) (109, 110). Methotrexate is well tolerated but may require dosing interval adjustment for elderly patients and should be given with daily folic acid. Hydroxychloroquine is also well tolerated, but its use must be monitored for macular toxicity, especially in light of the increased prevalence of macular degeneration in older patients. Penicillamine, sulfasalazine, gold, and cyclophosphamide are less well tolerated by elderly patients. Others suggest prednisone 5 to 15 mg daily as an adjunctive agent in management of seropositive RA and as the primary treatment for seronegative PMR-like disease and RS3PE syndrome. In contrast to classic PMR, late-onset RA may not respond promptly to low-dose prednisone.

Outcome and Prognosis

The development of extra-articular complications, including cutaneous vasculitis and gastrointestinal and neurologic disease, is probably related to duration of the disease and rarely is problematic for patients with LORA, even if seropositive. However, for older adults RA often results in early and progressive disability and loss of function beyond that seen in younger adults with RA. This in large part may be explained by comorbid illnesses that may work in synergy with arthritis to enhance disability in

Table 32.5

Slow-Acting and Disease-Modifying Antirheumatic Drugs and Their Use in the Elderly

Hydroxychloroquine	Start 200 mg po qd; increase to 200 mg bid daily maximum
	Time to effect: 2–6 months
	Elderly: reduced GFR, reduced plasma binding proteins may increase plasma levels; no adjustment for age recommended
	Toxicities: nausea, epigastric pain, rash, retinal damage (avoidable)
	Monitoring: visual fields and color vision monitoring q 6–12 mo
Aurothioglucose (Solganal) injectable	Test dose 10 mg; second dose 1 week later, 25 mg q wk × 2 wk; 50 mg q wk to 20 wk; if response, every other week, then q 3 wk, then q mo; maintain q mo; discontinuing maintenance therapy often results in recurrence of arthritis; may not remit when therapy reinstituted
	Time to effect: 3–6 months
	Elderly: efficacy and toxicity data conflict
	Toxicities: stomatitis, rash, proteinuria, leukopenia, thrombocytopenia; enterocolitis, aplastic anemia rare but potentially fatal; interstitial pneumonitis rare
	Monitor: CBC and urinalysis prior to each or every other injection
Methotrexate	5–20 mg po q wk; give folic acid 1 mg/daily; clinical improvement in 33/37 elderly patients with late-onset disease
	Time to effect: 6–8 wk
	Elderly: risk of toxicity may be high
	Toxicities: anorexia, nausea, vomiting, abdominal cramps, increased hepatic enzyme activity; rarely bone marrow suppression, pulmonary toxicity, hepatic fibrosis; hypersensitivity pneumonitis (1–4%) frequently severe; immunosuppressive (herpes zoster, PCP)
	Interactions: trimethoprim with sulfamethoxazole (Bactrim), possibly sulfasalazine (increased bone marrow suppression); increased methotrexate effect with probenecid; increased toxicity possible with NSAIDs
	Monitor: baseline CBC, urinalysis, liver profile, repeat after 1–2 wk of treatment, then q mo
Penicillamine (Depen, Cuprimine)	125 mg qd; increase by 125-mg increments q 1–3 mo to max 1 g daily; food delays absorption
	Time to effect: 4–8 wk
	Elderly: Increased severe skin reactions
	Toxicities: Some suggest more adverse effects in the elderly (proteinuria, stomatitis, rash, GI, leukopenia, thrombocytopenia; rarely: pemphigus, myasthenia, Goodpasture's syndrome, fever, lupuslike illness, polymyositis, dermatomyositis, cholestatic hepatitis, severe bone marrow depression, bronchiolitis
	Interactions: digoxin effect decreased; iron absorption decreased
	Monitor: baseline CBC, urinalysis, repeat in 1–2 wk, then q 4–6 wk
Sulfasalazine (enteric coated)	250 mg bid, increase by 500 mg q wk to 2 g qd
	Time to effect: 6–8 wk
	Elderly: not studied
	Toxicities: nausea, anorexia, and rash common; hepatitis and blood dyscrasias rare; fibrosing alveolitis, neuromuscular problems, aplastic anemia and agranulocytosis rare
	Monitor: baseline CBC, urinalysis, liver profile; repeat q 2–3 wk × 3 mo; repeat q 1–3 mo

(continued)

Table 32.5 (continued)

Slow-Acting and Disease-Modifying Antirheumatic Drugs and Their Use in the Elderly

Cyclophosphamide	1–2 mg/k/day; must be taken with at least 2 L of fluids qd to minimize toxicities
	Elderly: increased toxicity at high doses
	Toxicities: bone marrow suppression, hemorrhagic cystitis and malignancy, SIADH at high doses
	Interacts: barbiturates and steroids activate the drug
	Monitor: CBC, urinalysis
Azathioprine	1–2.5 mg/k/day (50 mg qd–tid); efficacy for elderly not established
	Time to effect: unknown
	Elderly: not studied
	Toxicities: nausea, vomiting, abdominal pain, hepatitis, reversible bone marrow suppression; increased risk of lymphoma
	Drug interactions: interferes with allopurinol metabolism
	Monitor: baseline CBC, urinalysis, liver profile; repeat in 1–2 wk, then q mo

Symptom-Modifying Drugs (No Disease Modification)

NSAIDs, including aspirin	All agents equally effective at the recommended dose
	Anti-inflammatory doses higher than analgesic doses
	Time to onset for analgesic: hours
	Time to onset for anti-inflammation: days-weeks
	Short half-life less hazardous than long half-life
Short half-life	Choline magnesium trisalicylate (Trilisate) 750 mg tid
	Ibuprofen (Motrin, Advil, Nuprin) 200–800 mg tid
	Etodolac (Lodine) 200 mg–300 mg tid
Prednisone	10–20 mg po AM to start, taper to 2.5–5 mg as tolerated by disease
	Time to inflammation reduction: 5–10 days; use intra-articular steroids when possible
	Toxicities: cataracts, poor wound healing, gastric ulcers, mental status change, hyperglycemia, hypertension, osteoporosis, immune suppression; risks less at low doses; full recovery of hypothalamic pituitary axis depends on duration and dose prescribed (up to a full year for chronic steroid use)

GFR, glomerular filtration rate; CBC, complete blood count; GI, gastrointestinal; PCP, *Pneumocystis carinii* pneumonia; SIADH, syndrome of inappropriate antidiuretic hormone secretion.

older adults. Late-onset seronegative RA is associated with a fairly good prognosis for most and remits spontaneously for some.

SJÖGREN'S SYNDROME

Primary Sjögren's syndrome (111–117) is a systemic autoimmune disease that results from lymphocytic infiltrates of the lacrimal and salivary glands (111, 112). Sjögren's syndrome may also accompany other rheumatic diseases including rheumatoid arthritis, scleroderma, and lupus.

The SICCA complex (xerophthalmia and xerostomia) is the most common manifestation of Sjögren's syndrome. SICCA complaints are common among elderly patients and more commonly arise from other causes, such as medications (particularly those with anticholinergic activity), autonomic neuropathy, and viral infections, including HIV (113). Approximately 3 to 4% of adults aged 60 and older have abnormal tests of lacrimal and/or salivary function, and even fewer have primary Sjögren's syndrome (dry eyes, xerostomia and autoantibody production; estimated prevalence 0.4%) (114).

Sjögren's syndrome can result in ocular, oral, and systemic complications. For elderly patients this may translate to compromised vision, difficulties with communication and swallowing, poor nutrition, and an increased risk of urinary tract infections. Extraglandular involvement is common in adults aged 50 and older; it may include pulmonary, renal, and central nervous systems. A nondeforming inflammatory arthritis that may be mistaken for rheumatoid arthritis accompanies 50 to 60% of cases of SS. Persistent parotid gland enlargement, adenopathy, monoclonal gammopathy, and cross-reactive idiotypes may all signal possible lymphomatous conversion, which occurs in approximately 10% of patients (115).

VASCULITIS

Vasculitis may involve blood vessels of any size and can occur independently or in the context of another rheumatic disease such as RA, lupus, Sjögren's syndrome, cryoglobulinemia, solid and hematologic malignancies, and myelodysplastic syndromes (118). In addition, other conditions such as cholesterol emboli syndrome, atrial myxoma, and endocarditis may be mistaken for vasculitis. Temporal arteritis (discussed in detail in the above sections) and a number of other vasculitides afflict elderly persons.

Although older adults are at increased risk for polypharmacy, the incidence of leukocytoclastic vasculitis in the older adult population is unknown. Leukocytoclastic vasculitis may follow drug exposure (hypersensitivity vasculitis). Purpuric or necrotic skin lesions maximally distributed over the lower legs and buttocks, appear 7 to 10 days after exposure. Since leukocytoclastic vasculitis may be the presenting feature of polyarteritis nodosa, Wegener's granulomatosis, lupus, rheumatoid vasculitis, and Sjögren's syndrome, it is important to exclude these other conditions. Although it is primarily a cutaneous disease, systemic manifestations may be present. Treatment decisions depend on the severity and extent of systemic involvement but should include removal of the offending agent (119).

Polyarteritis nodosa is a disease of medium-sized and small blood vessels. Its average age of di-

agnosis is from the mid 40s to 60s, and it can cause multisystem insufficiency or failure in the nervous, gastrointestinal, renal, cardiac, and pulmonary systems. Treatment should include an anti-inflammatory agent (prednisone 40 to 60 mg daily, cyclophosphamide, or chlorambucil), vasodilating agents, and antiplatelet medications (84).

Wegener's granulomatosis is an uncommon disease that classically involves the upper and lower respiratory tracts and kidneys. Persistent inflammatory nasal and sinus disease with fever, malaise, and migratory arthritis is typical of this disease. Although the mean age of onset is estimated at 40 years (120), this disease can develop in older adults. A retrospective cohort analysis suggests that in older adults, Wegener's is more likely to result in pulmonary infiltrates during the course of illness, and renal insufficiency is more commonly found at the time of diagnosis than in young adults. Central and peripheral nervous system involvement was also more common in late-onset Wegener's (121). The diagnosis of this life-threatening disorder is contingent on demonstration of vasculitis on biopsy. Circulating antineutrophilic cytoplasmic antibodies (c-ANCA) also support the diagnosis (120). Although older adults are as likely to respond to therapy with oral cyclophosphamide and prednisone as young adults, with response rates up to 85%, older patients are more prone to develop life-threatening infections following therapy (121).

Churg-Strauss syndrome also involves the small and medium-sized arteries with a granulomatous inflammatory process. Although age of onset can be as late as 70 years, this disease usually afflicts young adults. Its distinguishing features include asthma, eosinophilia, neuropathy, and pulmonary infiltrates (122). Studies suggest that prednisone and cyclophosphamide alone significantly affect survival of patients with Churg-Strauss syndrome and polyarteritis nodosa, without added clinical benefit with plasma exchange (123).

MALIGNANCY

The prevalence of malignant disease, primary, metastatic, and hematologic, increases with age. Most clinicians are familiar with hypertrophic osteoarthropathy (80). This condition results in digital clubbing and polyarthralgia. Painful sites include the wrists, knees, ankles, and elbows. Although sympathetic effusions are common, symptoms localize to the periarticular periosteum. Some 90% of patients with hypertrophic osteoarthropathy have or eventually develop malignancy, most commonly in the lung. However, the arthropathy may precede the discovery of malignancy by several months. Symptoms are responsive to anti-inflammatory agents and usually remit after the underlying malignancy has been eliminated.

Peripheral Arthritis

When arthritis is directly due to metastatic carcinoma, it most commonly involves a single joint, although not necessarily due to direct spread. Malignancy-associated polyarthritis can be easily mistaken for RA. However, in direct contrast to RA, the polyarthritis of malignancy is asymmetric. A malignancy-associated PMR-like illness causes asymmetric involvement at sites typical of PMR, is usually accompanied by characteristic abnormalities on radioisotope scanning, and is poorly responsive to prednisone (123). Carcinoma polyarthritis, PMR, and anti-inflammatory disease are poorly responsive to anti-inflammatory therapy.

The association with peripheral arthritis is not limited to solid tumors. The myelodysplastic syndromes are a group of common hematologic disorders that increase in incidence with age. A seronegative inflammatory arthritis, leukocytoclastic vasculitis, and a lupuslike illness have been described in association with myelodysplastic syndromes. The arthritis can precede the development of the bone marrow disorder and can be a guide to the diagnosis of this hematologic disorder in elderly patients presenting with an inflammatory arthritis and cytopenias (124).

Axial Manifestations

Back or bone pain that develops in adults aged 55 and older may be a presenting feature of malignancy. Pain with recumbency or pain that worsens at night, results in bilateral radiculopathy, or is accompanied by fever, weight loss, and night sweats is characteristic. Spinal tenderness, nerve root impingement above the first lumbar vertebrae, and neurologic deficits should be sought in those suspected of spinal metastases. Peripheral bone tenderness or signs of periostitis should be sought in patients with peripheral musculoskeletal complaints with a history of malignancy. Peripheral and axial skeletal involvement may follow breast, lung, thyroid, renal, and prostatic malignancies. Myeloma may result in similar symptoms and may be accompanied by anemia and renal impairment. The suspicion of bony malignancy, axial or peripheral, warrants prompt radiographic evaluation. Plain radiographs are a necessary part of early evaluation to exclude tumor and pathologic fractures. Nuclear imaging can demonstrate tumor (except for myeloma) and can identify lesions that may not yet be clinically apparent. CT provides the best sensitivity for cortical disruption but does not provide adequate sensitivity for intraosseous or intramedullary lesions, which are better visualized on MRI.

Systemic Rheumatic Illnesses

As discussed in earlier sections, weakness in older adults may be a manifestation of malignant disease. For patients with dermatomyositis, standard incidence ratios for malignancy is estimated to be 3.6 times the prevalence at the time of diagnosis of dermatomyositis and 26 times in the year following the diagnosis of dermatomyositis (125). This association also arises independently of treatment with cytotoxic agents. The association with malignancy is not as strong with polymyositis (126). Proximal muscle weakness may also develop without clinically apparent cutaneous or inflammatory muscle findings in the setting of malignancy (malignancy-associated myositis and Lambert-Eaton syndrome). Malignancy-associated weakness is less responsive to standard immunosuppressive therapies than dermatomyositis and polymyositis (126). As discussed earlier, electrodiagnostic and pathologic studies diagnose these conditions. At the time of diagnosis the primary malignancy is usually clinically apparent or can be revealed with standard radiographic procedures.

A number of reports have associated systemic sclerosis with breast, gastrointestinal, urogenital, and hematologic malignancies. Population-based studies estimate that patients with systemic sclerosis have 2.1 times the overall rate of malignancy of age-matched controls (127). The risk of malignancy is greatest for adults who are over 50 years old at the time of diagnosis and for those with pulmonary fibrosis (127).

Patients with Sjögren's syndrome are also at risk for malignancy. Persistent parotid gland enlargement, adenopathy, monoclonal gammopathy, and cross-reactive idiotypes may all signal lymphomatous conversion, which occurs in approximately 10% of patients (128).

Treatment-Associated Malignancy (129)

Cyclophosphamide use has been strongly implicated in bladder carcinoma and is a well-recognized complication of the treatment of lupus but is less frequent with aggressive hydration and mesna use. Patients with RA who have received treatment with oral cyclophosphamide are also at risk for malignancy (bladder and cutaneous) at 1.5 times that of adults who have not received this therapy. This association may be dose related (129). Azathioprine use can result in an increased risk of lymphoproliferative disease in patients with RA beyond that associated with the disease alone. Methotrexate use has also been associated with an increased risk but less so than azathioprine.

REFERENCES

1. Bagge E, Bjelle A, Eden S, Svanborg A. A longitudinal study of the occurrence of joint complaints in elderly people. Age Aging 1992;21:160–167.
2. Lawrence RC, Hochberg MC, Kelsey JL, et al. Estimates of the prevalence of selected arthritic and musculoskeletal diseases in the United States. J Rheumatol 1989;16:427–441.
3. Verbrugge L, Gates D, Ike R. Risk factors for disability among U.S. adults with arthritis. J Clin Epidemiol 1991;44:167–182.
4. Williamson JD, Fried LP. Characterization of older adults who attribute functional decrements to "old age." J Am Geriatr Soc 1996;44:1429–1434.
5. Hazzard WR, Bierman EL, Blass JP, et al. Principles of Geriatric Medicine & Gerontology. New York: McGraw-Hill, 1990.
6. Michet CJ, Evans JM, Fleming KC, et al. Common rheumatologic diseases in elderly patients. Mayo Clin Proc 1995;70:1205–1214.
7. Waller M, Toone EC, Vaughn E. Study of rheumatoid factor in a normal population. Arthritis Rheum 1964;7:513–520.
8. Lipsitz A, Jonsson PV, Kelley MM, Koestner JS. Causes and correlates of recurrent falls in ambulatory frail elderly. J Gerontology 1991;46:M114–122.
9. Sudarsky L. Current concepts—geriatrics: gait disorders in the elderly. N Engl J Med 1990;322:1441–1445.
10. Ensrud KE, Nevitt MC, Yunis C, et al. Correlates of impaired function in older women. J Am Geriatr Soc 1994;42:481–489.
11. Hughes SL, Gibbs J, Edelman P, et al. Joint impairment and hand function in the elderly. J Am Geriatr Soc 1992;40:871–877.
12. Fried LP, Guralnik JM. Disability in older adults: evidence regarding significance, etiology, and risk. J Am Geriatr Soc 1997;45:92–100.
13. Ettinger WH Jr, Fried LP, Harris T, et al. Self-reported causes of physical disability in older people: the Cardiovascular Health Study. CHS Collaborative Research Group. J Am Geriatr Soc 1994;42:1035–1044.
14. Gibbs J, Hughes S, Dunlop D, et al. Joint impairment and ambulation in the elderly. J Am Geriatr Soc 1993;41:1205–1211.
15. King MB, Tinetti ME. Falls in community-dwelling older persons. J Am Geriatr Soc 1995;43:1146–1154.
16. Nevitt MC, Cummings SR, Kidd S, Black D. Risk factors for recurrent nonsyncopal falls. A prospective study. JAMA 1989;261:2663–2668.
17. Campbell AJ, Borrie MJ, Spears GF. Risk factors for falls in a community-based prospective study of people 70 years and older. J Gerontol 1989;44:M112–M117.
18. Tinetti ME, Speechley M, Ginter SF. Risk factors for falls among elderly persons living in the community. N Engl J Med 1988;319:1701–1707.
19. Katz S, et al. Studies of illness in the aged: the index of ADL: a standardized measure of biological and psychological function. JAMA 1963;185:914–919.
20. Lawton MP, Brody EM. Assessment of older people: self-maintaining and instrumental activities of daily living. Gerontologist 1969;9:179–186.
21. Flemming KC, Evans JM, Weber DC, Chutka ES. Practical functional assessment of elderly persons: a primary-care approach, Mayo Clin Proc 1995;70:890–910.
22. Tinetti ME. Performance-oriented assessment of mobility problems on elderly patients. J Am Geriatr Soc 1986;34:119–126.
23. Mathias S, Nayak US, Isaacs B. Balance in elderly patients: the Get Up and Go test. Arch Phys Med Rehabil 1986;67:387–389.
24. Lachs MS, Feinstein AR, Cooney LM Jr, et al. A simple procedure for general screening functional disability in elderly patients. Ann Intern Med 1990;112:699–706.
25. Ling SM, Bathon JM. Osteoarthritis in older adults. J Am Geriatr Soc 1998;46:216–225.
26. Engel A. Osteoarthritis in adults by selected demographic characteristics, United States—1960–1962. Vital and Health Statistics 1966. Series 112.

27. Brandt KD, Fife RS. Ageing in relation to the pathogenesis of osteoarthritis. Clin Rheum Dis 1986;12:117–130.

28. Bagge E, Bjelle A, Eden S, Svanborg A. Osteoarthritis in the elderly: clinical and radiological findings in 79 and 85 year olds. Ann Rheum Dis 1991;50:535–539.

29. Oliveria SA, Felson DT, Reed JI, et al. Incidence of symptomatic hand, hip, and knee osteoarthritis among patients in a health maintenance organization. Arthritis Rheum 1995;38:1134–1141.

30. Lethbridge-Cejku M, Scott WW Jr, Reichle R, et al. Association of radiographic features of osteoarthritis of the knee with knee pain: data from the Baltimore Longitudinal Study of Aging. Arthritis Care Res 1995;8;182–188.

31. Felson DT, Zhang Y, Hannan MT, et al. The incidence and natural history of knee osteoarthritis in the elderly. Arthritis Rheum 1995;38:1500–1505.

32. Lawrence JJ, Bremner JM, Bier F. Osteo-arthrosis, prevalence in the population and relationship between symptoms and x-ray changes. Ann Rheum Dis 1966;25:1–24.

33. Egger P, Cooper C, Hart DJ, et al. Patterns of joint involvement in osteoarthritis of the hand: the Chingford Study. J Rheumatol 1995;22:1509–1513.

34. Mauer K. Basic data on arthritis knee, hip and sacroiliac joints in adults ages 25–74 years, United States 1971–1975. Vital Health Stat 1979. Series 11.

35. Tepper S, Hochberg MC., Factors associated with hip osteoarthritis: data from the first National Health and Nutrition Examination Survey (NHANES-I). Am J Epidemiol 1993;137:1081–1087.

36. Cooke TD, Dwosh IL. Clinical features of osteoarthritis in the elderly. Clin Rheum Dis 1986;12:155–174.

37. Hochberg MC, Altman RD, Brandt KD, et al. Guidelines for the medical management of osteoarthritis. Part I. Osteoarthritis of the hip. American College of Rheumatology. Arthritis Rheum 1995;38:1535–1540.

38. Hochberg MC, Altman RD, Brandt KD, et al. Guidelines for the medical management of osteoarthritis. Part II. Osteoarthritis of the knee. American College of Rheumatology. Arthritis Rheum 1995;38:1541–1546.

39. Altman R, Alarcon G, Appelrouth D, et al. The American College of Rheumatology criteria of the classification and reporting of osteoarthritis of the hand. Arthritis Rheum 1990;33:1601–1610.

40. Murphy WA, Altman RD. Updated osteoarthritis reference standard. J Rheumatol Suppl 1995;43:56–59.

41. Kellgren JH, Lawrence JS. Radiological assessment of osteoarthrosis. Ann Rheum Dis 1957;16:494–502.

42. Sartoris DJ, Resnick D. Radiological changes with ageing in relation to bone disease and arthritis. Clin Rheum Dis 1986;12:181–227.

43. Spiera H. Osteoarthritis as a misdiagnosis in elderly patients. Geriatrics 1987;42:37–42.

44. Schon L, Zuckerman JD. Hip pain in the elderly: evaluation and diagnosis. Geriatrics 1988;43:48–62.

45. Klippel JH, Dieppe PA. Rheumatology. St. Louis: Mosby, 1994.

46. Moskowitz RW, et al. Osteoarthritis: Diagnosis and Medical/Surgical Management. 2nd ed. Philadelphia: Saunders, 1992.

47. Pelletier JP, Howell DS. Etiopathogenesis of osteoarthritis. In: McCarty DJ, Koopman DJ, eds. A Textbook of Rheumatology. Philadelphia: Lea & Febiger 1993: 1723–1734.

48. Dieppe P, Altman R, Lequesne M, et al. Osteoarthritis of the knee: report of a task force of the Internal League of Associations for Rheumatology and Osteoarthritis Research Society. J Am Geriatr Soc 1997;45:850–852.

49. Palmoski MJ, Bolyer RA, Brandt KD. Joint motion in the absence of normal loading does not maintain normal articular cartilage. Arthritis Rheum 1980;23:325–334.

50. Ettinger WH Jr, et al. A randomized trial comparing aerobic exercise and resistance exercise with a health education program in older adults with knee osteoarthritis: the fitness arthritis and seniors trial (FAST). JAMA 1997; 277:25–31.

51. Schilke JM. Effects of muscle-strength training on the functional status of patients with osteoarthritis of the knee joint. Nurs Res 1996;45:68–72.

52. Judge JO, Underwood M, Gennosa T. Exercise to improve gait velocity in older persons. Arch Phys Med Rehab 1993;74:400–406.

53. Gerber LH. Exercise and arthritis. Bull Rheum Dis 1990;39:1–9.

54. Kovar PA, et al. Supervised fitness walking in patients with osteoarthritis of the knee: a randomized, controlled trial. Ann Intern Med 1992;116:529–534 (see comments).

55. Province MA, et al. The effects of exercise on falls in elderly patients. JAMA 1995;273:1341–1347.

56. Bradley DJ, et al. Comparison of an antiinflammatory dose of ibuprofen, an analgesic dose of ibuprofen, and acetaminophen in the treatment of patients with osteoarthritis of the knee. N Engl J Med 1994;325:87–91.

57. Blackburn WD. Management of osteoarthritis and rheumatoid arthritis: prospects and possibilities. Am J Med 1996;100(suppl 2A):24S–30S.

58. Polisson R. Nonsteroidal anti-inflammatory drugs: practical and theoretical considerations in their selection. Am J Med 1996;100:31S–36S.

59. Silverstein FE, Graham DY, Senior JR, et al. Misoprostol reduces serious gastrointestinal complications in patients with rheumatoid arthritis receiving nonsteroidal anti-inflammatory drugs. A randomized, double-blind, placebo-controlled trial. Ann Intern Med 1995;123: 241–249.

60. Morgan GJ, Poland M, DeLapp RE. Efficacy and safety of nabumetone versus diclofenac, naproxen, ibuprofen and piroxicam in the elderly. Am J Med 1993;95: 19S–72S.

61. Schnitzer TJ, Ballard IM, Constantine G, McDonald P. Double-blind, placebo-controlled comparison of the safety and efficacy of orally administered etodolac and nabumetone in patients with active osteoarthritis of the knee. Clin Ther 1995;17:602–612.

62. Rains C, Bryson H. Topical capsaicin: a review of its pharmacological properties and therapeutic potential in

post-herpetic neuralgia, diabetic neuropathy and osteoarthritis. Drugs Aging 1995;7:317–328.

63. McCarthy G, McCarthy D. Effect of topical capsaicin in the therapy of painful osteoarthritis of the hands. J Rheumatol 1992;19:604–607.

64. Frymoyer JW. Back pain and sciatica. N Engl J Med 1988;318:291–300.

65. Bornstein DG, Wiesel SW, eds. Low Back Pain: Medical Diagnosis and Comprehensive Management. 1st ed. Philadelphia: Saunders, 1989.

66. Bornstein DG, Burton JR. Lumbar spine disease in the elderly. J Am Geriatr Soc 1993;41:167.

67. Hall S, Bartleson JD, Onofrio BM, et al. Lumbar spinal stenosis: clinical features, diagnostic procedures, and results of surgical treatment in 68 patients. Ann Intern Med 1985;103:271–275.

68. Moreland LW, Lopez-Mendex A, Alarcon GS. Spinal stenosis: a comprehensive review of the literature. Semin Arthritis Rheum 1989;19:127–149.

69. Resnick D. Shapiro RF, Wiesner KB, et al. Diffuse idiopathic hyperostosis (DISH) (ankylosing hyperostosis of Forestier and Notes-Querol). Semin Arthritis Rheum 1978;7:153–187.

70. Deyo RA, Diehl AK, Rosenthal M. How many days of bed rest for acute low back pain? A randomized clinical trial. N Engl J Med 1986;315:1064–1070.

71. Deyo RA. Drug therapy for back pain: which drugs help which patients. Spine 1996;21:2840–2849.

72. Frost H, Klaber Moffett JA, Moser JS, Fairbank JC. Randomised controlled trial for evaluation of fitness programme for patients with chronic low back pain. BMJ 1995;310:151–154.

73. Garvey TA, Marks MR, Wiesel SW. A prospective, randomized double-blind evaluation of trigger-point injection therapy for low-back pain. Spine 1989;14:962–964.

74. Moore S, Shurman J. Combined neuromuscular electrical stimulation and transcutaneous electrical nerve stimulation for treatment of chronic back pain: a double-blind, repeated measures comparison. Arch Phys Med Rehabil 1997;78:55–60.

75. Thornhill TS. Shoulder pain. In: Kelly WN, Harris ED Jr, Ruddy S, Sledge CB, eds. Textbook of Rheumatology. Philadelphia: Saunders, 1993:417–440.

76. Katz RS, Zizic TM, Arnold WP, Stevens MB. The pseudothrombophlebitis syndrome. Medicine 1991;56: 151–164.

77. Ho G Jr, Tice AD, Kaplan SR. Septic bursitis in the prepatellar and olecranon bursae. Ann Intern Med 1978;89:21–27.

78. Doherty M, Dieppe P. Crystal deposition disease in the elderly. Clin Rheum Dis 1986;12:97–116.

79. McCarty D, ed. Crystalline deposition disease. In: Clinical Rheumatic Diseases. Philadelphia: Saunders, 1988:14.

80. Kelly WN, Schumacher R Jr. Gout. In: Kelly WN, Harris ED Jr, Ruddy S, Sledge CB, eds. Textbook of Rheumatology. Philadelphia: Saunders, 1993:1291–1336.

81. Hadler MM, Franck A, Bress M, Robinson R. Acute polyarticular gout. Am J Med 1974;56:715–719.

82. Roberts WM, Liang MH, Stern SH. Colchicine in acute gout. JAMA 1987;257:1920–1922.

83. McCarty DJ. Arthropathies associated with calcium-containing crystals. Hosp Pract 1986;21:109–120

84. Deleted in proof.

85. Gloth FM, et al. Functional improvement with vitamin D replenishment in a cohort of frail, vitamin D deficient older people. J Am Geriatr Soc 1995;3:1269–1271.

86. Reginato AJ. Musculoskeletal manifestations of osteomalacia. Rev Rhum Engl Ed 1997;64(6 suppl):107S–113S.

87. Wolfe F, Ross K, Anderson J, et al. The prevalence and characteristics of fibromyalgia in the general population. Arthritis Rheum 1995;38:19–28.

88. Chaung T, Hunder GG, Ilstrup PM, Kurland LT. Polymyalgia rheumatica. Ann Intern Med 1982;97: 672–680.

89. Cohen MD, Ginsburg WW. Polymyalgia rheumatica. Rheum Dis Clin North Am 1990;16:325–339.

90. Mody GM, Cassim B. Rheumatologic manifestations of malignancy. Curr Opin Rheumatol 1997;9:75–79.

91. Ayoub WT, Franklin CM, Torretti D. Polymyalgia rheumatica: duration of therapy and long-term outcome. Am J Med 1985;79:309–315.

92. Huston KA, Hunder GG, Lie JT, et al. Temporal arteritis: a 25-year epidemiologic, clinical, and pathologic study. Ann Intern Med 1978;88:162–167.

93. Chmelewski WL, McKnight KM, Agudelo CA, Wise CM. Presenting features and outcomes in patients undergoing temporal artery biopsy. Arch Intern Med 1992;152:1690–1695.

94. Hamilton CR, Shelley WM, Tumulty PA. Giant cell arteritis: including temporal arteritis and polymyalgia rheumatica. Medicine 1971;50:1–27.

95. Faulkner JA, Brooks SV, Zerba E. Muscle atrophy and weakness with aging: contraction-induced injury as an underlying mechanism. J Gerontol Series A, Biol Sci Med Sci 1995;50:124–129 (special issue).

96. Dalakas MC, Sivakumar K. The immunopathologic and inflammatory differences between dermatomyositis, polymyositis and sporadic inclusion body myositis. Curr Opin Neurol 1996;9:235–239.

97. Oddis CV, Medsger TA Jr. Inflammatory myopathies. Baillieres Clin Rheumatol 1995;9:497–514.

98. Griggs RC, Askanas V, DiMauro S, et al. Inclusion body myositis and myopathies. Ann Neurol 1995;38:705–713.

99. Plotz PH, Rider LG, Targoff IN, et al. NIH conference. Myositis: immunologic contributions to understanding cause, pathogenesis, and therapy. Ann Intern Med 1995;122:715–724.

100. Callen JP. Relationship of cancer to inflammatory muscle diseases: dermatomyositis, polymyositis, and inclusion body myositis. Rheum Dis Clin North Am 1994;20:943–953.

101. Chou SM. Inclusion body myositis. Baillieres Clin Neurol 1993;2:557–577.

102. Ling SM, Ling GSF. Autoimmune peripheral neuropathies. Resident Staff Physician 1994; suppl:26–31.

103. Baker SB, et al. Late onset systemic lupus erythematosus. Am J Med 1979;66:727–732.

104. Baer AN, Pincus T. Occult systemic lupus erythematosus in elderly men. JAMA 1983;249:3350–3352.

105. Slater CA, et al. Antinuclear antibody testing. Arch Intern Med 1996;156:1421–1425.

106. Sanchez-Guerrero J, et al. Postmenopausal estrogen therapy and the risk for developing systemic lupus erythematosus. Ann of Intern Med 1995;122:430–432.

107. Nesher G, Moore TL, Suckner J. Rheumatoid arthritis in the elderly. J Am Geriatr Soc 1991;39:284–294.

108. Drugs for rheumatoid arthritis. Med Lett 1995;36:101–106.

109. Dahl SL, Samuelson CO, Williams HJ, et al. Second-line antirheumatic drugs in the elderly with rheumatoid arthritis: a post hoc analysis of three controlled trials. Pharmacotherapy 1990;10:79–81.

110. Melnyk V. Geriatric rheumatology: safe use of potentially toxic antirheumatics. Geriatrics 1988;43:83–90.

111. Fox RI. Clinical features, pathogenesis, and treatment of Sjögren's syndrome. Curr Opin Rheumatol 1996;8:438–445.

112. Fox RI. Sjögren's syndrome. Curr Opin Rheumatol 1995;7:409–416.

113. Kompoliti A, Gage B, Sharma L, Daniels JC. Human T-cell lymphotropic virus type 1-associated myelopathy, Sjögren syndrome, and lymphocytic pneumonitis. Arch Neurol 1996;53:940–942.

114. Hochberg MC, Schein OD, Munoz B, et al. The prevalence of dry eye, dry mouth, autoimmunity and primary Sjögren's syndrome in the general population. Abstract presented at the annual meeting of the American College of Rheumatology, October 1996.

115. Anaya JM, McGuff HS, Banks PM. Talal N. Clinicopathological factors relating malignant lymphoma with Sjögren's syndrome. Semin Arthritis Rheum 1996;25:337–346.

116. St. Clair EW. New developments in Sjögren's syndrome. Curr Opin Rheumatol 1993;5:604–612.

117. Fox RI. V International Symposium on Sjögren's syndrome. Clinical aspects and therapy. Clin Rheumatol 1995;14(suppl 1):17–19.

118. Philippe B, Couderc LJ, Droz D, et al. Systemic vasculitis and myelodysplastic syndromes: a report of two cases. Arthritis Rheum 1997;40:179–182.

119. Arand M, Weingerger A. Leukocytoclastic vasculitis after use of acetaminophen: case presentation and approach to differential diagnosis. J Clin Rheumatol 1997;3:108–111.

120. Sneller MC. Wegener's granulomatosis. JAMA 1995;273:1288–1291.

121. Krafcik SS, Covin RB, Lynch JP, et al. Wegener's granulomatosis in the elderly. Chest 1996;109:430–437.

122. Guillevin L, Lhote F, Cohen P, et al. Corticosteroids plus pulse cyclophosphamide and plasma exchanges versus corticosteroids plus pulse cyclophosphamide alone in treatment of polyarteritis nodosa and Churg-Strauss syndrome patients with factors predicting poor prognosis: a prospective, randomized trial in sixty-two patients. Arthritis Rheum 1995;38:1638–1645.

123. Naschitz JE, Slobin G, Yeshurun D, et al. A polymyalgia rheumatica-like syndrome as a presentation of metastatic cancer. J Clin Rheumatol 1996;2:305–308.

124. Chandran G, Ahern MJ, Seshadri P, Coghlan D. Rheumatic manifestations of the myelodysplastic syndromes: a comparative study. Aust N Z J Med 1996;26:683–688.

125. Airio A, Pukkala E, Isomaki H. Elevated cancer incidence in patients with dermatomyositis: a population based study. J Rheumatol 1995;22:1300–1303.

126. Zantos D, Zhang Y, Felson D. The overall and temporal association of cancer with polymyositis and dermatomyositis. J Rheumatol 1994;21:1855–1859.

127. Abu-Shakra M, Guillemin F, Lee P. Cancer in systemic sclerosis. Arthritis Rheum 1993;36:460–464.

128. Anaya JM, McGuff HS, Banks PM, Talal N. Clinicopathological factors relating malignant lymphoma with Sjögren's syndrome. Semin Arthritis Rheum 1996;25:337–346.

129. Radis CD, Kahl LE, Baker GL, et al. Effects of cyclophosphamide on the development of malignancy and on long-term survival of patients with rheumatoid arthritis. Arthritis Rheum 1995;38:1120–1127.

CHAPTER 33

MICHELE F. BELLANTONI

Osteoporosis and Other Metabolic Disorders of the Skeleton in Aging

Table 33.1 lists the metabolic bone diseases that may first present in older adulthood. For all of these disorders, the goal of care is to prevent bony fractures. This chapter focuses on the management and where possible the prevention of the most common of the primary bone disorders of the elderly: osteoporosis, osteomalacia, hyperparathyroidism, and Paget's disease.

OSTEOPOROSIS
Pathophysiology

Adult bone is a metabolically active body tissue. At the cellular level, bone remodeling occurs at discrete foci in the skeleton called bone-remodeling units. Each cycle begins with activated osteoclasts lining the bone surface. Over about 2 weeks the osteoclasts excavate a lacuna on the surface of cancellous bone or a cavity within cortical bone. Bone formation occurs as osteoblasts secrete calcified matrix proteins. The effect of bone remodeling at the tissue level is determined by both the rate of bone turnover and the balance of the amount of bone resorbed and formed at each unit (1). When bone mass is maintained, resorption is coupled to formation. Osteoporosis is defined as low bone mass resulting from an excess of bone resorption over bone formation, with resultant bone fragility and increased risk of fracture. A population-based data model has estimated that 54% of 50-year-old women will sustain osteoporosis-related fractures during their remaining lifetime (2). Significant morbidity, mortality,

and medical expense result from osteoporosis-related fractures. Spinal fractures, which occur in 25% of white women by age 65, cause pain, deformity, and disability. Hip fractures result in at least short-term institutionalization in more than 50% of patients and are associated with a mortality rate of 5 to 20% within the first year of fracture (3). Moreover, it is estimated that more than 10% of women who sustain hip fractures become dependent in functional status, while many more never regain their full prefracture level of activity. The financial cost of osteoporosis in the United States each year exceeds $10 billion (4).

Risk Factors

Bone mineral density in the elderly is the result of a peak bone mass that occurs in late adolescence, the maintenance of bone mass during young adulthood, and subsequent bone loss over time. Family and twin studies suggest that a low peak bone mass can result from as yet unrecognized genetic defects (5), with other factors such as malnutrition, chronic disease states, and exogenous glucocorticoid use contributing to reductions in peak bone mass. The maintenance of bone mass during young adulthood depends on the maintenance of normal endocrine function, including ovarian, adrenal, and testicular function; adequate calcium intake; and weight-bearing exercise. Common conditions that result in the loss of bone mass in young adults include menstrual irregularities resulting from severe

Table 33.1

Metabolic Bone Disorders of the Elderly

Disorder	Metabolic Bone Defects	Common Risk Factors
Osteoporosis	Bone resorption predominates over formation	Postmenopausal women; hypogonadal men; chronic steroid, tobacco, or alcohol use
Osteomalacia	Mineralization defect associated with impaired or insufficient vitamin D metabolism	Homebound or institutionalized elderly; inadequate intake of dairy products; gastric surgery
Hyperparathyroidism	PTH-induced accelerated bone resorption	Postmenopausal women
Renal osteodystrophy	Secondary hyperparathyroidism resulting in accelerated bone resorption; osteomalacia related to impairment of vitamin D metabolism in the kidney; aluminum toxicity from phosphate buffers	Moderate to severe renal insufficiency; renal tubular defect; heavy metal exposures
Paget's disease	Increase in bone resorption and formation	Late manifestation of paramyxoviral infection (measles, respiratory syncytial virus)
Malignancies	Bone resorption related to ectopic hormonal production (lung and kidney); direct invasion of tumor causing either increased resorption (breast, thyroid, myeloma) or increased osteoblastic function (prostate)	Underlying malignancy
Infections	Accelerated bone resorption resulting from infection of bone (tuberculosis, osteomyelitis)	Diabetes mellitus, chronic wound overlying bone, vascular insufficiency
Genetic disorders		Genetic predisposition
Hypophosphatasia	Disorders of alkaline phosphatase activity	
Osteogenesis imperfecta	Type I collagen defects causing brittle bones	
Osteopetrosis	Impairment of bone resorption	
Pyknodysostosis	Sclerosing bone dysplasia	

weight loss or excessive exercise, gonadal dysfunction in women or men related to chronic disease, and the use of exogenous corticosteroids, cigarettes, or alcohol.

Estrogen deficiency results in accelerated bone loss at the time of menopause. It is likely that bone loss begins before the cessation of menses (6,7). The time course and magnitude of the perimenopausal bone loss appear to be variable, and the factors other than the loss of ovarian estrogen production that contribute to and modulate the bone loss during this period are not completely understood. For example, menopause is associated with a significant reduction in ovarian testosterone and adrenal androgen production. Bone loss during the menopausal transition can be up to 4% per year and may last 10 to 15 years (8). It is estimated that a third to half of bone loss in women may be attributable to menopause (1). While men do not have an easily identifiable menopause, hypogonadism in young men is associated with accelerated bone loss. In men over age 65, bone density is positively associated with serum estrogen levels but is not associated with serum testosterone levels within the normal range for young men (9).

Cross-sectional data suggest that bone loss continues in older women and men but that the degree of loss varies from site to site. In one study, decrements in bone density between women aged 65 to 69 and women aged 85 and older exceeded 16% in the distal and proximal radius, the calcaneus, and the proximal femur; the difference in bone mineral density of the lumbar spine between the two groups was 6% (10). The primary causes of bone loss in older adults are unknown; however, dietary interventions including calcium (11) and vitamin D (12) and weight-bearing exercise (13) have been shown to reduce the rate of bone loss and may to a small degree reverse bone loss in older adults. It is thought that estrogen deficiency plays little part in the continued bone loss in women over age 65; however, more recent epidemiologic data suggest that the bone mass of women who begin hormone replacement later in life can approach that of women who received long-term hormone replacement (14). Secondary osteoporosis can be caused by excessive exposure to endogenous or exogenous glucocorticoids and thyroid hormone as well as hyperparathyroidism and multiple myeloma. It is also possible that deficiencies in growth hormone and insulinlike growth factor I can contribute to bone loss in older men and women (15).

Screening

While osteopenia can be diagnosed with standard radiography, this technique is not reliably sensitive to losses less than 30% of bone mineral density. Thus, standard radiography is not an acceptable method to determine early or mild bone loss. Bone mineral densitometry is a useful technique for predicting the risk of fracture based on comparisons with age-matched controls. Single-photon absorptiometry, the first commercially available technique for the noninvasive measurement of bone mineral density, passes a beam of highly collimated monoenergetic photons from a radionuclide source through the area to be measured. The observed attenuation of the beam is a function of the density of the tissues through which the beam is passed.

Unlike single-photon absorptiometry, which requires a constant soft tissue path length, thereby limiting the technique to measurements of the peripheral skeleton, dual-energy absorptiometry uses two photon energies to allow the separation of bone and soft tissue mass attenuation. Dual-energy absorptiometry is used to measure bone mineral density of the lumbar spine and proximal femur. More recently, the radiation spectrum of gadolinium-153 has been simulated by radiographic techniques. Dual-energy x-ray absorptiometry scans now provide the most precise measurements of bone mineral density, with 1% precision for spine and 1 to 2% for femur scans, and with lowest radiation exposure, at doses per scan of less than 0.03% of the natural yearly radiation.

One criticism of bone densitometry is that the technique does not distinguish vertebral bone mass from fatty infiltrate. Also, degenerative changes that are common in the spinal column with aging, such as fatty infiltrate, result in falsely elevated bone mineral density measurements with absorptiometry techniques. In contrast, quantitative computed tomography allows the direct measurement of trabecular or total bone density; however, this technique is costly and entails greater radiation exposure than dual-energy x-ray absorptiometry. While studies have shown that single-photon absorptiometry of the appendicular skeleton equally predicts nonspine fracture risks as compared with dual-energy x-ray absorptiometry, it has been suggested that imaging of the trabecular component of the proximal femur using dual-energy techniques may better predict femoral fracture (16). More recent advances have led to the availability of portable devices that measure bone mineral density of the forearm or calcaneous using dual-energy x-ray technology, and ultrasound technologies may prove to be a nonradiographic method for bone mass measurement (17).

One study has documented that the results of bone densitometry substantially influence women's decisions about preventive measures for osteoporosis (18). There is considerable controversy about the appropriate use of bone densitometry as a screening test for osteoporosis. However, it is generally accepted that women who are at high risk for osteoporosis should be studied with a bone densitometry. Decreases in bone mineral density of more than 1% per year are considered clinically significant changes that may be corrected by the interventions described herein. Examples of patients who may benefit from such screening include a postmenopausal woman who has a strong family history of osteoporosis and who is not receiving estrogen replacement therapy, men and women who require long-term exogenous steroid therapy, and premenopausal women with menstrual irregularities. A single densitometry screen may be useful to a woman who is unwilling to take estrogen therapy without evidence of low bone mass.

Although densitometry provides an accurate assessment of bone mass, it does not provide information on the present rate of bone turnover. Bone-specific proteins and their metabolites can be measured in blood and urine specimens to estimate the current rates of bone formation and resorption (19). Serum procollagen peptide and Osteocalcin measurements reflect bone formation, while bone-specific alkaline phosphatase and the collagen metabolites of deoxypyridino-line cross-links and n-telopeptides reflect bone resorption. These biochemical markers combined with bone densitometry may be useful in determining which patients are at risk for osteoporosis-related fractures, such as a postmenopausal woman who has a low baseline bone mineral density and evidence of accelerated bone turnover. However, the role of biomarkers in the routine screening or treatment monitoring of osteoporosis requires further study.

Diagnostic Evaluation

Serum calcium and alkaline phosphatase levels are expected to be normal in osteoporosis but may be abnormal in other metabolic bone diseases, such as hyperparathyroidism and osteopenia caused by vitamin D deficiency (20, 21). A patient who has osteoporosis and elevated serum calcium and alkaline phosphatase level should be further evaluated with a serum measurement of intact molecule parathyroid hormone. The presentation of elevated alkaline phosphatase levels, muscle weakness, and osteoporosis in the setting of inadequate dietary intake of vitamin D or a predisposition to malabsorption should prompt an evaluation for vitamin D deficiency. It is suggested that a serum 25 vitamin D level be measured to assess the adequacy of vitamin D stores (22). Serum procollagen peptide and osteocalcin combined with the measurement of deoxypyridinoline cross-links or n-telopeptides provide evidence of the current rate of bone turnover.

Further diagnostic studies are recommended on the basis of the clinical presentation. For example, patients receiving thyroid supplements should be assessed for bone loss related to supraphysiologic thyroxine replacement. In this setting, a serum measurement of thyroid-stimulating hormone using a supersensitive assay technique is suggested. The finding of a suppressed hormone level indicates excessive replacement. Serum protein electrophoresis is appropriate in patients with elevated total protein in whom multiple myeloma is suspected. While the measurement of calcium excretion in a 24-hour collection of urine is used to identify those who have calcium wasting from the kidney that is reversed with thiazide diuretics, the practical difficulties of the test often preclude its use in the elderly.

Prevention and Treatment

Table 33.2 summarizes preventive strategies for various patients at risk for osteoporosis. There is well-documented evidence that estrogen replacement therapy prevents the accelerated bone loss attributed to menopause (23). The minimum fully effective dose of oral estrogens is 0.625 mg of conjugated equine estrogen, 1 mg 17β-estradiol orally or 50 to 100 μg transdermally per day. One study of daily low-dose estrogen, 0.3 mg conjugated equine estrogen combined with 2 g of calcium supplementation, showed efficacy of this regimen to prevent short-term bone loss (24). However, this has not been confirmed in long-term studies. In contrast, the 0.625-mg dose has been studied longitudinally with 20-year published data to support its efficacy as well as studies documenting the prevention of hip fractures (25).

Given the efficacy of estrogen in the prevention of osteoporosis, the routine use of perimenopausal hormone replacement is becoming commonplace. The maximum age or length of menopausal duration at which the initiation of estrogen is beneficial is controversial. The beneficial effects of estrogens on bone have been demonstrated on patients up to age 70 and in women with established osteoporosis (14); however, it appears that to achieve maximum benefit, estrogen replacement must begin at least at the time of cessation of menses. Frequent side effects of estrogens in older women include breast tenderness and bloating, both of which tend to peak by 6 weeks of therapy (26). The effects of postmenopausal estrogen replacement therapy on clotting factors are not clinically significant, unlike those of oral contraceptive treatments. A poorly studied potential side effect of long-term estrogens is biliary stone formation associated with the changes in cholesterol metabolism resulting from the relatively high levels of estrogens achieved in the portal circulation following oral estrogen therapy. The most controversial aspect of estrogen replacement remains the potential increase in breast cancer resulting from prolonged estrogen use. Data from the Nurses' Health Study suggest as much as a 25 to 30% increased risk of breast cancer with hormone replacement lasting 9 years or longer (27).

In light of these recent data supporting an increase in breast cancer risk with long-term use, the optimal duration of estrogen treatment is difficult to determine. Several factors must be considered in the decision to stop estrogen treatment. First, accelerated bone loss immediately follows estrogen withdrawal (28). Data obtained from the Framingham Study suggest that for the long-term preservation of bone mineral density, women should take estrogen for at least 7 years after menopause and that even this duration of therapy may have little residual effect on bone density in women aged 75 and older (29). A further consideration for the initiation and the maintenance of long-term estrogen replacement therapy is the potential protection against cardiovascular disease in postmenopausal women. It is estimated that the overall benefits of hormone replacement therapy in reducing the likelihood of developing coronary heart disease outweigh the risk of breast cancer for nearly all women in whom this treatment might be considered (30). A practical approach is to begin hormonal therapy during the menopausal transition and to maintain therapy until long-term prevention of osteoporosis is no longer an important aspect of health care for an individual woman or until the woman has a significant adverse event related to the therapy.

Progestins appear to enhance the effect of estrogen on bone (31); at the same time, they seem to antagonize the effects of estrogen on the endometrium to prevent endometrial hyperplasia. Recent studies suggest that low-dose daily progestin, such as medroxyprogesterone acetate 2.5 to 5 mg daily added to daily estrogen, may improve compliance by preventing monthly vaginal bleeding (32). However, a significant portion of women have unpredictable bleeding in the first 6 months of this treatment. An alternative therapy that results in predictable monthly vaginal bleeding is sequential progestin, medroxyprogesterone acetate 10 mg daily for 10 to 14 days at the beginning of each calendar month combined with daily estrogen.

In the past, progestins were added to estrogen therapy even for women who had undergone hysterectomy, under the assumption that progestins counterbalanced the effects of estrogen

Table 33.2

Patient-Oriented Prevention and Treatment Strategies for Osteoporosis

Common Clinical Presentations	Suggested Frequency of Diagnostic Evaluation[a]	Pharmacologic Interventions	Nonpharmacologic Interventions
Any perimenopausal woman; special emphasis if thin, smoker, sedentary, family history of fracture, early natural or surgical menopause	1 to 2 years if no estrogen therapy	Daily estrogen, cycled progestin[b] (low-dose contraceptives in nonsmoker until menopause complete); raloxifene as second-line therapy	Dietary calcium and vitamin D[c]; weight-bearing exercise; smoking cessation; modest alcohol and caffeine intake
Postmenopausal woman Aged up to 70 years	2 years if no estrogen therapy	Daily estrogen and progestin[b]; antiresorptive therapy[d]	As above
Aged above 70 years		Individual risk-benefit profile of estrogen and progestin; antiresorptive therapy[d]	As above
Postmenopausal woman with history of breast or endometrial cancer	1 to 2 years if no tamoxifen therapy	Profile of daily tamoxifen; antiresorptive therapy in high-risk patients[d]	As above
Symptomatic hypogonadism in an older man	1 to 2 years if no testosterone therapy	Individual risk-benefit profile of parenteral testosterone; antiresorptive therapy in high-risk patients[d]	As above
Chronic steroid use	1 to 2 years to monitor bone loss	Antiresorptive therapy prophylactically[d]	As above
Osteoporosis-related fracture	Initial evaluation and yearly to monitor therapy	Antiresorptive therapy[d]	As above; physical therapy to strengthen abdominal and paraspinal muscles; fall prevention

[a]Diagnostic evaluation includes bone mineral density scan of spine and hip. Osteoporosis: bone mineral density below normal peak bone mass by more than 2.5 standard deviations. Other laboratory studies according to clinical history.

[b]Hysterectomy obviates progestin cotherapy.

[c]Total daily intake of calcium 1–1.5 g/day and vitamin D 400–800 IU.

[d]Oral bisphosphonate is first-line choice; if patient is unable to use bisphosphonate, calcitonin nasal spray is first-line choice.

on breast tissue, analogous to the uterine effects. It is now known that both estrogens and progestins stimulate breast tissue growth. This effect on the breast, combined with the dose-related adverse effect on cholesterol profiles, precludes the use of progestins in women who are no longer at risk for endometrial cancer because of hysterectomy.

For women who have proven breast cancer, estrogen and progestin therapy are contraindicated. The synthetic estrogen receptor modulator tamoxifen, which is used in the treatment of breast cancer, has been shown in vitro to inhibit bone resorption and in a small clinical trial, to increase bone density (33). Tamoxifen also improves the lipid profile, yet there are potential adverse effects of therapy, such as thromboembolic disease and hepatic and endometrial tumors. A newer agent, raloxifene, recently has received U.S. Food and Drug Administration (FDA) approval for osteoporosis treatment, and it appears to offer additional benefit over tamoxifen in that there is no evidence of endometrial proliferation in short-term studies (34). However, as the long-term benefits versus the risks of synthetic estrogen receptor modulators as compared with older estrogen-progestin treatments are unknown, the current recommendation favors conventional hormone replacement as initial postmenopausal management. For women who are unwilling or unable to tolerate estrogen and progestin, raloxifene offers choice for hormone replacement.

Anabolic steroids increase bone mass in osteoporotic women; however, their adverse effects on lipid profiles and their potential to cause hepatic dysfunction make them inadequate substitutes for estrogen therapy. Testosterone replacement increases bone loss in hypogonadal men (35); however, the benefits of this therapy may be offset in elderly men by exacerbating both prostatic hypertrophy and cardiac risk factors such as lipoprotein profiles. Studies to establish a method of testosterone replacement that provides an overall health benefit to hypogonadal men are ongoing.

In addition to gender-appropriate sex hormone replacement therapy, calcium intake is important in maintaining bone mass. The recommended daily allowance of calcium was recently increased to 1 g daily for postmenopausal women receiving hormone replacement and to 1.5 g daily for all women and men over age 65 and for younger postmenopausal women not adequately treated with sex steroids. This is roughly equivalent to five 8-ounce glasses of milk daily. As most older American women do not consume a sufficient quantity of dairy products to meet their calcium needs, calcium supplementation is recommended. The most common side effect of calcium therapy is constipation. In women with normal renal function, no monitoring of electrolytes is needed to prevent hypercalcemia. In newly postmenopausal women, high calcium intake does not confer the same degree of osteoporosis prevention as estrogen replacement therapy, but it does potentiate the effect of estrogen and calcitonin on bone mass (36). In contrast, bone loss in elderly women whose dietary calcium intake is below 400 mg daily is retarded when calcium supplementation is provided to the level of 1 g daily (11).

Calcitonin was the first drug approved by the FDA for the treatment of established osteoporosis. While calcitonin deficiency is thought to have little effect on the development of osteoporosis, antiresorptive effects of exogenous calcitonin have been documented in patients with osteoporosis. However, the studies of calcitonin in osteoporotic patients are short term, 1 to 2 years. In addition, the current standard of efficacy for osteoporosis treatments is the ability to reduce fracture incidence. Calcitonin has been shown to reduce vertebral fractures but not hip fractures. Intranasal calcitonin 200 IU, or one metered puff daily, appears to be as efficacious as 100 IU of the salmon preparation or 0.5 mg of the recombinant human form subcutaneously 3 times weekly, with ease of administration and less nausea and facial flushing (37). Studies have combined calcitonin in a cyclical fashion with parathyroid hormone therapy to test the hypothesis that the combined therapy would stimulate bone formation and reduce resorption (38). Calcitonin has been studied in the setting of acute vertebral compression fracture and has been shown to be more effective than placebo in the short-term management of bone pain (39).

Bisphosphonates are a class of synthetic pyrophosphate analogs that bind strongly to hydroxyapatite crystals. They are adsorbed onto newly synthesized bone matrix and prevent bone resorption through inhibition of osteoclastic activity. Bisphosphonates also inhibit bone formation, but more recent compounds inhibit bone resorption more than bone formation. Drugs in this class are poorly absorbed and may cause gastrointestinal symptoms. To date, these drugs have been studied for efficacy in both the prevention of bone loss and the treatment of established osteoporosis. Cyclic etidronate was the first widely used treatment (40). However, alendronate 10 mg daily became the first FDA-approved bisphosphonate for the treatment of osteoporosis, based on 3-year data that showed a 50% reduction in vertebral and hip fractures (41). Short-term prevention of bone loss has been established for early postmenopausal women using alendronate 5 mg daily (42). Recent data suggest a role for bisphosphonate in the prevention and treatment of steroid-induced osteoporosis in men and women (43).

Bisphosphonates have low rates of gastrointestinal absorption and must be taken without food or drink other than water. They can cause nausea, dysmotility, and most worrisome, esophageal stricture from acid reflux. However, due to the reported reductions in fracture with bisphosphonates, they are the treatment of choice for osteoporosis, with intranasal calcitonin reserved for those who are unable to tolerate or at high risk of the gastrointestinal side effects of bisphosphonates.

Other antiresorptive agents include calcitriol, the active metabolite of vitamin D, and thiazide diuretics. Both agents improve calcium balance; calcitriol increases gastrointestinal absorption of calcium, while thiazides decrease renal excretion of calcium. Vitamin D replacement in deficient elders reverses secondary hyperparathyroidism (44). However, the therapeutic efficacy of calcitriol or synthetic analogs of calcitriol in the treatment of osteoporosis without vitamin D deficiency is unclear. Initial therapy with low-dose calcitriol can prevent hypercalcemia and renal stones, yet inactive metabolites of vitamin D may be associated with fewer adverse effects for patients who have dietary vitamin deficiency without metabolic defects caused by renal insuffi-

ciency. Thiazide diuretic use has been associated with reduced risk of fracture (45), but this is not a consistent observation. A randomized, placebo-controlled study is needed before thiazides can be recommended as antiresorptive therapy.

None of these therapies stimulates bone formation; they prevent bone resorption. Fluoride has been shown to stimulate osteoblast function. However, some studies of fluoride therapy have resulted in increased fracture incidence that was probably related to the dose-dependent effect of fluoride to impair mineralization of newly formed bone. Dosages of fluoride below 45 to 75 mg daily combined with calcium 1 g per day may offset the mineralization defects seen with higher-dose therapy (46). Other adverse effects include gastrointestinal side effects (nausea, dyspepsia, and hemorrhage) and rheumatic complaints, such as tendinitis and arthralgia, including lower extremity pain syndrome caused by incomplete fractures. These have been decreased by the use of extended-release formulations and by reducing the daily dose (47). However, one study of postmenopausal women with osteoporotic vertebral compression fractures, which used a maximum daily dose of 60 mg of enteric-coated tablets with dose reductions for adverse symptoms and serum fluoride levels above 15 lmol/L, reported that almost 40% of the subjects were intolerant of the drug within the first 18 months of treatment (48). Yet, patients who tolerated the therapy experienced a mean increase in vertebral bone mineral density of 8.4% per year, one of the highest achievable increases in bone density documented by therapeutic agents. Similar increases in lumbar density have been achieved in a second cohort of postmenopausal osteoporotic women, accompanied by 4% annual increases in proximal femur but 2% decreases in radial cortical bone (49). These changes persisted throughout 4 years of study. However, the most controversial aspect of fluoride treatment is the effect on fracture rates.

In summary, while fluoride has the potential to increase bone density, the potential abnormal structure and fragility of bone with excess fluoride content and the clinical side effects of fluoride preclude its use routinely in the management of patients with osteoporosis. However, ongoing studies of fluoride may determine safe and efficacious uses for this therapy in the future.

The effect of parathyroid hormone on bone metabolism is dose dependent. While sustained elevated circulating levels of parathyroid hormone result in osteoclast-mediated bone resorption, intermittent low-dose therapy, designed to mimic the endogenous pulsatile secretion of parathyroid hormone, has been shown to stimulate bone formation. In small groups of osteoporotic patients, sequential therapy with parathyroid hormone and calcitonin over 14 months increased trabecular vertebral bone by 12% (50). Combined therapy with calcitriol gave a similar result, but a plateau effect was reached after 12 months, followed by a decrease in mean bone mineral density. In addition, there was a concomitant decrease in cortical bone of the radius, raising concerns that prolonged therapy may result in increased fractures in appendicular bone. Research is under way to determine the mechanism for the different responses of trabecular and cortical bone to parathyroid hormone therapy.

Other potential stimulators of bone formation include the hormones of the somatotrophic axis: growth hormone-releasing hormone, growth hormone, insulinlike growth factor I, and more recently, small peptides that induce endogenous growth hormone secretion when taken orally. To date in small clinical trials, growth hormone replacement in deficient young adults increased cortical and trabecular bone density, and in healthy older men, increased lumbar bone density by 1.6% over 6 months (51). Bone-derived growth factors may prove useful to activate bone. Potential therapeutic agents include transforming growth factor-β, platelet-derived growth factor, fibroblast growth factors, and bone morphogenetic proteins.

Weight-bearing exercise is important in the maintenance of bone mass (52). Immobility, including bed rest and systemic illnesses, can cause rapid bone loss. Exercise prescriptions for elderly patients must minimize adverse events resulting from comorbid conditions such as cardiovascular disease and degenerative joint disease. Extension and isometric exercises minimize vertebral compression in patients with severe vertebral osteopenia (53). Fall prevention is paramount in

patients at risk for fractures because of severe osteoporosis. Other important behavioral interventions include smoking cessation and judicious alcohol and caffeine intake. Pain management of muscle spasms and the mechanical deformities of severe kyphosis include heat, massage, physical therapies, and analgesics.

In summary, osteoporosis is a common bone disorder, particularly of older women, with significant morbidity and mortality resulting from spinal deformity and hip fractures. Preventive strategies include adequate lifetime calcium intake and exercise, and postmenopausal hormone replacement. Treatment for osteoporosis is less well established, with each therapy posing potential difficulties including cost, side effects, and lack of long-term efficacy. Bisphosphonates offer the most reduction in fractures, but gastrointestinal side effects may limit their use.

OSTEOMALACIA

Vitamin D deficiency in the elderly can result in deep bone and muscle pain, muscle weakness, hyperesthesia, and fractures related to osteopenia and osteoporosis. The elderly are susceptible to vitamin D deficiency for several reasons. Less vitamin D is manufactured through the skin because aged skin has less precursor and converts these precursors more slowly. In addition, lotions and creams are applied topically to prevent skin cancer. These lotions filter out the ultraviolet (UV) light needed for the conversion of vitamin D precursors in the skin. Frail elderly are often physically unable to venture outdoors, and window glass filters out UV light. Restrictions of high-cholesterol foods, including dairy products and organ meats, result in insufficient dietary sources of vitamin D precursors. In addition, medications such as phenytoin may interfere with vitamin D metabolism. Studies of homebound elderly suggest that the recommended daily allowance of 400 IU of vitamin D may be insufficient to prevent osteomalacia and that vitamin D supplementation of 800 IU per day of ergocalciferol is needed in this population (22).

HYPERPARATHYROIDISM

Primary hyperparathyroidism is characterized by excessive production of parathyroid hormone that leads to hypercalcemia via two mechanisms: (a) osteoclast-mediated bone resorption and (b) calcium conservation at the level of the renal glomerulus. The recognized prevalence of mild forms of this condition has increased since the automation of serum chemistry analyzers and the routine use of blood work in medical evaluations. The incidence of hyperparathyroidism in men over age 60 is one new case per 1000 of population per year, with twice this frequency for women of similar age (54). Thus, this is a condition that primarily affects postmenopausal women. The disease course can vary in severity from the benign presentation of asymptomatic abnormal serum chemistries to a constellation of clinically relevant adverse events including constipation, hypertension, accelerated bone loss, peptic ulcer disease, pancreatitis, nephrocalcinosis, nephrolithiasis, and renal insufficiency. Added to this list are varied psychiatric symptoms including anxiety, depression, and cognitive impairment.

The diagnosis of hyperparathyroidism is considered when an elevation in serum calcium level is accompanied by a decreased or low normal serum phosphate level. Serum alkaline phosphatase may be either minimally or more strikingly elevated. Urinary calcium excretion is less than 250 mg/g of creatinine, while urinary cyclic adenosine monophosphate is typically elevated.

There are multiple radioimmunoassays for the measurement of serum parathyroid hormone levels. Assays that measure intact molecule, amino-terminal fragments, or midmolecule are recommended to confirm the diagnosis; measurements of carboxy-terminal fragments can give false elevations in the setting of renal insufficiency. Hypercalcemia accompanied by suppressed parathyroid hormone levels suggests either a malignancy or sarcoidosis, depending on the associated clinical findings. The measurement of parathyroid hormone-related protein may be clinically useful when no underlying malignancy is identifiable, although this assay is not widely available.

The radiographic findings, like the severity of the condition, are varied in hyperparathyroidism, ranging from diffuse osteopenia to more specific radiographic signs. The latter include extensive cortical bone resorption such as subperiosteal resorption of the radial aspect of the second and third phalanges, the distal clavicles, and the skull, that gives a salt and pepper appearance. In both cortical and trabecular bone, deep burrows resulting from resorption may be filled by fibrous tissue, giving a cystic appearance to the bone, termed osteitis fibrosa cystica. Bone tissue replaced by highly vascularized fibrous tissue, called brown tumors, may be misinterpreted as giant cell tumors of bone. Bone densitometry typically reflects more extensive involvement of cortical bone over trabecular bone, resulting in greater reductions in bone mineral density of the radius and hip than of the lumbar spine.

Definitive therapy for hyperparathyroidism is surgical resection of the adenoma; however, the indications for surgery in older patients are controversial. Probable indications for surgery include low bone mass (greater than 2 to 2.5 standard deviations below mean for age as assessed by densitometry), recurrent renal calculi, and pancreatitis (20). Hypercalcemia greater than 12 mg/dL, osteitis fibrosa, reduced and falling bone mass, and refractory ulcer disease are also targeted for surgical correction. Based on this strategy for surgical referrals, the appropriate evaluation should include a bone mineral density scan to assess for osteopenia. Hypertension, hypercalcemia less than 12 mg/dL, and psychiatric symptoms are thought not to be indications for surgical resection. Others have reported, however, that the psychiatric symptoms may be amenable to surgical correction. Also in question is the issue of a surgically correctable improvement in renal function in a patient with reduced creatinine clearance but with no prior history of renal calculi. The overall health status of the patient must be assessed in the decision for surgery, including the relative effect of hyperparathyroidism on function as compared with comorbid conditions.

Mild forms of the disease can be managed with estrogen replacement therapy in postmenopausal women. Daily doses of conjugated equine estrogen of 1.25 mg and ethinyl estradiol 50 μg have been shown to arrest accelerated bone turnover in postmenopausal women with hyperparathyroidism.

PAGET'S DISEASE

Osteitis deformans, or Paget's disease, was well described by Sir James Paget in 1877. It is common in older adults; studies have shown prevalence data ranging from 1 to 3% in areas of the United States to 10 to 15% of elderly Europeans, with a male to female ratio of 3:2. It is characterized by focal areas of active bone turnover that include both increased osteoclast-mediated resorption and excessive bone formation. The diseased bone is deformed, with thickened cortices and coarse trabeculations resulting in painful skeletal deformity, fragility, and fractures (55). The most commonly affected sites include the femur, spine, pelvis, humerus, tibia, cranium, and sternum. Clinical symptoms include bone pain, skeletal deformity, changes in skin temperature overlying areas of active bony involvement, pathologic fractures, and nerve compression syndromes, particularly of the thoracic and lumbar spine.

Degenerative disease is common in the joints adjoining affected weight-bearing bones. Complications include cranial nerve compression syndromes from basilar invagination, hearing loss related to alterations in the acoustic properties of bone, and alterations in blood flow related to metabolically active areas of bony involvement. Osteosarcomas, fibrosarcomas, and benign giant cell tumors develop in 2 to 4% of patients with symptomatic Paget's disease. The pathogenesis of Paget's disease is unknown, but it is hypothesized that the condition is a late manifestation of an earlier paramyxoviral infection such as measles, respiratory syncytial, or canine distemper virus. However, the viral type of inclusions identified on an ultrastructural level are not specific to Paget's disease.

It is estimated that perhaps 10 to 20% of patients with Paget's disease are asymptomatic and are diagnosed as a result of abnormal serum chemistries and radiographs performed for unrelated problems (56). Serum levels of alkaline phosphatase, Osteocalcin, and procollagen peptide are abnormal, particularly when bone formation is markedly increased. A second voided urine sample obtained following overnight fast should yield an elevation in the ratio of hydrox-yproline, deoxypyridinoline cross-links, or n-telopeptide to creatinine, particularly when bone resorption is markedly increased. Radiographic findings include cortical thickening and a mixture of lytic and sclerotic changes, although either presentation may predominate. Lytic areas of the skull are called osteoporosis circumscripta. Transverse lucencies of long bones, called pseudofractures, may progress to frank fractures. Nuclear bone scans using technetium-labeled polyphosphonate or diphosphonate scanning often reveal additional areas of asymptomatic or radiographically undetectable involvement.

Clinically, the radiographic changes of Paget's disease can be difficult to distinguish from those seen in metastatic prostate or breast cancer. The advent of serum markers such as prostate-specific antigen may help in the diagnosis; however, as both metastatic malignancy and Paget's are relatively common conditions in the elderly, they may coexist. Computed tomography may be helpful, with pagetoid lesions demonstrating bony expansion adjacent to areas of resorption. At times a therapeutic trial is performed as a first line of treatment, as biopsy confirmation of questionable lesions can be technically difficult and may require an open biopsy technique rather than a less invasive percutaneous approach.

The treatment of the asymptomatic patient is controversial (57). Treatment strategies range from no treatment other than baseline assessment of the extent of skeletal involvement with nuclear imaging to the treatment of asymptomatic patients with either active metabolic disease, as suggested by elevations of alkaline phosphatase levels to more than twice normal, or with involvement of the weight-bearing joints of the legs and spine to prevent bowing deformities. Pain syndromes must be carefully evaluated for potential nerve entrapment and joint manifestations, which may require management in addition to the treatment of the bone pain of Paget's disease.

Calcitonin therapy is effective in reducing osteoclast-mediated bone resorption in Paget's disease. It is recommended that an initial daily dose of 25 to 50 IU of salmon or 0.25 mg human calcitonin be given nightly, with an incremental increase in dose every 1 to 2 weeks until a clinical response is observed, with usual maintenance doses of 100 IU salmon and 0.5 mg human calcitonin (55). In the treatment of a pseudofracture, this dose is maintained until there is radiographic evidence of fracture healing and a reduction in the serum alkaline phosphatase level, at which time a dose reduction to 50 IU per day and then to 3 times weekly is suggested (56).

Bisphosphonates reduce bone resorption and have the advantage of oral administration. Etidronate dosing is 5 to 10 mg/kg per day. However, etidronate therapy should be limited to 3 to 6 months at a time because of adverse effects on bone mineralization. Calcium supplementation is suggested to improve mineralization. Combination calcitonin therapy for 6 weeks followed by low-dose daily etidronate, 5 mg/kg, for 6 months has been suggested (56). Relapses are treated in a similar fashion. Alternatively, pulse therapy with high-dose etidronate 20 mg/kg per day may be beneficial when given for a 1-month period every 4 months. The more recently developed bisphosphonates, such as pamidronate, alendronate, and tiludronate, appear to have no clinically significant effects on bone mineralization and may prove with further testing to be preferred for long-term therapy (57). Pamidronate intravenous infusions of 30 to 60 mg of every month when there is evidence of active bone turnover to 3 months to yearly for bone that is less metabolically active may be beneficial. The clinical goal on which the treatment interval is based is the maintenance of normal levels of the blood and urine markers of bone turnover. Options for lower-cost oral therapy include alendronate 40 mg and tiludronate 400 mg daily for 3 to 6 months; however, upper gastrointestinal side effects may limit oral therapy. Calcium and vitamin D repletion are recommended as adjuvant therapy with all antiresorptive treatments.

Some 15% of patients have an exacerbation in pain during the first 1 to 3 months, with marked increases in alkaline phosphatase levels and osteolytic progression noted on radiography. In this setting calcitonin should be substituted for bisphosphonate therapy. The chemotherapeutic agent mithramycin, while providing a rapid response, is reserved for the patient with impending paraplegia or one whose disease no longer responds to the standard therapies. Gallium nitrate is being tested for its effects on osteoclast activity.

REFERENCES

1. Riggs BL, Melton LJ III. The prevention and treatment of osteoporosis. N Engl J Med 1992;327:620–627.
2. Chrischilles EA, Butler CD, Davis CS, Wallace RB. A model of lifetime osteoporosis impact. Arch Intern Med 1991;151:2026–2032.
3. Cummings SR, Kelsey JL, Nevitt, et al. Epidemiology of osteoporosis and osteoporotic fractures. Epidemiol Rev 1985;7:178–208.
4. Christiansen C. Consensus development conference: prophylaxis and treatment of osteoporosis. Am J Med 1991;90:107–110.
5. Matkovic V, Fontana D, Tominac C, et al. Factors that influence peak bone formation: a study of calcium balance and the inheritance of bone mass in adolescent females. Am J Clin Nutr 1990;52:878–888.
6. Sowers MR, Clark MK, Hollis B, et al. Radial bone mineral density in pre- and perimenopausal women: a prospective study of rates and risk factors for loss. J Bone and Miner Res 1992;7:647–657.
7. Johnston CC, Hui SL, Witt RM, et al. Early menopausal changes in bone mass and sex steroids. J Clin Endocrinol Metab 1985;61:905–911.
8. Geusens P, Dequeker J, Verstraeten A, et al. Age-, sex-, and menopause-related changes of vertebral and peripheral bone: population study using dual and single photon absorptiometry and radiogrametry. J Nucl Med 1986;27:1540–1549.
9. Siemenda CW, Longcope C, Zhou L, et al. Sex steroids and bone mass in older men. J Clin Invest 1997;100: 1755–1759.
10. Seiger P, Cummings ST, Black DM, et al. Age-related decrements in bone mineral density in women over 65. J Bone Miner Res 1992;7:625–632.
11. Dawson-Hughes B, Harris SS, Krall EA, et al. Effect of calcium and vitamin D supplementation on bone density in men and women 65 years of age or older. N Engl J Med 1997;337:670–676.
12. Tilyard MW, Spears GF, Thomson J, Dovey S. Treatment of postmenopausal osteoporosis with calcitriol or calcium. N Engl J Med 1992;326:357–362.
13. Pocock NA, Eisman JA, Gwinn TH, et al. Muscle strength, physical fitness and weight but not age predict femoral neck bone mass. J Bone Miner Res 1989; 4:441–447.
14. Schneider DL, Barrett-Connor EL, Morton DJ. Timing of postmenopausal estrogen for optimal bone mineral density: the Rancho Bernardo Study. JAMA 1997;277:543–547.
15. Corpas E, Harman SM, Blackman MR. Human growth hormone and human aging. Endocrinol Rev 1993;14: 20–39.
16. Cummings SR, Black DM, Nevitt MC, et al. Bone density at various sites for prediction of hip fractures: the Study

of Osteoporotic Fractures Research Group. Lancet 1993; 341:72–75.

17. Cheng S, Tylavsky F, Carbone L. Utility of ultrasound to assess risk of fracture. J Am Geriatr Soc 45:1382–1394, 1997.
18. Rubin SM, Cummings SR. Results of bone densitometry affect women's decisions about taking measures to prevent fractures. Ann Intern Med 1992;116:990–995.
19. Ju HS, Leung S, Brown B, et al. Comparison of analytical performance and biological variability of three bone resorption assays. Clin Chem 1997;43:1570–1576.
20. Potts JT. Management of asymptomatic hyperparathyroidism. J Clin Endocrinol Metab 1990;70:1489–1493.
21. Demaux BB, Arlot ME, Chapuy MC. Serum osteocalcin is increased in patients with osteomalacia: correlations with biochemical and histomorphometric findings. J Clin Endocrinol Metab 1992;74:1146–1151.
22. Gloth FM, Tobin JD, Sherman SS, et al. Is the recommended daily allowance for vitamin D too low for the homebound elderly? J Am Geriatr Soc 1991;39:137–141.
23. Eastell R. Treatment of Postmenopausal Osteoporosis. N Engl J Med 1998;338:736–746.
24. Ettinger B, Genant H, et al. Postmenopausal bone loss is prevented by treatment with low-dosage estrogen with calcium. Ann Intern Med 1987;106:40–45.
25. Nachtigall LE, Nachtigall M J. Hormone replacement therapy. Obstet Gynecol 1992;4:907–913.
26. Bellantoni MF, Harman SM, Cullins VE, et al. Transdermal estradiol with oral progestin: biological and clinical effects in younger and older postmenopausal women. J Gerontol 1991;46:M216–222.
27. Colditz GA, Hankinson SE, Hunter DJ, et al. The use of estrogens and progestins and the risk of breast cancer in postmenopausal women. N Engl J Med 1995;332:1589–1593.
28. Christiansen C, Christiansen MS, Transbol I. Bone mass in postmenopausal women after withdrawal of oestrogen/gestagen replacement therapy. Lancet 1981;1:459–461.
29. Felson DT, Zhang Y, Hannan MT. The effect of postmenopausal estrogen therapy on bone density in elderly women. N Engl J Med 1993;329:1141–1146.
30. Col NF, Eckman MK, Karas RH, et al. Patient-specific decisions about hormone replacement therapy in postmenopausal women. JAMA 1997;277:1140–1147.
31. Gallagher JC, Kable WT, Goldgar D. Effect of progestin therapy on cortical and trabecular bone: comparison with estrogen. Am J Med 1991;90:171–178.
32. Effects of estrogen or estrogen/progestin regimens on heart disease risk factors in postmenopausal women. The Postmenopausal Estrogen/Progestin Interventions (PEPI) Trial. The Writing Group for the PEPI Trial. JAMA 1995;273:199–208.
33. Fornander T, Rutqvist LE, Sjöberg, et al. Long-term adjuvant tamoxifen in early breast cancer: effect on bone mineral density in postmenopausal women. J Clin Oncol 1990;8:1019–1024.

34. Delmas PD, Bjarnason NH, Mitlak BH, et al. Effects of raloxifene on bone mineral density, serum cholesterol concentrations, and uterine endometrium in postmenopausal women. N Engl J Med 1997;337:1641–1647.
35. Finkelstein JS, Klibanski A, Neer RM, et al. Increases in bone density during treatment of men with idiopathic hypogonadotropic hypogonadism. J Clin Endocrinol Metab 1989;69:776–783.
36. Nieves JW, Komar L, Cosman F, et al. Calcium potentiates the effect of estrogen and calcitonin on bone mass: review and analysis. Am J Clin Nutr 1998;67:18–24.
37. Overgaard K, Hansen MA, Jensen SB, et al. Effect of calcitonin given intranasally on bone mass and fracture rates in established osteoporosis: a dose-response study. BMJ 1992;305:556–561.
38. Hodsman AB, Fraher LJ, Ostbye T, et al. An evaluation of several biochemical markers for bone formation and resorption in a protocol utilizing cyclical parathyroid hormone and calcitonin therapy for osteoporosis. J Clin Invest 1993;91:1138–1148.
39. Lyritis GP, Tsakalakos N, Magiasis B, et al. Analgesic effect of salmon calcitonin in osteoporotic vertebral fractures: a double-blind placebo-controlled clinical study. Calcif Tissue Int 1991;49:369–372.
40. Storm T, Thamsborg G, Steiniche T, et al. Effect of intermittent cyclical etidronate therapy on bone mass and fracture rate in women with postmenopausal osteoporosis. N Engl J Med 1990;322:1265–1271.
41. Liberman UA, Weiss SR, Broll J, et al. Effect of oral alendronate on bone mineral density and the incidence of fractures in postmenopausal osteoporosis. N Engl J Med 1995;333:1437–1443.
42. McClung M, Clemmesen B, Daifotis A, et al. Alendronate prevents postmenopausal bone loss in women without osteoporosis. Ann Intern Med 1998;128:253–261.
43. Adachi JD, Bensen WG, Brown J, et al. Intermittent etidronate therapy to prevent corticosteroid-induced osteoporosis. N Engl J Med 1997;337:382–387.
44. Perry HM III, Miller DK, Morley JE, et al. A preliminary report of vitamin D and calcium metabolism in older African Americans. J Am Geriatr Soc 1993;41:612–616.
45. LaCroix AZ, Wienpahl J, White LR, et al. Thiazide diuretic agents and the incidence of hip fracture. N Engl J Med 1990;322:286–290.
46. Kleerekoper M, Balena R. Fluorides and osteoporosis. Annu Rev Nutr 1991;11:309–324.
47. Pak CY, Sakhaee K, Zerwekh JE, et al. Safe and effective treatment of osteoporosis with intermittent slow release sodium fluoride: augmentation of vertebral bone mass and inhibition of fractures. J Clin Endocrinol Metab 1989;68:150–159.
48. Hodsman AB, Drost DJ. The response of vertebral bone mineral density during the treatment of osteoporosis with sodium fluoride. J Clin Endocrinol Metab 1989;69:932–938.
49. Riggs BL, Hodgson SF, O'Fallon WM, et al. Effect of fluoride treatment on the fracture rate in postmenopausal

women with osteoporosis. N Engl J Med 1990;322:802–809.

50. Hesch RD, Rittinghaus EF, Harms HM, Delling G. Die Fruhtherapie der Osteoporose mit (1–38) Parathormon und Calcitonin Nasal Spray. Med Klin 1989;84:488–498.

51. Rudman D, Feller AG, Nagraj HS, et al. Effects of human growth hormone in men over 60 years old. N Engl J Med 1990;323(1):1–5.

52. Prince RL, Smith M, Dick IM, et al. Prevention of postmenopausal osteoporosis: a comparative study of exercise, calcium supplementation, and hormone replacement therapy. N Engl J Med 1991;325:1189–1195.

53. Sinaki M, Mikkelsen BA. Postmenopausal spinal osteoporosis: flexion versus extension exercises. Arch Phys Med Rehabil 1983;65:593–596.

54. Heath H, Hodgson SF, Kennedy MA. Primary hyperparathyroidism, incidence, morbidity, and potential economic impact in a community. N Engl J Med 1980;302:189–193.

55. Bone HG, Kleerekoper M. Paget's disease of bone. J Clin Endocrinol Metab 1992;75:1179–1185.

56. Delmas PD, Meunier PJ. The management of Paget's disease of bone. N Engl J Med 1997;336:558–566.

57. Siris ES. Management of Paget's disease of bone in the era of new and more potent bisphosphonates. Endocrine Pract 1997;3:264–266.

CHAPTER 34

MARK R. BELSKY, W. BRADLEY WHITE, KENNETH POLIVY, AND ALFRED HANMER

Musculoskeletal Injuries in the Elderly

Aches, pains, and injuries occur frequently in the elderly population. Often these non-life-threatening problems are set aside by the primary care physician to attend to the more serious medical problems related to the vital organs. However, the daily musculoskeletal complaints interfere with patients' routines, which affects their quality of living. Much of the aging population define the high points of their day by their physical accomplishments: how far I walked, how many games of tennis or holes of golf I played, that I was able to go shopping in the department store, that I can still drive myself.

As always, a complete and thorough history and physical examination are required to understand what is bothering the patient and how to help him or her. Some injuries that can be treated in the outpatient setting in younger patients require hospitalization in the elderly because of social reasons, such as not being able to care for themselves alone with a wrist fracture or shoulder injury. It is helpful to have a reasonable perspective in setting goals and expectations for the elderly. Relief of pain and return to function always remain the primary criteria for care. It is valuable to set the goals of care with the particular patient. The older patient is much more likely to accept less than full recovery and to have limited goals in rehabilitation. However, in some cases surgery (e.g., in treating impending pathologic fractures) is the more conservative approach to pain relief and early mobilization. The same is true for patients with hip fractures. Fairly minor levels of impaired function in any given extremity, coupled with various other medical problems such as weakness and gait abnormalities secondary to neurologic changes, may have a very dramatic effect on the whole person that would not be appreciated in the younger, healthier patient. It is reasonable to say that consideration for the entire patient is as important in treating musculoskeletal injuries in the elderly as it is in any other age group.

The primary care physician is in the best position to orchestrate the patient's care, even if he or she is not the primary physician managing the orthopaedic problem. The patient's family physician is most likely to be aware of the patient's medical problems, family situation, and psychosocial needs. It is important, though, that the orthopaedist be involved early on in the care of significant musculoskeletal problems, even as a one-time consultant. It is very common to have a seemingly minor soft tissue injury or affliction treated "conservatively" for months, until it is beyond benefit of optimal treatment by the orthopaedic surgeon, physiatrist, or rheumatologist. The primary care physician working with the musculoskeletal specialist early in the care of the injured elder is clearly in the patient's best interest. This approach often results in the cost-effective care desired in today's managed care environment.

This chapter discusses the most common injuries in the elderly. In addition, since often the patient is unaware of subtle injuries and complains of pain only, other afflictions that cause pain in the same region are included as an aid to differential diagnosis.

UPPER EXTREMITY

The upper extremity, shoulder to fingertip, is the part of the musculoskeletal system that enables us to interact with the world around us. When it is afflicted with injury or natural wear and tear, we are deprived of this interaction and greatly limited in our independence. Often for the elderly the loss of certain upper extremity function is the difference between being able to live independently and not.

Injuries to the neck and shoulder after falls and direct blows are common in the elderly. Some other shoulder injuries, such as neck strains, are more subtle. However, the diagnosis of the specific injured part can be elusive in the elderly because there is often a variable amount of underlying preexisting osteoarthritis and loss of motion of which the patient was not aware.

Neck

Symptoms and signs referable to the cervical spine are those most likely to be confused with or overlap with shoulder problems. In the older patient these conditions are likely to be cervical spondylosis (degenerative disc disease), cervical osteoarthritis, herniated nucleus pulposus (HNP, or ruptured disc), tumors, and traumatic injuries to the cervical spine. Neck problems frequently manifest as discomfort at the base of the cervical spine itself and/or in the periscapular region. Additionally, discomfort can be appreciated about the trapezia, and with radicular problems, at various places in the upper extremity down to the fingertips. In contradistinction, problems involving the shoulder generally do not radiate distally below elbow level nor medial to the acromioclavicular (AC) joint, unless that joint, the clavicle, or the scapula is involved.

During the evaluation of a patient with shoulder pain, it is important to make a brief evaluation of the cervical spine for gross range of motion, areas of focal tenderness, and masses. For patients whose shoulder pain is centered on the scapula and its attached muscles or radiates below the elbow, a more critical examination of the cervical spine is necessary. Older patients frequently have a loss of neck extension because of degenerative changes in the cervical spine, and attempts at neck extension, sometimes just to neutral, produce referred pain to these areas. If the patient is not too uncomfortable, he or she should first be evaluated by holding the neck in straight maximum extension, and then with the neck extended and tilted toward the affected shoulder. If symptoms are from radiculitis, this maneuver often reproduces the chief complaint in less than 20 seconds. Cervical spondylosis without frank nerve root impingement generally causes headaches, neck pain and stiffness, and referred pain to the upper back and periscapular region but not into the shoulder or more distal portions of the upper extremity. An isolated HNP without associated significant degenerative changes in the cervical spine is unusual in the older patient. Acute loss of strength in the shoulder or more distal portions of the upper extremity in association with dermatomal sensory changes or pain should immediately prompt a search for a cause of the nerve irritation. If the patient has pain and hypesthesia without gross motor weakness or gait abnormalities, there is no urgent reason to pursue a workup with expensive diagnostic studies such as myelograms and magnetic resonance imaging (MRI), since most patients improve with time, analgesics, and nonsteroidal or corticosteroid anti-inflammatory medications as tolerated. Even routine radiographs are not generally indicated in workup of neck or shoulder complaints in the elderly if there is no history of cancer or trauma and if symptoms have been present for less than 6 weeks. As mentioned, if there is a focal neurologic deficit, the workup should be more aggressive, even at initial presentation.

Shoulder

Primary problems of scapulothoracic articulation in the elderly are rare. Very active elders may have local pain and tenderness at this level from overuse and scapulothoracic (subscapular) bursitis. This problem is fairly common in the patient who has an established frozen shoulder, since most of the motion occurs at the scapulothoracic articulation in such patients. Each problem can usually be addressed with modification of activities, postural adjustments, a good stretching program, and anti-inflammatory medications or analgesics as needed. The bursa deep to the scapula can be approached medially or inferiorly, with the needle directed laterally anterior to the scapula and posterior to the rib cage.

This procedure can be made both diagnostic, and therapeutic, by injecting several milliliters of lidocaine (Xylocaine) along with the corticosteroid of choice (e.g., 4 mL 1% lidocaine and 1% betamethasone [Celestone]).

Sternoclavicular subluxation, a fairly common finding in the older patient, often appears without obvious antecedent trauma but can also be precipitated by pushing a heavy object, such as a door against the wind. Patients generally have a modestly tender prominence at the level of the sternoclavicular joint. There may be subtle erythema, deep ecchymosis, and warmth if the episode occurred within just a few days of presentation. Depending on the degree of subluxation, there may be crepitus at this level with elevation of the shoulder. Treatment is generally symptomatic. Only rarely is it necessary to perform a corticosteroid injection (l mL 1% lidocaine, 1 mL betamethasone), and then only if the patient has persistent discomfort at least 6 to 8 weeks after the initial injury. The patient can be reassured that this condition does not usually cause long-term functional problems, but in most cases a bump will remain. Surgery to correct this subluxation is fraught with complications and is only rarely recommended, and then only in those with significant pain or neurovascular compromise.

Separations of the AC joint are usually caused by a direct blow on the shoulder (Fig. 34.1). A fall onto the apex of the shoulder drives the acromion inferiorly (caudad), tearing the ligaments that attach it to the clavicle and more important, the coracoid (Fig. 34.2). The patient generally has a prominence of the distal clavicle and local tenderness at the AC joint. Initial treatment for all AC joint separations is symptomatic. Patients presenting with a gross deformity at the level of the AC joint (type III through VI separations [Fig. 34.1]), should be referred to the orthopaedist for consultation. Most of these more severe injuries are type III and can still be treated without surgery. For patients with an unacceptable cosmetic deformity, significant functional loss, or compromise of skin integrity because of tenting over the distal clavicle, a reconstructive procedure can be performed on an outpatient basis.

Osteoarthritis involving the AC joint is fairly common but in the older patient is not usually symptomatic without local trauma. Many patients present for other problems and are noted to have a very prominent AC joint, not from damage to the ligaments such as in an AC separation, but because of abutting osteophytes. The older patient with AC joint arthritis rarely has much if

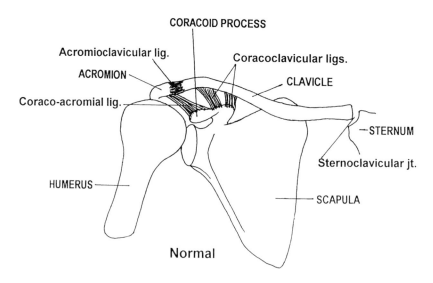

Figure 34.1.   Anterior view of the normal anatomy of a right shoulder. When a shoulder separation occurs, the coracoclavicular ligaments are in jeopardy.

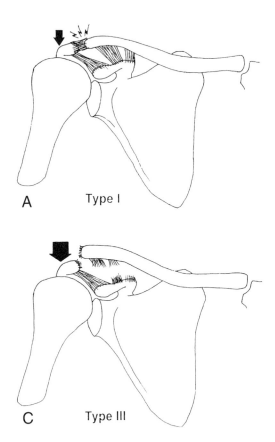

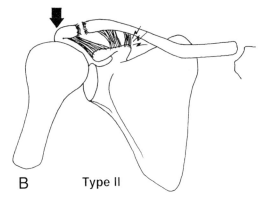

Figure 34.2. **A.** In a type I shoulder separation the AC ligaments are injured and tender. **B.** In a type II shoulder separation the AC ligaments are torn and the coracoclavicular ligaments are stretched, but the clavicle does not ride high. **C.** In a type III shoulder separation the coracoclavicular ligaments are torn and the clavicle rides high.

any motion remaining at that joint and thus even overhead activities are unlikely to induce the pain associated with osteoarthritis. Patients are more likely to have irritation from a shoulder strap, such as a bra strap, luggage, or camera bag strap. This can be addressed by eliminating the offending activity, and then if necessary, injecting a small amount of lidocaine and corticosteroid (0.5 mL betamethasone, 1 to 2 mL 1% lidocaine) into the subcutaneous area (bursa) of maximum tenderness. If the AC joint itself is to be injected, the needle generally has to be directed from lateral to medial to mimic the most common angulation of the joint. If radiographs are available, they can be helpful in determining the appropriate needle placement and angulation.

The clavicle attaches the upper extremity to the trunk at the sternoclavicular joint. It can be fractured with direct trauma to the bone itself, though more commonly a fall onto the lateral aspect or apex of the shoulder produces forces in the clavicle that break it. While in the younger patient the clavicle usually fractures in the middle, it is more common for fractures in the older patient to be more distal. Shaft fractures generally heal without difficulty and unless markedly angulated, can be treated by the primary care physician with a sling. If there is overlap of the fracture fragments, a figure-8 clavicular harness may provide more comfort. Caution must be exercised when using the clavicle strap, since to use the harness appropriately it must be fairly snug and frequently produces irritation in the axilla and occasionally even nerve damage from compression of the brachial plexus. Once the initial pain of the clavicle fracture subsides, the patient may start gentle pendulum exercises with the sling off (Fig. 34.3). Patients may advance activities as symptoms allow, but generally lifting above chest height should be avoided for the first month, since it increases both pain and the likelihood of a nonunion developing. Because of pain, patients find that sleeping can be difficult in the first week or so, but usually this is not as

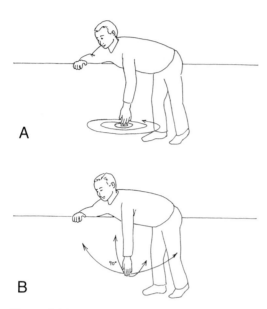

Figure 34.3. Pendulum exercises. **A.** Bend over, leaning on the back of a chair. Hang arm straight down and swing it in circles from the shoulder both clockwise and counterclockwise. **B.** Then swing arm north-south and east-west. Do each exercise for 1 minute; stand up and clear your head. Repeat several times a day.

much of a problem as is seen with fractures of the proximal humerus. They are encouraged to sleep semiupright at 45°, using pillows to support the head, neck, and shoulders. Getting in and out of bed is usually one of the more uncomfortable activities of the day, but once the patient is recumbent, the supporting musculature can relax, and the fracture ends assume a reasonable position.

Fractures involving the distal clavicle can be more problematic. Because the fracture is often just medial to the coracoclavicular ligaments, the bulk of the clavicle is pulled cephalad by the trapezius and the distal clavicle, caudad by the weight of the arm, and nonunions are a common result. Fortunately, even when a nonunion occurs, there can be a good functional result. If necessary a late ligamentous reconstruction can be carried out, as with the more severe types of AC separation. When nonunion is recognized early on, depending on the needs of the patient, pinning can be considered to stabilize the fracture and increase the likelihood of bone-to-bone healing.

Adhesive capsulitis, or frozen shoulder, occurs most commonly before the sixth decade of life but can affect the older patient. Adhesive capsulitis is essentially self-limited, and almost regardless of treatment, patients regain 90% or more of their motion and function. In the early stages pain can be quite significant, particularly at night, and symptomatic measures are appropriate. While it has not been shown to make any difference in the long run, a lidocaine and corticosteroid (1 mL betamethasone, 9 mL 1% lidocaine) injection can decrease the discomfort and help to sort out early adhesive capsulitis from rotator cuff tendinitis and bursitis. Subacromial injections in this condition result in a modest decrease in discomfort and no significant improvement in range of motion, while intra-articular injections yield a marked decrease in pain within minutes and yet a minimal improvement in range of motion. Patients with subacromial bursitis and rotator cuff tendinitis should have marked relief of pain with subacromial injection, and their motion should be essentially normal passively but may still be restricted actively if there is a rotator cuff tear. Primary adhesive capsulitis is an idiopathic condition of unknown cause, while secondary adhesive capsulitis, as the name implies, is secondary to another underlying condition. For example, patients with significant discomfort from subacromial bursitis or tendinitis or a contusion or nondisplaced fracture may restrict their motion for a long time because of pain and end up with a significant restriction of motion due to a secondary adhesive capsulitis.

Most studies have not shown physical therapy to offer significant benefit in the long run, but it can be helpful in the short term in getting patients over the painful stage and getting them started on a home program for range-of-motion exercises and gentle strengthening to facilitate functional restoration. Since this condition is usually very slow to resolve, some patients end up going to physical therapy for many months. This is not generally necessary, and it is important for the physician to stress to the patient that he or she should be doing the exercises several times a day at home, not relying on the therapist for prolonged sessions a few times a week in the office. The greatest role of the therapist, after educating patients, is reminding them how to do their exercises and providing an occasional checkup to see that they are doing the exercises properly and effectively. Avoiding the comfortable position of adduction with internal rotation (hand on lap or abdomen) for long periods, stretching for 5 to 10 minutes 6 times a day, and using the extremity for activities of daily living are most important.

Primary osteoarthritis of the shoulder is much less common and far less frequently symptomatic than that of the hip and knee. Patients usually have complaints of aching pain and insidious onset of restricted motion and often are aware of slipping or grinding within the shoulder. High-quality radiographs are important for an accurate diagnosis. A true anteroposterior (AP) view of the glenohumeral joint is taken tangential to that joint; in the normal patient it shows a 3- to 4-mm space between the humeral head and the glenoid. Most hospitals take an AP of the shoulder such that the glenoid and humeral head overlap, and this limits accurate assessment of the joint. With a good tangential projection that is not too light (i.e., underpenetrated) the space can be assessed for narrowing and the bony surfaces, for sclerosis, osteophyte formation, and cysts. Treatment should be individualized to severity of pain and loss of function. If the patient can tolerate them, nonsteroidal anti-inflammatory drugs (NSAIDs) are tried initially. Additionally, intra-articular injections with lidocaine and a corticosteroid can be very helpful. By maintaining range of motion with a stretching program and strengthening the muscles of the shoulder girdle, function can be maintained as long as possible. Shoulder arthroplasty, while less commonly performed than hip and knee arthroplasty, is very successful in relieving pain and improving function. Degenerative changes of the glenohumeral joint are seen with other processes as well; the two most common are rheumatoid arthritis and rotator cuff arthropathy. Regardless of the degenerative condition, management by the primary care physician is the same. Once the patient begins to have significant pain and/or functional limitations, referral should be made to the orthopaedist for evaluation and management. At end stage, all of the conditions that destroy the joint surfaces can be managed with various types of arthroplasty. The limiting factors often are the condition of the

muscles and rotator cuff, activity level, and expectations of the patient.

Fractures of the shoulder are quite common, with most involving the proximal humerus, usually the surgical neck of the humerus and a much smaller portion the anatomic neck. The former is at the junction of the diaphysis and the metaphysis, and the latter is in the immediate subcapital region, more proximal than the surgical neck. The relatively uncommon anatomic neck fractures usually have to be treated operatively unless they are not displaced. The great majority of fractures of the surgical neck of the humerus can be treated without operation, as even patients with fractures that heal in a position of marked displacement and angulation can end up with an acceptable functional result. The functional desires of the patient are critical in determining the appropriate treatment. Probably all but the completely nondisplaced proximal humerus fractures should be referred to the orthopaedist for management. A completely nondisplaced fracture can generally be treated with a sling for comfort for 7 to 10 days. During that time the patient often feels better sleeping in a recliner or propped upright in bed in a position similar to the one described for sleeping with a clavicle fracture. The sling should be removed several times a day to allow for active range of motion of the elbow, wrist, and digits while the shoulder is allowed to remain quiet. At the end of this first stage isometrics, shoulder shrugs, and pendulum exercises can be instituted. Patients can also begin to use the hand for activities of daily living limited by the level of discomfort. The sling can be discontinued as soon as patients are comfortable, which is usually not for 3 to 4 weeks. At that time they should be instructed on active range of motion exercises in all planes. They can also begin wall walking, stick or pulley exercises, or other stretches designed to restore functional motion. By 6 to 8 weeks, adequate bony healing has usually progressed, and patients, if able and willing, can proceed with a progressive resistance exercise (PRE) program. If physical therapy is used in care of patients with this fracture, it is extremely important not to let the therapist perform passive range-of-motion exercises for at least a month, as the nondisplaced fracture is likely to be displaced and can go on to a nonunion or more severe malunion.

Displaced fractures of the proximal humerus should be treated by the orthopaedist. If operation is selected, treatment options are numerous. In the more active elder patient it may be appropriate to attempt an open reduction internal fixation (ORIF) if functional needs are high and bone quality seems reasonable. In the more sedentary elder, particularly patients with significant osteoporosis (the majority), it is often prudent to proceed directly to hemiarthroplasty (partial replacement), since rehabilitation can begin fairly aggressively on the first postoperative day. Regardless of the method of treatment, most patients lose between 30 and 50% of their motion, though functional restoration is usually quite good in patients physically and mentally able to follow through with the rehabilitation.

Infections involving the shoulder joint are rare but are most commonly seen in the older patient. Since more than 50% of patients reaching age 70 have tears of the rotator cuff, infections of the glenohumeral joint or subacromial bursa generally communicate. These patients are generally debilitated, with various medical problems, such as diabetes mellitus and cancer, that cause relative immunocompromise. Presentation can be dramatic, with marked swelling, erythema, and systemic signs of infection, but usually the only complaint is of pain about the shoulder. Unless the physician has a high index of suspicion, the infection is missed, as the range of motion is often quite good, at least passively, and there may not be any overt signs of infection. Often there is subtle anterior swelling of the subacromial bursa (immediately anterior to the acromion), and a sterile tap of both the subacromial bursa and glenohumeral joint (through a separate stick) is necessary to rule out or confirm the diagnosis of septic arthritis. These infections are best managed with arthroscopic debridement and drainage. Arthroscopic debridement is much more extensive than can be carried out with an open procedure and thus only when there is suspicion of a myofasciitis should it be the first approach.

Primary tumors of the shoulder girdle are quite rare. The patient may simply have an enlarging mass but is more likely to come in with complaints of pain with or without a mass. Consequently, in the older patient who has had shoulder pain longer than 6 weeks, it is important to obtain screening radiographs of the shoulder joint and proximal humerus. Primary benign tumors of the shoulder presenting symptomatically in the older patient are quite uncommon, but occasionally subcutaneous or intramuscular lipomas are found. If these are greater than 5 cm in diameter, the patient should be referred for consultation and probable excision of the mass. Certain tumors (prostate, breast, lung, kidney, thyroid) have a predilection for spread to bone, and while the proximal humerus is sometimes involved, these lesions are much less likely to be symptomatic than those found in the weight-bearing lower extremity.

In a patient with a painful metastatic lesion in the humerus it is likely that symptoms be manifest early in the course of disease if the patient depends on ambulation aids, such as cane, crutches, or walker. It is particularly important to refer such patients for consultation early on, as it is much easier to perform a stabilization prophylactically than after a pathologic fracture. It is important to remember that once a lytic or blastic lesion is appreciated on radiography, very significant bony destruction has already occurred. Once the lesion approaches 2.5 cm or involves more than 30% of the cortex (which can be very difficult to determine) the patient is at high risk for pathologic fracture. While radiation can be very effective at decreasing pain, it is fairly common for the patient to fracture through the lesion. Prophylactic stabilization of such lesions in the humeral shaft is recommended. Large symptomatic lesions of the humeral head can be treated with a cemented hemiarthroplasty similar to that performed in the hip. Pathologic lesions and resulting fractures of the clavicle can usually be treated nonoperatively with symptomatic measures and radiation for pain control.

Soft Tissue Injuries

The subscapularis (internal rotation), supraspinatus (elevation in the plane of the scapula), and infraspinatus and teres minor (external rotation) muscles merge as the tendinous rotator cuff, inserting directly on the proximal humerus. Soft tissue injuries include contusions, strains (muscle-tendon unit) and sprains (ligaments). It is most important that motion be rapidly restored, and thus if immobilization is necessary to relieve pain, it is important to limit it to no more than a week. If there is any significant pain or swelling, cold packs should be applied to the injured area for 15 to 20 minutes several times per day for the first 48 to 72 hours. If the patient does not have reusable soft cold packs at home, a bag of frozen peas or corn works nicely, as it is inexpensive and reusable and readily molds to the injured body part. Motion exercises should be initiated no later than a week after injury with pendulums and active assisted stick exercises (Fig. 34.2). Opioid analgesics are not generally necessary for more than the first few days, and most commonly over-the-counter analgesics suffice. If the patient's gastrointestinal tract can tolerate an NSAID, naproxen or ibuprofen can be used for their analgesic and anti-inflammatory benefits. As pain subsides, gentle strengthening exercises should be instituted. Begin with isometrics (tightening and relaxing the muscle without moving the joint through a range of motion) and then progress with functional activities and a PRE program. If grossly normal motion and function do not return within 3 weeks, orthopaedic consultation is recommended.

Tears of the rotator cuff tendon or tendons are very commonly missed at the initial presentation. Tears that benefit from repair are most likely to have a satisfactory result if identified within 6 weeks of the injury. MRI reveals degenerative rotator cuff tears of some degree in 50% of seniors over age 70. If your patient presents after a fall (usually on the outstretched hand) with the primary complaint of inability to raise the arm, he or she has probably sustained a significant rotator cuff tear. Significant pain can often inhibit active motion, so the lidocaine injection test can be quite helpful in sorting out the cause of limitation. Instillation of 10 mL of 1% lidocaine into the subacromial space temporarily relieves most discomfort coming from the rotator cuff or the overlying bursa. If active motion is greatly improved after injection, such that the patient can easily raise the arm above the horizontal, it is unlikely that there is a large rotator cuff tear. If after eliminating most of the pain there is no improvement in active motion, a large tear is likely and immediate surgical consultation should be sought. While tears of the rotator cuff are usually caused by FOOSH (fall on outstretched hand) injuries, any dramatic fall resulting in loss of active shoulder motion (when radiographs are negative) should raise suspicion of a rotator cuff tear.

Tears of the proximal biceps tendon, which are usually associated with minimal pain and ecchymosis at the mid arm level anteriorly, are usually precipitated by lifting. Often the patient relates a history of shoulder "bursitis" or "tendinitis" when asked. Ruptures are usually caused by sudden overexertion, such as lifting heavy luggage or a trash can with dirt or sand in the bottom, or when the weight shifts and the muscle must suddenly contract against heavy resistance while carrying an awkward heavy object. The result is a Popeye appearance when the arm is viewed from the side, with a new bulge in the anterior surface of the arm in the biceps area. Since the proximal tendon of the biceps is only one of the two bellies of the muscle, the remainder of the biceps still functions. Only reassurance and symptomatic management are necessary. The patient can usually resume all activities without an appreciable loss of function.

A distal biceps tendon rupture is unusual in the older patient, but it can be more problematic, as both heads of the biceps tendon are rendered functionless with this injury. These patients should be referred for orthopaedic evaluation. With this injury pain, swelling, and ecchymosis are at the level of the antecubital fossa, and while there is some distortion of the contour of the anterior arm, the Popeye appearance is not noted. Unless the patient is very uncomfortable, resisted elbow flexion is mildly weakened and resisted forearm supination, with the elbow in flexion, is markedly diminished.

Diagnostic and Therapeutic Injections

The materials for diagnostic and therapeutic injections are a 10-mL syringe, 22-gauge needle for injecting, 18-gauge needle for drawing up medications, 1% lidocaine or other fast-acting anesthetic, betamethasone or corticosteroid of choice, alcohol or Betadine swabs, and ethyl chloride spray. The procedures are as follows:

Subacromial Space

The space can be approached either anteriorly or posteriorly. It is usually least painful to perform the injection from posterolaterally with the patient seated. With the hand on the thigh and the arm relaxed, the subacromial space opens up and a 22-gauge needle can be used to instill 1 mL of betamethasone and 9 mL of 1% lidocaine. The skin is prepped with alcohol or Betadine, depending on your preference. Ethyl chloride can be used to anesthetize the skin. The physician palpates the edge of the acromion and plans to inject just under the edge, aiming for the undersurface of the acromion. From immediately inferior to the posterolateral corner of the acromion the needle is directed anteriorly toward a point midway between the AC joint and anterolateral corner of the acromion. If observed closely, the bursal sac can usually be seen to fill with fluid anteriorly. When the injection is anterior, it is generally recommended that the needle be inserted immediately anterior to the acromion toward its lateral edge at a 45° angle until bone is encountered. The needle is then withdrawn a few millimeters until the fluid can be easily injected. With this technique, at its depth the needle tip is in the rotator cuff, and when withdrawn, it is in the subacromial bursa.

Glenohumeral Joint

Using a similar mixture, the glenohumeral joint can be approached anteriorly or posteriorly. The anterior approach is probably easier. With the patient seated, the coracoid is palpated (1 to 2 fingerbreadths distal to the AC joint); then the needle can be directed posteriorly 1 fingerbreadth lateral to the coracoid. If the tip of the needle is in the joint, there should not be significant resistance to injection. If the arm is gently rotated passively with the needle in place and the needle is seen to move back and forth, the needle is resting on the humeral head and should be directed a few millimeters to a centimeter more medially.

With all of these injections, if the medication is instilled into the vicinity of the painful focus, a 50% or better reduction of pain should be noted within 5 minutes. If not, consider an additional injection into the adjacent space (bursa or joint).

Elbow

The elbow's sole purpose in conjunction with the shoulder is to move the hand in space. Apart from needing to bear weight on the elbow and forearm when gait is impaired, the elbow functions as a hinge joint to allow the hand to reach both ends of the gastrointestinal tract as well as extending its reach. The most common affliction of the elbow is olecranon bursitis. This is a swelling directly behind the elbow, olecranon, that the patient may first notice in the mirror or when the spouse brings attention to it. Often it is painless and soft. The bursitis may be aggravated by leaning on the elbow or other blunt trauma. Occasionally the olecranon bursitis is painful, tender, and warm. This suggests an inflammatory component. The collection of fluid in the bursa may be quite large, often 10 to 50 mL (1) and tense. Although painful, the range of motion is minimally impaired by an inflamed olecranon bursitis. There may be a lack of the extremes of extension and/or flexion, but the rotation is not impaired. Even less commonly the olecranon bursitis becomes infected. Septic olecranon bursitis is a serious problem. It is often associated with tender swollen epitrochlear and/or axillary adenopathy. There is tender erythema (cellulitis) overlying the bursae, and elbow motion may be more limited.

Treatment of olecranon bursitis varies with severity (2, 3) and in certain conditions is controversial. The painless incidental appearance of olecranon bursitis in most cases is best treated with a protective elbow pad and avoidance of reinjury. A history of the patient's activity usually reveals the mechanism of injury. The trauma may occur while placing the elbow on the window when driving, on the table when eating or drinking, on the desk when on the phone, and so on. Avoiding these common daily traumas and a warm heating pad or compresses 10 to 20 minutes 3 times a day is usually all that is needed to resolve this problem. If the bursitis is painful and tender but obviously not infected, treatment includes repeated aspiration and NSAIDs. Aspiration is performed very carefully under sterile conditions. Although this can be performed with the patient seated, this position is awkward for the patient and the physician. If the patient lies supine and places the involved elbow across the chest, it is more easily approached. The area around the bursa is prepared and draped using sterile technique. Using sterile gloves, local anesthesia, usually 1% mepivacaine, is injected into the dermis and subcutaneous tissue. A large bore (18-gauge) needle on a 10- or 20-mL syringe facilitates removing as much fluid as possible. The fluid is sent for culture to assess for infection.

After aspiration, a gentle compressive dressing (i.e., Kerlix and elastic [Ace] bandage) are applied. If the bandage is too tight, it may create a venous tourniquet, which is to be avoided. Aspiration may be necessary every 4 to 10 days if the fluid reaccumulates. A sterile dressing is needed because the bursa may drain from the aspiration hole. If the bursitis is infected, treatment initially includes aspiration and intravenous antibiotics. Repeat aspirations may be necessary. Only in exceptional circumstances, such as failure to respond to aspirations, draining sinuses, and obviously necrotic tissue, is surgical debridement with excision of the bursae recommended.

What is controversial (3) is the use of cortisone preparations for injecting the inflamed but not infected bursitis. Although some authors have described the use of cortisone injection to treat olecranon bursitis, there is a risk of infection following this treatment. Cortisone injection should be reserved for painful uninfected olecranon bursitis due to severe rheumatoid arthritis, pseudogout, or other documented inflammatory arthritis that does not respond to appropriate systemic treatment.

Tendinitis, epicondylitis, and tennis elbow all are the same process, which gives rise to pain in the lateral or medial aspects of the elbow over the epicondyles. Although popularly called tennis and golfer's elbow respectively, these entities are more likely to manifest while the patient is reaching for a bottle of milk in the refrigerator or lifting a shopping bag off the counter. Pain on the lateral side of the elbow while lifting with the extended arm is the hallmark symptom of lateral epicondylitis.

In lateral epicondylitis the location of the pain overlies the epicondyle and may extend distally to the extensor mass of the forearm. Sometimes the pain is mostly in the extensor mass area. Pal-

pation may reveal a particular point of tenderness, but sometimes the soreness to palpation is diffuse. The pain may be elicited by resisted wrist dorsiflexion as well as resisting supination and pronation. Some authors emphasize that pain with resisted digital extension, particularly of the middle finger, suggests posterior interosseous nerve entrapment. This may not be a significant finding.

Patients with medial epicondylitis have pain and tenderness over the medial epicondyle that may be aggravated by resisted wrist palmar flexion. Lifting things off the floor or carrying heavy hand luggage may aggravate the symptoms, as may golf and tennis. With golf it is usually after playing the round or after practicing that the symptoms arise. These problems are best treated by temporarily avoiding the aggravating activity and stretching the involved muscle-tendon units (Fig. 34.4). When the epicondylitis is painful, resistive exercises are not helpful and can aggravate the condition. In most patients cortisone injections can be avoided and NSAIDs offer little help.

Only after an extended conservative course of careful stretching over several months should a

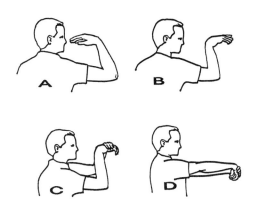

© Mark R. Belsky, MD

Figure 34.4.   Tennis elbow stretching exercises. **A.** Begin with elbow flexed, wrist flexed, and fingers pointing to nose. **B.** Pronate the forearm, pointing fingers away (making like a duck). **C.** Grasp hand with other hand, keeping wrist flexed. **D.** Gently and slowly extend elbow, keeping wrist flexed and fingers pointing at the floor. Exercise is a modification of a manipulation described by G. Percival Mills, F.R.C.S.

cortisone injection be considered to relieve the persistent severe pain. The pain and tenderness must be very focal, localized to an area on the epicondyle. For the lateral epicondyle, it is usually the anterior edge of the epicondyle where the pain and tenderness are most severe. The most successful cortisone injections are those with which the findings and the treatment are very local. When the symptoms and findings are diffuse, cortisone shots usually are not effective. The limit of two to three injections in the same tendon in the same year is considered a safe maximum.

It is recommended that 1 mL of triamcinolone acetonide 20 mg/mL and 1 mL of 1% mepivacaine be used together in the injection. The area is prepared with alcohol and sprayed with ethyl chloride to decrease some of the intense pain of the injection that follows. The point of maximum tenderness, often the anterior edge of the epicondyle, is sought with the point of the needle. The injection is made here and several millimeters to either side of this point. Inject slowly to diminish the severity of the pain and then cover with a small adhesive bandage.

The patient is advised that the cortisone takes 4 to 7 days to begin its effectiveness and is often more painful the first few days after injection. Ice packs and NSAIDs help to alleviate this pain. As the pain resolves, motion and activity are resumed. The cortisone is often effective for at least 3 months, and most patients find lasting relief after a single cortisone shot. The problem is to maintain the relief and resume activities such as golf and tennis. We recommend that patients resume the stretching exercises once they feel relief from the cortisone injection and maintain the stretching exercises (Fig. 34.4) for as long as they are active. It is not different from the walker or runner who is encouraged to stretch the Achilles tendons before daily activity.

Most significant trauma about the elbow can result in fractures and dislocations. Although these injuries are not common in the elderly, the most common types of injury are radial head fracture, olecranon fracture, and elbow dislocation. FOOSH is a common mechanism to cause these injuries. The radial head fracture is most common. Fracture can occur through the neck or intra-articularly through the head. The radial head articulates with the capitellum of the humerus. If the articular fracture is significantly displaced, it can interfere with forearm rotation. Radial head fractures are often nondisplaced or minimally displaced. After the elbow is rested in a sling for 4 to 5 days, the patient begins an early return to motion; flexion, extension, and rotation. Satisfactory motion is the goal of treatment. However, if the motion continues to be painful and the pain limits return of adequate motion and function, surgical care may be required.

Fractures of the olecranon are often displaced and necessitate surgical treatment to make the elbow stable and joint motion congruent. When the fractures are small at the tip of the olecranon, excision of the fragment and early return of motion and function is often preferable. More severe injuries to the elbow can result in dislocation and a combination of fractures. Although many of these injuries require surgical treatment, the guiding principle of care is an early return of motion and function.

Injuries to the wrist and hand are more common than elbow injury, and they may result in a significant loss of function. Often these injuries are not very severe, but the prolonged immobilization is a risk for leaving these patients with profound stiffness and loss of function. As emphasized earlier, the goal of treatment is preservation of and an early return to function.

The most common fracture in the upper extremity in the aging population is in the distal radius. After hip fracture, Colles' fracture and its variants account for most of the emergency room and hospital visits for elderly patients with fractures. Usually the result of FOOSH, there is often significant pain and deformity in the wrist. Distal radius fractures may be nondisplaced, impacted, displaced, or intra-articular. There are a number of very sophisticated classifications (4) that help the surgeon appreciate the extent of injury and plan of treatment.

Initially the patient has a swollen painful wrist. The hand and forearm are usually held against the body with the elbow flexed. Placing the hand down causes more throbbing pain. The patient may complain of tingling and numbness in the fingers, usually in the distribution of the median nerve. Physical examination initially excludes coincident injury of the shoulder, arm, elbow, and forearm. The classic silver fork deformity may be noted in the wrist. This is caused by a dorsal displacement of the distal radius fragment. The dorsally tilted and/or displaced fragment displaces the hand dorsally on the forearm, causing this classic deformity. The fracture line is tender. Thorough examination is performed to rule out the possibility of an adjacent intercarpal injury or compression of the median nerve. The carpal bones if injured are also tender. Median nerve compression at the wrist and sensibility are assessed by tapping over the carpal tunnel just proximal to the wrist flexion crease. Careful radiographic examination of the wrist with appropriate views to evaluate the carpal bones is performed. Just as it is with each regional examination, standard radiographs films are necessary to assess the extent of injury and displacement.

The elderly patient, usually a woman, often has significant osteoporosis. Such a distal radius has a very thin, eggshell-like cortex and minimal metaphyseal supporting structure. It does not take much force to crumble and impact the distal radius from a fall. Experience has taught orthopaedic surgeons that because of the nature of this bone, significant deformities are often accepted, with a focus on rapid return to satisfactory functional activity. The deformities that result with the radius shortened and impacted and the ulna prominent often permit most functions. However, the distinction between the patient who should accept the deformity and the one who would best benefit by reduction supplemented by external or internal fixation with a bone graft is often not obvious. Initial treatment necessitates splinting and elevation of the hand higher than the heart. If the fracture is nondisplaced, acceptably minimally displaced, or impacted, treatment is directed at splinting or casting the wrist until there is enough healing of the fracture to allow the patient to begin using the hand comfortably without support. Until that time, immobilization provides comfort while allowing shoulder, elbow, and hand motion and function.

The most common functional limitations that follow wrist fracture in the elderly are stiff shoulder, stiff fingers, and carpal tunnel syndrome. During the course of treatment of the elderly patient with a wrist fracture, maintenance of range of motion of the shoulder and fingers is very important. This can be done with specific exercises 3 minutes, 3 times a day.

The problem of carpal tunnel syndrome can be more subtle. Often these patients have a history of occasional night paresthesias in their hands. The effect of the change in the anatomy of the wrist because of the fracture, along with the bleeding and swelling that result, compromise the space in the carpal tunnel and can contribute to the compression of the median nerve. Although splinting and elevation often alleviate the symptoms, compression may be significant enough to cause anesthesia or severe burning in the hand that warrants emergency surgical decompression.

Skeletal injuries in the hand are usually fractures or sprains. Most phalangeal and metacarpal fractures are displaced minimally or not at all and require only splinting for 7 to 21 days, until comfortable. During the time of immobilization of the fractured fingers, range of motion exercises of the remaining digits and shoulder are encouraged to prevent loss of function. Certain displaced phalangeal and metacarpal fractures occur where the deformity significantly impairs function. In such cases there may be a malrotated shaft fracture or an angulated fracture with spikes impaling the tendon or the skin. Open reduction with internal fixation or closed reduction with percutaneous pin fixation allows the patient early return to active motion and use.

Proximal interphalangeal joint sprains are best treated with temporary dorsal splinting for 5 days and return to active use with buddy taping for a month. The same treatment is used following reduction of dorsal and lateral dislocations. During the first 5 days the splint is removed for bathing and gentle exercises when tolerated. The only purpose in the splinting is comfort. Loss of flexion after significant joint sprains and dislocation is common. The joint may stay swollen for 6 months or more. The patient is encouraged to do exercises that emphasize the extremes of motion of flexion and extension. A reasonable frequency of exercises is 3 minutes 5 times a day. These exercises should be active assisted range of motion.

Jam injury to the tip of a digit may result in a

mallet finger. As the patient actively extends the finger, the deforming force, such as a swinging door, forcibly flexes the finger tip. This may cause rupture of the terminal extensor tendon (soft tissue mallet) or the tendon may avulse a fragment of bone (bony mallet) from its dorsal attachment to the distal phalanx (Fig. 34.5). Both forms of injury are treated with the same method of dorsal splinting. An aluminum splint with the foam removed and covered with moleskin is taped to the dorsum of the finger from the base of the middle phalanx to the finger tip. The finger distal interphalangeal joint must be maintained in full extension for 6 weeks.

LOWER EXTREMITY

Pain, stiffness, and discomfort in the lower extremity can be caused by both traumatic and nontraumatic conditions. These conditions, quite common in the elderly, are aggravated by the fact that the lower extremities must bear weight and propel one through the environ-

ment. The inability of a person to walk significantly reduces the quality of life and can have a debilitating effect on general health, so the recognition and treatment of injury of the lower extremity is vitally important.

The successful care of a patient with a lower extremity problem often is determined by his or her ability to negotiate the immediate environment. These people frequently need assistance in performing their daily physical tasks, such as preparation of meals and transferring from the bed to a chair. Placing weight on the affected extremity may produce too much pain to allow normal functioning. The physician's role may be as simple as providing an ambulation aid, such as a cane, and helping a patient obtain a handicap placard for the car; or it may be as complex as reconstruction of severely arthritic weight-bearing joints and the organization of a multidisciplinary rehabilitation program. Postinjury treatment must include maintenance of the patient's physical condition to prevent loss of mus-

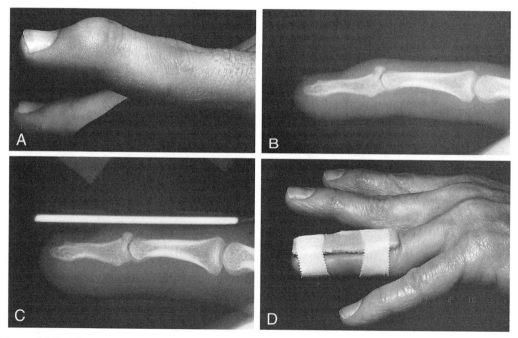

Figure 34.5.   **A.** Mallet deformity in a small finger. Note flexion of distal interphalangeal (DIP) joint and hyperextension of proximal interphalangeal (PIP) joint. **B.** Radiograph of an avulsion fracture of the distal phalanx, a bony mallet. **C.** Radiograph of the same fracture reduced by splinting. **D.** Proper dorsal splinting for a finger with a bony or soft tissue mallet injury. (Copyright Mark R. Belsky, M.D.)

cle mass during convalescence. This should include resistance exercises for the upper extremities as well as the uninvolved lower extremity in an effort to maintain muscle strength. Proper nutrition is essential for the normal healing of these injuries. Prevention of complications associated with lower extremity injuries has paramount importance. Many of these conditions are associated with a high incidence of deep vein thrombosis, and the prevention of this condition must be addressed in the treatment of lower extremity problems.

Hip

The hip joint connects the lower appendicular skeleton to the axial skeleton at the pelvis. Its range of motion along with the knee and ankle allow for locomotion, enabling people to propel themselves through their environment. Afflictions about any of these joints can severely limit a person's ability to perform these functions.

Trochanteric Bursitis

Trochanteric bursitis is characterized by pain over the lateral side of the hip at the level of the greater trochanter. Patients describe pain on weight bearing, pain when lying on the involved side, and occasionally the feeling of a snap with each step. The pain can be aggravated by rotation of the hip and is most often relieved by rest. There is rarely any observable swelling. Tenderness is elicited by palpating over the trochanter with the person lying on the uninvolved side. The condition is caused by tightness of the iliotibial band producing friction over the greater trochanter with resultant swelling of the bursa that lies between these two structures. This tightness may occur after sitting for long periods or after a sudden increase in exercise. Once produced, it can perpetuate itself indefinitely. Treatment includes rest, NSAIDs, and a stretching program for the iliotibial band. Physical therapy may be necessary, and occasionally a cortisone injection is needed to alleviate the symptoms.

Osteoarthritis

Osteoarthritis of the hip is a common problem in the elderly. It commonly has an insidious onset, and the discomfort that results can gradually decrease a person's ambulatory and functional capacity. It is characterized by aching discomfort, typically in the groin and buttock region, that is exacerbated by bearing weight and by rotation of the hip. Frequently people describe a stiffness in the hip region that preceded the pain. Early in the disease process the person may note difficulty rotating the hip to remove their socks and shoes or wash their feet. Family members may note a limp. As the disease progresses, people note that their ability to walk distances diminishes. Patients may begin walking up or down stairs one at a time. In more advanced cases, pain is noted with movements of the hip, even at night, which may affect sleep. There may be trouble lying on the involved side. The diagnostic procedure of choice is the plain radiograph, anteroposterior and frog lateral, which classically shows joint space narrowing, subchondral sclerosis, cyst formation, and often osteophyte formation. A weight-bearing radiograph is helpful in noting subtle joint space narrowing.

Initial treatment consists of anti-inflammatory medication, modification of activities, and stretching and strengthening exercises. If symptoms are not controlled through conservative measures, the treatment of choice is total hip arthroplasty. This procedure has an excellent track record and can dramatically improve the patient's quality of life. In the early stages of arthritis of the hip, the painful exacerbations are treated conservatively with a short course of protected weight bearing using a cane, crutches, or walker, as well as the gentle stretching, cutting back on weight-bearing activities, and anti-inflammatory medication. A steroid injection into the hip joint occasionally has some benefit, although it generally provides only temporary relief and must be performed under fluoroscopic control.

Traumatic Injuries of the Hip and Femur

Hip Fractures

Fractures of the hip in the elderly are extremely common. The incidence of hip fracture has reached epidemic proportions, resulting in a significant percentage of Medicare expenditure. The care of these fractures requires a multidisciplinary approach encompassing medical, nursing, and rehabilitation services. Hip fractures can result in profound changes in the patient's ability to remain independent and in significant stresses on the patient and the patient's family. Great effort is being expended in attempting to prevent these fractures through education of patients, and treatment of osteoporosis is an important predisposing factor.

Hip fractures can be broken down into two major categories: subcapital and intertrochanteric fractures. Subcapital fractures occur just below the femoral head in the neck region of the proximal femur. Intertrochanteric fractures occur along the intertrochanteric line, which lies distally. The intertrochanteric line corresponds to the attachment of the hip capsule. Thus subcapital hip fractures occur within the hip capsule and intertrochanteric fractures are extracapsular. These two fractures are lumped together as hip fractures but have significantly different treatments.

SUBCAPITAL HIP FRACTURES. Subcapital hip fractures generally occur when the patient falls, landing directly on the buttock of the involved side. A torque force on the leg has been implicated as a cause of these fractures as well. Patients generally have a painful hip with the leg shortened and externally rotated. Less commonly patients have pain in the groin or buttock and cannot bear weight on the involved side. Radiographs include AP and lateral views of the involved hip as well as an AP pelvis film to compare to the uninvolved side. Most often the diagnosis is obvious, with a displaced fracture that occurs just below the femoral head. The fracture may be impacted as well. At times radiographs appear normal.

Rapid diagnosis of this condition can be quite helpful in reducing the morbidity of the injury. One should consider this diagnosis in any elderly patient who has had a fall, and more important, cannot bear weight on the extremity. If the radiographs are not diagnostic and the diagnosis is suspected, further testing is indicated. If MRI is readily available, it can be used to diagnose an acute fracture and hasten treatment. If MRI is not readily available, the bone scan is the diagnostic procedure of choice. The disadvantage of the bone scan is that traditionally it is necessary to wait 2 to 3 days before scanning to increase the sensitivity of the test.

The treatment of subcapital hip fractures depends on the patient's medical status, functional status, and the amount of displacement at the fracture site. Displaced fractures are treated with hemiarthroplasty, in which the femoral head is replaced with a metallic implant. Some centers are attempting closed reduction and internal fixation of these fractures. Nondisplaced fractures are treated with stabilization using internal fixation techniques preserving the femoral head. These treatment principles apply to fully active patients living independently as well as to nonfunctional patients in chronic care facilities. In this situation the treatment becomes humanitarian in an attempt to relieve the pain of these fractures.

Preparing patients for the surgical treatment of this problem requires a team approach, including the orthopaedic surgeon and the patient's primary doctor. In general, rapid treatment of these fractures is associated with the fewest perioperative complications. The patient's medical condition should be stabilized as rapidly as possible. Hip fractures may result in a significant blood loss. This is particularly significant for the many elderly patients who are already chronically anemic; for them the blood loss after hip fracture can be catastrophic. Appropriate perioperative monitoring of cardiac and pulmonary status is necessary to diminish complications. It is optimal to perform surgery within 24 hours of admission. There is ample evidence that the sooner the patient with a hip fracture is stabilized medically and then operated on to have the hip fixed or replaced, the better the outcome. Postoperatively these patients progress to physical therapy once their medical condition stabilizes. Recovery from this condition is heavily dependent on the preoperative medical and functional status. After surgery, interim stays at a skilled nursing facility or an acute care rehabilitation facility are fairly common. In some settings, an effort is made to perform postoperative rehabilitation at home.

INTERTROCHANTERIC FRACTURES. The intertrochanteric fractures occur in much the same fashion as subcapital hip fractures. These fractures are somewhat more distal along the intertrochanteric line of the proximal femur. They have a similar history and similar physical examination. The leg is frequently shortened and externally rotated in displaced fractures. There is pain at the hip with attempts at internal or external rotation of the involved leg. Patients are unable to bear weight. Bruising over the greater trochanter may be noted.

As with subcapital hip fractures, the diagnostic procedure of choice is radiography of the hip and pelvis. Displaced fractures are well recognized, but nondisplaced fractures can be quite subtle. In suspected fractures with nondiagnostic radiographs, further testing may be necessary. MRI can be helpful in this case. In facilities that do not have MRI capability, the bone scan is the diagnostic procedure of choice. Treatment of this condition is to perform open reduction and internal fixation. The rationale for treatment and perioperative evaluation is similar to that for subcapital hip fractures.

These are major fractures that can have a profound effect on the life of the patient. The 1-year mortality of these fractures approaches 25%. This figure is a reflection of the magnitude of the injury and of the stresses that are placed on the patient's medical condition. Successful rehabilitation following these injuries is a team effort involving orthopaedists, the primary care physician, physical therapy, rehabilitation services, and often quality skilled nursing facilities. It is common for these injuries to result in a profound change in the patient's independence. One should not treat lightly the emotional ramifications of this injury with respect to the patient and family. It is important to keep all of these factors in mind if one is to treat these conditions effectively.

ACETABULUM FRACTURES. In the elderly, acetabulum fractures occur most frequently as a result of a fall onto the involved side. The femoral head is driven into the acetabulum, resulting in a fracture. These fractures are occasionally associated with fractures in other locations, such as the hip and pubic ramus. These fractures typically accompany complaints of groin and buttock pain and inability to bear weight. The radiograph is the diagnostic procedure of choice. These injuries usually show little displacement and are treated conservatively with a non-weight-bearing course using ambulation aids such as a walker or crutches. Healing may take 2 to 3 months. It is only with marked displacement of fracture fragments that more aggressive treatment is indicated in patients who can walk.

PUBIC RAMUS FRACTURES. Pubic ramus fractures are quite common. Their mechanism is similar to that of most other hip-related injuries in that they occur as a result of a fall onto the buttock or the involved side. The patient may complain of pain in the groin and tenderness high in the groin. Patients generally have difficulty bearing weight and have pain with range of motion of the hip. Plain radiographs, the diagnostic procedure of choice, often show the iliopubic ramus, the ischiopubic ramus, or both involved in the fracture. The treatment is conservative, with protected weight bearing using aids, gentle range-of-motion exercises of the hip as tolerated, and maintenance of lower extremity strength.

FEMORAL SHAFT AND SUPRACONDYLAR FEMORAL FRACTURES. Fractures of the mid or lower shaft of the femur occur in the elderly as a result of a fall or blunt trauma to the femur. These can be severe injuries that result in significant blood loss and debility. Restricted motion of the knee, as with patients who have osteoarthritis, may contribute to the production of femoral fractures. These patients typically give a history of a fall onto the involved side. Bedridden patients with osteoporotic bone may sustain these fractures during the act of transferring. This fracture occurs when those involved in the transfer grasp the patient's ankles and lift their lower extremities at that level. The torque applied to the lower extremity is transmitted through the extended knee to the supracondylar region of the femur and can result in fracture.

The patients have swelling about the thigh or knee region and complain of pain on weight bearing and inability to move the knee. There may be visible deformity with shortening of the involved leg. Radiographs are generally diagnostic. Treatment depends on the amount of displacement and the condition of the patient. Displaced fractures in a weight-bearing person are generally treated with surgical stabilization. Patients with nondisplaced fractures and patients who cannot walk are frequently treated with casting or bracing. In the case of bedridden patients, it is important for the caregiver to teach those who are providing day-to-day care the proper transferring techniques to reduce the risk of this type of injury.

Knee

Osteoarthritis

Osteoarthritis of the knee commonly affects a person's quality of life. Limited ability to walk decreases the patient's interaction with the environment, resulting in less independence and a poorer quality of life. The hallmark of osteoarthritis of the knee is pain on walking and weight bearing. This condition generally is associated with swelling and crepitation about the knee as well. There may be a previous injury, but the problem often presents insidiously. Initially patients complain of stiffness that is often worse toward the end of the day, when they have been on their feet. Pain may ensue along with episodes of swelling. These episodes are typically relieved with rest and may be adequately treated with anti-inflammatory medication. As the problem progresses, the patient's range of motion decreases. This may manifest as discomfort when squatting or when trying to straighten the leg. A flexion contracture of 5 to 10° is common in patients with osteoarthritis of the knee. The patient may limp on the involved side. If the arthritis is painful enough to cause a limp and favoring of the affected knee for a long enough period, there may be atrophy of the thigh and calf musculature. In later stages patients describe going up and down stairs one at a time, pain at night, and reliance on aids such as canes or crutches.

Plain radiographs are diagnostic for this condition; it is important to obtain a standing weight-bearing view. The best screening test is the standing weight-bearing view with the knees flexed approximately 40° and the beam shot from posterior to anterior. Typical radiographs reveal joint space narrowing, subchondral sclerosis, osteophyte formation, and subchondral cysts. Rarely is other testing necessary to confirm the diagnosis. A bone scan shows increased uptake in the region of the knee joint but does not contribute to the diagnosis. MRI often shows degenerative meniscal tears as well as thinning of the articular cartilage but is generally not necessary.

TREATMENT. Initially treatment is symptomatic, with the use of rest, anti-inflammatory medication, and quadriceps strengthening exercises. Stretching is helpful to decrease the risk of contractures. As the symptoms progress, walking aids such as a cane may be necessary. Physical therapy may improve the patient's strength and range of motion. Occasionally intra-articular steroid injection can be used to treat an acute flare-up of arthritic pain. Soft knee braces can be of some benefit.

The use of a custom molded knee brace designed to unload the arthritic joint has had some success. This is generally used in patients with arthritis in earlier stages who are physically active. These braces are generally worn during sports or physical activity. Arthroscopic treatment of an arthritic knee, which is designed to clean out torn cartilage and remove debris, is controversial. In some series 60% of people noted lasting relief after this procedure. Other series have not noted as much success, and most think it should only be used in specific circumstances in which a less invasive approach to knee arthritis is desirable.

The definitive treatment of an arthritic knee that has failed conservative management is total knee arthroplasty. The track record with this procedure has improved steadily and with current techniques can yield excellent long-term results. The decision to proceed with total knee arthroplasty entails consulting the patient, the patient's family, and the physicians. Factors taken into account must include the patient's desire to maintain normal activities, health status, and residential situation.

Baker's Cyst

Baker's cyst, which occurs in the posterior aspect of the knee, is usually a fluid-filled sac that communicates with the knee joint. Any condition that produces fluid in the knee can result in the formation of this cyst. It is generally thought that the cyst is a potential space that is present as a pouch off the back of the knee joint. The most common condition to produce a Baker's cyst is degenerative osteoarthritis of the knee. Other inflammatory conditions, such as rheumatoid arthritis, can result in similar bumps. In general, patients complain of fullness with discomfort in the posterior aspect of the knee that is worst with the knee in full extension. Patients may complain of related symptoms in the knee joint itself that are related to the underlying knee pathology. When these cysts are large, they can produce pressure on the neurovascular bundle in the posterior aspect of the knee, resulting in aching discomfort and tingling that radiates down the leg. These cysts have a tendency to rupture spontaneously, which may be the incident that brings the condition to the doctor's attention. Ecchymosis associated with swelling, fullness, and pitting edema may track down the leg below the knee. Plain radiographs of the knee may reveal arthritic change. MRI of the knee is diagnostic, showing the cyst and its relation to surrounding structures as well as the presence or absence of degenerative changes within the knee.

Treatment is aimed at controlling the underlying cause of the problem. This treatment may include use of anti-inflammatory medication, rest, and icing. Use of a soft knee brace may be helpful. Most of these conditions resolve spontaneously. Only occasionally is surgical excision of the mass necessary. Arthroscopic treatment of degenerative meniscal tears is quite successful in treating a common inciting cause of these cysts.

Pes Anserinus Bursitis

Pes anserinus bursitis is a painful condition of the knee that is characterized by pain along the medial side of the proximal tibia below the flare of the tibial condyle. The pes anserinus bursa, which lies in this area, is the friction-reducing tissue between the tibia itself and the collection of three tendons that wrap around the medial tibial condyle known as the pes anserinus. A number of conditions can produce this bursitis. Hamstring tightness caused by lack of exercise is

thought to be one cause. Direct injury from an inadvertent blow can produce swelling in the bursa as well. Arthritic conditions such as rheumatoid arthritis can manifest as pain in this bursal area. The patient may describe pain and swelling that is made worse by weight bearing and walking. The condition can be produced by excessive exercise. Patients typically display point tenderness over the pes anserinus bursa with discomfort on resistance to knee flexion and leg adduction. Only rarely is there crepitation in this area. Patients may display tight hamstrings on physical examination. Radiographs are done primarily to rule out any bony cause of the discomfort. Treatment consists of local modalities with ice and stretching exercises along with anti-inflammatory medication. A soft knee brace may be helpful. If these conservative measures fail, a steroid injection can be therapeutic.

Tendinitis of the Quadriceps and Patella

Quadriceps and patella tendinitis produces pain with exercise and walking. Patients describe pain and tenderness adjacent to the patella at the level of tendon insertion. The tenderness of quadriceps tendinitis manifests at the superior pole of the patella, whereas the tenderness in patella tendinitis is noted at the distal pole of the patella. These conditions are most common in those who exercise regularly or who are performing manual labor. Tightness of the quadriceps and hamstring musculature is thought to be a predisposing factor to the production of this condition. Generally there is minimal swelling, although in severe cases swelling may be prominent. This tendinitis is thought to be an overuse phenomenon. Radiographs of the knee are commonly normal, although in the case of quadriceps tendinitis one may see a traction spur off the superior pole of the patella.

The condition is treated conservatively, with the initial program including quadriceps and hamstring stretching exercises, ice, and anti-inflammatory medication. Exercises and activity are modified to reduce the stress on this area. A soft knee brace may be beneficial. If these initial measures fail, a course of physical therapy may be warranted to include further stretching and modalities such as ultrasound. Steroid injections are generally to be avoided in these conditions. Return to athletic or labor activities must be gradual to prevent recurrence.

Meniscus Tear

Meniscus tears in the elderly are quite common. In active patients doing exercise or manual labor, such a tear may be caused by a traumatic event such as a knee twist or fall. In the elderly it is also common as a result of normal activities of daily living. Patients may describe sudden pain in the knee after squatting or kneeling.

The location of discomfort depends on whether the lateral or medial meniscus is involved. The medial meniscus is involved most frequently; the tear manifests as pain along the medial joint line. Patients describe discomfort with twisting maneuvers and at the limits of flexion and extension of the knee. Weight bearing typically produces discomfort. Pain is described as achy and deep seated, occurring with weight bearing or knee motion. Pain may be absent at rest. There may be catching or locking, and an effusion is frequent. Physical examination reveals tenderness along either the medial or lateral joint line. There is typically pain at the limits of flexion and extension of the knee. Range of motion may be compromised, with lack of full flexion and extension. In some cases a large displaced cartilage tear locks the knee in place. The knee may lock going downstairs, giving out and causing the patient to fall. Radiographs may be normal, although in the elderly it is more frequent to see evidence of some degenerative changes or frank arthritis. A radiograph may show chondrocalcinosis with outlining of the cartilaginous structures by calcium deposition. In cases that do not respond to conservative management, MRI may be beneficial. This scan is quite accurate in showing meniscal pathology. In addition, it is helpful in delineating articular cartilage damage.

In the elderly, it is often difficult to determine whether knee pain is caused primarily by an acute event such as meniscal tear or by an exacerbation of a preexisting condition such as osteoarthritis. Acute onset of pain favors a new meniscal tear, whereas a more gradual onset of discomfort favors osteoarthritis. An effusion may be noted in both cases. The standing radiograph with the knees flexed at about 40° is helpful in determining the amount of joint space narrowing when considering osteoarthritis. Minimal narrowing rules out osteoarthritis and favors an acute meniscal injury. In any event, treatment of these conditions initially is conservative.

Initial treatment includes rest, ice, anti-inflammatory medication, a soft knee brace, and protected weight bearing if necessary. A sterile steroid injection may be quite helpful in patients who may have a degenerative meniscal tear. Physical therapy with modalities, lower extremity strengthening, and measures to improve range of motion is often quite helpful. If these measures fail and the evaluation has indicated that a meniscus tear is the primary problem, arthroscopic meniscectomy predictably improves the symptoms. Results of arthroscopic meniscectomy in the face of mild degenerative changes are somewhat less predictable. It is often difficult to determine the extent to which degenerative changes are affecting the symptoms. These changes are not changed by removal of a torn meniscus.

Traumatic Injury of the Knee and Leg

Tibial Plateau Fracture

Tibial plateau fractures are common in the elderly. Typically they are caused by a slip and fall. The lateral tibial plateau fracture, the most common, occurs when a valgus stress is placed on the knee. Osteoporosis is a common predisposing factor. The inward bending of the knee (valgus stress) that occurs with this type of slip and fall commonly produces a medial collateral ligament sprain in younger age groups. In the elderly the lateral tibial plateau fails in compression before the medial ligament tears. Elderly patients with a history of having twisted their knee should be considered to have a tibial plateau fracture until proven otherwise. Such fractures cause a swollen and painful knee with tenderness about the knee and proximal tibia most frequently on the lateral side. The patient frequently cannot bear weight and complains of pain with range of motion of the knee.

Radiographs of the knee are generally diagnostic, although subtle minimally displaced fractures are common. These fractures may be difficult to see on standard radiographs. Oblique films of the knee, in addition to the standard views, may help identify some subtle fractures. Sterile aspiration of the knee helps to decompress the tense effusion that frequently results from this injury. Aspiration also helps to diagnose subtle fracture, as this maneuver yields blood with diagnostic fat globules.

Initial treatment of these injuries includes splinting, pain control measures, and protected weight bearing. Subsequently, nondisplaced fractures may be treated with a brace and early range-of-motion exercises of the knee. Displaced fractures are treated surgically to recreate normal knee anatomy. In an effort to prevent posttraumatic arthritis of the knee, the goal of treatment is anatomic restoration of the articular surface.

Patella Fracture

Fractures of the patella generally occur as a result of one of two mechanisms. A fall with direct landing on the knees—a direct blow to the patella—can cause a fracture. A common second cause of patella fracture occurs with a slip or misstep and sudden contraction of the quadriceps on the weight-bearing leg. This sudden force on the flexed weight-bearing leg produces enough stress to fracture the patella. These fractures are typically transverse in the mid portion of the bone. Patients have severe pain, swelling, and tenderness about the knee. They cannot extend the knee. Physical examination reveals a tense knee effusion and tenderness about the patella. In the case of displaced fractures, crepitation and a palpable defect may be noted. Knee radiographs demonstrate the fracture. Treatment of these fractures initially entails splinting and sterile aspiration of the knee hematoma. Nondisplaced fractures are treated with bracing, protected weight bearing, and early range-of-motion exercises. Displaced fractures are treated with open reduction and internal fixation.

Tibial Shaft Fracture

Tibial shaft fractures are seen in two circumstances. The first is the standard traumatic event that is a result of a direct blow to the leg or fall. A twisting motion often accompanies the stresses that produce this fracture. The second circum-

stance involves debilitated patients who are osteoporotic and require transfers. The lifting of patients by the ankles produces a significant angular stress at the level of the tibia. This can lead to a fracture through osteoporotic bone. Prevention of this variation of tibial fracture requires correct lifting and transferring techniques. The patient's lower extremity should be supported near the knee to prevent overstress of the osteoporotic tibia.

A diagnosis is made by radiograph and is generally readily apparent. Nonambulatory patients are treated with closed methods with casting and/or splinting techniques. Patients who can walk are treated according to the displacement of the fracture. Nondisplaced fractures can be treated with casting or bracing. Displaced fractures are generally treated with internal fixation techniques, although patients with significant medical risks may be treated by closed methods. The goal of treatment is to stabilize the fracture and allow the patient to be as functional as possible.

Quadriceps and Patella Tendon Ruptures

The quadriceps muscles together insert on the patella. This is in continuity with the patella and the patella tendon, which in turn inserts into the tibial tubercle. Ruptures of the quadriceps tendon insertion and patella tendon are relatively common injuries. The quadriceps tendon ruptures much more commonly than the patella tendon. Mechanism of injury is typically a forceful resistance to a forceful contraction of the quadriceps tendon, such as a fall from a height or a slip. Patients typically complain of pain at the level of the knee and may provide a history of a tearing or popping sensation. There is typically a large amount of swelling that may be associated with ecchymosis. A palpable defect may be noted. The classic diagnostic test is the inability of the patient to raise the straightened leg. Radiographs of the knee may show altered position of the patella. In the case of a quadriceps tendon rupture, the patella appears lower (more distal) than usual; in the case of the patella tendon rupture, the patella is higher (more proximal) than usual. The treatment is operative, with reattachment of the tendon to its insertion point. Postoperative treatment requires the use of the brace and physical therapy to restore motion.

Ligament Sprains

Ligament sprains about the knee in the elderly are less common than tibial plateau fractures but have a similar mechanism of injury. Typically, valgus stress to the knee as a result of a slip and fall or a fall from a height produces this injury. The most common ligament to be injured is the medial collateral ligament. Patients typically have swelling and pain involving the medial side of the knee. Range of motion is diminished by pain. There is tenderness along the course of the medial collateral ligament. There may be laxity of the ligament on valgus stress testing. Radiographs of the knee are normal, with no evidence of a tibial plateau fracture. The treatment is conservative, with bracing, pain and edema control measures, and early range-of-motion exercises.

SPINE AND TRUNK INJURIES

Spinal and trunk injuries, frequent occurrences in the elderly patient, can vary from simple sprains to significant fractures with drastic consequences. The injuries occur primarily as a result of direct trauma and falls. This section deals with cervical, thoracic, and lumbar problems and injuries involving the trunk. Cervical injuries are quite common in the elderly. Cervical injuries to be discussed include simple strains, aggravated radiculopathy, and fractures.

Sprains and Strains

The simple sprains, or stretching of the cervical musculature or ligaments, are a result of flexion or extension injuries to the cervical spine most commonly associated with a fall. These problems are generally self-limited, lasting 1 to 5 days, and are usually helped by local use of heat, cold packs, and mild analgesics such as acetaminophen or mild muscle relaxants. Complaints include stiffness, loss of range of cervical motion, posterior occipital headaches radiating to the forehead, and quite frequently shoulder pain. There is generally no indication for imaging modalities, but physical therapy may be necessary to resolve symptoms.

Aggravated Radiculopathy

Because many elderly have degenerative osteoarthritis in the cervical facet joints and disc spaces, these problems frequently last longer or are associated with unilateral or bilateral radiculopathies. Especially with extension injuries to the neck, the foramina are narrowed, and if there is degenerative osteoarthritis in the facets, radiculopathy can occur. The radiculopathies can be purely sensory or motor, but they frequently involve both, with a significant radiating pain into the appropriate dermatome. When such injuries occur, the treatment again is supportive, including physical therapy. These problems generally resolve over 4 to 8 weeks with or without physical therapy. The use of a cervical supportive collar is generally beneficial. Rarely is surgery indicated. For persisting radiculopathies cervical spine films with obliques should be obtained, and MRI may be necessary to delineate any associated disc abnormalities.

Fractures

In significant falls associated with severe flexion and extension injuries, atlantoaxial fractures or instability (C1-C2) can go unrecognized. In any elderly patient with loss of consciousness associated with a fall, a complete cervical spine radiographic series should be performed to rule out odontoid (C2) fracture or instability. There are three types of fractures of the odontoid. The most common is a type II fracture at the base of the odontoid, which has a high nonunion rate in the elderly patient. It is necessary for the specific type of fracture to be identified, since treatments for the three types of fracture at C1-C2 can range from halo immobilization to hard cervical collar to open reduction and internal fixation. Unrecognized instability can lead to myelopathic developments and weakness in the lower extremities associated with long tract signs. With this type of fracture, the odontoid moves up against the spinal cord, causing an impingement. Symptoms can range from pain in the neck with movement to intermittent numbness and tingling in the lower extremities or weakness in the upper extremities. In rare instances significant flexion and extension injuries can also cause subluxation or fracture of other cervical vertebral bodies. These instances are rare but should not be overlooked, since surgical intervention is generally necessary. Acute injuries to the cervical spine can also lead to acute disc herniations. Once disc material protrudes from its annular confines, pressure on the spinal cord or nerve root causes neck, shoulder, or arm discomfort. In cases of significant disc herniations, lower extremity symptoms associated with bowel or bladder problems may also be present. Early recognition of these injuries is necessary, and MRI is an excellent means of evaluation.

Thoracic Spine

Injuries in the thoracic spine are generally limited to sprains and thoracic compression fractures. These sprains are similar to other sprains in the body. They are generally associated with lifting or twisting incidents, and they resolve with local treatments. The thoracic spine in the elderly is at risk for compression fractures, especially those associated with minimal trauma. With aging thoracic kyphosis can increase, and with the onset of osteoporosis the vertebral bodies also weaken. With a predisposition for osteoporotic compression fractures, any type of significant injury or fall places the thoracic spinal cord at increased risk for anterior compression fractures. Treatment modalities associated with this type of fracture include bed rest, analgesic medication, and hyperextension bracing if tolerated. The thoracic compression fractures generally take 1 to 3 months to heal but are not associated with catastrophic spinal cord symptoms. MRI is an excellent modality to visualize not only the compression fracture but also the spinal cord.

Lumbar Spine

The most frequent spinal injuries in the elderly occur in the lumbar spine. Trauma secondary to a fall is the most common cause. Problems associated with the lumbar spine include compression fractures, aggravated spondylolisthesis, acute disc herniation, sprains and strains, and coccyx and sacral fractures. Lumbar compression fractures occur in a high frequency secondary to the osteoporotic bone in the vertebral column. Any type of fall or axial compression can cause a vertebral column problem. MRI again is the single best way to visualize injuries in the lumbar spine. MRI is frequently necessary to determine whether the canal is compromised. In cases of severe canal compromise, leg weakness or bowel or bladder complaints are common, and it is necessary to decide whether to use surgical intervention for decompression of the spinal column. Osteoporotic compression fractures are clearly seen and can be differentiated from Paget's disease and metastatic lesions. Treatment for lumbar compression fractures includes inactivity until significant pain subsides. The advent of Velcro closure elasticized braces as opposed to the steel stay-laced corset has helped mobilize patients debilitated by significant lumbar pain. Lumbar spine compression fractures generally heal over 2 to 4 months; concurrent treatments include swimming, physical therapy, and pain medication. Associated abdominal complaints with lumbar compression fractures include ileus and in some instances may require either upper gastrointestinal or lower gastrointestinal tubes to relieve intra-abdominal pressures.

In addition to lumbar compression fractures, traumatic spondylolisthesis can occur with hyperextension injuries to the spine. Degenerative spondylolisthesis is common in the elderly, and it can be worsened by compression fractures or by herniation of the disc material into the spinal canal. Lifting or twisting injuries, in addition to falls, can cause asymptomatic spondylolisthesis to become problematic. Generally a course of conservative treatment including bracing, physical therapy, light analgesics, and an exercise and strengthening program is necessary to resolve the pain complaints. On occasion lumbar decompressive surgery proves fruitful. Acute disc herniations should not be overlooked in the differential diagnosis of musculoskeletal injuries. Axial compressions in osteoporosis can result in disc herniations protruding posteriorly against the nerve roots, causing a unilateral radicular component. Treatment includes a period of limited activity in association with physical therapy, lumbar epidural steroid injections if necessary, and occasionally microdiscectomy.

Sprains and strains can occur in a similar fashion to those of the cervical spine. Local modalities such as heat, ice, and physical therapy are generally used to eliminate pain associated with these common traumas. Spinal stenosis, or neurogenic claudication, can be aggravated by an injury, further narrowing the volume of the spinal canal and leading to radicular symptoms. Spinal stenosis is not the direct result of any musculoskeletal injury but rather can become symptomatic following an isolated injury to the lumbar spine. This is generally due to a disc protrusion as a result of a trauma and requires local treatments such as epidural steroids or in some occasions lumbar decompressive surgery.

Sacral and coccyx fractures result from a fall directly onto the buttocks. If a fracture occurs, it can become displaced, but these generally do not require any type of surgical intervention. Treatment for sacral and coccyx fractures is generally supportive, with a period of bed rest during which a fracture generally heals. The most common problem with this type of fracture or with a contusion to the bone is coccydynia, which is pain from the direct fall. Treatment of coccydynia can be very difficult. Pain often lasts for a year or two, and there are no magic treatments to improve the situation. Sitting on a pillow or soft seat in a high chair is generally helpful. Stretching exercises can also be performed for pain control. NSAIDs are frequently given, but the most common recommendation is for supportive care and patience. The surgical salvage procedure of coccygectomy produces equivocal results and is generally not indicated.

Trunk Injuries

Injuries to the trunk, which are very common in the elderly patient, include fractures of the ribs and the pelvis. The ribs can easily be fractured in osteoporosis as a result of blows to the chest wall, generally from falls. Fractures in the upper four ribs must be addressed with intensive study to ensure that no evidence of aortic dissection has occurred. Rib fractures, generally the result of a direct blow to the rib area, can be treated with intercostal blocks for pain relief as well as opioid pain medication. Strapping or wrapping of these rib fractures is not common these days. The pain generally lasts more than 2

weeks, but the ribs heal without any significant long-term sequela. Evaluation for rib fractures must include follow-up care to ensure that no pneumothorax has occurred. Serial chest radiographs may be needed, and these can also pinpoint pneumonia from splinting of the rib cage for pain. The use of incentive spirometers and deep breathing exercises, in addition to mild analgesics, is quite helpful.

Pelvic fractures are a frequent cause of trunk pain. Motor vehicle accidents and direct falls are the most common causes. The pelvic fractures are generally confined to the superior and inferior pubic rami. Most are nondisplaced, but some do have mild displacement, which can lead to local complications such as blood loss, significant swelling, and pain. In almost all instances they improve over a span of 2 to 3 weeks, with healing in approximately 5 to 8 weeks. With ligament disruption there can be prolonged pain. Treatment should include range-of-motion exercises of the affected hip and lower extremity to prevent contractures. Occasionally the fracture extends into the acetabulum, which makes weight bearing more difficult and prolongs the healing process. The patient can walk during healing with the use of a walker, which gives good stability as the patient gradually progresses from non-weight bearing to full weight bearing.

REFERENCES

1. Morrey BF. Bursitis. In: Morrey BF, ed. The Elbow and Its Disorders. 2nd ed. Philadelphia: Saunders, 1993: 872–880.
2. Canoso JJ. Idiopathic or traumatic olecranon bursitis. Clinical features and bursal fluid analysis. Arthritis Rheum 1977;20:1213–1216.
3. Weinstein PS, Canoso JJ, Wohlgethan JR. Long-term follow-up of corticosteroid injection for traumatic olecranon bursitis. Ann Rheum Dis 1984;43:44–46.
4. Fernandez DL, Jupiter JB. Fractures of the Distal Radius: A Practical Approach to Management. New York: Springer-Verlag, 1996.
5. Browner BD, Jupiter JB, Levine AM, Trafton PG, eds. Skeletal Trauma. Philadelphia: Saunders, 1998.

Foot Health for the Elderly

Considering the high prevalence of painful and debilitating foot disorders in the geriatric population, feet must be cared for so as to allow the elderly to remain ambulatory. Loss of the ability to walk may have a cascading effect on a person's self-respect, dignity, and desire to continue to contribute to society (1). The limiting factor in health and mobility for many elderly people is the condition of their feet, and appropriate foot care and treatment can prevent foot problems that lead to disability (2).

PHYSICAL EXAMINATION

In addition to a thorough history, the podiatric physical examination of the aging patient requires several areas of special attention; namely, assessment of vascular, neurologic, dermatologic, biomechanical, and musculoskeletal conditions.

VASCULAR ASSESSMENT

Prior to initiating a treatment plan for any form of podiatric disorder, the clinician must assess the level of arterial perfusion, especially in older patients. Aging is associated with a thickening of the intimal layer, along with less significant changes in the media and adventitious layers. Arterial walls stiffen and vessels elongate and become more tortuous with advancing age. The ability to perform a vascular examination is essential for a sound basis for making decisions that influence treatment options and affect outcomes. Sometimes there is enough blood flow to allow for conservative periodic trimming of an ingrown nail without consequence, but if permanent removal of the nail is attempted, the perfusion may be so tenuous that local swelling from the procedure overcomes the relatively low transluminal pressure, causing obstruction in capillary blood flow and ischemic necrosis. The need for accurate assessment of healing potential prior to initiating treatment is obvious.

In most cases, the physical examination alone yields sufficient information to assess vascular status. In borderline situations noninvasive testing may be necessary, and in others, vascular consultation and ultimately invasive angiography may be needed. Whenever there is any doubt, the wisest course of action is to seek vascular consultation before elective procedures. Exceptions occur in urgent circumstances, such as abscess formation. In the case of abscess, greater benefit may be gained by performing an immediate incision and drainage to decompress the area, limiting any additional tissue loss resulting from the effects of pressure and toxic necrosis. The elements of a vascular examination for the foot include documentation of the following: pedal pulses; capillary filling time; skin color, temperature, texture, and turgor; and elevation-dependent skin color changes and edema.

The absence of pulses is not a normal part of the aging process. The presence and quality of the dorsalis pedis and posterior tibial pulses should be documented. As in the examination of any pulse, allow for variations in anatomy and strength of the pulse by gently varying the pressure applied and by walking the fingers about the surrounding areas. The inability to palpate a pedal pulse may be because it is obscured by obesity or edema (3); also, in 10% of normal persons these pulses are absent (4). In such instances the lateral tibial artery, the terminal branch of the peroneal artery, lies inferior and medial to the lateral malleolus. The anterior tibial artery may be identified at the anterior aspect of the ankle.

Capillary filling time should be evaluated at the level of the digits. It is useful because capillary filling is the summation of the overall arterial perfusion into the toe. A delay longer than 3 seconds generally reflects diminished arterial perfusion; however, the test does not identify the level, location, or cause of the reduction in flow (5, 6). For example, a delayed refill time may be due to an organic process such as generalized atherosclerosis or atheromatous disease or to a functional abnormality such as high vasomotor tone (vasospasm, Raynaud's phenomenon). In the latter, a significant compromise in healing potential may exist even though pulses are present. The validity of this test may also be diminished by dependent rubor (6).

Rubor on dependency and pallor on elevation are serious indicators of arterial insufficiency. The foot is icy cold in patients with arterial insufficiency no matter the position of the foot. As the disease progresses, further changes affect the skin, nails, and muscles. With advanced peripheral vascular disease (PVD), the skin atrophies, becoming dry, scaly, shiny, and thin. While the absence of hair in and of itself is not specific for arterial insufficiency, the follicle is a delicate structure, and loss of hair usually mirrors the loss of arterial flow to the skin. The nails also grow more slowly and therefore thicken (6, 7). Just as the muscles may atrophy, so may the subcutaneous tissue, giving rise to the descriptive baked potato toe as the loss of resiliency on palpation to the distal aspect is noted (6).

Acute arterial occlusion is a podiatric emergency. Most acute arterial occlusions occur in the periphery because of emboli originating from the heart (atrial fibrillation, rheumatic heart disease, atherosclerotic heart disease). Other sources of emboli include ulcerated plaques from the aorta or proximal arteries or aneurysms. The presenta-

tion of acute arterial occlusion may lie along the course of a single digital artery or may be more diffuse, as in trash foot. In this condition a shower of emboli lodge in the smaller arteries of the foot, causing cyanosis, pain, and occasionally a diffuse petechial rash. A common finding is the acute onset of a dusky discoloration affecting the toes, findings that are often associated with palpable pulses (6).

The forces of gravity working against the relatively passive lymphatic and venous systems most profoundly affects the aging foot. Older patients sometimes are sedentary, and the lymphatic and venous systems rely heavily on the action of muscular pumping to facilitate proper function. Sitting compresses the venous and lymphatic vessels, raising the hydrostatic pressure at the venous side of the capillary bed. Elevated venous pressure slows the ingress of fluid back into the system, further aggravating the problem.

The elderly are likely to (*a*) have a tortuous venous system and incompetent valves, (*b*) have reduced cardiac and renal function, and (*c*) be on medications used to treat those conditions. It is no wonder that edema is such a common finding in the old patient. In addition to the local effect of edema on arterial perfusion, edema sets the stage for bacterial infection. Treatment of edema, along with elevation and compression, should address underlying causes (12).

NEUROLOGIC EXAMINATION

Balance, proprioception, muscle strength, and the protective sensory threshold are all areas of concern in evaluating the elderly patient. The challenge in evaluating the neurologic status lies in differentiating between normal deterioration associated with physiologic aging and a covert pathologic neurologic disorder. The most common clinical changes observed in the lower extremities of the aged adult are diminished Achilles reflex and vibratory sensation, decreased muscle mass and power, and compromised motor activity, including reduction in fine motor coordination and agility (9). With diminished muscle strength, flexibility, balance, and fine motor coordination, the elderly are prone to falls.

Vibratory sensation and the ability to perceive a 5.07 Semmes-Weinstein monofilament are the best means to assess the protective sensory threshold, particularly in the diabetic patient. Semmes-Weinstein monofilament devices are nylon strands available in various gauges. These filaments buckle at a reproducible force when applied at right angles to the skin. The 5.07 filament of nylon buckles when a force of 10 g is applied. The patient should be able to detect this light touch when it is applied and maintained in the buckled position for 1.5 seconds. Patients able to perceive a 5.07 Semmes-Weinstein monofilament are not likely to develop major neuropathic foot injuries (11).

BIOMECHANICS

The design requirements for a supportive device versus a mobile one are vastly different, yet the human foot must meet both of these needs. To make matters more difficult, ill-fitting or stylized footgear forces the foot to function in abnormal positions. Over the course of a lifetime, such factors have a dramatic effect on the architecture and alignment of the bones, joints, and surrounding soft tissue structures. The resulting alterations heighten the chance for acute, chronic and overuse injuries.

When the foot is pronated, the joints are unlocked or loose. This attitude is desirable only during the initial contact with the ground. It allows the foot to serve as a flexible adaptor to the terrain. It also allows for a degree of shock absorption. Beyond this stage, the foot must be more rigid to provide support and to serve as a lever across which the muscles may work efficiently to propel the body forward. It is the purpose of the supinated foot to fulfill this requirement. In this case, the bones of the foot are intrinsically locked, and the foot becomes an efficient lever. Pathology develops when the proper sequence of pronation and supination fails to occur.

Should a foot remain pronated past the contact phase of the gait cycle, muscles begin functioning out of phase, working longer and harder while attempting to provide the support that bones, joints, and ligaments were meant to provide. The patient with this type of pronated

foot is likely to develop tendinitis, shin splints, hallux valgus, and hammer toes as the dynamic balance between opposing muscle groups is disrupted. Premature fatigue and increased strain on fascial, ligamentous, and capsular tissues results as muscles attempt to propel the body forward through a yielding, flexible lever. Muscle cramping, fasciitis, and joint pain from capsulitis and synovitis develop. Ultimately degenerative joint changes may result from a lifetime of functioning in a compensated position.

Pes cavus, readily identified by a high arch, is usually associated with an inverted heel and adducted forefoot. These attitudes lend themselves to a rigid structure with impaired shock-absorbing capabilities and an increased chance of developing symptoms relating to compression. The inverted heel position is also likely to create an increased risk of lateral ankle instability and, in the elderly patient, sprains and falls.

COMMON FOOT PROBLEMS
Heel Pain

Causes of heel pain may be classified as any of the following: (*a*) inflammatory (rheumatoid and psoriatic arthritis, ankylosing spondylitis, Reiter's syndrome), (*b*) degenerative (Achilles tendinitis, retrocalcaneal bursitis, or inferior calcaneal bursitis), (*c*) nerve entrapment (medial or lateral plantar nerves, medial calcaneal nerve, tarsal tunnel syndrome, lumbosacral radiculopathy, peripheral neuropathy), (*d*) metabolic (gout, bone cyst, infection), and (*e*) traumatic and overuse syndromes (stress fractures, periostitis, plantar fasciitis) (14). In most cases of heel pain, the cause is related to heel spur syndrome or plantar fasciitis.

The typical presenting complaint of a patient with heel spur syndrome or plantar fasciitis is poststatic dyskinesia, particularly upon arising after a full night's rest. During the first steps the patient must grab objects for support and toe-walk to bear weight. Pain usually lessens or subside after a period of activity. On physical examination the pain is sharp and localized to the plantar medial aspect of the heel at the origin of the medial band of the plantar fascia. Radiographs may or may not confirm the presence of an inferior calcaneal spur (exostosis); indeed, the severity of the symptoms show little correlation with the presence or size of the exostosis.

The primary cause of this painful syndrome is believed to be biomechanical. The plantar fascia acts as nature's bowstring as it springs up the arch. Even under normal conditions the arch is under considerable tension, as it provides up to 25% of the strength of the longitudinal arch. Any factor that results in increased pressure on the arch adds to the tensile strain on the fascia. Weight gain, the diminution of elastin, atrophy of the plantar fat pad, reduced muscle mass, and diminished fidelity of the capsular and ligamentous structures that support the arch are also factors that predispose the older person to this condition.

Increased strain on the plantar fascia leads to a repetitive microavulsion injury at the proximal attachment of the fascia. The result is a local reparative process and an inflammatory response that causes the pain. Treatment must address the inflammation as well as the mechanical cause of pain. There are various alternatives. Primary care providers should initiate care with analgesics or nonsteroidal anti-inflammatory drugs (NSAIDs) as tolerated by the patient. Rest, ice, and flexibility and stretching exercises should be performed twice daily. Patients may derive great benefit from actively dorsiflexing the toes and ankle prior getting out of bed or upon attempting to bear weight after resting. Over-the-counter appliances such as Spenco Polysorb Orthotics and appropriate shoes should be tried. For exercise a good quality walking specialty shoe is mandatory. The shoe qualities desirable for daily use include a rigid shank, stiff heel counter, and when possible, an elevated heel. Sponge or foam heel cups and cushions usually offer little value for the relief of pain associated with plantar fasciitis, although they usually prove helpful for periostitis and inferior calcaneal bursitis.

Sometimes prefabricated supports are adequate to address problems related to abnormal mechanics. These devices may offer some shock absorption but very little in terms of support or control. For a mildly pronated foot or the minimally active older adult, a prefabricated appliance may be helpful. Over-the-counter appliances offer a good starting point and if nothing else provide a basis for evaluation as to the potential for response to a more costly custom orthosis.

Should these conservative measures fail, podiatric referral for local infiltration with a steroid, strappings, and orthotic devices are indicated. I have found that infiltration with betamethasone 4 mg in combination with lidocaine 10 mg through a medial approach is a safe way to administer this injection. One should avoid the more direct but painful route of plantar injection. Additional remedies include strappings, external splints such as a removable short leg immobilizer, and sometimes even fiberglass cast immobilization. Careful consideration must be given before immobilizing older persons because of the adverse sequelae that may result from an altered gait, not to mention the increased risk of falls, deep venous thrombosis, and muscular atrophy. Night splints are a worthwhile alternative to full-time immobilization. Only when conservative measures have been exhausted should surgical intervention be considered. This may take the form of endoscopic or open plantar fascial release or resection of the exostosis.

Tendinitis (Tenosynovitis, Peritendinitis)

In addition to collagen-vascular diseases and inflammatory arthropathies, trauma and repetitive stress expose tendons to injury. The most challenging types of tendinitis affecting the foot involve stance phase tendons such as the posterior tibial and the Achilles. These are difficult to resolve because the tendons are constantly battling the opposing force of gravity. The result is excessive tension on the tendon that leads to stretching and tearing followed by the reparative inflammatory response and pain. Adhesions may develop and limit the free flow of the tendon within its sheath (15). Persistence of these unchecked forces may lead to an attenuation or stretching of the tendon and eventual deformation and rupture.

In posterior tibial tendinitis the clinical presentation may include the subjective complaint of arch or ankle pain. Inspection reveals local warmth and tenderness at the insertion of the tendon to the navicular or extending proximally to the medial malleolus. Pain can also be reproduced by having the patient attempt to invert the foot against resistance. Chronic tenosynovitis can progress to fibrosis and scarring within the tendon sheath and eventually a limitation of motion. A plain radiograph readily identifies an accessory ossicle or bony hypertrophy of the navicular as well as dystrophic calcification of the tendon sheath. Magnetic resonance imaging (MRI) is not usually necessary unless a partial tear or rupture is suspected. Complete rupture can be strongly suspected if the patient has a newly acquired flatfoot.

Early treatment for tendinitis may include NSAIDs, rest, ice, contrast baths, and gentle stretching. In moderate cases modification to shoes and orthoses along with physical therapy may be necessary. For advanced cases, immobilization with removable ankle stirrup stabilizers or cast immobilization may be considered. The judicious use of steroids in combination with a local anesthetic may be considered in severe cases but should be accompanied by a protective immobilizer to reduce the chance of rupture while protective pain is blocked. Often the mere introduction of a local anesthetic into the sheath has the mechanical effect of breaking up adhesions. Rarely is surgery necessary, although it may be used to prevent the tendon from further degenerative changes that may result in rupture (15, 16).

Hammer Toes

Perhaps the most common pedal deformity is the hammer toe. This is a sagittal plane deformity, a dorsally positioned proximal phalanx and a plantarly contracted middle phalanx. It may affect one or more toes. Often believed to be related to ill-fitting shoes or short hose, the overwhelming majority have been found to have a biomechanical origin, loss of the stabilizing forces of the interossei and lumbricales muscles. Metabolic conditions such as rheumatoid arthritis and diabetes mellitus may result in atrophy of the intrinsic muscles of the foot. The ensuing disruption of tendon balance across the metatarsophalangeal (MTP) joint may likewise result in hammer toe formation.

Treatment is required when symptoms develop, usually in the form of local irritation from shoes. Initially, friction may cause blisters, and eventually continued shear forces applied over the skin result in the formation of painful hyperkeratotic lesions. Patients may use files or emery boards to remove excessive keratosis followed by the application of over-the-counter pads. These should be limited to unmedicated aperture pads, avoiding those that contain salicylic acid plasters. A considerable level of palliative relief may be achieved with professional debridement with a disposable number 20 scalpel blade on a number 4 handle. This can be accomplished with a gentle touch and no anesthetic.

Eventually, an exquisitely painful adventitious bursa may form below the lesion, confirmed by pain that is greater with indirect than direct palpation. At this point simple trimming and padding are inadequate. Sublesional infiltration with dexamethasone phosphate 1 mg in combination with lidocaine 5 mg with a 25-gauge needle on a tuberculin syringe yields significant relief.

In the aged patient the deformity may progress to a ulcerative process and even osteomyelitis, as this population is less likely to inspect or reach the affected toe or even perceive the pain that is associated with the early presentation. Additional recommendations include avoidance of constrictive shoes and possibly the purchase of footgear with a deep toe box or depth inlay oxfords. Many of the better-quality walking shoes have thick insole liners that can be removed to allow added room in the toe box. Developing a relationship with a local specialty shoe store is a good way to get service.

Recalcitrant deformities require surgical intervention. The procedures are varied, depending on whether the deformity is rigid, semirigid, or flexible, as well as on the underlying cause and medical status of the patient. The choices may range from a simple tenotomy or tendon transfer to arthroplasty and fusion. Rarely is digital amputation required.

Hallux Valgus

The cause of hallux valgus includes many of the same factors as that of hammer toe deformity. Excessive pronation removes the natural fulcrum effect that the cuboid provides for the peroneus longus tendon. This loss means the tendon cannot stabilize the first ray. Under load, the first metatarsal elevates and deviates medially, causing the hallux to drift laterally. The associated widening of the foot brings the first metatarsal head into a position of prominence. This results in additional shoe pressure and inflammatory changes to the overlying skin and soft tissue structures about the first metatarsal head, forming a common bunion. When these same findings are present at the lateral aspect of the fifth metatarsal head, the condition is called a tailor's bunion. In addition to bump pain, the first metatarsophalangeal joint itself may be the source of arthritic or joint pain. When range of motion is restricted, the condition is called hallux limitus, and when the toe is ankylosed, hallux rigidus. Treatment is similar to that for hammer toes.

Metatarsalgia

The term *metatarsalgia* is a description, not a diagnosis. Metatarsalgia comprises multiple maladies that affect the forefoot. These include plantar keratomas, plantar and intermetatarsal bursitis, synovitis, capsulitis, arthritis, neuroma, and anything else that may cause pain in the metatarsal region. All five metatarsals should function evenly across the transverse plane. Should one of the metatarsals be excessively long or plantigrade, it will bear more weight per time per step, leading to pressure related changes. For the elderly patient, symptoms may be secondary to loss or atrophy of the underlying metatarsal fat pad, plantar keratomas, bursitis, and so on. Similar difficulties are likely to develop adjacent to metatarsals that are excessively short or elevated. Debridement of plantar keratomas along with padding, shoe modifications, and orthotic devices is the recommended treatment. Conservative options are preferred, as surgical procedures that elevate plantarly prominent metatarsals may result in a shift of weight to an adjacent metatarsal, forming a new transfer lesion.

Morton's neuroma, intermetatarsal neuroma, and interdigital neuroma are synonyms for what is commonly called neuroma. The symptoms develop as a result of repetitive irritation of a common digital nerve. The accepted belief is that as the nerve courses below the deep transverse plantar metatarsal ligament, impingement occurs as pressure from the weight-bearing surface below compresses the nerve against the ligament above. This is compounded by shearing and compression forces from adjacent metatarsal heads, which occurs during the push-off stage of walking (17). High heels place further traction on the nerve, accentuating compression against the ligament along with side to side compression of the metatarsal heads. (18) Eventually a degenerative process including vascular congestion, edema, and perineural fibrosis results in enlargement of the nerve (19).

Diagnosis is based on clinical findings. The classic subjective description includes a clicking sensation accompanied by a sharp, excruciating, burning pain radiating from the plantar aspect of the third interspace into the third and fourth toes. This may also be associated with numbness of those digits. The pain occurs with weight bearing and walking and may be relieved by removing the shoes and massaging the foot.

Examination reveals pain and a palpable click (Mulder's click) with plantar pressure to the third interspace. This may or may not be associated with a reproduction of paresthesias into either of the affected digits. Manual compression of the forefoot by squeezing the first and fifth metatarsal heads together may also duplicate the symptoms. While the third interspace is most commonly affected, the condition less frequently affects the second or fourth spaces. Special diagnostic studies are not usually necessary, although standard radiographs should be obtained to rule out osseous or articular abnormalities, which may be considered in the differential diagnosis. Space-occupying or soft tissue masses within the interspace must also be ruled out.

Intermetatarsal bursitis is an inflammatory process that occurs between two adjacent metatarsal heads, presumably as a response to the excessive transverse plane motion of the forefoot resulting from excessive pronation. The symptoms may mimic intermetatarsal neuroma. Normally there are no associated paresthesias, but at times, if the inflammation is severe enough, a secondary neuritis may result.

Both intermetatarsal neuroma and bursitis may show a favorable response to infiltration of the interspace with a steroid (dexamethasone acetate or phosphate 1 to 2 mg) spaced 1 to 2 weeks apart depending on the patient's response. Since adverse sequelae such as atrophy of the plantar fat pad and weakening or loss of the attachment of the intrinsic insertions may result from excessive use of local steroids, this method should be limited to three injections. Flat shoes with thick rubber soles offer the best chance for relief. An alternative is the application of special pads or the insertion of a cushioned insole. Orthotic devices may be considered prior to surgical intervention, but for certain foot types they may actually worsen the condition by taking up room in the shoe. Neurectomy or surgical decompression should be performed when conservative treatment fails.

Exostosis

The extra-articular and periarticular manifestations of osteoarthritis are common in the elderly. They include the formation of hypertrophic bone at and about various joints. This new bone forms in response to excessive loading or motion across a joint. Pedal manifestations result from pressure and irritation from foot gear. Common areas of involvement include the dorsal aspect of the first metatarsophalangeal joint (dorsal bunion), first metatarsocuneiform joint (saddle bump deformity), posterior calcaneus (Haglund's deformity), and the medial and lateral aspects of the interphalangeal joints (similar to Heberden's nodes in the fingers). These spurs cause pressure-related problems, including the formation of painful hyperkeratotic lesions, bursitis, and ulcerations. They are treated through the avoidance of shoe pressure, or with pads, debridement, and surgical planing of the prominences.

The Diabetic Foot

Of the 120,000 nontraumatic amputations performed in the United States annually, 45 to 83% are diabetes related. In 40% of these cases the underlying cause is related not to ischemia but to neuropathy (20). Since neuropathy alone cannot lead to amputation, better screening and education of high-risk patients is needed to re-

duce this number. A recent 4-year study found that of a group of 255 patients admitted for the treatment of infected diabetic ulcerations, pedal pulses were not documented in 31.4% of the cases. The protective sensory threshold was not evaluated in 54.7% of admissions. These findings indicate that the infected diabetic foot is not properly evaluated on inpatients (21). Obviously, providers as well as patients need education if progress is to be made in reducing the number of lower extremity amputations.

Any attempt to treat a pedal ulceration must be deferred until an appropriate neurovascular and biomechanical examination has been performed. Adequate arterial perfusion must be established if not already present. The source of excessive pressure must be removed, particularly for the insensate patient. Infection must also be eliminated and the blood glucose controlled if one is to hope to gain closure of a diabetic ulcer (22). The existence or persistence of any of these elements may delay or prevent closure or result in recurrence.

Infection

In the absence of leukocytosis and systemic findings such as fever, chills, rigors, or malaise, the decision to treat an ulcer for infection should be based on local clinical findings. Erythema, swelling, drainage, odor, and pain are far better indicators of infection than identification of bacteria grown from a surface culture of an ulcer. It is expected that bacteria will be found on an open wound, but this does not confirm infection. A positive culture may be considered significant and requiring treatment when there are associated clinical findings. The assessment may be more difficult in the diabetic, in whom neuropathy, angiopathy, and a reduced immune response may obscure some of these important signs. When a wound fails to heal despite glycemic control, non-weight bearing, and adequate arterial perfusion, one should suspect infection. At this point, consideration should be given to obtaining a valid culture. Obtaining a valid culture can be achieved only by thoroughly debriding the wound, scrubbing away superficial contaminants, and obtaining a deep specimen. Should the wound still fail to improve despite appropriate antibiotics, non-weight bearing, and adequate arterial perfusion, deep infection or osteomyelitis should be suspected.

Osteomyelitis

Radiographs lag behind the clinical infection and may offer little value in diagnosing acute osteomyelitis. To further confuse matters, noninfective diabetic osteopathy may mimic osteomyelitis on radiograph, particularly when associated with an overlying ulceration. The most cost-effective and definitive means to diagnose osteomyelitis is bone biopsy, which can usually be performed under local anesthesia. A specimen of bone is removed from a separate incision so as to avoid contamination of the specimen from the wound. The biopsy may take one of two forms: diagnostic, in which a small specimen of bone is removed via needle biopsy, or definitive, in which an entire section of suspected bony involvement is resected. Specimens are submitted for histologic examination, culture, and sensitivity. Appropriate treatment can be based on accurate culture information. One must also be aware that biopsy is an invasive procedure and may be contraindicated in patients with PVD. For these patients, special noninvasive nuclear imaging techniques may be more appropriate.

Osteomyelitis Versus Diabetic Neuropathic Osteoarthropathy

Diabetic neuropathic osteoarthropathy (DNOA) is the broad description given to various disorders affecting the musculoskeletal system of the diabetic patient with peripheral autonomic, sensory, and motor neuropathy. DNOA includes diabetic osteolysis (both focal and diffuse), and Charcot joint disease. The clinical and radiographic appearance is often difficult to differentiate from infectious processes such as osteomyelitis. Presentation of a diabetic with an acutely swollen, red, and painful foot must be carefully evaluated. An acute Charcot joint may account for the symptoms. The acute Charcot foot requires immobilization and non-weight bearing, while the osteomyelitic foot requires antibiotics and possibly surgery. In the case of the insensate patient with an acute onset of an erythematous,

swollen, and sometimes painful foot, it is prudent to initiate treatment with non–weight bearing and antibiotics. If the condition fails to improve, one must consider DNOA in the differential diagnosis.

Bone scans are sensitive for detecting areas of increased bone metabolism, but they also are nonspecific, making it impossible to differentiate osteomyelitis from DNOA (23, 24). White blood cell (WBC) labeled scans (technetium-99m hexamethylpropyleneamine oxime [HMPAO] and indium-111) are much more specific for infection and therefore quite helpful in differentiating osteomyelitis from DNOA, although false-positive and false-negative findings may still occur. Active bleeding into a joint (in cases of acute DNOA), and incomplete labeling of the WBCs may lead to a false-positive and false-negative result respectively. When taking cost into account, the more sensitive three-phase bone scan may be used for initial screening. The more expensive WBC scanning can then be performed only if a positive test is identified on bone scanning. This sequence can reduce the need for more expensive WBC scanning by up to 50% (25). Cases that demonstrate positive studies in both the third phase of the bone scan and the WBC scan are compatible with osteomyelitis. DNOA is suspected when the bone scan is positive while the WBC scan is negative.

In the study of Newman et al. (23), 35 patients with 41 foot ulcers were followed. Radiographs, bone scans, and indium-111 WBC scans were compared with bone biopsy and culture. The study found that osteomyelitis was present below 68% of ulcers not exposing bone. Osteomyelitis was confirmed in all ulcers in which bone was exposed. In considering the risks of bone biopsy in ulcers that do not expose bone, they concluded that WBC scanning should be performed to diagnose osteomyelitis.

Treatment of Recurrent Ulceration

Patients with ulcers that have been determined to have an ischemic origin should be referred for revascularization. Once the ulcer has healed, causative bony deformities, such as bunions and hammer toes, may usually be surgically corrected. If adequate vascular supply cannot be reestablished, amputation at a level that will heal may be the only option. This is not the usual case in patients with neuropathic ulcerations, particularly those with an autonomic neuropathy. These persons have a loss of sympathetic tone resulting in vasodilation and increased blood flow. With the increase in blood flow to bone, demineralization causes a loss of resiliency. Taken in combination with insensitivity, bones and joints undergo massive destructive (Charcot) changes, including fracture, dislocation, and fragmentation (26). Early diagnosis and treatment are necessary to prevent collapse of the foot. Whether a neuropathic ulcer results from pressure due to a simple bony prominence or is the sequela of a gross deformity caused by destructive Charcot joint disease, the challenge in these patients is not so much obtaining closure but maintaining that closure.

In performing surgery on the diabetic foot, one must consider the effects of weight transfer in the creation of new lesions. For this reason it is important to reduce pressure through conservative means first. This can usually be accomplished through off-loading techniques, including total contact casts, short leg immobilizers, splints, crutches, walkers, wheelchairs, orthotic devices, balance padding, depth inlay, and custom-molded shoes. Should conservative treatment fail, surgical treatment of the high-risk deformity should not be held back from the well-controlled diabetic. "Failure to remove the source of the lesion is more dangerous than the judicious use of surgery to correct a deformity and relieve bony pressure" (27).

Instructing the Patient

The dividends received from the time spent in instructing patients are well worth the effort, especially for patients with diabetes. The intensity of instruction a diabetic patient has received about the disease is highly correlated with the development of foot lesions (28, 29). Patients should understand the importance of foot hygiene, appropriate footgear, styles, and fit. At least a daily inspection is needed for early detection of foot lesions. If identified, lesions require professional assessment. The patient should demonstrate an understanding of the role that insensitivity and

vascular insufficiency have in the development of serious complications affecting the lower extremities. Excellent printed materials for patients are available from the American Podiatric Medical Association, 9312 Old Georgetown Road, Bethesda, MD 20814-1621; 301-571-9200; or visit their website at http://www.apma.org.

DERMATOLOGIC EVALUATION

Cutaneous manifestations in the aging foot include changes that affect every function of the skin, with particular reference to its mechanical, thermoregulation, and microbial protective functions. Some of these problems are due to diminished vascular perfusion to the epidermis, dermis, and skin adnexa (30). In patients with autonomic neuropathy, similar diminished perfusion can be expected as blood is shunted through arteriovenous connections in the microcirculation (31). Mechanical protective function is affected as dermal thickness decreases, which in association with atrophy of the subcutaneous fat, provides less absorption and dissipation of shock. Sebaceous gland activity decreases. The reduced secretion of sebum accounts for the dryness of the skin of the elderly, leading to cracks or fissures offering a portal for bacterial invasion.

Decreased adhesion at the dermal epidermal junction between the rete ridges and pegs makes the skin susceptible to trauma. The epidermis sloughs easily in response to the shearing forces commonly encountered by the foot. An open wound is poorly defended by polymorphonuclear neutrophils, whose capacity for chemotaxis and phagocytosis is reduced. The older patient in particular becomes prone to infection by the gram-positive and gram-negative bacteria that normally colonize the skin (32). Fungi are particularly immune to the body's defenses because of the lack of skin sensitivity and reduced antigen-antibody response.

Fungal Infections of the Skin and Nails

As already described, a reduced host defense system allows for the increased susceptibility to opportunistic bacterial and fungal skin and nail infections. Until recently, fungal infections affecting the foot were thought to be limited to one of three dermatophytes: *Trichophyton, Microsporum,* or *Epidermophyton.* Formerly believed to be nonpathogenic, saprophytes are now implicated as the cause of 45 to 55% of fungal infections of the foot and nails. Podiatric Pathology Laboratory in Baltimore has performed two studies of 700 cases each, finding that in fungal infections involving the skin and nails of the foot, 55% were nondermatophyte or mixed fungal infection. Only 30% of fungal infections were found to be caused by dermatophytes in patients over age 45, in contrast to cultures from persons under age 40, more than 70% of whom had dermatophytic infection (Steven J Berlin, personal communication, 1997). This study is important because if these infections are treated with systemic antidermatophytic agents based on clinical appearance, one would expect a 55% failure rate. Only through culture and identification of the infecting agent can an appropriate antifungal be selected (32).

T. mentagrophytes often is the organism accounting for the acute presentation of tinea pedis as it affects the skin. This infection results in pruritus, maceration, erythema, and vesicles to the web spaces, digital sulcus, and non-weight-bearing surfaces of the sole of the foot. The more chronic form, presenting with asymptomatic dry scales and diffuse erythema in a moccasin distribution, is primarily attributed to *T. rubrum.*

Cutaneous manifestations can be treated with the application of a topical antifungal cream. Over-the-counter preparations such as clotrimazole (Lotrimin), miconazole (Micatin), and tolnaftate (Tinactin) are good first line choices. Resistant or recurrent infections often require the newer topical prescription antifungals, such as terbinafine (Lamisil) and itraconazole (Spectazole). These are very effective against dermatophytes, itraconazole being effective against yeast as well. Onychomycosis presents with four patterns: white superficial scaling, distal subungual, proximal subungual, and *Candida albicans.* With the exception of the white superficial scaling form, the response to local care is quite poor.

Failure of a skin infection to respond, or the presence of a symptomatic toe nail infection, may indicate the need for systemic treatment. Understanding the organism and the available

oral antifungals is important to effect a cure. A knowledge of the drugs used to treat fungal infections systemically is critical to prevent side effects and possible drug interactions. A positive fungal culture (identification of a sensitive dermatophyte or saprophyte) should be obtained along with a liver function study as a baseline prior to oral drug therapy with antifungal agents.

Itraconazole (Sporanox) may be or is commonly best prescribed in a pulsed dose: two 100-mg capsules twice a day for a week followed by 3 weeks off and repeat the cycle 3 times for toenail infections. Pulsed treatment for the skin is approved by the U.S. Food and Drug Administration (FDA), but even though common practice studies show pulsed treatment to be effective for nails, it has not yet been approved by the FDA. For skin infections, only a single week of therapy is required. Itraconazole is a broad-spectrum agent covering the dermatophytes, yeasts, and some saprophytes. Lamisil is more specific for dermatophytes; the regimen is one 250-mg capsule daily for a month for skin infection and at least 3 months for toenail infection. Improvement is noted in a short period for skin infections and longer for nail infection (6 to 12 months).

Hyperkeratosis, Xerosis, and Fissuring

Hyperkeratosis, or hypertrophy of the stratum corneum, may result from primary hereditary causes. More commonly, as is the case in podiatric presentations, hyperkeratosis is secondary to pressure or irritation (33). A thickened horny layer forms as the skin and subcutaneous tissue become impinged between the footgear and the underlying bone. The result is pain, and continued pressure may lead to adventitious bursa formation and ulceration. The dryness that is common to the aging foot is often exacerbated during winter, when the humidity is low, particularly in environments warmed by forced hot air. Frequent soaks and bathing also contribute to the pruritus associated with xerosis (30).

The formation of hyperkeratotic and xerotic skin about the margins of the foot, such as at the rim of the heel or the plantar medial aspect of the first metatarsal joint, are prone to fissuring. This dry, thickened layer of skin offers very little resilience to the forces encountered during walking. As pressure is applied during walking, the underlying subcutaneous tissue deforms and changes its shape to dissipate the load. The overlying brittle layer of skin is not supple enough to change its shape, causing the skin to crack. The crack acts as a stress riser as it focuses the forces that are shuttling back and forth across the skin to convene and tear the underlying tissue. The resulting fissure typically is painful and does not heal easily. Treatment entails removal of the hyperkeratotic and xerotic skin either mechanically (sharp debridement, electric sanding) or with keratolytics (10% salicylic acid with occlusion). (Keratolytics should be avoided in patients with diabetes, PVD, or open wounds). Topical antibiotic ointments can then be applied to the open areas, as much for the moisturizing as the antibacterial effect. Once healed, the patient should file the area regularly and keep the skin moisturized. Lactic acid- and urea-containing compounds (Lac-Hydrin 12% lotion and Ureacin cream) work especially well in hydrating the corneum, particularly when used in combination with a heel cup.

SUMMARY

This chapter examined the foot of the older patient and reviewed the presentation and treatment of common problems. An appreciation for the patient's overall health and activities, as well as the level of mobility, is necessary to determine the level of intervention most appropriate to restore that particular patient to an optimal level of function.

REFERENCES

1. Assessment of the geriatric patient. Clin Podiatr Med Surg 1993;10:47–57.
2. Crawford VL, Ashford RL, McPeake B, Stout RW. Conservative podiatric medicine and disability in elderly people. J Am Podiatr Med Assoc 1995;85:255–259.
3. Brewster DC. Evaluation of arterial insufficiency of the lower extremities. In: Goroll AH, May LA, Mulley AG, eds. Primary Care Medicine. 2nd ed. Philadelphia: Lippincott, 1987:74–75.
4. Rutherford RB. The surgical approach to vascular problems. In: Johnson, Kempczinski, Moore, et al. Vascular Surgery. Philadelphia: Saunders, 1989:1–16.
5. Bates B, Bickey LS, Hoekelmam RA, eds. Physical Examination and History Taking. 6th ed. Philadelphia: Lippincott, 1995.
6. Harkless LB, Dennis KJ. Role of the podiatrist. In: Levin ME, ed. The Diabetic Foot. St. Louis: Mosby 1992:507–530.
7. Whittemore AD, Donaldson MC, Mannick JA. Intermittent claudication. In: Branch WT, ed. Office Practice Medicine. 3rd ed. Philadelphia: Saunders, 1994:124–138.
8. Snow DA. Medical management. In: Abrahms C, McCarthy DJ, Rupp MJ, eds. Infectious Diseases of the Lower Extremities. Baltimore: Williams & Wilkins, 1991:331–339.
9. Katzman R, Terry RD. The Neurology of Aging. Philadelphia: Davis, 1983.
10. Weber GA, Cardile MA. Neurologic manifestations in the lower extremity in elderly persons. Clin Podiatr Med Surg 1993;10:161–178.
11. Birke JA, Sims DS. Plantar sensory threshold in the ulcerative foot. Lepr Rev 1986;57:261–267.
12. Snow DA. Medical management. In: Abrahams C, McCarthy DJ, Rupp MJ, eds. Infectious Diseases in the Lower Extremities. Baltimore: Williams & Wilkins, 1991;331–339.
13. Valmassy RL. The aging athlete. Podiatr Manage 1997:49–51.
14. Kwong PK, Kay D, Voner RT, et al. Plantar fasciitis: mechanics and pathomechanics of treatment. Clin Sports Med 1988;7:23.
15. Perlman M. Chronic ankle conditions. In: McGlamery ED, Banks AS, Downey MS, eds. Comprehensive Textbook of Foot Surgery. 2nd ed. Baltimore: Williams & Wilkins, 1992:989–1026.
16. Supple KM, Hanft JR, Janecki CJ. Posterior tibial tendon dysfunction. Semin Arthritis Rheum 1992;22:106–113.
17. Trevino S, Gould N, Korson R. Surgical treatment of stenosing tenosynovitis at the ankle. Foot Ankle 1981;2:37–45.
18. Wu KK. Morton's interdigital neuroma; a clinical review of its etiology, treatment, and results. J Foot Ankle Surg 1996;35:112–119.
19. Goldman F. Intermetatarsal neuroma: light microscopic observations. J Am Podiatr Assoc 1979;69:317–324.
20. Armstrong DG, Lavery LA, Harkless LB, Van Houtum WH. Amputation and reamputation of the diabetic foot. J Am Podiatr Med Assoc 1997;87:255–259.
21. Edelson GW, Armstrong DG, Lavery LA, Caicco G. The acutely infected diabetic foot is not adequately evaluated in an inpatient setting. J Am Podiatr Med Assoc 1997;87:260–265.
22. Habershaw GM, Lyons TE. Foot health for the elderly. In: Reichel W, ed. Care of the Elderly. 4th ed. Baltimore: Williams & Wilkins, 1995:356–364.
23. Newman LG, Waller J, Palestro CJ, et al. Unsuspected osteomyelitis in diabetic foot ulcers. Diagnosis and monitoring by leukocyte scanning with indium-111 oxyquinoline. JAMA 1991;226:1246–1251.
24. Harvey J, Cohen MM. Technetium-99-labeled leukocytes in diagnosing diabetic osteomyelitis in the foot. J Foot Ankle Surg 1997;36:209–214.

25. Copping C, Dalgliesh SM, Dudley NJ, et al. The role of ^{99} mTc-HMPAO white cell imaging in suspected orthopaedic infection. Br J Radiol 1992;65:309–312.

26. Giurini JM, Chrzan JS, Gibbons GW, Habershaw GM. Charcot's disease in diabetic patients. Correct diagnosis can prevent progressive deformity. Postgrad Med 1991; 89:163–169.

27. Catanzariti AR, Blitch EL, Karlock LG. Elective foot and ankle surgery in the diabetic patient. J Foot Ankle Surg 1995;34:23–41.

28. Delbridge L, Appleberg M, Reeve TS. Factors associated with development of foot lesions in the diabetic. Surgery 1983;93:78–82.

29. LoGerfo FW, Coffman JD. Current concepts. Vascular and microvascular disease of the foot in diabetes. Implications for foot care. N Engl J Med 1984;311:1615–1619.

30. Schiraldi FG. Common dermatologic manifestations in the older patient. Clin Podiatr Med Surg 1993;10:79–95.

31. Arora S, LoGerfo FW. Lower extremity macrovascular disease in diabetes. J Am Podiatr Med Assoc 1997;87:327–331.

32. Abramson C. Infection in the older patient. Clin Pod Med Surg 1993;10:249–269.

33. Domonkos AN, ed. Andrew's Diseases of the Skin. Philadelphia: Saunders, 1971.

The Endocrinology of Aging

ENDOCRINOLOGY OF AGING

Age-related physiologic changes, as well as those engendered by disease, have a major effect on the endocrine system. The delineation between health and disease states is not always clear-cut with aging. Aging of the endocrine system results in hormone levels that would be abnormal or borderline normal in a young adult, and these alterations from a youthful state may lead to a further decline of that person. Nor do changes in hormones necessarily occur at the same rate in all endocrine glands and their target tissues in an aging person. The synchronization or rhythmicity of glandular function and the concentration of the glandular output undergo age-related alterations. The loss of functional reserve that is seen with age is associated with an increased prevalence of endocrine deficiency diseases, such as hypothyroidism, hypogonadism, and diabetes. This chapter discusses the clinical implications and ramifications of the age-related alterations of the endocrine system.

The endocrine-deficient states may mimic other age-related changes or be nonspecific and thus may be misdiagnosed or missed altogether. For example, weight gain, cold intolerance, constipation, dry skin, hypercholesterolemia, and fatigue may be seen with aging per se as well as hypothyroidism. Apathetic hyperthyroidism may lead to delayed diagnosis of that disorder. Furthermore, complicating factors, such as concomitant disease that can alter hormone levels, such is as seen with euthyroid sick syndrome, can make evaluation and diagnosis of the older adult a true challenge.

HYPOTHALAMUS AND PITUITARY GLAND

While the pituitary gland may decrease in size with age from the maximal size of middle age, autopsy data suggest little change in pituitary weight (1, 2). Age-related fibrosis, diminished vascularity, and cyst formation occur. Magnetic resonance imaging (MRI) data reveal an increased frequency of empty sella (19%) but with no relation to pituitary size, volume, or basal anterior pituitary hormone concentration (3). This latter study found that posterior pituitary signals on T1-weighted MRI could not be detected in 29% of older subjects. This may be related to the depletion of neurosecretory granules due to the release of vasopressin in response to higher osmolarity seen in older adults.

The response of adrenocorticotropic hormone (ACTH) and cortisol to corticotropin-releasing hormone appears to be unimpaired by aging; however, sensitivity to glucocorticoid feedback is decreased with age and with delayed and blunted response of ACTH with cortisol administration (4). Diminished luteinizing hormone (LH) response to gonadotropin-releasing hormone (GnRH) has been found in older men, along with increased sensitivity to feedback inhibition of LH by testosterone (5). Age-related decreases in growth hormone-releasing hormone (GHRH) synthesis with release or binding to somatotrophs has been identified as one of the factors contributing to defective growth hormone secretion in older adults (6). The response to GHRH administration is also impaired with increasing age, though the response of growth hormone to insulin hypoglycemia is blunted in some older adults. Table 36.1 shows some common effects of aging on hormones.

ANTERIOR PITUITARY GLAND
Growth Hormone

Although basal levels of growth hormone may not alter dramatically, there is a well-recognized decrease in 24-hour growth hormone secretion and one of its mediators, insulinlike growth factor I (IGF-1) with age (7, 8). By age 70 to 80, about 50% of persons have no significant growth hormone secretion at night. The decrease in growth hormone tends to occur near age 40 in men and about a decade later in women. Factors other than age per se, such as obesity and hyperglycemia, also tend to affect growth hormone secretion.

Growth hormone deficiency with aging ("somatopause") has been implicated in changes in body composition with age, decreased lean body mass, increased body fat, and decreased muscle and bone mass. Growth hormone administration in older men has been associated with increased lean body mass and thicker skin but also with carpal tunnel syndrome, fluid retention, and gynecomastia (8–10). In malnourished elderly, the short-term administration of growth hormone increased body weight and midarm circumference and was associated with decreased urinary nitrogen loss, thus sparing protein (11). It is clear that further analysis of short- versus long-term administration of growth hormone, GHRH, their

Table 36.1

Aging and Hormones

Pituitary GH	Basal GH	N,↓↓
	24-hr secretion	↓↓
Prolactin	Basal	N,↑
TSH	Basal	N,↑
	Response to TRH	↑
ACTH	Basal	N
	Response to metyrapone	↑
	Response to hypoglycemia	↑
	Response to dexamethasone	↓
Gonadotropins	Basal LH (males)	N,↑
	Basal FSH	N,↑
	Response to GnRH	↓
AVP	Basal	?↑
	Response to stimuli	↑

analogues, and the risks and benefits should be ascertained.

Prolactin

There is a slight but significant increase in prolactin with increasing age (12). A small increase in prolactin response to thyrotropin-releasing hormone (TRH) also increases in prevalence with age (13). Whether this is directly due to the decreased dopaminergic activity seen with aging is unclear. In older adults, hyperprolactinemia may also be seen with diabetes, with renal dysfunction, and with the use of phenothiazines and H_2-blockers. The significance of these altered levels of prolactin is unclear. Elevations of prolactin are associated with decreased sex steroid production and diminished libido in both genders and perhaps with altered regulation of osmolality.

Thyroid-Stimulating Hormone

Sawin et al. (14) found 2.7% of elderly men and 7.1% of elderly women have thyroid-stimulating hormone (TSH) levels greater than 10 IU/L, perhaps indicating the verge of hypothyroidism. In the main, basal TSH does not undergo any marked change with age (15). Occasionally, levels of TSH that might be consistent with hyperthyroidism in young persons can be found in older adults, yet these persons are *not* hyperthyroid, and such overlap can cause confusion in the interpretation of thyroid tests (16). While a flat or diminished TSH response has been found with TRH administration in aging men and women, this can also be seen in the face of depression, fasting, nonthyroidal illness, uremia, and hypothalamic-pituitary dysfunction (17, 18). A normal response to TRH will rule out hyperthyroidism.

Adrenocorticotropic Hormone

No significant change in ACTH or the response to secretagogues occurs with aging. If anything, corticotropin-releasing factor, hypoglycemia, and metyrapone may elicit a higher and prolonged response in older adults than in younger persons (19). An ACTH stimulation test to assess adrenal insufficiency has a response unchanged by age. However, dexamethasone causes less ACTH suppression in older adults. Blunting of β-endorphin rhythmicity as well as lower levels in the cerebrospinal fluid (CSF) can be seen with age (20).

Male Gonadotropins

Although many past studies have shown an increase in LH and FSH with age in males, these studies have been reevaluated in light of other studies that have shown them to be normal (i.e., *not* elevated level of LH in response to low testosterone and bioavailable testosterone concentrations) (21–24). The sensitivity of the hypothalamic-pituitary axis to exogenous hormones rises, with testosterone suppressing LH to a greater extent in older rather than younger men (25). LH pulse characteristics also appear to change with age, with an apparent alteration of both amplitude and frequency (26). Bioactive LH may be variable, as studies have reported both high and low values. Longitudinal data have shown that nearly 50% of men have elevated LH concentrations over the course of a 14-year study (27). While LH appeared to rise above the upper limit of normal primarily in the oldest old, only 10% of subjects developed elevated LH concentrations over the course of the study.

Female Gonadotropins

In postmenopausal women, both LH and FSH increase in response to decreased ovarian estradiol and estrone concentrations. FSH increases to a far greater extent than LH (26). Illness may dramatically reduce FSH and LH levels and alter the response to GnRH (27). In the absence of illness, an exuberant rise of hormones in response to GnRH can be found in postmenopausal women because of the loss of negative feedback of ovarian hormones. Furthermore, the decrease in estrogen at menopause may be associated with decreased opioid inhibition of the GnRH response and/or decreased central nervous system (CNS) dopaminergic activity (28).

Posterior Pituitary Arginine Vasopressin

Altered fluid status is common in older adults, and arginine vasopressin (AVP) has a major role in water conservation. Older adults have impaired thirst response to dehydration and often limited access to fluid (altered mental status, mobility problems, iatrogenic fluid restriction) that lead to a tendency for dehydration. A relative vasopressin excess exists in older adults. For any level of osmolality, AVP tends to be higher in the elderly (29–31). However, other data have reported no change in AVP among young, middle-aged, and elderly healthy persons. In response to stimuli such as water deprivation and alcohol, older adults have a greater magnitude of effect on AVP than younger persons. Secretion of AVP responds to changes in blood volume, blood pressure, tonicity, nausea, stress, and pain. Impaired baroreceptor function may affect AVP, as input from the baroreceptor to the osmoreceptor is inhibitory and altered cholinergic function with age may alter AVP. With aging, the renal response to AVP is blunted, resulting in a loss of urinary concentrating ability. A variety of medications are also associated with either increased AVP secretion or enhanced renal AVP effect. Tricyclics, phenothiazines, chlorpropamide, and opioid analgesics may be associated with hyponatremia. Even nocturia may be due to a decrease of the rhythmicity of vasopressin at night.

THYROID

With aging, a decrease in thyroid hormone secretion by thyroxine appears balanced by a decrease in thyroid hormone clearance, such that the serum thyroxine (T_4) levels do not change with age (17). Nor are there major changes in thyroid-binding proteins or in the resin uptake test. Triiodothyronine (T_3) is generally low in older adults because of decreased production rate (without a concomitant decrease in clearance), but this is less marked when persons are chosen for optimal health (17, 32, 33). Since T_3 may decrease with fasting or illness, even nonthyroidal illness, this should be considered in evaluating thyroid hormone levels. As previously noted, elevated TSH concentrations (10 to 15 IU/L) may occur in older adults, including healthy persons. However, a level greater than 15 IU/L nearly always indicates hypothyroidism. Screening for thyroid illness in older adults is often appropriate, especially with deterioration of function or hospital admission. If one can do only a single test, usually a sensitive TSH is appropriate, but as noted, if the result is low (hyperthyroid), further evaluation should be performed prior to accepting a ready diagnosis of hyperthyroidism. Table 36.2 shows some common signs of both hyperthyroidism and hypothyroidism in older adults.

Table 36.2

Signs and Symptoms of Hyperthyroidism and Hypothyroidism in the Older Adult

Hyperthyroidism
- Flat affect
- Confusion
- Depression
- Weight loss
- Atrial fibrillation
- Constipation and/or diarrhea

Hypothyroidism
- Constipation
- Dry skin
- Cold intolerance
- Fatigue
- Ataxia
- Worsening congestive heart failure
- Cognitive impairment

Hyperthyroidism is fairly uncommon in older adults, with a prevalence of 0.7% in the nonhospitalized elderly (33). However, the presentation of hyperthyroidism may be quite different in older adults than in young persons. Tachycardia, heat intolerance, lack of energy, nervousness, tremor, and increased food intake are not as common in the older hyperthyroid patient as in younger persons. Indeed, apathetic hyperthyroidism with symptoms such as confusion, delirium, apathy, lethargy, constipation, and depression may occur. On the other hand, atrial fibrillation is far more common in the older hyperthyroid patient, as is exacerbation of angina, dyspnea, and other symptoms of congestive heart failure (34, 35). Anorexia, weight loss, and general malaise may suggest malignancy, but thyroidal status should be evaluated in anyone with unexplained weight loss or gain. In patients with Graves' disease, eye findings are less common in the young, as is goiter, but with age there is also an increase in the prevalence of toxic multinodular goiter. In fact, toxic multinodular goiter accounts for about 50% of the hyperthyroidism seen in older adults. Also, Graves' disease may be superimposed on a toxic multinodular goiter. Excessive iodine administration (Jod-Basedow disease), which may also result in hyperthyroidism, can be precipitated by iodine contrast, dietary ingestion of iodine, or amiodarone, which last item can cause hypothy-roidism or hyperthyroidism (36, 37). Iodine-induced thyrotoxicosis tends to be self-limited when the inciting cause is removed. Another pathogenetic factor in thyrotoxicosis is thyroiditis, which again tends to be self-limited. Euthyroid hyperthyroxinemia in an older person, who may have a low TSH, poses an interesting diagnostic challenge. The diagnosis of hyperthyroidism should begin with a supersensitive TSH test as a screen but, if the TSH level is low, should be confirmed with a free thyroxine index. As noted, euthyroid older adults may have low TSH levels. In some persons isolated T_3 toxicosis may occur, so high concentrations of T_3 are also helpful, as this is highly specific for hyperthyroidism in the elderly but not especially sensitive, often because of impaired T_4 to T_3 conversion, nonthyroidal illness, and/or medications. Euthyroid hyperthyroxinemia with a high T_4 may occur in the setting of acute psychiatric illness; elevation of thyroid-binding globulin, such as is seen with estrogen administration or hepatitis, or medications such as steroids may pose a true diagnostic dilemma. These patients truly appear euthyroid. A repeat of these tests in 2 to 3 weeks may resolve the issue, as they often normalize, especially with treatment of the underlying disorder. A normal response to TRH testing absolutely rules out hyperthyroidism. A subnormal or absent response does not assist in the diagnosis.

Treatment of Hyperthyroidism

Radioactive iodine is often the treatment of choice in the older adult unless problems such as hyperthyroid-induced atrial fibrillation or other urgent symptoms require a more immediate approach to therapy. Surgery is almost never indicated unless there is a phenomenon such as obstruction due to the mass of the thyroid interfering with swallowing. Often, although the intention to treat with radioactive iodine may be to achieve a euthyroid state, it is far easier to treat hypothyroidism, and in older persons, erring on the side of a larger dose of radioactive iodine is preferable to undertreating. However, the results of radioactive iodine administration may not take effect for up to 3 months, so the patient may need relief of symptoms in the meantime. Symptom control with β-blockers, propylthiouracil (PTU), or methimazole may be indicated. Nonradioactive iodine, such as contrast material, may also offer quick relief of symptoms but should not be given before radioactive iodine, since it impedes uptake of the radioactive iodine into the thyroid gland. Regardless of the therapy, patients should be monitored for evidence of hypothyroidism, which should be treated.

Hypothyroidism

Hypothyroidism tends to be overlooked and often underdiagnosed in older persons, since there is so much similarity to many symptoms associated with aging: constipation, dry skin, fatigue, muscle weakness, imbalance (ataxia), or the manifestations of comorbid disease: worsening of heart failure, arthritis, presbycusis, and depression. Cognition can certainly worsen in the face of hypothyroidism. Furthermore, hypothyroidism often evolves over a long time and progresses slowly. Indeed, it is rarely recognized on clinical examination (38). Most hypothyroidism is due to autoimmune thyroiditis. One can certainly make a strong case for thyroid screening when health status deteriorates or functional alteration occurs. The best test for hypothyroidism is a TSH concentration above 15 to 20 IU/L (39). Though some argue that lower concentrations may suffice for diagnosis, the values between 5 and 15 often constitute a gray zone that may be associated with nonthyroidal illness or medications that can lower TSH (steroids, dopamine, phenytoin). In persons with normal T_4 levels but elevated TSH concentrations, the presence of high concentrations of antimicrosomal antibodies makes hypothyroidism much more likely, and a third of these patients become hyperthyroid within 4 years (39). Rarely is hypothyroidism due to secondary (hypothalamic-pituitary) problems as would be seen in the context of other endocrine disorders. Treatment of hypothyroidism should follow the dictum of geriatrics (start low, go slow) in terms of replacement therapy with thyroxine. Too rapid or too great an increment in thyroxine replacement may be associated with the precipitation of angina when there is underlying coronary artery disease. A starting dose of 25 μg (0.025 mg) with a 25-mg increment as needed every 3 to 4 weeks until the optimal dose is reached (normalization of TSH without an elevation of the free thyroxine index) is appropriate. However, a patient who has been treated for hyperthyroidism and had subsequent hypothyroidism and who was able to tolerate the hyperthyroid state without significant cardiovascular difficulties can start replacement with a larger dose, such as 50 to 75 μg. The average replacement dose is lower in an older person (40). In patients on other medications, clearance may alter as hypothyroidism resolves, and thus drug doses should be reassessed.

ADRENAL HORMONE

Like many other hormones, cortisol undergoes some alterations with age, with a shift in rhythmicity (earlier peak and nadir) and reduction in clearance rate and secretion, but this still results in normal basal concentrations and normal urinary free cortisol (41, 42). Higher levels of cortisol in response to stress, ACTH, or depression tend to also remain elevated longer than in the young (43). Even dexamethasone results in less suppression of cortisol in older adults. Although basal levels of cortisol may not alter with aging, other hormones secreted by the adrenal do show marked changes with age. The size of the zona reticularis does appear to decrease with age relative to the other zones of the adrenal cortex, perhaps explaining the diminution of adrenal androgens such as dehydroepiandrosterone (DHEA) and its sulfate (DHEAS) (44, 45). There is much interest in these substances, but the effect of administration to humans (as opposed to animal models) has not turned back the clock. Neither immune function nor cognition improves with the administration of DHEA. It appears that there are other age-related hormones that have a better correlation to functional status than DHEA (46). Aging is also associated with lower basal and stimulated levels of aldosterone. The plasma renin response to upright posture also diminishes with age. This decrease in aldosterone leads to a state of relative hyporeninemic hypoaldosteronism, putting persons at risk for hyperkalemia due to medications such as potassium-sparing diuretics, especially if they have renal impairment. Adrenal medullary catecholamines also change with age, but unlike most secretory products, they increase. Basal plasma norepinephrine, and norepinephrine (NE) response to stimuli such as exercise and upright posture are higher in the older adult than in their younger counterparts. Responsiveness to both α- and β-receptor-mediated stimulation appears decreased with age.

Adrenal insufficiency in the older adult may have, like many other disease entities, a very nonspecific presentation. Weakness, fatigue, hypotension, failure to thrive, abdominal pain and weight loss with or without orthostasis, or just hypotension may occur and should be in the differential diagnosis. (Orthostasis can be due to hemorrhage or anticoagulation and certainly can be seen in many elderly who do not have hypoadrenalism.) Autoimmune causes of hypoadrenalism in late life are exceedingly rare. While previous steroid therapy with suppression of the hypothalamic-pituitary-adrenal axis is the most common cause of adrenal insufficiency in the elderly, other causes, such as metastatic disease, tuberculosis, and hemorrhage due to anticoagulation, should be considered in the differential diagnosis of these symptoms (47). An ACTH stimulation test should be performed if the adrenal insufficiency is thought to be primary.

Cushing's Syndrome

Many syndromes and diseases that occur commonly in older adults, such as diabetes, hypertension, osteoporosis, myopathy, and fragile skin, may not be linked to a consideration of hypercortisolemia. In the older person the most common cause of hypercortisolemia is the use of steroids. However, additional causes such as ectopic ACTH syndrome should be considered. Small cell tumors of the lung, pancreas, and liver; pheochromocytomas; and ovarian tumors have been associated with the ectopic production of ACTH. These patients may have none of the classic stigmata of Cushing's syndrome; rather, they are cachectic with hypokalemic alkalosis. These persons often have extremely high ACTH concentrations that do not suppress in response to high-dose dexamethasone.

Diabetes

The rate of diabetes per 1000 persons in the United States goes up nearly 10-fold when one compares those under 45 (10.6 cases) with those over age 65 (103.9 cases) (48). The prevalence is even higher among African-Americans. Nearly 20% of those 85 and older have diabetes. The diagnosis of diabetes carries with it increased risk of stroke, cardiac disease (especially coronary disease, cardiomyopathy, and hypertension), and amputations, among others; these risks are all greater in older diabetics. Older diabetics, especially those taking insulin (with presumably greater severity of disease) have 2 to nearly 3 times the number of hospital admissions as other diabetics; the morbidity and mortality are increased; and life expectancy even for an older diabetic is shorter than that of a nondiabetic (49, 50).

There are many reasons for the hyperglycemia of aging. Insulin resistance, impaired insulin secretion, decreased glucose transport, impairment in the inhibition of hepatic glucose output, and altered glucose disposal are only a few of the alterations associated with age and hyperglycemia (51–53). Much of the hyperglycemia of aging can be associated with factors such as obesity and sedentary lifestyle, rather than aging per se (54). Hemoglobin A1C tends to increase with age, regardless of the presence of diabetes, and thus may make this less useful in diagnosing diabetes. It is still a reasonable test for following diabetic control and intervention. The diagnostic criteria for diabetes, based on glucose values, are no different from those of young persons.

Atypical presentation of diabetes is quite common, and diabetes may go unrecognized for many years. Polyuria in an older man more often brings to mind prostate disease rather than diabetes, while in a woman, a urinary tract infection is more commonly thought of than diabetes. The anorexia of aging may cover any polyphagia, and feeling poorly, whether due to diabetes or another comorbid disease, may result in anorexia and weight loss. Polydipsia in older persons may actually be welcome in most elderly, for the hypodipsia of aging, with its inability to sense thirst even with a hyperosmolar load, makes dehydration likely. Silent myocardial infarction is more likely in the older diabetic.

In addition to the risk of accelerated atherosclerosis, nephropathy, and neuropathy, diabetes is associated with a high risk of glaucoma and cataracts (55). Cognitive impairment can also result from hyperglycemia, and memory can improve with a greater degree of glycemic control. Incontinence, confusion, weight loss, and falls are findings that should prompt consideration of diabetes. Special syndromes that occur commonly in older adults include diabetic cachexia (anorexia, painful myopathy, weight loss, and depression) and amyotrophy (wasting and weakness of the pelvic girdle and thigh muscles). These are diagnoses of exclusion but should be considered in the diabetic.

It is also clear that age does not mitigate the need for appropriate and tight control of diabetes. Relieving the symptoms of hyperglycemia, reducing the risk of complications and adding to quality of life as symptoms abate is certainly a good reason to seek glycemic control. In managing the older diabetic, awareness that malnutrition is more likely in the older adult may alter dietary regimens, but the addition of fiber along with water, moderating fat intake, and using a restricted diet in those more than 20 to 30% over ideal body weight according to an age-appropriate table is reasonable. Age-related changes in taste, smell, and dental issues, as well as issues related to access to food and its preparation, affect diet. In a nursing home setting, Coulston et al. (56) have shown that switching from an American Diabetes Association diet to a regular diet makes little difference in glycemic control. Exercise (even chair or bed exercise for the bedbound) improves more than glycemic control; it lowers lipids and often improves energy and mood. All modalities of therapy—diet, exercise, oral hypoglycemics, and insulin—should be considered. Underweight diabetics may not respond as well to oral agents as middle-aged overweight diabetics, as they may have insulin deficiency. Prolonged hypoglycemia with an oral hypoglycemic that has a long half-life (such as chlorpropamide) or the syndrome of inappropriate antidiuretic hormone secretion (SIADH) associated with chlorpropamide makes use of this agent inappropriate in older adults (57, 58). While second-generation and newer agents are used more often, both primary and secondary failures with oral agents may occur. Both glyburide and glipizide are effective in type

II diabetes. In a randomized crossover study of elderly type II diabetics treated for 8 weeks, equivalent control with 8.4 mg of glyburide and 11.9 mg of glipizide was obtained in diabetics with a mean age of 70 (59). Sulfonylureas work primarily by increasing insulin secretion and presumably increasing insulin sensitivity. The reintroduction of a biguanide (metformin) has also added to the therapeutic modalities. Biguanides reduce hepatic glucose output, decrease gluconeogenesis, improve glucose disposal, and increase the glucose transporter GLUT 1, but without significantly raising insulin secretion (60). The rare side effect lactic acidosis, which may be very insidious with its nonspecific symptoms of malaise, bradycardia, and muscle pains, can be lessened by not using a biguanide in anyone with a creatinine clearance less than 60 mL per minute or in those with hepatic dysfunction. α-Glucosidase inhibitors (acarbose) interfere with carbohydrate absorption, decreasing postprandial glucose excursion. However, possible gastrointestinal side effects such as flatulence, diarrhea, and transaminitis must be considered in its use. The thiazolidinediones (troglitazone) decrease hepatic glucose output and improve glucose sensitivity and binding to nuclear receptors, altering transcription of genes regulating glucose and lipid metabolism. They do not act as insulin secretagogues. Insulin must be present for this class of agents to be effective. The use of combination therapy of oral agents is becoming more common, with increasing use of sulfonylurea with biguanide and/or α-glucosidase inhibitor and/or thiazolidinedione and/or insulin. However, complicated, expensive regimens may also alter compliance and put patients at increased risk for hypoglycemia. The Veterans Affairs Cooperative Study on glycemic control has clearly shown that insulin is quite effective in improving glycemic control in persons with a mean age of 60 who have failed with oral agents without producing excessive hypoglycemia, hypertension, or dyslipidemia (61). Again, using a simple regimen is best, but once-daily insulin may not control blood sugar, and twice-daily therapy should be instituted. Additionally, there is no dawn phenomenon in the older diabetic (the rise in counterregulatory hormones such as

ACTH, growth hormone, epinephrine, and glucagon) that is associated with an early rise of blood sugar in the morning; therefore, a late evening dose of insulin may not be appropriate. For patients with declining renal function, aggressive control of blood pressure and the use of angiotensin-converting enzyme (ACE) inhibitors to reduce proteinuria should be undertaken when appropriate. The risks and benefits of each strategy and their effect on the patient should be assessed, and therapy must be individualized to achieve success.

MENOPAUSE

The average age of menopause in the United States is 51. Although menopause is certainly a developmental stage in life, not a disease, the cessation of ovarian production of hormones, the loss of estradiol, and decrease in estrone put women at risk for diseases and disorders such as cardiovascular disease, osteoporosis, incontinence, and dyspareunia. Until recently, many of the health implications incurred by the loss of estrogen at menopause were rarely considered by the medical profession, nor was there a groundswell of menopausal women who demanded information and choice in prevention and/or therapy. Table 36.3 lists common symptoms of menopause in both men and women.

Table 36.3

Signs and Symptoms of Male and Female Menopause

Male	Female
Decreased libido	Hot flashes
Alterations in mood	Atrophic vaginitis
Decreased muscle strength	Sleep disturbances
	Mood alterations
Osteoporosis	Incontinence
Increased anemia	Dyspareunia
Decreased appetite	Osteoporosis
Decreased energy	Cardiovascular disease
Decreased visual-spatial acuity	Skin changes (increased wrinkling, decreased turgor)
	Increased risk of falling

Menopause tends not to be an abrupt event, but rather is foreshadowed by perimenopause, in which the follicular phase of the menstrual cycle decreases (generally decreasing the length of the cycle), after which irregular cycling with long or shorter intervals between menses may be seen (26). Longer cycles tend to be anovulatory, lacking progesterone. The perimenopausal period may last for years and be accompanied by symptoms such as hot flashes. The decline in estrogen is accompanied by a rise in FSH that is far greater than that of LH. Androgens also decrease, but as estrogen levels fall far more dramatically, the ratio of androgen to estrogen increases. Menopause, or the permanent cessation of menses, is accompanied by hot flashes in about 70 to 80% of women. In approximately 15 to 20% of women these hot flashes last 5 years or more (62). Disruption of the sleep cycle does not enhance mood or performance, and emotional lability may occur. Difficulty concentrating even in the absence of a sleep disturbance has been noted by many women. Psychologic issues, however, appear often to relate to situational psychosocial issues rather than hormonal changes per se. Estrogen therapy actually improves REM sleep, the quality of sleep, and sleep latency (63). Other symptoms such as palpitations and vertigo may occur as part of menopause. Tissue changes due to lack of estrogen can result in decreased vaginal lubrication and symptoms of atrophic vaginitis, with itching, burning, and even bleeding. The loss of mucosal integrity may add to the risk of incontinence. The bladder and urethra may atrophy as well when estrogen is lost. See Chapter 33 for a discussion of osteoporosis.

The favorable status of women in terms of cardiovascular risk up to the time of menopause can be attributed to the positive effect on lipids along with other factors (increased high-density lipoprotein (HDL), decreased low-density lipoprotein (LDL), increased clearance of intermediate-density lipoprotein, up-regulation of the LDL receptor, inhibition of LDL oxidation, and reversal of endothelin-mediated vasoconstriction, perhaps due to enhanced nitric oxide concentration and function) (64–66). Hormone replacement therapy (HRT) may also improve the altered balance between fibrinolysis and coagulation, decrease central obesity, and diminish insulin resistance (67). The use of HRT is associated with approximately 50% reduction in the risk of coronary heart disease (68, 69). Stroke risk is also reduced (70). For women with an intact uterus, the use of a progestational agent is mandatory to prevent hyperplasia and reduce the risk of endometrial carcinoma. Although cyclic therapy (such as daily estrogen with 0.625 mg of conjugated estradiol or its equivalent plus 12 to 14 days of 5 mg of medroxyprogesterone acetate or its equivalent) may result in more withdrawal bleeding than the daily administration of estrogen and progesterone, at least one can tell whether the bleeding or spotting is in relation to the withdrawal of progesterone. Otherwise, such as with bleeding with a daily combined regimen of estrogen and progesterone, an endometrial biopsy might be needed to ascertain the cause of bleeding. For women who no longer have a uterus, progesterone is unnecessary. Bloating, breast tenderness, weight gain, mood changes, and increased frequency of migraines may occur with hormone replacement, and women should be told about these symptoms, but they can be lessened by altering the type of hormone, the dose, or the type of regimen for replacement. The risk of breast cancer and the duration of HRT remain controversial. Many of these women may undergo more intensive scrutiny, such as with mammography, because they are taking hormones. Everything from increased risk to reduced risk of breast cancer has been attributed to HRT (62). The risks and benefits of hormone therapy should be discussed, at the very least, with every woman at the time of menopause if not before.

ADAM: ANDROGEN DEFICIENCY IN THE AGING MAN

Women are not the only group to undergo reproductive hormonal changes with age. Although it was poorly recognized or even acknowledged for many years, testosterone levels do decline with age, and the testosterone production rate at age 80 is only 50% of that seen in a younger man (71–74). Testosterone drops by about 100 mg/dL per decade after age 60 (75). More striking than the decline in total testosterone and a better marker of clinical hypogonadism is the decrease

of bioavailable testosterone with age. This represents the portion of testosterone that is not bound by sex hormone-binding globulin (SHBG). This differs from the free testosterone, which measures both the non-SHBG-bound and non-albumin-bound fractions, but this is an underestimate of the testosterone that can be used by the body, since testosterone bound to albumin is only weakly bound, thus is free to unbind from albumin and be used. In many ways the decrement of testosterone and bioavailable testosterone, just as with estrogen in women, can be a harbinger of things to come. Low male hormone levels are associated with many factors that can lead to frailty, such as decreased muscle mass and strength, as well as osteoporosis. In addition, anemia, decreased libido, decreased sexual activity, and mood alterations may accompany hypogonadism (76, 77). Marked concern over the use of testosterone in older hypogonadal men has left many untreated. Tenover (78) noted that replacement of testosterone in older men resulted in increased lean body mass, decreased body fat, increased hematocrit, decreased cholesterol, and an elevation in prostate specific antigen (PSA). In preliminary short-term data with testosterone replacement, 3 months of therapy (in 8 men with a mean age of 78 receiving testosterone and 6 hypogonadal control subjects) increased dominant grip strength, increased hematocrit, decreased total cholesterol, and produced no change in PSA (79). More recently, longer-term studies (12 months and 2 years or more) of testosterone replacement in men have found that while polycythemia is a concern and must be monitored for, replacement is reasonably well tolerated (80, 81). No increase in cardiovascular risk, as evidenced by no increase in angina, myocardial infarction, or stroke occurred, nor did symptoms of benign prostatic hyperplasia worsen (81). Improvement in mood, libido, and strength; decreased bone loss and anemia; and improved appetite when therapy is given to hypogonadal men must weighed against the need for careful monitoring of hematocrit, prostate size, symptoms, and PSA. Other considerations, such as gynecomastia and accelerated prostate growth of carcinomatous focus, must be made in considering the risks and benefits of treatment. At this moment only testosterone injections or patch therapy should be considered. Oral testosterone that is available in the United States is 17a-alkylated and as such can be associated with significant hepatic dysfunction. Clearly, more and longer-term data will be helpful in addressing whether testosterone replacement can achieve the same level of benefit that replacement of estrogen clearly has in women.

REFERENCES

1. Everitt AV. Neuroendocrine function and aging. Adv Exp Med Biol 1980;129:233–242.
2. Andres R, Tobin TD. Endocrine systems. In: Finch CE, Hayflick L, eds. Handbook of the Biology of Aging. New York: Van Nostrand Reinhold, 1977:367.
3. Terano T, Seya A, Tamura Y, et al. Characteristics of the pituitary gland in elderly subjects from magnetic resonance images: relationship to pituitary hormone secretion. Clin Endocrinol 1996;45:273–279.
4. Wilkinson CW, Peskind ER, Raskind MA. Decreased hypothalamic-pituitary-adrenal axis sensitivity to cortisol feedback inhibition in human aging. Neuroendocrinology 1997;65:79–90.
5. Kaiser FE, Morley JE. Gonadotropins, testosterone and the aging male. Neurobiol Aging 1994;15:559–563.
6. degli Uberti EC, Ambrosio MR, Cella SG, et al. Defective hypothalamic growth hormone (GH)-releasing hormone activity may contribute to declining GH secretion in man. J Endocrinol Metab 1997;82:2885–2888.
7. Rudman D, Kutner MH, Rogers M, et al. Impaired growth hormone secretion in the adult population: relation to age and adiposity. J Clin Invest 1981;67:1361–1369.
8. Corpas E, Harman SM, Blackman MR. Human growth hormone and human aging. Endocrinol Rev 1993; 14:20–39.
9. Rudman D, Feller AG, Nagraj HS, et al. Effect of human growth hormone in men over 60 years old. N Engl J Med 1990;323:1–6.
10. Marcus R, Butterfield G, Holloway L, et al. Effects of short term administration of recombinant growth hormone to elderly people. J Clin Endocrinol Metab 1990;70:519–527.
11. Kaiser FE, Silver AJ, Morley JE. The effect of recombinant human growth hormone on malnourished older individuals. J Am Geriatr Soc 1991;39:235–240.
12. Sawin CT, Carlson HE, Geller A, et al. Serum prolactin and aging: basal values and changes with estrogen use and hypothyroidism. Gerontology 1989;44:131–135.
13. Blackman MR, Kowatch MA, Wehmann RE, Harman SM. Basal serum prolactin levels and prolactin responses to constant infusions of thyrotropin releasing hormone in healthy aging men. J Gerontol 1986;41:699–705.
14. Sawin CT, Chopra D, Azizi F, et al. The aging thyroid: increased prevalence of elevated serum thyrotropin in the elderly. JAMA 1979;242:247–250.
15. Hershman JM, Pekary AE, Berg L, et al. Serum thyrotropin and thyroid hormone levels in elderly and mid-
dle aged euthyroid persons. J Am Geriatr Soc 1993;41: 823–828.
16. Sawin CT, Geller A, Kaplan MM, et al. Low serum thyrotropin (thyroid stimulating hormone) in older persons without hyperthyroidism. Arch Intern Med 1991; 151:165–168.
17. Kaiser FE. Variability of response to thyroid releasing hormone in normal elderly. Age Aging 1997;16:345–354.
18. Prange AJ Jr, Lara PP, Wilson IC, et al. Effects of thyrotropin-releasing hormone in depression. Lancet 1972;2:999–1002.
19. Pavlov EP, Harman SM, Chrousos GP, et al. Responses of plasma adrenocorticotrophin, cortisol and dehydroepiandrosterone to avian corticotrophin releasing hormone in healthy aging men. J Clin Endocrinol Metab 1986;62:767–772.
20. Facchinetti F, Petraglia F, Nappi G, et al. Different patterns of central and peripheral beta endorphin, beta lipoprotein and ACTH throughout life. Peptides 1983; 4:469–474.
21. Baker HWG, Burger HG, DeKretser DM, et al. Changes in the pituitary testicular system with age. Clin Endocrinol 1967;5:349–372.
22. Neaves WB, Johnson L, Parker CR, Petty CS. Leydig cell numbers, daily sperm production and serum gonadotropin levels in aging men. J Clin Endocrinol Metab 1984;59:756–763.
23. Kaiser FE, Viosca SP, Morley JE, et al. Impotence and aging: clinical and hormonal factors. J Am Geriatr Soc 1988;36:511–519.
24. Korenman SG, Morley JE, Mooradian AD, et al. Secondary hypogonadism in older men: its relation to impotence. J Clin Endocrinol Metab 1990;71:963–969.
25. Winter SJ, Sheins RJ, Troen P. The gonadotropin suppressive activity of androgen is increased in elderly men. Metabolism 1984;33:1052–1059.
26. Kaiser FE, Morley JE. The menopause and beyond. In: Cassell CR, Reisenberg D, eds. Geriatric Medicine. New York: Springer-Verlag, 1990:279–290.
27. Quint AR, Kaiser FE. Gonadotropin determination and thyrotropin releasing hormone and luteinizing hormone-releasing hormone testing in critically ill postmenopausal women with hypothyroxinemia. J Clin Endocrinol Metab 1985;60:464–471.
28. D'Amico JF, Greendale GA, Lu JK, Judd HL. Induction of hypothalamic opioid activity with transdermal estrogen administration in postmenopausal women. Fertil Steril 1991;55:754–758.
29. Frolkis VV, Golovchenko SF, Medved VI, Frolkis RA. Vasopressin and cardiovascular system in aging. Gerontology 1982;28:290–302.
30. Crawford GA, Johnson AG, Gyory AZ, Kelly D.. Change in arginine vasopressin concentration with age. Clin Chem 1993;39:2023.
31. Helderman JH, Vestal JW, Rowe JW, et al. The response of arginine vasopressin to intravenous ethanol and hypertonic saline in man: the impact of aging. J. Gerontol 1978:33:39–47.

32. Olsen T, Laurberg P, Weeke J. Low serum triiodothyronine and high serum reverse triiodothyronine in old age: an effect of disease, not age. J Clin Endocrinol Metab 1978;47:1111–1115.

33. Mokshagundam S, Barzel US. Thyroid disease in the elderly. J Am Geriatr Soc 1991;41:1361–1369.

34. Davis PJ, Davis FB. Hyperthyroidism in patients over the age of 60. Medicine 1974;53:161–181.

35. Tibaldi JM, Barzel US, Albin J, Surks M. Thyrotoxicosis in the very old. Am J Med 1986;81:619–622.

36. Fradkin JE, Wolff J. Iodide induced thyrotoxicosis. Medicine 1983;62:1–20.

37. Broussolle C, Ducottet X, Martin C, et al. Rapid effectiveness of prednisone and thionamide combined therapy in severe amiodarone iodine-induced thyrotoxicosis. J Endocrinol Invest 1989;12:37–42.

38. Griffin JE. Review: Hypothyroidism in the elderly. Am J Med Sci 1990;299:334–345.

39. Rosenthal MJ, Hunt MC, Gary PJ, Goodwin JS. Thyroid failure in the elderly: microsomal antibodies as discriminant for therapy. JAMA 1987;258:209–213.

40. Rosenbaum RL, Barzel US. Levothyroxine replacement dose for primary hypothyroidism decreases with age. Ann Intern Med 1982;96:53–55.

41. Tsagarakis S, Grossman A. The hypothalamic pituitary adrenal axis in senescence. In: Morley JE, Korenman SG Endocrinology and Metabolism in the Elderly. Boston: Blackwell Scientific, 1992:70–91.

42. Barton RN, Horan MA, Weijers JW, et al. Cortisol production rate and the urinary excretion of 17-hydroxycorticosteroids, free cortisol, and 6 beta-hydroxycortisol in healthy elderly men and women. J Gerontol Med Sci 1993;48:M213.

43. Simpkins JW, Millard WJ. Influence of age on neurotransmitter function. Endocrinol Metab Clin N Am 1987;16:893–917.

44. Parker CR Jr, Mixon RL, Brissie RM, Grizzle WE. Aging alters zonation in the adrenal cortex of men. J Clin Endocrinol Metab 1997;82:3898–3901.

45. Orentreich N, Brind JL, Rizer RL, Vogelman JH. Age changes and sex differences in serum dehydroepiandrosterone sulfate concentrations through adulthood. J Clin Endocrinol Metab 1984;59:551–555.

46. Morley JE, Kaiser F, Raum WJ, et al. Potentially predictive and manipulable blood serum correlates of aging in the healthy human male: progressive decreases in bioavailable testosterone, dehydroepiandrosterone sulfate, and the ratio of insulin-like growth factor 1 to growth hormone. Proc Natl Acad Sci U S A 1997;9:7537–7542.

47. Anderson KC, Kuhajda FP, Bell WR. Diagnosis and treatment of anticoagulant-related adrenal hemorrhage. Am J Hematol 1981;11:379–385.

48. Gambert SR. Defining the problem: impact of diabetes mellitus on an aging society. In: Gambert SR, ed. Diabetes Mellitus in the Elderly: A Practical Guide. New York: Raven Press, 1990:1.

49. Harris MI. Epidemiology of diabetes mellitus among the elderly in the United States. Clin Geriatr Med 190;6:703–719.

50. Neil HA, Thompson AV, Thorogood M, et al. Diabetes in the elderly: the Oxford Community diabetes study. Diabet Med 1989;6:608–613.

51. Morley JE, Kaiser FE. Unique aspects of diabetes mellitus in the elderly. Clin Geriatr Med 1990;6:693–702.

52. Meneilly GS, Elahi D, Minaker KL, et al. Impairment of non-insulin mediated glucose disposal in the elderly. J Clin Endocrinol Metab 1989;63:566–571.

53. Porte DJ, Kahn SE. What geriatricians should know about diabetes mellitus. Diabetes Care 1990;23(suppl 2):47–50.

54. Zavaroni I, D'Aglio E, Bruschi F, et al. Effect of age and environmental factors on glucose tolerance and insulin secretion in a worker population. J Am Geriatr Soc 1986;34:271–275.

55. Rosenthal MJ, Morley JE. Diabetes and its complications in older people. In: Morley JE, Korenman SG, eds. Endocrinology and Metabolism in the Elderly. Boston: Blackwell Scientific, 1992:373–387.

56. Coulston AM, Mandelbaum D, Reaven GM. Dietary management of nursing home residents with non-insulin dependent diabetes mellitus. Am J Clin Nutr 1990;51:67–71.

57. Tanay A, Firemann Z, Yust I, et al. Chlorpropamide induced syndrome in inappropriate antidiuretic hormone excretion. J Am Geriatr Soc 1981;29:334–336.

58. Asplund K, Wiholm BE, Lithner F. Glibenclamide-associated hypoglycaemia: a report on 57 cases. Diabetologia 1983;24:412–417.

59. Brodows RG. Benefits and risks with glyburide and glipizide in elderly NIDDM patients. Diabetes Care 1992;15:75.

60. Hundal H. Cellular mechanism of metformin action involves glucose transporter translocation from an intracellular pool to the plasma membrane in L6 muscle cells. Endocrinology 1992;131:1165–1173.

61. Abraira C, Colwell JA, Nuttall FQ, et al. Veterans Affairs Cooperative Study on glycemic control and complications in type II diabetes (VA CSDM). Diabetes Care 1995;18:1113–1123.

62. Speroff L. Menopause and hormone replacement therapy. Clin Geriatr Med 1993;9:33–55.

63. Schiff I, Regenstein Q, Tulchinsky D, Ryan KJ. Effects of estrogens on sleep and psychological state of hypogonadal women. JAMA 1979;242:2405.

64. Knopp RH, Zhu X, Bonet B. Effects of estrogens on lipoprotein metabolism and cardiovascular disease in women. Atherosclerosis 1994;110(suppl):S83–S91.

65. Effects of estrogen or estrogen/progestin regimens on heart disease risk factors in postmenopausal women. The Postmenopausal Estrogen/Progestin Interventions (PEPI) Trial. The Writing Group for the PEPI Trial. JAMA 1995;273:199–208.

66. Nabulski AA, Folson AR, White A, et al. Association of hormone replacement therapy with various cardiovascular risk factors in postmenopausal women. N Engl J Med 1993;328:1069–1075.

67. Stevenson JC, Crook D, Godsland IF, et al. Hormone replacement therapy and the cardiovascular system. Drugs 1994;47(suppl 2):35–41.

68. Grady D, Rubin SM, Pettiti DB, et al. Hormone therapy to prevent disease and prolong life in postmenopausal women. Ann Intern Med 1992;117:1016–1037.

69. Stampfer MJ, Colditz GA. Estrogen replacement therapy and coronary heart disease: a quantitative assessment of the epidemiologic evidence. Prevent Med 1991;20: 47–63.

70. Finucane FF, Madans JH, Bush TL, et al. Decreased risk of stroke among postmenopausal hormone users. Arch Intern Med 1993;153:73–79.

71. Davidson J, Chen JJ, Crapo L, et al. Hormonal changes and sexual function in aging men. J Clin Endocrinol Metab 1983;57:71–77.

72. Kaiser FE, Viosca SP, Morley JE, et al. Impotence and aging: clinical and hormonal factors. J Am Geriatr Soc 1988;36:511–519.

73. Nankin HR, Calkin JG. Decreased bioavailable testosterone in aging normal and impotent men. J Clin Endocrinol Metab 1986;63:1418–1420.

74. Korenman SG, Morley JE, Mooradian AD, et al. Secondary hypogonadism in older men: its relation to impotence. J Clin Endocrinol Metab 1990;71:963–969.

75. Morley JE, Kaiser FE, Perry III HM, et al. Longitudinal changes in testosterone, luteinizing hormone and follicle stimulating hormone in healthy older men. Metabolism 1997;46:410–413.

76. Odell WD, Swerdloff RS. Male hypogonadism. West J Med 1976;124:446–475.

77. Stanley HL, Schmitt BP, Poses RM, Deiss WP. Does hypogonadism contribute to the occurrence of a minimal trauma hip fracture in elderly men. J Am Geriatr Soc 1991;39:766–771.

78. Tenover JS. Effects of testosterone supplementation in the aging male. J Clin Endocrinol Metab 1992;75:1092–1098.

79. Morley JE, Perry III HM, Kaiser FE, et al. Effects of testosterone replacement in old hypogonadal males: a preliminary study. J Am Geriatr Soc 1993;41:149–152.

80. Sih R, Morley JE, Kaiser FE, et al. Testosterone replacement in older hypogonadal men: a 12 month randomized controlled trial. J Clin Endocrinol Metab 1997;82:1661–1667.

81. Hajjar RR, Kaiser FE, Morley JE. Outcomes of long term testosterone replacement in older hypogonadal males: a retrospective analysis. J Clin Endocrinol Metab 1997; 82:3793–3796.

CHAPTER 37

LISA B. CARUSO AND REBECCA A. SILLIMAN

Diabetes Mellitus in the Elderly Patient

Diabetes mellitus increases in prevalence with age. In the United States, it is estimated that 3.6 million people aged 65 or older are afflicted with this disease, the majority of whom have type 2 disease (1). The costs of medical care are great; in 1992 approximately $38 billion were spent on medical care for elderly diabetics. The majority of this expense is for inpatient costs, with most being attributed to the care of cardiovascular complications (1, 2). Indeed, in the elderly diabetic patient, the challenges to the clinician are (a) to avoid symptoms and complications of hyperglycemia and hypoglycemia, (b) to minimize or delay microvascular and macrovascular complications if possible, and (c) to maximize daily function.

EPIDEMIOLOGY

Almost half of diabetics are age 65 or older, with an approximately even split between men and women. The absolute number of older persons with diabetes will continue to rise in the foreseeable future for at least two reasons: (a) the rate of diagnosed diabetes in persons 65 to 74 years of age and more than 75 years has increased about 2.5 times in the past 30 years, and (b) the number of older persons at risk is growing. Since about half of cases in older persons are undiagnosed, if methods of detection improve, the numbers of clinically recognized cases may rise even further (3).

DIAGNOSIS

Although the "poly" symptoms (polydipsia, polyuria, and polyphagia) are considered by many to be pathognomonic of diabetes, for several reasons this is often not true in older persons. First, these symptoms are nonspecific and may be due to other conditions. Second, they may be absent because of age-related or disease-related changes in organ function. Third, they may be masked by other conditions. Thus, relying on them results in both false-positives and false-negatives. The challenge to the clinician is to maintain a high level of suspicion yet be prudent with glucose testing.

The previously accepted criteria for diagnosing diabetes in asymptomatic adults as given by the World Health Organization (WHO) and the National Diabetes Data Group (NDDG) include an elevation in plasma glucose to more than 200 mg/dL 2 hours following a 75-g oral glucose tolerance test or a fasting plasma glucose of more than 140 mg/dL. In addition, glucose levels must be abnormal on more than one occasion (4). These criteria were recently revised by the Expert Committee on the Diagnosis and Classification of Diabetes Mellitus (5) to improve the predictive power of glucose testing. The new criteria are symptoms of diabetes and a random glucose level of more than 200 mg/dL, a fasting plasma glucose level of 126 mg/dL or greater, or an elevation in plasma glucose to more than 200 mg/dL 2 hours after a 75-g oral glucose tolerance test. As previously recommended by WHO and NDDG, the diagnosis must be confirmed by abnormal glucose levels on a different day.

Most elderly diabetics are classified as either

type 1 or type 2. Type 1 diabetics require insulin and are ketosis prone. Type 2 diabetics are insulin resistant and ketosis resistant. Many type 1 diabetics who started insulin in the 1930s are still alive, so when caring for a diabetic patient, it is important to establish when and how the diagnosis of diabetes was made to institute proper therapy and to anticipate the type of complications that are likely to develop.

SCREENING

As with other conditions, screening for diabetes would be indicated if the treatment of asymptomatic patients resulted in better outcomes, if the burden of suffering associated with it were high, and if the screening test were sensitive and specific, simple and inexpensive, safe, and acceptable for both patients and practitioners (6). Although no one would argue that the burdens associated with diabetes are great, there is no good evidence that early detection and treatment improve outcomes for patients with type 2 disease (7). The U.S. Preventive Services Task Force, however, suggests that clinicians may wish to screen persons aged 65 or over who are at high risk: the obese, those with a family history of diabetes, and persons of Native American, Hispanic, or African-American descent (7). Once diabetes has been detected clinically, screening for complications, specifically for retinopathy and foot lesions, can reduce morbidity, as is discussed later.

MANAGEMENT

To the elderly person, the diagnosis of diabetes may evoke multiple emotions, including dread, fear, and sadness. Not only are complications devastating, but following complex dietary, medication, and monitoring regimens may be overwhelming. Daily functional, nutritional, and medical assistance from professional and lay caregivers is often necessary when patients are physically and/or cognitively impaired. When developing a treatment plan for the elderly diabetic patient, it is important to involve the patient in his or her own care to the extent that this is possible and to be sensitive to the patient's perception of his or her quality of life as it is affected by various therapeutic interventions.

Recently the concept of *collaborative management* has received attention as a mechanism for better care of patients with such chronic diseases as diabetes. Collaborative management consists of (*a*) defining problems from the perspective of both patient and physician, (*b*) targeting key problems, setting goals, and planning methods to achieve goals, (*c*) teaching the patient and providing support services, and (*d*) evaluating the patient's progress in a frequent and regular follow-up plan (8). These elements can be implemented in a variety of practice models, ranging from the small group practice to the large health maintenance organization. It is important for all the members of the health care team to teach the patient as much as possible so as to make the patient an active participant in his or her own diabetic management.

Diet and Weight Loss

Most type 2 diabetics are overweight, although a subset of older patients are either normal weight or underweight (9). What constitutes an optimal diabetic diet for older persons has not yet been determined, although even modest weight loss in obese older persons can improve metabolic control, reducing symptoms of hyperglycemia. Achieving weight loss and metabolic control is not easy. Lifelong dietary habits are difficult to change, as are notions of what constitutes a healthful diet. This may be compounded by the fact that older patients frequently must rely on someone else for meals. They may live in households where food preferences are disparate. Furthermore, limited financial resources may interfere with patients' procuring appropriate foods, such as fresh fruits and vegetables.

Obese diabetics should attempt to lose weight, although for many it is not possible. For this group as well as those who are either underweight or of normal weight, the best strategy should be to help them achieve a balanced diet that includes fruit and legume sources of carbohydrate, restricts the amount of animal fat while maintaining the intake of protein at 0.8 to 1 g/kg of body weight, and incorporates fiber in moderate amounts (9). Adequate fluid intake of sucrose-free beverages is also important. This alone may help to reduce glucose levels and correct mild volume contraction related to osmotic diuresis. Elderly diabetic patients living in long-term care facilities must have diets appropriate to prevent or correct malnutrition. The American Diabetes Association recommends serving regular unrestricted meals to institutionalized diabetic patients (10). It is important for such patients to enjoy mealtime to satisfy nutritional needs and to contribute to their quality of life.

Exercise

If the elderly diabetic patient is able to exercise regularly, weight loss and glycemic control may be added benefits. Physical activity has been found to increase insulin sensitivity of muscle and of other tissues that have insulin receptors. Other cardiovascular risk factors, such as hyperlipidemia (11) and hypertension (12), may be reduced by regular exercise as well. Self-esteem and quality of life may also improve. However, exercise in the elderly diabetic may carry substantial risk. Exercise can exacerbate angina or ischemia in a patient with underlying cardiovascular disease. Peripheral neuropathy may result in soft tissue or musculoskeletal injuries. Symptomatic hypoglycemia can also occur, especially in patients taking oral hypoglycemic drugs. The American Diabetes Association recommends that type 2 diabetics who want to begin an exercise program undergo a "preexercise evaluation . . . to uncover previously undiagnosed hypertension, neuropathy, retinopathy, nephropathy, and, particularly, silent ischemic heart disease" (13). Elderly diabetics should have an exercise-stress electrocardiogram before beginning an exercise program, and they should monitor their glucose levels after any workout.

Drug Therapy

Unless the patient has significant symptoms of hyperglycemia, a 3-month trial of dietary modifications, exercise, and weight loss is generally warranted. As lifestyle modification is often difficult, especially for the elderly, engaging the help of a nutritionist and/or a nurse specialist improves the patient's chances for success. Drug therapy is indicated if the combination of diet, exercise, and weight loss is not successful in eliminating symptomatic hyperglycemia. An alternative strategy, particularly for patients whose plasma glucose levels are in the 300- to 400-

mg/dL range, is to begin drug therapy along with dietary and exercise programs. If the latter are successful, it may be possible to taper the patient off of medication later.

Whether glycemic control can assist in achieving long-term goals such as prevention of retinopathy and decreasing amputation rates is being addressed in a controlled trial of type 2 diabetic patients (14). In choosing among the antihyperglycemic therapies, concomitant liver disease, kidney disease, and obesity must be considered, as must the patient's preferences.

Oral hypoglycemic agents include the sulfonylureas, such as first-generation agents tolbutamide, chlorpropamide, acetohexamide, and tolazamide and second-generation agents glipizide, glyburide, and glimepiride; the biguanide metformin; the α-glucosidase inhibitor acarbose; and the first thiazolidinedione, troglitazone. Oral agents are easy to use and are frequently preferred by patients.

Sulfonylureas

The sulfonylurea drugs are the most frequently prescribed agents for treating hyperglycemia. They are generally efficacious, especially in patients who are not obese and in the first 2 to 5 years after diagnosis (15). Their loss of efficacy with time is probably due to a combination of patients' difficulty with dietary restrictions and a progressive diminution in β-cell function. The choice of sulfonylurea should take into account the following considerations. First, since all are metabolized at least in part by the liver, they should be used with care in patients with severe liver disease. Second, renal insufficiency prolongs the half-lives of the sulfonylureas. Tolbutamide has no active renal metabolism and the shortest duration of action (6 to 12 hours), so it is probably the best drug for patients with significant renal insufficiency (16). Third, because of its long half-life (36 hours), a risk factor for hypoglycemia, and its propensity to cause hyponatremia, chlorpropamide should be avoided in older persons. Fourth, since glyburide can also cause hypoglycemia in older persons, it also should be used with caution. Glipizide, the other second-generation agent, may be preferable because it does not have any active metabolites, although it must be taken 30 minutes before meals so as not to delay absorption, which may decrease compliance. The advantage of both of these newer agents over the older ones is that they are less likely to interact with other drugs. All sulfonylureas except for glimepiride are now available in generic form and are reasonably priced. For a 30-day supply of the lowest daily dose, wholesale costs range from $1.36 for chlorpropamide to $15.69 for glyburide (17).

Biguanides

The only biguanide available in the United States is metformin. It has recently been approved for oral treatment of type 2 diabetes, either alone or with a sulfonylurea. The most serious side effect is lactic acidosis, but this is a much less common problem than with the biguanide phenformin, which is no longer available. Since the biguanides inhibit lactate metabolism, increased concentrations of the drug due to renal insufficiency can cause lactic acidosis. Metformin therefore should be avoided by patients with conditions associated with renal insufficiency (e.g., hepatic or cardiac failure) and in patients with renal failure. It is contraindicated in men with a serum creatinine concentration above 1.5 mg/dL and in women with a serum creatinine concentration above 1.4 mg/dL (18). Drug clearance has also been shown to decrease with increases in age independent of renal function (19), so low doses should be used in the elderly.

The advantages of metformin are several. It has a positive effect on lipids by lowering triglycerides and low-density lipoprotein (LDL) cholesterol. It also does not contribute to weight gain in the obese patient. This effect may be due to significant gastrointestinal side effects, such as nausea, vomiting, anorexia, diarrhea, and a metallic taste in the mouth (20). While age is not a contraindication to its use, renal function should be monitored closely during treatment with metformin. The drug should be stopped 2 days prior to radiologic procedures involving contrast dyes.

α-Glucosidase Inhibitors

Acarbose reversibly binds to α-glucosidases on the upper intestinal brush border. This delays the digestion of disaccharides and complex carbohydrates and hence the absorption of glucose and other monosaccharides. Since only 1% of acarbose is absorbed, systemic effects are rare. However, flatulence, bloating, and diarrhea are common at high doses because of fermentation of unabsorbed carbohydrates in the large bowel. Acarbose has no effect on fasting glucose but has been shown to lower hemoglobin A1c values by 0.5 to 1% (21). It can be used alone with diet therapy or in addition to other hypoglycemics. Unfortunately, its gastrointestinal side effects and its cost ($41.32 per month) (17) may be prohibitive to the elderly diabetic patient.

Thiazolidinediones

The newest oral hypoglycemic is troglitazone, the first drug to improve peripheral insulin resistance in skeletal muscle. Its pharmacokinetics do not appear to be altered by age. Troglitazone has been used in trials alone and in combination with sulfonylureas and with insulin. It significantly decreases insulin requirements, fasting blood glucose, and hemoglobin A1c levels (22, 23). The benefits of this drug to elderly diabetic patients are that it causes no weight gain and no hypoglycemia, and it may reduce blood pressure (24). Unfortunately, hepatic injury and rare cases of hepatic failure have been reported in patients taking troglitazone. Therefore serum transaminase levels should be checked at the start of therapy, monthly for the first 6 months, every other month for the rest of the first year, and periodically thereafter. Further, troglitazone should not be used by patients with active liver disease. Therapy should be stopped if the patient exhibits signs or symptoms of liver disease or if the transaminases are elevated to 3 times normal (23). Its current cost at $160.20 per month makes it prohibitive to patients paying for their own medications.

Insulin

Insulin therapy may be needed to achieve metabolic control and may be preferable to oral agents in some patients. The decision to treat with insulin must include an assessment of the patient's beliefs about insulin and the potential for its safe use. For example, since most older patients have type 2 disease, they are likely to have had experiences with other family members or friends with diabetes. Insulin therapy is frequently instituted several years after diagnosis, when disease complications may be manifest. Thus, the worsening complications may be falsely attributed to the insulin itself. This and other fears should be explored with patients. In addition, visual and cognitive function and manual dexterity require careful evaluation if patients will be administering the insulin themselves. If not, the adequacy of informal or formal supports to manage insulin therapy consistently and safely must be evaluated.

Insulin therapy is frequently instituted in the hospital setting, when a diagnosis of diabetes is first made in conjunction with an admission for an acute infectious illness, a complication, or complicated hyperglycemia (e.g., for the diabetic hyperosmolar state or ketoacidosis). Given the differences in diet, physical activity, and stress levels between the hospital and the home, particular attention should be paid to monitoring the transition from hospital to home. This is a time when serious hyperglycemia or hypoglycemia is likely to occur, either because of changes in these factors or because of misunderstandings about dosing and the technical aspects of insulin administration.

When exogenous insulin is used as sole therapy for elderly diabetics, its dosage and injection schedule should be individualized. The ideal insulin regimen should have a low risk of hypoglycemia while controlling symptoms of hyperglycemia. After changing from oral therapy to insulin, most patients feel better, although some weight gain may occur with increasing insulin doses. A starting dose of 0.25 U/kg per day of intermediate-acting insulin (NPH) minimizes the risk of hypoglycemia. Adding a dose before dinner or at bedtime helps to reduce fasting blood glucose. Additional doses of short-acting insulin can be given with or between the NPH to control hyperglycemia. Insulin regimens should be tailored to the patient's response as well as to his or her acceptance of the regimen.

Insulin Plus Oral Agents

A recent meta-analysis of randomized, placebo-controlled trials comparing insulin plus sulfonylurea agents with insulin plus placebo demonstrated better metabolic control (lower fasting glucose values and lower glycohemoglobin concentrations) in patients on insulin plus a sulfonylurea (25). Furthermore, combination therapy required a smaller daily insulin dose to achieve better metabolic control. In common use is the regimen bedtime insulin, daytime sulfonylurea. Intermediate-acting insulin is given at night to suppress nocturnal hepatic gluconeogenesis and glycogenolysis and to lower fasting serum glucose. The sulfonylurea given during the day increases insulin secretion when stimulated by meals and decreases peripheral insulin resistance. This regimen requires the patient and/or caregivers to learn the techniques of insulin administration. The advantage is that lower doses of insulin may used, minimizing obesity and the atherosclerosis and hypertension that may result from hyperinsulinemia (26, 27).

Monitoring

Although self-monitoring of blood glucose is safe and relatively easy for most patients, its use has not been studied systematically in older persons. The main reasons to consider glucose monitoring in older patients are to prevent hypoglycemia in patients treated with hypoglycemic medications, particularly during illness and when medication changes are planned, and to guide adjustments of hypoglycemic therapy in conjunction with hemoglobin A1c levels. The hemoglobin A1c reflects glucose levels over the previous 8 to 12 weeks and is therefore useful in monitoring glycemic control over time.

Cardiovascular Risk Factors

The San Luis Valley Diabetes Study compared cardiovascular risk factor patterns in diabetic patients with such patterns in those who have impaired glucose tolerance. The findings suggest that the adverse risk factor profile seen so frequently in diabetics may develop either before or with diabetes (28). Regardless of when risk factors develop, diabetics are more likely to be hypertensive, to have elevated lipid levels, and to be obese (28, 29). These are equally strong risk factors for coronary disease in diabetics and in nondiabetics. Furthermore, diabetes itself is a risk factor for coronary heart disease (29, 30), and it not only negates the protective effect of female gender but confers a worse prognosis in women who develop myocardial infarctions and congestive heart failure (29).

There is no evidence that treating these risk factors confers the same or a greater benefit as in nondiabetics. Nonetheless, given the doubled or tripled risk of myocardial infarction and stroke in diabetics, it is prudent to try to modify cardiovascular risk factors, particularly in older persons, in whom additional comorbidities may cause important decrements in already compromised physical, social, and emotional function. Targeting obesity theoretically would improve clinical outcomes most, since it is a coronary heart disease risk factor and contributes to adverse lipid profiles and hypertension. However, the difficulties associated with achieving weight loss, as outlined earlier, are likely to impair the effectiveness of this approach in many older persons.

Although attempts at weight loss and diet modification should not be discounted or neglected, an equally important strategy for risk factor reduction is the treatment of any hypertension. Accumulating evidence suggests that treatment with angiotensin-converting enzyme (ACE) inhibitors can decrease proteinuria and preserve the glomerular filtration rate in patients with type 2 diabetes, whether or not they have hypertension (31, 32). This is an important observation, since at least 20% of type 2 patients develop nephropathy. Since many older diabetics have cardiac conditions that warrant the use of an ACE inhibitor, this class of antihypertensives is the drug of choice for treating hypertension in these patients. Careful attention should be paid to potassium levels when beginning therapy, since hyperkalemia may develop in those with even mild renal insufficiency. While cost and dry cough are other concerns, the additional advantage of these agents is that they do not cause or exacerbate urinary incontinence, constipation, lipid abnormalities, or hyperglycemia.

Given that the risk of cardiovascular disease in diabetics is increased and that two other independent risk factors for cardiovascular disease are age and hypercholesterolemia, it is recommended that all adults with diabetes be considered for aggressive treatment of dyslipidemia

(33). Further review of lipid abnormalities in the elderly can be found in Chapter 26. Once nutrition therapy and weight reduction have been attempted, drug therapy is indicated. The newer β-hydroxy-β-methyglutaryl coenzyme A (HMG-CoA) reductase inhibitors have few gastrointestinal side effects and minimal drug-drug interactions. Niacin should be avoided, since it can worsen glycemic control. The American Diabetes Association recommends lowering LDL cholesterol to less than 130 mg/dL in all diabetic patients and to less than 100 mg/dL in diabetic patients with known coronary heart disease.

Finally, although rates of cigarette smoking decline with age, an important subset of smokers survive to old age. Recent evidence suggests that the hazards of cigarette smoking for men and women, particularly with respect to cardiovascular mortality, extend into later life. Furthermore, the risk of death from cardiovascular disease for former smokers is similar to that of never smokers, independent of age at which people quit (34). Taken together, these data should compel clinicians to work with their older diabetic smokers to help them to quit.

Eye Disease

Data from the 1989 National Health Interview Survey indicate that among diabetics aged 65 and older, about 16% have serious trouble seeing, even with glasses (35). This is not only because of the ravages of diabetic retinopathy but also because older diabetics are likely to have cataracts and glaucoma. While 22% report that they have cataracts and 6% report that they have glaucoma (3), data from the Wisconsin Epidemiologic Study of Diabetic Retinopathy (WESDR) indicate that the prevalence of these conditions is actually much higher when based on physical examination. In that study of 1370 patients 30 years and older, over 95% of diabetics more than age 65 had evidence of cataracts; 7.5% had glaucoma. In comparison, between 35% and 40% in this age group who were not taking insulin had diabetic retinopathy; this rose to 50 to 70% in insulin users; about 8% had macular edema (36). Clearly, older diabetic patients have a considerable burden of eye disease. Given the critical importance of visual function to overall independence, eye disease in older diabetics deserves critical attention by clinicians.

The risk of developing diabetic retinopathy increases with duration of disease. Nearly all of type 1 diabetics and more than 60% of type 2 diabetics have retinopathy after 20 years. Because patients with type 2 disease frequently have had their disease for some time prior to diagnosis, they may already have retinopathy by the time they are diagnosed. Poor glucose control is also a risk factor for retinopathy.

Retinopathy may be manifested by preproliferative background changes, nonproliferative retinopathy, or more severe proliferative changes. Because of the high likelihood of finding preexisting retinopathy, all newly diagnosed diabetics should be referred for ophthalmologic evaluation, not only for retinopathy but also for cataracts and glaucoma. Ideally this evaluation should include stereoscopic fundus photography, since even in the best hands dilated ophthalmoscopy has a sensitivity of only about 80% for detecting proliferative retinopathy (37). The American College of Physicians, in conjunction with the American Diabetes Association and the American Academy of Ophthalmology, has published guidelines stating that if initial stereoscopic screening is negative, further screening need not occur until 4 years later, when annual screening with stereoscopic photographs or dilated ophthalmoscopy should begin. This strategy, of course, demands careful attention to ensuring that patients are followed carefully to avoid missing the 4-year anniversary. If stereoscopic photographic screening is not available, dilated ophthalmoscopy should be performed annually (38). The reasons for being compulsive about ophthalmologic screening are that one-third of the cases of blindness in diabetics are due to retinopathy; laser photocoagulation surgery has been shown to prevent visual loss in patients with proliferative retinopathy and macular edema; and treatment of comorbid eye disease may also help to preserve visual function.

Foot Care

For diabetic patients the risk of amputation increases with age. The estimated amputation rate in 1990 for those aged 65 to 74 was 1.4 times as high and for those aged 75 or older, 2.4 times as high as in diabetic patients under age 65 (39). In addition to the monetary costs of amputations is their profound effect on patients' mobility and the likelihood that they will precipitate institutionalization.

Peripheral vascular disease and sensory neuropathy are risk factors for lower extremity trauma and falls as well as for amputation. A recent case-control study has demonstrated that lack of patient education is an additional important risk factor for amputation (40). It is well known that most diabetic patients do not engage in preventive care of their feet and that physicians infrequently examine diabetics' feet. Improved self-care and physicians' attention to foot abnormalities, however, can be achieved relatively easily and inexpensively, improving outcomes (41). Patients should be instructed in self-examination methods, nail and callus care, washing techniques, and what constitutes appropriate footwear. Since many older persons have fungal infections of their nails and cannot safely cut them, referral to a podiatrist is prudent. Physicians should examine diabetic feet at each visit. This examination can be used to reinforce important foot care behaviors. At least annually, diabetics should also have a thorough vascular examination, which includes palpation of the lower extremity pulses, a neurologic examination to assess sensorimotor deficits, and a musculoskeletal examination to evaluate range of motion of the foot and ankle as well as bony abnormalities (42). Although there is still much to learn about the prevention and treatment of diabetic foot lesions, successful implementation of these strategies is a place to start.

Cognitive Function

There is evidence that older diabetic patients are more likely than their nondiabetic age-matched counterparts to perform poorly on cognitive tests. A recent literature review found consistently poorer verbal memory in diabetics than in nondiabetics despite significant heterogeneity among the methods of the studies reviewed (43). These changes are similar to those associated with normal aging, but whether they are manifestations of accelerated aging or occur via other mechanisms is not clear. Older diabetics are also more likely to have strokes and possibly adverse effects on cognition from hyperglycemia and hypoglycemia and hyperosmolar and hypoosmolar states. These are additional reasons for treating hypertension and for maintaining metabolic stability. Indeed, recent studies suggest that improved glycemic control improves some aspects of cognitive function in older patients with type 2 disease (44). There is also evidence for an association between diabetes and Alzheimer's disease, especially among those treated with insulin (45), although the mechanism is not yet known.

Because of diabetes-related changes in cognitive function and the increased likelihood of dementia, both age- and diabetes-related, periodic assessment of cognitive function in older diabetics is essential. This can reassure the worried well, who may have concerns about memory problems, and identify early those beginning to have subtle difficulties. Careful attention to these issues may uncover adverse drug effects, other metabolic derangements (e.g., hypothyroidism), and depression and identifies those who need additional help from clinicians and family or friends in adhering to complex treatment regimens.

Comorbidity

Because they have diabetes and manifestations of the complications thereof, as well as because of age, older type 2 diabetic patients are likely to have considerable coexisting disease. The fact that these patients take several medications and the likelihood that they have diminished organ function (especially renal function) and decreased physiologic reserve increase their risk of adverse drug effects. Careful attention therefore should be paid to avoiding drug-drug interactions. In addition, since compliance with medications is known to diminish as the number of medications and the complexity of the regimen increases, the physician should consider ways of decreasing the total number of medications (e.g., using one medication for more than one indication). This may also help with cost, which is frequently an issue for older persons on fixed incomes.

Family Considerations

There is growing evidence that families play significant roles in the management of older persons with chronic disease in addition to the well-known role that they play in the general daily care of frail older persons (46). A recent study of 357 family members of diabetic patients aged 70 or older demonstrated that over half (71% were spouses) participated in the patient's diabetes care (47). Although there is some evidence from studies involving younger patients with type 2 disease that regimen-specific family support is correlated with higher rates of adherence to regimens, no such studies have been done with older patients. If patients are having difficulty adhering to treatment regimens, if they rely on family members for certain activities (e.g., food preparation, managing medications), or if they have functional disabilities, their family members or other informal care providers must be taught about diabetes and receive instruction and support in methods of management.

SUMMARY AND CONCLUSIONS

Diabetes is common in older persons and is associated with considerable economic and personal costs. Attention to the prevention and management of cardiovascular, eye, and foot disease is therefore critical. Whether this can be achieved by maintaining tight glycemic control is not known. Although reducing blood glucose levels to values that eliminate hyperglycemic symptoms while minimizing the potential for hypoglycemic reactions should be attempted and cardiovascular risk factors treated, equal attention should be given to preventing eye and foot complications, in which screening and treatment have known efficacy.

REFERENCES

1. Rubin RJ, Altman WM, Mendelson DN. Health care expenditures for people with diabetes mellitus, 1992. J Clin Endocrin Metab 1994;78:809A–F.
2. Weinberger M, Cowper PA, Kirkman MS, Vinicor F. Economic impact of diabetes mellitus in the elderly. Clin Geriatr Med 1990;6:959–970.
3. Harris MI. Epidemiology of diabetes mellitus among the elderly in the United States. Clin Geriatr Med 1990; 6:703–719.
4. Harris MI. Undiagnosed NIDDM: clinical and public health issues. Diabetes Care 1993;16:642–652.
5. Report of the Expert Committee on the Diagnosis and Classification of Diabetes Mellitus. Diabetes Care 1997;20:1183–1197.

6. Fletcher RH, Fletcher SW, Wagner EH. Clinical Epidemiology: The Essentials. Baltimore: Williams & Wilkins, 1982.

7. Guide to Clinical Preventive Services. Report of the U.S. Preventive Services Task Force. 2nd ed. Baltimore: Williams & Wilkins, 1996.

8. Von Korff M, Gruman J, Schaefer J, et al. Collaborative management of chronic illness. Ann Intern Med 1997; 127:136–145.

9. Reed RL, Mooradian AD. Nutritional status and dietary management of elderly diabetic patients. Clin Geriatr Med 1990;6:883–901.

10. American Diabetes Association. Position statement: Translation of the diabetes nutrition recommendations for health care institutions. Diabetes Care 1997;20(suppl 1):S37–S39.

11. Goldberg L, Elliot DL. The effect of physical exercise on lipid and lipoprotein levels. Med Clin North Am 1985;69:41–45.

12. Seals DR, Hagberg JM. The effect of exercise training on human hypertension: a review. Med Sci Sports Exerc 1984;16:207–215.

13. American Diabetes Association. Position statement: Diabetes and exercise. Diabetes Care 1997;20(suppl 1)S51.

14. Turner R, Cull C, Hollman R. United Kingdom prospective diabetes study 17: a 9-year update of a randomized, controlled trial on the effect of improved metabolic control on complications in non-insulin-dependent diabetes mellitus. Ann Intern Med 1996;124:136–145.

15. Lebovitz HE. Physician's Guide to Non-Insulin-Dependent (Type II) Diabetes: Diagnosis and Treatment. Alexandria, VA: American Diabetes Association, 1988.

16. Peters AL, Davidson MB. Use of sulfonylurea agents in older diabetic patients. Clin Geriatr Med 1990;6:903–921.

17. Troglitazone for non-insulin-dependent diabetes mellitus. Med Lett Drugs Ther 1997;39:49–51.

18. McEvoy GK, ed. American Hospital Formulary Service Drug Information 97. Bethesda, MD: American Society of Health System Pharmacists, 1997.

19. Sambol NC, Chiang J, Lin ET, et al. Kidney function and age are both predictors of pharmacokinetics of metformin. J Clin Pharmacol 1995;35:1094–1102.

20. Bailey CJ. Biguanides and NIDDM. Diabetes Care 1992;15:755–772.

21. Hotta N, Kakata H, San T, et al. Long term effect of acarbose on glycemic control in NIDDM; a placebo-controlled double-blind trial. Diabetes Med 1993;10:134–138.

22. Kumar S, Boulton AJ, Beck-Nielsen H, et al. Troglitazone, an insulin action enhancer, improves metabolic control in NIDDM patients. Troglitazone Study Group. Diabetologia 1996;39:701–709.

23. Parke-Davis. Package literature for Rezulin. 1997.

24. Jennings PE. Oral antihyperglycaemics. Considerations in older patients with non-insulin-dependent diabetes mellitus. Drugs Aging 1997;10:323–331.

25. Johnson JL, Wolf SL, Kabadi UM. Efficacy of insulin and sulfonylurea combination therapy in type II diabetes. Arch Intern Med 1996;156:259–264.

26. Zavaroni I, Bonora E, Pagliara M, et al. Risk factors for coronary artery disease in healthy persons with hyperinsulinemia and normal glucose tolerance. N Engl J Med 1989;320:702–706.

27. Stout RW. Insulin and atheroma. Diabetes Care 1990;13:631–654.

28. Burchfiel CM, Hamman RF, Marshall JA, et al. Cardiovascular risk factors and impaired glucose tolerance: the San Luis Valley Diabetes Study. Am J Epidemiol 1990;131:57–70.

29. Kannel WB. Lipids, diabetes, and coronary heart disease: insights from the Framingham Study. Am Heart J 1985;110:1100–1107.

30. Koskinen P, Manttari M, Manninen V, et al. Coronary heart disease incidence in NIDDM patients in the Helsinki Heart Study. Diabetes Care 1992;15:820–825.

31. Kasiske BL, Kalil RS, Ma JZ, et al. Effect of antihypertensive therapy on the kidney in patients with diabetes: a meta-regression analysis. Ann Intern Med 1993;118: 129–138.

32. Ravid M, Savin H, Jutrin I, et al. Long-term stabilizing effect of angiotensin-converting enzyme inhibition on plasma creatinine and on proteinuria in normotensive type II diabetes patients. Ann Intern Med 1993;118: 577–581.

33. American Diabetes Association. Position statement: Standards of medical care for patients with diabetes mellitus. Diabetes Care 1997;20(suppl 1):S5–S13.

34. LaCroix AZ, Lang J, Scherr P, et al. Smoking and mortality among older men and women in three communities. N Engl J Med 1991;324:1619–1625.

35. National Diabetes Data Group. Diabetes in America. 2nd ed. Bethesda, MD: National Institutes of Health, 1995.

36. Klein BEK, Klein R. Ocular problems in older Americans with diabetes. Clin Geriatr Med 1990;6:827–837.

37. Singer DE, Nathan DM, Fogel HA, Schachat AP. Screening for diabetic retinopathy. Ann Intern Med 1992; 116:660–671.

38. American College of Physicians, American Diabetes Association, American Academy of Ophthalmology. Screening guidelines for diabetic retinopathy. Ann Intern Med 1992;116:683–685.

39. Centers for Disease Control and Prevention. Diabetes Surveillance. Atlanta: US Department of Health and Human Services, 1993.

40. Reiber GE, Pecoraro RE, Koepsell TD. Risk factors for amputation in patients with diabetes mellitus: a case-control study. Ann Intern Med 1992;117:97–105.

41. Litzelman DK, Slemenda CW, Langefeld CD, et al. Reduction of lower extremity clinical abnormalities in patients with non-insulin-dependent diabetes mellitus: a randomized, controlled trial. Ann Intern Med 1993; 119:36–41.

42. American Diabetes Association. Position statement: Foot care in patients with diabetes mellitus. Diabetes Care 1997;20(suppl 1):S31–S32.

43. Strachan MW, Deary IJ, Ewing FM, Frier BM. Is type II diabetes associated with an increased risk of cognitive dysfunction? A critical review of published studies. Diabetes Care 1997;20:438–445.

44. Meneilly GS, Cheung E, Tessier D, et al. The effect of improved glycemic control on cognitive functions in the elderly patient with diabetes. J Gerontol Med Sci 1993;48:M117–M121.

45. Ott A, Stolk RP, Hofman A, et al. Association of diabetes mellitus and dementia: the Rotterdam Study. Diabetologia 1996;39:1392–1397.

46. Stone R, Cafferata GL, Sangl J. Caregivers of the frail elderly: a national profile. Gerontologist 1987;27:616–626.

47. Silliman RA, Bhatti S, Khan A, et al. The care of older persons with diabetes mellitus: families and primary care physicians. J Am Geriatr Soc 1996;44:1314–1321.

CHAPTER 38

JANE F. DANAHY AND BARBARA A. GILCHREST

Geriatric Dermatology

Skin problems are common among the elderly and can interfere significantly with quality of life (1, 2). Over the past 15 years, clinical research has begun to clarify the prevalence and epidemiology of cutaneous disorders and complaints among the elderly. At the same time, basic research has begun to define the histologic and molecular changes in aging skin. Breakthroughs have occurred in the understanding of photoaging and its sequelae, ultraviolet-induced skin cancers, and pathophysiology of the most common blistering disorder of the elderly, bullous pemphigoid.

This chapter first reviews the clinical and histologic skin changes associated with aging, distinguishing between intrinsic aging and photoaging, then discusses skin tumors and dermatoses that commonly cause morbidity in the elderly. Emphasis is on recent advances relevant to the management of geriatric skin problems.

SKIN AGING: INTRINSIC AGING VERSUS PHOTOAGING

Skin aging has two components, intrinsic aging and photoaging. The recognition of the difference between these two processes permits analysis of their relative contributions to the appearance of aged skin and its predisposition to dermatologic disease. Intrinsic aging is best reflected by the clinical changes seen over time in sun-protected skin, whereas photoaging denotes in addition skin changes attributable to chronic sun exposure.

Intrinsically aged skin is thin, pale, and lax. Aged skin has decreased maximal function and reserve capacity, manifested as increased fragility and decreased immune responsiveness, thermoregulation, sweat responses, wound healing, and epidermal turnover. Structurally, intrinsically aged skin has a thinned epidermis, decreased vascularity, and marked thinning of the dermis. The most striking change is a flattening of the dermoepidermal junction with loss of the normal rete ridge pattern, an alteration that causes a loss of cohesion at the dermoepidermal interface and may account for the propensity of aged skin to blistering and blistering disorders.

In contrast, dermatoheliosis, or photoaging, accounts for the majority of the clinical changes seen in habitually sun-exposed skin. Coarseness, pigmentary changes, telangectasia, and deep wrinkling are all attributable to the cumulative effects of ultraviolet irradiation. The major morbidity of photoaging is the development of skin malignancies. The ultraviolet spectrum responsible for photodamage is UVA (320 to 400 nm) and UVB (290 to 320 nm) irradiation, as UVC (200 to 290 nm) radiation is effectively blocked by the ozone layer. While UVB radiation, the ultraviolet wavelengths primarily responsible for sunburning, was initially thought to be responsible for most of changes of photodamage, it is now understood that UVA also plays an important role, especially in the dermal changes of photoaging. Moreover, UVA wavelengths are responsible for virtually all drug photosensitivity reactions, such as those observed in patients taking thiazide diuretics, tricyclic antidepressants, certain hypoglycemic agents, and antibiotics.

The characteristic histologic changes seen in photoaged skin include keratinocytic heterogeneity, irregular distribution of melanocytes with increased melanization, a decreased Langerhans cell population, accumulation of abnormal elastotic material in the papillary dermis, dilated and tortuous blood vessels, and a low-grade inflammatory dermal infiltrate. The electron microscopic changes in photoaging are similarly specific (3). Some of the important clinical and histologic features of intrinsic and photoaging are compared in Table 38.1.

Strategies to prevent photodamage, hence prevent the morbidity and mortality of skin cancers, include sun avoidance, sun-protective clothing, and sunscreens. Physical sun blocks such as titanium dioxide protect against both UVA and UVB radiation. Most chemical sunscreen preparations protect against UVB irradiation preferentially, but newer broad-spectrum preparations absorb or reflect UVA irradiation also. Regular sun protection begun early in life should prevent photoaging and decrease the risk of skin cancer. In older patients with already damaged skin, regular sunscreen use has shown to decrease the frequency of new actinic keratoses, a common premalignancy of the skin, and to permit regression of established lesions (4).

Treatment for established photoaging is also available. The first agent firmly demonstrated clinically and histologically to improve photodamaged skin is topical tretinoin (all trans-retinoic acid), a derivative of vitamin A (5, 6). The observation that overall skin appearance improved in older women being treated with tretinoin for acne vulgaris led to controlled trials of the topical retinoid for photoaging that confirmed the initial observations and led to U.S.

Food and Drug Administration (FDA) approval of the drug for this indication. Within 4 to 6 months, daily tretinoin use improves photo-damage-associated hyperpigmentation, wrinkling, and roughness. Histologically, with the use of tretinoin, the epidermis thickens, melanin content decreases, the stratum corneum becomes more compact, and dermal mucin and collagen formation increase. Other studies have shown that topical tretinoin is also more effective than sun avoidance alone in preventing or reversing actinic keratoses. More recently tretinoin has been shown to ameliorate the changes associated with intrinsic aging also. Benefits of topical tretinoin therapy are relatively long-lasting even after discontinuation, and with one to three weekly applications, most users appear to maintain indefinitely the improvement gained after 6 to 12 months of daily application.

α-Hydroxy acids have also been shown to improve photoaged skin. Small studies of α-hydroxy acid use show mild clinical improvements in sallowness and wrinkling correlated with histologic thickening of the epidermis, a normalization of the rete ridge pattern of the dermoepidermal junction, decreases in the numbers of atypical basal cells, and increased dermal mucopolysaccharides (7). The mechanism of these effects is unclear, as is their duration. There are no data on the prevention of skin cancers with α-hydroxy acids. Skin atrophy, wrinkling, and dryness of aging skin in older women may also be improved by the use of postmenopausal estrogen replacement (8), although the effect on photodamage specifically has not been analyzed.

From a practical perspective, patients should be advised that daily sunscreen use prevents or arrests virtually all of the unwanted age-associated cosmetic changes in their skin and greatly reduces their risk of skin cancer. Topical tretinoin therapy provides additional benefit but entails greater cost and the likelihood of mild retinoid dermatitis (redness and scaling) at least initially. The very popular and numerous α-hydroxy acid-containing cosmetics may also improve skin appearance, although few data are available. Finally, improved skin comfort and appearance are likely to accompany skeletal and cardiovascular benefits in patients using estrogen replacement therapy.

Table 38.1

Aging Versus Photoaging: Clinical Aspects

Aging	Photoaging
Atrophic skin (epidermis and dermis)	Hypertrophic or atrophic skin
Decreased but uniform pigmentation	Irregular hyperpigmentation and hypopigmentation
Relatively smooth surface	Prominent fine and coarse wrinkling
	Skin malignancies

PREMALIGNANT LESIONS AND SKIN CANCERS

Ultraviolet-induced skin cancers are the most serious consequence of photodamage. The incidence of melanoma and nonmelanoma skin cancers has increased markedly over the past 20 years, with an exponential increase in age-specific incidence throughout adulthood. In 1994, the estimated incidence of nonmelanoma skin cancers, combined basal and squamous cell cancers, was 900,000 to 1.2 million (9) with estimated lifetime risks in the United States of developing a squamous cell or basal cell cancer 10 and 30% respectively (9). Deaths from squamous cell cancers are estimated at 1200 per year. Although still far less common than non-melanoma skin cancer, melanomas have increased in incidence far more rapidly over the past 20 years (10-12), with an estimated 40,300 new cases and 7300 expected deaths from melanoma in 1997 (13). Early recognition of premalignant and malignant skin lesions can thus prevent significant morbidity and mortality.

ACTINIC KERATOSES

Actinic keratoses, also called solar keratoses, are the most common premalignant skin lesions, affecting by some estimates 60% of light-complexioned persons over age 40. Actinic keratoses are important because they are direct precursors of invasive squamous cell carcinoma. Moreover, their presence is a risk factor for the other skin cancers, basal cell carcinoma and melanoma, and hence an indication that patients should be carefully monitored.

Actinic keratoses occur in light-skinned people in chronically sun-exposed areas such as the face, scalp, and forearms. They present as rough, gritty, or scaly papules or plaques, which are often more easily palpated than seen. Actinic keratoses can vary in size from 1 or 2 mm to several centimeters. They are sometimes slightly tender and occasionally have an overlying keratotic horny projection, a so-called cutaneous horn. Equivalent lesions on the lip are termed actinic cheilitis.

Although progression to invasive malignancy is uncommon to rare (14, 15), actinic keratoses are squamous cell carcinomas in situ. The histologic hallmark of an actinic keratosis is keratinocytic dysplasia, or disordered keratinocyte maturation. Not all squamous cell carcinomas develop from actinic keratoses, but the lifetime risk of an invasive squamous cell carcinoma in a person with multiple actinic keratoses may be significant.

All treatment modalities for actinic keratoses are locally destructive (16) and rely on reepithelialization with less-damaged keratinocytes, such as those from the hair follicles inaccessible to ultraviolet irradiation. Liquid nitrogen cryotherapy splits the skin at the dermoepidermal junction, removing the abnormal epidermal keratinocytes. Blistering or crusting at the treated sites typically resolves in a week. For extensively affected skin, topical 5-fluorouracil is another commonly used therapy. The cream is applied twice daily to the entire sun-damaged area rather than exclusively to discrete lesions and thus targets subclinical keratoses as well. After 2 to 3 weeks, sufficiently actinically damaged areas become tender, red, and often frankly eroded, at which point treatment is discontinued and healing occurs over an additional 2 to 3 weeks. Because of the severe irritation often associated with intensive topical 5-fluorouracil regimens, some practitioners favor less frequent applications over longer periods. Chemical peels, laser resurfacing, and curettage are other treatment options, for which the patient should be referred to a dermatologist familiar with these procedures.

SQUAMOUS CELL CARCINOMA

Risk factors for the development of squamous cell cancer (Fig. 38.1) include advanced age, light complexion, and sun exposure. As documented in studies of renal transplant recipients, chronic immunosuppression is also a risk factor for both squamous and basal cell cancers (17). Less commonly the development of squamous cell cancers is associated with environmental exposures to arsenic, thermal burns, x-rays, or chronic infection with oncogenic human papilloma virus subtypes.

Clinically a squamous cell carcinoma may have a variety of appearances, and any nonhealing nodule or plaque should arouse suspicion. It may occur as firm, indurated erythematous or pink scaling nodule or plaque. Its surface may be kera-

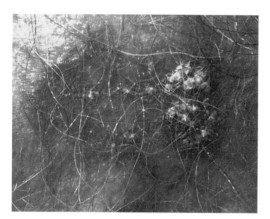

Figure 38.1. Squamous cell carcinoma in situ (Bowen's disease).

totic, ulcerated, or crusted. Typically squamous cell carcinomas are slow growing, but they can rapidly increase in size and metastasize. Squamous cell carcinomas of the head and neck have a particular propensity for invasion, and squamous cell carcinomas arising in scars are well described. Any nonhealing or newly ulcerated area within a scar merits evaluation. The association of squamous cell carcinoma with sun exposure is well documented. The accumulation of ultraviolet-induced mutations in the keratinocyte DNA first initiates and then promotes the malignant phenotype. Treatment either destroys or removes the tumors. Squamous cell carcinoma may respond to cryotherapy with liquid nitrogen or to carbon dioxide laser treatment. Radiation therapy is another treatment option, especially for tumors of certain locations or in patients too debilitated to undergo surgery. Surgical excision and Mohs' micrographic surgery are the most common treatment modalities.

BASAL CELL CARCINOMA

Basal cell carcinoma is the most common human malignancy. Ultraviolet damage is associated with the development of basal cell carcinomas but less strongly than with squamous cell carcinomas. Arsenic exposure and x-rays are also known risk factors. Although most basal cell skin cancers are easily curable, patients with a history of a basal cell carcinoma are at risk for subsequent skin cancers. Photoprotection and annual cutaneous examinations are recommended thereafter.

Basal cell carcinoma usually begins as a smooth firm papule in sun-exposed skin. Lesions are often described as pearly or translucent and often have overlying telangiectasias. They occur with great frequency on the face and especially over the nose. Clinical variants of basal cell carcinoma include the rodent ulcer (Fig. 38.2), which has a characteristic rolled firm border and a central crust; superficial basal cell carcinoma, which is usually a thin pink or erythematous plaque with a slightly elevated border and often an atrophic center; and the morpheaform basal cell carcinoma, which has a whitish almost scarlike appearance. Basal cell carcinomas are uncommonly pigmented.

Basal cell carcinomas are slow-growing tumors with very low metastatic potential. Local invasion into bony structures of the skull, for example, of large neglected tumors is seen but is uncommon. As with squamous cell carcinoma, treatment of basal cell carcinoma is tailored to the tumor size and location and the patient's comorbidities. Most tumors are surgically excised or removed with Mohs' micrographic surgery. Cryosurgery and radiotherapy are less commonly used therapies.

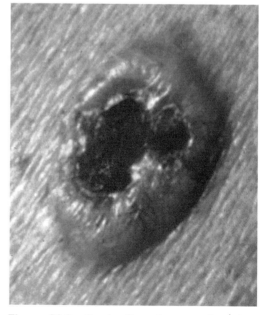

Figure 38.2. Basal cell carcinoma, rodent ulcer type. (Courtesy of Amal K. Kurban, M.D.)

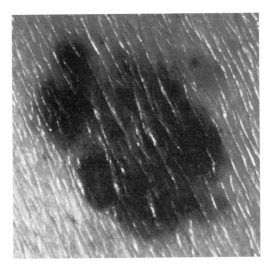

Figure 38.3. Malignant melanoma, superficial spreading type. (Courtesy of Thomas E. Rohrer, M.D.)

MELANOMA

As with squamous cell carcinoma (12), there is a statistically greater mortality rate for older men with melanoma than for women or for younger men, probably attributable to delayed diagnosis. Surgical cure of melanoma depends strongly on early diagnosis, with 5-year disease-free rates approaching 100% for very thin (less than 0.76 mm) lesions but less than 50% for thick primary lesions, even in the absence of clinically detectable spread at the time of diagnosis.

Risk factors for melanoma include a family history of melanoma, a history of dysplastic and congenital nevi, numerous nevi, fair complexion, and sun exposure. Whereas squamous cell cancer is associated with chronic sun exposure, melanoma seems more closely associated with intense intermittent sun exposure.

Melanomas usually begin as pigmented macules that spread and become more irregular in contour or color and may become elevated. Any new or changing pigmented lesion in the elderly deserves careful examination, and if any suspicion of melanoma exists, a biopsy should performed. As depth of invasion is critical prognostic information, shave biopsies of atypical pigmented lesions are not recommended.

The four clinical types of melanoma are superficial spreading melanoma (about 70% of cases) (Fig. 38.3), nodular melanoma (about 15 to 30%), acral lentiginous melanoma (about 2 to 10%) (Fig. 38.4), and lentigo maligna melanoma (about 5%). The last two types are relatively common in dark-skinned persons and in the elderly, respectively, and deserve special consideration in geriatric dermatology, as their incidence peaks in the 70s and 80s. However, as with other forms of skin cancer, age-specific incidence of all melanoma subtypes increases throughout adulthood.

Lentigo maligna is a type of in situ melanoma that occurs almost exclusively in elderly whites over areas of chronically sun-exposed skin such as the head, neck, and chest. Typically lentigo maligna begins as a pigmented macule that slowly grows. It may have variegated colors, with pink, tan, brown, and black seen in the same lesion.

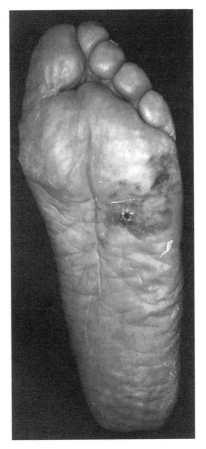

Figure 38.4. Acral lentiginous melanoma. (Courtesy of Thomas E. Rohrer, M.D.)

Chronic sun exposure is more closely linked with this form of melanoma than with other forms. The term lentigo maligna melanoma describes an invasive melanoma arising in a lentigo maligna. Although it was suggested that lentigo maligna melanoma conferred a better prognosis than other melanomas, multivariate analyses have shown that there is no difference in survival when the tumors are grouped by depth of invasion. Acral lentiginous melanoma denotes melanoma on the palms, soles, or nail beds. The most common form of melanoma in dark-skinned people, it is an irregular pigmented macule, papule, or plaque. It is often diagnosed later than other melanomas and hence has an unfavorable prognosis overall.

Pathologically all melanomas are proliferations of atypical melanocytes. All except nodular melanoma seem to begin with a radial growth phase, followed by an invasive or vertical growth phase. Melanoma is graded by depth of invasion, and depth correlates inversely with survival. The Breslow thickness of a tumor is measured from the top of the viable epidermis to the point of deepest invasion. Depth of less than 0.76 mm is associated with a 96% 5-year survival, whereas tumor depth of more than 4 mm is associated with 47% 5-year survival. In addition to depth, factors independently associated with poor prognosis in melanoma include advanced age, anatomic sites (scalp, hands, and feet are associated with worse prognoses), male sex, and ulceration.

There are two staging systems commonly used in melanoma. The traditional three-stage system divides disease according to its presence in the skin, nodes, and distant metastases. Stage I indicates disease limited to the skin and is further classified by Breslow thickness; stage II indicates nodal metastases; and stage III denotes distant metastases. The American Joint Committee on Cancer staging system divides patients into four stages in a classic tumor, node, metastasis (TNM) classification. Once melanoma is diagnosed, an appropriate staging evaluation should be done.

Although wide surgical margins were recommended in the past for all melanomas, the current recommendations are more conservative: melanoma less than 1 mm deep is excised with 1-cm margins; intermediate thickness, 2 to 4 mm, with 2-cm margins, and tumors deeper than 4 mm are excised with 3-cm margins. The benefit of elective lymph node dissections in the search for occult nodal disease has not been proved. Sentinel node dissection (selective lymph node dissection) intended to spare some of the morbidity of a complete lymph node dissection, is an experimental approach only.

Multiple chemotherapeutic and immune-modifying therapies have been used in the treatment of metastatic melanoma. Recently high-dose interferon A 2b has shown a survival benefit in a cohort of patients with metastatic disease (19).

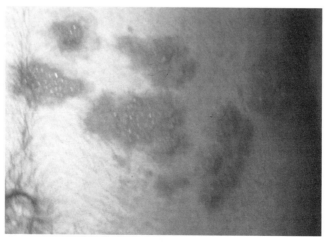

Figure 38.5. Herpes zoster. Dermatomal distribution of clustered vesicles. (Courtesy of Amal K. Kurban, M.D.)

HERPES ZOSTER

The major risk factor for herpes zoster (Fig. 38.5), an eruption due to reactivation of latent varicella zoster virus (VZV) infection, is advanced age. The morbidity of zoster also increases with age. A recent 2-year health maintenance organization (HMO) based survey of 1075 cases of zoster seen in 500,408 observed person years found 215 cases of herpes zoster per 100,000 person years overall, but among those over age 75, there were 1424 cases per 100,000 person years (20). This study also showed the incidence of zoster to be higher than previously reported, which may reflect true epidemiologic changes in the disease.

VZV is a DNA virus that shares with other herpesviruses the cardinal feature of latency. Varicella, the primary infection, is spread by respiratory secretions or direct skin contact and is responsible for chickenpox, the characteristic mild 1- to 3-week illness among children. Varicella is typically more severe as a primary infection in adults, with a higher rate of systemic complications. The decline in cell-mediated immunity that parallels aging is thought to account for the propensity for zoster in the elderly. In addition to age itself, predisposing factors for zoster include recent surgery or other trauma, and immunosuppression.

Zoster occurs equally in men and women, usually only once. More than two episodes of zoster in a lifetime is rare. Typically zoster presents with a prodrome with malaise, then pain and paresthesia centered around a dermatome. Pain is usually mild to moderate in younger people with zoster, but more often severe in older patients. Skin tenderness may precede the typical skin eruption, which evolves quickly from erythematous macules to papules into vesicles (Fig. 38.6) overlying a unilateral dermatomal distribution. Thoracic dermatomes are the most commonly affected. Typically zoster resolves in 2 to 3 weeks. As with varicella, herpes zoster can be complicated by bacterial superinfection of the skin lesions or systemic manifestations, including pneumonia, meningoencephalitis, arthritis, hepatitis, and cranial nerve palsies. Often a few vesicles are seen outside the primarily involved dermatome, but when more then 20 vesicles are

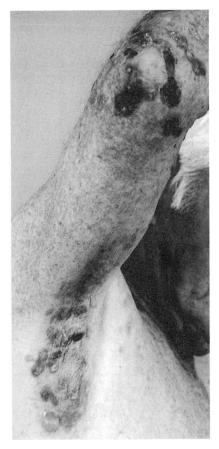

Figure 38.6.   Herpes zoster. A close-up of vesicles. (Courtesy of Amal K. Kurban, M.D.)

seen outside a dermatome, the illness is termed disseminated zoster. This has a higher rate of complications and usually warrants hospitalization for systemic treatment.

The diagnosis of zoster is usually made clinically. A Tzanck smear may help substantiate the suspicion of zoster. In this simple test a slide is prepared from the fluid and cells scraped from the base of a vesicle and stained with Wright's, Giemsa, or hematoxylin and eosin stains. Multinucleate giant cells help substantiate the diagnosis of zoster in the proper clinical setting, but they are not specific for zoster and can also be seen, for example, in herpes simplex infections. Viral cultures from the vesicle fluid can distinguish zoster from other herpetic infections but are technically difficult, and often no virus is identified. An immunoperoxidase or immunofluorescence test or enzyme immunoassay can also distinguish among herpes virus infections.

The differential diagnosis of zoster includes herpes simplex and other localized skin infections, contact dermatitis, burns, and insect bites. During the prodrome, zoster may mimic biliary disease, sciatica, and a wide variety of other pain syndromes.

Complications

The complications of zoster can be divided into the complications of the acute infection, such as cranial nerve palsies and ocular involvement, and those occurring subsequently, the prototype being postherpetic neuralgia. Zoster occurring in the distribution of certain cranial nerves can cause distinct clinical syndromes. Facial palsies and associated tinnitus, vertigo, deafness, loss of hearing, or loss of taste should alert one to the possibility of zoster and prompt an examination of the ear, nose, and mouth for the vesicular eruption.

Zoster occurring in the V1 dermatome can be complicated by ocular involvement and a range of ocular pathology: corneal ulcers, keratitis, scleritis, uveitis, neuritis, glaucoma. When zoster presents on the face, especially in the trigeminal nerve distribution V1, an ophthalmologic evaluation is warranted. A clinical sign that may correlate with eye involvement is the so-called Hutchinson's sign. Skin lesions occurring over the tip and side of the nose may indicate ophthalmic involvement, as the nerve area is supplied by the nasociliary branch of the ophthalmic nerve.

Postherpetic neuralgia is variously defined as pain that persists after the skin eruption of zoster has resolved or for an arbitrary length of time, such as 3 months. The incidence of postherpetic neuralgia increases with age, and some estimate that 20 to 40% of those over 60 have it. Patients at particular risk are those with ophthalmic zoster, very severe initial pain, severe skin lesions, or very high VZV antibody titers. The pathophysiology is unknown. In about half of patients it resolves spontaneously in 1 to 3 months, but in others it is persistent and disabling.

Treatment

Antiviral therapy in zoster has been shown to limit the extent of zoster acutely and to limit its complications. Acyclovir, a nucleoside analog that inhibits viral DNA polymerase, has been shown to decrease pain and the duration of viral shedding and to speed the time to healing of skin lesions if therapy is begun within 72 hours of disease onset. Importantly, acyclovir has also been shown to reduce the risk and duration of postherpetic neuralgia. The effective dose of acyclovir is 800 mg orally 5 times a day for 7 days.

Two related antivirals are also approved for the treatment of zoster: famciclovir, the prodrug of penciclovir, and valacyclovir, the prodrug for acyclovir. The approved dosing for famciclovir is 500 mg and for valacyclovir 1 g, both given orally 3 times a day for 7 days. In clinical trials the three drugs are similar in their effects on healing of skin lesions, duration of acute pain, and risk of development of postherpetic neuralgia, although valacyclovir may be most effective with regard to the latter two parameters (21). Famciclovir requires dose adjustment for creatinine clearances of less than 60 mL per minute. Although initial reports suggested an effect, corticosteroids administered orally during the acute zoster episode have not consistently proven beneficial in preventing postherpetic neuralgia (22).

In the future, use of the live attenuated VZV vaccine may reduce the morbidity associated with zoster. This vaccine has been used safely in some elderly populations, but no randomized controlled trials have been completed, nor is it clear that the immunity conferred by this vaccine protects against reactivation of the virus (23).

BULLOUS PEMPHIGOID

Bullous pemphigoid (Fig. 38.7) is a relatively common autoimmune blistering disorder (24), usually in patients between ages 60 and 80. Bullous pemphigoid is characterized by tense clear or hemorrhagic bullae usually distributed preferentially over flexural areas, the abdomen, or intertriginous areas. A localized variant occurs over the lower extremities. Lesions can arise on normal-appearing or erythematous skin, and sometimes papules or urticarial plaques predominate over frank blisters. Often pruritus is a cardinal

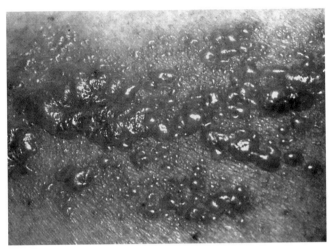

Figure 38.7.   Bullous pemphigoid. Note the hemorrhagic crusts and intact bullae. (Courtesy of Jill R. Slater-Freedberg, M.D.)

feature, and this may precede other findings. The blisters of bullous pemphigoid may evolve into erosions and crusts; these typically heal with postinflammatory pigment changes but without scarring. Mucous membrane involvement occurs in an estimated 30% of patients but is rarely a presenting feature. Administration of drugs such as captopril, furosemide, phenacetin, and aldosterone antagonists as well as exposure to ultraviolet light have been associated with the development of the disease.

Skin biopsy is diagnostic in almost all patients. Histologically, bullous pemphigoid is characterized by a subepidermal blister with a normal overlying epidermis and an inflammatory, predominantly eosinophilic dermal infiltrate of variable extent. The extent of this infiltrate varies. Immunofluorescence reveals the deposition of immunoglobulin-τ (IgG) and C3 at the dermoepidermal junction, the site of discohesion between the dermis and epidermis. Indirect immunofluorescence reveals circulating autoantibodies in 60 to 70% of patients, but titers do not correlate with disease activity. The pathogenic antibodies responsible for bullous pemphigoid are directed against the hemidesmosome-associated proteins located in the lamina lucida region of the basement membrane zone. The differential diagnosis of bullous pemphigoid includes other less common blistering diseases, such as epider-molysis bullosa acquisita, linear immunoglobu-lin-α (IgA) bullous disease, and dermatitis herpetiformis.

Typically, bullous pemphigoid is self-limited, with most cases resolving over the course of several months or years (26). Treatment depends largely on the extent of the disease. Sometimes limited involvement can be managed with topical corticosteroids only, but most patients require oral glucocorticoids for adequate disease control, and in the presteroid era death from sepsis was common. A typical regimen of 1 mg/kg of prednisone is continued until no new blisters form; the dose is then gradually tapered. Dermatologic referral is strongly advised for the management of bullous pemphigoid. Azathioprine is used commonly as a steroid-sparing agent. Other effective but less commonly used treatments include cyclophosphamide, methotrexate, dapsone, pulse corticosteroids, and cyclosporine. The combination of tetracycline and nicotinamide is reported to be efficacious, especially in limited disease (27).

Although previous literature suggested a relation between bullous pemphigoid and internal malignancy, when patients are stratified by age, no excess malignancies are found among the patients with bullous pemphigoid. Hence, development of this disease is not itself an indication for a malignancy workup.

PRURITUS

Pruritus is common in the elderly (1, 28, 29). It is typically classified as pruritus with a known cause, either dermatologic or systemic disease, or idiopathic pruritus. Before the diagnosis of idiopathic pruritus is made, known causes of itching must be excluded. A thorough history may uncover medications or topical contactants that may be responsible. A directed physical examination may reveal scabies or a systemic disease such as hepatic or renal disease, thyroid disease, lymphoma, anemia, or paraproteinemia as a cause for the pruritus. In a survey study of dermatologists, most supplemented their clinical evaluation of pruritic elderly patients with laboratory tests (29).

Idiopathic pruritus tends to be general and to worsen with age. There are no primary skin lesions, and even secondary skin changes, such as excoriations or lichenification, may be absent. Skin biopsy is unrevealing. Pruritus associated with detectable systemic disease is characteristically severe and responds best to amelioration of the underlying disease. Idiopathic pruritus is often associated with xerosis and in any case often responds at least partially to regular use of emollients. Some patients find emollients containing phenol or menthol particularly soothing, perhaps because of the alternative skin sensations imparted by these additives. Topical corticosteroids are generally ineffective. Oral antihistamines may be prescribed, particularly at bedtime, but must be used with caution in the elderly. Sedative effects and drug interactions of antihistamine preparations should be reviewed carefully with each patient.

ONYCHOMYCOSIS

The development of new and more efficacious antifungal medications has focused attention on the previously recalcitrant problem of onychomycosis, fungal infection of the nails (Fig. 38.8). An estimated 20% of people aged 40 to 60 have onychomycosis, and this frequency is certainly greater among older people (2). Recent reviews have emphasized the morbidity associated with onychomycosis: ill-fitting shoes, pain associated with walking, compromised tactile function of the nails, and difficulty with routine nail care (30).

Onychomycosis usually presents as nail dystrophy with thickening, yellowing, and subungual debris. Predisposing factors include tinea pedis, slower growth of the nails with age, tight-fitting or occlusive footwear, and increased trauma to the foot. Age-associated decreases in immune function and decreased circulation to the distal foot have also been postulated as contributing factors. Toenails are more commonly affected than fingernails. Although onychomycosis is the most common reason for thickened, yellowed nails, differential diagnosis includes psoriasis and changes of the nail due to trauma.

Because the treatment for onychomycosis entails months of systemic therapy and considerable expense, confirming the diagnosis before initiating therapy is strongly advised. The presence of hyphae on a potassium hydroxide (KOH) preparation or on pathologic examination of the nail stained with periodic acid Schiff (PAS) confirms the diagnosis. Fungal culture may take a few weeks to grow, but it has the advantage of identifying the fungal pathogen. The most common organisms causing onychomycosis in the United States are the dermatophytes *Trichophyton rubrum* and *Trichophyton mentagrophytes*.

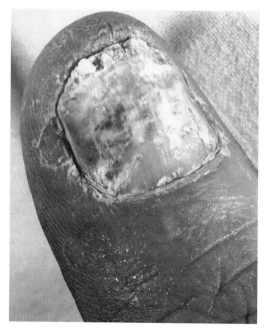

Figure 38.8.   Onychomycosis. (Courtesy of Amal K. Kurban, M.D.)

Yeasts and nondermatophytic molds are less common causes of onychomycosis.

The newer oral antifungal drugs are safer and more efficacious than previously used griseofulvin and ketoconazole, whose utility were limited because of the long duration of treatment required (often a year or longer), high relapse rates, and drug interactions and other side effects. In contrast itraconazole, terbinafine, and fluconazole have excellent safety records, require usually only 3 months of therapy, and have long-term mycologic cure rates up to 65 to 85%. Itraconazole and terbinafine are FDA-approved for the treatment of onychomycosis, with recommended doses of 200 mg and 250 mg per day respectively. Both drugs have a high affinity for keratinized structures, creating a reservoir of drug in the nail plate that provides continuous delivery of the drug with intermittent dosing. Fluconazole has been used extensively, but the optimal dosing for onychomycosis has yet to be determined. Each of the agents is effective against most dermatophytes that cause onychomycosis, although their efficacy against other fungi differs slightly.

The administration of itraconazole with terfenadine, astemizole, or cisapride is contraindicated because of the associated fatal ventricular arrhythmias, prolonged QT intervals, and torsades de points associated. Itraconazole is an inhibitor of the P450 cytochrome oxidase system, and coadministration may alter the drug levels of medications commonly used by the elderly, such as digoxin, warfarin, and oral hypoglycemics.

BENIGN PROLIFERATIVE LESIONS ASSOCIATED WITH AGING

Certain benign proliferative lesions occur frequently in the elderly. These include seborrheic keratoses, cherry angiomas, sebaceous hyperplasia, and acrochordons. Their importance lies in the possible confusion with malignant lesions and with the cosmetic distress they sometimes cause older persons. Seborrheic keratoses are pink to darkly hyperpigmented warty papules and plaques with a characteristic stuck-on appearance. If bothersome, seborrheic keratoses can be treated with liquid nitrogen, curettage, or light electrocautery; otherwise they require no therapy. Rarely, a biopsy is indicated to exclude melanoma. Cherry angiomas are bright red smooth papules, usually 2 to 4 mm, that consist of a proliferation of vessels in the papillary dermis. They can occur anywhere on the skin but are most common over the trunk. Histologically they are a proliferation of vessels and endothelial cells in the papillary dermis. Cherry angiomas may be removed with shave excisions, a tunable dye laser, or electrocautery.

Sebaceous hyperplasia usually presents as firm yellowish lobulated facial papules with a central dell. These sometimes resemble basal cell carcinomas, although a dermatologist can almost always differentiate the two conditions without biopsy. Acrochordons, or skin tags, are flesh-colored or slightly hyperpigmented pedunculated papules, often found in the axillae, groin, around the neck, or over the upper eyelids. These are common in women and in obese persons. An experienced clinician can easily excise bothersome skin tags.

SEBORRHEIC DERMATITIS

Seborrheic dermatitis is a common inflammatory condition of unknown causation consisting of erythema with overlying waxy scale preferentially involving the scalp, eyebrows, nasolabial folds, and postauricular areas. Sometimes the central chest is also involved. It tends to be more severe in patients with HIV disease and certain neurologic disorders. Most patients clear within days using hydrocortisone 1 or 2.5% cream twice a day. This therapy can then be used intermittently and indefinitely as needed to suppress the dermatitis. The frequent improvement observed with topical antifungal preparations suggests a role for the yeast *Pityrosporum ovale* in pathogenesis of seborrheic dermatitis. In stubborn cases, ketoconazole 2% cream twice a day may be added or substituted for hydrocortisone.

REFERENCES

1. Beauregard S, Gilchrest BA. A survey of skin problems and skin care regimens in the elderly. Arch Dermatol 1987;123:1638–1643.
2. Fleischer AB Jr, McFarlane M, Hinds MA, Mittlemark MB. Skin conditions and symptoms are common in the elderly: the prevalence of skin symptoms and conditions in an elderly population. J Geriatr Dermatol 1996;4:78–87.
3. Toyoda M, Bhawan J. Electron-microscopic observations of cutaneous photoaging versus intrinsic aging. J Geriatr Dermatol 1995;3:131-143.

4. Thompson SC, Jolley D, Marks R. Reduction of solar keratoses by regular sunscreen use. N Engl J Med 1993; 329:1147–1151.

5. Gilchrest B. Treatment of photodamage with tretinoin: an overview. J Am Acad Dermatol 1997;36:S27–S36.

6. Topical drugs for aging skin. Med Lett Drugs Ther 1997;39:78–79.

7. Ditre CM, Griffin TD, Murphy GF, et al. Effects of alpha-hydroxy acids on photoaged skin: a pilot clinical, histologic, and ultrastructural study. J Am Acad Dermatol 1996;34:187–195.

8. Dunn LB, Damesyn M, Moore AA, et al. Does estrogen prevent skin aging? Results from the first national health and nutrition examination survey (NHANES 1). Arch Dermatol 1997;133:339–342.

9. Miller DL, Weinstock MA. Nonmelanoma skin cancer in the United States: incidence. J Am Acad Dermatol 1994;30:774–778.

10. Gallagher RP, Ma B, McLean DI, et al. Trends in basal cell carcinoma, squamous cell carcinoma, and melanoma of the skin from 1973 through 1987. J Am Acad Dermatol 1990;23:413–421.

11. Glass AG, Hoover RN. The emerging epidemic of melanoma and squamous cell skin cancer. JAMA 1989; 262:2097–2100.

12. Weinstock M. Death from skin cancer among the elderly: epidemiologic patterns. Arch Dermatol 1997; 133:1207–1209.

13. Parker SL, Tong T, Bolden S, Wingo PA. Cancer Statistics, 1997. CA Cancer J Clin 1997;47:8–9.

14. Dodson JM, DeSpain J, Hewett JE, Clark DP. Malignant potential of actinic keratoses and the controversy over treatment. Arch Dermatol 1991;127:1029–1031.

15. Marks R. The role of treatment of actinic keratoses in the prevention of morbidity and mortality due to squamous cell carcinoma. Arch Dermatol 1991;127:1031–1033.

16. Drake LA, Ceilley RI, Cornelison RL, et al. Guidelines of care for actinic keratoses. J Am Acad Dermatol 1995; 32:95–98.

17. Webb M, Compton F, Andrews P, Koffman C. Skin tumors posttransplantation: a retrospective analysis of 28 years' experience at a single center. Transplant Proc 1997;129:828–830.

18. Johnson TM, Smith JW, Nelson BR, Chang A. Current therapy for cutaneous melanoma. J Am Acad Dermatol 1995;32:689–707.

19. Kirkwood JM, Strawderman MH, Ernstoff MS, et al. Interferon alfa-2b adjuvant therapy of high-risk resected cutaneous melanoma: the Eastern Cooperative Oncology Group trial EST 1684. J Clin Oncol 1996;14: 7–17.

20. Donahue JG, Choo PW, Manson JE, Platt R. The incidence of herpes zoster. Arch Intern Med 1995;155: 1605–1609.

21. Beutner KR, Friedman DJ, Forszpaniak C, et al. Valacyclovir compared with acyclovir for improved therapy for herpes zoster in immunocompetent adults. Antimicrob Agents Chemother 1995;39:1546–1553.

22. Whitley RJ, Weiss H, Gnann JW, et al. Acyclovir with and without prednisone for the treatment of herpes zoster. Ann Intern Med 1996;125:376–383.

23. Levin MJ, Hayward AR. Prevention of herpes zoster. Infect Dis Clin North Am 1996;10:657–675.

24. Bernard P, Vaillon L, Labeille B, et al. Incidence and distribution of subepidermal autoimmune bullous skin diseases in three French regions. Arch Dermatol 1995; 131:48–52.

25. Bastuji-Garin S, Pascal J, Picard-Dahan C, et al. Drugs associated with bullous pemphigoid: a case-control study. Arch Dermatol 1996;132:272–276.

26. Ahmed AR, Maize JC, Provost TT. Bullous pemphigoid: Clinical and immunologic follow-up after successful therapy. Arch Dermatol 1977;113:1043–1046.

27. Fivenson DP, Breneman DL, Rosen GB, et al. Nicotinamide and tetracycline therapy of bullous pemphigoid. Arch Dermatol 1994;130:753–758.

28. Gilchrest BA. Pruritus in the elderly. Semin Dermatol 1995;14:317–319.

29. Fleischer Jr AB. Pruritus in the elderly: management by senior dermatologists. J Am Acad Dermatol 1993;28: 603–609.

30. Scher R. Onychomycosis is more than a cosmetic problem. Br J Dermatol 1994;130:15.

Anemia and Other Hematologic Problems of the Elderly

ANEMIA

Anemia is the most common hematologic disorder encountered by physicians caring for elderly patients. It occurs when the quantity or quality of circulating erythrocytes falls below normal. It has been suggested that an age-related decline in hematologic parameters occurs, and therefore, that hematologic norms should be lowered for the elderly (1). Opponents of this belief suggest that while anemia is prevalent, it should not be regarded as a normal concomitant of aging and caution against establishing lower hematologic norms for elderly persons (2). Defining hematologic norms for the elderly is difficult, since studies of "normal" elderly populations often include large numbers of persons with chronic and inapparent underlying diseases that may affect hematopoietic function.

The concentration of hematopoietic stem cells and bone marrow stroma function is preserved in healthy elderly persons. More committed bone marrow red blood cell precursor concentrations are reduced in normal elderly persons, suggesting that marrow proliferative capacity becomes attenuated (3). Hematopoietic reserve and the capability to respond to a major stressor, such as sepsis or significant blood loss, is variable. It is suggested that the common low-grade anemia in elderly persons may be a result of a chronic low-grade nutritional deficiency or a chronic disease that is not clinically apparent (4). There is consensus that an evaluation of anemia is indicated in elderly persons and when the hemoglobin concentration is 12 g/dL or less for men and 11.5 g/dL or less for women or when a recent fall in hemoglobin concentration (1 g/dL or more over a year) has occurred (5–7).

Anemia is most commonly found among hospitalized patients (8), institutionalized patients, persons of low socioeconomic classes, persons of African-American descent (9), patients with concomitant disease or poor nutritional status, patients who have had a recent gastrectomy (10, 11), and elderly men. The symptoms of anemia, fatigue, light-headedness, shortness of breath at rest or with mild exercise, and angina, rarely occur until hemoglobin levels have fallen below 8 g/dL in otherwise healthy persons.

Classification of Anemias

Anemia may be classified into three types of disorders: (a) decreased red blood cell production (hypoproliferative or hyporegenerative anemias), (b) ineffective hematopoiesis (the megaloblastic anemias, thalassemias, and myelodysplastic syndromes), and (c) red blood cell destruction (hemolysis) (12, 13).

Hypoproliferative Anemias

IRON DEFICIENCY ANEMIA. Iron deficiency anemia occurs when there is a reduced iron supply for hemoglobin synthesis as a result of blood loss, malnutrition, or chronic inflammation. Iron requirements do not change with age, and iron absorption is unchanged in the elderly (14). Tea and coffee consumption reduce absorption, and vitamin C enhances it (15). There is minimal daily loss of iron in stool, sweat, urine, and other secretions. Dietary iron deficiency can occur in elderly patients with atrophic gastritis and hypochlorhydria, since an acidic milieu enhances absorption. Iron storage in the form of ferritin and hemosiderin in general increases with age. Most total body iron exists in circulating hemoglobin.

The main cause of iron deficiency anemia is blood loss, most commonly through the gastrointestinal tract, frequently as a result of using nonsteroidal anti-inflammatory drugs and steroids or because of cancer; ulcers; polyps; angiodysplasia; more rarely, neoplasms of the genitourinary tract; bleeding disorders; and chronic intravascular hemolysis (16). The laboratory diagnosis of iron deficiency anemia may be suggested by a reduced serum ferritin concentration (no more than 50 mg/L in association with transferrin saturation below 15%) (17, 18). The peripheral blood smear usually contains hypochromic and microcytic red blood cells. The blood findings in iron deficiency anemia may be altered in elderly persons with anemia of chronic diseases (normal or high ferritin levels with low transferrin levels), and when both conditions coexist, the only definitive test may be a bone marrow examination (19). Iron deficiency anemia is diagnosed with certainty by lack of bone marrow iron stores.

The investigation of patients with iron deficiency anemia should focus on identifying the source of blood loss. Stool should be examined for occult blood. Further investigation, including colonoscopy and esophagogastroduodenoscopy, may also be indicated to identify any upper and lower gastrointestinal bleeding sources. Concomitant lesions of both the upper and lower gastrointestinal tract are rare, such that detection of the likely source of blood loss during the initial examination may obviate further investigations (20). Symptoms related to a specific site in the gastrointestinal tract usually predict disease in the corresponding portion of the bowel. The positive predictive value of symptoms in the lower gastrointestinal tract and positive fecal occult blood tests is very high (86%) for detecting lesions of the lower gastrointestinal tract (21). If neither colonoscopy nor esophagogastroduodeno-

scopy identifies a source of blood loss, a reasonable approach is to observe the patient over time and provide supplemental iron. Patients who fail to respond to iron may require further evaluation, including a small-bowel series. Intravascular hemolysis may be detected by examining the blood smear.

The management of patients with iron deficiency anemia requires identifying and treating the source of blood loss and providing iron supplementation. Patients with iron deficiency anemia show rapid improvements once taking iron therapy. A 2 g/dL rise in hemoglobin should occur within 2 weeks of therapy, and a reticulocytosis response should occur within a week. Iron supplementation should be continued for 6 months to replenish iron stores. Gastrointestinal side effects (constipation, cramping, diarrhea, and nausea) may occur in patients taking supplemental iron preparations. At 325 mg of ferrous sulfate per day, side effects are less likely to occur. Ferrous gluconate, ferrous fumarate, and pediatric iron suspensions are well tolerated. Parenteral iron therapy may be useful for patients with poor absorption (inflammatory bowel disease, malabsorption) and in rare patients who are intolerant of all oral iron preparations. Iron dextran may be given intramuscularly or intravenously. Side effects, such as arthralgia, myalgia, fever, itching, and rarely, anaphylaxis, may occur. Red blood cell transfusion is indicated only for severe hemorrhage, for patients with symptoms of anemia, and for patients with hemoglobin levels below 8 g/dL who are asymptomatic (22, 23). Blood transfusion is indicated for hemoglobin levels below 10 g/dL who have significant coronary artery disease.

ANEMIA OF CHRONIC DISEASES. The anemia associated with chronic disease (ACD) is the most common form of anemia in older persons (24). It is usually mild, stable, and related to the severity of the underlying disease (Table 39.1). Typically, red blood cells are normochromic and normocytic, although occasionally red blood cells are microcytic. Several mechanisms have been proposed to account for the development of anemia in these conditions. The net effect is an impaired ability of the reticuloendothelial cell to recruit iron derived from phagocytosed red blood

Table 39.1

Disorders Associated With the Anemia of Chronic Diseases

Chronic renal failure
Liver failure
Chronic infections
    Bacterial endocarditis
    Chronic pyelonephritis
    Chronic fungal infections
    Tuberculosis
Neoplasms
    Lymphoma
    Leukemia
    Multiple myeloma
Collagen-vascular diseases
    Rheumatoid arthritis
    Osteoarthritis
    Polymyalgia rheumatica
    Systemic lupus erythematosus
Endocrine disorders
    Hypothyroidism
    Addison's disease
    Hypopituitarism
Chronic bed sores (stages 3 and 4)

cells. Iron released from the phagocytosed red cell is diverted to iron stores in the form of ferritin and hemosiderin instead of being delivered to the cell membrane for uptake by circulating transferrin.

Evidence suggests that the erythropoietic abnormalities of ACD are caused by the secretion by macrophages of the endogenous pyrogens, interleukin-1, and tumor necrosis factor (25). These pyrogens may be responsible for the decreased ability of the reticuloendothelial system to release iron. Secretion of interleukin-1 and tumor necrosis factor occurs in neoplasia, chronic infections, and chronic or acute inflammatory disorders (chronic renal failure, rheumatoid arthritis, osteomyelitis). Other mechanisms may affect development of the ACDs, including a reduction in erythropoietin production relative to the degree of anemia, a reduction in red cell survival, blood loss, immune hemolysis, and sideroblastic anemia (26).

Multiple myeloma should be considered as a possible cause in elderly patients who present with a low-grade normochromic normocytic anemia and no obvious underlying causative chronic disorder (27). A combination of anemia, fatigue, and an elevation of the erythrocyte sedimentation rate should prompt the physician to order a serum protein electrophoresis and immunoelectrophoresis.

In patients with ACD, the hemoglobin level is usually above 10 mg/dL, the serum iron level is usually reduced (not more than 60 mg/dL), and serum transferrin levels are below 250 μg/dL. In contrast to iron deficiency anemia, the serum ferritin level is normal or increased (28). A bone marrow evaluation reveals abundant iron stores but reduced iron incorporated into maturing erythroblasts. The management of patients with ACD should focus on identifying and treating the underlying disorder. In patients with chronic renal disease, erythropoietin 50 to 100 U/kg given parenterally 3 times per week, with doses increasing to 150 U/kg if there is no response in 2 to 3 weeks, reduces the need for red blood cell transfusions (29–31). Concomitant iron therapy is usually necessary when treating with erythropoietin.

HYPOPLASTIC BONE MARROW. Rarely intrinsic bone marrow failure selectively affects red blood cell production. The most common causes of red blood cell stem cell dysfunction are bone marrow invasion by tumor, bone marrow fibrosis, medications, autoimmune disorders, and rarely, infections (32). Most commonly implicated medications include penicillamine, chloramphenicol, gold, phenylbutazone, anticonvulsants, propylthiouracil, chloroquine, sulfonamides, and quinidine (33). Effects may be mediated by dose-related, idiosyncratic, or hypersensitivity reactions. Tuberculosis, brucellosis, hepatitis A and B, and rarely, mumps, rubella, mononucleosis, and influenza infections may cause intrinsic bone marrow failure affecting red blood cell production. Aplastic anemia and hairy cell leukemia should be considered in the differential diagnosis of bone marrow hypoplasia. When these conditions are suspected, a bone marrow aspiration and biopsy are always indicated, and patients should be evaluated by a hematologist.

Ineffective Erythropoiesis

Ineffective erythropoiesis may occur because of abnormalities of either nuclear or cytoplasmic maturation of red blood cells. Megaloblastic anemia, which occurs when nuclear maturation becomes impaired, is almost always due to vitamin B_{12} or folic acid deficiency (Table 39.2). The megaloblastic anemias are characterized by macrocytosis (mean corpuscular volume above 100), hypersegmented granulocytes, indirect hyperbilirubinemia, and a bone marrow that shows megaloblastoid erythrocyte precursors, band forms, and giant metamyelocytes. Normoblastic macrocytosis may occur in elderly patients who are chronic tobacco and alcohol abusers, also in patients with hypothyroidism, leukemia, and among patients taking anticonvulsant medications.

VITAMIN B_{12} DEFICIENCY. The normal diet contains 5 to 30 μg of vitamin B_{12} per day, with most dietary vitamin B_{12} coming from animal tissues. Pure vegetarians who also avoid dairy products can become vitamin B_{12} deficient on a dietary basis, but this is uncommon. Most elderly persons have adequate stores of vitamin B_{12}, and enterohepatic absorption ensures that stores are not depleted. No changes in vitamin B_{12} absorption occur in the elderly. Low levels of vitamin B_{12} have

Table 39.2

Causes of Folic Acid Deficiency

Dietary
  Alcoholism
  Malabsorption
  Coeliac disease
  Tropical sprue
Increased use, cell turnover states
  Neoplasms
  Hemolysis
  Blood dyscrasias
Drugs
  Anticonvulsants
  Trimethoprim
  Pyrimethamine
  Methotrexate
  Sulfasalazine
Loss
  Skin exfoliation
  Dialysis
  Liver damage
  Biliary loss
Reduced effectiveness
Vitamin C deficiency

been described in the elderly without any hematologic or neurologic complications (34). Low serum levels of vitamin B_{12} can also be seen among patients with iron deficiency and folic acid deficiency even when vitamin B_{12} stores are normal (35).

The prevalence of vitamin B_{12} deficiency increases with age, and the most common cause is malabsorption (36). Pernicious anemia, atrophic gastritis, small-bowel bacterial overgrowth, ileal malfunction, and certain medications (neomycin, potassium chloride, para-amino salicylic acid, and alcohol) may result in vitamin B_{12} deficiency. Other causes include surgical removal of the gastric antrum (postgastrectomy patients), chronic treatment with histamine blockers or proton pump inhibitors, *Helicobacter* infections, and inadequate ability to hydrolyze food-bound vitamin B_{12} (37). While most elderly patients have some degree of atrophic gastritis, most secrete enough intrinsic factor to ensure adequate absorption of vitamin B_{12}.

Pernicious anemia is the most common cause of vitamin B_{12} deficiency. It is a systemic familial disorder characterized by megaloblastic hematopoiesis and neuropathy. After age 70, 0.1 to 0.2% of persons are affected; it is most common in persons of northern European descent (38). It is an autoimmune disorder characterized by gastric parietal cell atrophy resulting in an inability to secrete intrinsic factor. Some 80% of patients with pernicious anemia have anti–parietal cell antibodies and close to 60% have anti–intrinsic factor antibodies. Intrinsic factor is required to bind specifically with cobalamin (vitamin B_{12}) extracted from foods for transport to the terminal ileum where absorption occurs. Patients with pernicious anemia frequently have other autoimmune disorders, including vitiligo, psoriasis, hypothyroidism, diabetes mellitus, and hypoparathyroidism.

Patients may present with fatigue, anorexia, anergia, glossitis, and weight loss. Neurologic symptoms may be subtle and may occur even when the patient is not anemic (30%). Common neurologic symptoms include paresthesia, gait abnormalities, psychologic symptoms (delirium, paranoia, psychosis, personality changes, and depression) (39), visual problems, impotence, urinary incontinence, sensory ataxia, and peripheral neuropathy. The full-blown subacute combined degeneration of the spinal cord syndrome has been well described in patients with pernicious anemia.

The diagnosis is made by measuring serum vitamin B_{12} levels, and the cause may be more clearly defined by the Schilling test, which tests a patient's ability to absorb radioactive labeled cyanocobalamin. Elevated serum or urine levels of methylmalonic acid and homocysteine may help confirm the diagnosis (40). A food Schilling test can help diagnose inability to extract vitamin B_{12} from dietary sources. Treatment, which consists of monthly administration of parenteral hydroxocobalamin, should be continued for life. Hematologic function improves almost immediately, but neurologic symptoms rarely improve, especially if they have been present for more than 6 months. Macrocytosis may persist for months, and peripheral hypersegmented polymorphonucleocytes may be still present up to a year after treatment.

FOLIC ACID DEFICIENCY. The anemia associated with folic acid deficiency is secondary only to iron deficiency as a nutritional cause for anemia. Older people are likely to be deficient in folic acid because of poverty, reduced dietary intake of vegetables, or overcooking of foods. Body stores folic acid can deplete in 4 months. The diagnosis of folic acid deficiency anemia should be suspected when anemia together with an increased mean corpuscular volume, leukopenia, and thrombocytopenia is found. The peripheral blood smear may show hypersegmented neutrophils (containing more than 5 nuclear lobes), anisocytosis, and macroovalocytes. The serum lactate dehydrogenase and indirect bilirubin may be elevated, reflecting ineffective erythropoiesis and premature destruction of red blood cells. The diagnosis is confirmed by demonstrating low serum folic acid or red blood cell folate concentration (less than 150 μg/mL). Serum red blood cell folic acid levels more accurately reflect deficiency of folic acid stores.

Before beginning treatment, it is important to exclude concomitant vitamin B_{12} deficiency, since administering folic acid to a patient with vitamin B_{12} deficiency may result in neurologic complications. Treatment is directed at replacing folic acid. Blood transfusions are rarely required. Folic acid

may be given at doses of 1 mg per day until the deficiency is corrected. Higher doses may be required in patients with malabsorption syndromes.

ABNORMALITIES OF CYTOPLASMIC MATURATION. *Myelodysplastic Syndromes.* Myelodysplastic syndromes are clonal disorders of bone marrow precursor cell maturation that result in abnormal development of red blood cell lines (41). Five forms of myelodysplasia have been described according to findings seen on examination of the peripheral blood smear and bone marrow biopsies. These include (*a*) refractory anemia (RA), (*b*) refractory anemia with ringed sideroblasts (RARS), (*c*) refractory anemia with excess blasts (RAEB), (*d*) chronic myelomonocytic leukemia (CML), and (*e*) refractory anemia with excessive blasts in transformation (RAEBT). RA and RARS have a better prognosis than the others. Patients with RA and RARS may have mild anemias and are as symptomatic, but some progress to bone marrow failure or acute leukemia, usually acute myeloid leukemia. Occasionally patients develop myelodysplastic syndromes as a result of chemotherapy or radiotherapy, but the most common cause is idiopathic. The diagnosis is suggested by anemia associated with macrocytosis, anisocytosis, and poikilocytosis. Serum iron and transferrin levels are usually normal or elevated (42).

The treatment of myelodysplasia is mostly supportive. Pyridoxine 50 to 200 mg per day may be effective in some patients with RARS. Erythropoietin may lessen the severity of the anemia and decrease the need for red blood cell transfusions in some patients, if serum erythropoietin levels are below 200 mU/mL. Chemotherapy is indicated if the patient progresses to acute leukemia. Recent studies suggest that a combination of hematopoietic growth factors, especially G-CSF and erythropoietin, may be more beneficial than traditional chemotherapy in prolonging the survival of patients who have progressed to the acute leukemic phase.

Sideroblastic Anemias. The sideroblastic anemias are a group of acquired or hereditary disorders characterized by abnormal red blood cell iron metabolism. These disorders are characterized by findings on the peripheral blood smear of microcytosis that is not due to iron deficiency.

The underlying abnormality is that of porphyrin synthesis. The cause is usually idiopathic, but sideroblastic anemia may be secondary to alcohol abuse, medications (phenacetin, paracetamol, chloramphenicol, and antituberculosis agents), and certain chronic diseases (neoplasia, rheumatoid arthritis, systemic lupus erythematosus, lead toxicity), chronic infections, and multiple myeloma. The diagnosis should be considered in patients with microcytic anemia and normal or increased serum iron and ferritin levels. It is confirmed by the finding of ringed sideroblasts on bone marrow examination. The idiopathic type is usually benign, self-limited, and not progressive. When abnormalities in platelet or white blood cell production are found, acquired idiopathic sideroblastic anemia is considered to be a myelodysplastic syndrome and often indicates a preleukemic state. Some patients may respond to combinations of pyridoxine, folic acid, vitamin C, and tryptophan.

THALASSEMIAS. The thalassemias are inherited disorders characterized by underproduction by either the α- or β-globin chains of the hemoglobin molecule. These disorders most commonly occur in persons of Mediterranean, African, Middle Eastern, or Asian descent. Occasionally, thalassemias remain undiagnosed until the later years. Most commonly newly diagnosed in the elderly is thalassemia trait, which is caused by diminished or absent β-globin chain synthesis. These patients are usually asymptomatic and have mild hypochromic microcytic anemia. Patients may be suspected as having iron deficiency anemia but be distinguished by findings of normal red blood cell counts, profound microcytosis, normal serum iron levels, and normal red cell distribution widths.

Increased Red Blood Cell Destruction (Hemolytic Anemias)

The hemolytic anemias, which are uncommon in the elderly, result from autoimmune disorders, intrinsic red blood cell membrane defects, abnormal hemoglobins or red blood cell enzyme defects, and extrinsic mechanical or lytic factors that reduce the life of red blood cells (43). Of these causes, autoimmune hemolysis and mechanical red blood cell destruction are most commonly seen in the elderly. The cardinal diagnostic feature of hemolytic anemia is reticulocytosis. The reticulocyte production index (RPI), which takes into consideration the maturation time of immature red blood cells (reticulocytes) at different hematocrit levels can be determined using this formula:

$$RPI = (Reticulocytes \div Maturation\ time) + Observed\ hematocrit \div 45$$

Where 45% is considered to be a "normal" hematocrit (Hct), a reticulocyte maturation time of 1 day is associated with a hematocrit of 45%, 1.5 days at Hct of 35%, 2 days at Hct of 25%, 2.5 days at 15%, and so on. If the RPI is above 3, the diagnosis of hemolytic anemia is likely. Other common findings in patients with hemolysis are elevations of the serum indirect bilirubin, reduction in serum plasma haptoglobin levels, hemoglobinuria, hemosiderinuria, and in severe cases, finding of nucleated red blood cells in the circulation.

IMMUNOLOGIC HEMOLYTIC ANEMIA. Immunologic hemolytic anemia may be an autoimmune disorder. This most commonly develops in association with lymphomas, paraproteinemias, collagen-vascular disease, ulcerative colitis, and myelofibrosis. Immunologic hemolytic anemia may also be secondary to the use of some medications, most commonly α-methyldopa, high-dose penicillin, cephalosporins, quinidine, and phenacetin. Autoantibodies may be warm reacting immunoglobulin-γ (IgG) or cold reacting (IgM [immunoglobulin-μ] or, more rarely, IgG). *Mycoplasma* pneumonia, *Haemophilus influenzae, Clostridium,* meningococcemia, malaria, and parvovirus infections may cause severe hemolysis mediated by antibodies complement or enzymatic destruction of red blood cells.

A hematologist should be consulted to assist in treating patients with immunologic hemolytic anemia. These anemias may respond to a regimen that includes high-dose steroids, immunoglobulins, and in patients with warm-antibody hemolytic anemia, splenectomy. For patients with cold-antibody hemolytic anemia, avoidance of cold, elimination of any offending medications if possible, and plasmapheresis may be beneficial. Red blood cell transfusions are usually not indicated, and transfusion antibody-mediated reactions are common.

INTRINSIC RED BLOOD CELL ABNORMALITIES. Intrinsic red blood cell abnormalities, which include abnormalities of red blood cell membranes, abnormal hemoglobins (thalassemias, sickle cell anemia), and red blood cell enzyme defects (glucose-6-phosphate dehydrogenase deficiency, pyruvate kinase deficiency) are uncommon in the elderly. Paroxysmal nocturnal hemoglobinuria is a rare acquired mutation of stem cells that results in an increased susceptibility of red blood cell membrane to the activation of complement and may cause a severe hemolytic anemia. It most commonly occurs in the 50s. Sickle cell anemia and the other hemoglobinopathies are rarely newly diagnosed in elderly patients. Hemoglobin electrophoresis confirms the diagnosis, and typically hemoglobin S compromises 80 to 90% of hemoglobin.

MECHANICAL CAUSES OF HEMOLYTIC ANEMIA. Mechanical heart valves, severe vascular occlusive disease, and collagen-vascular diseases can cause microangiopathic hemolytic anemia on a purely mechanical basis. These anemias are characterized by findings of fragmented red blood cells, helmet cells, schistocytes, hemoglobinemia, and hemoglobinuria. Treatment, which is mostly supportive, includes supplementing iron and folic acid. Blood transfusions may be necessary depending on the severity of the anemia.

ANEMIA OF AUTONOMIC DYSFUNCTION. A normochromic normocytic anemia has been recently described in association with primary autonomic failure (44). This anemia has unknown causation, but a component of it may be dilutional secondary to relative fluid retention. Associated findings include an impaired ability to mount an adequate blood pressure response to standing, associated with no increased heart rate response to sitting or standing. In some patients the anemia can be corrected by administering erythropoietin in doses of 25 to 75 U/kg 3 times per week subcutaneously. Simultaneous iron therapy may be required as the hematocrit normalizes.

POLYCYTHEMIA VERA. Polycythemia vera is a disease of later life characterized by excessive proliferation of erythrocyte, myeloid, and platelet cell lines within the bone marrow, resulting in a massively increased red blood cell mass and often increased white blood cell and platelet counts (45). Other disorders may cause an increase in the red blood cell mass as a result of increased production of erythropoietin (e.g., chronic obstructive lung disease, renal cell carcinoma), but in polycyth-emia vera, serum erythropoietin levels are low or absent.

Symptoms are attributed to increased blood viscosity and thrombosis. Frequent symptoms include light-headedness, blurred vision, spontaneous bleeding, and arterial and venous occlusive events. Laboratory data typically reveal an elevation of the hemoglobin concentration, hematocrit, and red blood cell count. Red blood cells are usually hypochromic and microcytic, suggesting low serum iron levels (46). The red blood cell life span is usually normal early in the course of the disease but becomes reduced later as a result of ineffective erythropoiesis. Leukocytosis and thrombocytosis are frequent findings. Hyperuricemia, increased serum levels of lactate dehydrogenase, and bilirubin levels are other common abnormalities. The diagnosis is made by demonstrating an increased red blood cell mass, not associated with excessive erythropoietin production.

The treatment of polycythemia vera is directed at maintaining peripheral blood counts and red blood cell mass close to normal. Many patients for whom this can be achieved live for 10 or more years. Most patients shift from a proliferative to a stable phase, probably as a result of progressive bone marrow myelofibrosis. The initial treatment of a newly diagnosed patient with polycythemia vera is phlebotomy. Hematocrit levels should be maintained ideally at approximately 50%. Chemotherapeutic agents such as hydroxyurea, chlorambucil, and busulfan are effective in the management of polycythemia vera and can extend life expectancy up to 20 years (47). Aspirin and dipyridamole do not reduce the incidence of thrombotic events.

MYELOPROLIFERATIVE DISORDERS
Chronic Myelogenous Leukemia

Chronic myelogenous leukemia (CML) accounts for 20% of cases of leukemia in the United States. The incidence of CML increases with age, and patients who are over age 60 have a poor prognosis. The cardinal feature in CML is the Philadelphia chromosome in bone marrow cells of more than 95% of patients. Most patients are asymptomatic and are diagnosed by hematologic studies ordered for other reasons. These patients' white blood count may be relatively low at the time of diagnosis. Symptoms are usually nonspecific and secondary to anemia (fatigue, malaise) and splenomegaly (a sense of left upper quadrant fullness) (48). Late in the course of the disease, symptoms such as shortness of breath, drowsiness, or confusion may occur as a result of sludging of white blood cells in blood vessels.

Most patients present with CML in a benign chronic phase. Blast crises characterized by abrupt elevations in the white blood cell count, hepatomegaly, splenomegaly, and lymphadenopathy occur in up to 20% of patients per year. All patients with CML have elevations in white blood cell counts ranging from 10,000 to more than 1 million per microliter. Most are of the neutrophil series with a left shift, often extending to blast cells. Other associated laboratory findings include anemia, thrombocytosis, decreased leukocyte alkaline phosphatase, and increased serum lactate dehydrogenase and uric acid levels.

Treatment of CML is not necessary unless the white blood cell count exceeds $200,000/\mu L$ or there are severe symptoms such as painful splenomegaly, suggestive of splenic infarction. Hyperuricemia should be treated with allopurinol. CML has been successfully treated with chemotherapeutic agents such as busulfan and hydroxyurea. More recently, human leukocyte interferon and recombinant α-interferon have induced hematologic and cytogenic remissions in CML (49).

Acute Myelogenous Leukemia

The incidence of acute myelogenous leukemia (AML) increases with age, and it is the most common acute leukemia occurring in the elderly (50). Patients often develop a myelodysplastic syndrome before full-blown AML. Elderly patients may have symptoms and signs resulting from decreased bone marrow function, including fatigue, angina, heart failure, ecchymoses, bleeding gums, and sometimes life-threatening infections. The diagnosis of AML is made by bone marrow aspiration and biopsy. Blast cells largely replace the nor-

mal bone marrow. Combination chemotherapy may result in remission, but younger patients have a greater likelihood of complete remission (51). A regimen of mitoxantrone plus etoposide has recently been shown to be an effective and well-tolerated first-line induction regimen for AML in the elderly (52). This regimen should be studied further and compared with the standard regimen of cytarabine and anthracycline. Since the incidence of graft-versus-host disease increases with age, most centers limit bone marrow transplantation to patients below age 50 (53).

Chronic Lymphocytic Leukemia

Chronic lymphocytic leukemia (CLL) is characterized by the accumulation of monoclonal lymphocytes, usually B cells. These cells accumulate in the bone marrow, liver, spleen, and lymph nodes. CLL, is the most common leukemia in the world, is largely a disease of the elderly (54). Most patients with CLL are asymptomatic and are diagnosed when lymphocytosis is noted on a peripheral blood smear examination. Symptoms are nonspecific and are related to the degree of anemia or tumor burden. Enlarged lymph nodes may be found on examination. Hepatosplenomegaly is less common, as is soft tissue or solid organ infiltration. Late in the disease, massive lymph node enlargement may cause obstruction of the bowel or biliary tree. The diagnosis is made when an absolute lymphocytosis is found on examination of a peripheral blood smear. Levels are usually in the range of 40,000 to $150,000/\mu L$. Anemia and thrombocytopenia are secondary to bone marrow replacement and hypersplenism. Autoimmune hemolytic anemia occurs in up to 10% of cases.

The prognosis is variable, with many patients living for up to 20 years or dying of other causes. The median survival of patients with CLL is 4 to 5 years after treatment is initiated. Patients tend to progress through stages, and eventually the bone marrow fails. Tumor burden and bone marrow function are the most important prognostic indicators. Early treatment with chemotherapy has not been shown to prolong survival significantly. Intermediate-stage disease (lymphadenopathy, hepatosplenomegaly) if accompanied by symptoms (sweats, weight loss, fatigue) is an indication for treatment. Chlorambucil and corticosteroids are usually the first agents used. Fludarabine and pentostatin have been shown to induce complete remission in some patients with CLL, but these agents are associated with greater toxicity (55).

Thrombocytopenias

Low platelet counts can be caused by disturbances in platelet production, sequestration, or destruction. Qualitative platelet disorders may occur in patients with chronic liver disease, alcoholism, leukemia, or dysproteinemia. Decreased production of platelets may result from replacement of the normal bone marrow by tumor (breast, lymphoma, prostate), leukemias, or myelofibrosis. A deficiency of either vitamin B_{12} or folic acid can cause thrombocytopenia mediated by ineffective thrombocytopoiesis. Aplastic anemia or bone marrow damage as a result of drugs, radiation, alcohol, infections, medications, or chemicals may result in hypoplasia of platelet stem cells. Certain medications have been reported to cause thrombocytopenia, most commonly quinidine, sulfa compounds, thiazide diuretics, heparin, digitalis, ranitidine, and carbamazepine. The mechanism of medication-induced thrombocytopenia is usually immunologic. Other medications may alter platelet function and prolong the bleeding time by reversibly or irreversibly inhibiting cyclo-oxygenase while platelet counts are normal. These include aspirin, dipyridamole, ticlopidine, and nonsteroidal anti-inflammatory agents.

Hypersplenism results in both sequestration and premature destruction of red blood cells and platelets. Patients with hepatic cirrhosis and portal hypertension may develop anemia, thrombocytopenia, and leukopenia as a result. Platelet transfusions are indicated when serious bleeding is associated with thrombocytopenia, but only when the cause of thrombocytopenia is decreased production.

Autoimmune Thrombocytopenia

Autoimmune thrombocytopenia causes accelerated platelet destruction mediated by antibodies directed against platelets. The disease may be idiopathic (ITP) or may occur in association with lymphoma, chronic lymphocytic leukemia, or systemic lupus erythematosus. ITP occurs most commonly in younger adults but is frequently seen as a "chronic" condition in the elderly (56). In most cases of ITP, the diagnosis is clear-cut, with manifestations of severe thrombocytopenia (platelet counts below 50,000) associated with normal red and white blood cell morphologies.

Most ITP in adults is chronic and is not commonly associated with a specific precipitating cause (e.g., a viral infection) (57). In elderly patients, chronic ITP is usually associated with a benign clinical course. Indications for treating ITP include bleeding and severe thrombocytopenia. If bleeding is associated with ITP, high-dose prednisone should be administered until the platelet count has become stable. Splenectomy is usually indicated for patients who do not respond to steroids. Other therapeutic modalities that may be effective include immunoglobulin infusion, immunosuppressive drugs (cyclophosphamide, azathioprine), and danazol.

Thrombotic Thrombocytopenia Purpura

Thrombotic thrombocytopenia purpura (TTP) is rare, but the incidence increases with age. It is characterized by severe thrombocytopenia, hemolytic anemia, and neurologic abnormalities (58). Fever and kidney involvement (proteinuria, hematuria, and azotemia) are universal. Disseminated intravascular coagulation should be considered in the differential diagnosis; however, patients with TTP have normal coagulation tests. The treatment of choice for patients with TTP is large-volume plasmapheresis. Platelet transfusions should be avoided because of the danger of accelerating thrombosis. Plasmapheresis should be continued until the platelet count is normal or stable. Resolution of anemia and clinical neurologic signs usually follows normalization of the platelet count.

REFERENCES

1. Freedman ML, Marcus DL. Anemia in the elderly: Is it physiology or pathology? Am J Med Sci 1980;280: 81–85.
2. Zauber NP, Zauber AG. Hematologic data of healthy very old people. JAMA 1997;257:2181–2184.
3. Lipschitz DA, Udupa KB. Age and the hematopoietic system. J Am Geriatr Soc 1996;34:448–454.

4. Herbert V. Nutritional anemias in the elderly. Prog Clin Biol Res 1990;326:203–227.

5. Baker WF. Clinical evaluation of the patient with anemia. In: Bick RL, ed. Hematology: Clinical and Laboratory Practice. St. Louis: Mosby, 1993:203–229.

6. Brown RG. Determining the cause of anemia. Postgrad Med 1991;89:161–170.

7. Daly MP, Sobal J. Anemia in the elderly: a survey of physicians' approaches to diagnosis and workup. J Fam Pract 1989;28:524–528.

8. Joosten E, Pellemans W, Hiele M, et al. Prevalence and causes of anemia in a geriatric hospitalized population. Gerontology 1992;38:111–117.

9. Johnson-Spear MA, Yip R. Hemoglobin difference between black and white women with comparable iron status: justification for race-specific anemia criteria. Am J Clin Nutr 1994;60:117–121.

10. Ania BJ, Suman VJ, Fairbanks VF, et al. Incidence of anemia in older people: an epidemiologic study in a well-defined population. J Am Geriatr Soc 1997 45:825–831.

11. Ania BJ, Suman VJ, Fairbanks VF, et al. Prevalence of anemia in medical practice: community versus referral patients. Mayo Clin Proc 1994;69:730–735.

12. Mansouri A, Lipschitz DA. Anemia in the elderly patient. Med Clin North Am 1992;76:619–630.

13. Lipschitz DA. Anemia. In: Exton-Smith AN, Weksler ME, eds. Practical Geriatric Medicine. New York: Churchill Livingstone, 1985:290–296.

14. Johnson MA, Fischer JG, Bowman BA, Gunter EW. Iron nutriture in elderly individuals. FASEB J 1994;8:609–621.

15. Garry PJ, Goodwin JS, Hunt WC. Iron status and anemia in the elderly: new findings and a review of previous studies. J Am Geriatr Soc 1993;31:389–399.

16. Smieja MJ, Cook DJ, Hunt DL, et al. Recognizing and recognizing iron deficiency anemia in hospitalized elderly people. Can Med Assoc J 1996;155:691–696.

17. Guyatt GH, Patteson C, Ali M, et al. Diagnosis of iron-deficiency anemia in the elderly. Am J Med 1990;88:205–209.

18. Joosten E, Hiele M, Ghoos Y, et al. Diagnosis of iron-deficiency anemia in a hospitalized geriatric population. Am J Med 1991;90:653–654.

19. Yip R, Johnson C, Dallman PR. Age-related changes in laboratory values used in the diagnosis of anemia and iron deficiency. Am J Clin Nutr 1994;39:427–436.

20. Rocky DC, Cello JP. Evaluation of the gastrointestinal tract in patients with iron deficiency anemia. N Engl J Med 1993;329:1691–1695.

21. Moses PL, Smith RE. Endoscopic evaluation of iron deficiency anemia: a guide to diagnostic strategy in older patients. Postgrad Med 1995;98:213–224.

22. Welch HG, Meehan KR, Goodnough LT. Prudent strategies for elective red blood cell transfusion. Ann Intern Med 1992;116:393–402.

23. Clinical Practice Guideline. Practice strategies for elective red blood cell transfusion. Ann Intern Med 1992;116:403–406.

24. Sears DA. Anemia of chronic disease. Med Clin North Am 1992;76:567–579.

25. Lipschitz DA. The anemia of chronic diseases. J Am Geriatr Soc 1990;38:1258–1264.

26. Krantz SB. Pathogenesis and treatment of the anemia of chronic disease. Am J Med Sci 1994;307:353–359.

27. Gautier M, Cohen HJ. Multiple myeloma in the elderly. J Am Geriatr Soc 1994;42:653–664.

28. Chiari MM, Bagnoli R, DeLuca PD, et al. Influence of acute inflammation on iron and nutritional status indexes in older inpatients. J Am Geriatr Soc 1995;43:767–771.

29. Eschbach JW, Kelly MR, Hayley NR, et al. Treatment of the anemia of progressive renal failure with recombinant human erythropoietin. N Engl J Med 1989;321:158–163.

30. Krantz S. Erythropoietin. J Am Soc Hematol 1991;77:419–434.

31. Moreno F, Aracil FJ, Perez R, Valderrabano F. Controlled study on the improvement of quality of life in elderly hemodialysis patients after correcting end-stage renal disease-related anemia with erythropoietin. Am J Kidney Dis 1996;27:548–556.

32. Rappeport JM, Bunn HF. Bone marrow failure: aplastic anemia and other primary bone marrow disorders. In: Isselbacher KJ, Braunwald E, Wilson JD, et al., eds. Harrison's Principles of Internal Medicine. 13th ed. New York: McGraw-Hill, 1994:1754–1757.

33. Murphy PT, Hutchinson RM. Identification and treatment of anemia in older patients. Drugs Aging 1994;4:113–127.

34. Carmel R. Pernicious anemia: the expected findings of very low serum cobalamin levels, anemia, and macrocytosis are often lacking. Arch Intern Med 1988;148:1712–1714.

35. Carmel R. Subtle and atypical cobalamin deficiency states. Am J Hematol 1990;34:108–114.

36. Carmel R. Prevalence of undiagnosed pernicious anemia in the elderly. Arch Intern Med 1996;156:P1097–1100.

37. Carmel R, Sinow RM, Siegel ME, Samloff IM. Food cobalamin malabsorption occurs frequently in patients with unexplained low serum cobalamin levels. Arch Intern Med 1988;148:1715–1719.

38. Pruthi RK, Tefferi A. Pernicious anemia revisited. Mayo Clin Proc 1994;69:144–150.

39. Lindenbaum J, Healton EB, Savage DG, et al. Neuropsychiatric disorders caused by cobalamin deficiency in the absence of anemia or macrocytosis. N Engl J Med 1988;318:1720–1728.

40. Savage DG, Lindenbaum J, Stabler SP, Allen RH. Sensitivity of serum methylmalonic acid and total homocysteine determinations for diagnosing cobalamin and folate deficiencies. Am J Med 1994;96:239–246.

41. Saba HI. Myelodysplastic syndromes in the elderly: the role of growth factors in management. Leuk Res 1996;20:203–219.

42. Jandl JH. Blood: Textbook of Hematology. Boston: Little Brown, 1987.

43. Rosse W, Bunn HF. Hemolytic anemias. In: Isselbacher KJ, Braunwald E, Wilson JD, et al., eds. Harrison's Prin-

ciples of Internal Medicine. 13th ed. New York: Mc-Graw-Hill, 1994:1743–1754.

44. Biaggioni I, Robertson D, Krantz S, et al. The anemia of primary autonomic failure and its reversal with recombinant erythropoietin. Ann Intern Med 1994;121:181–186.

45. Abyad A, Kligman E. Primary polycythaemia vera in the elderly. J Int Med Res 1994;22:121–129.

46. Murphy S. Polycythemia vera. In: Williams WJ, Beutler E, Erslev AJ, et al., eds. Hematology. 4th ed. New York: McGraw-Hill, 1990.

47. Conley CL. Polycythemia vera, diagnosis and treatment. Hosp Pract 1987;22:107–114.

48. Rosenthal DS. Clinical aspects of chronic myeloproliferative diseases. Am J Med Sci 1992;304:109–124.

49. Ziegler-Heitbrock HW, Schlag R, Flieger D, et al. Favorable response of early stage B CML patients to treatment with IFN-alpha2. Blood 1989;73:1426–1430.

50. Ballester O, Moscinski LC, Morris D, Balducci L. Acute myelogenous anemia in the elderly. J Am Geriatr Soc 1992;40:277–284.

51. Lowenberg B. Treatment of the elderly patient with acute myeloid leukemia. Baillieres Clin Haematol 1996;9:147–159.

52. Bow EJ, Sutherland JA, Kilpatrick MG. Therapy of untreated acute myeloid leukemia in the elderly: remission-induction using a non-cytarabine-containing regimen of mitoxantrone plus etoposide. J Clin Oncol 1996;14:1345–1352.

53. Acute Leukemia Forum '95: advances and controversies in induction therapy and treatment of older adults with AML. Symposium proceedings. San Francisco, California, USA, November 10, 1995. Leukemia 1996(suppl 1):S1–S48.

54. Foon KA, Rai KR, Gale RP. Chronic lymphocytic leukemia: new insights into biology and therapy. Ann Intern Med 1990;113:525–539.

55. Keating MJ, Kantarjian H, Talpaz M, et al. Fludarabine: a new agent with major activity against chronic lymphocytic leukemia. Blood 1989;74:19–25.

56. Linares M, Servero A, Colomina P, et al. Chronic idiopathic thrombocytopenic purpura in the elderly. Acta Hematol 1995;93:80–82.

57. McMillan R. Chronic idiopathic thrombocytopenic purpura. N Engl J Med 1981;304:1135–1147.

58. Ruggenenti P, Remuzzi G. Thrombotic thrombocytopenia purpura and related disorders. Hematol Oncol Clin North Am 1990;4:219–241.

Surgical Principles in the Aged

IMPORTANCE OF PREOPERATIVE ASSESSMENT IN THE ELDERLY

The high probability that older patients will require surgery and the increased risk of morbidity and mortality in the elderly necessitate a thorough preoperative assessment in older adults. Surgical rates are 50% higher in persons over age 65 than in younger groups, and 40% of admissions of older patients at general hospitals are to surgical services (1, 2). Generally, older patients account for 75% of postoperative deaths compared with 25% of patients under age 65. However, these generalizations, as is shown in the remainder of this chapter, are subject to tremendous variation depending on risk factors identified during the preoperative period and the management of those risk factors.

Surgery involving the thoracic or abdominal cavity confers the greatest postoperative risks. Typical postoperative mortality rates of older patients undergoing major intra-abdominal surgery range from 3 to 5%, about twice that of persons under age 65. Cardiac and peripheral vascular procedures such as abdominal aortic aneurysm repair confer a higher risk, ranging from 3 to 10%. Low-risk surgeries with mortality rates substantially less than 1% include cataract surgery, hernia repair, and transurethral resection of the prostate (1).

ROLE OF THE CONSULTING PHYSICIAN

An often mistaken impression is that the consultant should clear the patient for surgery. The concept of clearing the patient is misleading: one cannot provide absolute assurance of no adverse events. On the contrary, the role of the consulting physician is to identify any significant risk factors of adverse outcomes and to provide recommendations for the evaluation and management of these risk factors. The consultant should advise the patient and the surgeon of the procedure's consequences to functional status. For example, an elderly person with multiple chronic disorders may be sufficiently compromised after surgery that he or she can no longer live independently. This loss of independent living status and other deficits in quality of life and function should be considered, along with other traditional clinical outcomes.

GENERAL APPROACH TO RISK ASSESSMENT

Many studies of postoperative outcomes in the elderly derive mortality data from combinations of low-risk persons undergoing elective procedures and persons at high risk because of emergency procedures or multiple coexisting diseases (3). Chronologic age should not be viewed as an independent risk factor based on these data because the risk of adverse consequences varies considerably among these strata.

The most important predictors of postoperative morbidity and mortality in the elderly are the urgency of the procedure and the presence of coexisting illness, particularly cardiac and pulmonary disease. Irrespective of the operation, patients who undergo urgent or emergency procedures (procedures having to be performed within 24 hours of an unscheduled admission) carry an increased risk of an adverse outcome that can be as high as 2 to 4 times that of persons electively undergoing the same procedure. Cardiac and pulmonary complications deserve particular attention because of the potential magnitude of the adverse effects and the potential to ameliorate these outcomes if they are identified before the surgery. Thromboembolic events, distal and proximal deep venous thrombi and pulmonary embolism, are another important general issue that should be considered in all cases. Persons undergoing major surgery of the hip or knee, persons undergoing surgery for cancer in the pelvis or abdomen, or persons with a history of a deep venous thrombus or pulmonary embolism are in a high-risk category. These persons have a risk of a distal deep venous thrombosis (DVT) ranging from 40 to 80% and a risk of a proximal DVT of 20 to 40%, and 20% have at least one pulmonary embolism (4).

SPECIAL ISSUES AND COMMON COMPLICATIONS OF SURGERY IN THE ELDERLY

In addition to the acute medical problem such as cardiac or pulmonary complications, the consultant should also screen for common problems seen in older adults. Diabetes and atherosclerosis affecting the heart, brain, or extremities are common although certainly not restricted to the elderly. Decreased mobility or exercise tolerance is an important nonspecific predictor in the elderly, not only associated with cardiac adverse outcomes but also with mortality in general. Dementia predisposes to delirium, which can lead to a cycle of dehydration and malnutrition. However, although it is cited as a risk factor, investigators have not studied dementia as an independent risk factor for postoperative death or morbidity (1). Depression, when occurring as a major depressive disorder or a minor depression, can dispose to dehydration and deconditioning. Malnutrition or undernutrition have been shown in several studies to be associated with significantly high mortality among patients with 20% weight loss preoperatively. However, there is considerable controversy as to whether nutritional supplements in the preoperative phase improve surgical outcome. Most experts agree that delaying surgery to provide preoperative nutrition is not warranted except possibly for the severely malnourished. Parkinsonism, another subtle chronic disorder, can lead to deconditioning, falls, aspiration pneumonia, and prolonged recovery. Prostate disease can lead to urinary retention and subsequent infections. Most of these chronic disorders predispose the patient to develop pressure ulcers.

THE MEDICAL HISTORY AND PREOPERATIVE PHYSICAL EXAMINATION

The high prevalence of multiple comorbidities in the elderly necessitates a comprehensive history and physical examination. The type of procedure as well as the presence of several risk factors can be identified by a review of the patient's medical history. In general, a comprehensive physical examination should be conducted. Several neuropsychiatric problems easily overlooked in the elderly must be included: delirium, dementia, depression, and idiopathic or drug-induced parkinsonism.

The cardiac history should attempt to identify any past incidents of coronary artery disease or congestive heart failure. A myocardial infarction in the previous 6 months, active heart failure, and unstable angina confer substantial risks of postoperative cardiac complications (5). With the exception of extreme levels (diastolic blood pressure over 110), chronic hypertension does not increase the risk of postoperative complications. However, evidence of recent fluctuations in blood pressure or the new onset of hypertension may predict unstable blood pressure during the procedure. The pulmonary history should attempt to identify any chronic obstructive pulmonary disease (COPD) or asthma. Similarly, a medical history can reveal past thromboembolic events involving the lower extremities or lungs.

The cardiac examination should aim to detect any active heart failure or cardiac murmur, particularly aortic stenosis, the most common valvular disease in the elderly. Bradycardia, tachycardia, and irregularities suggesting ectopic beats can also be detected by physical examination. Peripheral pulses should be examined carefully, and any evidence of edema should be recorded. The physician should note decreased breath sounds, which may suggest COPD, rales or broncho-spasm, suggesting pulmonary disease or heart failure. The neuropsychiatric examination is aimed at detecting acute or chronic cognitive impairment, depressed mood, or other symptoms of depression; extrapyramidal signs (bradykinesia, cog-wheel rigidity, and tremor) suggestive of parkin-sonism; and focal weakness. Swallowing function should be assessed by examination. The patient should be observed walking for evidence of de-conditioning and gait instability, which may be exacerbated during the postoperative period.

PRINCIPLES OF PREOPERATIVE SCREENING

For purposes of this discussion, screening refers to tests of asymptomatic persons. In persons with symptoms, such as shortness of breath or chest pain, testing is designed to establish a di-agnosis rather than to discover whether there is a disorder. In either case, the value of a given test is based on its marginal benefit above and be-yond the information that one obtains through clinical means (the medical history and physical examination). This marginal benefit plus the side effects of the test dictate whether it should be performed. Also, the benefit of testing must be evaluated in relation to potential outcomes in the postoperative period, not to general or long-term outcomes. Using hypertension as an example, al-though it is known that mild and moderate high blood pressure confer a risk of long-term com-plications, mild to moderate hypertension (with diastolic less than 110) has not been shown to be a predictor of postoperative cardiac outcomes. Moreover, screening of asymptomatic patients implies that the problem to be screened is preva-lent or that its outcomes are severe and effective treatment is available. Many tests, e.g., the pro-thrombin time and urinalysis, fail to meet the cri-teria for screening in asymptomatic persons be-cause of their lack of relevance to postoperative outcomes or the minimal addition that these val-ues add to clinical information. For the same rea-son, routine use of other tests, such as thallium screening for coronary artery disease, which is discussed later, may not be as useful as once assumed.

APPLICATION OF CLINICAL INDEXES TO PREOPERATIVE ASSESSMENT

Anesthesiologists have long used the Dripps' Physical Status Scale, which classifies patients in five groups from class I, healthy persons, to class V, patients who are not expected to survive 24 hours with or without the operation. This scale, useful in predicting outcomes for patients in the extreme classes, does less well in predicting the in-termediate classes II, III, and IV. Furthermore, it gives no insight into the correctability of specific risk factors.

Perhaps the most commonly applied index by consulting physicians is the Cardiac Risk Index (5), a predictor of postoperative cardiac outcome in noncardiac surgery. Nine independent risk fac-tors of adverse outcomes have been identified and assigned points, as shown in Table 40.1. The nine components of the Cardiac Risk Index are scored to classify patients into four risk categories with regard to life-threatening cardiac complications (myocardial infarction, pulmonary edema, or ventricular tachycardia) and death from cardiac causes. Class I, from 0 to 5 points, is associated with 0.7% risk of complications and 0.2% risk of cardiac death. Intermediate classes are associated with increasing risk: class II, from 6 to 12 points, 5% risk of complications and 2% risk of cardiac death; class III, from 13 to 25 points, 11% risk of

Table 40.1

Cardiac Risk Index

Risk Factor	Points
Third heart sound	11
Elevated jugulovenous pressure	11
Myocardial infarction past 6 mo	10
ECG: premature atrial contractions or any rhythm other than sinus	7
ECG greater than 5 premature atrial contractions per minute	7
Age > 70 years	5
Emergency procedure	4
Intrathoracic, intra-abdominal, or aortic surgery	3
Poor general status (metabolic disorders or bedridden state)	3

complications and 2% risk of cardiac death. Class IV, 26 points or more, confers the most risk (22% risk of complications and 56% risk of cardiac death). Subsequent studies (6) have shown that class I, as defined by this index, may underestimate the risk of cardiac complications in patients undergoing peripheral vascular procedures. Most important, persons over age 70 who undergo an intra-abdominal, intrathoracic, or aortic procedure and who have any of the first five risk factors have a total of 13 points, sufficient to place them in one of the two highest risks by this scale.

ROUTINE PREOPERATIVE TESTS

Whereas symptoms can guide the selection of ancillary tests in persons under age 40, the prevalence of acute illness with a nonspecific presentation in the elderly dictates a lower threshold for screening. Elderly persons undergoing surgery should have the following routine tests: a fasting glucose to screen for diabetes; a complete blood count to indicate any infection or anemia; electrolytes; blood urea nitrogen; creatinine to determine risk of cardiac arrhythmias and postoperative renal failure; chest radiograph to screen for pulmonary disease; and an electrocardiogram (ECG) to detect any ischemia or arrhythmia. Studies have shown that if these tests have been performed within 3 months prior to admission in persons without new symptoms, they need not be repeated. Nevertheless, most practicing physicians and surgeons repeat the tests within a few days of surgery as a matter of habit.

PULMONARY FUNCTION TESTING

Not all procedures confer an increased risk of pulmonary complications. Thus age greater than 65 or 70 is not an absolute indication for pulmonary function testing (7, 8). Patients undergoing lung resection should always undergo pulmonary function testing. Procedures that entail incisions of the upper abdomen or thorax should also undergo pulmonary function tests, especially if any of the following factors are present: cough, known COPD, cigarette smoking, dyspnea, or known pulmonary disease (8). On the other hand, orthopaedic procedures and procedures of the lower abdomen confer minimal risk of pulmonary compromise, so pulmonary function tests are not indicated in asymptomatic persons. Because body size and age affect pulmonary function tests, there is uncertainty as what age-adjusted spirometric measures are appropriate in the elderly as predictors of respiratory complications. Nevertheless, existing data suggest the following cutoff as predictors of complications: PCO_2 above 45 mm Hg, forced expiratory volume in 1 second (FEV_1) less than 2 L and particularly less than 1 L; maximal ventilatory volume less than 50% of predicted value (8).

CARDIAC PREOPERATIVE TESTING

Cardiac preoperative testing aims to detect the presence or the likelihood of developing heart failure, a cardiac arrhythmia or an acute coronary ischemic event during the postoperative period. Known risk factors for heart failure include previous myocardial infarction, mitral regurgitation, preoperative heart failure, and age above 70 even in the absence of known heart disease (5). A low ejection traction on cardiac echo has also been shown to predict postoperative heart failure, but this knowledge adds little to clinical data (9). Thus it is unnecessary to conduct cardiac imaging for the sole purpose of predicting postoperative heart failure in noncardiac surgery. However, persons with systolic murmurs suggesting aortic stenosis should undergo imaging studies, because severe aortic stenosis may predispose to hypotension and heart failure.

Because of the concern about postoperative ischemic events, thallium testing, particularly with dipyridamole, has become almost a routine procedure before surgery in the elderly (10). Such a routine approach is not indicated. The impetus to obtain thallium or other similar imaging studies derives from evidence that myocardial infarction (MI) occurs in 1 to 10% of noncardiac procedures, with a 1 to 5% risk of death (11, 12). However, the reinfarction rate can be predicted largely by clinical data. For example, persons with an MI during the 6 months prior to surgery have a risk of 2 to 5%. Ashton (11), in one of the few studies that used consecutive patients to assess incidence of ischemic events, determined that 1.7% (15 of 835) of persons undergoing surgery had an MI. However, among the patients with postoperative events, clinical data further defined postoperative risk. An MI occurred in 4.1% of high-risk patients, defined as those with known coronary disease; in 0.8% of intermediate-risk patients, defined as those with other vascular disease but not involving the heart; and in no low-risk patients, defined as persons with known atherogenic risk factors such as hypertension, diabetes, and old age but without any cardiac or other vascular symptoms. In this study the principal independent risk factors were age above 75, signs of heart failure, known coronary artery disease, and vascular operation.

One of the shortcomings of studies of preoperative cardiac testing is that for the most part the studies were conducted not in consecutive patients undergoing cardiac procedures but in persons selected for the study because they had undergone imaging studies. A study by Eagle et al. (6) suggests that cardiac imaging studies with dipyridamole thallium scanning should be considered in persons with Q waves on the resting electrocardiogram, history of ventricular ectopy requiring treatment, diabetes, angina, and age over 70. If only one of these risk factors is present, the likelihood of a postoperative cardiac event is so low as to militate against testing. If three or more are present, the likelihood is so high that testing again does not add much to the clinical data. However,, if one or two of the risk factors are present, imaging is useful in distinguishing those who may or may not suffer a postoperative ischemic event. By contrast, Baron (9) conducted a prospective study of thallium scanning and radionuclide studies in 457 consecutive patients (202 over age 65) undergoing elective abdominal aortic aneurysm surgery. The best predictors of cardiac complications were definite clinical evidence of coronary disease and age over 65. Left ventricular ejection fraction predicted heart failure. Age over 65 was the only independent predictor of postoperative death.

Studies of other preoperative tests, including Holter monitoring, exercise testing, and others, have not been consistently useful. In summary, patients should be stratified by type of procedure and clinical evidence of coronary disease (13–16). If patients fall into a very low risk category as defined by Ashton et al. (11), no testing is indicated, and if very high risk, no testing is indicated either, since one knows the tests will be positive.

PREOPERATIVE MANAGEMENT: WHAT TO DO WITH THE INFORMATION

Cessation of smoking prior to surgery is helpful but must be undertaken at least 2 weeks prior to surgery (7). Training in coughing and deep breathing exercise should be undertaken prior to surgery. If COPD is present, aggressive use of bronchodilators should be implemented both before and after the operation. Prophylaxis of thromboembolic events is based on the type of procedure and level of risk of the patient (4). In high-risk general surgical patients, e.g., those undergoing surgery because of an intra-abdominal pelvic malignancy, heparin 5000 to 7500 U every 12 hours begun on the day of surgery is effective. Low-molecular-weight heparin twice a day with or without intermittent pneumatic compression is also effective. Among orthopaedic surgery patients undergoing procedures of the hip or knee, anticoagulation is ideally started on the day of surgery. Three successful approaches have been documented in the medical literature: (*a*) warfarin 2 mg the night before surgery and 5 mg the first postoperative day and on separate days, adjusting the dose to prolong the prothrombin time by 3 to 4 seconds; (*b*) warfarin 2 mg on the evening of surgery followed by daily warfarin to maintain an international normalized ratio (INR) of 2 to 3; (*c*) low-molecular-weight heparin administered subcutaneously twice a day. Minidose heparin (1 mg) daily and aspirin provide little or no benefit in preventing postoperative thromboembolic phenomena in orthopaedic patients. Pneumatic compression stockings should be used in patients undergoing neurosurgery.

Recommendations for the perioperative management of anticoagulation in patients who are already taking oral anticoagulants have been discussed at length (17). Patients at highest risk for a venous or arterial embolism are those with an embolus in the past month. There is no good evidence that surgery increases the risk of arterial emboli, although it certainly increases the risk of venous emboli. Presurgery heparin is unlikely to cause bleeding, but the same cannot be said for heparin begun immediately postoperatively. Elective surgery should be avoided in the first month after an acute episode of venous thromboembolism. When oral anticoagulants are withheld in the absence of heparin replacement therapy, the person is likely to be subtherapeutic for 2 days prior and 2 days after therapy. If used, heparin should not be restarted until 12 hours after major surgery and should be delayed even longer if there is any evidence of bleeding. Heparin should be restarted without a bolus. Other specific recommendations for a variety of common clinical scenarios are discussed along with their rationale.

All metabolic problems should be corrected and nutrition should be replete if possible. Application of routine testing, pulmonary function testing, and thallium scans should be used as discussed earlier. Hemodynamic monitoring with a right ventricular catheterization is indicated in patients undergoing major vascular procedures and in those with active heart failure, significant aortic stenosis, unstable angina, or recent MI. Right heart catheterization should not be used simply because of old age.

In patients at risk for postoperative ischemia, antianginal medications should be maximized. Heart failure should be corrected preoperatively. Antihypertensives should be continued at the preoperative dose. Most importantly, Mangano et al. (18, 19) have shown that β-blockers should be given preoperatively and up to 7 days postoperatively if the preoperative heart rate is above 55 beats per minute or systolic blood pressure over 100 mm Hg. In this study, patients tolerated the use of β-blockers without significant adverse consequences. Most of the benefit was achieved over 2 years rather than in the typical 30-day postoperative period, raising some questions about the usefulness of this intervention.

Prophylactic coronary artery bypass grafting for the sole purpose of preventing a perioperative ischemic event is unwarranted. Cohort studies have shown that patients who survived coronary artery bypass grafting have a decreased risk during subsequent noncardiac surgery. However, these data on patients who have already survived a coronary procedure do not apply to persons in whom one is considering a prophylactic procedure. No randomized clinical trials have studied prophylactic revascularization or

angioplasty in the preoperative period. To warrant such a decision such a study would have to show that the morbidity and mortality of the prophylactic coronary procedure and the primary operation (e.g., the peripheral vascular procedure) combined is less than the morbidity and mortality of the primary procedure alone (12). Furthermore, Bodenheimer (13) presents two other factors arguing against prophylactic surgery: the likelihood of increased mortality of coronary bypass surgery in this particular setting compared with routine bypass surgery and the increased mortality due to the delay of the primary procedure. In general, the physician should ask whether the patient would be revascularized in the absence of the planned surgical procedure. If yes, then it is reasonable to perform the prophylactic revascularization.

POSTOPERATIVE CARE

The most important postoperative problems are ischemic heart disease, heart failure, arrhythmia, thromboembolic events, respiratory complications, delirium, and general deconditioning. In general preoperative management should be continued, with particular emphasis on anticoagulants. It is important to monitor the patient for heart failure clinically and for ischemia with an ECG. ECGs on days 1 and 2 identify 96% of postoperative MIs (20). Postoperative Holter monitoring detects silent ischemia during the postoperative period, but the value of the information is questionable (18). Judicious use of opioid medications is vital, but sometimes these agents must be discontinued because of delirium. Exercise is important for general reconditioning as well as prevention of thromboembolic events. An individualized exercise program under the direction of a physical therapist is warranted for most patients.

REFERENCES

1. Johnson J. Surgical assessment in the elderly. Geriatrics 1988;43(suppl):83–90.
2. Thomas DR, Ritchie CS. Preoperative assessment of older adults. J Am Geriatr Soc 1995;43:811–821.
3. Kroenke-May K. Pre-operative evaluation: the assessment and management of surgical risk. J Gen Intern Med 1987;2:257–269.
4. 4th American College of Chest Physicians Consensus Conference on Antithrombotic Therapy. Tucson, Ari-

zona, April 1995. Proceedings. Chest 1995;108(suppl): 225S–522S.

5. Goldman L, Caldera D, Southwick F, et al. Multifactorial index of cardiac risk in non-cardiac surgical procedures. N Engl J Med 1977;297:845–850.

6. Eagle KA, Coley CM, Newell JB, et al. Combining clinical and thallium data optimizes preoperative assessment of cardiac risk before major vascular surgery. Ann Intern Med 1989;110:859–886.

7. Jackson MC. Preoperative pulmonary evaluation. Arch Intern Med 1988;148:2120–2127.

8. Zibrak JD, O'Donnell CK, Morton K. Indications for pulmonary function testing. Ann Intern Med 1990;112:763.

9. Baron J, Mundler O. Dipyridamole-thallium scintigraphy and gated radionuclide angiography to assess cardiac risk before abdominal aortic surgery. N Engl J Med 1994;330:663–660.

10. Eagle KA, Brundage BH, Chaitman BR, et al. Guidelines for perioperative cardiovascular evaluation for noncardiac surgery. Report of the American College of Cardiology/American Heart Association Task Force on Practice Guidelines (Committee on Perioperative Cardiovascular Evaluation for Noncardiac Surgery). J Am Coll Cardiol 1996;27:910–948.

11. Ashton C, Petersen N, Wray N, et al. The incidence of perioperative myocardial infarction in men undergoing noncardiac surgery. Ann Intern Med 1993;118:504–510.

12. Goldman L. Assessment of perioperative cardiac risk. N Engl J Med 1994;330:707–709.

13. Bodenheimer M. Noncardiac surgery in the cardiac patient: what is the question? Ann Intern Med 1996;124: 763–766.

14. Fleisher L, Eagle K. Screening for cardiac disease in patients having noncardiac surgery. Ann Intern Med 1996; 124:767–772.

15. Halm E, Warren B, Tubau J, et al. Echocardiography for assessing cardiac risk in patients having noncardiac surgery. Ann Intern Med 1996;125:433–441.

16. Wong T, Detsky A. Preoperative cardiac risk assessment for patients having peripheral vascular surgery. Ann Intern Med 1992;116:743–752.

17. Kearon C, Hirsh J. Management of anticoagulation before and after elective surgery. N Engl J Med 1997;336: 1506–1511.

18. Mangano D, Browner W, Hollenberg M, et al. Association of perioperative myocardial ischemia with cardiac morbidity and mortality in men undergoing noncardiac surgery. N Engl J Med 1990;323:1781–1788.

19. Mangano D, Layug E, Wallace A, Tateo I. Effect of atenolol on mortality and cardiovascular morbidity after noncardiac surgery. N Engl J Med 1996;335:1713–1720.

20. Charlson M, Peterson J, Szatrowski TP, et al. Long-term prognosis after peri-operative cardiac complications. J Clin Epidemiol 1994;12:1389–1400.

Pressure Ulcers: Practical Considerations in Prevention and Treatment

A pressure ulcer is a "lesion caused by unrelieved pressure resulting in damage of underlying tissue" (1). Elders are particularly prone to pressure sores because of the predispositions of physiologic aging changes and common diseases. Although many areas of medicine have advanced over the past several decades, the prevention and treatment of pressure ulcers remains a significant area of medical ignorance. At present there are few good scientific data on the most effective preventive and therapeutic regimens for pressure sores, and many anecdotal treatments are in common practice. However, the Agency for Health Care Policy and Research (AHCPR) has published guidelines for the prevention and treatment of pressure ulcers (1, 2). Distressingly, despite the publication of these guidelines, a recent survey of physicians showed that 70% were unaware of the guidelines and up to 20% of respondents were still recommending treatments that have clearly been shown to be harmful (e.g., doughnut cushions) (3).

Pressure ulcers are a concern for anyone involved in the treatment of elders because of the consequent morbidity, suffering, and the cost of care (4). Although the development of a pressure sore in a high-risk patient is not necessarily associated with poor care, this is often assumed to be the case (4). There are more than 17,000 lawsuits a year related to pressure ulcers, with settlements as high as $4 million (4).

EPIDEMIOLOGY

Approximately 3 million persons are affected by pressure sores in the United States (4). More than 50% of pressure ulcers occur in patients aged 70 or older (4–7), and more than 60% develop in the acute care setting (4). Actual occurrence rates for pressure sores have been difficult to determine because of methodologic problems with the data (1). In-hospital incidence rates vary from 2.7 to 29.5%, while prevalence rates range from 3 to 30% (8). The best estimate of the hospital prevalence rate is 9.2% (1). Pressure ulcers are a frequent reason for nursing home placement and remain a common problem in that setting. In long-term care the 1-year incidence rate is 13%, while the prevalence rate varies from 2 to 25% (9–11). Pressure ulcers increase in frequency with length of nursing home stay (1). Some 20 to 22% of patients develop pressure ulcers within 2 years of admission to a long-term care facility (9, 10). The focus of care in a nursing home often makes this setting preferable for healing pressure sores, and in general, staff of long-term care facilities are quite skilled in application of preventive skin care. However, the serious coexisting illnesses of nursing home residents can make skin breakdown almost inevitable at times. Little is known about occurrence rates in the home care setting, and more research is needed in this area. Pressure sores are also common with certain illnesses. There is a

60% prevalence in quadriplegic patients and a 66% incidence in elderly patients with femoral fracture (1).

The development of a pressure ulcer is a poor prognostic sign and is associated with a fourfold increase in in-hospital mortality (10–12). Non-healing sores are associated with a sixfold increase in mortality (11). Some 23 to 37% of patients with pressure ulcers die during hospitalization; most of these deaths are the result of severe underlying illnesses (7, 13). Pressure ulcers are very costly. In 1984 the treatment cost for a stage IV pressure sore was $40,000 (14, 15). In the United States, annual expenditures for the prevention and treatment of pressure ulcers exceeds $5 billion (16).

PATHOGENESIS

It is thought that pressure ulcers can develop when the skin is subjected to four mechanical forces: pressure, shearing force, friction, and maceration (10, 17, 18). Of these four forces, pressure must be present for skin breakdown (18–20), although the intensity and duration of pressure that is damaging varies with several intrinsic and extrinsic factors (19, 21). Skin does not respond well to pressure forces; the only skin area capable of withstanding substantial pressure for long periods is the soles of the feet. The epidermis is more resistant to pressure damage than is muscle (10, 19). Pressure effects on skin and muscle have been well studied in animal models (20, 22). The studies done with pigskin are most relevant, as porcine skin is very similar to the human integument (22). When skin is compressed between a contact surface and a bony prominence, pressure effects are concentrated over the bone. In comparison with the skin surface, pressure effects are more widely dispersed at the level of the bone, producing a cone-shaped area of tissue damage (10, 18). As capillary pressure (32 mm Hg) is exceeded, local tissue ischemia develops. Theoretically 2 hours of pressure greater than 32 mm Hg should damage skin and muscle, but clinical evidence indicates much greater skin tolerance (19). In porcine studies, no skin breakdown developed with 200 mm Hg of pressure for 15 hours (19); 200 mm Hg pressure for 16 hours or 600 mm Hg

pressure for 11 hours was needed for full-thickness skin breakdown (7). As a point of reference, a 70-kg person produces approximately 150 mm Hg of pressure over the greater trochanter when lying on his or her side on a regular mattress (22). Seated pressure over the ischium is 500 mm Hg (22). The pressure threshold for ulcer development is decreased by the soft tissue changes seen with paraplegia (muscle atrophy), local infection (tissue necrosis), and repetitive trauma (muscle scarring) and by any additional adverse mechanical factors (7, 19). Along with the absolute amount of pressure, its duration is significant (20). Muscle tolerates pressure applied intermittently (relieved every 5 minutes) better than the same amount of pressure applied continuously (20).

The cycle of pressure-induced skin damage is the following: when capillary pressure is exceeded, capillaries and lymphatics occlude, producing ischemia. These blood vessels leak, leading to interstitial edema and hemorrhage. Because of the lack of circulation, metabolic wastes accumulate, causing bacterial deposition and tissue necrosis (11, 17–19).

Shearing force is "the sliding of adjacent surfaces of laminar elements providing a progressive relative displacement" (18). This mechanical force is especially relevant to the sacral area. The sitting patient on a reclining chair or a semirecumbent patient in bed can slide forward, during which the sacral skin remains stationary while the deeper tissues shift. These forces undermine dermal tissues and stretch and angulate dermal blood vessels, causing thrombosis and occlusion (18, 22). In older persons, sacral shearing forces can reduce blood flow in the sacral vessels by two thirds (7). Whereas shearing forces occur more at the dermal level, frictional forces are most important in the development of superficial lesions (7). Strong abrasive forces are placed on the epidermis when a patient is pulled across bed linens or repositions himself or herself using elbows and heels (22). These frictional forces remove the stratum corneum and cause epidermal blistering (7, 18). At pressures of less than 500 mm Hg these frictional forces increase the incidence of pressure ulcers (22). As a further example of the additive effect of these mechanical forces to pressure damage, friction and repetitive pressure of as little as 45 mm Hg lead to pressure ulcers (22). Such minimal pressures are easily exceeded in the at-risk elderly patient.

The final factor in skin breakdown is maceration. As with friction, maceration is most important in the development of shallow lesions (7). Maceration leads to epidermal injury (1). In addition, both moderate moisture and excessive dryness lead to an increase in friction (23). Dry skin is further associated with fissuring of the stratum corneum, which reduces its effectiveness as a barrier to mechanical injury (1).

RISK FACTORS

Pressure ulcers occur because of a combination of extrinsic (adverse mechanical forces) and intrinsic (susceptibility) factors (21). Each elderly person has a different risk for skin breakdown, necessitating an individualized approach to prevention. More than 100 risk factors have been associated with the development of pressure ulcers (24); the most common ones are listed in Table 41.1. Immobility is the most important factor in the breakdown of skin (7). One study revealed that hospital patients who made 50 or more spontaneous movements a night developed no pressure sores, whereas 90% of patients who moved 20 or fewer times per night developed skin breakdown (25). The risk of pressure ulcers may be highest in the newly immobile patient. Some 56 to 92% of elders who develop pressure sores do so in the first 2 weeks of their hospital stay (26, 27). Age is also a significant risk factor because of age-related skin changes. These changes include epidermal thinning; an increase in skin permeability; and decreases in dermal vessel number, skin elasticity, wound repair rate, and dermal and subcutaneous tissue mass; and a flattening of rete pegs, which predisposes to friction and shear force injury (7, 17).

One cross-sectional study found that only three of the factors listed in Table 41.1 are independently associated with the development of pressure ulcers in a bedridden patient. These factors are low serum albumin, fecal incontinence, and fracture (28). In a separate analysis with a cohort design, a history of stroke, bed- or chair-bound status, and impaired nutritional status were independent predictors of new pressure sore development (29).

Table 41.1

Risk Factors for Pressure Ulcers

Advanced age
Anemia
Corticosteroid therapy
Decreased level of consciousness
Dehydration
Dementia
Edema
Extremes of weight (high and low)
Fecal incontinence
Foley catheter use
Fracture
Immobility
Increased or decreased skin temperature
Insensate skin
Low serum albumin
Major surgery
Malnutrition
Paralysis
Peripheral vascular disease
Urinary Incontinence

Adapted from Olson B. Effects of massage for prevention of pressure ulcers. Decubitus 1989;2:32–37. Inman KJ, Sibbald WJ, Rutledge SS, Clark BJ. Clinical utility and cost-effectiveness of air suspension bed in the prevention of pressure ulcers. JAMA 1993;269:1139–1143. Allman RM, Laprade CA, Noel LB, et al. Pressure sores among hospitalized patients. Ann Intern Med 1986;105:337–342. Robson MC, Phillips LG, Lawrence WT, et al. The safety and effect of topically applied recombinant basic fibroblast growth factor on the healing of chronic pressure sores. Ann Surg 1992;216:401–408.

PRESENTATION AND COURSE

When presented with an ulcerative lesion, the clinician should first think of all possible causes. This differential diagnosis includes stasis ulcer, ischemic ulcer, vasculitides, cancer, radiation injury, early ischial-rectal abscess, deep mycotic infection, pyoderma gangrenosum, and other ulcerative dermatologic conditions (7, 18). Location is also helpful in differential diagnosis; pressure sores are commonly distributed over bony pressure points (18). Some 80% of pressure ulcers occur over the sacrum, ischia, greater trochanters, heels, and lateral malleoli (7).

Once a pressure ulcer is diagnosed, staging of the lesion is imperative. Staging is helpful in the selection of appropriate therapy and also allows generalizability of research data. A commonly accepted pressure ulcer staging system was developed at a consensus conference of the National Pressure Ulcer Advisory Panel in March 1989. This system, an adaptation of a model proposed by Shea, is presented in Table 41.2 (30). Stage I ulcers (nonblanching erythema) may be difficult to diagnosis in a dark-skinned person (1). In these persons, signs may include local skin discoloration, warmth, edema, or induration. Reactive, or blanching, erythema is produced by the restoration of blood flow to an area previously under pressure and is different from and less concerning than nonblanching erythema. Checks for blanching erythema should be used to identify skin areas at particular risk for breakdown. Lesions cannot be staged unless eschar and all necrotic debris are removed (10). A dark eschar often signifies a full-thickness skin lesion (7, 10). Deep lesions may look deceptively benign because of undermining secondary to the cone-shaped pattern of pressure damage mentioned in the section on pathogenesis (18). The healing process also differs by stage. Stage I and II lesions heal by epithelial cell migration from the ulcer edges. With appropriate treatment this healing process should occur in a matter of days to weeks (7, 17). Stage III and IV lesions heal from the buildup of granulation tissue at the wound base. This process typically requires many months (7, 17). With appropriate treatment, some evidence of ulcer healing should be seen within 2 to 4 weeks (2).

PREVENTION

Prevention of pressure ulcers is both time and cost effective (4, 31). Several studies show that institution of preventive measures for high-risk patients in an acute care setting can decrease the rate of pressure sore development by more than 50% (4, 7). Prevention of pressure ulcers begins with a risk factor assessment of the patient. Those at highest risk should receive the most substantial preventive interventions. Indiscriminate use of resources just increases cost. Two well-tested, standardized scales have been developed to assist in identification of patients at high risk for skin breakdown. Although these scales are somewhat lacking in specificity (8, 10, 32), their use does promote systematic evaluation of patients. The Norton Scale assesses five factors, physical condition, mental state, activity, mobility, and incontinence, each graded from 1 to 4, with 4 reflecting the highest function (11, 33). Low scores (12 or below) are associated with higher risk of pressure ulcer development. The Norton scale has been tested in the acute care setting. The

Table 41.2

Staging System for Pressure Ulcers

Stage	Description
I	Nonblanching erythema of intact skin
II	Partial thickness skin loss involving the epidermis and/or dermis; clinically abrasion, blister, or shallow crater
III	Full-thickness skin loss to but not through underlying fascia; clinically deep crater that may be undermined
IV	Full-thickness skin loss with extensive tissue destruction and necrosis; may include damage to muscle, bone, supporting structures; may be undermined, have sinus tracts

Adapted from Panel for the Prediction and Prevention of Pressure Ulcers in Adults. Pressure Ulcer in Adults: Prediction and Prevention. Clinical Practice Guideline 3 (AHCPR 92–0047). Rockville, MD: US Department of Health and Human Services, Public Health Service, Agency for Health Care Policy and Research, 1992. Goode PS, Allman RM. The prevention and management of pressure ulcers. Med Clin North Am 1989;73:1511–1524. Shea JD. Pressure sores. Classification and management. Clin Orthop 1975;112:89–100.

Braden Scale contains six subscales: sensory perception, skin moisture, activity level, mobility, nutritional status, and friction and shear (32, 34). Each subscale is scored 1 to 4 except friction and shear, which is scored 1 to 3. Again, the highest subscale score indicates the most intact state (32, 34). A low score (16 or below) predicts pressure sore development with a reported sensitivity of 100% and specificity ranging from 64 to 90% (10, 32). The Braden Scale has good interrater reliability and has been used in acute hospitals and long-term care facilities (32). Upon admission to a health care facility or home care agency, a patient should be assessed for skin breakdown potential with a standardized scale (1). Assessment should recur at a frequency determined by the patient's risk status (1).

Prevention should address the four mechanical forces causal in pressure ulcer development (see Pathophysiology section). Treatable risk factors (Table 41.1) should be sought and remedied as possible. Table 41.3 contains a summary of AHCPR recommendations that was published as a clinical practice guideline in May of 1992 (1). At-risk patients should receive care according to a standardized protocol. Not all of the recommended preventive interventions may be relevant for each patient. For some elders, the goal of medical treatment may be comfort and not cure, and in this situation more limited intervention may be appropriate.

The following discussion explains and augments the guidelines presented in Table 41.3. Initial recommendations improve skin tolerance to pressure and prevent other forms of skin injury. The skin should be kept well hydrated and treated gently in all therapeutic interventions. For years skin massage to promote blood flow has been recommended; however, recent evidence suggests that massage is damaging, as it tears dermal tissues (8, 14). Extrinsic factors, such as catheter tubing, food particles, and wrinkled sheets, can irritate and break down the skin (35). A well-padded footboard prevents sliding and shear force injury, especially if the head of the bed is elevated less than 20° or more than 70° (24).

Pressure-relieving overlays for a standard mattress are appropriate, but the use of these and other gadgets will never supplant good basic skin care. All at-risk patients should be placed on a pressure-relieving mattress surface. There are many pressure-relieving devices on the market. There is no evidence that one device is better than another for prevention of pressure ulcers (1). Regular 2-inch egg crate foam pads do not substantially decrease local pressure. Other differently constructed foam pads are inexpensive and decrease local pressure below capillary pressure (36). Sheets should be left somewhat loose over foam mattresses so as not to detract from their pressure-distributing characteristics. Air mattresses are more expensive but also effective (15). Doughnut devices should not be used, as they may decrease circulation to the central area and promote venous congestion and edema (7). Sheepskin is not a pressure-relieving device but is somewhat compressible, so it may distribute pressure more evenly. The main purpose of sheepskin is to reduce friction between surfaces and absorb moisture (37). The heels are very susceptible to pressure-induced skin damage and must be well protected in the bed-bound person. There are several prefabricated products that elevate the heel off the bed (38), but an effective and less expensive alternative is the placement of a thick pillow lengthwise under the calf.

The clinical practice guideline puts a strong emphasis on structured teaching of the multidisciplinary health care team, the patient, and any other caretakers about appropriate skin care (1). In addition, the formal introduction of facility-wide protocols for skin care is promoted. There is good research evidence that such protocols decrease the incidence of pressure ulcers (8, 17).

TREATMENT

Any patient with a pressure ulcer requires a comprehensive evaluation that includes an assessment of physical health and psychosocial status. This identifies patient-specific factors that should be addressed in the treatment plan. Treatment of a pressure ulcer depends on the wound's characteristics. For any ulcer, the first part of treatment should be to review all aspects of the preventive skin care protocol (Table 41.3) to determine areas for improvement. The characteristics of the pressure ulcer should be documented:

Table 41.3

Guidelines for Pressure Ulcer Prevention

1. Document and perform daily, comprehensive, skin inspection.[a]
2. Keep skin clean using mild soap and water. Minimize the application of pressure and frictional forces during cleansing.[a]
3. Avoid ambient low humidity (less than 40%) and cold. Use moisturizers on dry skin.[a]
4. Do not massage the skin over bony prominences.[b]
5. Minimize skin exposure to moisture. Assess and manage any urinary or fecal incontinence. Use absorbent underpants when necessary to help keep skin dry. Topical agents that produce a moisture barrier can be used.[a]
6. Lessen frictional and shearing force injury through proper positioning, transferring, and turning.[a]
7. Friction may be decreased through the use of lubricants (cornstarch, creams), protective films (transparent film dressings, skin sealants), protective dressings (e.g., hydrocolloids), and protective padding.[a]
8. While the patient is in bed, use a written, systemic turning schedule to reposition the patient approximately every 2 hours if consistent with overall patient treatment goals.[b]
9. Use foam and/or pillows for bed positioning. Keep bony prominences from contact with each other.[a]
10. Any at-risk patient should be placed on a pressure-relieving surface (foam, static air or alternating air mattress, gel or water mattress).[b]
11. The bed-bound patient requires positioning to provide complete heel pressure relief.[a]
12. Avoid the use of doughnut cushions.[a]
13. Avoid positioning directly on the greater trochanter.[a]
14. Use lifting devices (sheets, bed trapeze) to alleviate frictional forces.[a]
15. Maintain the head of the bed as flat as possible consistent with medical restrictions. The head of the bed should be elevated for as little time as possible.[a]
16. A patient in a chair should reposition every hour and weight shift every 15 minutes.[a]
17. Positioning of chair-bound patients should include consideration of pressure relief, postural alignment, weight distribution, and balance. Use a pressure-relieving seat cushion.[a]
18. Provide appropriate nutritional assessment and support.[a]
19. Maintain or improve mobility as possible.[a]
20. A structured comprehensive educational program should be developed for all health care providers (doctors, nurses, therapists), patients, and caregivers. The program should be evaluated as to its effectiveness.[c]
21. A written skin care plan should be used to document risk assessment and preventive interventions. Responsible caretakers should be clearly stated. The patient's response to preventive interventions should be monitored and documented. The skin care plan should be adjusted to the patient's response to treatment.[a]

Adapted from Panel for the Prediction and Prevention of Pressure Ulcers in Adults. Pressure Ulcer in Adults: Prediction and Prevention. Clinical Practice Guideline 3 (AHCPR 92–0047). Rockville, MD: US Department of Health and Human Services, Public Health Service, Agency for Health Care Policy and Research, 1992.
[a]Based on expert opinion and panel consensus.
[b]Based on modest research-based evidence.
[c]Based on good research-based evidence.

location, dimension, signs of infection, and any granulation tissue, undermining, sinus tracts, necrotic tissue, and exudate (39).

Wound treatment entails debridement as needed, followed by cleansing and application of the dressing. For stage III and IV lesions, the ulcer cavity should be loosely packed with the chosen dressing to eliminate dead space, which may lead to abscess formation (2). In general, any new therapy should be used for at least 2 to 4 weeks before therapeutic effectiveness is judged (8). The use of any therapeutic agent should be reassessed once the intended goal of treatment is accomplished.

Mattresses and Overlays That Reduce or Relieve Pressure

If a patient is not on a pressure-relieving mattress, the development of a sore is an indication of the need for such a surface (17). Pressure relief can be provided by a variety of devices at varying cost. The selection of a support surface depends on characteristics of the patient. No support surface is clearly superior to all others in all circumstances (2). Deep-cut foam cube mattress overlays improve healing time of pressure ulcers (40). However, the height added to the standard bed by these devices poses a safety risk for some patients. Also, these surfaces (along with static air, water, or gel overlays) may bottom out when used for heavy (more than 250 pounds) persons. Bottoming out is the compression of the support surface material to less than 1 inch thick; when this occurs, the surface has lost optimal pressure-relieving capacity. Bottoming out is detected by placing a hand, palm up, under the support surface at the point below the pressure ulcer or the body part at risk. A patient who bottoms out or has not shown any evidence of healing on a static device may be considered for a dynamic air overlay. These overlays consist of multiple air-filled tubes that alternately inflate and deflate with air. Low-air-loss and air-fluidized beds are effective but costly (9, 12) and should be reserved for the patient who has multiple deep lesions on more than one turning surface and for the person who has not responded to less aggressive treatment (2). The air-fluidized bed consists of a woven fabric sheet covering ceramic beads through which warm, pressurized air is circulated. Air-fluidized beds do decrease local pressure below capillary pressure. They also provide a clearly movable contact surface for the skin that may decrease friction and shearing force and reduce skin moisture (12). However, these beds have drawbacks, which include the promotion of insensible fluid loss and ineffective cough. Repositioning and transfers of the patient are also difficult on an air-fluidized bed. The combination of limited positioning options and impaired cough mechanism may increase the risk of aspiration pneumonia (12). These problems do not occur on a low-air-loss bed system consisting of multiple inflatable fabric pillows attached to a modified hospital bed frame (9). Perhaps the best device for ultimate cost savings is a reusable pressure-reduction mattress, which can be purchased as a replacement for a standard hospital bed mattress.

No pressure-relieving mattress surface replaces the need for regular turning and repositioning of the patient. No randomized controlled trials on optimal turning frequency have been conducted in humans, so no hard and fast rules can be made regarding turning frequency (17). Although turning every 2 hours is generally recommended, this may be insufficient or excessive for an individual patient based on particular skin tolerance and risk factor profiles (7). The patient should always be positioned off the pressure ulcer.

Debridement

Sharp or surgical debridement is often necessary when necrotic tissue can be seen. Necrotic tissue is associated with high bacterial counts, so successful debridement also promotes wound disinfection. The bacteremia rate during debridement may be as much as 50%, necessitating antibiotic prophylaxis for patients at risk for endocarditis (10). Mechanical debriding methods include wet to dry saline dressings (changed every 8 hours) and whirlpool baths, but both are nonselective (17, 24, 41), as new granulation tissue may be removed along with necrotic debris. Chemical enzymatic agents for debridement are available, but there are no good studies on the utility of these agents, and their continued use may damage healthy tissue (18). New wound dressing products induce autolytic debridement because the covering dressing promotes release of self-degradative enzymes from underlying necrotic tissue.

Antiseptic and Antibacterial Agents

The reduction of bacterial counts to less than 10^5/g of tissue and the removal of necrotic material, including eschar, are two key points in successful healing of pressure ulcers (7, 42). Numerous antiseptic agents are in common use. Wound cleansers (e.g., Shur Chens, Safclens) are also available. Although bactericidal, these products are cytotoxic in certain concentrations and may therefore delay wound healing (43). In fibroblast studies, 1% povidone-iodine, 0.25% acetic acid, 3% hydrogen peroxide, and 0.5% sodium hypochlorite (Dakin's solution) were all 100% cytotoxic to fibroblasts; in animal models, all but hydrogen peroxide delayed wound healing (43). Hydrogen peroxide was found to be minimally bactericidal (42).

Antibacterial agents appear to be noncytotoxic (43) but may select for resistant organisms (44). Pressure ulcers can then serve as a reservoir of antibiotic-resistant bacteria and nosocomial infection (7, 12). There is also the potential for contact dermatitis or a hypersensitivity reaction with topical antibacterial agents. Sulfadiazine cream 1% reduces bacterial counts quickly and is 100% effective in lowering counts below 10^5/g of tissue after 3 weeks of use (42). In this same study, cleansing with sterile 0.9% normal saline was 78.6% effective in reducing bacterial colony counts below 10^5/g of tissue within 3 weeks (42). Therefore, the role of topical antibiotics is not entirely clear. Use of these agents should probably be reserved for the locally infected wound unresponsive to more aggressive cleansing and debridement and for the ulcer without any evidence of healing despite 2 to 4 weeks of treatment (2). Topical antibiotics should be discontinued when signs of infection (purulence, odor) have abated (35, 42) and should not be used for more than 2 weeks (2).

Therefore, normal saline irrigation is the cleansing agent and procedure of choice. Irrigation pressure between 4 and 15 pounds per square inch optimally cleanse tissue without additional traumatic damage (2). This irrigation pressure can be provided by several devices, including a 35-mL syringe with 19-gauge angiocatheter or a dental irrigator (Water Pik) at the lowest setting (2).

Wound Dressings

Almost every concoction known has been placed on or into pressure ulcers in an attempt to heal them. Few data are available to support the efficacy of most of these therapies. With a stage II, III, or IV ulcer, some form of wound dressing is appropriate to keep the ulcer base clean and moist and to maintain dryness of the periulcer skin. Wound characteristics dictate dressing selection (Table 41.4). The moist saline dressing (changed or remoistened with 3 mL of saline every 4 hours) is the old standard dressing of choice (17, 24), but it is quite labor intensive and impractical for nonhospital settings.

In the past few years there has been an explosion of wound care products. The annual market

for such products is as much as $1 billion (6). All of these dressings have comparable healing times but overall may be less costly than moist saline dressings because of decreased nursing time for treatment (41, 45, 46). The clean stage II lesion may be best treated by a transparent thin film or hydrocolloid dressing (10, 41, 45, 46). Transparent thin film dressings are sterile polyurethane sheets that are impermeable to water and bacteria but permeable to moisture vapor and oxygen. This dressing should be changed when it stops adhering, usually in 3 to 7 days. The contact surface of a hydrocolloid dressing mixes with wound fluid to form a gel that allows migration of epithelial cells onto the ulcer surface (17, 45). Hydrocolloid dressings should also be changed when they stop sticking, typically every 3 to 7 days. Hydrogels are hydrophilic polymers that absorb water to form a water-soluble gelatinous substance on the wound surface. Depending on the amount of wound exudate, hydrogel dressings are changed every 1 to 3 days. Polyurethane foam dressings absorb up to a moderate amount of wound exudate and may remain in place for up to 7 days. For a lesion with copious exudate, calcium alginate dressings absorb wound fluid without desiccating the ulcer bed.

Nutrition

Adequate nutrition is imperative to healing of all pressure ulcers (24, 41). A patient requires 30 to 35 calories per kilogram per day with 1.5 g protein per kilogram per day along with 25 to 35 mL of fluid per kilogram per day. One randomized placebo-controlled trial suggested vitamin C supplementation (500 mg twice a day) is helpful (7). There is insufficient information on the role, if any, of zinc supplementation in the patient who is not zinc deficient (17).

Surgery

Surgical closure is rarely considered for older persons but may be appropriate in the medically stable, vigorous patient in whom rapid healing would improve functional status and quality of life (47). Aggressive local debridement and disinfection must precede definitive surgery (48). Candidates for surgery must be medically stable, adequately nourished, and able to tolerate operative

Table 41.4

Pressure Ulcer Dressings

Type	Formulations	Use by Stage	Use With Local Infection	Exudate Control	Debriding Action
Moist saline-soaked gauze	Cavity filler	II, III, IV	Yes	No	None
Wet to dry saline-soaked gauze	Cavity filler	II, III, IV	Yes	Yes	Mechanical
Transparent thin film	Surface wafer	I,[a] II	No	No	Autolytic
Hydrocolloid	Surface wafer, cavity filler	I,[a] II, III, IV	No	Minimal to mild amounts	Autolytic
Hydrogel	Surface wafer, cavity filler	II, III, IV	Yes; cavity filler only; change dressing daily	Minimal to mild amounts	Autolytic
Polyurethane foam	Surface wafer, cavity filler	II, III, IV	Yes; change dressing daily	Mild to moderate amounts	Autolytic
Calcium alginate	Cavity filler	II, III, IV	Yes; change dressing daily	Moderate to heavy amounts	Autolytic

Adapted from Findlay D. Practical management of pressure ulcers. Am Fam Physician 1996;54:1519–1528. Evans JM, Andrews KL, Chutka DS, et al. Pressure ulcers: prevention and management. Mayo Clin Proc 1995;70:789–799.

[a] For stage I ulcers, dressing forms protective layer to reduce friction.

blood loss and the expected postoperative immobility (2). Four surgical options are available: simple secondary closure, skin graft, local rotation skin graft, and facial or muscle flap (48). Muscle flap closure is especially good for large wounds. Because of the retained vascular supply, healing time is often improved with muscle flap procedures (48). Surgery is not a panacea, however. Of patients who initially healed after surgery, 61% had breakdown of their surgical sites within 9.3 months (49). The breakdown rate after a flap procedure can be as high as 79% (50).

COMPLICATIONS

Every year 60,000 people die of pressure ulcer-related complications (24). Several types of complication occur. The first category, which is due to direct extension of the ulcer into neighboring tissues, includes erosion into the bowel or bladder and joint disarticulation and infection. The second type of complication is infectious, including cellulitis, generalized sepsis (which may lead to endocarditis or meningitis), osteomyelitis, and tetanus.

Cellulitis is suggested by fever, wound erythema, purulent drainage, and odor (7, 10). Because of surface contamination with many organisms, swab surface wound cultures correlate poorly with the actual infecting bacteria (5). Quantitative tissue culture is more appropriate for identification of these organisms (5, 11). Stage III and IV ulcers are likely to be infected with polymicrobial flora (gram-positive, gram-negative, and anaerobic organisms). A foul-smelling ulcer suggests anaerobic infection (7). In nursing homes especially, methicillin-resistant *Staphylococcus aureus* may be a problem. Treatment of cellulitis includes local aggressive wound cleansing and debridement as well as systemic antibiotics. Pressure ulcers almost by definition have poor circulation, so some antibiotics, e.g., first-generation cephalosporins, may not penetrate well into the tissues (7, 42). Appropriate presumptive antibiotic therapy, pending culture results, includes cefoxitin with an antipseudomonal aminoglycoside or imipenem cilastin.

Sepsis (bacteremia) related to pressure ulcers has a greater than 50% in-hospital mortality rate among patients 60 years of age or older (17).

Pressure ulcer-related sepsis occurs at 1.7 cases per 10,000 hospital discharges (41). Some 20 to 38% of patients with pressure sore-related bacteremia have polymicrobial (including anaerobic) sepsis (7) necessitating broad antibiotic coverage. Wound debridement to remove necrotic tissue, which is often the source of the bacteremia, is imperative (7).

Osteomyelitis is not a particularly common complication of pressure ulcers, but it can be difficult to diagnose. Osteomyelitis is seen in approximately 33% of stage IV ulcers (47) and 26% of nonhealing sores (4, 7). Usual organisms are gram-negative rods and anaerobes. These bacteria are frequently multidrug resistant (51). The diagnosis of osteomyelitis should be considered when a pressure ulcer does not heal well or there is surgical breakdown after a repair (51). No radiologic test is particularly specific for the diagnosis of osteomyelitis. The gold standard for diagnosis is histologic changes on bone biopsy (51). Plain radiographs are often abnormal in osteomyelitis, but it can be difficult to differentiate actual osteomyelitis from pressure-induced bone changes (51). Radiographs may be helpful in identifying appropriate areas for biopsy (51). Bone scans are sensitive (65 to 100%) but again not specific (30 to 57%) for osteomyelitis (51). Therefore, a negative bone scan makes the diagnosis of osteomyelitis very unlikely (51). The predictive value of a positive triple-phase bone scan is only 18% in patients with pressure ulcers who are suspected of having osteomyelitis (6). Computed tomography (CT) detects areas of bone destruction and allows CT-guided bone biopsy. Magnetic resonance imaging (MRI) has not found a clinical place in the diagnosis of osteomyelitis as yet. Bone cultures are usually done at the time of biopsy. Preceding debridement and disinfection of the ulcer decrease the chance of a false-positive culture (51). One study has suggested that at least one positive response from a specific combination of laboratory tests has a sensitivity of 89% and a specificity of 88% for the diagnosis of osteomyelitis (52). These same tests have a positive predictive value of 69% when all three parameters are positive (2). The positive results are a white blood cell count of 15,000/mm^3 or greater, an abnormal plain radiograph, and an erythrocyte sedimentation rate of 120 mm/hour or greater (52).

An uncommon but important complication of pressure ulcers is tetanus infection. Deep, indolent sores can lead to heterotopic calcifications, which may be associated with the development of tetanus (18). Elders as a group have low immunization rates against tetanus (53). In the surveillance year 1989 to 1990, several of the 117 diagnosed cases of tetanus were associated with pressure ulcers (53). It is recommended that elderly patients without evidence of up-to-date tetanus immunization receive appropriate wound prophylaxis and immunization.

Pressure sores are an important and common problem among elders. Although much is yet to be known about the prevention and treatment of these lesions, we do know enough to prevent or heal the majority of pressure ulcers.

REFERENCES

1. Panel for the Prediction and Prevention of Pressure Ulcers in Adults. Pressure Ulcer in Adults: Prediction and Prevention. Clinical Practice Guideline 3 (AHCPR 92–0047). Rockville, MD: US Department of Health and Human Services, Public Health Service, Agency for Health Care Policy and Research, 1992.
2. Panel for the Prediction and Prevention of Pressure Ulcers in Adults. Pressure Ulcer Treatment. Clinical Practice Guideline 15 (AHCPR 95–0653). Rockville, MD: US Department of Health and Human Services, Public Health Service, Agency for Health Care Policy and Research, 1994.
3. Kimura S, Pacala JT. Pressure 3 in adults: family physicians' knowledge, attitudes, practice preferences, and awareness of AHCPR guidelines. J Fam Pract 1997;44: 361–368.
4. Moss RJ, LaPuma J. The ethics of pressure sore prevention and treatment in the elderly: a practical approach. J Am Geriatr Soc 1991;39:905–908.
5. Findlay D. Practical management of pressure ulcers. Am Fam Physician 1996;54:1519–1528.
6. Patterson JA, Bennett R G. Prevention and treatment of pressure sores. J Am Geriatr Soc 1995;43:919–927.
7. Allman RM. Pressure ulcers among the elderly. N Engl J Med 1989;320:850–853.
8. Xakellis GC. Guidelines for the prediction and prevention of pressure ulcers. J Am Board Fam Pract 1993;6: 269–278.
9. Ferrell BA, Osterweil D, Christenson P. A randomized trial of low-air-loss beds for treatment of pressure ulcers. JAMA 1993;269:494–497.
10. Spoelhof GD, Ide K. Pressure ulcers in nursing home patients. Am Fam Physician 1993;47:1207–1215.
11. Emanuele JA, Katz T, Levien DH. Pressure sores: how to prevent and treat them. Postgrad Med 1992;91:113–118, 120.
12. Allman RM, Walker JM, Hart MK, et al. Air-fluidized beds or conventional therapy for pressure sores. Ann Intern Med 1987;107:641–648.
13. Thomas DR, Goode PS, Tarquine PH, Allman RM. Hospital-acquired pressure ulcers and risk of death. J Am Geriatr Soc 1996;44:1435–1440.
14. Olson B. Effects of massage for prevention of pressure ulcers. Decubitus 1989;2:32–37.
15. Inman KJ, Sibbald WJ, Rutledge SS, Clark BJ. Clinical utility and cost-effectiveness of air suspension bed in the prevention of pressure ulcers. JAMA 1993;269:1139–1143.
16. Evans JM, Andrews KL, Chutka DS, et al. Pressure ulcers: prevention and management. Mayo Clin Proc 1995;70:789–799.
17. Goode PS, Allman RM. The prevention and management of pressure ulcers. Med Clin North Am 1989;73: 1511–1524.
18. Reuler JB, Cooney TG. The pressure sore: pathophysiology and principles of management. Ann Intern Med 1981;94:661–666.
19. Daniel RK, Priest DL, Wheatley DC. Etiologic factors in pressure sores: an experimental model. Arch Phys Med Rehabil 1981;62:492–498.
20. Kosiak M. Etiology of decubitus ulcers. Arch Phys Med Rehabil 1961;42:19–29.
21. Versluysen M. Pressure sores in elderly patients. The epidemiology related to hip operations. J Bone Joint Surg [Br] 1985;67:10–13.
22. Dinsdale SM. Decubitus ulcers: role of pressure and friction in causation. Arch Phys Med Rehabil 1974;55:147–152.
23. Sultzberger MB. Studies on blisters produced by friction: 1. Results of linear rubbing and twisting techniques. J Invest Dermatol 1966;47:456–465.
24. Perez ED. Pressure ulcers: updated guidelines for treatment and prevention. Geriatrics 1993;48:39–41, 43–44.
25. Exton-Smith AN, Sherwin RW. The prevention of pressure sores: significance of spontaneous bodily movements. Lancet 1961;2:1124–1126.
26. Allman RM, Goode PS, Patrick MM, et al. Pressure ulcer risk factors among hospitalized patients with activity limitation. JAMA 1995;273:865–870.
27. Smith DM, Winsemius DK, Besdine RW. Pressure sores in the elderly: can this outcome be improved? J Gen Intern Med 1991;6:81–93.
28. Allman RM, Laprade CA, Noel LB, et al. Pressure sores among hospitalized patients. Ann Intern Med 1986;105: 337–342.
29. Berlowitz DR, Wilking SV. Risk factors for pressure sores. A comparison of cross-sectional and cohort-derived data. J Am Geriatr Soc 1989;37:1043–1050.
30. Shea JD. Pressure sores. Classification and management. Clin Orthop 1975;112:89–100.
31. Oot-Giromini B, Bidwell FC, Heller NB, et al. Pressure

ulcer prevention versus treatment, comparative product cost study. Decubitus 1989;2:52–54.

32. Bergstrom N, Braden BJ, Laguzza A, Holman V. The Braden Scale for predicting pressure sore risk. Nurs Res 1987;36:205–210.

33. Norton D. Calculating the risk: reflections on the Norton Scale. Decubitus 1989;2:24–31 (erratum 1989;2:10).

34. Braden BJ. Clinical utility of the Braden Scale for predicting pressure sore risk. Decubitus 1989;2:44–46, 50–51.

35. Guggisberg E, Terumalai K, Carron JM, Rapin CH. New perspectives in the treatment of decubitus ulcers. J Palliat Care 1992;8:5–10.

36. Treatment of pressure ulcers. Med Lett Drug Ther 1990;32:17–18.

37. Denne WA. An objective assessment of the sheepskins used for decubitus sore prophylaxis. Rheumatol Rehabil 1979;18:23–29.

38. Pinzur MS, Schumacher D, Reddy N, et al. Preventing heel ulcers: a comparison of prophylactic body-support systems. Arch Phys Med Rehabil 1991;72:508–510.

39. Pieper B, Mikols C, Mance B, Adams W. Nurses' documentation about pressure ulcers. Decubitus 1990;3:32–34.

40. Andrews J, Balai R. The prevention and treatment of pressure sores by use of pressure distributing mattresses. Decubitus 1988;1:14–21.

41. Gorse GT, Messner RL. Improved pressure sore healing with hydrocolloid dressings. Arch Dermatol 1987;123:766–771.

42. Kucan JO, Robson MC, Heggers JP, Ko F. Comparison of silver sulfadiazine, povidone-iodine and physiologic saline in the treatment of chronic pressure ulcers. J Am Geriatr Soc 1981;29:232–235.

43. Lineaweaver W, Howard R, Soucy D, et al. Topical antimicrobial toxicity. Arch Surg 1985;120:267–270.

44. Hirschmann JV. Topical antibiotics in dermatology. Arch Dermatol 1988;124:1691–1700.

45. Xakellis GC, Chrischilles EA. Hydrocolloid versus saline-gauze dressings in treating pressure ulcers: a cost-effectiveness analysis. Arch Phys Med Rehabil 1992;73:463–469.

46. Sebern MD. Pressure ulcer management in home health care: efficacy and cost effectiveness of moisture vapor permeable dressing. Arch Phys Med Rehabil 1986;67:726–729.

47. Siegler EL, Lavizzo-Mourey R. Management of stage III pressure ulcers in moderately demented nursing home residents. J Gen Intern Med 1991;6:507–513.

48. Anthony JP, Huntsman WT, Mathes SJ. Changing trends in the management of pelvic pressure ulcers: a twelve-year review. Decubitus 1992;5:44–47, 50–51.

49. Robson MC, Phillips LG, Lawrence WT, et al. The safety and effect of topically applied recombinant basic fibroblast growth factor on the healing of chronic pressure sores. Ann Surg 1992;216:401–408.

50. Robson MC, Phillips LG, Thomason A, et al. Recombinant human platelet-derived growth factor-BB for the treatment of chronic pressure ulcers. Ann Plast Surg 1992;29:193–201.

51. Sugarman B. Pressure sores and underlying bone infection. Arch Intern Med 1987;147:553–555.

52. Lewis VL, Bailey MH, Pulawski G, et al. The diagnosis of osteomyelitides in patients with pressure sores. Plast Reconstr Surg 1988;81:229–232.

53. Prevots R, Sutter RW, Strebel PM, et al. Tetanus surveillance—United States, 1989–1990. MMWR Morb Mortal Wkly Rep 1992;41:1–9.

CHAPTER 42

CYNTHIA MATTOX, HELEN K. WU, AND JOEL S. SCHUMAN

Ocular Disorders of Aging

Some 80 million Americans have a medical or surgical disease of the eye and visual system (1, 2). More than 1 million Americans are legally blind, and Americans over age 65 constitute 50% of the U.S. blind population (2). Furthermore, 13% of Americans over age 85 are blind (3, 4). Many more Americans, nearly 3 million, are visually impaired. In a population-based study, the rate of visual impairment in subjects 80 years and older was 15 to 30 times that of subjects aged 40 to 50 (3). In addition, many are unaware of their eye disease. A thorough ophthalmologic evaluation allows for diagnosis and possible treatment of many common and uncommon eye diseases. Persons 65 and older, in the absence of symptoms or other indications, should have a comprehensive eye examination every 1 to 2 years (5). Ophthalmologists are in the unique position of being able to provide not only primary eye care for the elderly but also comprehensive medical and surgical eye care, as well as understanding the other medical conditions that afflict the older population.

EYELIDS AND LACRIMAL SYSTEM

The function of the eyelids is to protect and lubricate the surface of the globe. The eyelids are composed of an anterior lamella consisting of the cilia, the dermis, the orbicularis oculi muscle, and the lid retractors (Fig. 42.1A). The tarsal plate, which is composed of dense connective tissue, and the palpebral conjunctiva constitute the posterior lamella (Fig. 42.1B).

The meibomian glands, the sebaceous glands of Zeis, and the apocrine glands of Moll contribute to the lipid layer of the tear film. The lacrimal and accessory lacrimal glands supply the aqueous portion of the tears, and the conjunctival goblet cells produce the mucinous layer of the tear film, which adheres to the superficial conjunctival and corneal surfaces. The tears drain through the upper and lower lid puncta, through the canaliculi, into the nasolacrimal sac, and into the nose. The nasolacrimal duct extends from the sac and opens into the nose below and beside the inferior turbinate.

STRUCTURAL CHANGES ASSOCIATED WITH AGING

Dermatochalasis is the progressive laxity of the delicate eyelid skin, which may cause visual impairment by obstructing the superior visual field. This may be associated with *blepharoptosis,* the drooping of the upper lid due to either levator aponeurotic dehiscence or disinsertion; less commonly, myogenic disorders such as myasthenia gravis may be associated with ptosis.

The lids may develop horizontal laxity with *lagophthalmos,* or inability to close the lids completely. *Entropion,* the inward rotation of the eyelid margins, may be due to involutional changes or cicatrizing processes in the posterior lamella, such as Stevens-Johnson syndrome or ocular cicatricial pemphigoid. *Trichiasis* (malpositioned eyelashes) may be alone or accompany entropion. *Ectropion,* the outward rotation of the lid margin, may be a consequence of involutional, cicatricial, or inflammatory processes of the anterior lamella or of paralytic sequelae of seventh nerve palsies. These eyelid malpositions may produce tearing and ocular discomfort secondary to mechanical irritation or exposure keratopathy.

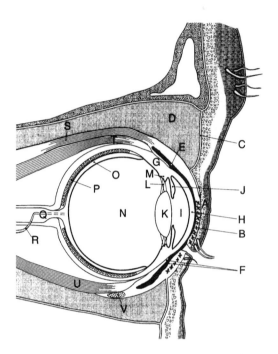

Figure 42.1.   Cross-section anatomy of the eye, orbit, and eyelids. *A*, anterior lamellae of the eyelid; *B*, posterior lamellae of the eyelid; *C*, orbital septum; *D*, conjunctiva; *E*, orbital fat; *F*, cornea; *G*, anterior chamber; *H*, iris; *I*, lens; *J*, ciliary body; *K*, vitreous; *L*, retina; *M*, choroid; *N*, optic nerve; *O*, ophthalmic artery; *P*, superior rectus muscle; *Q*, inferior rectus muscle; *R*, inferior oblique muscle; *S*, sclera.

The treatment of these structural changes is generally surgical.

Obstruction of any portion of the lacrimal tract may lead to abnormal tearing. The most common reason for tearing, however, is aqueous hyposecretion or tear film abnormalities. The proper workup for tearing should thus include examination of the lids and tear film for dry eyes, blepharitis, and mechanical irritation from trichiasis or lid malpositions. Stenotic puncta or lacrimal sac obstruction should be evident with inspection and palpation. *Involutional stenosis of the nasolacrimal duct* is the most common form of nasolacrimal duct obstruction in elderly persons, and is twice as common in women as in men (6). The treatment for lacrimal tract obstruction depends on its anatomic location. Stenotic puncta may be enlarged with a simple snip procedure, while lacrimal sac and nasolacrimal duct obstructions usually require silicone intubation and dacryocystorhinostomy, in which a bony ostium is created between the sac and the nasal cavity.

EYELID NEOPLASMS

Basal cell carcinoma is the most common malignancy of the eyelid skin, accounting for more than 90% of tumors (7). It is most likely to be associated with ultraviolet exposure, and it is most common in southern climates and in persons with fair skin. It occurs with the greatest frequency on the upper lids and medial canthus and has the worst prognosis in the medial canthal area. Typically, the lesion is painless, grows slowly, and has the appearance of a nodular ulcer with raised rolled edges (rodent ulcer). Its color ranges from light to dark brown. It may also appear as a diffuse indurated tan plaque-like lesion (morpheaform) with ulcerated areas or nodules interspersed throughout the lesion. The diagnosis is made with an excisional biopsy.

The treatment of basal cell carcinoma is generally surgical. The technique of Mohs' micrographic surgery, with careful stepwise excision and microscopic monitoring of the surgical margins, has a lower recurrence rate than other methods (8). Chemotherapy may be used in unresectable tumors.

Squamous cell carcinoma of the eyelid is much less common than basal cell carcinoma, accounting for fewer than 5% of malignant eyelid tumors. It too occurs in areas of actinic exposure, most commonly in the lower lid. Squamous cell tumors grow more rapidly than basal cell carcinomas and are locally destructive, with extension into surrounding structures. They may arise in areas of actinic keratosis and may resemble other benign lid lesions or basal cell carcinomas. Metastasis occurs in only 0.5% of squamous cell carcinomas that arise from sun-damaged skin, although metastasis may be more common in tumors from chronically inflamed areas (9). Clinically the tumor is flat and mildly erythematous, with overlying telangiectasias and scaling. As the tumor grows, it often develops an ulcer with surrounding induration and loss of the eyelashes. Surgical excision with frozen section examination of the margins is the treatment of choice for squamous cell carcinomas of the eyelid.

Sebaceous cell carcinoma, like the superficial variant of basal cell carcinoma, is thought to be multicentric in origin, and it exhibits pagetoid or horizontal spread. Found most frequently in elderly people, it has a variable clinical presentation. It may present as a chronic unilateral blepharitis, for which a high degree of clinical suspicion is necessary. It arises from the meibomian glands, glands of Zeis, and sebaceous glands from the caruncle. It is diagnosed with a full-thickness lid biopsy. The prognosis for sebaceous cell carcinoma is worse than that of basal or squamous cell carcinoma, with a mortality rate of 20% or more because of metastasis (10). The treatment includes surgical excision, including possible orbital exenteration, and radiation therapy.

Nonmalignant tumors of the eyelids include seborrheic and actinic keratosis and keratoacanthoma, among others. *Seborrheic keratosis,* which is quite common, appears as an elevated, light brown, greasy plaque on the skin. The tendency to develop these lesions is inherited as a dominant trait. *Actinic keratosis* is considered a premalignant lesion; it develops in persons who have had excessive sun exposure. It is associated with surrounding inflammatory changes in the skin and may progress to squamous cell carcinoma (11). *Keratoacanthoma* develops rapidly over several weeks and may be mistaken for a squamous cell carcinoma. It is a large, round, elevated lesion with a central depressed core of keratin. These lesions are treated with simple excision and should always be examined histopathologically.

Blepharitis is a common condition characterized by inflammation of the anterior eyelid margin or by meibomian gland dysfunction in the posterior lids. It is frequently associated with *dry eye syndrome,* which is aqueous hyposecretion and/or tear film dysfunction leading to ocular surface irritation. Both entities occur most commonly in elderly patients, and dry eye syndrome is more common in women than in men. Patients with blepharitis and dry eyes complain of burning, foreign-body sensation, redness, mild itching, and tearing. These symptoms worsen in the evening and are exacerbated by prolonged reading and by wind. Patients with keratoconjunctivitis sicca associated with autoimmune processes such as Sjögren's syndrome may have severe pain, photophobia, and blurry vision.

Blepharitis may be secondary to staphylococcal infection, but noninfectious blepharitis is equally common. Infectious organisms that inhabit the eyelids may produce infections or inflammation of the lids and cornea or even lead to endophthalmitis after intraocular surgery. It is therefore important to recognize and treat significant blepharitis.

The signs of *anterior staphylococcal blepharitis* include collarettes, or material deposited at the base of the eyelashes, as well as broken or absent cilia (madarosis). A mucopurulent discharge, hordeolum, chronic conjunctivitis, and sometimes corneal changes are associated clinical signs. The clinical course of blepharitis waxes and wanes. The treatment for staphylococcal blepharitis includes lid hygiene and topical antibiotics. Patients should be instructed to scrub the eyelid margins with dilute baby shampoo or a commercial preparation using the fingers or a washcloth to loosen the crusts from the lashes, followed by a thorough rinsing with warm water. Warm compresses may be applied to the lids with a clean washcloth. Lid hygiene should be performed each morning as part of the patient's daily routine. An antibiotic ointment, such as erythromycin or bacitracin, may be applied to the lids before bedtime for at least 6 weeks. Eyelid cultures are usually unnecessary unless the condition is severe.

Noninfectious types of blepharitis include seborrheic blepharitis and meibomitis. Patients with *seborrheic blepharitis* may exhibit oily lid margins, crusting of the lashes, conjunctivitis, and an associated seborrheic dermatitis. *Meibomitis* involves the posterior eyelid surface and is characterized by thickened irregular lid margins with inflammation around the orifices of the glands. The material within the glands, when expressed, may have a thick consistency. Chalazion formation can also be associated. Many patients with meibomitis have acne rosacea. The treatment for noninfectious blepharitis includes lid hygiene, warm compresses, and systemic tetracycline or its derivatives for 6 to 8 weeks, longer if necessary.

Patients with *dry eye syndrome* may have mild conjunctival injection, a low tear meniscus, and an abnormal tear breakup time, which is the interval between the blink and the separation of the tear film. In patients with *keratoconjunctivitis sicca,* rose bengal stains the desiccated conjunctival and corneal surfaces and mucus strands in the tear film. The Schirmer test quantifies tear production by measuring the millimeters of wetting of a strip of filter paper inserted into the inferior fornix. Topical anesthesia is used to measure basic tear secretion; less than 10 mm of wetting is considered abnormal. Treatment includes artificial tear preparations, lubricating ointment at bedtime, punctal occlusion, and the use of humidifiers and side shields on glasses. A tarsorrhaphy can minimize exposure in patients with severe disease.

CONJUNCTIVA AND CORNEA

Conjunctivitis is a common condition in all age groups; it may be classified as acute or chronic and may be due to infection or a noninfectious cause. It generally does not cause structural damage to the eye, but certain organisms, such as *Neisseria gonorrhoeae,* may invade the cornea and cause blindness if untreated. The symptoms, which are usually nonspecific, include irritation, discharge, photophobia, and itching. The conjunctiva is typically diffusely erythematous, and

a follicular or papillary response may be discernible in the palpebral conjunctiva by slit-lamp examination.

Patients with *bacterial conjunctivitis* have a mucopurulent discharge. Although the disease is generally self-limited, cultures should be obtained if a bacterial infection is suspected. Treatment includes a topical broad-spectrum antibiotic agent, such as erythromycin or bacitracin ointment, for 5 to 7 days. The antibiotic regimen may be modified according to results from culture and sensitivity testing. Any patient with gonococcal or meningococcal infection should be hospitalized and treated systemically with intravenous antibiotic therapy because of the rapid and destructive clinical course of these infections.

Patients with *adenoviral conjunctivitis,* the most common of the viral infections, may have associated upper respiratory tract flulike symptoms. The discharge is more watery than that associated with bacterial infections. The disease is self-limited, typically lasting up to a week. Preauricular lymphadenopathy and rapid progression with bilateral spread are characteristic of epidemic keratoconjunctivitis, caused by adenovirus types 8 and 19. This condition affects the corneal epithelium, with subsequent photophobia and blurry vision. It is highly contagious and may be contracted in health care environments, such as physicians' offices. Viral conjunctivitis does not require therapy except lubricants and topical vasoconstricting agents for relief of symptoms.

Allergic conjunctivitis is characterized by itching, which may be severe, and a stringy white mucous discharge. These patients commonly have concurrent seasonal allergic symptoms. Cold compresses and topical nonsteroidal agents or antihistamine preparations help to relieve itching. Environmental control of the offending allergen is the most effective therapy; in addition, systemic antihistamines, topical sodium cromolyn, and topical steroid medication may be required. Topical steroids are a last resort and should always be administered by an ophthalmologist, as these agents may induce glaucoma and cataract formation.

The differential diagnosis of conjunctivitis includes primary conjunctival conditions as discussed; in addition, patients with systemic diseases such as Stevens-Johnson syndrome or ocular cicatricial pemphigoid may exhibit chronic conjunctival inflammation. Other causes of chronic conjunctivitis include occult neoplasm (squamous or sebaceous cell carcinoma), retained foreign body, eyelid abnormalities, chronic dacryocystitis, or orbital processes such as arteriovenous shunt or thyroid disease. Topical medications, such as antiglaucoma agents, may also cause chronic irritation. If a neoplastic or cicatricial systemic process is suspected, a conjunctival biopsy should always be performed.

The *cornea* (Fig. 42.1*H*) is the major refracting surface of the eye. Its transparency allows transmission of light to the retina, and it provides structural integrity to the globe. The cornea consists of five layers: epithelium, Bowman's membrane, stroma, Descemet's membrane, and endothelium. The endothelium functions as a metabolic pump, transporting fluid across its surface, keeping the cornea dehydrated and clear. The number of endothelial cells and the pumping action of the endothelium decrease with age. Corneal edema may result from the loss of endothelial cells. The normal decrease in endothelial cells due to aging is usually insufficient to cause corneal edema, unless there is an underlying dystrophy or trauma due to intraocular surgery.

Fuchs' dystrophy, first described in 1910, is characterized by corneal epithelial and stromal edema associated with endothelial changes called guttata, which are warty excrescences of Descemet's membrane. The endothelial cells overlying the guttata are abnormal or absent, producing a thickened basement membrane. It is more common in women than in men and is bilateral, although it may be asymmetric. Initially these persons are asymptomatic. Symptoms of early stromal edema include blurry vision in the morning that clears throughout the day as the evaporation from the ocular surface leads to stromal dehydration. As the endothelial function decreases over time, the visual acuity decreases and epithelial edema or bullae may occur, causing pain and tearing. The treatment of Fuchs' endothelial dystrophy begins with topical hyperosmotic agents for morning stromal edema and may progress to therapeutic contact lens use for pain relief from corneal epithelial edema and ruptured bullae. If further corneal decompensation occurs and vi-

sual rehabilitation is required, corneal transplantation may be very successful.

Persons who have had cataract extraction with intraocular lens implantation may develop progressive corneal stromal edema with epithelial swelling similar to the changes seen in Fuchs' dystrophy. This condition, known as *pseudophakic bullous keratopathy,* may also be seen in aphakic persons. It requires corneal transplantation for improvement of vision. The development of improved cataract surgical techniques and intraocular lens implants has decreased the incidence of pseudophakic bullous keratopathy in recent years (12).

Infectious diseases of the cornea are another cause of decreased vision and pain and should always be suspected in persons who complain of a sudden onset of red eye, photophobia, and tearing. Contact lens wearers in particular are susceptible to microbial keratitis, including *Pseudomonas* and *Acanthamoeba* infections. *Staphylococcal infections* may lead to peripheral corneal infiltrates that progress slowly, while *gram-negative bacterial infections* progress rapidly and may lead to corneal perforation. *Acanthamoeba* is a ubiquitous protozoan organism found in soil, swimming pools, hot tubs, and lake water. It is also associated with homemade saline solution. *Fungal keratitis* is most common in southern climates and in immunocompromised persons. *Herpes simplex* and *varicella zoster* viral infections may cause corneal anesthesia and scarring. Varicella zoster infections also produce pain and vesicular skin lesions in a dermatomal distribution and may involve all the structures of the eye and surrounding orbit.

The management of most corneal infections includes Gram and Giemsa staining of material obtained by scraping the bed of the ulcer, as well as culture and sensitivity testing. Fortified broad-spectrum antibiotics that are normally used for intravenous therapy and/or topical fluoroquinolones may be applied topically up to every 15 minutes initially. Modification of the treatment regimen is based on culture results and clinical response. Corneal biopsy may be necessary to diagnose fungal or acanthamoeba infections. Prolonged topical therapy is usually successful, but surgical treatment may be necessary in severe cases. Herpes simplex keratitis is treated with topical antiviral agents. Oral acyclovir may be helpful in treating and preventing recurrent keratitis. Acute varicella zoster infections are treated for 7 to 10 days with acyclovir 800 mg orally 5 times daily, famciclovir 500 mg 3 times daily, or valacyclovir 1g 3 times daily to minimize ocular complications (13).

Indications for *corneal transplantation* include corneal scarring due to trauma or herpetic infections, severe keratoconus, and corneal dystrophies involving the deeper layers of the stroma. Corneal grafts have a success rate approaching 90%. The success rate decreases markedly, however, if the underlying pathology includes inflammatory or infectious diseases, such as herpes simplex keratitis, which may induce corneal neovascularization (14). Superficial corneal scarring or anterior basement membrane corneal dystrophies may be an indication for phototherapeutic keratectomy, superficial keratectomy, or partial-thickness lamellar corneal transplantation.

Presbyopia is the most common ocular condition affecting the aging population. Presbyopia develops in the aging eye when accommodation for near focusing becomes so weak that visual aids (bifocals) are required. This usually begins in the mid-40s and progresses with aging. Accommodation of the normal eye is produced by the ciliary muscle, which contracts and causes a change in the shape and therefore the power of the crystalline lens (Fig. 42.2A). A rigid lens from metabolic aging may play a part in the decreased ability to accommodate with aging. However, in recent years, experimental evidence in aged monkeys has suggested that a loss of ciliary muscle contractility and/or innervation may play a large role in the development of presbyopia (15). As yet there is no chemical or surgical remedy for the loss of accommodation.

The lens lies behind the iris and is supported by zonular fibers that arise from the internal layers of the eye (Fig. 42.1*K* and *L*). By adulthood, the lens measures 9 mm in equatorial diameter and 5 mm in anteroposterior thickness. The lens consists of several layers and becomes thicker with age. *Cataract* is defined as an opacity in the lens. Epidemiologically, cataract is age-related. At present there is no medical therapy to prevent the formation or progression of cataract in an other-

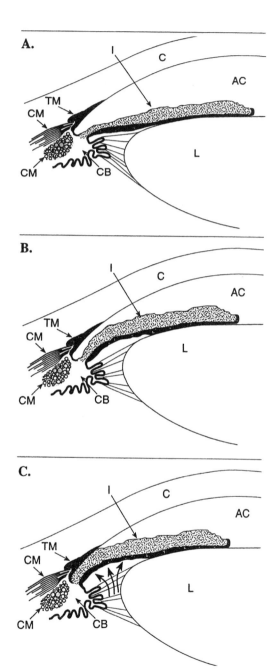

Figure 42.2. Detail of the anterior chamber angle. **A.** Open angle. **B.** Narrow angle. **C.** Angle closure. *C,* cornea; *AC,* anterior chamber; *I,* iris; *L,* lens; *CB,* ciliary body; *TM,* trabecular meshwork; *CM,* ciliary muscle.

wise healthy eye. The production of cataractous changes is a multifaceted progressive process, and the precise sequence of events has yet to be elucidated. Two fundamental processes seem to occur in the lens to produce cataract. The lens cortex may become overhydrated, and the lens nucleus proteins become aggregated. The resulting changes cause a deterioration in the highly organized structure of the lens and opacification results. Oxidative damage and photo-oxidation over decades of chronic exposure may contribute to the development of cataract (16). The lens has high concentrations of the antioxidants glutathione and ascorbic acid that decrease with age. However, there is no concrete evidence in humans that supplemental antioxidants will slow the progression of cataract formation. Poor nutrition producing deficiencies of trace minerals and certain vitamins has also been found to cause experimental cataract in animals, but the role in human cataractogenesis is uncertain.

Other than aging, some specific entities may cause cataract in the older patient. Blunt trauma, electrical shock, or ionizing radiation may cause cataract to develop acutely or with a delayed onset. Large osmotic shifts in a patient's fluid balance may produce reversible or irreversible cataracts due to swelling of the lens fibers. Systemic conditions may predispose to the development of cataract. Diabetes mellitus is associated with early onset and high incidence of cataract. Many drugs have been reported to cause cataract. Corticosteroids given over the long term often produce posterior subcapsular cataract changes. Chlorpromazine, naphthalene, dinitrophenol, p-dichlorobenzene, and others have been implicated in cataract formation.

Most patients with cataract changes have a combination of opacities in the nuclear and cortical layers. Nuclear sclerosis, which occurs as the increase in number and density of lens fibers accrues, produces a gradual decline in visual acuity. Initially the change may manifest as an increase in myopia, in which patients find that they can read without glasses or that a change in the eyeglass prescription is necessary. The progressive yellowing of the lens causes poor hue discrimination. Cortical cataract changes often appear as spoke-shaped opacities; they impair vision to varying degrees. Posterior subcapsular cataract tends to be more prevalent in a somewhat younger population and in patients chronically taking corticosteroids. Visual difficulty is found in bright light because of severe glare once the central axis of the pupil is affected.

CATARACT SURGERY

The prevalence of cataract in Americans between ages 65 and 74 is about 50% (17, 18). The prevalence increases to 70% in Americans over age 75. In 1995, about 1.4 million cataract extractions were performed in the United States Medicare population, and the visual disability associated with cataract accounts for more than 8 million office visits per year (17, 19). Nonsurgical management of cataract entails accurate refraction and changes of eyeglass correction. Eventually the vision does not improve significantly with a change in lens prescription. Once optical modalities no longer meet the patient's needs, the patient may be offered cataract surgery based on the ophthalmologist's full evaluation.

The technologic advances in cataract surgery over the past 2 decades have been enormous. Extracapsular cataract extraction and phacoemulsification are microsurgical techniques that remove the cataract and leave the posterior lens capsule intact so that an intraocular lens may be implanted. Intraocular lens implants are small disc-shaped pieces of polymethylmethacrylate, acrylic, silicone, or hydrogel that are manufactured with differing powers. The power of the implant is determined by the optical properties of each patient's eye, measured with sophisticated instruments. Almost all cataract surgery is done on an outpatient basis with local anesthesia and mild intravenous sedation. Adequate wound healing and stabilization occur by 4 to 8 weeks, and the patient is then prescribed new eyeglasses, if necessary.

Visual acuity after cataract surgery is 20/40 or better in 97% of patients without coexisting ocular pathology. Patients have significant improvement in their quality of life functions, such as nighttime and daytime driving, community and home activities, mental health, and life satisfaction, along with the improvement in their visual function (20). In addition, patients who undergo necessary cataract surgery in both eyes report greater subjective improvement than patients who undergo surgery in one eye alone (21).

Complications may follow cataract surgery, however (22). The lifetime incidence of retinal detachment increases after cataract surgery and may be as high as 0.7%. Opacification of the remaining posterior capsule of the lens is fairly common and may necessitate opening with a laser months to years later. Cystoid macular edema following cataract surgery may cause temporary and sometimes permanent visual impairment. Less common but sight-threatening complications include secondary glaucoma, hyphema, intraocular lens dislocation, endophthalmitis, and expulsive choroidal hemorrhage.

Glaucoma is the second most common cause of blindness in the United States. Among black Americans it is the leading cause of blindness. Of the 2 million people who have glaucoma, nearly half are unaware of their disease (23, 24). Up to 15 million people have characteristics that put them at risk for developing glaucoma (25). Glaucoma increases markedly in prevalence with age. In the United States 1 in 10 elderly blacks and 1 in 50 elderly whites have glaucoma (24). Glaucoma is not a single disease but rather a group of diseases with common findings. Glaucoma is intraocular pressure that is too high for the health of the optic nerve, which develops a characteristic optic atrophy and pattern of visual field loss. The damage, once it occurs, is irreversible. The goal, therefore, is early identification and treatment to prevent further loss of visual function.

Intraocular pressure is the function of three features of the eye: the rate of aqueous fluid production by the ciliary body (Fig. 42.1*M*), the resistance to aqueous outflow through the trabecular meshwork in the anterior chamber angle (Fig. 42.2*A*), and the venous pressure of the episcleral veins. In most eyes with elevated intraocular pressure, increased resistance to outflow through the trabecular meshwork is at fault. The intraocular pressure is not the only cause of the disease, however. Some patients are predisposed to develop glaucoma for reasons that are not clear. It is likely a multifactorial genetic tendency that makes a person susceptible to glaucoma. The known risk factors for glaucoma are high intraocular pressure, black race, old age, family history, myopia, high hyperopia, diabetes, and vascular disease.

Routine direct ophthalmoscopy of the optic disc in all adult patients by the primary care physician identifies possible glaucoma. Although the ratio of cup to disc varies, usually a ratio of 0.3 in whites and 0.5 in blacks is considered normal. The optic discs should be symmetric. Larger cups, especially vertically oval ones that have a ratio of cup to disc greater than 0.6, are suspicious (Fig. 42.3). The disc rim should have uniform thickness throughout its temporal portion, without notches, localized atrophy, or splinter-like hemorrhages. Intraocular pressure measurements should be a part of a routine physical examination of adults over 40. The population "normal" level of intraocular pressure is 21 mm Hg or less. However, glaucoma may develop with levels of intraocular pressure in the "normal" range. Primary care physicians should become facile in the use of a Schiötz tonometer for routine examinations as well as for eye emergencies. Other hand-held devices are available, but most cost more. If the primary care physician does not routinely include measurement of intraocular pressure and evaluation of the optic disc cup, the patient should be referred to an ophthalmologist.

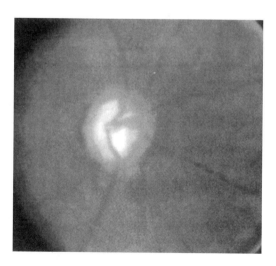

Figure 42.3. Clinical photograph of a glaucomatous optic disc with characteristic enlargement of the optic disc cup. Note the thin optic disc rim, especially inferiorly.

During routine comprehensive examinations, the ophthalmologist takes a medical and family history and performs an examination that includes several tests to screen for glaucoma. This includes Goldmann applanation tonometry, gonioscopy (a mirrored lens examination of the anterior chamber angle), and dilated fundus examination with detailed evaluation of the optic discs and nerve fiber layer. Patients who have risk factors for glaucoma may undergo visual field testing by automated or manual methods.

Open-angle glaucoma has no obvious macroscopic mechanical restriction to outflow, while angle-closure glaucoma has an impediment to outflow from mechanical blockage by the peripheral iris (Fig. 42.2). Open-angle glaucoma accounts for most glaucoma in the United States, and primary open-angle glaucoma constitutes 70% of glaucoma in adults.

Primary open-angle glaucoma does not cause any symptoms until late in the course of the disease, when near total loss of the visual field becomes obvious to the patient. The elevated intraocular pressure often found is a chronic condition and does not produce any sensation of fullness or pain. The early visual field loss develops slowly and affects the peripheral and paracentral fields without affecting the central visual acuity, so the patient may not detect any visual change until the disease is far advanced. The diagnosis is made by finding characteristic optic disc cupping and typical visual field changes in the presence of an open, normal-appearing angle. The intraocular pressure may or may not be elevated beyond what is considered the population normal of 21 mm Hg.

Pigmentary glaucoma, pseudoexfoliation glaucoma, and steroid-induced glaucoma are other types of open-angle glaucoma. Patients who are taking systemic or topical steroids for any condition may develop steroid-induced high intraocular pressure and glaucoma. Even skin creams containing steroids that are used near the eye may cause steroid-induced glaucoma if used on a continuing basis. The steroids modify the intracellular structure of the trabecular meshwork cells and increase the resistance to outflow. The effect may or may not be reversible.

Although it occurs in only 0.1% of people over age 40 in the United States, *acute angle-closure glaucoma* is a true emergency. A patient who develops acute angle-closure glaucoma is already predisposed by an anatomically narrowed anterior chamber angle depth (Fig. 42.2B). Many patients who are moderately to highly hyperopic have a narrow angle. Acute angle closure occurs more frequently in women than men and in whites than in blacks, with an intermediate occurrence in Asians. The peak prevalence is between ages 55 and 70 (26).

The anterior chamber depth decreases normally with age because of the growth of the lens. In patients who already have a narrow chamber angle, the iris becomes apposed to the anterior surface of the lens. This impedes the normal flow of aqueous fluid from its production site behind the iris to the drainage site in the trabecular meshwork. The pressure builds up behind the iris, causing the peripheral iris to bow forward, further obstructing aqueous outflow (Fig. 42.2C). The fluid production continues and an acute rise in pressure ensues. It is this rapid rise in intraocular pressure that is responsible for the severe pain that accompanies this condition.

The unilateral presentation of pain and redness is sudden, can be excruciating, and may be attributed to sinus pain or headache. It is fairly common for nausea and vomiting to occur. Fewer than 5% of patients have bilateral attacks, although the narrow angle is a bilateral condition. The vision becomes blurred as the cornea swells and becomes edematous. Corneal edema is responsible for patient complaints of halos or rainbows around lights. The anterior chamber may appear shallow, and the pupil is moderately dilated and nonreactive.

The attack often occurs in the evening during periods of dim illumination or during physical or emotional stress or excitement, when the pupil becomes moderately dilated and has the greatest surface contact with the anterior lens. Rarely, a dense, swollen neglected cataract precipitates an angle-closure glaucoma. Patients who have narrow angles and have undergone pharmacologic dilation may develop angle-closure glaucoma as the dilation slowly wanes and the iris becomes arrested in mid-dilation. Certain common medications predispose patients with narrow angles to angle closure, including any with anticholinergic side effects, such as decongestants, tricyclic antidepressants, and antispasmodics.

The diagnosis is made by the clinical appearance of the eye and a usually severely elevated intraocular pressure. The ophthalmologist uses gonioscopy to confirm the closed angle in the involved eye and the narrow angle in the other eye. Treatment should be started immediately. The goals of treatment are first to lower the intraocular pressure as rapidly as possible with medical treatment and then to relieve the angle obstruction definitively with a laser iridectomy. The hole in the iris provides a channel for aqueous to flow to the anterior chamber, and the iris settles back, relieving the outflow obstruction. It protects against further attacks of angle-closure glaucoma and should be performed in both eyes.

Chronic angle-closure glaucoma may develop in patients who have chronic apposition of the iris against the trabecular meshwork for anatomic reasons or in patients who are chronically treated with medications that have anticholinergic side effects, such as decongestants, tricyclic antidepressants, and antispasmodics. Asians and blacks seem to be at high risk for this type of glaucoma. Laser iridectomies may relieve the iris apposition, but damage to the delicate trabecular meshwork cells may have produced a mixed open- and closed-angle form of glaucoma.

The goal of *glaucoma treatment* is to lower intraocular pressure to a safe level and prevent further damage to the optic nerve and visual field. Medical therapy is usually the initial treatment in the United States. Topical glaucoma medications all have the potential for systemic side effects, because they are drained through the nasolacrimal duct system and absorbed by the nasal mucosa. Nevertheless, patients often do not attribute systemic symptoms to their eyedrops. Primary care physicians should question their patients about ophthalmic medications (Table 42.1).

β-Adrenergic antagonists have been the first line of therapy since their introduction in 1978 (Table 42.1). The β-blockers lower intraocular pressure by reducing aqueous fluid production. They can be given once or twice a day and are usually well tolerated but are contraindicated in

patients with congestive heart failure, bradycardia, or pulmonary disease. Newer medications with less potential for systemic side effects are becoming more popular.

Adrenergic α$_2$-agonists are approved for long-term use and perioperatively during laser surgery. Apraclonidine and brimonidine have minimal systemic side effects and are potent inhibitors of aqueous fluid production. They have greatly increased the safety of ocular laser procedures by reducing the risk of postoperative pressure elevations. They are not contraindicated in patients with cardiovascular or pulmonary disease and may be safer than β-blockers in the geriatric population.

Latanoprost, a once-a-day drop, is the first prostaglandin analog approved for glaucoma treatment. It lowers intraocular pressure by increasing uveoscleral outflow, and. it has minimal systemic side effects. A topical carbonic anhydrase inhibitor, dorzolamide, has fewer systemic side effects than the oral medications. The oral carbonic anhydrase inhibitors acetazolamide (Diamox) and methazolamide (Neptazane) lower intraocular pressure by reducing aqueous fluid production up to 50%. The systemic side effects of the oral drugs often limit their use, especially in older patients.

For decades miotics have been used to treat glaucoma by increasing the outflow of aqueous. They have few systemic side effects but many ocular side effects. They cause miosis and may produce eye and brow ache from ciliary spasm, induce some myopia, and may cause unacceptable dimness in the presence of cataract. Pilocarpine has the mildest of these discomforts but requires administration 4 times a day in its drop form. A gel and an extended-release device preparation are available, but older patients often have difficulty using them. An adrenergic agonist, epinephrine, enhances outflow from the eye, but local side effects limit its use. Dipivefrin (Propine) is cleaved into epinephrine once inside the eye. It tends to have fewer local side effects, although it is usually not as effective as other agents. These agents are rarely used today.

Laser trabeculoplasty is applied with an argon or diode laser by directing small, focused spots of light energy at the trabecular meshwork. The desired result is an improvement in outflow fa-

Table 42.1

Systemic Side Effects of Glaucoma Medications

Drugs	Side Effects

Topical β-blockers
  Timolol (Timoptic, Betimol)
  Levobunolol (Betagan)
  Betaxolol (Betoptic-S)
  Metipranolol (Optipranolol)
  Carteolol (Ocupress)
	Exacerbate COPD or asthma
	Exacerbate congestive heart failure
	Bradycardia
	CNS disturbances and depression
	Impotence
	Worsen myasthenia gravis

Adrenergic α₂-agonists
  Apraclonidine (Iopidine)
  Brimonidine (Alphagan)
	Dry mouth
	Fatigue

Adrenergic agonists
  Epinephrine
  Dipivefrin (Propine)
	Hypertension
	Dysrhythmias

Cholinergic agents (miotics)
  Anticholinesterases
    Echothiophate iodide,
      demecarium bromide,
      physostigmine
	Acute poisoning by overdose: sweating, GI disturbances, defecation, bradycardia, respiratory paralysis

Direct acting Pilocarpine, carbachol	Acute poisoning by overdose: sweating, salivation, nausea, tremor, hypotension

Carbonic anhydrase inhibitors
  Topical
    Dorzolamide (Trusopt)
    Brinzolamide (Azopt)
	All more common with oral, IV dosing than topical
	Lethargy
	Anorexia

Oral, IV
    Acetazolamide (Diamox)
    Methazolamide (Neptazane)
	Paresthesias
	Metabolic acidosis
	Hypokalemia
	Renal lithiasis
	Blood dyscrasias: aplastic anemia, agranulocytosis, thrombocytopenia

cility and reduced intraocular pressure. Studies in patients with primary open-angle glaucoma have shown laser trabeculoplasty to be safe and effective, although approximately 50% of patients show a loss of effect by 5 years (27). Current practice in the United States is to offer laser trabeculoplasty prior to glaucoma filtration surgery.

Glaucoma filtration surgery is usually offered after medical and laser therapies fail to provide adequate control of the glaucoma. The surgery entails the creation of a fistula from the anterior chamber of the eye to the subconjunctival space.

Eyes that have failed multiple surgeries may undergo cyclodestructive procedures or the implantation of an artificial aqueous drainage device.

REFERENCES

1. Sommer A. Disabling Visual Disorders. Maxcy-Rosenau Public Health and Preventive Medicine. East Norwalk, CT: Appleton-Century-Crofts, 1986.
2. American Academy of Ophthalmology. Eye Care for the American People. San Francisco: American Academy of Ophthalmology, 1987.
3. Tielsch JM, Sommer A, Witt K, Katz J. Blindness and visual impairment in the urban population: the Baltimore Eye Survey. Arch Ophthalmol 1990;108:286–290.

4. Klein R, Klein BE, Linton KL, DeMets DL. The Beaver Dam Eye Study: visual acuity. Ophthalmology 1991;98: 1310–1315.

5. American Academy of Ophthalmology. Comprehensive Adult Eye Examination. San Francisco: American Academy of Ophthalmology, 1996.

6. McCord DC. The lacrimal drainage system. In: Tasman W, Jaeger EA, eds. Duane's Clinical Ophthalmology, vol 4. Philadelphia: Lippincott, Chapter 13, 1989.

7. Ferry A. The eye lids. In: Sorsby A, ed. Modern Ophthalmology, vol 4. Philadelphia: Lippincott, 1972:833–853.

8. Margo CE, Waltz K. Basal cell carcinoma of the eyelid and periocular skin. Surv Ophthalmol 1993;38:169–192.

9. Dryden RM, Wilkes TD. Periocular squamous cell carcinoma. In: Fraunfelder F, Roy F, eds. Current Ocular Therapy 2. Philadelphia: Saunders, 1985:213–214.

10. Jacobiec FA. Sebaceous tumors of the ocular adnexa. In: Albert DA, Jacobiec FA, eds. Principles and Practice of Ophthalmology, vol 3. Philadelphia: Saunders, 1994: 1745–1770.

11. Doxana MT, Iliff WJ, Iliff NT, Green WR. Squamous cell carcinoma of the eyelids. Ophthalmology 1987;94:538–541.

12. Mamalis N, Anderson CW, Kreisler KR, et al. Changing trends in the indications for penetrating keratoplasty. Arch Ophthalmol 1992;110:1409–1411.

13. Pepose JS. The potential impact of the varicella vaccine and new antivirals on ocular disease related to varicella-zoster virus. Am J Ophthalmol 1997;123:243–251.

14. Vail A, Fore SM, Bradley BA, et al. Corneal graft survival and visual outcome. Ophthalmology 1994;101:120–127.

15. Bito LZ, DeRousseau CJ, Kaufman PL, Bito LZ. Age-dependent loss of accommodative amplitude in rhesus monkeys: an animal model for presbyopia. Invest Ophthalmol Vis Sci 1982;23:23–31.

16. Datiles MB, Kinoshita JH. Pathogenesis of cataracts. In: Tasman W, Jaeger EA, eds. Duane's Clinical Ophthalmology. Philadelphia: Lippincott, Chapter 72B, 1991.

17. National Advisory Eye Council. Vision Research: A National Plan: 1983–1987. U.S. Department of Health and Human Services Pub 87–2755, 1987.

18. Leibowitz HM, Krueger DE, Maunder LR, et al. The Framingham Eye Study monograph: an ophthalmological and epidemiological study of cataract, glaucoma, diabetic retinopathy, macular degeneration, and visual acuity in a general population of 2631 adults, 1973–1975. Surv Ophthalmol 1980;24(suppl):335–610.

19. Office of the Inspector General. Medicare Cataract Implant Surgery (DHHS OAI85IX046). Washington: US Department of Health and Human Services, 1986.

20. Brenner MH, Curbow B, Javitt JC, et al. Vision change and quality of life in the elderly. Arch Ophthalmol 1993;111:680–685.

21. Javitt JC, Brenner H, Curbow B, et al. Outcomes of cataract surgery: improvement in visual acuity and subjective visual function after surgery in the first, second, and both eyes. Arch Ophthalmol 1993;111:686–691.

22. Powe NR, Schein OD, Gieser SC, et al. Synthesis of the literature on visual acuity and complications following cataract extraction with intraocular lens implantation. Cataract Patient Outcome Research Team. Arch Ophthalmol 1994;112:239–252.

23. Bankes JL, Perkins ES, Tsolakis S, Wright JE. Bedford glaucoma survey. BMJ 1968;1:791–796.

24. American Academy of Ophthalmology Practice Pattern Committee. Primary Open Angle Glaucoma. San Francisco: American Academy of Ophthalmology, 1996.

25. Tielsch JM, Sommer A, Katz J, et al. Racial variations in the prevalence of primary open angle glaucoma: The Baltimore Eye Survey. JAMA 1991;266:369–374.

25. Lowe RF, Ritch R. Angle closure glaucoma. In: Ritch R, Shields MB, Krupin T, eds. The Glaucomas. St. Louis: Mosby, 1989:825–853.

27. Shingleton BJ, Richter CU, Bellows AR, et al. Long-term efficacy of argon laser trabeculoplasty. Ophthalmology 1987;94:1513–1518.

Retinal Disorders of Aging

As the eye ages, a host of conditions can affect the vitreoretinal interface, the retinal circulation, the retinal pigment epithelial-choroidal complex, and the optic nerve. Most of these conditions may result in moderate to severe visual loss. The rapid identification of retinal emergencies (Table 43.1) and the early recognition of conditions that may be amenable to laser photocoagulation (Table 43.2) can result in the prevention of severe visual loss. Preventing blindness is an important factor in improving the elderly's ability to function autonomously and lead productive lives. The personal, familial, and societal burdens that are the result of retinal blinding disorders are significant and can be profound.

VITREORETINAL DISORDERS
Rhegmatogenous Retinal Detachment

Retinal detachment secondary to a tear or hole (rhegma) in the retina is typically seen in persons over age 50. The incidence of occurrence is highest in patients who have had cataract extraction or myopia. Some 25,000 people in the United States have retinal detachment each year. The mechanism of hole or tear formation is detachment of the posterior vitreous from the surface of the retina, which is common in persons over age 55.

Symptoms of posterior vitreous detachment include floaters and flashing lights. Floaters may be found with retinal holes or tears or vitreous hemorrhage secondary to avulsion of a retinal blood vessel. Symptoms of retinal detachment include a decline in central vision if the macula

is involved; more commonly, a peripheral visual field defect is detected by the patient. Examination of the retina by binocular indirect ophthalmoscopy and including scleral depression is the most important way to identify retinal tears and detachment. Techniques for repair of retinal detachments include photocoagulation, pneumatic retinopexy, scleral buckling, and pars plana vitrectomy (removal of the vitreous gel). Rapid referral to an ophthalmologist is indicated if retinal detachment is suspected, so that intervention may improve the chances of saving central and peripheral vision.

Macular Hole

Idiopathic macular holes result in loss of central vision to the 20/60 to 20/400 range. A partial or complete hole in the neurosensory retina located in the fovea is observed clinically. This condition typically occurs in the 50s to 70s. The prevalence of this condition is 1 in 3000. Formation of macular holes may be due to vitreoretinal traction caused by the separation of the posterior vitreous. The chance of a bilateral condition is 5%. Vitrectomy surgery may improve central visual acuity in patients affected with this disorder (1).

Idiopathic Epiretinal Membrane

Epiretinal membranes (cellophane maculopathy) are typically seen in patients over age 50. Bilaterality occurs 20% of the time. Posterior vitreous detachment is thought to result in small dehiscences of the internal limiting membrane of the retina, causing glial cells to proliferate on the surface of the retina. Retinal distortion may re-

Table 43.1

Retinal Emergencies

Bacterial endophthalmitis
Central retinal artery occlusion
Choroidal neovascularization
Retinal detachment
Giant cell arteritis

Table 43.2

**Retinal Disorders Amenable
to Laser Treatment**

Choroidal neovascularization
Macular edema secondary to branch retinal vein
    occlusion or diabetes
Proliferative diabetic retinopathy or severe
    nonproliferative diabetic retinopathy
Retinal neovascularization associated with branch or
    central retinal vein occlusion
Retinal tears or holes

sult from contraction of the epiretinal membrane. Loss of normal retinal capillary integrity may cause cystoid macular edema. In general, when visual acuity drops to 20/100 or worse, surgical removal of the epiretinal membrane can be performed by pars plana vitrectomy in an attempt to improve vision (2).

RETINAL VASCULAR DISORDERS
Diabetic Retinopathy

After 15 years of type II diabetes mellitus there is a significant risk of diabetic retinopathy or maculopathy. Type II diabetes is typically diagnosed in middle age; therefore, retinopathy is usually a problem in persons over age 50. Persons diagnosed with diabetes should be examined yearly by an ophthalmologist or expert in retinal diseases for evidence of retinopathy. Background changes, the earliest signs of diabetic retinopathy, include microaneurysms, dot and blot hemorrhages, cotton wool spots, and venous beading (Fig. 43.1). Proliferative diabetic retinopathy is evidenced by the formation of new retinal blood vessels on the surface of the retina and in the vitreous cavity. These abnormal blood vessels can hemorrhage within the

vitreous cavity and exert traction on the retina, detaching it.

Diabetes can affect central visual acuity as well. Abnormal retinal capillaries can form microaneurysms. These microaneurysms leak serous or lipid exudate into the retina, and this can result in macular edema. Macular edema is the most common cause of loss of vision in type II diabetics. Fluorescein angiography aids in the diagnosis and treatment of macular edema. The prompt identification of proliferative diabetic retinopathy or maculopathy is critical to the visual well-being of the diabetic patient, because both of these problems have proved treatable by laser photocoagulation (3,4). The goal of laser photocoagulation in proliferative diabetic retinopathy is to halt the progression of new blood vessels that can result in vitreous hemorrhage and provide a scaffold for retinal detachment. Pars plana vitrectomy is an important technique for clearing the vitreous cavity of blood and removing the fibrovascular scaffold that allows retinal detachment by traction (5).

Branch Retinal Vein Occlusion

Branch retinal vein occlusion (BRVO) typically occurs in persons over age 60. Symptoms include loss of central vision and visual field defects. Associated systemic conditions include hypertension (approximately 75% of the time), diabetes

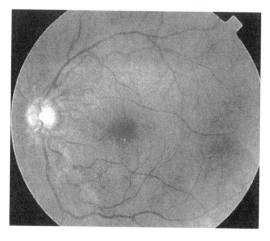

Figure 43.1. Dot hemorrhages, microaneurysms, and exudate in a patient with background diabetic retinopathy.

(10%), and arteriosclerosis. Acute changes on fundus examination show superficial hemorrhages, retinal edema, and cotton wool spots in a sector of the retina. An obstructed vein that is dilated and tortuous can be seen. Fluorescein angiography typically shows slow filling of the obstructed vein. Invariably the site of occlusion is an arteriovenous crossing site. Loss of vision is typically due to macular edema. Retinal neovascularization also occurs, with the possibility of vitreous hemorrhage. Laser photocoagulation offers proven benefit for the two major complications, macular edema and retinal neovascularization (6, 7).

Central Retinal Vein Occlusion

Some 90% of patients with occlusion of the central retinal vein are older than 50 years. Systemic associations include cardiovascular disease (75%), systemic hypertension (60%), and diabetes (35%). Blood dyscrasias, dysproteinemias, and vasculitides all may result in central retinal vein occlusion (CRVO). CRVO is characterized on fundus examination as displaying tortuous retinal veins, retinal edema, intraretinal hemorrhage, and cotton wool spots throughout the entire retina. The retinopathy of carotid occlusive disease has some characteristics similar to those of CRVO.

CRVO may be nonischemic or ischemic. Capillary perfusion in the nonischemic group is normal or nearly normal as determined by fluorescein angiography. Retinal or anterior segment neovascularization is unusual in this group of patients. Ischemic CRVO is characterized by widespread capillary nonperfusion on fluorescein angiography. The prognosis for vision is poor in this group of patients, and only 10% of eyes with ischemia end up with better than 20/400 visual acuity. Anterior segment neovascularization is a frequent complication, and retinal neovascularization may be seen as well. Management of patients with this disorder includes diagnosing and treating any underlying medical condition that may predispose to CRVO. Laser photocoagulation plays a role in the treatment of retinal and anterior segment neovascularization.

Branch Retinal Artery Occlusion

Acute branch retinal artery occlusion (BRAO) results in an edematous white retina caused by infarction of the inner retina at a branch retinal arteriole secondary to an embolus. Patients typically have visual field defects and/or loss of central vision. Cholesterol emboli arise from the carotid arteries, platelet-fibrin emboli are associated with large vessel arteriosclerosis, and calcific emboli originate from cardiac valves. Evaluation and management of patients is geared to determining the specific systemic causation of the emboli. Carotid noninvasive testing and cardiac echography are important tests in determining causation. There is no specific treatment for BRAO.

Central Retinal Artery Occlusion

Central retinal artery occlusion (CRAO) is characterized by a sudden, severe, painless loss of vision. Acuity is typically worse than 20/400. CRAO is generally caused by emboli or intraluminal thrombosis of the central retinal artery. A cherry spot can be seen with mild to severe degrees of retinal whitening. Systemic causes of CRAO are similar to those of BRAO. Giant cell arteritis is another possible cause of CRAO and a very rare cause of BRAO. A sedimentation rate should be obtained in patients with CRAO and BRAO. Signs of embolic disease affecting other organ systems (e.g., stroke) should be sought if retinal emboli are suspected as causing the retinal infarct. Carotid noninvasive studies and color Doppler imaging are useful in assessing flow through the carotid, ophthalmic, and retinal circulations.

CRAO is recognized as an ophthalmic emergency, and therapy should be instituted promptly, including measures to reduce intraocular pressure and to dilate the arterial bed by inhalation of 95% oxygen and 5% carbon dioxide. There may also be a role for thrombolytic agents. Even with immediate treatment, the prognosis for good visual acuity is poor. Long-term complications of CRAO include anterior and posterior segment neovascularization (8).

CHOROIDAL DISORDERS
Age-Related Macular Degeneration

Age-related macular degeneration is the leading cause of blindness in the United States. Affected persons are typically over age 60; the prevalence of this disorder rises with age. Approximately 2% of patients over age 65 have severe loss of vision (worse than 20/200) due to this disorder. Its hallmark is the sudden loss of central vision, which is typically associated with the wet, or exudative, form. Choroidal neovascularization results in hemorrhage, lipid exudate or serous exudate that is typically observed in the macula (Fig. 43.2). Prompt referral to an ophthalmologist for fluorescein angiography is necessary to define the location and extent of the abnormal choroidal blood vessels that result in visual loss. Indocyanine green angiography is a new technique that may also help to determine the extent and location of the abnormal blood vessels under the retina (9). Early signs of age-related macular degeneration include drusen (excrescences underneath the retina that contain cellular debris). Only a minority of patients who have drusen lose vision to the exudative changes of age-related macular degeneration.

Laser photocoagulation is the only treatment with proven benefit for the choroidal neovascular sequelae of this disorder (10). Low-vision aids, particularly magnifiers, telescopes, and computers, can be useful for persons with loss of central vision.

Vitreoretinal Complications of Cataract Surgery

Cataract surgery is typically performed in elderly persons. Two important vision-threaten-

ing complications are acute bacterial endophthalmitis and cystoid macular edema. Identification of these problems and referral to an ophthalmologist is extremely important to preserve vision.

Bacterial Endophthalmitis

Bacterial endophthalmitis is a true emergency and one of the most feared complications of intraocular surgery (11). The most common occasion is after cataract surgery, and typically it occurs within 2 weeks after surgery. Approximately 1 in 1000 surgeries are complicated by acute bacterial endophthalmitis (12). The most common causative organism is *Staphylococcus epidermidis.* Less commonly, *Staphylococcus aureus,* streptococcal species, and gram-negative bacteria are identified. In most cases the bacteria come from the patients' own conjunctival flora.

Patients typically have eye pain and loss of vision. Anterior chamber inflammation may be associated with a hypopyon (layered leukocytes). The vitreous is cloudy, and there is a poor view of the retina. Immediate referral to an ophthalmologist is necessary if this condition is suspected. Pars plana vitrectomy with instillation of intravitreal antibiotics and steroids has been successful in treating this condition.

Cystoid Macular Edema

Cystoid macular edema (CME) is characterized by intraretinal edema. A decline in central vision is its hallmark. The most common occasion for CME is after cataract surgery (13). The incidence of visually symptomatic CME retina can be seen within the perifoveal area of the macula. Typically CME occurs 6 to 10 weeks after cataract surgery, and it spontaneously improves approximately 75% of the time. Fluorescein angiography is used to diagnose this condition. Steroid drops, nonsteroidal anti-inflammatory drops, and periocular steroids may be useful in cases that do not spontaneously improve.

OPTIC NERVE DISORDERS
Giant Cell Arteritis

Giant cell arteritis has a multitude of systemic complications. The primary vision-threatening disorder is one that affects the optic nerve and

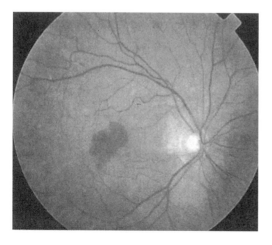

Figure 43.2.   Retinal hemorrhage associated with age-related macular degeneration.

causes an anterior (arteritic) optic neuropathy. Visual loss is rapid. There may be concomitant systemic complaints, including headache, weight loss, malaise, jaw claudication, and proximal muscle weakness. Preauricular tenderness or an enlarged temporal artery may be signs of temporal arteritis. An erythrocyte sedimentation rate (ESR) should be performed stat on any patient suspected of having this condition. The general rule is that any patient who is over age 50, who is suspected to have giant cell arteritis, and who has an ESR greater than 50 should have immediate biopsy of a temporal artery (14). Biopsy should also be performed if the diagnosis of giant cell arteritis is entertained, even if the ESR is normal, as 10% of patients with this condition have a normal ESR.

If the diagnosis is suspected, high-dose steroids should be administered immediately. The role of steroids is to protect the person from the sequelae of other organ disease (e.g., prevent loss of vision in the unaffected eye). Temporal artery biopsy should be performed within 3 days of initiating steroid treatment, because steroid treatment reverses the pathologic signs of this condition when administered longer. High-dose intravenous administration is preferred to oral use.

Anterior (Nonarteritic) Ischemic Optic Neuropathy

Infarction of the optic nerve usually occurs in patients over age 50. It is associated with hypertension and diabetes mellitus. There is an acute loss of vision not associated with pain. Vision may vary from normal to no light perception. Altitudinal or arcuate visual field defects are seen. On ophthalmoscopy, the optic disk is partially swollen, and there may be hemorrhages within the nerve fiber layer. Vision is rarely recovered. There is no proven treatment for this condition. The role of optic nerve sheath fenestration is controversial in the treatment of infarction of the optic nerve.

REFERENCES

1. Kelly NE, Wendel RT. Vitreous surgery for idiopathic macular holes: results of a pilot study. Arch Ophthalmol 1991;109:654–659.
2. Michels RG. Vitrectomy for macular pucker. Ophthalmology 1984;91:1384–1388.
3. Diabetic Retinopathy Study Research Group. Photocoagulation treatment of proliferative diabetic retinopathy: the second report of Diabetic Retinopathy Study findings. Ophthalmology 1978;85:82–106.
4. Early Treatment of Diabetic Retinopathy Study Research Group. Photocoagulation for diabetic macular edema. Arch Ophthalmol 1985;103:1796–1805.
5. Diabetic Retinopathy Vitrectomy Study Research Group. Early vitrectomy for severe vitreous hemorrhage in diabetic retinopathy. Arch Ophthalmol 1985;103:1644–1651.
6. Branch Vein Occlusion Study Group. Argon laser photocoagulation for macular edema in branch vein occlusion. Am J Ophthalmol 1984;98:271–282.
7. Branch Vein Occlusion Study Group. Argon laser scatter photocoagulation for prevention of neovascularization and vitreous hemorrhage in branch vein occlusion. Arch Ophthalmol 1986;104:34–41.
8. Duker JS, Sivalingam A, Brown GC, Reber R. A prospective study of acute central retinal artery obstruction. Arch Ophthalmol 1991;109:339–343.
9. Reichel E, Puliafito CA. ICG-enhanced diagnosis and treatment of choroidal neovascularization in age-related macular degeneration. In: Lewis H, Ryan SJ, eds. Medical and Surgical Retina. Philadelphia: Mosby-Year Book, 1993.
10. Macular Photocoagulation Study Group. Argon laser photocoagulation for senile macular degeneration: results of a randomized clinical trial. Arch Ophthalmol 1982;100:912–918.
11. Puliafito CA, Baker AS, Haaf J, Foster CS. Infectious endophthalmitis: a review of 36 cases. Ophthalmology 1982;89:921–929.
12. Javitt JC, Vitale S, Canner JK, et al. National outcomes of cataract extraction: endophthalmitis following outpatient surgery. Arch Ophthalmol 1991;109:1082–1089.
13. Gass JD, Norton EW. Cystoid macular edema and papilledema following cataract extraction. A fluorescein, funduscopic and angiographic study. Arch Ophthalmol 1966;76:646–661.
14. Hedges TR, Gieger GL, Albert DM. The clinical value of negative temporal artery biopsy specimens. Arch Ophthalmol 1983;101:1251–1254.

Geriatric Ear, Nose, and Throat Problems

Ear, nose, and throat problems, ranging from impacted cerumen and postnasal drip to malignancies and epistaxis, are often neglected by older people. They deny the existence of these problems, and sometimes the symptoms are dismissed by older people because they assume that discomfort, loss of function, and changes in structure are obvious consequences of aging. Sometimes these problems are totally ignored for reasons associated with the stigma surrounding old age: fears of complaining too much, of beginning to fail, or of becoming senile. The same ear, nose, and throat problems that affect the young patient also affect the elderly patient. However, the emotional, mental, and physical needs of an elderly patient may be quite different from those of a younger person. Accordingly, the prescribed course of treatment should be developed with an understanding of the special needs for this age group (1, 2).

The sequelae of otorhinolaryngologic diseases are especially serious because they disrupt an important human function, verbal communication. The inability to hear others and/or to speak to others may be the most devastating handicap of old age. This handicap isolates a person who otherwise would have the physical and mental capacity to lead a happy and useful life. Persons with communication handicaps may withdraw from both the environment and social stimulation, increasing their debilitation, depression, and lack of motivation for living (3).

A speech therapist or speech pathologist and/or an audiologist may be needed to assist the otolaryngologist in the diagnosis and treatment of communicative disorders. The audiologist is a nonmedical professionally trained person who specializes in the measurement of hearing loss, in the nonmedical rehabilitation aspects of the hearing impaired, and in the diagnosis of vestibular or balance disorders. The audiologist has either a master's degree or a PhD and must meet certification or licensure requirement. The speech therapist or speech pathologist, who must meet the same academic and certification or licensure requirements as the audiologist, is concerned with the diagnosis and treatment of speech and language disorders.

EAR

Hearing impairment is classified as conductive, sensorineural, or mixed. Conductive hearing loss may be caused by anything that precludes the normal transmission of sound through the external auditory canal, tympanic membrane, or middle ear ossicles. Various conditions that frequently result in conductive hearing loss include impacted cerumen, tympanic membrane perforation, otitis media, and discontinuity or fixation of the middle ear ossicles. Sensorineural hearing loss occurs when the inner ear, auditory nerve (cranial nerve VIII), brainstem, or cortical auditory pathways are not functioning properly. Mixed hearing loss is a conductive hearing loss superimposed on a sensorineural hearing loss (4).

External Auditory Canal

Aging affects all portions of the otologic mechanism, the external auditory canal, middle ear ossicles, cochlear apparatus, and vestibular system. The external auditory canal is affected by a decrease in both the number and the activity of ceruminal glands. These glands occupy only the outer half of the external auditory canal. Cerumen is never present in the inner half or osseous portion of the external auditory canal unless it is pushed there or accumulates as a result of pressure from the use of headphones or telephones. The cerumen can be intimately adherent to the skin of the external canal in elderly patients. The hearing loss from impacted cerumen is insidious and can result in difficulty with communication. Careful, slow, time-consuming efforts are necessary to separate the cerumen from the intact skin without causing otalgia (pain) or bloody otorrhea. These efforts include curettage, suctioning, and irrigation with room temperature water. Irrigation should not be performed if the tympanic membrane has not been examined before or if there is a history of perforation of the tympanic membrane (5).

The skin of the external auditory canal may become atrophic and dry as a result of atrophy of the epithelium and the sebaceous glands. In elderly persons, itching can be attributed to the dryness, but pruritus sometimes is a major complaint even when no apparent clinically significant abnormality is discovered by the examining physician. This itching is a frequent but unwelcome symptom associated with senile skin. This problem can be exacerbated by vigorous efforts to remove accumulated dry cerumen with cotton-tipped applicators and other foreign instruments. This self-induced trauma further increases the problem. Bathing with hot water, especially in the winter when the air is dry, removes moisture from the skin. Drying the external canal with rubbing alcohol or alcohol-acetic acid mixture may help prevent otitis externa; however, it removes fat and increases the dryness, leading to further irritation and itching of the external auditory canal. Efforts must be directed toward breaking the cycle by avoiding moisture, trauma, and defatting agents in the external auditory canal.

Emollients, such as glycerin, act as an epidermal seal to slow the loss of moisture from the skin.

There is no increased incidence of infections in the external auditory canal. However, there does seem to be an increased amount of otalgia and tenderness in the ear canal when there is a disease process. One aggressive external ear disease is malignant otitis externa, which is a *Pseudomonas* osteitis and osteomyelitis of the temporal bone. This life-threatening disease is usually seen in elderly diabetic patients.

Mild dermatoses, furunculosis, and occasionally infected sebaceous cysts sometimes involve the outer half of the external auditory canal. These infections should be treated early with topical medication in a cream vehicle. These may contain an antibiotic or steroid compound, depending upon the disease process. Adjunctive oral antibiotics may be needed (6).

Benign bony growths that narrow the external auditory canal can also predispose patients to impacted cerumen. These bony growths consist of either benign osteophytes, which may narrow the canal medially, or benign lateral osteomas. Although malignant changes occur infrequently in the external auditory canal, persistent bloody otorrhea or an increased amount of granulation-appearing tissue should arouse suspicion of a neoplastic process. It is imperative to obtain a biopsy early to establish the correct diagnosis. Most carcinomas of the external auditory canal are squamous cell carcinomas. Basal cell carcinomas and ceruminomas (including adenomas, pleomorphic adenomas, adenoid cystic carcinomas, and adenocarcinomas) should be considered in all patients who complain of chronic otalgia with or without otorrhea, hearing loss, vertigo, or facial nerve paralysis (7).

Middle Ear

In 1974, Etholm and Belal (8) reported arthritic changes of the ossicular articulations within the middle ear. There is a hyalinization of the joint capsules, calcification of the articular cartilage, and calcification of the joint capsule itself. These changes are strictly age related, with no sexual predilection. Surprisingly, there is almost no conductive hearing loss associated with these changes.

Atrophic or sclerotic changes of the tympanic membrane are common in the aged, but these changes do not usually cause appreciable losses of hearing. If there is marked retraction of the tympanic membrane or malfunction of the ossicular chain, there is accompanying moderate to severe conductive hearing loss. If there is a serous middle ear effusion, eustachian tube inflation with proper medication usually effectively treats it. Occasionally myringotomy with aspiration of the fluid and possible placement of a tympanostomy tube is required to restore eustachian tube function.

Perforations of the tympanic membrane occur in various locations and in various sizes. These may be due to direct injury from a foreign object, such as cotton-tipped applicators, pencils, or pens. These perforations also may be sustained from a blow to the ear from a fall or a hand slap to the side of the head; the pressure changes in the middle or external ear are barotraumatic. Bleeding, vertigo, and secondary infection may accompany these. Otologic examination and audiologic evaluation are necessary for perforated tympanic membranes. If there are no middle ear complications, simple patching with tissue paper, temporalis fascia, or sclera (banked) may close a small perforation to restore the hearing. A larger perforation may require tympanoplasty or a myringoplasty, depending upon the status of the middle ear ossicles.

Otosclerosis is a bony disease causing conductive hearing loss as a result of fixation of the footplate of the stapes. Otosclerosis also may affect other parts of the labyrinth and otic capsule, causing a sensorineural hearing loss. It affects approximately 10% of the population and is usually bilateral. Otosclerosis most commonly starts in early adult life; however, it may not be recognized until secondary presbycusis sets in. The aging sensorineural hearing loss added to a previously unrecognized borderline conductive hearing loss then becomes evident. The diagnosis of otosclerosis is made by the patient's medical history, otologic examination, and audiologic evaluation.

There are three possible approaches to treatment. The patient may choose surgical correction, a hearing aid, or both. The combination may be the most desirable with severe hearing loss, as the surgery may improve it to the point that a hearing aid can be used to greater advantage. In older medical literature, arguments have been made against ear surgery for the elderly patient. However, there is no age limitation as long as the general condition of the patient is good. As with younger patients, each candidate for surgery must be evaluated on an individual basis. Klotz and Kilbane (9) reported postoperative results of stapedectomies in elderly patients after 2 years of observation. They found that elderly patients did just as well as younger patients. Goodhill (10) reported excellent results from stapedectomy, averaging a 34.6-dB gain for patients over 70 years of age with profound mixed type of hearing loss.

In older patients with larger perforations, cotton should be worn in the ear canal during exposure to cold temperatures or cold wind to avoid vertigo. Middle ear and mastoid tumors do occur in the aged population. These malignancies must be considered when there is a chronically draining ear and an abundance of granulation tissue. However, the most common tumor in the middle ear and mastoid area is cholesteatoma. After thorough audiologic, otologic, and radiologic evaluation and medical therapy failure, chronic otorrhea may require mastoid and/or tympanic membrane surgery (11).

Inner Ear

Presbycusis

In the United States hearing loss constitutes one of the most common physical disabilities; 25% of those between 65 and 74 and 50% of those 75 or older have hearing difficulties. For older adults, the major auditory dysfunction is the result of presbycusis. Presbycusis is a diagnosis made by exclusion, by taking a complete history of the patient and by having a thorough audiologic, otologic, and, if necessary, radiologic evaluation. Variables associated with presbycusis include metabolism, arteriosclerosis, smoking, noise exposure, genetic factors, diet, and stress. According to Schuknecht (12), there are four categories of presbycusis: (a) sensory, (b) metabolic or strial, (c) neural, and (d) mechanical or cochlear conductive.

As a result of the imbalance in hearing for low and high frequencies, speech may be heard as distorted or even unintelligible. Presbycusis patients usually know when they are being spoken to, but they may not always understand what is said. The words are distorted by the patient's imperfect auditory system. When the distortion problem is compounded by a difficult listening situation, such as several people talking at once, patients with presbycusis have an especially difficult time. More reliance on visual cues, such as reading lips, is important. The presbycusis patient who has difficulty with vision has an even worse problem.

There is no known prevention for presbycusis. However, the amount of hearing loss in the geriatric patient is usually the result of a combination of factors. The most serious complicating factor for most men is that they have spent a lifetime in a noisy working environment. The effects of prolonged exposure to loud noise are similar to the effects of presbycusis in that the hearing for higher frequencies is usually affected first. There is no effective treatment for noise-induced hearing loss after the fact. It can be prevented by avoiding excessively noisy environments and by wearing ear protective devices when exposed to noise levels above 80 dB.

Treatment of presbycusis with vasodilators, vitamins, diuretics, steroids, hormones, and so on has been attempted with little evidence of success. Because the possibility of improving presbycusis by medical therapy is limited, other approaches are often needed to assist the geriatric patient. The primary source of help is auditory rehabilitation. This includes the use of hearing aids, auditory training, assistive listening devices, and training in lip-reading. The task of the otorhinolaryngologist and audiologist is to examine patients thoroughly, evaluate their auditory function, assess their ability to benefit from amplification, and counsel them and their families.

Hearing Aids and Amplification

Although a relatively large number of geriatric patients wear hearing aids, many elderly persons deny a hearing loss, refuse to get their hearing evaluated, and refuse to consider wearing a hearing aid. The decision to evaluate the hearing and to consider wearing a hearing aid

must be made by the patient, but family and friends should be made aware and encourage the patient if there is a possibility of a hearing loss and/or lost communicative skills. If a hearing aid can help the elderly person, the family and close friends should be counseled about the hearing aid itself, assistive listening devices, training in lip-reading, and auditory training.

The hearing aid is a small, personalized loudspeaker system consisting of a battery-operated microphone, amplifier, and speaker. The net effect of passing a sound through a hearing aid is to make the sound louder through amplification. The hearing aid cannot correct discrimination or differentiation of words; it can only make sounds louder. Therefore, the hearing aid is most useful in face-to-face conversation, as lip-reading can aid in discriminating or differentiating the word. When the distance from the source of the desired sound increases, so does interference from ambient noise and reverberant sound.

Many elderly patients purchase and wear a hearing aid for a while, then complain about it and even may stop using it. The most common complaints are squealing, excessive background noise, uncomfortable loudness at certain pitches, and ineffectiveness in group conversations. Adjustments to the hearing aid usually can correct these complaints.

The elderly hearing-impaired person whose vision is also impaired is doubly handicapped because of decreased ability to lip-read. As blind persons are more dependent on their sense of hearing, hearing-impaired persons are more dependent on their sense of sight. Light-flashing door bells, telephones, and fire alarm systems are used by many hearing-impaired persons. Other home assistive listening devices include special telephone devices and television and radio earpiece receivers. It is important for the hearing-impaired person to be aware of the assistive listening devices available in the community. These include the infrared and loop systems that may be found in places of worship, movie theaters, and other public places.

Patients may find that they gain 15 dB by the use of ear cupping, or placing a hand directly behind the auricle and deflecting the sound. Patients may prefer the hearing aid in the ear canal itself or behind the ear, depending on their situation. If for cosmetic reasons a patient does not want a hearing aid that can be seen, an implantable hearing aid may be the solution. Implantable hearing aids give better sound and appear more natural and attractive, but they require operation for implantation near the mastoid bone.

Rules and regulations regarding the evaluation and issuance of hearing aids vary from state to state, as they are the results of certain problems and policies in those states. Most areas now require a complete audiogram by an audiologist or certified hearing aid dealer, medical evaluation by an otolaryngologist, and the opportunity for the person to try the hearing aid before purchasing it.

Although there are many auditory function tests, the audiogram is the basic test to evaluate hearing loss. Pure-tone levels at individual frequencies can be tested, as can discrimination of words. In general, there are three types of hearing loss: neurosensory, conductive, and mixed (combination of neurosensory and conductive). Figure 44.1 shows these three types of hearing loss.

Hearing impairment presents in many different ways. The patient may be aware of a sudden, gradual, or questionable hearing loss. Sometimes persons are not aware of a hearing loss and deny the existence of such a problem, although their family and friends are aware of it. When oral communication between two persons decreases, there is a possibility of hearing loss, and an audiogram should be considered. Because of the increased incidence of hearing loss in the elderly, screening of elderly people has been encouraged.

Tinnitus

Tinnitus, a major problem for the geriatric patient, is a buzzing, ringing, hissing, or similar type of sound that usually is related to hearing loss in the higher frequencies. This may be related to presbycusis or prolonged noise exposure. Aspirin and other medications may cause hearing loss and tinnitus. Tinnitus is a bothersome and troubling symptom that may or may not originate in the ear. Sometimes there is an objective cause, and sometimes the cause cannot be found. Subjective tinnitus occurs when the patient is aware of the ringing, buzzing, humming, whistling,

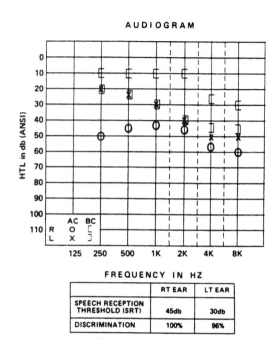

AUDIOGRAM

	RT EAR	LT EAR
SPEECH RECEPTION THRESHOLD (SRT)	45db	30db
DISCRIMINATION	100%	96%

Left ear (X, ⊐) demonstrates neurosensory loss. Right ear (O, ⊏) demonstrates conductive loss with a mixed loss at 4K and 8K.

Figure 44.1. Audiogram of elderly person demonstrating both neurosensory and conductive hearing losses.

roaring, or clicking sound; however, the examiner cannot hear it. Objective tinnitus is a bruit that can be heard by the examining physician. There are two types, ear tinnitus (tinnitus aurium) and head tinnitus (tinnitus cranii). Cochlear and retrocochlear lesions can produce unilateral tinnitus. Ménière's disease is frequently accompanied by an ipsilateral tinnitus on the side with the hearing loss and vertigo. Acoustic neuroma and cerebellar pontine-angle tumors also are characterized by an ipsilateral tinnitus. Unilateral tinnitus is a bothersome symptom that requires a thorough diagnostic evaluation.

There is no specific treatment for tinnitus aurium. Tinnitus is difficult to treat, and the patient must understand that it may persist forever. Treatment of tinnitus may include therapy for the underlying condition, such as a psychosomatic problem. Elimination of aspirin or similar medication may reduce the tinnitus. There is hope of converting the decompensated tinnitus into a compensated state. Acoustic sedation is helpful, as patients usually are most bothered at quiet times, such as when they are trying to fall asleep at night. The use of a bedside radio or tape recorder frequently helps provide an artificial source of ambient noise to mask out this objective tinnitus. Some people require the use of tinnitus maskers that give them a sound constantly throughout the day. As there is no specific medical therapy for ear tinnitus, there is no effective surgery for tinnitus per se. If the tinnitus becomes a major factor and is a unilateral process, only as a last resort would a unilateral obliterative operation be considered.

Sudden Hearing Loss

Sudden hearing loss is a topic unto its own. Vascular changes can involve branches of the internal auditory artery. This type of loss is due to constriction or occlusion of the blood vessels or hemorrhage within the organ of Corti. Several medical regimens have been tried; however, no one form of therapy has been proved to be most effective.

Vestibular System

Vestibular complaints have been recorded in more than 50% of elderly patients living alone. Vertigo is a specific term used to describe the symptoms of the vestibular system, including the peripheral labyrinthine, retrolabyrinthine, and central nervous system vestibular components. Dizziness is a vague term that may include giddiness, imbalance, faintness, wooziness, and fainting. Dizziness may be used to describe cortical or visual disorientation, altered states of consciousness, and limb incoordinations. Balance depends on the input and proper functioning from the vestibular, visual, and proprioceptive pathways. Impaired function in any one of these three components may yield symptoms of dizziness (11). In the vestibular system, the disease process is usually in the sensory epithelium, the primary afferent fibers, and the vestibular apparatus.

Histopathology of the aged vestibule reveals a decrease of up to 40% in myelinated nerve fibers, with myelinated fibers of the cristae being affected most often. The otoconia of the saccule degenerate progressively from the posterior to the anterior end, and the saccular membranes rupture frequently in the elderly. Tissue between the endolymphatic duct and the bony vestibular aqueduct becomes fibrotic (13). Finally, postural vertigo (cupulolithiasis) is associated with dense deposits of insoluble particles in the pars superior at the ampule of the posterior semicircular canal (2). In addition to the general decrease of vestibular sensitivity, Schuknecht (14) has described four age-related conditions of dysequilibrium: (*a*) cupulolithiasis, (*b*) ampullary dysequilibrium, (*c*) macular dysequilibrium, and (*d*) vestibular ataxia.

Nystagmus

Nystagmus is an objective finding that accompanies vertigo. It is characterized by a slow movement of the eye to one side with a corrective fast return movement to the other side. By convention, nystagmus is identified by the direction of the quick component. Thus, a nystagmus to the left means a nystagmus that has a slow movement to the right and a quick corrective component to the left. The direction of the nystagmus may be horizontal, vertical, diagonal, or rotary. Manifest nystagmus can be observed with the naked eye under ordinary conditions. Occult nystagmus can be observed by using a +20 Fresnel lens to abolish fixation or by electronystagmography, a diagnostic test that allows differentiation between central nervous disorders and peripheral disorders within the labyrinth.

Vertical nystagmus can be produced either by peripheral labyrinth or by central nervous system disorders. Peripheral vertical nystagmus can originate from the semicircular canals, utricle, or saccule of the labyrinth. The vertigo may be accompanied by nausea, vomiting, and general malaise. Common causes of peripheral vertigo include labyrinthitis, Ménière's disease, and labyrinthine fistula. Central vertical nystagmus may be caused by tumor in the temporal lobe (transverse gyrus of Heschl), by cerebral arteriosclerosis, and by lesions of the midbrain, pons, cerebellum, and brainstem. Lesions of the posterior inferior cerebellar artery involve vestibular nuclei and their connections to the medial longitudinal fasciculus. Peripheral and central pathways can interact also.

NOSE

In aging, the nose loses its internal moisture, as mucus production is decreased. The mucus is thicker, and the patient may complain of a thickness in the nose. Aging also brings on absorption of the adipose tissue and atrophy of muscle within the nose itself. The most significant nasal finding in the aged patient is the increased fragility and sclerosis of blood vessels, contributing to epistaxis.

Cartilaginous changes show that the elderly person's nasal dorsum is convex, with a retracted columella and a downward rotation of the lobule. These changes are accentuated by loss of muscle mass of the orbiculus oris, absorption of facial adipose tissue, loss of teeth, and absorption of the maxilla and the mandible, causing a loss in the vertical dimension of the lower third of the face. The patient's nasal airway is decreased as the tip droops and the columella becomes retracted. There can be some fragmentation between the upper lateral cartilage and the lower lateral cartilage, causing collapse in the nasal valve area. Sometimes septoplasty and a tip rhinoplasty are done for elevation of the nasal tip to improve the airway. A resection of 2 to 4 mm of the lower lateral cartilage rotates the tip upward to improve the nasal airway.

In the elderly, the most distressing nasal condition is epistaxis. A nosebleed can be severe enough to threaten the life of the patient; furthermore, epistaxis can be challenging to treat because elderly patients have a higher percentage of posterior nasal bleeding than other patients. Typically, posterior epistaxis occurs in the middle of the night, causing the patient to wake up gagging on a mouthful of blood, which requires emergency treatment. Epistaxis can be caused by any of several factors, but certainly aging, with increased fragility and sclerosis of the blood vessels, is the most important factor. Hypertension and sicca (dryness) accentuated by the loss of internal moisture contribute to epistaxis among the elderly. Other causes are trauma, septal perforation, blood dyscrasias, use of medications (aspirin, warfarin, and so on), benign or malignant tumors of the nose and sinus, atrophic rhinitis, Wegener's granulomatosis, and mucormycosis.

Atrophic rhinitis is a progressive chronic disease in which the nasal fossae are greatly enlarged as a result of atrophic changes in the mucosa and underlying bone. Thick, smelly, adherent crusts are formed in the nasal passages. Atrophic rhinitis is also known as ozena, derived from the Greek word for stench. The infecting organisms of mucormycosis are species of *Absidia, Mucor,* or *Rhizopus.* It is associated with facial cellulitis, acute rhinosinusitis, and gangrenous mucosal changes. It occurs in diabetic patients and in patients who have received immunosuppressive therapy for lymphomas, leukemias, or connective tissue disorders. Intranasal examination is diagnostic with the finding of a black inferior turbinate resulting from necrosis of the inferior turbinate. The disease process can progress rapidly and may cause death by extension into the intracranial area.

Acne rosacea is a pustular dermatologic condition that may affect the nose. If it becomes advanced, it develops into a rhinophyma, which is hypertrophy of the underlying sebaceous glands in the affected area, giving rise to a very bulbous nasal tip. Acne rosacea can be controlled by the application of mild steroid cream to the affected areas. If the lesion advances to rhinophyma, surgical removal should be done by dermabrasion or carbon dioxide laser resection (15, 16).

Postnasal drip, one of the frequent symptoms in the elderly patient, usually is accompanied by a sinusitis, and of course, it has to do with thickening of the mucus. The key to this diagnosis is to elicit a history of the color and type of drainage, to do a thorough nasopharyngeal and nasal examination, to document with sinus radiographs or computed tomography, and to consider diagnostic nasal and/or sinus endoscopy. Furthermore, the postnasal drip may cause a chronic cough, clearing of the throat, a catch in the throat, and/or hoarseness. If the medical treatment of chronic sinusitis is unsuccessful, surgical sinus endoscopy ise needed to correct the osteomeatal complex blockage causing the maxillary, ethmoid, frontal, and/or sphenoid sinusitis. The techniques of endoscopic sinus surgery continue to be refined and expanded to relieve chronic sinusitis and its pulmonary sequelae (17, 18).

Taste and smell are related chemical senses. It is possible to have malfunction of one or both of them. However, more complaints center on the loss of olfaction. An acute loss of sense of smell (anosmia) can be related to an upper respiratory infection. Because of the short-term effect, the patient is rarely seen for this condition. Chronic anosmia occurs after blockage of the air currents through the nose, such as with nasal obstruction. Losses of taste and smell are common in the elderly, resulting from normal aging, medications, surgical interventions, closed head trauma, environmental exposure, benign tumors, malignant tumors, and certain diseases, such as Alzheimer's disease, cancer, hyperthyroidism, hepatitis, and liver disease (15, 19).

ORAL CAVITY

Aging significantly alters the dentition, oral cavity mucosa, and salivary glands. The mucosa has thinner epithelium (especially tunica propria), blunted rete pegs, decreased collagen and water content, and reduced numbers of functioning capillaries. Arteriosclerosis delays and reduces healing; also, the tissue is more prone to injury. Salivary gland production is diminished 25% by loss of secretory parenchymal volume, acinar hyalinization, and salivary ductal adhesions. The result is an increase in dental caries, mucosal atrophy, and mucosal burning, with a decrease in the sensitivity of the taste buds.

Glossodynia (burning pain in the tongue) may be caused by anemia (folic acid, iron, or B_{12} deficiency), candidiasis, denture irritation, lichen planus, xerostomia, neuropathy of diabetes mellitus, postviral neuropathy, or carcinoma. Sometimes it affects the entire mouth to cause a burning mouth syndrome. Usually the patient does not demonstrate any lesion. If no cause can be found and psychosomatic conversion can be eliminated, the patient may require a lemon and glycerin mouthwash and possibly a tranquilizer.

Geographic tongue is also known as migratory glossitis. This can be secondary to a minor viral infection; however, it usually is of no consequence. Some people in their normal state have geographic tongue.

Fordyce granules, which are the fourth most common oral lesions in the elderly, are ectopic sebaceous glands that are benign raised yellow to white areas on the buccal or lip mucosa. No treatment is required.

Angular cheilitis is most evident at the oral commissures, which are fissured, macerated, erythematous, and tender. Loss of connective tissue support causing redundant skin folds allows pooling of saliva and resulting candidiasis. Application of nystatin cream to the oral commissure usually corrects angular cheilitis; however, correction of ill-fitting dentures and management of iron or vitamin B deficiency may be required.

Candidiasis appears to be more common in the elderly than in other age groups. It occurs after prolonged and/or intensive antibiotic therapy and also in debilitated persons. A typical clinical picture consists of white patches on the throat and hypopharynx with mild inflammatory reaction to the underlying tissue. Mycostatin mouthwash suspension is usually effective. For advanced cases, the patient may need systemic treatment with intravenous amphotericin B.

Lichen planus is a benign chronic disease usually caused by emotional or physical stress. Nonerosive lichen planus has a roughened, asymptomatic, hyperkeratotic leukoplakia on the mucosa; the painful erosive type has vesicles and bullae. There is no definite correlation between lichen planus and oral cavity carcinoma.

Temporomandibular joint (TMJ) syndrome, or Costen's syndrome, is a dysfunction of the temporomandibular joint with severe pain in the joint itself, the ear, or adjacent structures. Causes can be dental malocclusion, acute trauma to the mandible, clenching of the teeth with muscular contraction, arthritis, or tumors in the area. TMJ can cause vertigo, a ringing type of tinnitus, or a clicking or popping sensation when the jaw is opened. Nonsurgical treatment includes use of topical heat, soft diet, physical therapy, analgesics, steroids, dental splints, bite blocks, biofeedback, and psychotherapy. In the event that these are unsatisfactory, exploratory surgery of the joint should be considered (20).

Speech Alterations

Hoarseness, difficulty swallowing, and painful swallowing increase with the patient's age. If any of these symptoms persist, the patient must have an indirect laryngoscopy mirror examination. If a thorough mirror examination cannot be done, fiberoptic laryngoscopy can be carried out. Sometimes a barium swallow is also needed for aid in diagnosis. Causes range from benign vocal cord nodules and diverticulum to aggressive malignant tumors. Gastroesophageal reflux is one of the more common disorders causing hoarseness, catch in the throat, or dysphagia.

Vocal strain occurs frequently in the geriatric patient. The aging process affects the voice pitch, quality, and volume and the rate of speech to varying degrees in different persons. The voice intermittently changes to what is described as a tired, failing, and faltering type of voice. A wavering tone and decreased volume reduce the ability to communicate. Articulation also may be significantly distorted by missing teeth, dentures, or stroke. Chronic vocal strain can result from voice misuse.

The elderly voice has a change in pitch after age 50 years. According to data obtained by Honjo and Isshiki (21), men have a vocal fold atrophy causing an increase in fundamental frequency, whereas women have a vocal fold edema causing decreased fundamental frequency. The muscles of the larynx, especially the thyroarytenoid muscle, become atrophic. The voice becomes drier as the false vocal cords have a reduction in mucous glandular production and may actually show some squamous metaplasia. The cricoarytenoid joint and the cricothyroid joint may develop a relaxation of the joint capsule or partially become fixed.

As a result of some of these changes, the patient may develop a spastic dysphonia type of voice. The patient develops a tight and squeezed voice sound with extreme tension and a strained, creaking, choking type of vocal attack. The patient complains of reduction in clarity and volume with no pathologic findings evident on indirect or direct laryngoscopy. Speech therapy is most helpful. For true documented spastic dysphonia, recurrent laryngeal nerve sectioning should be considered only after intensive speech therapy has been deemed a failure.

Laryngeal dysfunction secondary to vocal cord paralysis engenders special problems. Unilateral vocal cord paralysis can be due to many factors ranging from laryngeal carcinoma to left chest dis-

ease to central nervous system disorders. Of patients developing unilateral vocal cord paralysis, 30% never have the cause determined. After allowing about 6 months for spontaneous resolution of the paralysis, it may be desirable to eliminate aspiration of liquids and foods and to attempt to improve the voice and the effectiveness of the cough reflex by injecting polytetrafluoroethylene (Teflon) lateral to the paralyzed cord.

Bilateral abductor vocal cord paralysis does not affect the voice quality so much. However, it affects the inspiratory function of the larynx, requiring corrective surgery. The patient benefits from a lateralizing procedure of the vocal cord, such as arytenoidectomy, or perhaps a valved tracheostomy tube.

Dysphonia secondary to gastroesophageal reflux is usually found in obese patients who have a chronic sore throat and a globus sensation with possible pain over the thyrohyoid membrane. Physical examination reveals erythema of the arytenoid mucosa. If the problem is advanced enough, contact granuloma or hyperkeratosis of the true vocal cords can be seen. Treatment includes diet, elevation of the head of the bed, antacids, and H_2-receptor blocking agents (1, 2).

Senile bowing of the vocal cords is secondary to muscle atrophy and loss of connective tissue. Dryness of the laryngeal mucosa (laryngitis sicca) results from atrophy of the mucous glands. Voice tremor can be associated with other tremors in the head and neck area and may be a solitary finding. The voice quivers with sudden abrupt changes similar to those found in spastic dysphonia. Dysarthria also may cause inarticulation or problems in communication. Dysarthria may be found in patients suffering from cerebral vascular accidents, trauma, Parkinson's disease, Huntington's chorea, or lower or upper motor neuron disease.

Tracheostomy

If a short- or long-term tracheostomy is necessary, the patient and the family should have proper preoperative counseling. It is necessary to explain the purpose of the procedure and make it clear that the patient will probably be without a voice until the tracheostomy tube can be occluded. Humidification of the patient's immediate environment is very important. Suctioning and cleaning of the airway with saline solution is also very important in limiting crusting and thinning the secretions. Suctioning should be reduced to a minimum as soon as possible so as not to remove any more cilia from the trachea than is absolutely necessary.

Facial Nerve Palsy

Facial nerve palsies are usually idiopathic. Bell's palsy is a diagnosis by exclusion of all other causes of the facial nerve palsy. Herpes zoster oticus (Ramsay Hunt's syndrome), cholesteatoma in a chronic suppurative otitis media, carcinoma of the middle ear, and parotid tumor are a few of the causes of a facial palsy. The most important step in the initial assessment of facial palsy is exclusion of any middle ear pathology or tumors along the distribution of the facial nerve.

Otalgia

Otalgia may originate within the ear itself or may be referred from numerous structures in the head and neck. Pain originating within the ear is usually due to an acute inflammation of the outer or middle ear. Referred pain is a common important phenomenon. A number of cranial nerve sensory components to the external and middle ear are also sensory components to the pharynx, hypopharynx, and larynx; a lesion elsewhere in the head and neck area may manifest as otalgia. Otalgia may be a symptom of a carcinoma on the base of the tongue, pharynx, or larynx. Furthermore, ordinary common causes of such referred pain include cervical osteoarthrosis and TMJ dysfunction. In both, pain may be centered on the ear, but they usually show differing radiations, with osteoarthrosis having a cervical root distribution and TMJ having a preauricular, maxillary, and mandibular pattern.

HEAD AND NECK CANCERS

Head and neck cancers constitute 5% of malignancies in the body. They occur more frequently in the elderly than in the younger population. Because of the possible pronounced functional and cosmetic deformities from ablative surgery, early diagnosis to allow the least destructive therapy is important. Poor oral hygiene, alcohol, and smoking are prime factors in the formation of these head and neck tumors.

Common geriatric complaints that should be investigated for possible malignancy include neck masses, hoarseness, dysphagia, dyspnea, hearing alterations, painful teeth, swollen face, bad breath, otalgia, and hemoptysis. Common presenting symptoms include proptosis due to tumors of the orbit or ethmoid, frontal, or maxillary sinuses; epistaxis associated with cancer of the paranasal sinuses or nose; ulceration of the mouth; hoarseness associated with laryngeal carcinoma; and dysphagia resulting from laryngeal and esophageal tumors. Facial swelling also can result from tumors of the parotid gland, floor of the mouth, maxillary sinus, palate, or mandible.

The most common malignancy in the head and neck area is epidermoid squamous cell carcinoma. If the laryngeal lesions are found early, a cure rate greater than 95% can be achieved. The early lesions are treated with radiation, carbon dioxide laser resection, or partial laryngectomy. While still providing a possible cure rate, advances in surgical techniques of partial laryngectomy can preserve the voice and deglutition to many moderately advanced cases. Total laryngectomy is still required in advanced tumors, and this sometimes is done in combination with irradiation (1, 2).

Carcinoma of the oral cavity occurs most commonly in the older age groups. Age itself is not a contraindication to surgery, as extensive head and neck surgery is generally well tolerated by the elderly patient. Johnson et al. (22) reported that in 27 cases of composite resection in patients more than 65 years of age, the surgical complications were equivalent to or less than those of an equally paired younger age group. There was an increase in associated medical complications for the elderly population; however, the head and neck complications were fewer. Rehabilitation time for oral alimentation and for discharge of the patient was essentially the same in both age groups. Age also is no contraindication to partial laryngeal surgery, as it seems to be tolerated relatively well in the elderly patient. Tucker (23) reviewed 27 cases of conservation laryngeal surgery in the elderly age group. His 11% complication rate with no deaths compared favorably with the rates for total laryngectomy and radiotherapy alone. McGuirt et al. (24) reported no increased incidents of surgical complications in the group above 70 years of age. His series also had a slight increase in medical complications; however, the head and neck complications were equal.

Thyroid malignancies act more aggressively in the elderly because more anaplastic or undifferentiated carcinomas occur. Hoarseness, dysphagia, dyspnea, and enlarging neck mass are symptoms of thyroid cancer. The most useful diagnostic techniques are fine-needle aspiration and radioactive imaging. Surgical resection is the initial treatment of choice for thyroid malignancies. For follicular or papillary carcinoma, radioactive iodine ablation and thyroid supplementation are recommended after total or near-total thyroidectomy (with a modified neck dissection for positive lymphatic involvement). For medullary carcinoma, external radiation to the neck and mediastinum and thyroid supplementation should be given after total thyroidectomy and regional lymphatic resection. For anaplastic carcinoma, external radiation, possibly chemotherapy, and thyroid supplementation should be given after total thyroidectomy and regional lymphatic resection (25). Old persons have skin changes that are significant to the otolaryngologist. Basal cell carcinoma, squamous cell carcinoma, malignant melanoma, and the numerous premalignant skin lesions are discussed elsewhere in this textbook.

In summary, it appears that age alone is not a criterion for withholding curative surgery from an elderly patient. Instead, postponing an operative procedure is unwise. Consequently, the head and neck surgeon should evaluate each patient on the basis of other medical problems, the psychologic and mental condition, the type of surgery required with possible reconstructive procedure, probable postoperative functional state, and the support facilities available where the operation will be done. Only after weighing all of these considerations should the surgeon make recommendations regarding major head and neck surgery.

There has been significant improvement in rehabilitation after total laryngectomy. In addition to an electrolarynx and esophageal speech, there are now multiple approaches to the surgical re-

construction of the speaking mechanism. Cosmetic and reconstructive facial surgery has growing importance to the aging population. The physician must pay careful attention to the patient's desires, needs, and physical capabilities. Reconstructive surgery is crucial in the rehabilitation of a cancer patient. The postsurgical defect following removal of a malignancy may require both functional and cosmetic surgery. Recent developments with microsurgery, regional flaps, free flaps, and myocutaneous flaps have improved reconstructive surgery significantly (6, 27).

REFERENCES

1. Cummings CW, Fredrickson JM, Harker LA, et al., eds. Otolaryngology: Head and Neck Surgery. 2nd ed. Baltimore: Williams & Wilkins, 1993.
2. Paparella MM, Shumrick DA, eds. Otolaryngology. 3rd ed. Philadelphia: Saunders, 1991.
3. Boone DR, Bayles KA, Koopmann CF Jr. Communicative aspects of aging. Otolaryngol Clin North Am 1982; 15:313–327.
4. English GM, ed. Otolaryngology. 2nd ed. Philadelphia: Harper & Row, 1986.
5. Anderson RG, Meyerhoff WL. Otologic manifestations of aging. Otolaryngol Clin North Am 1982;15:353–370.
6. Gates G, ed. Current Therapy in Otolaryngology-Head and Neck Surgery. 5th ed. St. Louis: Mosby, 1994.
7. Senturia BH. Diseases of the External Ear. New York: Grune & Stratton, 1980.
8. Etholm B, Belal A. Senile changes in the middle ear joints. Ann Otol Rhinol Laryngol 1974;83:49–54.
9. Klotz RE, Kilbane M. Hearing in an aging population, preliminary report. N Engl J Med 1962;266:277–280.
10. Goodhill V. Diseases, Deafness, and Dizziness. New York: Harper & Row, 1979.
11. Ballenger JJ. Diseases of the Nose, Throat, Ear, Head, and Neck. 13th ed. Philadelphia: Lea & Febiger, 1985.
12. Schuknecht HF. Further observations on the pathology of presbycusis. Arch Otolaryngol 1964;80:369–382.
13. Johnsson LG. Degenerative changes and anomalies of the vestibular system. Laryngoscope 1971;81:1682–1693.
14. Schuknecht HF. Pathology of the Ear. Cambridge, MA: Harvard University Press, 1974.
15. Patterson CN. The aging nose: characteristics and correction. Otolaryngol Clin North Am 1980;13:275–278.
16. Edelstein DR. Aging of the normal nose in adults. Laryngoscope 1996;106:1–25.
17. Lamear WR, Davis WE, Templer JW, et al. Partial endoscopic middle turbinectomy augmenting functional endoscopic sinus surgery. Otolaryngol Head Neck Surg 1992;107:79–84.
18. Metson R. Endoscopic treatment of frontal sinusitis. Laryngoscope 1992;102:712–716.
19. Schiffman SS. Taste and smell losses in normal aging and disease. JAMA 1997;278:1357–1361.

20. Koopmann CF Jr, Coulthard SW. The oral cavity and aging. Otolaryngol Clin North Am 1982;15:293–312.
21. Honjo I, Isshiki N. Laryngoscopic and voice characteristics of aged persons. Arch Otolaryngol 1980;106:149–150.
22. Johnson JT, Rabuzzi DD, Tucker HM. Composite resection in the elderly: a well tolerated procedure. Laryngoscope 1977;87:1509–1515.
23. Tucker HM. Conservation laryngeal surgery in the elderly patient. Laryngoscope 1977;87:1995–1999.
24. McGuirt WF, Loevy S, McCabe BF, Krause CJ. The risks of major head and neck surgery in the aged population. Laryngoscope 1977;87:1378–1382.
25. Holt GR, Mattox DE. Decision making in otolaryngology. St. Louis: Mosby, 1984.
26. Chvapil M, Koopmann CF Jr. Age and other factors regulating wound healing. Otolaryngol Clin North Am 1982;15:259–270.
27. Koopmann CF Jr. Special considerations in managing geriatric patients. In: Gates G, ed. Current Therapy in Otolaryngology-Head and Neck Surgery. St. Louis: Mosby, 1987.

Geriatric Dentistry

Geriatric dentistry has evolved dramatically as a result of demographic trends, changes in oral disease prevalence, and research findings linking oral health and systemic disease. In turn, the focus of geriatric dental care has shifted from predominant attention to the replacement of missing teeth in the edentulous patient and the special needs of elders in long-term care settings to the provision of comprehensive oral health care to the growing population of community-dwelling elders. Moreover, the need for such comprehensive care, encompassing all of the dental specialties, is projected to grow as more elders retain their natural dentition throughout life (1). As persons over 65 typically see physicians more regularly and more often than they see a dentist, there is also an important need for nondentist health care providers to identify oral problems early, undertake appropriate interventions, and make timely referrals for further evaluation and treatment. In particular, elders frequently seen by physicians are often those who have a great burden of comorbidities of aging and who are at highest risk for developing oral problems. While there is growing recognition that aging per se is not a major risk factor for oral diseases, development of age-related systemic diseases, such as osteoporosis (2) and diabetes (3), place elders at risk for oral problems. Furthermore, there is mounting evidence that oral conditions may also be significant predictors of important medical outcomes in elders (4, 5).

AGING AND CHANGES IN ORAL STRUCTURES AND FUNCTION
Dental Caries, Periodontal Diseases, and Tooth Loss

Perhaps the most significant oral health-related change taking place in the population is the decline in tooth loss and edentulism. In the United States there are now more elders with teeth than without (6, 7). Comparison of national data over the past 4 decades clearly shows declines over time in the number of missing teeth per person. The trends for the prevalence of complete edentulism are similar (Table 45.1). In the most recent U.S. national survey, only one third of those 65 and older were completely edentulous, a reverse of the situation just 30 years earlier. Even in the northeastern United States, an area historically known for its high prevalence of dental disease and tooth loss, secular trends toward better oral health and tooth retention are evident. In 1991 a random sample of New England elders found that more than two thirds had teeth (1). More important, of elders with teeth, more than 80% had kept most of their teeth.

This decreasing rate of edentulism is expected to continue into the future, as younger cohorts in the population demonstrate a similar trend regarding tooth retention. Important factors in this trend include a decline in incidence of dental caries related in large part to widespread availability of fluoride (8), a change in professional

Table 45.1

Prevalence of Tooth Loss in the United States, 1957–1986: Percent of Adults Without Teeth

Survey Year	Type	Ages Sampled	% Edentulous, Overall Population	% Edentulous, Ages 65–74
1957–1958	NHIS-I	All ages	13	55
1960–1962	NHES-I	18–74	17	50
1971	NHIS-II	All ages	11	45
1971–1974	NHANES-I	18–74	15	46
1985–1986	NIDR	All ages	4	37

NHANES-I, National Health and Nutrition Examination Survey I; NHES-I,; NHIS-I, National Health Interview Survey I; NHIS-II, National Health Interview Survey II; NIDR, National Institute of Dental Research.

philosophy concerning retention of the natural dentition, and a concomitant change in the public's expectations regarding keeping their teeth for a lifetime (9). In addition, the acceptance of preventive dentistry and the improvement in oral hygiene by adults have also led to declines in the prevalence of periodontal diseases in elders (6). It is becoming recognized that any disproportionate levels of oral disease or dysfunction found in elders are related more to comorbid conditions than to any normative age-related changes in the oral cavity. Tooth loss is thus not an inevitable consequence of aging. Rather, it is an end point of a complex interaction among dental diseases (caries and periodontitis) and behavioral and attitudinal factors toward tooth retention and treatment preferences on the part of both patient and provider (7).

Periodontal disease, manifested as gingival inflammation and loss of tooth-supporting alveolar bone, has been traditionally viewed as the predominant cause of tooth loss in adults. However, recent data from longitudinal epidemiologic studies have not confirmed this long-held belief, instead indicating that dental caries is more important. Using data from the Rand Health Insurance Experiment, Bailit et al. (10) analyzed the causes of tooth extraction in a sample of 1210 young and middle-aged adults and found that fewer than 4% of extractions could be ascribed to periodontal disease. In a community-based sample of elders in rural Iowa, Hand et al. (11) found that root and coronal caries were significantly more important predictors of tooth loss than was periodontal condition. Longitudinal results from

the Veterans Affairs Normative Aging Study also show that dental caries is a more important predictor of tooth loss than periodontal disease (12). A repeated observation from many of these studies is that health care providers' decisions to remove otherwise healthy teeth to facilitate a prosthetic treatment plan is the major contribution to tooth loss (13). It has become clear that factors other than caries and periodontitis are important to understanding tooth loss, including sociocultural and economic factors, access to and availability of care, and care providers' treatment preferences (14).

Dental caries, both coronal and root decay, remain major problems in elders (6), with the annual incidence in elders being equivalent to that seen in high-risk populations of children and adolescents, when incidence rates are adjusted by the number of tooth surfaces present at risk for decay. As has been found to be the case with tooth loss, multiple risk factors are at play. Specific groups of elders are at dramatically high risk for caries, including those with Alzheimer's disease (15) and salivary gland dysfunction (16).

Certain changes do occur with aging in the adult dentition. There is a tendency toward mesial, or forward, drift of the teeth that may result in anterior crowding. With advancing years tooth enamel typically exhibits attrition on the occlusal and incisal surfaces of the teeth. The severity of such attrition is highly variable and due to masticatory forces, coarseness of the diet, and oral habits such as bruxism or grinding. Fracture lines may also develop in the enamel over time. Internal to the enamel is the dentin layer, which continues to be formed throughout life by an odontoblastic cell layer within the dental pulp. With age, the dentin layer thickens while the dental pulp narrows. Gingival recession, a common finding in elders, exposes root surfaces. The tooth root may be abraded at the cementoenamel junction because of a mechanical process, such as excessive tooth brushing, or erosion. Cementum, the mineral layer that covers tooth roots, is less dense than enamel, so it is also much more susceptible to decay, leading to the increased risk of root surface caries noted in elders.

Periodontal changes typical of aging include not only gingival recession with root exposure but also loss of the attachment apparatus, including the tooth-supporting alveolar bone (17). While severe and extensive periodontal destruction is limited to a small proportion of the total population, the rate of periodontal attachment loss and alveolar bone loss can be particularly great in elders with specific risk factors (18). Cigarette smoking has been identified as a major risk factor for periodontal disease (19), tooth loss (20), and other oral problems in elders (21, 22). Cigarette smokers have also been shown to have low bone mineral density at various skeletal sites and are at high risk for osteoporosis (23). Oral bone changes may also reflect systemic bone metabolism (24). In turn, persons with low bone mineral at various skeletal sites (e.g., hip, spine, radius) are also at high risk for tooth loss (2).

In addition to osteoporosis, the other major comorbidity of aging with important oral consequences is non–insulin-dependent diabetes mellitus (NIDDM). With more than 10% of elders affected by NIDDM and an equivalent number having impaired glucose tolerance, the influence of these conditions as risk factors for oral disease is quite large. Both the prevalence and the severity of periodontal disease have been found to be increased in persons with NIDDM, and they are also at high risk for tooth loss (3, 25, 26). Adult diabetics report dry mouth (xerostomia) at high rates (27), although subjective reports do not appear to correlate well with objectively measured stimulated or unstimulated salivary flow (28). Changes in the composition of saliva in diabetics, rather than changes in the flow rates, have been hypothesized to account for the dry mouth re-

ported by patients and may also explain in part the increased incidence of oral mucosal candidal infections in diabetics (29).

Salivary Gland Function, Xerostomia, and Oral Candidiasis

Salivary gland function, as measured by salivary flow rates, remains essentially unchanged with age in the absence of systemic disease or certain medication usage (30). Minor changes with age in the electrolyte composition of parotid saliva have been noted (31). Decreases in saliva secretion are well correlated with a number of specific medical disorders and have also been related to the use of certain common medications (27–30, 32–35). Interestingly, most studies show poor correlations between patient-reported symptoms of xerostomia and objective measures of salivary flow rates (36). Elders with diminished salivary flow, but not those with subjective complaints, have been found to have high salivary yeast counts and to be at high risk for oral candidiasis (37). Yeasts are normal commensals in the oral cavity but may cause oral lesions under certain conditions, including use of antibiotics, salivary dysfunction, inadequate prostheses, and more rarely use of inhaled corticosteroids by asthmatics (38). Such infections present in various forms (39), including acute pseudomembranous candidiasis (thrush), raised whitish plaques that may be scraped off, leaving an erythematous and often ulcerated base; chronic hyperplastic candidiasis; and chronic atrophic candidiasis. The last is often accompanied by angular cheilitis, linear ulcerated fissures at the corners of the mouth that may be superinfected with bacteria.

Nutrition, Oral Health, and Mastication

Longitudinal research findings clearly demonstrate that masticatory function and food selection do not change as a direct result of aging (40). Stable dentition and the absence of medical problems or medication usage affecting salivary function or taste allow normal function and diet over time. However, the worse one's dental status is, the more compromised is one's ability to chew adequately and swallow food, and oral problems, missing teeth, and inadequate prosthetic replacements may lead to severe compromises in nutrition (41). This may in turn significantly impair general health and well-being (42), including involuntary weight loss in frail elders (43). Given the remaining high prevalence in elders of missing teeth, ill-fitting dentures, and their associated problems, improvements in oral health could significantly improve the nutritional status of elders.

Dietary preferences of elders may change as masticatory function decreases because of progressive tooth loss or is compromised by inadequate replacements of missing teeth. Under such conditions patients may prefer soft and easily chewed foods, including a shift to packaged, processed foods, and may also select foods that are sweet, or salty, inasmuch as gustatory sensation diminishes in the presence of poorer oral health status. In turn, such shifts in food selection may have systemic health consequences and affect the medical management of comorbid conditions, such as hypertension and diabetes. In parallel to the apparent stability of masticatory function with aging, there appear to be no major changes in taste perception with aging (44). When alterations in taste and smell are noted in elders, they are related to underlying disease rather than to normative age changes in chemosensation. In contrast, there is evidence that swallowing ability may change with aging because of altered oropharyngeal proprioception.

Oral Cancer

Oral cancer has a high incidence in older patients and is more common in men than women. As with other aspects of oral health in elders, oral cancer is not an inevitable consequence of aging but is significantly associated with specific preventable risk factors, primarily alcohol and tobacco use. Approximately 4 to 5% of cancers occur in the oral cavity and adjacent tissues. Oral carcinomas, typically squamous cell type, occur at different sites with varying frequency. Carcinoma of the lip is chiefly associated with pipe smoking and exposure to sunlight. Carcinoma of the tongue may present as ulceration, leukoplakia, or an erythematous patch (erythroplakia), often with a hyperkeratotic periphery. The lateral borders of the tongue are the most common intraoral sites of

dysplastic and neoplastic lesions. On the buccal mucosa and gingiva, lesions may have a highly variable appearance, including an ulcerated, indurated mass with leukoplakia. Adenocarcinomas may arise from the minor salivary glands, where they may appear as a painless, firm, or fluctuant mass, most frequently near the juncture of the hard and soft palate. All patients who are to receive head and neck radiotherapy should receive a comprehensive oral evaluation before treatment begins. Elimination of oral infection, maintenance of optimal oral hygiene, and a daily topical fluoride regimen must be established to prevent rampant dental caries and oral mucositis, which can be important sequelae to salivary gland dysfunction resulting from irradiation. All necessary dental extractions should be performed before therapy to avoid osteoradionecrosis following extractions.

ORAL HEALTH ASSESSMENT
Self-Assessment and the DENTAL Screening Initiative

Oral problems, as with other health problems, are best managed if identified early. However, neither patients nor non-dental health care professionals are often comfortable in their abilities to diagnose oral diseases, and problems may thus go unrecognized until they progress significantly. The DENTAL screening initiative (Table 45.2) is a simple self-administered questionnaire for a patient's assessment of his or her oral health status to facilitate obtaining needed consultation and follow-up care (45). This simple instrument also lends itself readily to use by physicians, nurses, dietitians, and other health care providers for easy identification of oral problems in their elder patients. The goals of this screen are to identify and treat sources of potential oral infection, to improve the ability to eat a balanced diet comfortably, and to facilitate social interactions by improving appearance and self-esteem and permitting ease of eating and speaking. Other simple instruments for use in elders include the Geriatric Oral Health Assessment Index (46, 47).

Clinical Examination

A simple visual and digital oral examination should identify the presence of or potential for

Table 45.2

The DENTAL Screening Initiative

Determine Your Oral Health

Warning signs of poor oral health are often overlooked. You can use the answers to the following six statements to evaluate your own oral health. Read each statement below. If you answer yes to one or more statements, you should contact your dental or medical provider and ask him or her for assistance.

D   I have a **D**ry mouth.

E   I have **E**ating or swallowing problems, or my **E**ating habits have changed in the past year as a result of problems with my teeth or mouth.

N   I have **N**ot had a dental examination in the past year.

T   I have frequent **T**ooth or mouth pain, or **T**ender, bleeding gums.

A   Problems with my teeth or gums have **A**ffected my **A**ppearance or my social interactions with family, friends, or coworkers.

L   I have **L**esions or sores in my mouth.

These warning signs do not represent the diagnosis of any condition. Instead they suggest that you may be at risk of poor oral health and that you should visit a professional who can help you determine the best course of action to enhance your dental health.

---

oral infection and screen for oral cancer and precancerous lesions. Teeth should be noted and counted. The hygiene of remaining teeth and of any dentures should also be noted. Problems needing immediate attention include grossly decayed or fractured teeth, teeth that move laterally or vertically to finger pressure, purulence from the gingiva or other soft tissues, and areas of ulceration or desquamation. In addition, areas of leukoplakia and erythroplakia may be noted for referral to a dentist for oral cancer evaluation.

Oral hygiene is also a major concern in the edentulous patient. Even the best-fitting dentures may cause mucosal irritation in areas of constant contact and may be reservoirs for oral yeasts and bacteria. In patients with chronic oropharyngeal candidiasis, dentures must be treated to eliminate an important source of reinfection. All dentures should be removed from the mouth at bedtime and should not be worn when asleep. Dentures should be brushed daily for proper plaque removal. An appropriate oral hygiene regimen should be followed daily to promote optimal cleansing of oral tissues and dental prostheses. Modification of cleansing aids can be designed to make patients with physical limitations more self-reliant and responsible for their own care. Providers for patients unable to care for them-

selves and for those under long-term care should make a point to set a simple goal that every day their patients will go to sleep with a clean mouth. Daily brushing with a topical fluoride gel may prevent dental decay and also may prevent progression of gingivitis and periodontal disease. A variety of other highly effective products, including oral rinses, are readily available as adjuncts to routine oral hygiene (48).

This basic clinical screening should be performed on all patients as a simple oral and soft tissue examination of the head and neck:

1. Observe face and neck for any swelling, asymmetry, lesions, or unusual pigmentation, and palpate lymph nodes and glands of the face and neck.

2. Observe and palpate the lips, buccal mucosa, floor of the mouth, palate, and tongue. When observing the tongue, grasp the tip with gauze pad, gently extend it, and view both of the lateral borders and the ventrum.

3. Check salivary duct patency for any signs of blockage, purulence or inflammation, and note the adequacy of the saliva.

4. Check the teeth for decay, mobility, and level of oral hygiene.

5. Check the gingiva (gums) for inflammation, purulence, and bleeding.

MANAGEMENT OF COMMON ORAL PROBLEMS

As elders often see physicians and other health care providers more frequently than they see dentists, recognition of oral problems by these health care providers plays a key role in providing comprehensive care by facilitating early intervention and appropriate referrals for more definitive treatment. The diagnosis of dysplastic and neoplastic lesions (leukoplakia, erythroplakia) and the identification and treatment of caries and periodontal infections have primary importance. Prompt referral to a dentist is indicated.

Dry mouth (xerostomia) is often reported by elders and may be managed by the use of various commercially available saliva substitutes and oral lubricants. Severe xerostomia has been treated with some success with secretagogues, including pilocarpine and carbocholine, in patients with some residual salivary gland function (49, 50). Such patients can also benefit from the use of oral rinses containing fluoride or chlorhexidine (48).

Burning mouth (stomatodynia) and burning tongue (glossodynia) are other common complaints that may be reported together with dry mouth. Pain can be mild to severe. Vitamin deficiencies, especially vitamin B complex, may be implicated. Other conditions, such as anemias, Sjögren's, Mikulcz's, and Plummer-Vinson syndromes may also be associated with xerostomia and burning or itching sensations, and such symptoms may be brought about by side effects of medications used to manage psychiatric problems. Treatment may consist of drug substitution or modification of dosage of the implicated medication, use of vitamin supplements when a deficiency is identified, or use of salivary gland stimulants or saliva substitutes. In addition, subclinical oral candidiasis must be ruled out as a cause of burning mouth. A course of treatment with an oral antifungal agent may be appropriate.

Denture sores (denture stomatitis) are common in patients who wear dentures. They may appear as reddened, inflamed areas, noted on the palate, mandibular ridges, or vestibular mucosa, corresponding with the denture base. Denture sores are also often the result of poor oral hygiene and failure to cleanse dentures properly. Papillary hyperplasia is often seen in patients wearing dentures for extended periods without removal. This condition appears as a raised papular lesion in the mucosa or gingiva under or alongside the edge of complete dentures. Ulcerations due to trauma or inadequate dentures occasionally appear on any mucosa in older adults. The ulceration caused by an overextended denture on examination is consistent with the margin of the denture or site of irritation. If left unadjusted, the area of the ulceration may eventually lead to a reactive hypertrophy of epithelial tissue known as an epulis fissuratum. Fibroepithelial polyps, or irritation fibromas, are frequently observed in the buccal mucosa of the tongue, the vestibular mucosa, or the lips. They may be either sessile or pedunculated and are generally smooth-surfaced and firm upon palpation. Causative factors include ill-fitting dentures, irritation from fractured dental restorations or teeth, and oral habits such as cheek or lip biting. They are remarkable only if they are a source of discomfort or interfere with function.

Candida albicans, normally resident in healthy persons, may proliferate in certain patients as the result of malnutrition, antibiotic therapy, steroid therapy, diabetes, or xerostomia. Antifungal oral rinse-and-swallow suspensions used for 2 weeks are usually the first treatment of choice in uncomplicated cases. Also appropriate are clotrimazole troches and ketoconazole and fluconazole tablets systemically for 14 days.

Angular cheilitis, an inflammatory fissuring and ulceration at the commissures (corners) of the lips, may occur either unilaterally or bilaterally. Causes include loss of vertical dimension due to overclosure of the jaws in edentulous persons, vitamin deficiencies, and xerostomia. Infection with *C. albicans* may also be present. Treatment may include fabrication of appropriately fitting dentures, and/or use of antifungal ointments, such as nystatin (Mycostatin), when a diagnosis of candidiasis is made.

Temporomandibular (TMJ) disorders are articulation dysfunctions of the TMJ, between the glenoid fossa of the skull and the condylar process of the mandible. Studies have generally been inconclusive in correlating physical changes, such as internal derangements of the

TMJ, with symptoms. Patients may have pain, tenderness, swelling, limited movement, and clicking in the area of the joint. Pain may also be referred to the ears or temporal region and may be earaches or temporal headaches. Initial treatment usually is symptomatic with the use of analgesic and anti-inflammatory medications. Radiographic evaluation is indicated for patients with persistent or progressive symptoms.

Idiosyncratic oral manifestations of pharmacologic therapy, particularly with psychotropic drugs, are a common reason for dental consultation. In particular, polypharmacy in older persons may lead to a variety of side effects that have oral manifestations, including xerostomia, mucositis, glossodynia, stomatodynia, desquamation of the oral mucosa, and gingival bleeding.

ETHICAL ISSUES IN ORAL HEALTH CARE FOR ELDERS

Oral health care may be viewed as a value in its own right but must also be viewed as an integral part of comprehensive patient care. Important as it is to the nutritional, psychologic, and physical well-being of elders, oral health care plays a key role in geriatric health assessment and treatment. Under ideal circumstances, in which social, economic, and medical contraindications do not present significant barriers to treatment, health care providers reach clinical decisions about appropriate levels of care with some confidence about the long-term outcomes of the chosen interventions. Such decisions become more difficult in certain categories of older patients, particularly those with a high burden of comorbidities, those with dementia, and those with especially limited life expectancies. Ethical considerations also come into play regarding issues of decision making and informed consent to treatment in patients with certain conditions, while at the same time the dentist wishes to carry out ideal high-quality treatment in all patients (51). In geriatric dentistry, we must accept a premise that age per se should not be a determinant of treatment. As we are learning that normative aging processes do not represent a major risk factor for oral disease, we have also learned that comprehensive dental care, including implant dentistry, is highly appropriate in certain elders and even

beneficial to their health, nutrition, and feelings of general well-being. Nevertheless, treatment decisions in the majority of elders requires consideration of many factors, medical, dental, psychological, social, and economic, to determine the appropriate level of care. Appropriate care may be viewed as the level of intervention that considers the patient's physical and mental ability to tolerate or accept treatment, with the goal of restoration and maintenance of function, and that best corresponds to the patient's own perception of need and quality of life (52, 53).

The management of the oral health care needs of residents in long-term nursing care facilities and of frail elders in general presents particular dilemmas regarding comprehensive and appropriate dental care for elders who may be severely compromised. The oral health status of the patient is often not a priority in the geriatric evaluation. While the medical and nursing staff may be aware of oral problems, there may not be a clear understanding of how such problems can be managed or how oral problems affect the general health and well-being of the patient (54). One simple triage scheme by which to approach the issue of appropriateness is an initial level of basic interventions, involving the elimination of sources of infection and relief of pain through extraction, dental cleaning, antibiotic therapy, and so on. The restoration of teeth to establish optimal oral function constitutes a subsequent stage of care. Last, advanced care encompasses the full range of specialty dental services, including endodontic and periodontal surgical care and comprehensive prosthetic dentistry. A basic set of preventive interventions, such as daily oral hygiene (self-care or assisted), topical fluorides, and oral rinses, could be made available to all patients to prevent the recurrence and progression of oral diseases. Difficult judgments must still be made as to what intensity of care is to be considered appropriate for a particular patient at any particular time. For example, should extensive dental restorative and prosthetic care be provided to patients with dementia? Should decayed teeth be extracted or aggressively treated with restorative, endodontic (root canal), and periodontal therapy in the patient with a short life expectancy? Should dentures be provided to long-term nursing care residents who did not have them before admission? Are there any circumstances in which no treatment, or watchful waiting, is an appropriate option in geriatric dentistry?

CONCLUSION

The better we can identify elders at highest risk for oral problems, the better we can target our preventive and therapeutic interventions. Changes in geriatric dental practice have come about in great part because of research findings that debunked a number of old myths about the oral health of elders. The seemingly simple question what are the effects of aging on oral health? has proved to be quite complex and difficult to answer. The formulation of testable hypotheses has often been complicated by the large number of confounders for which the available data are often inadequate. Furthermore, needed information pertaining to the medical and psychosocial factors that can affect specific outcome measures of oral health status frequently is unavailable. Most studies dealing with the effects of aging on oral health had cross-sectional study designs, comparing old with young and attempting to correlate age with various oral health outcomes. An alternative approach by which the relation of aging and oral health has been investigated is use of longitudinal studies (55). Such studies are helping to identify risk factors associated with oral health changes in aging and to understand the interplay between oral health and systemic diseases and the influence of oral conditions on health-related quality of life. However, there are still many important questions about the relation of aging and oral health status. While great progress has been made in the biomedical domain, there is much to do in the psychosocial domain. How do we determine appropriateness of oral health care for different groups of elders? Do attitudes about oral health and preventive health behaviors change with aging? What are the relations between health behaviors and attitudes and specific oral health outcomes? How do self-assessments of elders' oral health affect their behavioral functioning, social interactions, and sense of well-being? What interventions most improve elders' oral hygiene and in turn their oral health and function? Finally, we need to learn to what extent improving access to and use of com-prehensive dental care services by elders can significantly improve their oral health, systemic health, and quality of life.

REFERENCES

1. Douglass CW, Jette AM, Fox CH, et al. Oral health status of the elderly in New England. J Gerontol 1993;48:M39–M46.
2. Krall EA, Garcia RI, Dawson-Hughes B. Increased risk of tooth loss is related to bone loss at the whole body, hip, and spine. Calcif Tissue Int 1996;59:433–437.
3. Taylor GW, Burt BA, Becker MP, et al. Glycemic control and alveolar bone loss progression in type 2 diabetes. Ann Periodontol 1998;3:30–39.
4. Appollonio I, Carabellese C, Frattola A, Trabucchi M. Dental status, quality of life, and mortality in an older community population: a multivariate approach. J Am Geriatr Soc 1997;45:1315–1323.
5. Sullivan DH, Martin W, Flaxman N, Hagen JE. Oral health problems and involuntary weight loss in a population of frail elderly. J Am Geriatr Soc 1993;41:725–731.
6. National Institute of Dental Research. Oral Health of United States Adults: The National Survey of Oral Health in U.S. Employed Adults and Seniors: 1985–86, National Findings. National Institutes of Health pub 87–2868. Hyattsville, MD: U.S. Dept. of Health and Human Services, 1987.
7. Weintraub JA, Burt BA. Oral health status in the U.S.: tooth loss and edentulism. J Dent Educ 1985;49:368–376.
8. Ripa L. A half-century of community water fluoridation in the U.S.: review and commentary. J Public Health Dent 1993;53:17–44.
9. Burt BA. The oral health of older Americans. Am J Public Health 1985;75:1133–1134.
10. Bailit HL, Braun R, Maryniuk GA, Camp P. Is periodontal disease the primary cause of tooth extraction in adults? J Am Dent Assoc 1987;14:40–44.
11. Hand JS, Hunt RJ, Kohout FJ. Five-year incidence of tooth loss in Iowans aged 65 and older. Community Dent Oral Epidemiol 1991;19:48–51.
12. Chauncey HH, Glass RL, Alman JE. Dental caries: principal cause of tooth extraction in a sample of U.S. male adults. Caries Res 1989;23:200–205.
13. Niessen LC, Weyant RJ. Cause of tooth loss in a veteran population. J Public Health Dent 1989;49:19–23.
14. Gilbert GH. Access to and patterns of use of oral health care among elderly veterans. Med Care 1995;33:NS78–NS89.
15. Jones JA, Lavallee N, Alman J, et al. Caries incidence in patients with dementia. Gerodontology 1993;10:76–82.
16. Fox PC, van der Ven P, Sonies BC, et al. Xerostomia: evaluation of a symptom with increasing significance. J Am Dent Assoc 1985;110:519–525.
17. Brown LJ, Oliver RC, Loe H. Periodontal diseases in the US in 1981: prevalence, severity, extent and role in tooth mortality. J Periodontol 1989;60:363–370.
18. Beck JD, Koch GG, Rizier RG, Tudor GE. Prevalence and

risk indicators for periodontal attachment loss in a population of older community-dwelling blacks and whites. J Periodontol 1990;61:521–528.

19. Haber J, Wattles J, Crowley M, et al. Evidence for cigarette smoking as a major risk factor for periodontitis. J Periodontol 1993;64:16–23.

20. Krall EA, Dawson-Hughes B, Garvey AJ, Garcia RI. Smoking, smoking cessation, and tooth loss. J Dent Res 1997;76:1653–1659.

21. National Cancer Institute and National Institute of Dental Research. Tobacco effects in the mouth. National Institutes of Health pub 92–3330. Washington: Government Printing Office, 1992.

22. Jette AM, Feldman HA, Tennstedt SL. Tobacco use: a modifiable risk factor for dental disease among the elderly. Am J Public Health 1993;83:1271–1276.

23. Krall EA, Dawson-Hughes B. Smoking and bone loss among postmenopausal women. J Bone Miner Res 1991;6:331–337.

24. Jeffcoat MK, Chestnut CH. Systemic osteoporosis and oral bone loss. J Am Dent Assoc 1993;124:49–56.

25. Schlossman M, Knowler WC, Pettit DJ, Genco RJ. Type II diabetes and periodontal disease. J Am Dent Assoc 1990;121:532–536.

26. Nelson RG, Schlossman M, Budding LM, et al. Periodontal disease and glucose tolerance in Pima Indians. Diabetes Care 1990;13:836–840.

27. Sreebny LM, Yu A, Green A, Valdini A. Xerostomia in diabetes mellitus. Diabetes Care 1992;15:900–904.

28. Cherry-Peppers G, Sorkin J, Andres R, et al. Salivary gland function and glucose metabolic status. J Gerontol 1992;47:M130–M134.

29. Sreebny LM, Valdini A, Yu A. Xerostomia part 2: Relationship to nonoral symptoms, drugs and diseases. Oral Surg Oral Med Oral Pathol 1989;68:419–427.

30. Baum BJ. Salivary gland fluid secretion during aging. J Am Geriatr Soc 1989;37:453–458.

31. Chauncey HH, Feller RP, Kapur KK. Longitudinal age-related changes in human parotid saliva composition. J Dent Res 1987;66:599–602.

32. Navazesh M. Xerostomia in the aged. Dent Clin North Am 1989;33:75–95.

33. Atkinson JC, Travis WD, Pillemer SR, et al. Major salivary gland function in primary Sjögren's syndrome and its relation to clinical features. J Rheumatol 1990;17:318–322.

34. Ship JA, DeCarli C, Friedland RP, Baum BJ. Diminished submandibular salivary flow in dementia of the Alzheimer type. J Gerontol Med Soc 1990;45:M61–M66.

35. Narhi TO, Meurman JH, Ainamo A, et al. Associations between salivary flow rate and the use of systemic medication among 76-, 81-, and 86-year-old inhabitants in Helsinki, Finland. J Dent Res 1992;71:1875–1880.

36. Fox PC, Busch KA, Baum BJ. Subjective reports of xerostomia and objective measures of salivary gland performance. J Am Dent Assoc 1987;115:581–584.

37. Narhi TO, Ainamo A, Meurman JH. Salivary yeasts, saliva, and oral mucosa in the elderly. J Dent Res 1993;72:1009–1014.

38. Stead RJ, Cooke NJ. Adverse effects of inhaled corticosteroids. BMJ 1989;298:403–404.

39. Holmstrup P, Axell T. Classification and clinical manifestations of oral yeast infections. Acta Odontol Scand 1990;48:57–59.

40. Chauncey HH. Longitudinal changes in masticatory performance and food acceptability observed with stable and altered dentition. In: Chauncey HH, ed. Geriatric Dentistry: Biomedical and Psychosocial Aspects. Chicago: American Dental Association Health Foundation, 1985:60–69.

41. Krall EA, Hayes C, Garcia RI. Dentition status, masticatory function, and nutrient intake. J Am Dent Assoc 1998;129:1261–1269.

42. Gordon SR, Kelley SL, Sybyl JR, et al. Relationship in very elderly veterans of nutritional status, self-perceived chewing ability, dental status, and social isolation. J Am Geriatr Soc 1985;33:334.

43. Sullivan DH, Martin W, Flaxman N, Hagen JE. Oral health problems and involuntary weight loss in a population of frail elderly. J Am Geriatr Soc 1993;41:725–731.

44. Weiffenbach JM, Cowart BJ, Baum BJ. Taste intensity perception in aging. J Gerontol 1986;41:460–464.

45. Bush LA, Hornekamp N, Morley JE, Spiro A. D-E-N-T-A-L: a rapid self-administered screening instrument to assess perceived need of dental problems in the older adult. J Am Geriatr Soc 1996;44:979–981.

46. Atchison KA, Dolan TA. Development of the Geriatric Oral Health Assessment Index. J Dent Educ 1990;54:680–687.

47. Kressin NR. Associations among different assessments of oral health outcomes. J Dent Educ 1996;60:501–507.

48. Cianco SG. Agents for the management of plaque and gingivitis. J Dent Res 1992;71:1450–1454.

49. Johnson JT, Ferretti GA, Nethery WJ, et al. Oral pilocarpine for post-irradiation xerostomia in patients with head and neck cancer. N Engl J Med 1993;329:390–395.

50. Joensuu H, Bostrom P, Makkonen T. Pilocarpine and carbocholine in treatment of radiation-induced xerostomia. Radiother Oncol 1993;26:33–37.

51. Antczak-Bouckoms A. Quality and effectiveness issues related to oral health. Med Care 1995;33:S123–S142.

52. Gift HC, Redford M. Oral health and the quality of life. Clin Geriatr Med 1992;8:673–683.

53. Kressin NR, Spiro A III, Bosse R, et al. Assessing oral health related quality of life: findings from the Normative Aging Study. Med Care 1996;34:16–427.

54. Calabrese JM, Friedman PK, Rose L, Jones JA. Using the GOHAI to assess oral health status of frail homebound elders. Spec Care Dent (in press).

55. Garcia RI, Chauncey HH. Longitudinal studies of aging and oral health. J Dent Res 1991;70:865–866.

Care of the Elderly Patient
Other Considerations

CHAPTER 46

CHARLES P. MOUTON AND DAVID V. ESPINO

Ethnic Diversity of the Aged

Diversity is a central feature of the aging U.S. population. The aging minority population shows proportionate increases in percentages and absolute numbers. According to 1995 census estimates, African-Americans make up 7.8% of the population older than 65 (2.5 million people), a figure expected to grow to 8.6% by 2010 and 15% by 2050 (1, 2). Hispanic-Americans make up about 4.4% (1.4 million), and this proportion is expected to triple to 15% (12 million) by 2050. Asian-Americans make up about 1.6% (513,000) and expect to be just under 9% (7 million) by 2050. In particular, Asian elders showed a significant rise in absolute numbers, going from 200,000 to 500,000 between the 1980 and 1990 censuses, and also showed a rise as a percentage of the population, doubling from 0.78% in 1980. Native Americans make up about 0.35% (114,306) and are expected to grow to 0.71% (562,000) by 2050. Similar to their white counterparts, older members of minority groups will become an increasingly important proportion of the average clinician's daily practice. Each group brings a unique set of life experiences to the doctor-patient relationship.

The Census Bureau classification of minority groups is a broad, sweeping definition, and within particular racial and ethnic classifications there is a large amount of diversity. This means that in some situations the provision of medical care will require special attention to group-specific concerns. Also, because of this diversity, no study or series of studies can fit every older minority group. Clinicians should evaluate each older minority person as an individual. Therefore, those remarks should be used as general guidelines or points to consider when managing the care of an older member of a minority group. This chapter is divided into two parts; the first concentrates on group-specific concerns regarding mortality, geriatric syndromes, and selected disease entities. The second focuses on socioeconomic and caregiving issues and the doctor-patient relationship.

LIFE EXPECTANCY

The projected increase in age-specific life expectancy of the older members of minority groups is astonishing. In every group that has had growth in the population of elders, two trends in life expectancy have been observed. First, there has been an increase in life expectancy from birth. Second, there has been an increase in the life expectancy once a person has attained the age of 65 years. The same is true for this country.

Specific data on racial and ethnic groups show crossover of life expectancy as they age. Half of African-Americans will live an average of 15.5 additional years once they reach age 65 (3). Once they reach age 85, African-Americans' longevity increases to 8.2 years for men and 10.6 years for women compared with 5.5 and 7.2 years for white men and women, respectively (2). For other minority subpopulations the figures are less clear, but earlier studies suggest that life expectancy for Hispanic-Americans is 14.1 years for men and 17.4 for women once they reach 65 (4, 5).

MORTALITY DATA

For older African-Americans, mortality rates are far beyond that of their white counterparts. Total age-adjusted mortality rates were 785/100,000 for African-Americans compared with 485/100,000 for whites in 1995. However, death rates were lower for Mexican-Americans over age 65 than for whites, African-Americans, and mainland Puerto Ricans. Only Cuban-Americans had lower death rates than the Mexican-American cohort (6). Asian-Americans had mortality rates of 294/100,000 as of 1993.

As for the cause of death, heart disease and malignancies continue to be the leading causes of death for all older subpopulations (1, 7). Heart disease accounted for 305/100,000 deaths in whites compared to 246/100,000 in African-Americans. Malignant neoplasms accounted for 215/100,000 deaths in whites compared with 186/100,000 in African-Americans. While these overall mortality rates are higher for whites, African-Americans over 65 have a higher expected death rate from cardiac arrests (115% higher for men, 95% higher for women), cancer (26% higher for men, 3% higher for women), and diabetes mellitus (11% for men, 90% for women) (8). As for Hispanic elders, more of them die of diabetes mellitus and complications of diabetes than whites (9). Asian-Americans tend to have higher death rates from liver disease and gastrointestinal cancers than whites. Because of their increasing numbers in the population and the larger number of older adults being seen in medical practice, clinicians should be aware of some of the unique features in the care of older minority members.

COGNITIVE AND PSYCHOLOGIC FUNCTION
Dementia

The prevalence of dementia in minority populations is not well documented, but there are some clues to the disease burden in this community. The Duke Longitudinal Aging Study suggests the prevalence of Alzheimer's disease is higher among African-Americans than whites (10). However, the frequency of Alzheimer's disease in African-Americans is controversial, with some studies reporting greater frequency, some reporting lower frequency, and others showing no difference in Alzheimer's disease compared with whites. These discrepancies may be partly due to the diagnostic bias of the instruments used to screen for dementia (11). Regarding other types of dementia, there is evidence that multi-infarct and alcohol-related dementias may be more common in African-Americans than in other subgroups (12). Multi-infarct dementia has been reported to have a relative risk in African-Americans up to 5.6 times that of whites, and alcohol-related dementia, up to 8.44 times that of whites (12, 13).

The Hispanic Established Populations for Epidemiologic Studies in the Elderly (EPESE) indicated that when a Folstein Mini-Mental State Examination (MMSE) cutoff score of 24 is used, 22.3% of Mexican-American elders demonstrated cognitive impairment (14). Only minimal research has been conducted on elder Asians and Pacific Islanders. Studies suggested that the prevalence of vascular dementia among Japanese elders living in Hawaii is lower than among similar cohorts in Japan and that the prevalence of Alzheimer's disease is higher, approaching a level seen in whites. The Honolulu Asia Aging Study shows a prevalence of all-cause dementia of 9.3%, Alzheimer's disease, 5.4%, and vascular dementia, 4.2% in older Japanese-American men (15). However, Graves et al. (16) found that the prevalence rate for all dementias was 6.3% in older Japanese-Americans and rose with each 5-year age increment. Lin (17) reported the incidence of senile psychosis among elderly Chinese to be lower than that of the general population of the United States. Published data on the incidence of cognitive impairment among elder Native Americans are markedly deficient.

Depression

Major depression is less common in African-American elders than in their white counterparts (18). About 2% of elders from the general African-American population were found to be depressed (11). In fact, the highest suicide rates for older adults is in white men, while the lowest is in African-American women (19). However, in family practice and general medicine clinics, 11 to

33% of older African-American patients were found to be depressed, a rate approaching that of white elders (20).

Major depression was also found to be less common in older Mexican-Americans than in whites. Rates of depression in Mexican-Americans are reported to be 20 to 28% (21, 22). In a large study of community-dwelling residents, 38% of the whites compared with 28.5% of the Mexican-Americans reported more than 2 weeks of dysphoria. Only 7.9% of the Mexican-Americans had suicidal ideation, compared with 20.7% of the whites (22). Kemp et al. (22) showed that 26% of Hispanic elders in Los Angeles County met the criteria of *Diagnostic and Statistical Manual of Mental Disorders* (DSM-III-R) for these two mood disorders. Furthermore, the Los Angeles Epidemiologic Catchment Area survey suggests that depressive illness may occur in Mexican-Americans more often than in non-Hispanics (23).

In Asian-Americans, there are some differences in depression based on sex. In older Chinese women, the suicide rate is 3 to 7 times higher than in white women (24, 25). Japanese women also have higher suicide rates than whites (25). In Koreans, 2.6% of older men and 6.7% of older women manifest depressive symptoms (24).

PHYSICAL IMPAIRMENT

Maintaining function is one of the main reasons that older members of minority groups seek medical care. As African-Americans age, their functional status declines more rapidly than that of whites. In the North Carolina EPESE, 9.6% of African-Americans older than 65 reported difficulty with two or more activities of daily living (ADLs); 19% reported two or more difficulties on instrumental ADLs (IADLs) (3, 26). Older African-Americans are 1.38 times as likely to have trouble getting around and more than 1.5 times as likely to be confined to their homes than non-Hispanic whites (27). However, as they reach their 80s and 90s, older African-Americans seem to function better, possibly because of a selection bias in the aging process, but some authors suggest that they live with higher rates of poor health (3).

Comparative data on community-based assessments of functional status of elderly Hispanics are lacking. A nationwide telephone survey conducted by the Commonwealth Fund found that elderly Hispanics were more functionally impaired than whites (28). This impairment was manifested by difficulties across all ADLs and IADLs. Markides et al. (29) reported that the chances for functional impairment related to specific medical conditions such as diabetes mellitus, stroke, myocardial infarction, arthritis, and hip fracture were higher than in white populations. Finally, there are comparative data demonstrating that institutionalized Hispanic elders are more functionally and mentally disabled than their white counterparts (30, 31). Likewise, Rudkin et al. (32) demonstrated that functional limitations of Mexican-Americans elders were higher than those of non-Hispanic whites and lower than those of African-Americans. Comparative data on function impairment and disability in Asian-Americans are also lacking. Asian-Americans who have high socioeconomic status and/or are from early immigrant groups are probably similar to whites in level of function. Further data on function in Asian-Americans are limited.

Measurement Issues

Because of the importance that function plays in the health of older adults, several instruments have been adapted for use in older members of minority groups, including self-report questionnaires, such as the ADL and IADL scales, as well as performance-based measures (33–35). The assessment of function using the ADL scale has proved to be fairly reliable and valid in African-Americans and Hispanic-Americans (35). It measures self-reports of behavior that are considered to predict the independent living ability of older adults. Clinicians can use this instrument to identify those who may benefit from assisted living or a greater level of caregiving. Another instrument, the IADL, assessing a higher level of function than the ADL scale (36), has been used in minority populations, but there are limited data on its reliability and validity in these groups.

Since the ADL and IADL scales rely on self-report and thus are limited, performance-based assessments of function have been developed to provide a more objective measurement. Performance-based measures include the gait and balance evaluation, the Timed Manual Performance test, and the Get Up and Go test (34, 37, 38). No data on the validity of these instruments in minority elders are available, but some clinicians find them helpful in assessing patients.

COMMON DISEASES IN ETHNIC MINORITY GROUPS

Chronic health conditions affecting the elder minority population include osteoarthritis, diabetes mellitus, cardiovascular disease, cerebrovascular disease, cancer, osteoporosis, and fractures. Because of the increased frequency of these conditions in older adults, clinicians should understand some of the racial and ethnic differences that may be encountered.

Arthritis

Osteoarthritis, a degenerative process of articular cartilage, is a major cause of morbidity in both African-American and white elders, leading to more than 7 million office visits annually (39). In a study of African-American elders, 52.8 to 66.4% had been diagnosed with osteoarthritis (39). Special considerations in choosing a treatment should include the risk of drug side effects, especially gastrointestinal hemorrhage, nephrotoxicity, and the degree that osteoarthritis impairs daily function.

The incidence of osteoarthritis may be lower in elder Mexican-Americans. Espino et al. (40) using data from the Hispanic Health and Nutrition Examination Survey (HANES) Southwestern sample found that the prevalence of arthritis was significantly lower than in the general population. Likewise, Markides et al. (41) found that 41% of Mexican-American elders reported having arthritis, compared with 50% of the general population.

Osteoporosis and Fractures

There are important differences in bone mass and the rate of osteoporosis among the minority subpopulation. African-Americans have higher bone mass than whites at all ages (42, 43). As for hip fractures, white women have the highest incidence of hip fractures (807/100,000), followed by white men (428/100,000), African-American women (306/100,000), and African-American men (238/100,000) (44). In the National Hospi-

tal Discharge Survey, older white women have relative risks of hip fracture that were 2 to 3.2 times those of older African-Americans. The rates for white and African-American men were similar to those for women (45). Little is known about the incidence of hip fractures in Hispanics. However, it seems that Mexican-Americans and African-Americans of both sexes have lower risks of hip fractures than whites (46, 47). Bone mineral density has also been reported to be lower in Asian-American and white adults than in Hispanic and African-American adults. The rates of osteoporosis and osteoporosis-related fractures are similar for whites and Asian-Americans.

Non–Insulin-Dependent Diabetes Mellitus

Diabetes mellitus is the seventh leading cause of death in the United States. While incidence of diabetes increases with age, it disproportionately affects African-Americans, Mexican-Americans, and Native Americans. The prevalence of diabetes in older African-Americans (age 65 to 74 years) was 25.9 to 26.4 per 1000 (29.4 for men and 23.1 to 24.1 for women) compared with 16.9 to 17.9 per 1000 for whites (48). As for the age-specific mortality, diabetes accounted for 129/100,000 African-American deaths in those 65 to 74 years old and 283/100,000 deaths in those 75 or older. This is 1.78 and 2.8 times as many deaths as their white counterparts (49, 50).

Non–insulin-dependent diabetes mellitus (NIDDM) has a major effect on the older Hispanic population. Espino et al. (40) found that 21.6% of older Mexican-Americans in the Southwestern United States had diabetes mellitus as compared with 9.8% of the general population (40). Other studies have found the risk of diabetes in Hispanics to be 2 to 5 times that of whites (51).

About 20% of Native Americans overall are diabetic (52). The mortality rates of diabetes for Native Americans exceeds those of all other racial and ethnic groups in the United States (53). The age-adjusted rate is 4.3 times that of whites and 2 times that of African-Americans (54). Although progress has been made, NIDDM continues to be a problem for older Native Americans. Through its effects on the vascular system and kidneys, NIDDM is a major cause of morbidity and mortality for Native Americans.

Although rates are not as high as among other minority populations, Japanese have a higher prevalence of diabetes mellitus and impaired glucose tolerance than whites. The incidence of "possible" diabetes was 12.8% for Japanese-American men, and the incidence of NIDDM was 1.25 times as high in men as in women (55, 56). The prevalence of diabetes in Chinese men from Boston was 13.3% (57). The rise of diabetes in Asians and Pacific Islanders can be traced to the adoption of an "American" diet (58).

Hypertension, Cardiovascular Disease, and Stroke

As with younger minority adults, hypertension is a common problem for older members of minority groups. Hypertension affects approximately 71% of African-Americans, 61% of Mexican-Americans, and 60% of whites who are age 60 or older. Hypertension is a major contributor to the "60,000 annual excess deaths" (59) of African-Americans (60). Because of hypertension, African-Americans have a 1.3-fold rate of nonfatal stroke, a 1.8-fold rate of fatal stroke, a 1.5-fold rate of heart disease deaths, and a 5-fold rate of end-stage renal disease than whites. Their higher prevalence of salt sensitivity, obesity, and cigarette smoking also contributes to these risks. However, if adequate therapy is provided, older African-Americans can achieve similar blood pressure declines and lower their incidence of cardiovascular disease.

Guidelines for treating hypertension in older members of minority groups are extrapolated from the general recommendations for special populations. For patients with stage 1 hypertension without evidence of end organ damage, an attempt to control blood pressure with lifestyle modification (weight loss, reduced dietary sodium intake, increased physical activity, and moderation of alcohol intake) should be tried for at least 6 months prior to initiating pharmacologic therapy. For pharmacologic treatment, diuretic agents are recommended as first-line therapy in African-American older adults. Also, young and older African-Americans respond well to calcium channel blockers (61, 62). Monotherapy with α-

blockers or αβ-blockers seem to be as effective in African-Americans as in whites, while β-blockers and angiotensin-converting enzyme (ACE) inhibitors may be less effective. Starting doses and increases in dose should be smaller for older patients. Changes in dosing should be spaced at longer intervals.

As in younger Hispanics, the elderly cohort has rates of hypertension, cardiovascular disease, and stroke similar to or less than those of whites in the same age group (63). The ethnic advantage may be due to positive risk factor profiles, such as lower serum cholesterol, lower rates of smoking, and lower rates of alcohol consumption (64). Although they have lower rates of stroke, older Hispanics have been found to have twice the risk of intracerebral hemorrhage as non-Hispanic whites (64, 65).

Data about prevalence rates and therapeutic efficacy for hypertension in older Asian-Americans are limited. One study showed that older Chinese-Americans in the Boston area had a 39% prevalence of hypertension (57). In Native Americans, there is strong regional variation in hypertension and cardiovascular disease. As a whole, hypertension in Native Americans is less prevalent than in whites and other ethnic populations. Ischemic heart disease is relatively high in the Northern Plains tribes and low in Alaskan natives and Southwestern tribes.

Neoplasms

When matched for age, African-Americans have greater incidence rates and mortality for certain cancers than whites. The overall 5-year cancer survival rate for African-Americans is 12 percentage points below that of whites. Of 25 primary cancer sites, African-Americans had lower survival in all but 3. Breast and prostate cancer are two of the leading cancers in which older African-Americans show poor survival.

Epidemiologic data for the overall Hispanic population in the United States are lacking. Data for New Mexico and Texas indicate that the incidence of neoplasms is consistently lower in Hispanics than in whites and African-Americans. Hispanics have lower incidences of lung, colon, breast, and prostate malignancies and higher incidences of stomach, liver, gallbladder, and cervical malignancies, although cervical malignancies may be decreasing (5, 66, 67).

The 5-year breast cancer survival rates between 1978 and 1982 were 73.5 to 76.4% for white women compared with 60.5 to 64.1% for African-American women, despite their lower incidence rates. This difference is related to the large number of African-American women presenting with lymph node involvement or direct extension of their cancer (stage IIIB), lower rates of screening in African-American women, and poorer socioeconomic status (68–72). Early detection through mammography, clinical breast examination, and encouraging breast self-examination is the major way that family physicians can improve the health of these women. Survival rates in African-American women improve as they gain information about breast cancer screening (73, 74). The prevalence of breast cancer in Asian-American women born in China or Japan and their U.S.-born counterparts is about 50% and 75% that of non-Hispanic whites. Breast cancer in Filipino-Americans is 40% of whites (75).

Prostate cancer rates are 30% higher in African-American men over 65 than in same-age whites. Older African-American men also face lower survival rates for prostate cancer, 64% compared with 79% for whites, possibly because of their later stage of detection. As for screening, African-American men had higher prostate-specific antigen (PSA) levels across all stages, grades, and age categories and were 2.2 times as likely to have values above 10 ng/mL (76). How and why men should be screened for prostate cancer is controversial, but, screening with digital rectal examination and PSA levels in African-American men over 40 may be appropriate (76–80). In Los Angeles County, prostate cancer mortality was constant between 1976 and 1988 for Hispanics, non-Hispanic whites, and Asians but increased by 1.6% in African-Americans (81). African- and Hispanic-Americans were at a significantly higher risk of being diagnosed with prostate cancer (odds of being diagnosed 1.39 and 1.24, respectively, compared with whites). Although older Hispanics have a lower incidence of prostate malignancies, they are more likely than whites to have spreading disease at diagnosis (81).

Asian-Americans tend to have higher rates of incidence of nasopharyngeal and liver cancer than whites (82). Filipinos have substantially lower rates of cancer than whites, but liver, nasopharyngeal, and thyroid cancer rates are higher (83). This implies that efforts to diminish hepatitis B virus transmission would be helpful in preventing disease.

PREVENTION PRACTICES

Some suggest that the ethnic and racial disadvantage for some health problems may result from underuse of health strategies for disease prevention (84, 85). Some 29% of minority elders versus 26% of white elders do not receive preventive care services such as blood pressure monitoring, Pap smears, or cholesterol screening (86). Vietnamese (47%) (87), Mexican-Americans (39%), and Puerto Rican-Americans (38%) were even less likely to receive preventive care than African-Americans.

For cancer prevention, the lack of preventive services is particularly distressing. About 70% of cancer mortality and morbidity is related to major remediable risk factors, such as diet, tobacco, and alcohol abuse. Proportionately, more African-Americans smoke than whites, though whites proportionately smoke more cigarettes per day. Also, the numbers of African-Americans who consume alcohol is predicted to worsen, especially considering large increases in alcohol consumption by African-American youths. Unfortunately, many investigators believe that the urban members of minority groups are one of the hardest groups to reach with traditional techniques to change health behaviors (85). Both African-Americans and Hispanic-Americans are more obese and less physically active than whites.

One issue may be a sense of powerlessness regarding health promotion. This sense of powerlessness leads to dependency on someone else (i.e., the physician) to take responsibility for health and poses a barrier to behavior change. The attitude of powerlessness also leads to poorer adherence to treatments that require active behaviors. These factors may make it more difficult for the primary care physician to manage and provide the best care for these groups. Educational efforts addressed at alleviating this sense of powerlessness while simultaneously developing healthy behaviors in the minority elders would strengthen the health of the entire community and make the clinician's job easier and more fulfilling.

SOCIAL FUNCTION AND ECONOMICS

Socioeconomic factors, probably more than race and ethnicity, have a great effect on longevity and functional decline. In fact, when socioeconomic forces are controlled, many of the differences between older members of minority groups and other older adults disappear or narrow. As a whole, minority elders show greater levels of financial strain than their white counterparts (88, 89). Older members of minority groups also may face what some have termed double jeopardy. Their age and minority status lead to a greater burden of illness and greater limitation on their financial resources (90–92). Physicians should consider the financial constraints of their older minority patients as they develop recommendations for treatment. While direct questioning about finances may be offensive to some older adults, presenting the possibility of a less expensive but equally effective treatment shows a depth of understanding that is appreciated.

Family Issues

Family structure and dynamics must be taken into account when managing the care of all patients. It has been estimated that families provide as much as 80% of the needed home care for the frail elderly, and although underacknowledged, family members are usually the primary caregivers for older demented patients (93). This is true especially within minority households. The primary caregiver of the older minority patient is a member of the family, and studies have demonstrated that Native Americans and Hispanics provide significant levels of interactive care for these persons (94, 95). It is important for the health care provider to be aware that long-term care placement of a minority elder may not be a viable option for the family.

African-American elders are often in a family structure that promotes support between genera-

tions (88, 96, 97). Older African-Americans seem to rely more on these larger, more supportive informal networks than on formal service providers (98). Much of this support may arise from other socioeconomic factors, such as marital status and number of other persons living in the household, rather than race (97, 99). As for the characteristics of caregiving, African-Americans show more favorable attitudes toward caregiving even though they tend to care for persons with greater functional and cognitive impairment (100, 101). However, support for filial norms of caregiving may be lower in African-Americans than in whites (102).

Older Hispanics have strong family ties and family interactions. The extended family continues to provide significant support for the Hispanic elder. Even those with high degrees of disability may be attended to at home for long periods (30, 103–106). The designated primary caregiver is usually the elderly spouse, adult daughter, or daughter-in-law. However, family caregiving entails a high cost to the caregivers. Family caregivers of elderly Hispanics have high levels of stress and depression (107). Also, older Hispanics with chronic illnesses are less likely than those without such illnesses to perceive that they have an available caregiver. Lower socioeconomic status is also associated with lack of a perceived caregiver (108). Although there is a reliance on nuclear and extended family members as the primary advocates and gatekeepers for Hispanic elders, family caregivers do use community supportive services (107). Hispanic cultural traditions, as with many minority groups, express different values and customs. Most Hispanics place a great deal of value on family relations. They are trained to believe that the family as a whole or another family member's needs are more important than one's own needs. This places the emphasis on cooperation and sharing, which leads to the family as the most important support system for its older members. But as each generation becomes acculturated to the "American" value system in which fewer people live in extended-family households, the expectations of older Hispanics are often left unmet. Besides emphasizing mutual social responsibility, the Hispanic family structure also tends to be patriarchal. The oldest man tends to be the decision maker and authority figure, as with the Asian cultures. Another value centers on dealing with other persons on a basis of trust, respect, and dignity. Hispanics expect to be treated with respect and dignity regardless of job or social status. These values are earned over time.

Rural Native American populations tend to live with families (three fourths of the rural population), whereas only half the urban Native American population lives with the family (109). Again, socioeconomic factors, especially poverty, may be a greater determinant of this social arrangement.

Asian-Americans as a group tend to have strong family ties and a supportive relationship in the care of the older adults. In the Chinese-American and Japanese-American communities, the filial obligation of children to care for their aging parents is still strong. Ross et al. (93) suggest that Japanese-American women may deny cognitive or memory problems out of respect for their elder husbands or fathers (93). Some studies suggest, however, that with the acculturation of each successive generation, this filial responsibility is becoming weaker. Korean-Americans seem to depart from these two Asian-American communities; there is less of a tendency for Korean elders to live with their children, and many prefer to live independently apart from their children (110).

ECONOMICS

Studies have shown a racial disparity in economic well-being (111, 112). Older African-Americans have 50% of the economic resources of older whites. This has been called cumulative disadvantage, since it represents the accumulation of early economic deficits over the life of African-Americans (112).

Poverty continues to be a growing problem for older members of minority groups. In 1989, 11.4% of all elders lived in poverty, with 9.6% of whites, 30.8% of African-Americans, 20.6% of Hispanics, and 7.4% of Asian-Americans living in poverty. In 1990, 12.2% of all elders were poor, with whites making up 10.1%, African-Americans 33.8%, Hispanic-Americans 22.5%, and Asian-Americans 12.1%. Within the Hispanic subpopulation, Mexican-Americans made up 23.1% of those in poverty, and Puerto Ricans

made up 31.7% (111). Native Americans' poverty ranged from 21 to 41% for urban elders to as high as 57% for rural and reservation elders. Some 93% of whites, 89% of African-Americans, and 77% of Hispanic-Americans receive their income from Social Security. Equal numbers of African-Americans and Hispanic-Americans (22%) were on public assistance. White elders had 4 times the wealth of African-Americans and twice the wealth of Hispanic-Americans.

Financial Burdens

Several studies have identified that one of the strongest predictors of poor health and access to health care among minority elders is the lack of health insurance (21, 112–115). Among elderly minority groups, nearly 47% of Hispanics and 70% of African-Americans are at or below the poverty level, compared with 25% of the white elders (116–118). The limitation of financial resources among aged minority groups restricts their ability to use services such as mental health or long-term care (119). Additionally, third-party payers often do not provide reimbursement for items such as mental health and dental care, hearing aids, prescription lenses, home nursing, podiatric care, and numerous laboratory or radiologic tests (120). These inadequate funding sources necessitate increased monetary as well as caregiver support by family members, and this often imposes economic stress on the family that precludes appropriate care and creates substantial financial burdens (121). This financial strain often results in decreased family support, neglect, and possibly elder abuse.

Communication Issues

The recognition of the use of nonverbal communication among older ethnic minority groups is critical to the development of a care plan (122). While they may vary in their preference for autonomy, African-Americans generally expect to be given information about their illness. Unfortunately, studies show that African-Americans are less likely to receive health information than whites (88). Among minority elder populations such as Asians, Pacific Islanders, and Native Americans, the use of nonverbal communication is common (123).

Problems in communication can also lead to diagnosis difficulties. Diagnostic discrepancies have been observed between standardized and subjective assessment techniques, and it has been suggested that social distance, racism, unconscious fears, and similar concerns may contribute to this problem (120). Older members of minority groups are also less likely to be referred to specialists or to receive surgical and diagnostic procedures (124).

Because of their experience with discrimination, minority elders may be reluctant to adopt a collegial relationship with a nonminority physician (88, 125–127). This tendency may possibly change as the baby boomers mature and with the acculturation of successive generations, since they are living in a different historical context, largely due to the civil rights movement and enhanced opportunities. Physicians can foster a more collegial doctor-patient relationship by spending extra time discussing values, understanding patients' perceptions of health and illness, and developing trust with their older minority patients.

Medication Usage

Health professionals supervising the care of frail or demented minority elders must be attentive to the administration of prescribed medications by family caregivers. Caregivers may have difficulty understanding instructions, and this can lead to incorrect medication administration and the suggestion of noncompliance. Many elderly patients within traveling distance of Mexico may purchase Mexican over-the-counter pharmaceuticals (105). These medications are not always bioequivalent to U.S. pharmaceuticals, and complications such as erratic absorption, poor distribution, and adverse interactions are possible. Also, traditional folk remedies and health beliefs play an influential role in the health maintenance of elder Mexican-Americans (106). As a result, Hispanic elders may rely on unconventional therapies to a greater extent than non-Hispanics, even when socioeconomic factors are controlled (90, 128). The use of herbs, home remedies, and faith healers (curanderos) is common in many minority populations and is prevalent in the Hispanic culture (129). However, as pointed out by Trotter and Hixon (43), the use of specific herb teas or compounds such as azarzon (which contains a large concentration of lead tetroxide) may exacerbate memory loss and behavioral disturbances in the patient (130).

DECISION MAKING AND ETHICS

The paucity of research on the influence of race and ethnicity on doctor-patient interaction among elderly members of minority groups forces us to extrapolate from the research in older adults from the majority population and in younger minority adults. The dialog between a clinician and an older minority adult may be affected by demographic variables such as age, gender, and race. Doctors who are 65 and over are in similar birth cohorts as their patients and have witnessed comparable historical events. This suggests a sense of commonality that should lead to better communication, but this effect has not been thoroughly studied. Younger doctors are apt to be more ageist than their older colleagues and spend less consultation time with older adults (131, 132).

As for the patients, those over age 60 are most likely to accept the physician's authority (133, 134). These findings were confirmed by Beisecker (135) and Beisecker and Beisecker (136), who found older patients less likely than young ones to believe in patients' rights to make medical decisions or to challenge a doctor's authority. Patients who had challenging attitudes were likely to be well informed about health issues (133, 137). Conversely, other studies have found that patient age had a positive relation to the amount of information given by health providers; this may indicate an improving doctor-patient relationship (124).

Carp (125) states that the old, the poor, and members of ethnic minority groups have relatively little in common with the mainstream of society and are in poor communication with it. This poor communication spills over into doctor–ethnic minority patient relations for both young and older patients. African-American elders may be less likely to adopt or desire a collegial relationship with a physician not from the same ethnic background (85, 126). Similarly, studies show that doctors tend to give less time and less complete information to persons viewed as belonging to a lower class. These tendencies can produce adverse effects on outcomes (124).

Physicians should understand the patient's health goals and treatment preferences, which play a major role in the medical decision making. Also, physicians should encourage clear communication through written advance directives and family discussions. Although African-American elders may be less inclined to complete written advance directives, they are often willing to discuss their preferences with family (138). Appropriately involving family members as informed participants in decision making can facilitate this discussion. Furthermore, understanding health preferences is important in developing strategies to maintain health and physical function. Acculturation may be an important factor in relation to disease processes regardless of socioeconomic status. Older Hispanics who are more acculturated have higher rates of hypertension than Hispanic elders who are less acculturated (139). Further investigation is needed in this area, however.

Language

Individual characteristics among elderly minority populations can create problems in diagnosing dementia, and one of the most prevalent of these is language. Gilman et al. (140) reported that among Asian older populations language differences is one of the 60 most common reasons for avoidance of health care services as well as errors in diagnosis. Lacayo (141) found that in the older populations, 94% of Cuban-Americans, 91% of mainland Puerto Ricans, 86% of Mexican-Americans, and 76% of Hispanics speak Spanish as their principal language. These persons usually have difficulty communicating with primarily English-speaking health care providers, and this often makes it difficult for the provider to use standard screening instruments. Language barriers can lead to diagnostic errors and misinterpretation of the symptoms of dementia (142). Language problems are compounded when untrained translators such as family members are used: translator bias, poor understanding of terminology, and inaccurate paraphrasing are but a few of the possible difficulties (143). However, because of the diversity of languages and sub-

tleties of language groups such as those found in Asians and Pacific Islanders, there are often few alternatives to using younger family members as translators (144).

Education

The United States Census reported that the population of Hispanics aged 65 and older has the highest proportion of persons (63%) with 8 years or less of formal education (2). This compares with 52% of elderly African-Americans, 46% of Native Americans, and contrasts with 24% of elderly whites and 32% of Asians and Pacific Islanders. Furthermore, it has been estimated that nearly two in five Spanish- and Asian-language-speaking elders are linguistically isolated; i.e., in their households no one aged 14 or over speaks English fluently. Therefore, standard written or verbal questions and phrases used by health professionals to assess health status may elicit inaccurate responses from elderly Hispanics, African-Americans, and Native Americans. Also, the educational bias of many dementia screening instruments such as the MMSE may compound these problems by eliciting inappropriate responses from the patient who is subject to language barriers (144–146).

CONCLUSION

Understanding the features of an ethnically diverse group of older adults provides a basis for the care of older members of minority groups. The diversity in the older population presents a challenge in understanding the differences in mortality and morbidity, especially from chronic diseases. Special attention to the differences in dementia screening, functional assessment, and treatment allows physicians to handle the challenges in caring for this population.

REFERENCES

1. US Bureau of the Census. Statistical Abstract of the United States, 1996. 116th ed. Washington: US Bureau of the Census, 1996.
2. US Bureau of the Census. Population Projections of the United States, by Age, Sex, Race and Hispanic Origin: 1992–2050. Current Population Reports, Series p25–1092. Washington: US Government Printing Office, 1993.
3. Miles TP, Bernard MA. Morbidity, disability, and the

health status of black American elderly: a new look at the oldest-old. J Am Geriatr Soc 1992;40:1047–1054.

4. Markides KS. Mortality among minority populations: a review of recent patterns and trends. Public Health Rep 1983;98:252–260.

5. US Bureau of the Census. Coverage of the Hispanic Population of the United States in the 1970 Census: Current Population Reports. Special Studies. Series p23, no 82. Washington: US Government Printing Office, 1979.

6. Rosenwaike I. Mortality differentials among persons born in Cuba, Mexico, and Puerto Rico residing in the United States, 1979–81. Am J Public Health 1987;77:603–606.

7. Wild SH, Laws A, Fortmann SP, et al. Mortality for coronary heart disease and stroke for six ethnic groups in California, 1985 to 1990. Ann Epidemiol 1995;5:432–439.

8. Rogot E, Sorlie PD, Johnson NJ, Schmitt C. A Mortality Study of 1.3 Million Persons by Demographic, Social and Economic Factors: 1979–1985 Follow-up. U.S. National Longitudinal Mortality Study (NIH 92–3297). Washington: National Institutes of Health, July 1992.

9. Espino DV, Parra EO, Kriehbiel R. Mortality differences between elderly Mexican Americans and non-Hispanic whites in San Antonio, Texas: 1989. J Am Geriatr Soc 1994;42:604–608.

10. Fillenbaum GG, Hughes GC, Heyman A, et al. Relationship of health and demographic characteristics to Mini-Mental State Examination score among community residents. Psychol Med 1988;18:719–726.

11. Baker FM. Mental health issues in elderly African-Americans. Clin Geriat Med 1995;11:1–13.

12. de la Monte SM, Hutchins GM, Moore GW. Racial differences in the etiology of dementia and frequency of Alzheimer lesion in the brain. J Natl Med Assoc 1989; 81:644–652.

13. Advisory Panel on Alzheimer's Disease. Fourth Report on the Advisory Panel on Alzheimer's Disease, 1992 (National Institutes of Health 93–3520). Washington: US Government Printing Office, 1993.

14. Majurin R, Espino DV, Lichtenstein MJ, et al. Point-prevalence of cognitive impairment in the Southwest U.S. Mexican American elderly population: a large scale community survey using the Mini-Mental State Examination. J Gerontol (in press).

15. White L, Petrovich H, Ross GW, et al. Prevalence of dementia in older Japanese-American men in Hawaii: The Honolulu-Asia aging study. JAMA 1996;276:955–960.

16. Graves AB, Larson EB, Edland SD, et al. Prevalence of dementia and its subtypes in the Japanese American population of King County, Washington state: the KAME project. Am J Epidemiol 1996;144:760–771.

17. Lin TY. Psychiatry and Chinese culture. West J Med 1983;139:862–867.

18. Robins LN, Reiger DA, eds. Psychiatric disorders in America: the epidemiologic catchment area study. New York: Free Press, 1991.

19. Gardner P, Hudson BL. Advance Report of Final Mortality Statistics, 1995. In: Monthly Vital Statistics Report. Hyattsville, MD: National Center for Health Statistics, 1996;44 (7):12–28.

20. Rosenthal MP, Goldfarb NJ, Carlson BL, et al. Assessment of depression in a family practice center. J Fam Pract 1987;25:143–148.

21. Munoz E. Care for the Hispanic poor: a growing segment of American society. JAMA 1988;260:2711–2712.

22. Kemp BS, Staples FR, Lopez-Aqueres W. Epidemiology of depression and dysphoria in an elderly Hispanic population. J Am Geriatr Soc 1987;35:920–926.

23. Regier DA, Burke JD. Psychiatric disorders in the community: the epidemiologic catchment area study. In: Psychiatry Update: The American Psychiatric Association Annual Review. Washington: American Psychiatric Press, 1987;6:610–624.

24. Liu WT, Yu E. Asian/Pacific American Elderly: mortality differentials, health status and the use of health services. J Appl Gerontol 1985;4:35–64.

25. Lum OM. Health status of Asians and Pacific Islanders. Clin Geriatr Med 1995;11:53–67.

26. Foley DJ, Fillenbaum G, Service C. Physical functioning. In: Cornoni-Huntley JC, Blazer DG, et al., eds. Established Populations for Epidemiologic Studies of the Elderly, vol 2: Resource Data Book (NIH 90–495). Washington: National Institutes of Health, 1990:34–50.

27. Edmonds MK. Physical health. In: Jackson LS, Chatters LM, Taylor RJ, eds. Aging in Black America. Newbury Park, CA: Sage, 1993:151–167.

28. Andrews J. Poverty and Poor Health Among Elderly Hispanic Americans. Baltimore: Commonwealth Fund Commission, 1989.

29. Markides KS, Stroup-Benham, CA, Goodwin JS, et al. The effect of medical conditions on the functional limitations of Mexican American elderly. Ann Epidemiol 1996;6:386–391.

30. Espino DV, Neufeld RR, Mulvihill MK, Libow LS. Hispanic and non-Hispanic elderly on admission to the nursing home: a pilot study. Gerontologist 1988;28:821–824.

31. Chiodo LK, Karren DW, Gerety MB, et al. Functional status of Mexican American nursing home residents. J Am Geriatr Soc 1994;42:293–296.

32. Rudkin L, Markides KS, Espino DV. Functional limitations in elderly Mexican Americans. Top Geriatr Rehab 1997;12:38–46.

33. Katz S, Ford AB, Moskowitz RW, et al. Studies of illness in the aged: the index of ADL: a standardized measure of biological and psychosocial function. JAMA 1963: 185:914–919.

34. Katz S, Downs TD, Cash HR, Grotz RC. Progress in the development of the index of ADL. Gerontologist 1970; 10:20–30.

35. Tinetti ME. Performance-oriented assessment of mobility problems in elderly patients. J Am Geriatr Soc 1986;34:119–126.

36. Lawton MP, Brody EM. Assessment of older people: self-maintaining and instrumental activities of daily living. Gerontologist 1969;9:179–186.

37. Spector WD. Functional disability scales. In: Spilker B, ed. Quality of Life Assessments in Clinical Trial. New York: Raven, 1990.

38. Williams ME, Hornberger JC. A quantitative method of

identifying older persons at risk for increasing long-term care services. J Chronic Cis 1984;37:705–711.

39. Schappert SM. National Ambulatory Medical Care Survey: 1992 summary. Division of Health Statistics, National Center for Health Statistics. Advance Data 1994; 253:1–20.

40. Espino DV, Burge SK, Moreno CA. The prevalence of selected chronic diseases among Mexican-American elderly: data from 1982–84 Hispanic Health and Nutrition Examination Survey. J Am Board Fam Pract 1991; 5:319–321.

41. Markides KS, Rudkin L, Angel RJ, Espino DV. Health status of Hispanic elderly in the United States. In: Martin LG, Soldo BJ, Foote KA, eds. Racial and Ethnic Differences in Late Life in the United States. Washington: National Academy of Sciences, 1996 (in press).

42. Garn SM, Pozanski AK, Larsen K. Metacarpal length, cortical diameters and areas from the 10-state nutrition survey. In: Jaworski ZFG, ed. Proceedings of the First Workshop on Bone Morphology. Ottawa: University of Ottawa Press, 1976:367–391.

43. Trotter M, Hixon BB. Sequential analysis in weight, density, and percentage ash weight of human skeletons from an early fetal period through old age. Anat Rec 1974;179:1–18.

44. Jacobsen SJ, Goldberg J. Miles TP, et al. Hip fracture incidence among the old and very old: a population-based study of 745,435 cases. Am J Public Health 1990;80: 871–873.

45. Farmer ME, White LR, Brody JA, Bailey KR. Race and sex differences in hip fracture incidence. Am J Public Health 1984;74:1374–1380.

46. Bauer RL. Ethnic differences in hip fractures: a reduced incidence in Mexican Americans. Am J Epidemiol 1988; 127:145–149.

47. Bauer RL, Diehl AK, Barton SA, et al. Risk of postmenopausal hip fractures in Mexican American women. Am J Public Health 1986;76:1020–1021.

48. Harris MI, Hadden WC, Knowler WC, Bennett PH. Prevalence of diabetes and impaired glucose tolerance and plasma glucose levels in US population aged 20–74 yrs. Diabetes 1987;36:523–534.

49. Polednak AP. Mortality from diabetes mellitus and ischemic heart disease among blacks in a higher income area. Public Health Rep 1990;105:393–399.

50. Trends in diabetes mellitus mortality. MMWR Morbid Mortal Wkly Rep 1988;37:769–773.

51. Markides KS, Coreil J. The health of Hispanics in the southwestern United States: an epidemiologic paradox. Public Health Rep 1986;101:253–265.

52. Gohdes D, Kaufman S, Valway SE. Diabetes in American Indians. Diabetes Care 1993;16(suppl):239–245.

53. Heath SW, Orneal R, Marquat C. An action plan for American Indian and Alaska Native Elders. IHS Primary Care Provider 1993;18:81–83.

54. Newman JM, DeStefano F, Valway SE, et al. Diabetes-associated mortality in Native Americans. Diabetes Care 1993;16:297–304.

55. Burchfiel CM, Curb JD, Rodriquez BL, et al. Incidence and predictors of diabetes in Japanese American men: the Honolulu Heart Program. Ann Epidemiol 1995;5:33–43.

56. Hara H, Egusa G, Yamakido M. Incidence of non-insulin-dependent diabetes mellitus and its risk factors in Japanese-Americans living in Hawaii and Los Angeles. Diabet Med 1996;13(suppl 6):S133–S142.

57. Choi ES, McGandy RB, Dallal GE, et al. The prevalence of cardiovascular risk factors among elderly Chinese Americans. Arch Intern Med 1990;150:413–418.

58. Lipson LG, Kato-Palmer S. Asian Americans. Diabetes Forecast 1988;41:48–51.

59. Birrer RB. Urban family medicine: lost horizon or last frontier? Am Fam Pract 1992;46:1074–1076.

60. Wassertheil-Smoller S, Apostolides A, Miller M, et al. Recent status of detection, treatment, and control of hypertension in the community. J Community Health 1979;5:82–93.

61. Materson BJ, Reda DJ, Cushman WC, et al. Single-drug therapy for hypertension in men: a comparison of six antihypertensive agents with placebo. N Engl J Med 1993;328:914–921.

62. Hypertension prevalence and status of awareness, treatment, and control in the United States: final report of the subcommittee on the definition and prevalence of the 1984 joint national committee. Hypertension 1985;7: 457–468.

63. Shetterly SM, Rewers M, Hamman RF, Marshall JA. Patterns and predictors of hypertension incidence among Hispanics and non-Hispanic whites: the San Luis Valley Diabetes Study. J Hypertension 1994;12:1095–1712.

64. Gillum RF. Epidemiology of stroke in Hispanic Americans. Stroke 1995;26:1707–1712.

65. Bruno A, Carter S, Qualls C, Nolte KB. Incidence of intracerebral hemorrhage among Hispanics and non-Hispanic whites in New Mexico. Ethnicity Dis 1997;7:27–33.

66. Chao A, Becker TM, Jordan SW, Darling R, Gilliland FD, Key CR. Decreasing rates of cervical cancer among American Indians and Hispanics in New Mexico (United States). Cancer Causes Control 1996;7:205–213.

67. Cubillos, H, Prieto M. The Hispanic Elderly: A Demographic Profile. Washington: National Council of La Raza, 1978.

68. Douglass M, Bartolucci A, Waterbor J, Sirles A. Breast cancer early detection: differences between African-American and White women's health beliefs and detection practices. Oncol Nurs Forum 1995;22:835–837.

69. Ansell D, Whitman S, Lipton R, Cooper R. Race, income, and survival from breast cancer at two public hospitals. Cancer 1993;72:2974–2978.

70. Wells BL, Horm JW. Stage at diagnosis in breast cancer: race and socioeconomic factors. Am J Public Health 1992;82:1383–1385.

71. Gordon NH, Crowe JP, Brumberg DJ, Berger NA. Socioeconomic factors and race in breast cancer recurrence and survival. Am J Epidemiol 1992;135:609–618.

72. Cella DF, Orav EJ, Kornblith AB, et al. Socioeconomic status and cancer survival. J Clin Oncol 1991;9:1500–1509.

73. Foster RS, Costanza MC. Breast self-examination and breast cancer survival. Cancer 1984;53:999–1005.

74. Fox SA, Stein JA. The effect of physician-patient communication on mammography utilization by different ethnic groups. Med Care 1991;29:1065–1082.

75. Stanford JL, Herrington LJ, Schwartz SM, Weiss NS. Breast cancer incidence in Asian migrants to the United States and their descendants. Epidemiology 1995;6: 181–183.

76. Moul JW, Sesterhern IA, Connelly RR, et al. Prostate-specific antigen values at the time of prostate cancer diagnosis in African-American men. JAMA 1995;274: 1277–1281.

77. Woolf SH, Lawrence RS. The physical examination: where to look for preclinical disease. In: Woolf SH, Jonas S, Lawrence RS, eds. Health Promotion and Disease Prevention in Clinical Practice. Baltimore: Williams & Wilkins, 1996.

78. An assessment of the effectiveness of 169 interventions. In: Guide to Clinical Preventive Services. Report to the U.S. Preventive Services Task Force. Baltimore: Williams & Wilkins, 1989.

79. American Cancer Society. Guidelines for the cancer-related checkup: recommendations and rationale. Cancer 1980;30:4.

80. National Cancer Institute. Working Guidelines for Early Detection: Rationale and Supportive Evidence to Decrease Mortality. Bethesda, MD: National Cancer Institute, 1987.

81. Danley KL, Richardson JL, Bernstein L, et al. Prostate cancer: trends in mortality and stage-specific incidence rates by racial/ethnic group in Los Angeles County, California. Cancer Cause Control 1995;6:492–498.

82. Yu ES. Health on the Chinese elderly in America. Res Aging 1986;8:84–109.

83. Bernstein L, Miu A, Monroe K, et al. Cancer incidence among Filipinos in Los Angeles County, 1972–1991. Int J Cancer 1995;63:345–348.

84. Krause N, Wray LA. Psychosocial correlates of health and illness among minority elders. In: Stanton EP, Torres-Gil FM, eds. Diversity: New Approaches to Ethnic Minority Aging. Amityville, NY: Baywood, 1992.

85. Mouton CP, Johnson MS, Cole DR. Ethical considerations with African-American elders. Clin Geriatr Med 1995;11:113–129.

86. National Comparative Survey of Minority Health Care. New York: Commonwealth Fund, 1995.

87. Die AH, Seelbach WE. Problems, sources assistance and knowledge of services among elderly Vietnamese immigrants. Gerontologist 1988;28:448.

88. Jackson LS, Chatters LM, Taylor RJ. Aging in African-American America. Newbury Park, CA: Sage, 1993.

89. Reed W. Health care needs and services. In: Harel Z, McKinney EA, Williams M, eds. African-American Aged: Understanding Diversity and Service Needs. Newbury Park, CA: Sage, 1990.

90. Dowd JJ, Bengston VL. Aging in minority populations: an examination of the double jeopardy hypothesis. J Gerontol 1978;33:427–436.

91. Jackson M, Kolody B, Wood JL. To be old and African-American: the case for the double jeopardy on income and health. In: Manuel RC, ed. Minority Aging: Sociological and Social Psychological Issues. Westport, CT: Greenwood, 1982.

92. Ferraro KF. Double jeopardy to health for African-American older adults? J Gerontol 1987;42:528–533.

93. Ross GW, Abbott RD, Petrovitch H, et al. Frequency and characteristics of silent dementia among elderly Japanese-American men. JAMA 1997;277:800–805.

94. Brody SJ, Poulshock SW, Masciocchi CF. The family caring unit: a major consideration in the long-term support system. Gerontology 1978;18:556–561.

95. Strong C. Stress and caring for elderly relatives: Interpretations and coping strategies in an American Indian and white sample. Gerontologist 1984;24:251–256.

96. Cantor M. The informal support system of New York's inner city elderly: is ethnicity a factor? In: Gelfand DE, Kutsik AJ, eds. Ethnicity and Aging: Theory, Research and Policy. New York: Springer, 1979:153–174.

97. Mutran E. Intergenerational family support among blacks and whites: response to culture or socioeconomic differences. J Gerontol 1985;40:382–389.

98. Miner S. Racial differences in family support and formal service utilization among older persons: a nonrecursive model. J Gerontol Soc Sci 1995;50B:S143–S153.

99. Chatters LM, Taylor RJ, Jackson JS. Aged blacks' choices for an informal helper network. J Gerontol 1986;41:94–100.

100. Lawton MP, Rajagopal D, Brody E, Kleban MH. The dynamics of caregiving for a demented elder among black and white families. J Gerontol Soc Sci 1992;47:S156–S164.

101. Fredman L, Daly MP, Lazur AM. Burden among white and black caregivers to elderly adults. J Gerontol Soc Sci 1995;50B:S110–S118.

102. Hanson SL, Sauer WJ, Seelbach WC. Racial and cohort variations in filial responsibility norms. Gerontologist 1983;23:626–631.

103. Montiel M. Chicanos in the United States: An overview of socio-historical context and emerging perspectives. In: Montiel M, ed. Hispanic Families. Washington: National Coalition of Hispanic Mental Health and Human Service Organizations, 1978.

104. Erbes RA, Bradley-Rawls M. The underutilization of nursing home facilities by Mexican-American elderly in the Southwest. Gerontologist 1978;18:363–371.

105. Greene VL, Monahan DJ. Comparative utilization of community based long term care services by Hispanic and Anglo elderly in a case management system. J Gerontol 1984;39:730–735.

106. Espino DV. Medication usage in elderly Hispanics: what we need to know. In: Sotomayor M, Ascencio NR, eds. Proceedings on Improving Drug Use Among Hispanic Elderly. Washington: National Hispanic Council on Aging, 1988:7–11.

107. Cox C, Monk A. Minority caregivers of dementia victims: a comparison of black and Hispanic families. J Appl Gerontol 1990;9:340–354.

108. Talamantes MA, Cornell J, Espino DV, et al. SES and ethnic differences in perceived caregiver availability

among young-old Mexican Americans and Non-Hispanic whites. Gerontologist 1996;36:88–99.

109. Manson S, Gallaway DG. Health and aging among
American Indians. In: Harper MS, ed. Minority Aging:
Essential Curricula Content for Selected Health and Al-
lied Health Professions (DHHS HRS P-DK-90-4).
Washington: US Government Printing Office, 1990.

110. Koh JY, Bell WG. Korean elders in the United States: intergenerational relations and living arrangements.
Gerontologist 1987;27:66–71.

111. Crystal, S, Shea D. The economic well-being of the elderly. Rev Income Wealth 1990;36:227–247.

112. Shea DG, Miles TP, Hayward M. The health-wealth
connection: racial differences. Gerontologist 1996;36:
342–349.

113. Minority Elders: Longevity, Economics, and Health.
Building a Public Policy Base. Washington: Gerontological Society of America, 1991.

114. Hubbell FA, Waitzkin H, Mishra SI, Dombrink J. Evaluating health-care needs of the poor: a community-oriented approach. Am J Med 1989;87:127–131.

115. Freeman HE, Aiken LH, Blendon RJ, Corey CR. Uninsured working-age adults: characteristics and consequences. Health Serv Res 1990;24:811–823.

116. Lopez-Aqueres W, Kemp B, Plopper M, et al. Health
needs of the Hispanic elderly. J Am Geriatr Soc 1984;
32:191–198.

117. Churchill LR. Health care, social justice and the elderly.
N C Med J 1987;48:587.

118. Maldonado D. The Hispanic Elderly: Vulnerability in
Old Age. Draft, Southern Methodist University, 1988.

119. Baker FM. Psychiatric treatment of older African Americans. Hosp Community Psychiatry 1994;45:32–37.

120. Brangman SA. African-American elders: Implications for
health care providers. Clin Geriatr Med 1995;11:15–23.

121. Health and Public Policy Committee. Long-term care of
the elderly. American College of Physicians. Ann Intern
Med 1984;100:760–763.

122. Miranda M, Ruiz RA. Chicano Aging and Mental Health.
Washington: US Department of Health and Human Services, 1981;273–274.

123. Rhoades ER. Profile of American Indians and Alaska Natives. In: MS Harper, ed. Minority Aging: Essential Curricula Content for Selected Health and Allied Health
Professions (DHHS HRS P-DV-90-4). Washington: US
Government Printing Office, 1990:45–62.

124. Beisecker AE. Aging and the desire for information and
input in medical decisions: patient-consumerism in
medical encounters. Gerontologist 1988;28:330–335.

125. Carp FM. Communicating with elderly Mexican Americans. Gerontologist 1970;10:126–134.

126. Satcher D. Does race interfere with the doctor-patient
relationship? JAMA 1973;223:1498–1499.

127. Marsh WW, Hentges K. Mexican folk remedies and
conventional medical care. Am Fam Pract 1988;37:
257–262.

128. Valle R, Martinez C. Natural Network of Elderly Latinos
of Mexican Heritage: Implications for Mental Health in
Chicano Aging and Mental. Washington: US Department of Health, Education and Welfare, 1980:27–31.

129. Kreisman JJ. The curandero's apprentice: a therapeutic
integration of folk and medical healing. Am J Psychiatry 1975;132:81–83.

130. Gratton B, Wilson V. Family support systems and the
minority elderly; a cautionary analysis. J Gerontol Soc
Work 1988;13:81–93.

131. Adelman RD, Greene MG, Charon R, Friedmann E.
The content of physician and elderly patient interaction
in the medical primary care encounter. Community
Res 1992;19:370–380.

132. Clark JA, Potter DA, McKinlay JB. Bringing social structure back into clinical decision making. Soc Sci Med
1991;32:853–866.

133. Haug MR. Doctor-patient relationships and the older
patient. J Gerontol 1979;34:852–860.

134. Haug MR, Ory MG. Issues in elder patient-provider interactions. Res Aging 1987;9:39–44.

135. Beisecker AE. Aging and the desire for information and
input in medical decisions: patient consumerism in
medical encounter. Gerontologist 1988;28:330–335.

136. Beisecker AE, Beisecker TD. Patient information-seeking
behaviors when communicating with doctors. Medical
Care 1990;28:19–28.

137. Hall JA, Roter DL, Katz NR. Meta-analysis of correlates
of provider behavior in medical encounters. Med Care
1988;26:657–675.

138. Adams PL. Black patients and white doctors. Urban
Health 1977;1:21–23.

139. Espino DV, Maldonado D. Hypertension and acculturation in elderly Mexican Americans: results from 1982–
84 Hispanic HANES. J Gerontol 1990;45:M209–
M213.

140. Gilman SC, Justice J, Saepharn K, et al. Use of traditional and modern health services by Laotian refugees.
West J Med 1992;157:310.

141. Lacayo CG. A national study to assess the service of the
Hispanic elderly. Los Angeles: Asociación Nacional Por
Personas Mayores, 1980.

142. Lum O. Health status of Asians and Pacific Islanders.
Clin Geriatr Med 1995;11:53–67.

143. Putsch RW. Cross-cultural communication: The special case for interpreters in health care. JAMA 1985;
254:3344–3348.

144. Haffner L. Translation is not enough: interpreting in a
medical setting. West J Med 1992;157:255.

145. Escobar JI, Burnam A, Karno M, et al. Use of Mini-Mental State Examination (MMSE) in a community population of mixed ethnicity. Cultural and linguistic arti-
facts. J Nerv Ment Dis 1986;174:607–614.

146. Murden RA, McRae TD, Kaner S, et al. Mini-Mental
State Examination scores vary with education in blacks
and whites. J Am Geriatr Soc 1991;39:149–155.

CHAPTER 47

STEVE ILIFFE (THE UNITED KINGDOM), DUNCAN ROBERTSON (CANADA),
MASAKI YOSHIKAWA (JAPAN), AND WILLIAM REICHEL (COMMENTARY ON JAPAN)

Care of the Elderly in Three Nations

THE UNITED KINGDOM

The medical and social care of older people in the community in Britain depends on six agencies, each with its own perspectives, work cultures, and agendas. In order of importance, they are as follows:

1. Older people themselves, their families, and their social networks of friends and neighbors
2. Social services organized and financed by local government
3. Community nursing and other clinical services provided by the National Health Service (NHS)
4. General practitioners working under contract with the NHS
5. Hospital specialists in medicine for the elderly (geriatrics) and old-age psychiatry (psychogeriatrics)
6. Commercial residential and nursing homes operating a mixed economy of individual payment and state subsidy

This chapter explains how these services collaborate for the benefit of their patients and clients and points to new developments that may overcome remaining problems in the care of older people. First, is a brief introduction of each of the key agencies.

OLDER PEOPLE THEMSELVES

Older people themselves, with their families, their neighbors, their social and cultural organizations (especially churches, mosques, and temples) and voluntary organizations such as Age Concern, Help the Aged, and the Alzheimer's Disease Society, make the greatest contribution of all of the key agencies to the medical and nursing care of ill or disabled older people. Families are the traditional caregivers for ill older people (1) and remain so, often at great cost to themselves (2). Although disability increases in prevalence during the eighth decade of life (3), the majority of older people are relatively well. Among those aged 75 and over, one quarter take no medication on a regular basis, about a third need medication regularly to control medical problems, and the remainder have multiple medical problems and use three or more medicines on a regular basis (4). About 80% can get out of their homes without assistance from others, and 95% can move about within their own homes independently. Their main difficulties are with bathing and foot care, particularly cutting nails (5). This large group of retired citizens plays an important social and economic role in providing care for others, including child care, voluntary work in hospitals and in the community, and care for ill family members or neighbors. The economic relation between older people and their social networks is not simple dependency of old on young, but instead a complex pattern of exchanges that only sometimes shifts toward younger people being the predominant givers (6). Their importance has been recognized—belatedly—by government, which has focused the attention of social and medical services through the Carers Act of 1995. That law offers special support to older people caring for others, giving them a statutory right to have their needs assessed by social services alongside those for whom they care.

Voluntary organizations are particularly powerful sources of information, education, and support. The Alzheimer's Disease Society, for example, has local branches that work to increase public awareness of Alzheimer's disease, raise funds for research, contribute to training of professionals working with Alzheimer patients, run support groups for people caring for persons with dementia, and in some places provide assistance in the home for families. Age Concern has a similar role in providing care at the local level, initiating user involvement in the development of local services and campaigning on behalf of older people.

SOCIAL SERVICES

Social services are provided by local government according to defined criteria of need, usually with some financial contribution from the older person who uses them. Their history is well documented elsewhere (7). These services provide home care, sources of information, and institutional support of the frail elderly:

- Help with work in the home (cleaning, shopping)
- Help with personal care (especially bathing)
- Aids to daily living (adaptations to the home, such as stair rails, showers in place of baths, elevated chairs that assist people to rise to their feet)
- Communication systems and alarms that allow people living alone to contact emergency services easily
- Financial benefits to those who have low incomes or are looking after ill or disabled relatives
- Clubs and social activities, including physical activity programs (fitness classes)
- Access to residential care in nursing homes for short-term relief of caregivers or for longer-term care

- Places in day care centers mainly for disabled people wanting social and sometimes therapeutic activities

Local government also controls access to subsidized transport: cheap bus fares, use of taxis at subsidized costs, and dedicated bus services for disabled people. Local governments have had less and less money to spend during the past decade, with the result that these services have decreased or have been means tested, making older people pay for some services, such as home help and personal care. The organization of social care has also been moved onto a market basis, so that local government social service departments now buy services for older people from private agencies instead of providing services directly. As a consequence there is increasing geographic variability in the quantity and quality of social care available to older people and emerging evidence of underprovision (8).

COMMUNITY NURSING

Community nurses work for the National Health Service and are employed by local organizations (hospital or community trusts) that are separate from local government. They provide nursing care in the home at the request of general practitioners or hospital specialists. This home nursing care may be complex, providing care at a level comparable with that of a hospital ward (hospital at home), or very specialized, providing care for those who are dying (terminal care nurses are called Macmillan nurses, and the service they provide is hospice at home) or for those with mental health problems (community psychiatric nurses).

The workload of community nurses, which is focused on older people, includes daily care for those with disabilities so severe that they are unable to look after themselves unaided. Community nurses also care for patients discharged from hospital after operations, and this task is increasing in importance because patients do not stay long in hospital, 6 to 7 days on average after emergency admission for major illnesses, up to 11 days after hip replacement. Community nurses are well trained in assessment of disability and usually have good working relations with social services, unlike their general practitioner colleagues.

GENERAL PRACTITIONERS

General practitioners are doctors who provide medical care for people of all ages within a small locality. They are not employed by the National Health Service, but they have contracts with it. People register with a general practitioner, who acts as a gatekeeper to medical specialists. General practitioners must have 3 years' special training in a wide range of medical disciplines, including care of older people, before they can work in the community. There are 33,000 general practitioners, and on average each general practitioner has 1,900 registered patients, of whom on average about 130 are aged 75 and over. Most general practitioners work in groups, with the average group size being three or four. General practitioners must provide services for their patients 24 hours a day, every day of the year, and at nights and weekends many transfer their responsibility of care to a local cooperative of doctors. This general medical care is provided in a clinic or in the patient's home if he or she cannot come to the clinic, and the doctor may be assisted by nurses and psychologists. General practitioners are paid a fixed sum each year for each person who is registered with them, which is higher for those aged 65 and over than for younger people. Each year every general practitioner must invite every patient aged 75 and over to have a health review in the patient's home. This review must include assessment of *sensory functions, especially sight and hearing; mobility and the need for aids to mobility; mental condition; physical condition, including continence; social support and environment; and medication use.*

Unfortunately the majority of general practitioners are ill-equipped do this very well, so the potential for improving the health of older people and their quality of life is not realized. Where these assessments are done at all, they are delegated to nurses and given relatively low priority. There is little evidence of innovative, imaginative service development (10). The reasons for this reluctance are complex but include among some doctors the belief that nothing much can be done for disabling problems such as depression, dementia, and ar-

thritis. As a whole general practitioners have limited contact with and understanding of social services, which results in avoidable inefficiencies in providing and coordinating care (11). This assessment program has not been given high priority by the NHS, and little effort is made to help general practitioners to carry it out (12).

HOSPITAL SPECIALISTS

Older people have access through their general practitioners to specialists in the care of the elderly (geriatricians) in every district. Many (but not yet all) districts also have psychiatrists who specialize in old age psychiatry (psycho-geriatricians). Hospital specialists in medicine for older people head multidisciplinary teams and run outpatient clinics, wards for acutely ill older people, rehabilitation services, and in some cases also have some long-stay beds for those who cannot be looked after at home (13). They may visit ill people in their home, but only at the request of the general practitioner, and may also run day hospitals for assessment of ill older people and for their rehabilitation after acute illnesses (14).

NURSING HOMES

Commercial residential and nursing homes provide care for older people with long-term illness and disability. They have taken over the main role of providing continuing care for very frail old people from NHS hospitals, most of which have closed their wards for long-term care, and from local governments, which have reduced the number of long-stay homes (15). The costs of care in commercial nursing homes may be paid in part by the government and in part by the patient or his or her family. This has created a problem for some older people, who have been forced to sell their house to pay for their own care instead of passing the house to their children, and this in turn has fueled debate about how best to provide long-term care for frail older people (16).

RECENT SUCCESSES

Recent successes in providing care for older people in Britain include the emergence of geriatric medicine as a powerful specialty and the replacement of large, impersonal institutions for the frail elderly with smaller community-based residential homes. The rapid growth of high-quality specialist medical services in hospitals during the 1970s and 1980s brought effective curative medicine to older people on a wider scale than previously and is helping to overcome the still widespread belief that older people cannot benefit from advanced and high-technology medicine and surgery (17). Age barriers to treatment are being removed, and health promotion activities are being designed for people up to the early or mid 80s in hypertension control, smoking cessation, and physical activity.

An increase in the number of community-based residential homes for frail elderly people has occurred in the same period. Most of these homes are small, allowing frail and chronically ill people to stay close to their family and neighborhood instead of being moved to a large hospital some distance away, although the continuing concerns about their funding may undermine the benefits of their human scale. The successes have enormously helped older people with serious illness and disability and cannot be underestimated. However, those with less severe but still significant problems, who remain in their own homes and do not need so much specialist medical care, have not benefited so much. The remaining problems in the provision of medical and social services for older people in Britain are mainly problems of caring for people in the community.

The limitation in resources of local government is leading to rationing of care and the introduction of charges to patients by social services. These may prevent older people with low incomes or with relatively moderate problems from obtaining services. Such people may seek help from the NHS because it is free, only to find that it cannot meet their needs. Frail older people may be admitted to hospitals when they could be cared for at home, but lack of resources in local government prevents the deployment of the necessary social services. The result is bed blocking in acute hospital wards for lack of affordable long-term care facilities. The slow, uneven development of quality care for older people in general practice has been slow and uneven. General practitioners provide services according to public demand, and older people may be less demanding than younger for the following reasons:

- Many elders have low expectations and believe that their illness or disability is normal for their age.
- Many elders are more respectful toward doctors and nurses than younger people and believe that there is "always someone worse off than I am."
- Many elders are less mobile and have more communication difficulties than the young and middle-aged because of arthritis, cardiovascular disease, deafness, and so on.

This results in bias toward younger, relatively well people and against older people. A change in approach is under way in general practice, with attention to need rather than demand being emphasized, but such change is necessarily slow. The rate of change could increase if greater political priority were to be given to the health of older people living in the community by the NHS.

The different organization of services can cause inefficiencies in organization and poor coordination, so that the quality of service deteriorates. Innovative mechanisms, or possibly even a single organizational structure for all provider agencies, are needed to allow general practitioners, community nurse, social services, and medical specialists to work together efficiently for the maximum benefit of their patients.

CONCLUSIONS

Many attempts are being made to overcome these problems, making work with older people one of the most dynamic and exciting areas of medical care. The biggest obstacle to high-quality, efficient, and humane care for ill older people is probably the limited funding of local government, and this must be overcome in the next decade if the problems of an aging population are to be dealt with effectively. The issue of coordination of services is being approached from different directions, with experiments to bring together social care workers and general practitioners and to extend health promotion through collaborative work between general practitioners, specialists, and community nurses. Although we are beginning to understand that the health of older people has great importance to the whole of society, we do not yet understand how much change must take place in the attitudes of professionals, in the way in which money is spent on health and social care, and in the ways that we work together on a daily basis. Britain has a good track record in developing medical care for an aging population, but we still have much to do.

REFERENCES

1. Townsend P, Wedderburn D. The Aged in the Welfare State. London: Bell, 1996.
2. Jones DA. A survey of carers of elderly dependents living in the community. Cardiff: University College of Wales, College of Medicine, 1986.
3. Martin J, Meltzer H, Elliot D. The Prevalence of Disability Among Adults. London: Her Majesty's Stationery Office, 1989 (OPCS Surveys of Disability in Great Britain, report 1).
4. Iliffe S. Medication review for older people in general practice. J R Soc Med 1994;87(suppl 23):11–13.
5. Victor C. Old Age in Modern Society: A Textbook of Social Gerontology. Beckenham, UK: Croom Helm, 1987.
6. Arber S. Is living longer a cause for celebration? Health Serv J 1996;106:28–31.
7. Lawson R, Davies B, Bebbington A. The home help service in England and Wales. In: Jamieson A, ed. Home Care for Older People in Europe: A Comparison of Policies and Practices. Oxford: Oxford Medical, 1991:63–98.
8. Walker A. Community care: past, present and future. In: Munro J, Iliffe S. Healthy Choices: Future Options for the NHS. London: Lawrence & Wishart, 1997:178–200.
9. Idris Williams E. Caring for Elderly People in the Community. London: Chapman and Hall, 1989.
10. Iliffe S, Gould MM, Wallace P. Evaluation of the 75 and over checks in general practice: Report to the NHS Executive. London: Department of Primary Care & Population Sciences, Royal Freel Hospital School of Medicine, 1996.
11. Huntington J. Social work and general medical practice: collaboration or conflict? London: George Allen & Unwin, 1991.
12. Glendenning C, Chew C, Wilkin D. GP Assessments of Patients Aged 75 and Over: the Views of FHSA Managers. Manchester, UK: Centre for Primary Care Research, University of Manchester, 1997.
13. Ensuring Equity and Equality of Care for Elderly People. London: Royal College of Physicians, 1994.
14. Geriatric Day Hospitals: Their Role and Guidelines for Good Practice. London: Royal College of Physicians/British Geriatrics Society, 1994.
15. Health Committee third report, volume 1. Long-Term Care, Future Provision and Funding, London: Her Majesty's Stationery Office, 1996.
16. Joseph Rowntree Foundation. Meeting the Costs of Continuing Care: Public Views and Perceptions. London: Social Care Research 84, 1996.
17. The Health of the UK's Elderly Population. London: Medical Research Council, 1994.

CANADA

Canada occupies nearly 4 million square miles (almost 10 million square kilometers) and has a population of about 30 million, more than 85% of whom live within 200 miles (320 kilometers) of Canada's border with the United States. The people of Canada include native North Americans (First Nations and Inuit) and immigrants from all parts of the world. Migration between the 17th and mid 20th centuries was largely from Europe, initially from France and later from Great Britain, and from the United States. Immediately following World War II many migrants came from other European countries, and more recently immigrants and refugees from all parts of the world have added to Canada's ethnic mix. Canada is officially bilingual and multicultural. Of the present elderly population, about 70% speak English and 15% French with 5% speaking neither English, nor French (1). Recent immigration policy has encouraged family reunification, resulting in relocation of older family members of migrants to Canada; this challenges providers of health care to make health and social services accessible to recent older immigrants who may not speak one of the official languages and whose health beliefs and practices may differ from those of other older citizens. In 1967, the centennial year of confederation, Canada was a young country, with half the population aged 25 or under. In Canada, as in most Western nations, declining fertility after the baby boom and increasing life expectancy have resulted in rapid population aging. Population projections that make "medium" assumptions for fertility, mortality, and immigration anticipate that Canada's population will increase from 30 million in 1996 to 40 million in 2041 and that the population aged 65 and older will increase almost threefold in absolute terms. It is projected that by 2041 those over 75 will constitute 14.2% of the population (5.1% in 1991) and those over 85, 4.5% (1.2% in 1991) (1).

Since hospital and medical services fall under provincial rather than federal jurisdiction, one cannot with accuracy speak of a single Canadian health care system. Rather, each of the 10 provinces and 2 territories has its own system of care. The federal Canada Health Act (1984) outlines the principles that govern all provincial and territorial health care services. These principles include universality, accessibility, comprehensiveness, portability, and public administration. Hospital services, primary medical care, and care by specialists are equally accessible to all citizens at no direct cost. In most provinces the costs are covered through general taxation, although some provinces levy modest health care premiums. Several provincial health care plans include chiropractic and other nonmedical services. In some provinces partial coverage of drugs and medical devices is included. Home care support services and long-term care services are not included under the provisions of the Canada Health Act, and no provincial plan covers the full cost of home care or long-term residential care. Most Canadians can get access to some form of home support or home nursing care by making a means-tested personal contribution. The costs of long-term care in a facility such as a chronic hospital or a nursing home in most cases is subsidized by provincial governments, and copayment is required. Long-term care facilities are called by various names in various jurisdictions, and they do not necessarily compare in function with equivalent facilities in the United Kingdom and United States (2). The most commonly used terms are nursing home and chronic (extended care) hospital. Ownership of long-term care facilities may be municipal, denominational, charitable, or private. The private for-profit sector, which is much smaller than in the United States, predominates at the residential or minimal support level of care. In most provinces assessment procedures for admission to a long-term care facility are coordinated at a regional level, and eligible citizens receive subsidized long-term residential care and home nursing care. Individuals may bypass these procedures by paying the full cost of care in private facilities or by contracting directly with private community care providers. Some groups, such as veterans, have access to enhanced community services funded by the federal Veterans Affairs Canada. Income security for older Canadians includes federal old age pensions and income supplements, which until recently were universal programs, i.e., paid to all seniors irrespective of income. Proposed legislation will replace universal pensions with a seniors' benefit that is means tested to direct payments to low-income elders. Seniors who were employed during and after the 1960s have contributed to the Canada Pension or Quebec Pension Plans and receive pensions based on their contributions. Many younger seniors and those approaching retirement have contributed to company or individual pension plans. The very old and women, especially those who have not been employed, are relatively disadvantaged with respect to income.

Most Canadians have a primary care physician, usually a family physician, who manages their primary care and arranges access to specialists by referral. In general, specialists do not engage in primary medical care. The role of the primary care physician in Canadian health care and in care of the elderly warrants particular mention, since it differs from that in other countries (3–5). Family physicians receive certification by the College of Family Physicians of Canada after 2 years of postmedical doctor training. In contrast with the United States, family physicians are numerous, accounting for more than half of medical school graduates. In contrast with some European countries, family physicians usually have hospital admitting privileges, conduct office-based and hospital-based practices, and provide continuing care for their patients when they are admitted to long-term care facilities. This can be a challenge in large urban areas where the patient's choice of long-term care facility may result in a physician having patients resident in 10 or more nursing homes. In some parts of the country family physicians restrict their practices to one or a few long-term care facilities and transfer care of their patients to other doctors when they are admitted elsewhere. Many physicians also act as part-time medical directors or medical coordinators in nursing homes and extended-care hospitals.

Specialists in Canada are certified by the Royal College of Physicians and Surgeons of Canada after 4 to 7 years of postgraduate training. In academic centers some specialists are exclusively hospital based, but most have both hospital- and office-based practices. Elderly patients constitute a large part of the referral practices of many internists, psychiatrists, and subspecialists. Patients are referred to specialists by their family physician, to whom they return for care after consultation and treatment (4).

In 1981 the Royal College of Physicians and Surgeons of Canada recognized geriatric medicine as an area of special competence, based on prior certification in internal medicine. There are now about 150 specialists in geriatric medicine in Canada. Until recently, geriatricians practiced almost exclusively in academic health science centers and large urban areas, but in recent years geriatric services have been established in smaller centers, and a number of geriatric centers provide outreach consultation to remote rural areas. Some specialists in geriatric medicine practice exclusively with the frail elderly, while others also practice general internal medicine. Geriatric psychiatry is now a recognized subspecialty, and an increasing number of psychiatrists practice geriatric psychiatry on a full-time or part-time basis. Most general practitioners and specialists work on a fee-for-service basis and bill provincial medical care plans directly for office and hospital services. Some provincial health care plans provide for higher fees for patients aged 75 and over to take account of additional time required for interviewing and examining older patients. No copayment is required for any medically necessary services, and there is no limit to the number of services a patient may receive. The Canada Health Act prohibits physicians from billing patients greater amounts than the fee negotiated between provincial governments and provincial medical associations. The health status of Canada's elderly population has been reported recently in a National Population Health Survey undertaken in 1994–1995. Self-assessment of overall health, prevalence of chronic illness, and level of activity limitations were included. In general, people under age 75 differ little from the remainder of the adult population with respect to their self-reported health status. Persons over age 75 are increasingly likely to have multiple health problems, and use of medical services increased rapidly after age 75 (5). Since older age groups within the population, those with the greatest levels of illness and disability, are projected to increase disproportionately in the coming decades, attention has been directed toward specialized services that meet the needs of the frail elderly (6).

SPECIALIZED GERIATRIC SERVICES

Specialized services for the assessment, treatment, and rehabilitation of older people first appeared in Canada in the 1970s. The federal government provided early impetus for the development of specialized geriatric services by developing guidelines for geriatric assessment units and geriatric day hospitals (7) and by enabling the development of special geriatric units in several veterans' hospitals. Responsibility for medical and hospital care of veterans was subsequently transferred to provincial governments, and the ownership and operation of veterans' hospitals was transferred to various universities and provinces. Since then Veterans Affairs Canada has not played a role in developing specialized geriatric services that is comparable with that of its counterpart in the United States. These and other early initiatives in specialized geriatric services in Canada have already been described (2). Universities and university-affiliated teaching hospitals played a major role in the evolution of geriatric medicine in Canada with the first acute care geriatric assessment unit being opened at the University Hospital, University of Saskatchewan, in 1979. There and elsewhere funding support was provided for geriatricians who had both academic and clinical roles. The presence of geriatricians with academic appointments in university and teaching hospitals fostered the inclusion of gerontology and geriatrics in undergraduate and postgraduate curricula. In the late 1970s few Canadian medical schools had any specific geriatric content in their curricula; however, by the mid 1990s all 16 medical schools had integrated aging and care of the elderly into modules of the curriculum, and several universities required undergraduates to undertake clinical rotations through geriatric assessment units and other specialized services. Postgraduate programs in family medicine and internal medicine also included mandatory and elective rotations in geriatrics.

In Canada's largest province, Ontario, guidelines for the development of regional geriatric programs in teaching hospitals in the five health science centers of the provinces were published (8). In each of these centers the Ministry of Health provided additional funding to develop new services and enhance existing geriatric services, creating a network of specialized services encompassing six program components. These comprise three community-oriented services and three hospital-based programs. Services directed to elderly persons living in the community include the following: multidisciplinary outreach teams that provide comprehensive assessment in an older person's place of residence; geriatric specialty clinics for assessment, treatment, and monitoring of elderly persons who can travel to the clinic site; and geriatric day hospitals for delivering short-term diagnostic, rehabilitative, and therapeutic services to older persons living at home or in long-term care facilities.

Hospital-based programs include acute inpatient units, hospital consultation teams, and geriatric rehabilitation units. Acute geriatric units for short-term assessment and treatment of elderly persons were developed in several teaching hospitals. These units are entered directly from home or day hospitals or by transfer from other units within the hospital. Interdisciplinary teams were also established to provide consultation services to inpatients of medical and surgical units, and in some cases these teams also provide urgent response for frail elderly persons in emergency departments. It was recognized that an essential component of the network of services is geriatric rehabilitation. Postacute units were developed in chronic hospital units linked to acute geriatric units for patients who required continued treatment and rehabilitation for up to 3 months before returning home or entering long-term facility care.

The continuum of specialized geriatric services just described enables many frail older persons to receive appropriate diagnostic and functional assessment, treatment, and rehabilitation, thereby avoiding or delaying admission to a long-term care facility and minimizing inappropriate hospital bed use. Referrals to each regional program are managed through an intake office that provides overall coordination, matches clinical need to the appropriate service, and avoids unnecessary duplication of referrals. Regional geriatric programs work in close collaboration with the patient's primary care physician, who remains the responsible physician except when patients are admitted to a hospital. The family physician resumes care when patients return home or are admitted to a long-term care facility. Patients use individual program components as appropriate, and their individualized care plans may include, for example, sequential use of in-home consulting, acute hospital care, and post-discharge day hospital attendance according to individual circumstances. Close working relations with providers of community-based home support services and home nursing and rehabilitative services have been achieved to enable smooth transition to home-based care. Specialized geriatric services in university-affiliated teaching hospitals are not accessible to all seniors who might benefit from referral; however, physicians and other health professionals in training receive clinical training in these model units and can apply their knowledge and skills in their practices elsewhere. Similar networks of specialized services have been developed elsewhere in Canada. In some regions these resources are under common governance and operate in an integrated fashion, while in other regions working arrangements have developed between component parts of the network that are operated by separate agencies.

HEALTH CARE RESTRUCTURING

Unlike many other Western nations, the organization of health care in Canada escaped fundamental restructuring through the 1970s and 80s. In the past decade, pressures common to other industrialized countries—the forces of demographic change, emerging technologies, new diseases, and increasing consumer expectations—have converged at a point when governments are attempting to eliminate budget deficits and reduce public debt. Since health care services account for about a third of the provincial budget, each province is examining how to reduce health care costs and has either restructured the health care system or is planning to do so.

Efforts to reduce health care costs have included measures to reduce the cost of physicians' services. Since fees are already controlled by agreements between provincial governments and medical associations, attention has been directed to the supply of physicians and the number of services provided. Alternative payment mechanisms for physicians have also been proposed, but most physicians continue to be reimbursed by fee for service. Nurse practitioners and physicians-extenders (physician's assistants) do not at present have a substantial role in Canadian health care. Significant reduction of hospital stays has been achieved through management techniques that include case mix funding formulas for acute care hospitals. Greater success has been achieved in reducing surgical inpatient use than in medical care. Long-stay medical patients are typically frail older persons for whom suitable discharge plans cannot easily be made. As yet, few postacute or subacute programs, such as restorative or convalescent care, which reduce medically unnecessary hospital stay and improve outcomes for frail elderly medical patients, have been developed.

Of 10 provinces, 9 have recently created regional structures for health care decision making and administration of hospitals and institutional and community-based health and support services. Regions typically include several hundred thousand people and incorporate most publicly funded health services except medical care. There are now 123 such regions in Canada. Each is governed by a board that replaces the boards of hospitals, facilities, and agencies that were disbanded to form the region. In the province of Saskatchewan, for example, 30 district boards replaced 435 previously autonomous boards of gov-

ernance (9). As responsibility for health care planning and funding is devolved from provinces to regions, it is likely that the system effects of inadequate service provision for frail elderly persons will become apparent and that specialized geriatric services and subacute and postacute programs of rehabilitative convalescent and palliative care will be expanded. Lomas (9), commenting on regionalization of health care service in Canada, asserts that "central to the creation of a health care system is the devolved authorities' ability to rationalize, integrate and coordinate previously autonomous and sometimes competing services." How devolution of power from provinces to regional authorities will affect the health of the frail elderly and the services they receive is uncertain. Regionalization does, however, offer geriatricians and others concerned with population health an unprecedented opportunity to influence ways the health and well-being of older citizens can be maintained and to participate in systemwide approaches to preventing and treating illness and disability. The growing evidence base that demonstrates effectiveness of preventive and treatment and rehabilitative interventions in improving the health, function, and quality of life of frail older persons is essential ammunition for those advancing the case for improved medical care for the frail elderly in Canada.

REFERENCES

1. The Future Population of Canada and Its Age Distribution. IESOP Research Paper 3. Hamilton, Ontario, Canada: Faculty of Social Sciences, McMaster University Press, 1996.
2. Robertson D. Establishing new services: Canada as a case study. In: Coakley D, ed. Establishing a Geriatric Service. London: Croom Helm, 1982:121–145.
3. Canadian Medical Association. The Role of the Physician in Primary Health Care in Canada. Ottawa: CMA, 1994.
4. Relationship between Family Physicians and Specialists/Consultants. Ottawa: College of Family Physicians of Canada, Royal College of Physicians and Surgeons of Canada, 1993.
5. Rosenberg MW, Moore EG. The health of Canada's elderly population: current status and future implications. Can Med Assoc J 1997;157:1025–1032.
6. Robertson D. Alternative models for health care delivery. In: Aging With Limited Health Resources. Ottawa, Canada: Economic Council of Canada. Minister of Supply & Services Canada, 1987.
7. Minister of Supply & Services Canada, Report of the Sub-

committee on Institutional Program Guidelines: Geriatric Services in Acute Care Hospitals. Health Services & Promotions Branch, Health & Welfare Canada, 1979 and 1990.

8. Ministry of Health Guidelines for the Establishment of

Regional Geriatric Programs in Teaching Hospitals. Ontario Ministry of Health. Toronto: Queens Printer, 1988.

9. Lomas J. Devolving authority for health care in Canada's provinces: 4 emerging issues and prospects. Can Med Assoc J 1997;156:817–823.

JAPAN

This discussion reviews demographic trends, including life expectancy, aspects of contemporary medical care, and how culture affects care of the elderly in Japan.

DEMOGRAPHIC TRENDS IN POPULATION AGING

Population aging has become one of the best-known terms in contemporary Japan. The general trend of population aging shows a demographic transition from high birth and death rates to lower rates, as evidenced by the change in age distribution of the Japanese population from 1920 to 1994. In 1920 the population age distribution looked like a pyramid or Mount Fuji, with many people at younger ages. In 1994, the demographic pyramid was shaped more like a tall pot because of the increased numbers of persons in the middle and late years of life. Projections for 2025 and 2050 show a rectangular demographic profile, with continued growth and then stabilization of the age distribution of the population.

Demographic trends are often expressed as the percentage of persons aged 65 years and older in the population. For Japan the percentage of older persons was 7.1% in 1971, 9.1% in 1980, 12% in 1990, and 14.1% in 1994. Compared with many European countries, Japan is a late starter with respect to population aging. However, the future pace of aging in Japan will be rapid, and by 2025 the proportion of persons aged 65 and older will be 25.8%. The rapidity of population aging in Japan can be traced to the unprecedented steepness of the decline in the birth rate and a continued low level of fertility. Along with population aging, the decrease in the

number of children has become recognized as a national trend.

LIFE EXPECTANCY

Life expectancy at birth is also important to population aging. In 1960 the life expectancy in Japan was 65.3 years for men and 70.2 years for women. However, in a relatively short period, namely by 1984, life expectancy had reached 74.2 years for men and 79.8 years for women, the longest life expectancy of any country in the world. The increase in life expectancy that occurred in the postwar years was largely attributable to the rapid decline in the mortality of children and young adults. The decline in the mortality rate for children was due mainly to control of infections by better hygiene and the introduction of antibiotics. While tuberculosis killed many young people in the first half of the century, it is no longer the threat it once was because of better public health control measures and the use of chemotherapeutic agents. In contrast, mortality among older persons is not as easily reduced as in younger people. Even so, there have been appreciable recent declines in the mortality among older persons in Japan. More meticulous analysis of population data will be necessary for full appreciation of new trends in mortality among the old in Japan.

In discussing life expectancy in Japan, the aging of the aged population itself warrants special attention. The proportion of those aged 75 and older has grown since the turn of the century. The ratio of persons aged 75 and older to persons aged 65 and older in Japan is projected to rise from 39.9% in the year 2000 to 56.6% in the year 2025. Population projections prepared by the United Nations (1984) reveal that the proportion of older persons in Japan in the year 2025 is likely to be by far the highest in the world, followed by Sweden (at 51.1%). Obviously, this marked age shift of the Japanese population will generate a substantial effect on the pattern and level of demand for medical care and welfare services, discussed later. This trend of increasing numbers of older persons is also clearly demonstrated even in older age groups. The number of centenarians has increased every year for the past 27 years, and 8491 centenarians were listed in Japan in 1997 (81.5% women, 18.5% men). The trend for women to outnumber men becomes more marked as one moves from septuagenarian to octogenarian to nonagenarian to centenarian.

There are differences in age distribution among the prefectures in Japan. Some central prefectures, such as Tokyo, Saitama, Chiba, Kanagawa, and Osaka, have younger populations, while the relatively rural, agricultural, and forestry- and fishery-oriented prefectures far from metropolitan areas have older populations. The most important cause of this age difference is differences in the rates of in- and out-migration across prefectures. Both central and local government have made great efforts to prevent and reverse the tendency to exaggerate these age differences. However, differences in aging of the population in the various prefectures is deeply rooted in the culture of each prefecture.

POPULATION AGING AND CHANGES IN THE FAMILY AND HOUSEHOLD

The family or household is the primary unit for social and economic activities. Family composition and mores have undergone marked change during the 20th century. In the Showa era, population aging was a deep influence on the family in Japan. The size of household, family structure, and three-generation households among the elderly are well known by demographers. The many older women as the population ages, in a society in which virtually everyone marries, means that the number of widows will grow dramatically in Japan in the coming decades.

Older people are no longer rare, and living to a ripe old age is the norm. The wish of older people in Japan to continue working is very strong, but maintaining a job is not always easy for older persons in Japan. The century-old seniority system is changing. Debate on these issues is active, and the public system of support will continue to evolve.

MEDICINE AND MEDICAL CARE IN JAPAN

Medicine has tended to concentrate on clinical observation, diagnosis, and treatment of individual patients. The scientific tradition in medicine goes back to the 16th century, the Renaissance, and is the basis for public trust in medical care throughout the world, including Japan, especially since the Meiji era. The concept of health includes the following components: (*a*) Structure and function of the body are correctly maintained. (*b*) Supply of energy to organs of the body is consistent. (*c*) Homeostasis of the body is well maintained. (*d*) The immune and repair mechanisms of the body function well. (*e*) Mobility and sensory functioning are good. (*f*) Mental status is normal. (*g*) The reproduction systems are functioning normally. The emphasis on maintenance of good health is in contrast to medicine's focus on diseases. In Japan, a Clinical Classification of Diseases, Tokyo (CCDT), was reported at the 39th Congress of the Japan Geriatrics Society in June 1997 (president, Professor Syunsaku Hirai). CCDT has made it possible for Japanese clinicians to diagnose the person as a whole, following the model of the ICD-10 (*International Classification of Diseases,* volume 10, published by the World Health Organization).

In geriatric treatment in Japan, dietary prescriptions have special importance. Dietary practices are imbued with Japanese culture and are becoming more popular in the West as well. A great deal of research is being carried out on nutritional aspects of treatment in Japan using principles of the scientific method of Western medicine.

JAPAN AS A WELFARE NATION

The history of welfare in Japan is similar to that of Western countries, except that the welfare system of Japan has its own identity imposed by culture and tradition. The public notion of a stable and fulfilled life during one's elderly years is very strongly held. The welfare nation, which includes the concepts of social security, medical care, comfortable housing, and welfare services, is expected and demanded by most people. The demand has been stimulating the government and other influential members of the society to hasten the development of the welfare system in Japan. Needless to say, the cost has drawn much attention from officials, the public, and others in Japan.

With regard to the socioeconomic consequences of population aging in Japan, in 1963 the Law for the Welfare of the Elderly was enacted. In 1982 the Law for Health and Medical Services for the Elderly was passed. In July 1996, the Japanese government published the Cabinet Decision on the General Principles Concerning Measures on the Aging Society. These principles included ideas in the domains of income, health, learning and social involvement, living environment, and promotion of research on aging. The Ministry of Health and Welfare proposed the new Gold Plan in Welfare Work in 1995. The concept of normalization and integration of the disabled person into society proposed by the United Nations and the World Health Organization was adopted. The practical plan is now being formulated in active discussion. Concept of the international classification of impairments, disabilities, and handicaps (ICIDH) was also adopted, and the cooperation of medical and welfare staff was emphasized to maximize the ability of people to work.

Institutionalization poses special challenges. The life of the elderly who have been admitted to the old age home supported by the Welfare Law and the intermediate home supported by the Law for Health and Medical Services has been studied from a gerontologic viewpoint, namely, the sociologic, psychologic, and biomedical dimensions. In my experience with clinical studies on nursing home and intermediate home care, older persons admitted to these facilities have multiple diseases of various organs of the body. However, the clinical features of these diseases are often stable, enabling small numbers of clinical and other staff to provide medical care, living assistance, and recreation without much difficulty. Over time, changes in disease condition or some acute complications can occur. In these cases, the responsibility of clinical and welfare staff means that they must have the knowledge of geriatric care and welfare work to respond to changing conditions. Using the CCDT, we expect to have more data about older persons in institutions in the near future.

HUMANITIES AND HUMANISM

Mental health is fundamental to our humanity. In Asia, the problem of the soul and spiritual matters has been shaped by different cultures in the traditions of every nation. While Japanese people of course have an Oriental way of thinking (influenced greatly by the distinct religious beliefs and language of the Japanese), many Japanese adopted a Western lifestyle and way of thinking in the Meiji era. Among 120 million Japanese, illiteracy is very rare; almost everyone can read, write, and calculate easily. Science and technology have penetrated every aspect of Japanese life. Newspapers, radio, and television, as well as print media such as books and journals, have done a great deal to promote the different cultures of the Japanese people. The University of the Air has an excellent curriculum and teaching staff and will be broadcast over all regions of Japan. The open university will play an important role in the education of Japanese people, integrating media and universities, so that educational opportunities will be available to all, including lifelong learners.

COMMENTARY ON JAPAN

The United States and countries around the world have much to learn from Japan. Japan is known for having the world's longest life expectancy and has a high percentage of the oldest old. Over the years, the Japanese tradition of elders being taken care of by their children and the highly developed pension and health care systems appeared to be the role model for the world. And yet we need to examine the care of the elderly with our colleagues in Japan, because there are difficulties that we all face. Even poor nations are now burdened by rising populations of the old. A graying of developing nations is being witnessed around the world. So the experience in Japan, the United States, Great Britain, Canada, Germany, Australia, Scandinavia, and other nations has practical importance around the world.

In Japan, we read news reports of changes in family systems. With greater mobility of the Japanese population, fewer elders live with their children than 40 years ago. Also, the role of Japanese women has changed, with many more working outside of home. The Japanese family in this way resembles the family in the United States and elsewhere. And the oldest old in Japan have children who themselves are old, and there is great stress on the caregiver. The chapter part on demographic trends in populations aging in Japan provides a glimpse of these trends. What is also critical is that pension and health care systems are under tremendous financial stress, as they are in the United States. The need for long-term care, including nursing homes and home care, is striking. Professor Yoshikawa describes the systems that have been put in place, and yet

there is still a shortage of services for many elders. This shortage has numerous consequences, including many women leaving their employment to stay home and care for elderly relatives. And many hospitalizations in Japan are "social admissions" to fill the need for nursing home care and community care.

As with the United States and many other countries, in Japan we can project a significant rise in the numbers of elderly who will require care. All of this may mean more financial burden on those in the workforce who are supporting the pension system. Japan, like the United States and other countries, will have to solve major economic, political, and family and cultural problems as it enters the next millennium. There are many hurdles to be leaped in caring for the people with the longest life expectancy. Professor Yoshikawa provides not only a glimpse into the Japanese system of caring for the elderly but a glimpse of what the entire world faces with the graying of populations around the world.

CHAPTER 48

GEORGE W. REBOK AND JOSEPH J. GALLO

Successful Aging: Optimizing Strategies for Primary Care Geriatrics

How is it that one individual may seem able to integrate painful conditions of old age into a new form of psychosocial strength, while another may respond to similar conditions in a fashion that seems to inhibit effective integration and healthy, ongoing development?
—Erikson et al. (1)

Physicians and other health care professionals who care for the elderly may find it difficult to consider that aging could ever be described as successful or that the notion of successful aging could have any relevance to their practice. Older persons must deal with an increasing burden of functional symptoms and disability from chronic illness (2, 3). Aging persons also have progressive increases in age-specific mortality rates and face declines in measurable perceptual and cognitive abilities, such as a slowing of reaction time and reduced working memory capacity. Important social and emotional supports are lost as spouse, friends, and family move away or die. Given the universal, progressive, and largely irreversible losses of late life, it is important to understand why more elderly people, especially the oldest old, do not eventually succumb to despair. How do older people adapt to and compensate for age-related losses in mental and physical reserves? What personal and environmental factors allow them to optimize their resources to achieve a truly successful old age? How can the physician assist older patients with the advice, skills, and treatments that prevent age-related declines

and disease and that promote healthy, productive aging?

This chapter focuses on several themes that influence how we describe and understand successful aging. The first section defines successful aging, with particular focus on developmental aspects of it. The second section deals with ways that older adults maintain their sense of self and well-being and maintain vital involvement in old age despite declines in physical and mental capacity. The third section considers successful aging within the context of care and considers specific strategies to prevent age-linked losses and promote healthy, productive aging.

DEFINING SUCCESSFUL AGING

We believe that it is a mistake to construe successful aging only in terms of ability to carry out the activities of daily living. Instead, it is more fruitful to consider success in aging along multiple dimensions and multiple domains. The psychologic aspect of successful aging suggests processes that might best be considered as developmental. Successful aging is very much related to the opportunity to accomplish the developmental tasks of late life. Erikson's stage model (1, 4) suggests that a major task of old age is acceptance and resolution of one's life. Described as a crisis between ego integrity and despair, the challenge in old age is to accept oneself and one's deeds, both good and bad, to achieve a sense of psychologic well-being and ultimately acceptance of one's life as one that could have been lived in no other way. Defining and ensuring one's legacy is a core part of this task. According to Erikson, this is essential to psychologic well-being in late life and thus to successful aging. It also appears that under certain conditions meeting these developmental needs may confer health and functional benefits (5).

Theoretic models of mental health have also contributed to the definition of successful aging (6). For example, models of self-actualization (7), the healthy personality (8), and the trusting, meaningful life (9) all implicitly suggest that successful aging is the realization of one's full human potential. From the perspective of personality and positive mental health, the more recent work by Ryff (10, 11) is perhaps the most encompassing. Ryff has proposed an integrative model of successful aging that is based in developmental, clinical, and mental health criteria for positive function:

- Self-acceptance
- Positive relations with others
- Autonomy
- Environmental mastery
- Purpose in life
- Personal growth

The concept of successful aging discussed by Rowe and Kahn (3) focuses on function, namely, (*a*) low probability of disease and disease-related disability, (*b*) high functional capability, including cognitive and physical components, and (*c*) active engagement with life. According to their model, successful aging is more than the absence of disease or severity of risk factors for disease and more than the maintenance of functional capacities, important as they are. It is the combination of these factors with active engagement in life that represents the concept of successful aging most fully. "Successful aging goes beyond potential; it involves activity" (3). In the Rowe and Kahn paradigm, engagement with life has two major components: maintenance of interpersonal relations and productive activity. Active participation in family and social relations can continue even in the face of physical illness. An activity is viewed as productive if it creates societal value, whether or not it is reimbursed. A person who cares for a disabled family member or works as a volunteer in a local church or hospital is productive, although unpaid (3). So successful aging encompasses an internal psychologic development that accepts one's own life, good and bad, as well as external engagement with the world to the fullest extent possible.

MAINTAINING ACTIVE INVOLVEMENT IN OLD AGE

Most older adults express a clear desire to continue to make contributions to society and to future generations. When asked to describe what successful aging means, the most frequent response focused on making a contribution, helping others, and having a sense of purpose, and the second most frequent response focused on having opportunities to learn new things and having a sense of personal growth (12). Surveys such as these indicate that older adults by and large are not interested in pursuing a life of relaxation and leisure. Contrary to the stereotype of an unproductive old age, most older people make productive contributions of some kind, especially as informal helping and volunteer work rather than paid employment. When all forms of productive activity are combined, the amount of work done by older men and women is substantial (13, 14).

Older people are not considered old by family and friends, nor do older persons think of themselves as old, as long as they remain active and make productive contributions of some kind (3, 5, 15). Concerns about meaningful productivity, or to borrow Erikson's term, "generativity," are likely to be highly salient to older adults. A number of studies indicate that levels of self-reported generativity tend to increase through middle age and then appear to decline somewhat at advanced ages (16–18). This decline in self-reported generativity may reflect the lack of normative social roles at older ages that provide the sense of making socially valued contributions—of being generative—that are provided by the clear social norms for full-time employment and raising one's children that are dominant in middle adulthood. Recent analyses of data from the MacArthur Studies of Successful Aging indicate that a general measure of productivity (based on reports of volunteer and other activities) protects against short-term mortality independent of health status and physical and cognitive functioning (19). Generativity thus promotes psychologic and social well-being.

One type of productive activity that has been receiving increased attention is volunteering. Programs to foster volunteering among the elderly have grown rapidly in the past decade. This rise has been attributed not only to demographic changes in older populations and the changing meaning of later life but also the initiation of public and private programs to promote volunteer opportunities (20). Programs include the Service Core of Retired Executives, Foster Grandparents, Retired Senior Volunteer Program, and the Widowed Persons Service. One recent demonstration program that may serve as a model for attracting older volunteers is called the Experience Corps (5). This program places teams of 10 to 15 retirees in public elementary schools, where they carry out various activities, such as tutoring students who need extra help, developing enrichment programs, and resolving conflicts. Pilot results from the Experience Corps program show promise for increasing activity, generativity, and social support for older adults, as well as opportunities to use existing skills and to gain new ones. As Monk (21) points out, it has been taken for granted that volunteering is good for older adults, but empiric testing is limited and inconsistent. Several studies have documented that volunteering is associated with higher life satisfaction and increased health (20, 22, 23). However, methodologic constraints prevent conclusions that volunteering produced these gains; these findings may result from the selection of healthier, better-educated persons into volunteer roles. For example, men and women functioning at high physical and cognitive levels are 3 times as likely to be doing some paid work and more than twice as likely to be doing volunteer work as their impaired age-related cohorts (3).

On a societal scale, the concept of a connection between the aging person's sense of self and active engagement with the broader sociohistorical context is important to consider for successful aging. Clinical experience suggests that the degree to which a person feels that he or she has been actively involved in the march of history has at least some connection with a sense of self and well-being in later life. Successful aging could well be enhanced by increased opportunity for work that will outlive the self and activities that create a legacy (24).

Remaining active in other ways also has health benefits important to successful aging. Physical and cognitive activity, along with social supports and networks, are related to improved health and function with aging. Some early research supports the use-it-or-lose-it notion for cognition and for physical activity. It may be that staying cognitively active helps to protect memory as people age (25, 26). Lifelong activity, physical, cognitive, and social, appears to be important to health and well-being in later life.

Continued physical activity provides one of the most important hedges on development of frailty (27). Randomized trials have demonstrated the ability of exercise programs to increase the functional status of the full range of older adults, including at-risk elderly adults (28), institutionalized nonagenarians (29), and those suffering from arthritis (30). Even when initiated in advanced old age, improved functioning ability and morale result from exercise programs. Such exercise regimens, especially when carefully initiated and supervised, can be expected to diminish cardiovascular disease morbidity and mortality to a substantial extent even among those older than 75 years (31). Physicians play an important role in acknowledging and promoting exercise and physical activity in older patients. One of the major recommendations from Healthy People 2000 is that 50% or more of primary health care providers inquire about the frequency, duration, type, and intensity of exercise habits in most new patients (32). One mechanism to ensure that exercise counseling occurs is to provide a written prescription. A formal exercise prescription should include specific advice about frequency, intensity, duration, type, and progression of physical activity. Injury prevention and program maintenance also should be addressed (33). Programs to help maintain flexibility and strength can be recommended to most older patients (34, 35).

PERCEIVED CONTROL AND SUCCESSFUL AGING

A growing body of literature suggests that perceiving oneself as in control of one's life and environment is an important factor in successful aging (36). More specifically, perception of a high degree of control contributes to happiness and to a positive outlook on the future, makes one willing to face challenges, and leads to persistence in coping with stress and loss. In addition, those who believe strongly in their ability to affect health outcomes are likely to seek health information and participate in health maintenance activities. Research on control beliefs demonstrates that internal control beliefs remain relatively stable throughout life and continue to be adaptive in late life (37, 38). On the other hand, beliefs about the power of others over one's life increase with age as internal resources diminish (39). This increase in external control beliefs, however, may be viewed as an adaptive response rather than a loss, since it implies that others are part of one's resources. Therefore, the belief that circumstances and people in one's environment become more important than one's own ability to control events is not necessarily synonymous with giving up responsibility over one's life.

Although it is now widely held that having a high perception of control over one's life leads to positive outcomes (36), this notion may not be valid. Eizenman et al. (40) have presented data suggesting that most people have considerable variations in control perceptions and that high perceived control does not predict longevity. They reasoned that short-term variation in control perceptions and other psychologic and physiologic characteristics may reflect a loss of underlying physiologic reserve capacity and represent a risk factor for the development of disease or disability. Their research indicated that holding one's control beliefs *consistently,* at whatever level, is a critical part of achieving a positive outcome in old age. Feeling a loss of control does not lead to disease per se, but it alters the physiologic state of the person and leads to increased physical and mental vulnerability.

THE AGELESS QUALITY OF WISDOM

No account of the quality of wisdom in old age is likely to be complete. For Jung, successful aging entailed life review, psychologic growth, and growth toward full humanity and wisdom.

The emerging research on wisdom has demonstrated that certain facets of wisdom are measurable; moreover, in favorable life circumstances, wisdom-related pragmatic knowledge is part of the potential of the aging mind (41). Although wisdom has historically been closely linked with age, age itself does not guarantee wisdom. In addition to general factors of cognitive, personal, and social efficacy, three life conditions are potentially relevant for the development of wisdom: (*a*) extensive experience with a wide range of human conditions, (*b*) tutor- or mentor-guided practice, and (*c*) motivational dispositions such as generativity (1, 42) or the continuing motivation to expand one's insights into matters of life and their mastery (43). Research focusing on beliefs about wisdom shows that people in general identify wisdom as one of the very few positive goals in later life. Wisdom, on average, is expected to emerge during the 50s and continue into old age.

Knowledge about the pragmatics of life, or wisdom-related knowledge, includes knowledge about the structure and function of the self, how we conceive our identity, and how we feel and think about life in general, about our past and about our future (44). In social psychologic research, several processes of cognitive pragmatics dealing with self-management function as immunizing conditions, protective factors, and coping strategies, but also as ways by which persons can developmentally move forward in personality growth (i.e., toward wisdom). These processes include: (*a*) activation and changing use of different possible selves, (*b*) changes in levels of aspiration and expectations, (*c*) changes in goals and goal structures, and (*d*) changes in processes of social comparisons and use of social norms (45). From research on the personality correlates of wisdom, it has been suggested that those who have a high degree of *openness to experience* (46) and an intermediate degree of extroversion also display high levels of wisdom-related performance (47). These characteristics appear to operate as protective factors for the management of self-related changes in old age. Those who are open to new experiences appear to be well equipped to adapt to age-related changes and to devise innovative strategies to deal with them.

A MODEL OF SUCCESSFUL DEVELOPMENT AND AGING

Clinicians know older persons who compensate for age-related physical, cognitive, and functional declines through various adaptive mechanisms that make such declines less debilitating and less general than otherwise might be expected. Baltes (41), Baltes et al. (43), and Baltes and Baltes (45) have formulated these observations into a useful model of development and aging called *selective optimization with compensation* (SOC) to describe this adaptive process. The assumption of the SOC model is that the three elements (selection, optimization, and compensation) constitute the basic component processes for age-related change in adaptive capacity (development). It is also assumed that the three components always interact. Through selection, a person might focus on a smaller set of daily activities while not pursuing alternative options. Compensation might involve acquiring new strategies (means) or replacing goals to deal with actual or anticipated age-related losses. Finally, optimization denotes the means of achieving a goal or higher levels of functioning in a selected domain through enhancing existing strategies and searching for enriching environments. Baltes et al. (48) note the strategies used by the late pianist Arthur Rubenstein as an illustration of selective optimization with compensation. Rubenstein selected a limited repertoire, rehearsed frequently, and slowed down before fast segments to the give the impression of faster play. SOC is a useful framework for good or successful aging that has practical application.

More generally, the SOC model is viewed as one conceptualization of adaptation to the conditions of old age that includes mastery and progress despite an age-related shift toward a less positive balance between gains and losses in later life. The primary reason for this shift in the dynamics between gains and losses lies in the fact that old age brings with it a higher probability of pathology and a definite reduction in the scope and range of adaptive or reserve capacity. Baltes maintains that SOC is a general metalevel strategy of adaptation that holds across functional domains (cognitive, social, physical) and across cultural contexts. At the same time, while the general process of SOC is posited to be universal, its specific phenotypic expressions depend on the cultural context, individual life histories, and the personal circumstances that individuals face as they grow older.

With regard to geriatric practice, it is important to inquire whether the SOC strategies can be taught. Age-related processes that interfere with compensation and selection mechanisms result in functional decline. Especially in later life, the ability to compensate for deficits due to loss of functioning seems to be an important predictor of continued personal efficacy and the ability to live independently in the community (49). It thus is important to identify the personal resources or capacities of the aging person and to try to maximize those resources by teaching compensatory strategies. The more resources a person has, the easier it is to anticipate, confront, and adapt to aging losses. One strategy might involve compensatory selection, as in selective restrictions in participation in discretionary tasks. Another strategy may be teaching reliance on other means of performance maintenance in later life, such as mnemonic aids for memory problems, dependency in personal and household care, or social and caregiving support from others (50).

As already indicated, selection processes refer to putting one's efforts into activities that are most important or most pleasurable. The selection process can entail actively or passively reducing the number of goals and domains to free and conserve energy for more important goals or to select new goals in the service of new developmental tasks. Optimization refers to maximizing the chosen activities through practice and accommodation of the environment to one's abilities. Optimization can be viewed as the fundamental component of enhancing or maintaining the means and strategies for goal attainment. To facilitate optimization, cognitive, motivational, and goal-appropriate means must be brought to convergence. The most explicit example of this type of selective optimization is deliberate practice of the chosen activity. The geriatrician must address the older person's physical and mental status to identify processes that interfere with

SOC. When considering the aging person in context as a whole, optimization can also imply generalization and transfer of skills. For example, the acquisition and enhancement of basic cognitive skills such as memory and problem-solving ability may generalize or transfer to many domains of everyday life activity (51, 52). Similarly, enhancement of an older person's level of optimism and sense of personal control can improve function in a number of everyday domains. Older patients can be introduced to the strategy of SOC to incorporate the paradigm into their view of the balance between age-related losses and gains.

SUCCESSFUL AGING IN THE CONTEXT OF CARE

Successful aging does not mean that an older person has not encountered difficulties with health or family life, but instead implies something about the elder's response to challenging life circumstances. In addition, some persons move in and out of success, just as people move in and out of illness (3), and older people differ in resilience to challenges. As Art Linkletter points out, "Old age is not for sissies"; being old is hard work (53). We opened this chapter by asking why some persons appear to negotiate difficulties and emerge stronger while others fail to progress, and then we reviewed the concept of successful aging and its developmental aspects. We cannot be sure the extent to which these developmental processes are malleable, but it seems that in the primary care setting there are opportunities to encourage older adults to employ the strategies of successful agers. The geriatrician can review activities and encourage the older patient to participate in life to his or her fullest capability. We have presented a model of successful aging that is characterized as selective optimization with compensation, which may be a guiding principle in interactions with older adults.

Research has shown that intervention that entails cognitively restructuring or reframing problems can be effective in old age. In other words, the way we think about circumstances affects how we feel. Cognitive-behavioral, brief psychodynamic, and interpersonal therapies have been applied to the mental disturbances of late life, such as depression, anxiety, and sleep distur-

bance (54). Cognitive-behavioral approaches rely on the notion that it is the personal meaning and interpretation of events that initiate and perpetuate depression, and if the cognitive distortions are addressed, persons feel less depressed (55). Increasing pleasant activities, supportive listening, and problem-solving discussions can also help with depression and promote successful aging (56). Reframing problems means helping the patient put problems in perspective, readjusting expectations, or focusing on coping strategies and resources. Other psychologic studies report that older adults find it beneficial to engage in reminiscence or life review, in which past problems and successes are the focus of reflection (57). The goal of life review is to help the older person come to full terms with the many threads of his or her own developmental history, with an aim of better psychologic integration and emotional resiliency.

Interventions to improve self-efficacy or mastery in the face of chronic illness appear to be effective among older persons. Loring et al. (58) reviewed 76 studies on arthritis patient education published between 1976 and 1986 and 45 studies published between 1987 and 1991 (59). They found that most studies show some benefit of interventions with regard to self-care behaviors and psychologic variables, such as depression and anxiety. Notably, studies that included coping skills, self-efficacy, and problem-solving skills tended to be more effective than programs that emphasized range-of-motion exercises. A program to improve self-care skills among older persons with arthritis reduced health care costs and medical care visits as well as pain and disability (60). Patient education programs have similar effects on pain and disability as do NSAIDs (61). Glasgow et al. (62) reported on a program to improve self-care among older adults with diabetes mellitus. In that study, 100 patients were randomized to immediate or delayed intervention. The intervention focused on diet, exercise, and glucose monitoring in 10 group sessions. The intervention was associated with significant improvement in self-care activities, objective measures of diabetic control, and problem-solving ability (62). Lustman et al. (63) found that among adults with non-insulin-dependent diabetes, intensive behavioral diabetes management alone was not as effective in dealing with depressive symptoms, self-care activities, and glycemic control as when combined with cognitive therapy. In the area of heart disease, self-management programs help older adults deal with chronic heart disease. For example, Clark et al. (64, 65) described a program called PRIDE, based on problem solving therapy (*p*roblem solving, *r*esearching, *i*dentifying a goal, *d*eveloping a management plan, *e*stablishing a reward for yourself for making progress). The PRIDE program included a workbook, videotape, and four group sessions. Among 246 persons for whom complete data were available at 12-month follow-up, persons in the intervention group were more likely to show declines in anxiety and feelings of hopelessness than those in the comparison group (65). Self-efficacy appears to be related to successful behavioral change across a range of behaviors, such as smoking cessation, weight loss, exercise, and consistency of contraception use (66).

CONCLUSION

In this chapter, successful aging is conceptualized as selective optimization with compensation. Successful older adults therefore are seen as those who can employ or be taught to employ compensatory strategies in the face of age-related declines to optimize their developmental potential. In light of the physical, cognitive, and functional changes that often occur with age, the key challenge is to help the elderly develop compensatory strategies that draw on their own selective reserve capacities. Clearly, one prescription does not suit all. Considerable research suggests that there is more reserve capacity, even among the oldest old, than was previously assumed. Randomized controlled intervention trials show that physical, cognitive, and functional performance can be restored to previous levels or even raised to higher levels by powerful new intervention procedures. We should also keep in mind that successful aging may be as much a matter of creating communities in which, despite functional impairment, older people can maintain involvement.

Primary care physicians have a strategic role in promoting successful aging, not only in physical health and functioning but also in cognition and mental health (67). Many risk factors are modifiable, which opens up the stage to prevention and intervention. It is clear that we know a great deal more about successful and unsuccessful aging than we did at the last edition of this book. The best prescription for older patients is to share the accumulating knowledge that holds great promise for optimization of function and quality of life.

REFERENCES

1. Erikson EH, Erikson JM, Kivnick H. Vital Involvement in Old Age: The Experience of Old Age in Our Time. New York: Norton, 1986.
2. Sullivan MD. Maintaining good morale in old age. West J Med 1997;167:276–284.
3. Rowe JW, Kahn RL. Successful aging. Gerontologist 1997;37:433–440.
4. Erikson EH. The Life Cycle Completed. New York: Norton, 1982.
5. Fried LP, Freedman M, Endres TE, Wasik B. Building communities that promote successful aging. West J Med 1997;167:216–219.
6. Bandura A. Self-efficacy: The Exercise of Control. New York: W. H. Freeman, 1997.
7. Maslow A. Toward a Psychology of Being. 2nd ed. Princeton: Van Nostrand, 1968.
8. Jahoda M. Current Concepts of Positive Mental Health. New York: Basic Books, 1958.
9. Rogers C. On Becoming a Person. Boston: Houghton Mifflin, 1961.
10. Ryff CD. Successful aging: a developmental approach. Gerontologist 1982;22:209–214.
11. Ryff CD. Beyond Ponce de Leon and life satisfaction: new direction in quest of successful aging. Int J Behav Dev 1989;12:35–55.
12. Fischer LR, Mueller DP, Cooper PW. Older volunteers: a discussion of the Minnesota Senior Study. Gerontologist 1992;31:183–194.
13. Herzog AR, Kahn RL, Morgan JN, et al. Age differences in productive activities. J Gerontol 1989;44:129–138.
14. Herzog AR, Morgan JN. Age and gender differences in the value of productive activitities: four different approaches. Res Aging 1992;14:169–198.
15. Kaufman SR. The Ageless Self: Sources of Meaning in Life. Madison: University of Wisconsin Press, 1986.
16. McAdams DP, St. Aubin ED, Logan RL. Generativity among young, midlife, and older adults. Psychol Aging 1993;8:221–230.
17. Heidrich SM, Ryff CD. Physical and mental health in later life: the self-system as mediator. Psychol Aging 1993;8:327–338.
18. Heidrich SM, Ryff CD. The role of social comparisons in the psychological adaptation of elderly adults. J Gerontol Psychol Sci 1993;48:127–136.

19. Glass TA, Seeman TE, Herzog AR, et al. Change in productive activity in late adulthood: MacArthur Studies of Successful Aging. J Gerontol Soc Sci 1995;50B:565–576.

20. Chambre SM. Good Deeds in Old Age: Volunteering by the New Leisure Class. Lexington, MA: Lexington Books, 1987.

21. Monk A. Volunteerism. In: Maddox GL, ed. Encyclopedia on Aging. New York: Springer, 1995:958–960.

22. Hunter K, Linn M. Psychosocial differences between elderly volunteers and non-volunteers. Int J Aging Hum Dev 1980–81;12:205–213.

23. Farkas KJ. Volunteers tell of benefits from service to others. Perspect Aging 1991;Nov-Dec:26–29.

24. Kotre J. Outliving the Self. Dearborn, MI: Norton, 1996.

25. Arbuckle TY, Gold D, Andres D. Cognitive functioning of elderly people in relation to social and personality variables. Psychol Aging 1986;1:55–62.

26. Craik FI, Byrd M, Swanson JM. Patterns of memory loss in three elderly samples. Psychol Aging 1987;2:79–86.

27. Fried LP, Guralnik JM. Disability in older adults: evidence regarding significance, etiology, and risk. J Am Geriatr Soc 1997;45:92–100.

28. Buchner DM, Cress ME, de Lateur BJ, et al. The effect of strength and endurance training on gait, balance, fall risk, and health services use in community-living older adults. J Gerontol Med Sci 1997;52:218–224.

29. Fiatarone MA, O'Neill EF, Ryan ND, et al. Exercise training and nutritional supplementation for physical frailty in very elderly people. N Engl J Med 1994;330:1769–1775.

30. Ettinger WH, Burns R, Messier SP, et al. A randomized trial comparing aerobic exercise and resistance exercise with a health education program in older adults with knee osteoarthritis. JAMA 1997;277:25–31.

31. Paffenberger RS, Hyde RT, Wing AL, et al. The association of changes in physical activity and other lifestyle characteristics with mortality among men. N Engl J Med 1993;328:538–545.

32. US Department of Health and Human Services. Healthy People 2000: Review and 1995 Revision. Washington: US Government Printing Office, 1995.

33. Jones TF, Eaton CB. Exercise prescription. Am Fam Physician 1995;52:543–550.

34. Lorig K, Fries JF. The Arthritis Helpbook. 4th ed. New York: Addison-Wesley, 1995.

35. Nelson M, Wernick S. Strong Women Stay Young. New York: Bantam, 1997.

36. Rowe JW, Kahn RL. Human aging: usual and successful. Science 1987;237:143–149.

37. Lachman ME, Weaver SL, Bandura M, et al. Improving memory and control beliefs through cognitive restructuring and self-generated strategies. J Gerontol Psychol Sci 1992;47:293–299.

38. Lachman ME, Ziff M, Spiro A. Maintaining a sense of control in later life. In: Abeles RP, Gift HG, Ory MG, eds. Aging and Quality of Life. New York: Springer, 1994: 116–132.

39. Baltes MM, Lang FR. Everyday functioning and successful aging: the impact of resources. Psychol Aging 1997; 12:433–443.

40. Eizenman DR, Nesselroade JR, Featherman DL, Rowe JW. Intraindividual variability in perceived control in an older sample: the MacArthur Successful Aging Studies. Psychol Aging 1997;12:489–502.

41. Baltes PB. The aging mind: potential and limits. Gerontologist 1993;33:580–594.

42. Erikson EH. Childhood and Society. New York: Norton, 1963.

43. Baltes PB, Lindenberger U, Staudinger UM. Life-span theory in developmental psychology. In: Lerner RM, ed. Handbook of Child Psychology. 5th ed. Vol 1: Theoretical Models of Human Development. New York: Wiley, 1998:1029–1143.

44. Sternberg RJ. Wisdom: Its Nature, Origins, and Development. New York: Cambridge University Press, 1990.

45. Baltes PB, Baltes MM. Psychological perspectives on successful aging: the model of selective optimization with compensation. In: Baltes PB, Baltes MM, eds. Successful Aging: Perspectives From the Behavioral Sciences. New York: Cambridge University Press, 1990:1–34.

46. Costa PT, McRae RR. The NEO Personality Inventory. Odessa, FL: Psychological Assessment Resources, 1985.

47. Baltes PB, Staudinger UM. The search for a psychology of wisdom. Curr Direct Psychol Sci 1993;2:1–6.

48. Baltes MM, Wald HW, Reichert M. Successful aging in institutions? In: Schaie KW, Lawton MP, eds. Annual Review of Gerontology and Geriatrics. New York: Springer, 1991:311–337.

49. Wolinsky FD, Callahan CM, Fitzgerald JF, Johnson RJ. The risk of nursing home placement and subsequent death among older adults. J Gerontol Soc Sci 1992;47: 173–182.

50. Marsiske M, Lang FR, Baltes PB, Baltes MM. Selective optimization with compensation: life-span perspectives on successful human development. In: Dixon RA, Backman I, eds. Compensating for Psychological Deficits and Declines: Managing Losses and Promoting Gains. Mahwah, NJ: Erlbaum, 1995:35–79.

51. Willis SL. Cognition and everyday competence. Annu Rev Gerontol Geriatr 1991;11:80–109.

52. Willis SL, Rebok GW, Ball K. From educational training on basic cognitive abilities to everyday activities. Gerontologist 1997;37:182 (157).

53. Linkletter A. Old Age Is Not for Sissies: Choices for Senior Americans. New York: Viking, 1988.

54. Abeles N. What Practitioners Should Know About Working With Older Adults. Washington: American Psychological Association, 1997.

55. Shearer SL, Adams GK. Nonpharmacologic aids in the treatment of depression. Am Fam Physician 1993;47: 435–443.

56. Brody DS, Thompson TL, Larson DB, et al. Strategies for counseling depressed patients by primary care physicians. J Gen Intern Med 1994;9:569–575.

57. Butler RN, Lewis M, Sunderland T. Aging and Mental Health: Positive Psychosocial Approaches. 4th ed. New York: Macmillan, 1991.

58. Lorig K, Konkol L, Gonzalez V. Arthritis patient educa-

tion: a review of the literature. Patient Educ Counsel 1987;10:207–252.

59. Hirano PC, Laurent DD, Lorig K. Arthritis patient education studies, 1987–1991: A review of the literature. Patient Educ Counsel 1994;24:9–54.

60. Lorig KR, Mazonson PD, Holman HR. Evidence suggesting that health education for self-management in patients with chronic arthritis has sustained health benefits while reducing health care costs. Arthritis Rheum 1993;36:439–446.

61. Superio-Cabuslay E, Ward MM, Lorig KR. Patient education interventions in osteoarthritis and rheumatoid arthritis: a meta-analytic comparison with nonsteroidal antiinflammatory drug treatment. Arthritis Care Res 1996;9:292–301.

62. Glasgow RE, Toobert DJ, Hampson SE, et al. Improving self-care among older patients with type II diabetes: the "sixty something. . ." study. Patient Educ Counsel 1992;19:61–74.

63. Lustman PJ, Griffith LS, Clouse RE, et al. Efficacy of cognitive therapy for depression in NIDDM: results of a controlled trial. Presented at the American Diabetes Association annual meeting, June 21, 1997 (abstract).

64. Clark NM, Rakowski W, Wheeler JR, et al. Development of self-management education for elderly heart patients. Gerontologist 1988;28:491–494.

65. Clark NM, Janz NK, Becker MH, et al. Impact of self-management education on the functional health status of older adults with heart disease. Gerontologist 1992; 32:438–443.

66. Strecher VJ, McEvoy DE, Vellas B, et al. The role of self-efficacy in achieving health behavior change. Health Educ Q 1986;13:73–91.

67. Gallo JJ, Rabins PV, Iliffe S. The 'research magnificent' in late life: psychiatric epidemiology and the primary health care of older adults. Int J Psychiatry Med 1997; 27:185–204.

Cell Biology and Physiology of Aging

The colloquial term of aging in organisms carries connotations of both longevity and senescence; longevity implies a period that an organism can normally be expected to live and senescence is a process of progressive degenerative change with time (1, 2). Aging in humans, however, is a universal biologic and psychologic phenomenon that is associated with positive and negative connotations determined by the cultural environment. In physical terms, normal aging may be considered as the time-related differential decline in biologic functions of both the whole organism and its parts, ultimately resulting in death. In psychologic terms, normal aging may be considered as the development of the person accompanied by age-specific culturally determined roles and expectations.

A distinction should be made between loss of function because of aging and loss of function because of disease. Normal aging may be accompanied by a decline of the number or capacity of cells needed for optimal functioning of the person. Disease states of individual components, while often age-related, imply a potential for reversibility of pathology or for retardation of aging. An example of aging is the age-related loss of neurons in the brain, while disease states include severe memory impairment, malignancy, cataracts, presbycusis, and marked skin wrinkling. Whether aging itself can be slowed is unknown, although genetic and dietary experiments with fruit flies and primates suggest that is possible.

The dual action of the loss of cells and gradual decline in function combined with the accumulation of abnormal changes has promoted a distorted view of aging. The functional decline of

a critical organ such as the brain due to Alzheimer's disease or Parkinson's disease is often misconstrued as the result of an aging process, even though other organs may still be normal. Thus "old age" becomes synonymous with diseases such as osteoporosis, atherosclerosis, and cancer. Medical advances and diagnostic technology that make prevention, diagnosis, and treatment of disease increasingly possible also blur the distinction between nonpathologic aging and pathology-related aging.

To define the known biologic and molecular changes more clearly, potentially influential factors related to aging can be divided into intrinsic and extrinsic factors (Table 49.1). Intrinsic factors include the person's genetic constitution, which determines maximum longevity; extrinsic factors are environmental exposures that impinge on the person's survival in the environment.

Both overfeeding and starvation shorten life in many animal species, and the ability of these and other extrinsic factors to influence expression of genetic potential has been studied extensively in the past decade, although not specifically in humans. A distinction has to be made between a substantial deprivation of food intake (starvation) and chronic partial reduction (i.e., 30 to 60%) in daily food consumption. In the former case, deterioration of survival capacity is accelerated, whereas in the latter case, biologic adaptation to diminished oxygen demands (lower metabolic rate) slows deterioration in laboratory animals. The effect of such dietary reduction to retard aging in humans remains to be seen, although substantial progress has been made with Rhesus monkeys used as a model (3). Whether lowered metabolic rate or

Table 49.1

Biologic Factors in Human Aging

Intrinsic Factors	Biologic Role
Genetics	Genes acquired to retard the damage of endogenous metabolic toxins, to regulate the rate of cellular maturation and metabolic rate, to suppress the tendency toward unlimited cell proliferation
Basal metabolism	Maintenance of energy-generating capacity by mitochondrial DNA and its decline because of damage from oxygen-derived free radicals
Endocrine system	Progressive decline in reproductive and homeostatic functions beyond age 30; menopause
Immune system	Gradual loss of immune responses needed for protection against pathology induced by extrinsic pathogens
Extrinsic Factors	
Exercise	Protection against chronologic decline of organ systems
Diet	Retardation of functional loss by balanced food intake; excessive or unbalanced dietary intake leading to cardiovascular disease
Mutagens	Accelerated decline of orderly function of genetic expression
Radiation	Destruction of genetic control of tissue functions

generally reduced physical activity is the primary reason for diminished age-related deterioration was resolved. The study shows that lowered metabolic rate is the major factor in longevity enhancement when physical activity is maintained at a level similar to that of unrestricted animals (4).

GENETIC FACTORS

The existence of genes associated with the aging process is indicated by the wide variation in maximal survival times among different organisms (5). These times vary from 4600 years for the bristlecone pine to 4 to 6 weeks for the fruit fly. Among mammals the average longevity ranges from a low of 12 months for the shrew to 70 to 80 years for humans. Studies on longevity in fruit flies show that their average lifespan can be extended by inbreeding of long-lived individuals. The health and activity of these long-lived progeny also seem to be more youthful than age-matched normals (6). Similar inbreeding experiments with mice gave the same result, extended lifespan. Moreover, it is known that human longevity is enhanced in people who have long-lived parents that lived under similar lifestyle and economic conditions (7). These findings raise a question: is longevity controlled by a set

of genes that regulate the rate of cell maturation and development (clock genes) or by a set of genes that suppress the damage inflicted on chromosomes by metabolic toxins by means of protective enzymes such as superoxide dismutase? Answers to this question are emerging from studies of the genetic control of aging in organisms such as the worm (*Caenorhabditis*), the fruit fly (*Drosophila*) and yeast (*Saccharomyces*). Genetic analysis of the genomes of these organisms has provided a role for aging-related or longevity genes designated as *age-1*, *clk-1*, and *daf* (8). *Age-1* specifically confers longevity on the worm, whereas *daf* promotes worm survival by inducing a sporelike nonvegetative state when crowding or nutrient restriction stresses its development. The *clk-1* gene appears to control early embryonic development and metabolic rate in various organisms (9). The model that seems to define the interaction of these "gerontogenes" is one that allows for short life by delayed onset of damage repair systems to chromosomes or long life by early onset of chromosomal damage-repair systems (9). Werner's syndrome, which results in accelerated aging in humans, has been attributed to a mutation in the gene for the enzyme helicase required for normal chromosomal replication (10). It seems likely that homologs of these gerontogenes in the animal species discussed earlier are also expressed in mammals to exert similar effects on the aging process.

Early studies by Hayflick (11) on the mitotic capacity of isolated human fibroblasts to reproduce in cell culture show that such cells can reproduce only a limited number of times. When skin fibroblasts from persons of different ages were cultured, a calculation of the maximum number of mitoses that remained in these cells showed a net decline of mitotic capacity with age. Starting with a maximum of 61 mitoses remaining for cells from newborns, the numbers decline by three mitotic divisions per decade (6, 12). Extrapolation of this value to an age for zero remaining divisions suggests a maximal reproductive life for fibroblasts from normal humans of somewhat more than 200 years. This restricted mitotic potential has been confirmed for similar cells derived from many other species and is found to have a unique value for each species (12).

The existence of a finite number of cell doublings in differentiated cells is accounted for by a molecular mechanism in chromosomes that prevents terminal ends of the chromosomes (telomeres) from being replicated completely in each mitotic cycle (13). Each successive cell division causes a progressive shortening of a repeating nucleotide sequence (TTAGGG) in the telomere to a point at which DNA replication is no longer possible (14). Malignant cells, sperm, and ova express a gene, not active in cells with limited mitotic potential, that produces the enzyme telomerase to correct the mitotic shortening of telomeres and thus confer immortality on these and other cells. The HeLa cell line is an example of an immortal human cell line that expresses this gene (13).

Immortalization or malignant transformation of cells can arise from other genetic mechanisms as well, such as through the action of genes that control cell proliferation in normal growth. Cells produce protective enzymes to counteract metabolic toxins that otherwise might lead to genetic and cellular damage and induce malignant transformation. These protective components, derived from both internal and external sources, are listed in Table 49.2. If these protective mechanisms fail, cell transformation may result.

BASAL METABOLISM

The cellular basis for energy production from oxygen resides in the mitochondria. As a result of normal metabolic activity, reactive free radical derivatives of oxygen such as superoxide anion (O_2^-), hydrogen peroxide (H_2O_2), and nitric oxide (NO) are generated and produce destructive oxidation of membranes, proteins, and DNA. The major defenses against such destruction are the protective enzymes superoxide dismutase and catalase, which remove the reactive free radicals derived from O_2^- and H_2O_2, and others that convert NO to nitrite or nitrate ions (15). Re-

Table 49.2

Aging Resistance Factors in Cells

Endogenous Protection (Cellular Origins)	
Enzymes that degrade free radicals and peroxides	Superoxide dismutase, catalase, glutathione peroxidase
Enzymes that facilitate replacement of damaged cellular components	Proteases, peptidases (proteins); phospholipases (membranes); nucleases, polymerases (DNA)
Exogenous Protection (Dietary Origins)	
Compounds that act as free radical scavengers	Viitamin E (tocopherol); vitamin A (retinol); vitamin C (ascorbate); BHT (butylated hydroxytoluene)
Factors that reduce free radical production	Diminished food consumption by 30 to 60% of optimal caloric intake

generative systems such as the enzymes associated with the removal, repair, and replacement of biologic constituents then restore damaged components. Components that turn over slowly or not at all, such as proteins and DNA, accumulate damage over time. This damage eventually leads to the cell's demise or impairment of cellular function (16). The lipofuscin pigment found in aged neurons as a result of their high metabolic activity is typical of the oxidative debris found in cells. DNA in neuronal mitochondria is particularly vulnerable to oxidative damage because these cells do not multiply after birth. Oxidative debris is also seen in other tissues, and a general measure for aging dependent metabolic loss is seen in the decline in VO_{2max}, the maximal oxygen extraction capacity of the lungs (17, 18).

Cross-sectional studies of the aging population show that several physiologic parameters such as body weight, basal metabolism, renal clearance, and cardiovascular function decline with age (19, 20). Longitudinal studies, however, suggest that specific persons show gains rather than losses with age (20). Buskirk and Hodgson (18) found that the VO_{2max} in some older exercising people was elevated relative to generally sedentary peers, even though the slopes for decline for both groups were parallel. Aging, as measured by loss of physiologic function, thus should be defined more precisely in terms that distinguish between usual, normal, and successful changes. Usual aging may be considered the culturally and genetically defined biologic and psychologic losses with age that vary with degrees of pathology. Normal aging is associated with nonpathologic longitudinal changes in biologic function beyond age 35. In successful aging, biologic capacity is optimized for overall function with exercise, nutrition, and other factors in the absence of pathology (21).

Reduction in the levels of superoxide dismutase caused by progressive loss of expression of its gene with age may account for many of the age-related declines in physiologic functions. Fruit flies endowed with increased longevity had higher levels of superoxide dismutase activity in their cells (22). Mechanisms for reducing free radical damage in cells can be found in the ac-

tivities of dietary antioxidants such as vitamin E, vitamin A, vitamin C, and butylated hydroxytoluene (BHT) (22). Experiments have demonstrated that diets high in vitamin E or BHT have the capacity to prolong the lifespan of mice or chickens (23). Whether similar modification of the diet will also prolong the lifespan of humans remains to be seen.

ENDOCRINE AND IMMUNE SYSTEMS

Maturation of reproductive organs is influenced by hormones with both cellular and genetic effects. Cellular factors that activate cell mitosis are mediated by a class of genes designated as proto-oncogenes in the normal state or oncogenes in the mutated condition. The cellular proto-oncogenes are expressed early during cellular development and differentiation to allow control of functions that are expressed in the mature cell. Estrogens and androgens stimulate cell growth and function by modulating expression of the proto-oncogenes. This in turn promotes or suppresses growth regulatory mechanisms within specific cells. In humans an age-specific determinant of cessation of reproductive potential in women is found in the onset of menopause. Onset of menopause, commonly around 50 years, is the time when ovulation ceases because of changes in the pituitary secretion of follicle-stimulating hormone (FSH) required for the maturation and release of ovarian follicles in the menstrual cycle. The timing of this event is thought to be initiated by age-related changes in biologic pacemakers in the suprachiasmatic nuclei of the hypothalamus that desynchronize the rhythmic release of FSH and other gonadotrophins by the pituitary (24).

Aging is associated with the accumulation of somatic mutations in regulatory genes that lead to the loss of coordinated control of cell growth and function. Several tumor suppressor genes damp the activity of the oncogenes that otherwise would cause mature cells to undergo abnormal mitosis, resulting in tumors (25). During normal maturation, steroid hormones serve as activators for specific genes that stimulate mitosis and growth of reproductive organs. All the while, metabolic suppression of the action of tumor suppressor genes permits controlled cell proliferation to take place. When hormone levels decline with age, the tumor suppressor genes become active again unless they have mutated so that suppressor function is lost. These mutational changes probably account for the increased probability of tumors with advanced age.

The loss of a tumor suppressor gene is, in fact, the most common somatic mutation of human cancer (26). The normal cellular process for the suppression of mitotic activity elicited by mutated DNA is to eliminate the mutated cell by the induction of programed cell death, or apoptosis. This occurs when a cellular protein recognizes mutated DNA and activates a gene for the induction of apoptosis, eliminating the tumor-producing cell. The programed death and peeling of mutated skin cells after exposure to sunlight is characteristic of this protective process (27, 28). The frequency of somatic mutations in oncogenes and tumor suppressor genes increases with age. This is a result of exposures to various mutagens, including dietary mutagens, radiation, and transforming viruses such as papillomavirus, immunodeficiency virus (HIV), and T-cell lymphotropic virus (HTLV) (29, 30). Such mutational events perturb the mitotic inhibition state of mature cells, allowing activation of mitotic factors from oncogenes.

Immune system cells such as T and B lymphocytes are regulated by specific hormones such as interleukin-1, interleukin-2, tumor necrosis factor, and interferon, all of which control proliferation and differentiation in lymphocytes in response to antigenic exposure. When excessive stimulation of interleukin-2 secretion by T lymphocytes is caused by abnormal antigen signaling, the resultant stimulation of T cells may lead to activation of autoimmune responses found in age-related diseases such as arthritis (31, 32).

In the aging process the normal functional responses of the immune system mediated by T lymphocytes are diminished by cumulative defects in the receptor signaling process whereby they recognize foreign antigens. These changes can also raise the level of serum autoantibodies (33, 34).

SUMMARY

It has been established that aging and associated pathology result from the decline in homeostasis of genetic and metabolic factors that regulate cellular proliferation and maintenance. These factors are mediated by genes that regulate the rate of cellular oxygen use and that confer protection against age-dependent damage induced by exposure to oxygen free radicals. Mutational changes that accumulate in DNA with time are less efficiently suppressed with age, when cell mechanisms involved in the control of cellular proliferation in the immune, endocrine, and reproductive systems may lead to pathology. Future attempts to retard the cellular aging process must manipulate genes at many levels of metabolism and mutation protection. A better understanding of aging versus disease will emerge from longitudinal studies of aging that include a search for mutable risk factors as well as intervention by means of long-term dietary restriction, physical activity, and cognitive enhancement studies in humans (35).

REFERENCES

1. Hayflick L. How and Why We Age. New York: Ballantine Books, 1994:15–18.
2. Ricklefs RE, Finch CE. Aging: A Natural History. New York: Scientific American Library, 1995:3–7.
3. Finch CE. Longevity, Senescence and the Genome. Chicago: University of Chicago Press, 1990:504.
4. Ramsey JJ, Roecker EB, Weindruch R, Kemnitz JW. Energy expenditure of adult male rhesus monkeys during the first 30 mo of dietary restriction. Am J Physiol 1997;272:E901–E907.
5. Reichel W. The biology of aging. J Am Geriatr Soc 1966;14:431–446.
6. Rose MR. Evolutionary Biology of Aging. New York: Oxford University Press, 1991:130.
7. Goldstein S, Gallo JJ, Reichel W. Biologic theories of aging. Am Fam Pract 1989;40:195–200.
8. Jazwinski SM. Longevity, genes and aging. Science 1996;273:54–59.
9. Guarente L. What makes us tick? Science 1997;275:943–944.
10. Yu CE, Oshima J, Ying-Hui F, et al. Positional cloning of the Werner's syndrome gene. Science 1996;272:258–262.
11. Hayflick L. The limited in vitro lifetime of human diploid cell strains. Exp Cell Res 1965;37:614–636.
12. Goldstein S, Reichel W. Care of the Elderly: Clinical Aspects of Aging. 2nd ed. Baltimore: Williams & Wilkins, 1983:511–517.
13. Levy MZ, Allsop RC, Futcher AB, et al. Telomere end-replication problem and cell aging. J Mol Biol 1992;225:951–960.
14. Moyzis RK. The human telomere. Sci Am 1991;265:48–55.

15. Ambs S, Hussain SP, Harris CC. Interactive effects of nitric oxide and the p53 tumor suppressor gene in carcinogenesis and tumor progression. FASEB J 1997;11: 443–448.

16. Sohal RS, Weindruch R. Oxidative stress, caloric restriction and aging. Science 1996;273:59–63.

17. Hagberg JM. The effect of training on the decline of VO_{2max} with aging. Fed Proc 1987;46:1830–1833.

18. Buskirk ER, Hodgson JL. Age and aerobic power: the rate of change in men and women. Fed Proc 1987;46: 1824–1829.

19. Shock NW. The Science of Gerontology. Council on Gerontology Seminar Proceedings, 1959-61. Durham, NC: Duke University Press, 1962:123–140.

20. Shock NW, Greulich RC, Andres R, et al. Normal Human Aging: The Baltimore Longitudinal Study of Aging. Washington: US Government Printing Office, 1984:174–179.

21. Rowe JW, Kahn RL. Successful aging. Gerontologist 1997;37:433–440.

22. Rusting RL. Why do we age? Sci Am 1992;267:130–141.

23. Young VR. Diet as a modulator of aging and longevity. Fed Proc 1979;38:1994–2000.

24. Wise PM, Krajnak KM, Kashon ML. Menopause: the aging of multiple pacemakers. Science 1996;273:67–70.

25. Aaronson SA. Growth factors and cancer. Science 1991; 254:1146–1153.

26. Weinberg RA. Tumor suppressor genes. Science 1991; 254:1138–1146.

27. Steller H. Mechanisms and genes of cellular suicide. Science 1995;267:1445–1449.

28. Thompson CB. Apoptosis in the pathogenesis and treatment of disease. Science 1995;267:1456–1462.

29. Hausen H. Viruses in human cancers. Science 1991; 254:1157–1163.

30. Smith JR, Pereira-Smith OM. Replicative senescence: implications for in vivo aging and tumor suppression. Science 1996;273:63–67.

31. Johnson HM, Russell JK, Pontzer CH. Superantigens in human disease. Sci Am 1992;266:92–101.

32. Miller RA. Gerontology as oncology. Cancer 1991;68: 2496–2501.

33. Miller RA. The aging immune system: primer and prospectus. Science 1996;273:70–73.

34. Report of the Task Force on Immunology and Aging (NIH 96–4018). Bethesda, MD: National Institutes of Health, 1996:9–77.

35. Gilchrest BA, Bohr VA. Aging processes, DNA damage, and repair. FASEB J 1997;11:322–330.

CHAPTER 50

LODOVICO BALDUCCI AND MARTINE EXTERMANN

Principles of Cancer Prevention and Cancer Treatment in the Older Person

Older persons do benefit from appropriate cancer management. The mortality related to common neoplasms, such as colorectal, breast, and prostate cancer, has declined among persons aged 65 and over in the past 5 years (1). Seemingly, lifestyle changes with elimination of environmental carcinogens, early detection of cancer from screening asymptomatic persons, and safer and more effective treatment of advanced cancer have improved cancer control of the aged.

Appropriate cancer management requires understanding the unique interactions of cancer and aging. This chapter outlines principles of cancer prevention and treatment in the older person after exploring the influence of age on the incidence and prevalence of cancer, the biology of neoplasia, and the risk of therapeutic complications.

EPIDEMIOLOGY

Approximately 50% of neoplasms occur in the age window 65 to 90 (2). Presumably the relative prevalence of cancer among older persons will increase with the growth of the population in that age range. Figure 50.1 illustrates the relation of age with the incidence of various neoplasms. The incidence of lung cancer rises until age 65 and declines thereafter, that of breast cancer levels out between ages 80 and 85, and that of prostate cancer and of nonmelanomatous skin cancer rises even after age 85. These incidence patterns may reflect differences both in the duration of carcinogenesis and in age-related susceptibility to various neoplasms.

The prevalence of other serious diseases also increases with age; approximately 50% of cancer patients aged 85 and older have comorbid conditions that compete with cancer as causes of death (3). At autopsy, comorbidity is similar among older cancer patients and persons of the same age without cancer (4). The clinical diagnosis of cancer, however, is disproportionately more common among community-dwelling elderly than among nursing home residents (5). Symptoms of other diseases and functional and cognitive limitations may delay or prevent the recognition of cancer among the frail elderly. In these persons, cancer may be an incidental finding with no effects on life expectancy or quality of life. The recognition of malignancies that threaten the life and the function of older persons is pivotal in treatment-related decisions.

During the past 20 years the incidence of nonmelanomatous skin cancers, non-Hodgkin's lymphomas, and brain tumors (anaplastic astrocytomas and glioblastoma multiforme) has increased disproportionately among older persons (6). The significance of these findings is uncertain. It is possible that older persons develop cancer earlier than younger persons after exposure to new environmental carcinogens because they are more susceptible to carcinogenesis. Older persons may represent a natural monitor system of the environment that predicts cancer epidemics.

CARCINOGENESIS AND AGE

Two non–mutually exclusive mechanisms may explain the association of cancer and age.

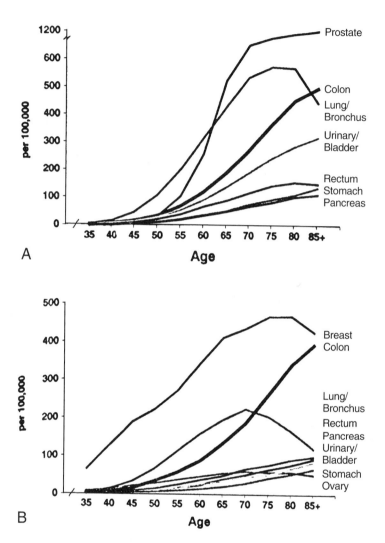

Figure 50.1. Age-related incidence of different forms of cancer in men **(A)** and women **(B).** (Reprinted with permission from Yancik R, Ries LA. Cancer in older persons. Cancer 1994;74:1995–2003.)

First, carcinogenesis is a time-consuming process whose end product, cancer, becomes manifest more commonly at advanced ages. Second, when exposed to these carcinogens, older persons are more susceptible to environmental carcinogens and develop cancer at higher rate than younger ones. Experimental and epidemiologic data support both mechanisms (7). An overview of carcinogenesis may help understand why age enhances the susceptibility to some carcinogens. Carcinogenesis is a stepwise process, requiring the serial action of different carcinogens. A useful classification distinguishes early carcinogens

(mutagens), which effect the initial stages of neoplastic transformation, and late carcinogens (promoters), which effect the late stages. Late carcinogens are effective only on cells already primed by early carcinogens. Increased concentration of cells that underwent early carcinogenic changes may increase the susceptibility of older tissues to late-stage carcinogens. The effects of late-stage carcinogens, unlike those of early-stage carcinogens, may be chemically reversed (chemoprevention).

The molecular interactions of carcinogenesis and aging are complex. Carcinogenesis entails alterations in tissue homeostasis, with increased cellular proliferation, and decreased cellular differentiation and cellular death (Fig. 50.2). These effects entail a number of genetic changes. The expression of proto-oncogenes is abnormally enhanced and that of tumor-suppressing genes (antioncogenes) is abnormally reduced. Proto-oncogenes encode substances involved in cell proliferation, such as growth factors, growth factor receptors, and enzymes modulating signal transduction and DNA replication. Antioncogenes encode substances that inhibit cell proliferation. The best characterized of the antioncogenes, the P53 gene on the short arm of chromosome 17, encodes a phosphoprotein that blocks the proliferation of transformed cells and allows repair of cancer-prone genetic abnormalities (8). Clearly, alterations of the P53 function facilitate the development of various malignancies. Cytogenetics and molecular changes of aging involving chromosomal translocation, formation of DNA adducts, and DNA hypomethylation may lead to activation of proto-oncogenes and deactivation of antioncogenes (7). Although some molecular changes of aging may favor carcinogenesis, it is important to highlight the differences between aging and cancer in terms of cellular and molecular biology (Fig. 50.2). Aging of tissues capable of self-renewal appears associated with changes opposed to those of cancer, including a reduced pool of stem cells capable of self-replication, enhanced cellular differentiation, and programed cell death (apoptosis). At least three molecular changes epitomize the differences between aging and cancer. Cellular aging is associated with progressive decline in the concentration of telomerases that maintain the terminal DNA sequences (telomeres) (9). Loss of telomerases is associated with loss of self-replication. In some neoplastic cells, telomerases are maintained and the cellular replicative ability is preserved. In some neoplasms, such as follicular lymphomas, the Bcl-2 gene, whose product prevents apoptosis, is activated (10). Cellular aging is associated with increased expression of the P16 antioncogenes, which encode a substance that inactivates cyclin-dependent kinases, while the P16 expression is reduced in neoplastic cells (11).

Cancer Biology and Age

Age may influence the natural history and the therapeutic response of some tumors. The natural history of cancer may become more indolent in the aged: lung cancer is diagnosed at an earlier stage in persons over 65 than in younger persons (12), and the prevalence of hormone receptor-rich, well-differentiated breast cancer rises among aging women (13). Natural selection may account in part for these changes: slowly growing tumors take longer to become detectable and consequently are diagnosed predominantly among older persons (14). Seemingly, changes in the patient may also modulate tumor growth: these include endocrine and nutritional status, immunosenescence, decreased production of tumor growth factors, and increased production of cytokines, which inhibit tumor growth. In the case

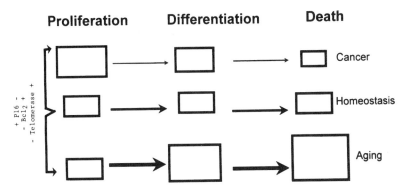

Figure 50.2.   Cellular and molecular differences of homeostasis, aging, and cancer.

of lung cancer the possibility of a selection bias should also be entertained. It is possible that among elderly patients with lung cancer, those with early disease were preferentially referred to academic cancer centers.

The response to antineoplastic chemotherapy is less likely and less durable in persons over 60 with acute myelogenous leukemia (AML), acute lymphoblastic leukemia, large cell non-Hodgkin's lymphoma, and epithelial cancer of the ovary (15–17). In the case of AML, a number of factors concur to produce chemotherapy resistance. The multidrug resistance (MDR1) gene expressed in 71% of older patients (versus 30% of those younger) prevents access of active drugs to the cell; involvement of the pluripotent hemopoietic stem cell in the disease process compromises the normal hemopoietic reserve and prevents hemopoietic recovery after marrow ablation; and higher prevalence of unfavorable cytogenetics results in early relapse after treatment (Cheryl Willman, American Society of Hematology, personal communication, December, 7, 1996).

While age may be associated with changes in cancer biology, age itself is a poor predictor of the natural history of cancer in individual patients. Older persons may develop very aggressive forms of breast cancer needing intensive treatment, and they may obtain excellent responses to the chemotherapy for AML, non-Hodgkin's lymphoma, or epithelial cancer of the ovary. The treatment of cancer in the aged should be determined by the characteristics of the neoplasm and by the patient's life expectancy and ability to tolerate treatment, not by the patient's age.

From this brief review we may draw three conclusions: that cancer control should target persons aged 65 to 90, because these persons manifest an increasing risk of cancer and of dying of cancer; that age may influence the natural history and the treatment of cancer; and that cancer prevention and treatment should be tailored to individual clinical situations.

PRINCIPLES OF CANCER PREVENTION

Primary prevention of cancer entails elimination of environmental carcinogens and administration of substances that offset late carcinogenic stages (chemoprevention). Chemoprevention appears particularly promising for older persons, who have heightened susceptibility to late-stage carcinogens. At least three groups of substances, estrogen antagonists, retinoids, and nonsteroidal anti-inflammatory drugs, demonstrated chemopreventive activity in humans (18). Of the estrogen antagonists, tamoxifen prevents contralateral breast cancer in women with history of breast cancer. *cis*-Retinoic acid has a wide range of cancer-preventive activity, including squamous cell carcinoma of the head and neck area and nonmelanomatous skin cancer. A new and less toxic synthetic retinoid, the fenretinide, is undergoing intensive clinical trials. Aspirin may prevent deaths from cancer of the large bowel; aspirin and other nonsteroidal drugs, including sulindac and indomethacin, may cause regression of colonic polyps. A number of other substances oppose the development of cancer in experimental systems. Antioxidants may be particularly promising for older persons, as enhanced formation of free radicals may cause molecular aging (18). Chemoprevention of cancer should be considered experimental until the balance of benefits and risks has been clarified in clinical trials. Secondary prevention of cancer entails early detection of cancer by screening asymptomatic persons. Secondary prevention of breast cancer, cervical cancer, and colorectal cancer has reduced the cancer-specific mortality of these diseases, but the benefits of screening have not been conclusively demonstrated in elders (19). Age-related factors may both favor and disfavor screening of elders. In favor of screening, the positive predictive value of screening tests may improve as the prevalence of cancer increases with age and the sensitivity of some tests, such as physical examination of the breast, also improves. Also, detection of colorectal cancer at early stages may avoid emergency surgery for intestinal obstruction, particularly risky in the aged. On the other side, the limited life expectancy of older persons may lessen the life-saving potential of screening, and screening tests performed at younger ages may have eliminated all prevalence cases of cancer. The benefit of detecting incidence cases in face of reduced life expectancy is not clear.

As a matter of practicality, we recommend screening for breast and colorectal cancer in persons aged 70 to 85 with a life expectancy of at least 3 years. For breast cancer we recommend yearly examination of the breast and mammography every 2 years; for colorectal cancer, yearly examination of the stools for fecal occult blood.

CANCER TREATMENT

Cancer treatment includes surgery and radiotherapy, which are local forms of treatment, and cytotoxic chemotherapy, hormone therapy, and biologic therapy, which are systemic forms of treatment. Elective cancer surgery is as safe and effective in persons in their 80s with adequate pulmonary and cardiac reserve as it is in younger persons, with the possible exceptions of hepatic and gastric resections (20, 21). The mortality of emergency surgery increases with the age of the patient, mainly because of sepsis from gram-negative organisms. The safety of radiotherapy has been extensively studied in older persons, including the oldest old (22). Radiotherapy proved safe even in patients of poor performance status, so that one should conclude that nobody is too old or too sick to benefit from it (23). The issues related to cytotoxic chemotherapy include changes in pharmacokinetics and pharmacodynamics of antineoplastic agents and increased susceptibility of several organ systems to therapeutic toxicity. The most consistent changes are decreased elimination of renally excretable drugs; increased prevalence of drug resistance; and increased risk of drug-induced myelosuppression, mucositis, and cardiac and nervous toxicity (24–26). The risks of chemotherapy may be ameliorated by a number of provisions (Table 50.1). The dose of renally excretable drugs should be adjusted to the estimated creatinine clearance of the older person. Toxicity may also be modulated by changing the modality of administration. For example, the cardiotoxicity of doxorubicin is markedly reduced when the drug is administered by continuous intravenous infusion. A number of new agents offer effective alternatives to previous drugs. Mitoxantrone may take the place of doxorubicin in the management of breast cancer and possibly lymphoma; vinorelbine, a semisynthetic alkaloid, is effective in breast cancer, prostate cancer, and non–small cell cancer of the lung; gemcitabine, an analog of cytidine, is effective in

Table 50.1

Prevention of Chemotherapy-Related Complications in Older Persons

Dosing of chemotherapy
  Dose adjustment for renally excretable drugs
    Methotrexate
    Carboplatin
    Bleomycin
    Fludarabine
    Cladribine
  Changes in administration schedule
Use of new and safer agents
  Mitoxantrone
  Oral etoposide
  Vinorelbine
  Gemcitabine
  Liposomal anthracyclines
Antidotes to drug-related toxicity
  Myelosuppression
    Hemopoietic growth factors
  Anthracycline cardiotoxicity
    Dexrazoxane
  Cisplatin nephrotoxicity
    Amifostine

pancreatic cancer, non–small cell cancer of the lung, and breast cancer. Liposomal doxorubicin and daunorubicin minimize the cardiotoxic effect of the anthracyclines. Perhaps the most important advance in the protection of normal tissues from cytotoxic chemotherapy has been the development of antidotes to drug toxicity. Hemopoietic growth factors include granulocyte colony-stimulating factor (G-CSF), granulocyte-macrophage colony-stimulating factor (GM-CSF), and erythropoietin (27). G-CSF and GM-CSF reduce the duration of neutropenia and the incidence of neutropenic infection and may prolong the survival of older persons with acute myelogenous leukemia. GM-CSF is preferred to G-CSF in acute leukemia, as it may prevent fungal infection more effectively and may also ameliorate mucositis. Erythropoietin may obviate red blood cell transfusion and maintain the energy level of older persons. Dexrazoxane prevents the formation of free radicals in the sarcomere of the myocardium by chelating cellular iron (28). Amifostine, a prodrug metabolized to a free thiol in normal but not in cancer cells, prevents nephro-toxicity, myelotoxicity, and neurotoxicity from cisplatin (29). Evidence is accumulating that am-ifostine may also prevent toxicity from alkylating agents (29).

Hormone therapy of cancer is well tolerated by patients of all ages; biologic therapy involves interferon alfa (IFN) and interleukin-2. At low doses (up to 5 MU daily), IFN is well tolerated by patients of all ages; at higher doses IFN may be associated with myelosuppression, peripheral neuropathy, hepatotoxicity, and nephrotoxicity. The use of interleukin-2 has been associated with serious complications, including anaphy-laxis, nephrotoxicity, and adult respiratory dis-tress syndrome (24).

New modalities of cancer treatment of special interest to older persons include endoscopic tu-mor ablation for cancer of the gastrointestinal tract, radiosurgery for small tumors of the cen-tral nervous system, and organ preservation with combined radiotherapy and chemotherapy for cancers of the larynx, anus, esophagus, and bladder (30).

In conclusion, with proper precautions, can-cer treatment may be beneficial to older persons. The decision to treat must balance potential gains in survival and quality of life with the risks of treatment-induced morbidity. Even in the case of advanced cancer, cytotoxic chemother-apy may improve the patient's overall survival, delay disability from tumor metastases, and ulti-mately reduce the cost of palliative care.

REFERENCES

1. Cole P, Rodu B. Declining cancer mortality in the United States. Cancer 1996;78:2045–2048.
2. Yancik R, Ries LA. Cancer in older persons. Cancer 1994;74:1995–2003.
3. Extermann M, Balducci L. Practical proposals for clini-cal protocols in elderly patients with cancer. In: Balducci L, Lyman GH, Ershler WB, eds. Comprehensive Geri-atric Oncology. London: Hardwood Academic Press, 1997:263–269.
4. Stanta G, Campagner L, Cavalieri F, et al. Cancer in the oldest old: what we have learned from autopsy studies. Clin Geriatr Med 1997;13:55–69.
5. Caranasos GJ. Prevalence of cancer in older persons liv-ing at home and in institutions. Clin Geriatr Med 1997; 13:15–32.
6. Balducci L. Cancer and age: issues and perspectives. In: Vellas BJ, Albarede JL, Garry PJ, eds. Facts and Research in Gerontology, 1994. New York: Springer, 1994:173–178.
7. Anisimov VN. Age as a risk factor in multistage carcino-genesis. In: Balducci L, Lyman GH, Ershler WB, eds. Comprehensive Geriatric Oncology. London: Hardwood Press, 1997:157–178.
8. Harris CC. p53: at the crossroad of molecular carcino-genesis and risk assessment. Science 1993;262:1980–1981.
9. Bestilny LJ, Brown CB, Miura Y, et al. Selective inhibition of telomerase activity during terminal differentiation of terminal cell lines. Cancer Res 1996;56:3796–3802.
10. Yang E, Korsmeyer SJ. Molecular thanatopsis: a dis-course on the BCL2 family and cell death. Blood 1996; 88:386–401.
11. Hannon GJ, Beach D. P15 is a potential effector of TGF-beta induced cell cycle arrest. Nature 1994;371:257–261.
12. Goodwin JS, Samet JM, Key CR, et al. Stage at diagnosis of cancer varies with the age of the patient. J Am Geriatr Soc 1986;34:20–26.
13. Balducci L, Silliman RA, Baekae P. Breast cancer in the older woman: an oncological perspective. In: Balducci L, Lyman GH, Ershler WB, eds. Comprehensive Geri-atric Oncology. London: Hardwood Academic Press, 1997:629–660.
14. Ershler WB. A gerontologist's perspective on cancer bi-ology and treatment. Cancer Control JMCC 1994;1:103–106.
15. Extermann M. Acute leukemia in the elderly. Clin Geri-atr Med 1997;13:227–244.
16. International Non-Hodgkin's Lymphoma Prognostic Factor Project: a predictive model for aggressive non-Hodgkin's lymphoma. N Engl J Med 1993;329:987–994.
17. Omura GA, Brady MF, Homesley HH, et al. Long-term follow-up and prognostic factor analysis in advanced ovarian carcinoma: the Gynecologic Oncology Group experience. J Clin Oncol 1991;9:1138–1150.
18. Lippman S, Benner SE, Hong WK. Cancer chemopre-vention. J Clin Oncol 1994;12:851–873.
19. Robinson B, Beghé C. Cancer screening in the older pa-tient. Clin Geriatr Med 1997,13:97–118.
20. Berger DH, Roslyn JJ. Cancer surgery in the elderly. Clin Geriatr Med 1997;13:119–142.
21. Balducci L, Cox CE, Greenberg H, et al. Management of cancer in the older aged person. Cancer Control JMCC 1994;1:132–137.
22. Olmi P, Ausili-Cefaro GP, Balzi M, et al. Radiotherapy in the aged. Clin Geriatr Med 1997;13:143–168.
23. Zachariah B, Casey L, Balducci L. Radiotherapy of the oldest old cancer patients: a study of effectiveness and toxicity. J Am Geriatr Soc 1995;43:793–795.
24. Cova D, Beretta G, Balducci L. Cancer chemotherapy in the elderly. In: Balducci L, Lyman GH, Ershler WB, eds. Comprehensive Geriatric Oncology. London: Hardwood Academic Press, 1997:429–442.
25. Kimmik G, Fleming R, Muss H, Balducci L. Cancer

chemotherapy in the older adults. Drugs Age 1997;10: 34–49.

26. Baker SD, Grochow LB. Pharmacology of cancer chemotherapy in the older person. Clin Geriatr Med 1997;13: 169–184.

27. Geller RB. Use of cytokines in the treatment of acute myelocytic leukemia: a critical review. J Clin Oncol 1996;14:1371–1382.

28. Hellman K. Anthracycline cardiotoxicity prevention by dexrazoxane: breakthrough of a barrier sharpens antitumor profile and therapeutic index. J Clin Oncol 1996; 14:332–333.

29. Kemp G, Rose P, Lourain J, et al. Amifostine pretreatment for protection against cyclophosphamide-induced and cisplatin-induced toxicities: results of a randomized controlled trial in patients with advanced ovarian cancer. J Clin Oncol 1996;14:2101–2112.

30. Balducci L, Trotti A. Organ preservation: an effective and safe form of cancer treatment. Clin Geriatr Med 1997;13:185–202.

CHAPTER 51

JAMES G. O'BRIEN AND JACOB CLIMO

The Elderly and Their Families

At present the family continues to be the single most important entity in ensuring that most older adults can live independently in their homes. Given the continuing increase in life expectancy, the duration of the relationship between parents and children is likely to increase. More adult children, including septuagenarians, are caregivers for disabled and infirm elderly parents for a wide variety of illnesses and for longer periods than ever before (1).

Despite the major support that home care agencies and various other social services contribute to the subsistence of older adults at home, these efforts are dwarfed by family contributions, particularly to personal care. Even for elderly who are institutionalized, the family continues to be the single most important outside source of support. Along with the basic goal of improving health care to prolong life itself, a corollary is that successful aging increasingly means sustaining a satisfying quality of personal life and social relationships.

THE PAST

Some of the efforts of contemporary families are demeaned when they are compared with the supposed outstanding efforts of families in former times to care for their elderly parents in an extended family context. Much of this idealized notion of family care in the past is more myth than reality. In the 18th and 19th centuries, short life expectancy ensured that most elderly spent very little time in multigeneration families because the average person died shortly after becoming a grandparent (2). In many instances the elderly parent lived nearby; if the parent lived with an adult child, this may have been in the elders' home, which possibly the child hoped to inherit. In many instances an explicit contract may have obligated the child to provide care in return for the inheritance. Thus it was fairly common for children to delay marriage to fulfill this obligation (3). Even though the elderly in the past were accorded greater respect and revered more than today, many were unsure of family commitment and support. The preferred arrangement was living close by (intimacy from a distance), not dissimilar to arrangements we witness today. Elders who lacked family or whose children were remote often took in boarders, which provided income, company, and perhaps safety and security (4).

The empty nest syndrome was not unknown in the past. When a child returned home, it was likely to be in response to a parent's need or perceived obligation. Today, when children return to the parents' home, it is likely to be in response to the child's need, such as a failed career or a divorce, rather than a parent's need. The returning child may be accompanied by his or her children, which adds to the burden of the elderly parent.

Gradually over this century the family has relinquished responsibility to various social agencies to care for elderly parents. In contrast with the past, total care can now be delegated from family to institution, as in the case of nursing home placement, although most families retain an overview responsibility when that occurs.

THE PRESENT

The elderly population in the United States is in transition. In 1996 almost 33.5 million persons, or 12.8% of the population, was age 65 or older. It is predicted that by the year 2020 55 million, or 20% of the population, will be 65 or older (5). The changes in composition of the American population will encompass not only quantitative differences but qualitative differences as well. A low fertility rate, high divorce rate, and the return of women to the workforce have changed the structure of the family and its ability to deal with the needs of an elderly population. In addition, a great deal of uncertainty surrounds the projected changes. The average life span is projected to increase, but the amount of the increase is unknown. Furthermore, the condition of those long-lived persons cannot be predicted: persons living longer in independence and good health may substantially add to society's well-being, whereas increased morbidity of the aged may pose an intolerable burden on the health care system. Recent data suggest that perhaps overall the health of the elderly population is improving. If sustained, this trend may result in fewer demands on the health care system. These questions and others add to the uncertainty about the future of the American elderly.

In 1994, 28% of older persons assessed their health as fair or poor (compared with 10% for all persons). There was little difference between the sexes on this measure, but older African-Americans were much more likely to rate their health as fair or poor (43%) than were older whites (27%) (5). About 12% of older Americans were in the workforce in 1995 (working actively or seeking work), including about 17% of men and 9% of women. About half were employed part-time. The educational level of older Americans improved dramatically between 1970 and 1994. The percentage of older Americans who had completed high school rose from 28% to 62%. In terms of ethnic groups, 65% of whites had completed high school, while only 37% of African-Americans and 30% of Hispanics had managed to do so.

In 1994, 81% of older men and 58% of older women lived in families. About 13% did not live with a spouse but lived with children, siblings, or other relatives. Approximately 30% of all non-institutionalized elderly (40% of women and 16% of men) lived alone.

The combined effects of a remarkable growth in the older population, a decreased birth rate, the effects of divorce, geographic scatter, and more caregivers in the workforce are likely to lead to a decrease in informal support. In Japan, the ratio of elders to caregivers is likely to reach 91 elders per 100 women aged 50 to 64 (the typical caregiver age range) by year 2025. This phenomenon is likely to occur in a less extreme form in most developed countries, including the United States, in the near future.

This chapter presents a series of clinical case studies in which older adults and their familial relationships are described in the context of a clinical practice from the perspective of a primary care physician.

THE WELL-ADJUSTED FAMILY

Dr. S., an 82-year-old retired PhD physiologist, and his wife, a retired elementary school teacher aged 79, live in their original home in a Midwestern university community where they both taught. They are both independent in all activities of daily living (ADLs) and instrumental ADLs (IADLs), and they require no assistance to manage their affairs. Dr. S. has had some health problems, including hypertension for 40 years and an irregular heartbeat secondary to premature ventricular contractions not requiring any treatment. He also recently had a transient ischemic attack and has decreasing vision in one eye because of macular degeneration and a retinal hemorrhage. He can still drive during daylight. Mrs. S. can drive at night, but she is reluctant to do so.

Mrs. S.'s health is relatively good. She has degenerative arthritis of her knees and hips, but her symptoms are controllable with acetaminophen and occasional use of nonsteroidal anti-inflammatory medications. She also has irritable bowel syndrome and is lactose intolerant, with occasional bouts of sudden diarrhea. This has resulted in accidents, limiting her comfort with long-distance traveling.

They have one son, a surgeon, who lives with his wife and two children in the South. He and his family usually visit at least once a year, and he telephones every week. He is supportive and has been helpful when a parent had some medical problem. Dr. and Mrs. S. are particularly attentive to their two grandchildren and enjoy a special relationship with them. They are each firmly committed to maintaining health and independence. They see their physician regularly for ongoing care of their chronic problems; participate in regular preventive activities, such as annual vaccinations and cancer screening; and maintain a daily regimen of walking. Neither one smokes and they have a very modest ingestion of alcohol.

Both are active in their community, particularly with the faculty retirees group, which promotes many educational activities for emeritus faculty. They are frequent travelers with Elder Hostel. They enjoy a wide circle of friends, and both volunteer at the library and at a local hospital. They have discussed moving to be closer to their son and his family and have also considered selling their home and moving to a retirement community in the area but have been unable to agree on this.

A small but increasing number of retired Americans migrate seasonally or permanently to national amenity areas such as California, Arizona, and Florida, which are known for their pleasant climates and desirable retirement lifestyle communities (6). Although only 5% of Americans move to another state for retirement, such amenity migrations are increasingly common among healthy, active people who seek to improve the quality of their lives and can afford migration (7). When aging parents discuss moving, adult children's reactions reveal their perceptions of their parents' ability to live and make decisions independently.

Living as a couple is a satisfying and successful arrangement for the elderly because it can provide for the emotional, social, and instrumental needs of the partners. A growing awareness of increasing difficulty keeping house or the anticipation of an increasing need for services may motivate an elderly couple or widow to move to a retirement center that provides domestic services, health care, safety, and an attractive social environment. Such discussion may be regarded as anticipatory preparation for the eventual late-life moves. To the extent that aging parents can discuss anticipated changes openly with their families, they may prevent the trauma of unexpected rapid and dramatic changes.

Approximately 10 million elderly parents live too far away from their adult children for frequent face-to-face relationships. Despite the limitations of geographic separations, such persons in general remain in close contact and maintain strong bonds of affection through regular telephone calls, seasonal visits, and assistance in health crises (8).

A more complex situation occurs when either the parents or children are divorced. In these situations it may be much more difficult to identify family members who accept responsibility for care. With parental divorce, the children frequently take sides and form allegiance with one parent. For some children it is impossible to respond to the needs of an estranged parent. Compounding this problem may be issues of inheritance and conflicting values. Sometimes one child agrees to help; unfortunately, sometimes families refuse to help, which results in dependence on friends, other networks, and agencies.

Increasingly, distant family members wish to be more involved in decision making and assisting their disabled and infirm elderly parents. With the recent development and diffusion of high technologies, such as video phones in the home, this trend will flourish. Distant relatives can participate in their family members' health regimen and provide important assistance in everyday living through communication with health care professionals. Of course many domestic services must be performed by someone nearby. An important part of the S. family's routine is regular contacts with their children and grandchildren. For most people, maintaining social networks and emotional bonds to family, friends, and community is basic to physical and mental health. Both Dr. and Mrs. S. exemplify the most effective treatment of chronic conditions: self-management of their illnesses at home in consultation with their physician.

FAMILY OF A PATIENT WITH DEMENTIA OF THE ALZHEIMER TYPE

Mrs. K. is a 79-year-old woman whose son recently moved her to his community because she could not manage in her own home in a distant state. She has been widowed for 8 years and managed independently until about a year ago, when a number of changes began to occur. She bounced a number of checks because she had failed to deposit pension income in that account. She got lost while driving within a mile of her home and had to be taken home by the police. Her son was also concerned that she might have been drinking to excess, compounding the memory problem. Subsequently she was evaluated and determined to have progressive dementia of the Alzheimer type.

The son moved her to his home, where he lives with his wife and two children, aged 8 and 12 years. The introduction of Mrs. K. to the home has been very difficult. The stress of relocation, coupled with the new environment and the presence of children, has caused sensory overload that is manifested by increasing confusion and acting out. The daughter-in-law in particular resents the entry of her mother-in-law into the household. She does not feel it is her obligation to provide care. She feels her husband should not have agreed to this arrangement but should have asked one of his other two siblings to care for Mrs. K. In fact, her son is the child who was least favored by the mother in the past, but the other two siblings are very domineering and exerted pressure that resulted in this arrangement.

Dementia is a chronic progressive disease that is common in older age. It is irreversible, has physical and emotional consequences, and may have significant social and economic effects that intrude on all aspects of living. Usually when there is functional decline resulting from this disease, families are involved in some aspect of care, from oversight responsibilities to direct provision of care. The effect on families is often devastating, and given the increasing prevalence of dementia with aging, it is likely that most families in the future will have a demented member. Population studies suggest that almost 50% of those over age 85 may have dementia (9).

Today almost three quarters of all elderly Americans live with a spouse (40%) or alone (35%). An important minority still live with their own aging parents or their adult children in nuclear two-generation households (12%) and/or with their parents, children, and grandchildren in three-generation households (6%). Patients' preferences for remaining at home often require creative solutions, including formal and informal collaboration, to achieve this.

The bulk of care of the elderly is provided by informal networks of family and friends, with almost three fourths of the care provided by women (10). Spouses "provide the bulk of the care required by their impaired partner" (11). While there has been a decrease in the number of parents and adult children living together, data show that more than half of the children living with elderly parents do so to benefit themselves (12).

Caregiving is composed of two components: personal burden to the caretaker, such as loss of independence and limited personal activity, and interpersonal burden, such as difficulties dealing with the behaviors of the elderly person (13). "Daughters and wives were more likely to report such limitations than sons and husbands" (14). Caregivers who quit work to provide care were likely to be less healthy than those who continued to work (12). Overall, social isolation increases with the progressive frailty of the elderly person, and social network becomes a major factor in caregiver reactions to the burden of caregiving (12).

After age 85, elderly women continue to outnumber men 5 to 2 (15), but the proportion of widows is expected to decrease as men continue to gain in life expectancy. One of two major changes in the elderly population is the delineation of women in the middle, who must fulfill three or more simultaneous life roles, such as child rearing, working for a living, and caring for frail or disabled parents (16). Since women assume more caregiving responsibilities than men, the proportion of women in this situation grows with the elderly population.

The physician may play several roles in the care of the elderly demented person and the family. That role should be flexible and adapted to the stage of the disease and the needs of the patient and family. In the early stages of the disease the emphasis is on making a precise diagnosis, which is not always easy. Standard algorithms, if used appropriately, should result in diagnostic accuracy exceeding 80% (17). Atypical cases should be referred to consultants in neurology or geropsychiatry or special memory disorder diagnostic centers.

Families can use many resources to learn about the disease and the assistance necessary in managing the disease, such as *The 36 Hour Day* (18) and assistance from the local Alzheimer's Association.

Given the insidious nature of the disease and the waxing and waning of the mental impairment, families may disagree about the time of onset and severity, hence about when safety measures such as discontinuing driving should be instituted. Many families are in denial and reject the diagnosis initially. Follow-up visits that verify the progression of the disease and allow for continued dialog with the family generally help shift the family to a more reasonable and accepting position. The family may have fears about the risk of inheriting the disease, whether the disease is infectious, or whether the behaviors are deliberate. Each of these issues has to be addressed. Given the demands of a busy practice, many practitioners do not have the time to respond to all of these needs but can link families with other community resources such as an Alzheimer's Association, a geriatric assessment program, and various home health agencies. The physician can recommend that a family member or friend assume durable power of attorney before the patient becomes so impaired that such an arrangement cannot legally be executed.

It is helpful to discuss goals and expectations with the family. The emphasis should be on quality of life rather than life extension, given that this is a terminal illness. As the disease progresses and the elderly parent becomes more impaired, the demands on the family members typically increase. A particularly painful experience for family members occurs if the patient enters a paranoid phase and accuses caregivers of misusing funds or stealing from him or her. Sometimes family members are not even recognized. These behaviors may signal the need to consider placement outside the home. The types of settings available vary by community; some communities have special Alzheimer units or specialized assisted living facilities; others will have very limited options.

The physician may be able to help if guilt is the dominant family theme regarding placement, perhaps because of a previous commitment not to place a parent in a nursing home. The physician may have to balance responsibility to the patient against the desire to assist an overwhelmed family. Acknowledging the inability of the family to meet the increasing need of the Alzheimer's patient in the home and pointing out the potential for resulting harm may help the family decide to institutionalize. When the patient is no longer able to recognize the home, a move may be negotiated fairly easily.

In the final stages of the disease the family frequently must decide how aggressive the medical care should be. It is very helpful to have documented preferences expressed by the patient in the form of an advance directive. Issues regarding feeding tubes, ventilators, and other extraordinary means require careful discussion. The family needs to understand the immediate and short-term benefits and burdens of such decisions. Any action should be guided primarily by the prior expressed wishes (if known) of the patient. If the patient is placed in an institution, the family can still contribute greatly to the quality of life of the patient by supporting nursing home staff, monitoring the quality of care, and acting as advocate.

UNCOOPERATIVE FAMILY OF A FRAIL ELDER

Mrs. B., a widow of many years in her late 60s, recently moved to this community with her 41-year-old son, his wife, and their teenage daughter. Her son was not successful in real estate and made a major midlife career change to enter law school. The family rented two apartments in the same building, with plans to build a house with a mother-in-law suite. After an unsuccessful year in law school, the son became manager of the housing complex they were living in. He later bought a house, but his remodeling plans did not consider his mother.

Mrs. B was in frail health. She had hypertension, arthritis, and cirrhosis of the liver; on an early visit she admitted she was a recovering alcoholic. In addition, she had anxiety attacks. Mrs. B. was capable of basic self-care and managed her own finances but depended on her son and daughter-in-law for shopping, transportation, and social supports.

The family generally, and Mrs. B. in particular, have not made a satisfactory adjustment to the community. After 4 years they have few friends and virtually no social involvements. Relations within the family were also poor. Mrs. B. was openly critical of her son and daughter-in-law's discipline of her granddaughter. Mrs. B. did not get along with her daughter-in-law; when the daughter-in-law took her to the doctor's office, she would leave her, never speak to the doctor, and only return when summoned from the office.

Mrs. B. was a difficult patient. Periodically she would ask the doctor why she wasn't being referred to specialists for her arthritis or liver, but when referred, she would refuse to go. She contracted with the physician for a limited supply of diazepam for her anxiety. After 1 week of upper respiratory symptoms, she telephoned for a refill of diazepam and for a cough medicine that worked the previous year. One day later she died suddenly.

Following her death, the family were threatening and intimidating; they also revealed some disturbing information. First, they wanted to know why she died suddenly and blamed the physician when he said he wasn't sure. The daughter-in-law claimed that Mrs. B. had been having fainting spells, which "I'm sure she told you about. Couldn't you have done some cardiac tests with a dye?" they asked. The physician agreed to an autopsy, but ultimately the family decided against it. At the funeral home, which was attended by virtually no one, the son volunteered to the physician that he had been providing his mother with beer for many years. The physician's attendance at the funeral home allowed an open discussion that otherwise would not have occurred.

This is an isolated family that uprooted itself and made a poor adjustment to the new community. The son and daughter-in-law were apparently uninvolved in their mother's health care but enabled her alcoholism and possibly frightened her by planning to leave her in the apartment when they moved to their home.

This is a particularly difficult situation for the physician, and given the family dynamics, the potential for the physician to become a scapegoat for any bad outcome is great. The survivors are probably angry, perhaps feeling guilty and remorseful yet unwilling to acknowledge their contributions to the patient's problems. Certainly they enabled the continuation of her alcoholism and failed to inform the physicians of her continued drinking, knowing full well that she was also taking diazepam.

Alcoholism among the elderly is a major problem and may be even less likely to be detected in this age group than in younger persons. Many older adults do not have work obligations and may not be visited or called on at night, which may allow the problem to be overlooked. Many of the symptoms and signs of alcoholism, such as hypertension, falling, insomnia, and confusion, may be attributed to aging (19). Most physicians have a low index of suspicion when dealing with elderly patients who don't fit the stereotype.

Sometimes the physician can be only as good as he is allowed to be by patient and family. The physician in this situation is disadvantaged by not knowing the family situation. They never asked him to make a home visit, and he had very limited opportunity to discuss the patient with any other family members. Similarly, the patient was adamant in her refusal to acknowledge she was drinking.

CHALLENGES TO THE FAMILY WITH A DYING PATIENT

Mrs. O. was a 79-year-old African-American woman admitted to the hospital with pneumonia. She was living independently until about 3 months ago, when she began to fail. She was not eating as well as before and had lost weight. Her interest in socializing had diminished, and she complained of fatigue and just generally not feeling well. She had eight living children, most of whom reside in the community where she lived. The family is very close and she was the matriarch, especially since the death of her husband 10 years previously.

Before she was admitted with the pneumonia, a number of measures were instituted by her family physician in an attempt to explain her decline; diagnostic laboratory work had failed to yield a diagnosis. A trial of an antidepressant did not help. Increasing attention by family members, including the provision of meals, failed to increase her appetite or weight. After admission to the hospital, she failed to improve with antibiotic therapy. A pulmonologist was consulted. Bronchoscopy failed to provide any additional diagnostic clues. Her chest radiographs and clinical status deteriorated over the next few days, leading to intubation and assisted ventilation, which was consistent with the desires of the family and expressed by her daughter, who had durable power of attorney.

She continued to decline, and 7 days after admission to the hospital, at the request of her physician and with the agreement of the family except her youngest son, the ventilator was discontinued and the patient died. Her autopsy revealed a rare malignant histiocytosis. The autopsy results, which became available some weeks after her death, were discussed with the family. Although death is most likely to occur in old age, the older person does not necessarily accept death, nor are the family members necessarily prepared for the demise of a parent.

It is estimated that 72% of deaths in the United States occur among persons aged 65 or older; this amounts to approximately 1.7 million deaths annually (5). Many are the culmination of multiple chronic diseases over time with accompanying functional decline. This scenario often prepares or allows family members to anticipate death. Conversely, death may be sudden and unanticipated, leaving family members to cope with the sequelae of an unexpected loss.

When death is expected, the family members can begin grieving, especially when there is open discussion of death between the patient and family. In most instances when discussion does take place, it is initiated by the older adult. If this open discussion has not already taken place, it allows consideration of advance directives, allowing the older adult the autonomy to dictate how death and dying may be managed. But given the high prevalence of dementia, particularly in octogenarians, the older adult may not be able to participate in decisions about medical treatment.

Many families are uncomfortable with the topic of death and unwilling to discuss it. Others want to conceal the fact that death is imminent and not discuss it with the parent, which can place the physician in an untenable position. Knowing the family's motives in making such a request may allow the physician to negotiate a reasonable course of action with the dying person. Data from researchers in this subject, including Kubler-Ross (20), indicate that the dying person usually knows that he or she is dying, and children can be reassured that the topic can be gradually broached with the older adult. The physician frequently can assist by eliciting the older adult's understanding of the disease state and expectations for treatment.

Because of the likelihood that older adults are likely to die in institutions, the net result is to isolate the parent from direct family care. If death takes place in the hospital, particularly in intensive care, the ability to talk with the parent is greatly impeded, particularly if the person is intubated. If death is inevitable, moving the older person to a site in the hospital where comfort care rather than curative care is emphasized allows more open access and an opportunity for personal care by the family. Ideally the physician, in collaboration with nurses, clergy, and hospice or at a minimum applying hospice principles, aggressively pursues relief of symptoms and attempts to ensure the best quality of life for the dying patient.

Older adults who die in long-term care facilities or nursing homes benefit when the family can have ready access and contribute as much personal care as they can without being overburdened by providing total care. If death is expected and hospice is involved, the patient and family may prefer home care, which is often a most gratifying experience for the patient's family and providers.

When death is sudden and unexpected, the spouse or family has little time to prepare; there is no opportunity to say good-bye or time for those with guilt feelings to attempt to resolve old issues and attain forgiveness. This may be a particular problem for children who live at a distance and have not had the opportunity to interact with a parent as much as they might desire.

An older adult who is dying may not accept death and the fact that life will continue after the event; he or she may attempt to cling to life by demanding excessive and futile medical care (21). Because of feelings of guilt or lack of knowledge, the family may also demand futile care. A personal relationship with a trusted physician is vital during these situations, and occasionally an ethics committee may help with the process. In other instances families may just need to witness recurrent failure to restore quality of life before accepting the inevitability of death and allowing the transition to comfort care.

There is a general perception that the loss of an older adult is less significant than the loss of a child or a younger adult; this notion makes it particularly difficult for a spouse or child to grieve appropriately for a loved one (22). This may lead to grief in isolation, without support or assistance from others (23). This problem should be acknowledged and the bereavement legitimized. The death of a parent or spouse is an event of great importance and is a time of transition and a time for families to retrench, cope, and learn how to continue in the absence of an influential elder.

REFERENCES

1. Brody EM. Parent care as a normative family stress. Gerontologist 1985;25:19–29.
2. Hareven TK. Historical perspectives on the family and aging. In: Blieszner R, Hilkevitch Bedford V, eds. Handbook of Aging and the Family. Westport, CT: Greenwood Press, 1995:13–31.
3. Smith DS. Parental power and marriage patterns: analysis of historical trends in Hingham, Massachusetts. J Marriage Fam 1993;35:419–428.
4. Ruggles S. Prolonged Connections: The Case of the Extended Family in Nineteenth Century England and America. Madison: University of Wisconsin Press, 1987.
5. A Profile of Older Americans: 1995, PF 3049 (1296). D 996. Washington: AARP, 1995.
6. Litwak E, Longino CF. Migration patterns among the elderly: a developmental perspective. Gerontologist 1987; 27:266–272.
7. Morrison PA. Demographic factors reshaping ties to family and place. Res Aging 1990;12:399–408.
8. Climo J. Distant Parents. New Brunswick, NJ: Rutgers Press, 1992.
9. Evans DA, Funkenstein HH, Albert MS, et al. Prevalence of Alzheimer's disease in a community population of older persons. Higher than previously reported. JAMA 1989;262:2551–2556.
10. Collins C, Stommel M, King S, Given CW. Assessment of the attitudes of family caregivers toward community services. Gerontologist 1991;31:756–761.
11. Pruchno RA. The effects of health patterns on the mental health of spouse caregivers. Res Aging 1990;12:57–71.
12. Crimmins E, Ingegneri D. Interaction and living arrangements of older parents and their children. Res Aging 1990;12:3–35.
13. Miller B, McFall S. Caregiver burden and the continuum of care. Res Aging 1992;16:376–398.
14. Miller B, Montgomery A. Family caregivers and limitations in social activities. Res Aging 1990;12:72–93.
15. Fowles D. A Profile of Older Americans. Washington: The Program Resources Department AARP, AOA. US Department of Health and Human Services, 1992.
16. Spitze G, Logan J. More evidence on women (and men) in the middle. Res Aging 1990;12:182–198.
17. Emery V, Oxman T, eds. Dementia: Presentations, Differential Diagnosis and Nosology. Baltimore: Johns Hopkins University Press, 1994.
18. Mace N, Rabins P. The 36 Hour Day: A Family Guide to Caring for Persons With Alzheimer's Disease, Related Dementing Illnesses and Memory Loss in Later Life. Baltimore: Johns Hopkins University Press, 1982.
19. Adams WL, Yuan Z, Barboriak JJ, Rimm AA. Alcohol related hospitalizations of elderly people. Prevalence and geographic variation in the United States. JAMA 1993; 270:1222–1225.
20. Kubler-Ross E. On Death & Dying. New York: Collier Books, 1993.
21. Sullender R. Losses in Later Life: A New Way of Walking With God. New York: Paulist Press, 1989.
22. Hargrave T, Anderson W. Finishing Well: Aging and Reparation in the Intergenerational Family. New York: Brunner/Mazel, 1992.
23. Moss M, Moss S. Death and bereavement. In: Blieszner R, Hilkevitch Bedford V, eds. Handbook of Aging and the Family. Westport, CT: Greenwood Press, 1995:459–473.

CHAPTER 52

MARY C. SENGSTOCK AND JAMES G. O'BRIEN

The Mistreatment of Older Adults

INTRODUCTION AND DEFINITIONS

Maltreatment of older adults is not a new problem. Like other forms of family abuse, however, it has only recently been recognized as a social problem. The mistreatment of older adults includes several types of abuse. *Physical abuse* includes direct physical assaults, from slapping to homicide. This also includes sexual assaults, which some authorities place in a separate category. *Physical neglect* is the failure to provide a dependent older adult with the necessities of life, such as food, clothing, medicine, a safe living environment, and assistive devices. *Psychologic abuse and neglect* include verbal abuse, isolating the person from social contact, and threats, a common one being the threat to place the elder in a nursing home. *Exploitation* includes actions taken against an older adult's property or other items and forcing an older adult to make decisions against his or her will, such as forcing a change in residence or a will or preventing a marriage or divorce.

These categories are often interrelated. Most cases of victimization involve more than one type, and the less severe types, such as psychologic abuse or neglect and exploitation, are often precursors of the more life-threatening physical abuse and neglect (1). Most laws focus on mistreatment at the hands of others, but some also focus on *self-neglect,* which is being reported with increasing frequency in most states and is frustrating to deal with.

It is difficult to obtain accurate data on the prevalence of elder mistreatment, since victims and their families are prone to hide such behavior. Official statistics fail to include large numbers of cases, and studies tend to employ small, biased samples. The most frequently quoted study, using a community sample of households of persons over 65, found a rate of 32 per 1000, or approximately 3% (2). Since this study excluded some types of elder mistreatment, this figure should be considered to be a minimum.

Mistreatment can occur in the older adult's own home, the homes of relatives, and in institutional facilities. Not all elder mistreatment is a deliberate action taken to injure the victim. Families often face serious dilemmas in caring for an aged member. For example, older adults often fail to recognize their failing capacities and may insist on living alone when they no longer are capable of caring for themselves. Their children must either violate their rights by forcing them to move or worry that they may later be charged with neglect if the older adult should fall or otherwise be injured.

THE PHYSICIAN'S ROLE

The unique position of physicians gives them a particularly important role with regard to exposing elder abuse. Most older adults see a physician regularly. Hence physicians are in a position to identify many cases of mistreatment that would not otherwise come to public attention. Older adults also trust physicians and are likely to confide in them. In many instances, doctors also have contact with the older adult's family and may understand the factors surrounding the mistreatment. Physicians also have access to critical tests needed by other professionals to verify abuse.

Legal Requirements

As a means to deal with mistreatment of older adults, as of 1990 all states had passed legislation requiring reporting of this problem. These laws vary somewhat from state to state. All are designed to protect "vulnerable" adults, which includes adults who because of advanced age and/or physical or mental disability are not able to protect themselves. In such instances, the state intervenes on their behalf. Mandatory reporting laws require health and social service professionals to report suspected cases of elder mistreatment to an adult protective services agency. Physicians are usually among those required to report and should determine the specific reporting requirements for their particular state and county. State laws generally provide protection for reporters, keeping the identity of the reporter confidential and guaranteeing immunity from litigation to those who report.

Adult protective service workers investigate the reports, document whether mistreatment has indeed occurred, and provide assistance. This may include referral to police or other authorities to protect the victim from the abuser. Laws also require that the independence of mentally competent elders be protected and that their decision not to receive services will be respected.

Who Is at Risk?

Mistreatment of older adults can occur among all economic, racial, and religious categories. Since most older adults are women, most victims of elder mistreatment are also women. However, there is some indication that older men may be at greater risk. Physicians should never assume that any segment of their patient population is free from risk. At particularly high risk, however, are patients who are isolated; are highly dependent on others for their care; have been dependent for an extended period; have dementia, depression, or other psychiatric problems; or engage in behaviors, such as wandering or aggressiveness, that make caregiving difficult.

Certain characteristics of the family and caregiver are also associated with a high risk of abuse, such as elders in families with a history of poor relationships, especially those involving conflict, abuse, or violence. If the caregiver or other family members have mental or psychologic problems or are substance abusers, the older adult is at greater risk. Many older adults are alone; they are often at the mercy of caregivers or neighbors.

Even in families with a high level of cohesion and resourcefulness, long-term care of an older adult can stretch resources to the breaking point. Care of an aged adult is highly disruptive of normal family status and power relationships. A parent who is dependent on an adult son or daughter may attempt to maintain his or her former authority, resulting in tension, conflict, and possible violence. If the older adult requires extensive personal care from a son or daughter, this may violate some of society's strongest taboos, which prohibit parents and adult children from seeing each other naked. Whenever a caregiver is under a particularly heavy burden, either from patient care alone or from a combination of patient care and other problems and tasks, the patient is at risk for mistreatment.

Clinical Identification of Mistreatment

Since physicians are more likely to observe the older adult than any other professional, they are likely to be better able to identify persons at risk or actually victims of mistreatment (3). Since mistreatment frequently escalates over time, early identification may allow intervention to prevent the more life-threatening types which may occur later.

There are several medical indicators of high risk for mistreatment. Protocols for assessment and screening are outlined in Figure 52.1. When injury from abuse or neglect has occurred, families are likely to take the victim to different medical facilities, particularly emergency centers, in the hope that health care providers will not see a pattern and recognize the mistreatment. Other indicators include a sudden decline in function; failure to thrive; frequent use of medical facilities; noncompliance with medical advice; failure to appear for appointments; and delay in seeking treatment. Table 52.1 provides a summary of such factors. In addition, specific indicators can be delineated for each type of mistreatment.

Physical abuse can be identified by observing

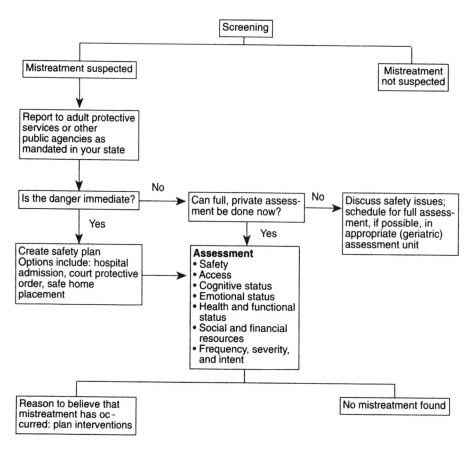

Figure 52.1. Screening and assessment for elder abuse and neglect should be based on an algorithm such as this one, developed and recommended by the American Medical Association. (Adapted from American Medical Association Department of Mental Health. Diagnostic and Treatment Guidelines on Elder Abuse and Neglect. Chicago: American Medical Association, 1992.)

repeated or unusually placed injuries. For example, physical examinations or radiographs may indicate previous injuries that have been neglected. A radiograph may show a spiral fracture, an injury caused by a twisting motion, which is inconsistent with the description of the accident described by the patient or family.

Bruises should be carefully examined for special patterns. These may include bruises that take the pattern of the object inflicting them, such as a belt, electric cord, hanger, or the fingers of the human hand. Bruises should also be examined to determine whether they are consistent with the explanation given. New bruises tend to be red, blue, or purple; after several days or a few weeks, they turn green, yellow, or brown. If bruises are not all the same age, the explanation should reflect this rather than attribute all to a single incident.

These examples illustrate the importance of a thorough history and physical examination. Careful attention should be paid to any injuries that do not match the patient's history. Particular attention should be paid to injuries in the breast or perineal areas, which may indicate that sexual abuse should be investigated.

Physical neglect may be present if the patient exhibits a lack of any necessities. Unexplained weight loss, not following prescribed medical protocols, or lacking such aids as dentures, eyeglasses, or hearing aids may indicate that a dependent patient is not receiving proper care. Patients may also exhibit evidence of being improperly restrained, with bruises or burns on the wrists or elsewhere. Overmedicating and symptoms of alcohol or drug overdose may also be signs that a caregiver is using these as methods of restraint.

Table 52.1

Warning Signs of Possible Elder Mistreatment

History
  Pattern of "physician hopping"
  Unexplained delay in seeking treatment
  Previous unexplained injuries or injuries inconsistent with medical findings
  Previous reports of injuries similar to the current ones
  Conflicting accounts between patient and potential abuser
Physical findings
  Fractures, falls, dislocations
  Evidence of physical restraint
  Bruises, hematomas, welts, lacerations, abrasions, punctures
  Burns of unusual shape or in unusual locations
  Injuries that are bilateral, clustered, or in various stages of healing
  Evidence of overmedication or undermedication
  Unexplained sexually transmitted disease or genital infection
  Pain, itching, bruising, or bleeding in genital area
  Signs of poor personal hygiene, decubitus ulcers, dehydration, malnutrition
  Inadequate or inappropriate clothing
  Absence of needed eyeglasses, hearing aids, dentures, prostheses
  Poor walking indicating hidden injuries or sexual assault
  Evidence of substance abuse in patient or caregiver
Clinical observations
  Signs of withdrawal, depression, agitation, low self-esteem
  Infantile behavior
  Mental status changes from previous examination
  Evidence of sleep disorder or deprivation
  Ambivalence, resignation, fearfulness toward caregiver or family members
  Substandard care despite adequate financial resources
  Confusion over or lack of knowledge of financial situation
  Sudden transfer of assets to a family member
  Sudden inability to meet financial needs
  Caregiver refusing to let patient see physician alone
  Unusual behavior patterns between patient and caregiver

Adapted from AMA Department of Mental Health. Diagnostic and Treatment Guidelines on Elder Abuse and Neglect. Chicago, 1992; The Mount Sinai Victim Services Agency Elder Abuse Project. Elder Mistreatment Guidelines for Health Care Professionals: Detection, Assessment and Intervention. New York, 1988; The Harborview Medical Center Department of Social Work. Protocol for Identification and Assessment of Elder Mistreatment. Seattle, 1992; Beth Israel Hospital Elder Abuse/Neglect Protocol. Boston, 1991; and Bloom JS, Ansell P, Bloom MN. Detecting elder abuse: a guide for physicians. Geriatrics 1969;44:40–56.

Psychologic abuse and neglect are more difficult to identify. Depression, withdrawal, fear of the caregiver, or isolation from others may be indicators.

Exploitation can often be observed in the medical setting by noting whether a mentally competent older adult is in control of his or her health care and finances. If a caregiver or others try to prevent a patient from consulting a physician alone or make decisions for him or her, this may be evidence of mistreatment. If a patient is unable to pay for treatment or prescribed medications, especially if this is a change from an earlier pattern, the patient's funds may have been misappropriated. Identification of the problem at this point may prevent an escalation at a later time. Medical facilities sometimes facilitate exploitation by inviting family members to provide information or make decisions, rather than allowing older adults to do these things for themselves;

Table 52.2

Guidelines for Interviewing Victims

Ensure privacy.

Separate victims from caregivers.

Ensure confidentiality.

Allow adequate time for response.

Progress from general (screening) to specific (direct) questions.

Keep questions simple and appropriate for educational level.

Respect cultural and ethnic differences.

Do not blame victims.

Do not blame or confront perpetrators.

Do not show frustration.

Acknowledge that this process may require multiple interviews.

Determine whether cognitive impairment is present.

Use other people, such as office or emergency room nurses, to conduct the interview if this is less threatening to victims.

Reprinted with permission from O'Brien JG. A primary care clinician's perspective. In: Baumhover LA, Beall SC, eds. Abuse, Neglect, and Exploitation of Older Persons. Baltimore: Health Professions Press, 1996:51–64.

e.g., an admissions clerk who asks someone other than the older adult to find his or her Medicare card is, in effect, giving that person permission to search the older adult's wallet or purse.

Interviewing Victims and Possible Perpetrators

As has been noted, a critical component of identifying elder mistreatment is obtaining an accurate case history. A number of techniques may help to accomplish this, as noted in Table 52.2 (4). First, it is essential that the older adult be interviewed apart from the suspected abuser or any other family member; during this period another staff member may interview family members to obtain additional information. Both should be interviewed in a quiet, private, nonthreatening setting. Both should be assured of confidentiality: never tell the family what the older adult has said or vice versa. In both instances, the interviewer should make an effort at the outset to develop rapport.

The interviewer can assist the interview by judicious questioning (Table 52.3) (5, 6). Questions should proceed from the general to the spe-

cific. In this private setting, do not be afraid to ask the older adult directly if he or she has been injured or threatened. Ask the respondent to describe a typical day. Both the older adult and the family members are likely to describe stresses and problems, as well as defenses. The abuser and even the victim may defend the abuser's behavior; interviewers should allow them to maintain these defenses.

As indicated, a thorough physical examination of the older adult is also critical; the physician should explain the need for this and ask the patient's permission. All findings in both history and physical should be clearly documented in the event of a later investigation. It is important at this point to determine the degree of danger or urgency of the situation. Patients whose lives may be in danger must be handled differently from those to whom the threat is less serious or immediate.

In interviewing the alleged abuser or other family members, attempt to determine both stresses and possible supports. What caregiving problems exist? What other personal or family problems are present? Are there resources in the family that can be called upon for support?

A number of approaches should be avoided in these interviews. Always avoid blaming the victim for his or her situation. Also avoid confronting the suspected abuser with his or her actions. In most instances confrontation is not useful; and in any event, this is the role of protective services or legal authorities, not the physician. If a report is mandatory, avoid using it as a threat. Rather present it as a means of protection and assistance, but do not suggest that protective services can solve all problems. However, good data from a thorough history and physical can have considerable value to protective services in any further action on the case.

Case Management

Assistance to older patients who have suffered mistreatment is a long-term process. There are short- and long-term management goals. *Short-term management* includes actions that must occur within the 24- or 48-hour period immediately following the discovery of mistreatment. During this period it is critical to assess the degree of danger to the older adult. If physical abuse has already occurred or is threatened and

Table 52.3

Suggested Questions from the Hwalek-Sengstock Elder Abuse Screening Test[a]

Items indicating violation of personal rights or direct abuse

4. Who makes decisions about your life, like how or where you should live?
9. Does someone in your family make you stay in bed or tell you you're sick when you know you're not?
10. Has anyone forced you to do things you didn't want to do?
11. Has anyone taken things that belong to you without your permission?
15. Has anyone close to you threatened to hurt you or harm you recently?

Items indicating characteristics of vulnerability

1. Do you have anyone who spends time with you, taking you shopping or to the doctor?
3. Are you sad or lonely often?
6. Can you take your own medication and get around by yourself?

Items indicating a potentially abusive situation

2. Are you helping to support someone?
5. Do you feel uncomfortable with anyone in your family?
7. Do you feel that nobody wants you around?
8. Does anyone in your family drink a lot?
12. Do you trust most of the people in your family?
13. Does anyone tell you that you give them too much trouble?
14. Do you have enough privacy at home?

Adapted from Hwalek MA, Sengstock MC. The Elder Abuse Screening Test ("EAST"). Detroit: SPEC Associates, 1986. Neale VA, Hwalek MA, Scott RO, et al. Validation of the Hwalek-Sengstock Elder Abuse Screening Test. J Appl Gerontol 1991;10:40–418.

[a]A response of "no" on items 1, 6, 12, and 14 and a response of "someone else" on item 4 are associated with abuse. On all other items, a response of "yes" is associated with abuse. Item numbers refer to their order in the questionnaire.

the alleged abuser still has access to the patient, immediate separation of victim and abuser is imperative. Experts have determined that risk is particularly high if there are guns or other weapons in the home, if drug or alcohol abuse is present, or if there has been previous serious injury or threats of homicide or suicide (7).

Ideally the abuser, rather than the victim, should be removed from the home. Often this is not possible, and placement of the older adult in other living arrangements may be necessary for his or her own protection. Sometimes another relative or friend is available or the patient may be placed in foster care or a nursing home. Temporary hospitalization under the abuse-related diagnosis-related groups (DRGs 454 and 455) may be an option, particularly if there are other diagnoses that justify the admission. For example, a vulnerable demented victim could be admitted to a geropsychiatry unit, if available. Consultation with your hospital's utilization review department can be useful.

Financial abuse may also require speedy action. If a person's assets are being misappropriated, a great deal of mischief can be done in only a few hours. Legal action may be required to change a guardian or conservator, eliminate a power of attorney, and so on. Referring the patient to an attorney or legal services agency may assist with these problems. When the patient or his or her assets do not appear to be in immediate danger, the physician, staff, and protective services agency can take somewhat longer to develop a plan of action.

Long-term case management is necessary in all cases of elder mistreatment, because these situations involve ongoing family patterns that are rarely resolved in a short time. Patients who suffer from mistreatment generally require a great many services, not only for the older adult, but also for the family, to prevent further mistreatment. These services are rarely within the scope of any single professional and often require interdisciplinary involvement. The physician's role in these cases varies with the physician's relationship with the patient. An emergency physician's role differs from that of a physician who has an ongoing relationship with the patient and family.

When the patient or family are continuing patients, the physician should continue to be involved in case management. Because the physician is trusted, his or her continuing role can be particularly helpful. The involvement of a case manager who identifies and locates needed services and coordinates their implementation has been found to be critically important in these cases. When no single person is in charge, the older adult is likely to become confused or discouraged and terminate services. Some physicians prefer to retain this role in their own office or clinic. Another option is to refer the case management role to a formal case management agency.

The types of services that should be involved vary with a wide variety of factors, including, among others, the degree of dependence of the patient, health insurance, financial resources, the supports available in the family, and the intention of the alleged abuser. For example, a fully functioning older adult who is being mistreated may alter the situation by means of a change of residence or social contacts, while a dependent patient may require extensive help in changing caregiving arrangements.

The intention of the suspected abuser is a critical factor in determining services. Where the mistreatment appears to be an intentional act, separation of the victim and the abuser is usually necessary and may require criminal prosecution or civil action to force the abuser to avoid the patient.

In many instances, however, the mistreatment is not a deliberate act. It may result from lack of knowledge of proper care techniques on the part of the caregiver or from extreme stress. In such instances, providing services to alleviate these stresses may resolve the situation. Visiting nurses, respite care, or home health aids, for example, may provide needed caregiving information or help a caregiver cope. A family coping with marital or unemployment problems may be more effective in caregiving once these difficulties have been alleviated. Some caregivers have physical or mental impairments that render them incapable of providing proper care. The knowledgeable case manager can identify these situations and make appropriate referrals.

Elder Abuse Management in a Managed Care Setting

The current emphasis on efficiency and volume in the managed care setting discourages physicians from engaging in the time-consuming detection and management of conditions such as abuse. On the other hand, not dealing with the problem is likely to result in greater cost, with abuse and neglect causing increased visits to emergency facilities, hospitalizations, and increased mental and physical problems, such as fractures, skin breakdown, malnutrition, depression, and noncompliance with treatments. The interest of many health maintenance organizations (HMOs) in maintaining the older patient outside of institutions should make the detection of abuse and neglect a priority. Furthermore, the interdisciplinary style of practice in HMOs, with the incorporation of other providers such as nurses, nurse practitioners, home health nurses, social workers, and case managers, provides an ideal setting for efficient management of abuse cases.

CONCLUSION

Mistreatment of an elder at a minimum compromises quality of life during the remaining years and may in fact result in his or her premature death. As such, it should be a matter of concern to physicians and other health care providers. Considering the physician's unique opportunities in terms of knowledge of patient and family, access to diagnostic and management strategies, and general influence, intervention in such cases may achieve an outcome that rivals the successful treatment of a medical condition. How we treat and care about our elders is thought by many to be a measure of our success or failure as a society.

REFERENCES

1. Sengstock MC, Barrett SA. Abuse and neglect of the elderly in family settings. In: Campbell J, Humphreys J, eds. Nursing Care of Survivors of Family Violence. St. Louis: Mosby, 1993:173–208.
2. Pillemer K, Finkelhor D. The prevalence of elder abuse: a random sample survey. Gerontologist 1988;28:51–57.
3. American Medical Association Department of Mental Health. Diagnostic and Treatment Guidelines on Elder Abuse and Neglect. Chicago: American Medical Association, 1992.
4. O'Brien JG. A Primary care clinician's perspective. In: Baumhover LA, Beall SC, eds. Abuse, Neglect, and Exploitation of Older Persons. Baltimore: Health Professions Press, 1996:51–64.
5. Hwalek MA, Sengstock MC. The Elder Abuse Screening Test ("EAST"). Detroit: SPEC Associates, 1986.
6. Neale VA, Hwalek MA, Scott RO, et al. Validation of the Hwalek-Sengstock Elder Abuse Screening Test. J Appl Gerontol 1991;10:406–418.
7. Campbell JC. Prediction of homicide of and by battered women. In: Campbell JC, ed. Assessing Dangerousness. Thousand Oaks, CA: Sage, 1995:96–113.

CHAPTER 53

EMILY M. AGREE AND VICKI A. FREEDMAN

Implications of Population Aging for Geriatric Health

Aging is both an individual and a population-level process. Just as each additional year of life marks the aging of a person, increases in the absolute numbers of older persons and a rise in the relative share of the population that is considered old reflect the aging of a population. Whereas older persons face increased risks of death, disease, and impairment, aging populations are marked by a higher prevalence of chronic disease and disability and rising age at death.

The U.S. population has been aging for more than a century, though the pace has accelerated over the past 20 to 30 years. As recently as 1970 less than 10% of the population was 65 and older; by 1997 this figure had grown to 12.7%; and conservative estimates suggest that it will exceed 20% by 2050 (1). During the same period, life expectancy at birth has increased from 67 to 72.5 years for males and from 75 to 79 years for females (2). Projections suggest that by 2050 men and women will live on average to age 80 and 84, respectively (1).

The elderly population itself also is aging rapidly. There are 34 million persons aged 65 or older, and more than 11% of these are considered the oldest old (aged 85 or older). By 2050 this proportion is expected to rise to almost one in four. In numbers this means an increase from about 3.8 million persons aged 85 or older today to more than 18 million in 2050 (1).

Population aging is driven by the three basic components of population growth: fertility, mortality, and migration. In the first half of the 20th century, declines in fertility were responsible for increasing the relative share of elderly persons in the U.S. population, though the baby boom slowed this trend for a while. Since the 1960s, however, reductions in mortality among the aged (Fig. 53.1) have accelerated population aging (3, 4). These declines are largely attributable to reductions in cardiovascular and cerebrovascular mortality (5, 6). The National Center for Health Statistics reports that changes in the mortality of diseases of the heart, cerebrovascular disease, and atherosclerosis were responsible for 80% of the increase in life expectancy between 1984 and 1989 (6). In contrast, migration has had a minimal influence on the rate of population aging, since the amount of net migration in any year is far less than the number of births and deaths. Nevertheless, migration has contributed to the changing composition of America's elderly, particularly in terms of increasing racial and ethnic diversity.

Because of the prominent role of mortality trends in explaining population aging in recent years and the strong links between mortality and morbidity, population aging in the United States can be expected to have important consequences for the health of the older population. Yet the linkages between population aging and geriatric health are complex. Theories abound about how morbidity rates change in concert with declining mortality; each perspective lends itself to a different interpretation about the future of geriatric medicine. At one extreme, if all persons were to live their lives in good health and die of "natural"

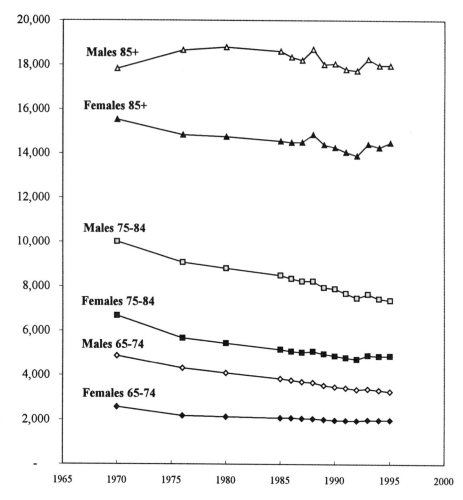

Figure 53.1.   Trends in age-specific death rates 1970–1995 by sex. (Data are from National Center for Health Statistics (NCHS). Report of Final Mortality Statistics, 1995. Monthly Vital Statistics Reports, vol 45, no 11, suppl 2 (PHS 97–1120), 1997.)

causes at a very old age, geriatric practice would be reduced to routine monitoring of general health. At the other extreme, if increased longevity were to add only years of frailty, geriatric practitioners would by necessity focus more on palliative care for chronic conditions.

The purpose of this chapter is to provide insight into the implications of population aging for geriatric health. The next section begins with a conceptual model of population health. This discussion sets the stage for a review of the major theories of linkages between morbidity and mortality. To evaluate these theories, we present evidence regarding recent changes in morbidity,

disability, and mortality in the United States and discuss the likely implications of population aging for the future of geriatric health.

MODELING POPULATION HEALTH

The changes in health that accompany increasing longevity have been characterized by competing theories that rest upon assumptions about the relations among old-age mortality, morbidity, and disability. A useful model for thinking about these linkages was developed by the World Health Organization (WHO) (7) and is shown in Figure 53.2. Extrapolating from the basic survival function of the life table, this model

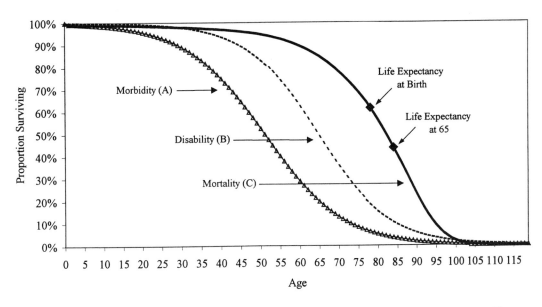

Figure 53.2.   Survival curve for U.S. females, 1990, and hypothetical disability and morbidity curves. (Data are from Bell FC, Wade AH, Goss SC. Life Tables for the United States Social Security Area. Actuarial Study 107 (SSA 11–11536). Washington: Social Security Administration, 1992.)

represents graphically the age structure of morbidity, disability, and mortality in a population. The X-axis is age in years and the Y-axis shows the proportion of a cohort that survives to a specific age without experiencing a particular event, either the onset of disease (A), disablement (B), or death (C). Curve C is the survival function derived from U.S. age-specific mortality rates for females in 1990. Curves A and B represent the *hypothetical* distribution of survival to each age without disease or disability, respectively.

This formulation lends itself to the calculation of summary measures of the health and mortality of the population in the form of expectations (or averages). For example, life expectancy at birth (LE⁰) and at age 65 (LE⁶⁵) are shown as points on curve C. Comparable measures of healthy and active life expectancy, which represent the average number of years lived before the onset of chronic morbidity and disability, respectively, also can be represented. Healthy life expectancy is described by the area under curve A, representing the total number of person-years of good health in the population. Active life expectancy is the area under curve B, and the difference between the two curves shows the aver-

age amount of time spent with illness but without disability.

THEORIES ON THE RELATION BETWEEN MORBIDITY AND MORTALITY

The WHO model formalizes the relationships among morbidity, disability, and mortality and provides a useful framework for describing and evaluating theories about the morbidity and disability changes that accompany increases in longevity. In this section we describe in detail the four most prominent theories of morbidity-mortality linkages.

Pandemic of Chronic Disease

One of the first theories relating mortality changes in the 20th century to patterns of morbidity was Gruenberg's pandemic of chronic disease theory (8, 9). This model asserts that the invention of anti-infectious drugs, such as sulfa drugs and antibiotics, and insulin in the early part of this century led to the increased survival of persons with chronic morbid conditions. That is, frail persons with reduced immune function who would have died of pneumonia or other opportunistic infections before the invention of such drugs were now able to survive longer, though in relatively poor health. Conditions that "benefited" from the elimination of fatal sequelae include arteriosclerosis, hypertension, diabetes, Down's syndrome, and organic brain disease. Such gains in survival also may have increased the prevalence of mental disorders, such as dementia, which have a higher incidence at older ages (9). This theory assumes that the age at onset of chronic diseases will remain the same but that mortality will be postponed. Consequently, the number of years spent morbid or disabled will expand with increases in longevity. In terms of Figure 53.2, we would expect to see the mortality curve shift outward as improvements in survival take place but would observe no changes in the disability or morbidity curves, because the onset of disease and disability are assumed to remain the same.

Compression of Morbidity

Probably the best-known theory inspired by increases in longevity is the compression of morbidity theory espoused by James Fries. Fries (10, 11) argues that the average length of the human life is fixed according to some predetermined biologic endowment. In his original description of the theory, he assumes life expectancy is fixed at 85 (10). In more recent articles, he has allowed this maximum to move up as far as 86.9 years but has not entertained further increases in maximum average life span (12). Furthermore, he contends that the age of onset of chronic disease will of necessity increase as we approach a time when all causes of premature mortality are eliminated. In terms of Figure 53.2, the mortality curve does not shift outward but instead becomes rectangular as more deaths occur close to the maximum average life span. The morbidity and disability curves follow a similar course as the infirm period of life is deferred. As the area between the mortality and morbidity curves decreases, a compression of morbidity takes place.

Life Span Expansion

Several researchers, including Roy Walford (13), have proposed that Fries's contention of a fixed maximum life span resulting from an unalterable rate of aging is biologically inaccurate and encourages fatalism among medical practitioners. He argues that it is possible to intervene in the underlying process of senescence, increasing life expectancy by as much as 25 years. In this theory, slowing the aging process and therefore pushing back the age at onset of disease and disability would expand the proportion of active life. Walford in particular expects that these changes could result from dietary manipulations, especially from restriction of calories, which has been related to longevity in mice. He argues that animals reared with dietary restriction not only live longer but experience a shift toward later ages in the onset of diseases such as cancer, cardiovascular disease, and autoimmune disorders (13).

The interventions envisioned by Walford would affect the risk of onset of disease but not necessarily the disease process itself. The onset of morbidity (curve A) would shift to later ages, but the years lived with morbidity and disability would remain unchanged. In other words, all three curves in Figure 53.2 would shift proportionately to later ages, with the area between the curves remaining the same.

Dynamic Equilibrium

Manton (14, 15) has proposed a fourth perspective on these relationships, dynamic equilibrium. Manton's view makes explicit the complex interactions among morbidity, disability, and mortality. A fundamental assumption of his approach is that all three processes are mutable. That is, if there is a limit to life expectancy, we have not yet come close enough to observe evidence of it. Furthermore, he argues that the three processes are interrelated, so that interventions designed to affect one of the processes inevitably alter all three. For example, in the late 1970s and early 1980s, interventions to control hypertension not only reduced disability due to the disease but also may have contributed to reductions in the incidence of myocardial infarction and consequent mortality. Declines in heart disease mortality in turn may have lead to increases in the prevalence of related disabling diseases, such as congestive heart failure (16).

The dynamic equilibrium theory differs from the other described approaches in that it assumes that years of life are gained through a combination of postponement of disease onset, reductions in severity of disease and speed of progression, and improved techniques for clinical management. It is also distinguished in assuming that chronic disease and mortality are related. For example, Manton (14) suggests that decreasing or eliminating atherogenesis would not only decrease mortality by reducing the risk of acute incidents such as stroke and myocardial infarction but also strengthen the cardiovascular system in its ability to withstand other diseases of later life, such as cancer.

Within the WHO framework, dynamic equilibrium anticipates that all three curves will shift and change in shape as the cascading effects of changes in the disease process manifest themselves. Because all three curves shift, no conclusions can be drawn about the necessary relationships among the curves.

EVALUATING EVIDENCE OF LINKAGES BETWEEN MORBIDITY AND MORTALITY

When the WHO model was developed, empirical evidence was not available to test these theories, but in recent years, many longitudinal and time-series studies have been undertaken to assess the implications of increases in longevity for population health. To evaluate the competing theories of morbidity-mortality linkages, we summarize studies in three areas. First, we review studies focusing on the rectangularization of mortality. Second, we review studies of trends in chronic disease and disability. Finally, we examine trends in life expectancy and active life expectancy in the United States.

The Rectangularization of Mortality

Of the four theories we have reviewed, only Fries's view asserts a limit to longevity. A number of studies have attempted to address whether the U.S. population is indeed reaching such a limit. Such studies are predicated on the assumption that even if we do not know the exact limit to human life span, we would expect to see certain patterns in mortality if the older population is approaching such a limit. First we would expect mortality reductions in old age, but these reductions would be smaller for subgroups close to the limit. That is, for very old subgroups with particularly high life expectancy, such as very old white women, we would expect to see improvements in mortality to be smaller than for the rest of the population, who have not yet approached the limit. Second, if we were approaching the limit to longevity, we would expect to see less variation around the average age at death. That is, as more people approach the biologic limit to life and causes of death not related to senescence are eliminated, the variation around the average age at death should decline.

What evidence is there for the rectangularization of mortality? Manton (14) shows that from 1950 to 1977 white women had larger gains in life expectancy than white men, suggesting that they had not yet reached the biologic limits of life. Even white women aged 85 and older—those most likely to have reached the limit—had improvements in mortality over the same period. More recently, Manton and Singer (16) also show patterns of mortality change that are inconsistent with a rectangularization of the survival curve. They compared the age to which the last 5% and last 1% of the population survived using Social Security Administration survival curves from 1900 to 1992. If compression had been occurring over this period, the age to which the last 5% survived should have increased more than the age to which the last 1% survived; yet both measures increased by the same amount.

Several researchers also have addressed the issue of the variability of age at death among the older population (14, 17, 18). Mean age at death for persons aged 50 and over for 1960 and 1978 for standard U.S. life tables show that the variance of the age at death had increased by 16.5%, more than 75% faster than the mean age at death had increased (14). Even when deaths are disaggregated by both underlying and mentioned causes of death, the means and standard deviations for all conditions are increasing (17). Such patterns are inconsistent with a rectangularization of mortality, though it may be that we have not yet approached the maximum possible human age.

Trends in Chronic Disease and Disability

Even if the geriatric population has not reached the limit of average life span, the morbid or disabled period could change because of shifts in the morbidity and disability curves. What evidence do we have about the trend in chronic disease and disability among older Americans? Evidence from the 1970s and early 1980s suggested that older Americans had longer periods of morbidity and disability than previous cohorts. Verbrugge (19) and Waidmann et al. (20), for example, found increases in self-reported chronic diseases by older Americans during the 1970s. Studies also showed increases in self-reported disability (19), even within 5-year age groups (21). Whether such trends reflect actual changes in the underlying health of the older population is subject to debate. Waidmann et al. (20) attribute increases in hypertension during the 1970s and 1980s to a trend toward earlier detection rather than actual changes in the prevalence of the disease. Similarly, they attribute increases in the numbers identifying themselves as unable to carry out activities to increased awareness of social programs with disability benefits.

Evidence from more recent years suggests that longer life does not necessarily imply worsening health. Table 53.1 shows the prevalence of a variety of morbidity and disability measures as reported by older Americans from the 1984 and 1994 National Health Interview Survey. Overall, the comparisons across years paints a more benign picture of changes in the health of older Americans than earlier studies, even without controlling for differences in the age structure of the older population over time.

Over the 10-year period, fewer older men reported having cerebrovascular disease, diabetes, emphysema, hardening of the arteries, and visual impairments, and fewer older women reported diabetes, hardening of the arteries, heart disease, hypertension, and hearing, visual, and osteopathic impairments. These findings are consistent with those reported by Waidmann et al. (20) and Manton et al. (22), who show declines or no change in most self-reported chronic diseases during the 1980s. Analysis of medical records of elderly HMO enrollees over two 9-year periods also suggests the incidence of heart disease was no greater from 1980 to 1989 than from 1970 to 1979 (23).

Table 53.1

Rates for Select Chronic Conditions, Impairments, and Activity Limitations of the Population 65 and Older, 1984 and 1994

	Men		Women	
	1984	1994	1984	1994
Selected Chronic Conditions[a]				
Arthritis	405.7	428.6	547.7	553.5
Cataracts	101.5	129.6	183.6	192.4
Cerebrovascular disease	82.6	53.1	53.8	60.5
Diabetes	194.7	107.3	108.5	96.9
Emphysema	73.7	67.9	20.1	29.6
Hardening of arteries	93.0	69.1	84.8	41.3
Heart disease	334.9	360.5	309.7	299.4
Hypertension	311.2	319.5	471.9	395.8
Impairments[a]				
Hearing	352.1	354.1	283.3	238.0
Vision	114.9	94.6	91.3	75.5
Osteopathy, deformity	142.7	153.7	193.2	174.1
Activity limitation (% reporting)	38.9	36.9	39.0	39.1

Source: Tables 58, 68, and 70 (34, 35).
[a]Per 1000 population.

Nevertheless, some chronic diseases have increased in recent years. For women, cerebrovascular disease and emphysema increased from 1984 to 1994 (Table 53.1). At the same time, reports of heart disease and hypertension have increased for men. Furthermore, both older men and older women are more likely to report arthritis and cataracts in 1994 than in 1984. Such increases in chronic disease are driven in part by the aging of the population, i.e., the fact that the age of the average geriatric patient has increased substantially over the past decade. Also, in some cases, changes in the detection and treatment of the specific disease in question may be fueling an increase. The increase in reports of cataracts at the same time vision impairment has declined is an obvious example of how changes in treatment (in this case cataract surgery) can have apparently contradictory effects on self-reported trends in health. In other cases, increases in disease may reflect changes in the risk factors for older men and women earlier in their lives; e.g., the increase in emphysema in women is likely due at least in part to smoking trends among younger cohorts of women earlier in the century.

Irrespective of the trends in self-reported disease, Table 53.1 shows that in 1994 fewer older men describe themselves as having a limitation in their major activity than in 1984. Women, on the other hand, have not changed their reports of activity limitations. The lack of increase in disability is consistent with other studies focusing on older Americans' ability to carry out personal care activities, such as bathing, dressing, and feeding, and routine care activities, such as shopping, using the telephone, and managing money. Crimmins et al. (24), for example, show no trend in the prevalence of needing help with personal care but show declines in prevalence of needing help with routine care and declines in the incidence of both personal and routine care needs. Manton et al. (25, 26) have put forth even stronger evidence for a decline in prevalence and incidence of old-age disability, describing a difference of 1.4 million in the number of older Americans who would have been disabled in 1996 if disability rates had not declined since 1982.

Trends in Active Life Expectancy

Evidence of declines in mortality, morbidity, and disability in isolation are insufficient to distinguish among theories of morbidity-mortality linkages. If the mortality curve shifts outward but is not matched by shifts in the morbidity and disability incidence curves, for example, an expansion in morbidity and disability will occur along the lines of Gruenberg's pandemic of chronic disease scenario. Alternatively, if shifts in the morbidity curve are matched by similar changes in disability and mortality, no change in the morbid period will come about, as predicted by the life span expansion theory.

Competing theories can be distinguished, however, according to their predictions about absolute changes in life expectancy and the number of years and relative amount of the life span expected to be spent in healthy or active states. In practice, measures of disability have been more readily available than measures of morbidity, so we focus on *active* (rather than *healthy*) life expectancy measures here. Measures of active life expectancy are most often calculated from prevalence rates and may therefore be interpreted as the experience of a hypothetical cohort subject to rates prevailing during the period in question, usually a single year. Period estimates, because they merge the experience of different cohorts, cannot tell us whether persons are living more years in ill or good health and can lead to pessimistic conclusions about health at a given time (27). However, they provide a useful portrait of the trends in the health of a population over successive periods (28). Measures of disability used to calculate active life expectancy vary widely from study to study, although measures of inability in carrying out roles or activities are used most frequently (29).

Table 53.2 shows the expected direction of changes in four summary measures of population health for each of the four theories of morbidity-mortality linkages. The first column shows the expected direction of total life expectancy, or the average number of years of life. The second and third columns show expected directions of the average number of years spent in disabled and active states, respectively. Estimates of the average number of years spent in disabled and active states

Table 53.2

Expected Changes in Population Health Measures Under Four Theoretic Perspectives

Theory	Total Life Expectancy	Disabled Life Expectancy	Active Life Expectancy	Active Life Expectancy as a Percentage of Total Life Expectancy
Pandemic of chronic diseases	↑	↑	0	↓
Compression of morbidity	0	↓	↑	↑
Life span expansion	↑	0	↑	↑
Dynamic equilibrium	↑	↑	↑	?

↑, increase; ↓, decrease; 0, no change; ?, unknown.

sum to total life expectancy. Column four shows the expected change over time in the *proportion* of total life expectancy that is active (active life expectancy divided by life expectancy); this measure is particularly useful because it takes into account changes in both active and disabled years.

In terms of anticipated changes in active life expectancy, the rows of the table may be interpreted as follows: Gruenberg's pandemic of chronic diseases implies increases in life expectancy and disabled life expectancy but no change in active life expectancy. Consequently, we would expect to observe declines in the proportion of active life. Fries's theory of compression of morbidity is consistent with little or no change in life expectancy but anticipates increases in active life expectancy offset by declines in disabled life expectancy. This theory also is consistent with expected increases in the relative amount of active life. If Walford's life span expansion theory holds true, we would expect to see increases in life expectancy and active life expectancy but no change in disabled life expectancy, also leading to an increase in the proportion of years spent in active life. Only Manton's theory of dynamic equilibrium asserts that increases in all three—life expectancy, active life expectancy, and disabled life expectancy—will occur. Unlike the three previous theories, this model can offer no prediction about changes in active life as a proportion of total life expectancy, as such forecasts can only be made when one of the three parameters is assumed to be fixed.

Table 53.3 presents evidence on the direction these four summary measures of population health have taken in recent decades. Our estimates

of change are calculated from the longest available time-series of life expectancy and active life expectancy for the United States (30), which are based on cross-sectional disability prevalence rates from the National Health Interview Survey for 1970, 1980, and 1990. In this table disability is defined broadly to include persons in the community with long- and short-term limitations in their ability to carry out their normal activities because of a health condition and persons institutionalized for the care of a mental or physical condition. The top panel shows changes for the earlier decade (1970 to 1980) and the bottom panel presents estimates for more recent changes (1980 to 1990). For each period we show changes in expectations calculated at birth and at age 65, for men and women separately. We focus on the measures for age 65, as they are less susceptible to the effects of changes in survival and health at the younger ages.

From 1970 to 1980 total life expectancy at age 65 increased for both men and women (1.2 and 1.6 years). Most of this increase was in disabled years: men had an additional 1 and women 1.4 years of disabled life after age 65. Years of active life expectancy also increased, but the increase was much smaller (0.2 years for both men and women). Despite increases in all three measures, the *proportion* of total life spent in an active state declined by 2.9 and 3.7 percentage points for men and women during this decade.

These trends may mask important variation over time in the distribution of older persons across different levels of disability. Multinational comparisons of trends in the 1970s show that when calculations of disabled life include only

Table 53.3

Changes in U.S. Population Health Measures, 1970–1980 and 1980–1990

	Change in Total Life Expectancy (years)	Change in Disabled Life Expectancy (years)	Change in Active Life Expectancy (years)	Change in Active Life as a Percentage of Total Life Expectancy
1970–1980				
At birth				
Males	3.1	2.4	0.7	-2.7
Females	3.0	2.9	0.1	-3.1
At age 65				
Males	1.2	1.0	0.2	-2.9
Females	1.6	1.4	0.2	-3.7
1980–1990				
At birth				
Males	1.7	0.1	1.6	0.3
Females	1.2	0.1	1.1	0.2
At age 65				
Males	0.9	0.3	0.6	1.1
Females	0.5	0.0	0.5	1.4

Adapted from Crimmins EM, Saito Y, Ingegneri D. Trends in disability-free life expectancy in the United States, 1970–1990. Pop Dev Rev 1997;23:555–572.

the most severely disabled, increases in life expectancy were matched by increases in active life expectancy (31). That is, the proportion of life spent in a severely disabled state did not increase during this period. Thus the declines in the proportion of life spent in a nondisabled state during the 1970s can be attributed to increases in moderate or light disability.

The second decade shows smaller increases in total life expectancy at age 65 than the earlier period: an additional 0.9 and 0.5 years for men and women, respectively. Increases also were observed in both disabled and active life expectancy at age 65; however, in contrast to the earlier period, a greater share of the increase in total life was due to increases in active life expectancy. As a result, the percent of total life expectancy spent in an active state actually *increased* by 1.1 and 1.4 percentage points for men and women, respectively, from 1980 to 1990.

Although at face value this evidence appears contradictory, suggesting an expansion of disability in the earlier period and a compression more recently, these results are consistent with Manton's theory of dynamic equilibrium. During

both periods increases in total, active, and disabled life expectancy were observed, and such changes did not have a predetermined effect on the proportion of remaining life spent in an active state.

IMPLICATIONS

Taken together, recent trends in mortality, disability, and life expectancy offer little evidence that Fries's compression of morbidity is taking place. Although evidence from the 1970s suggests that morbidity may have been expanding, the trend has not been unidirectional, and it was followed in the 1980s by improvements in morbidity and disability at the oldest ages. Instead, existing evidence suggests that increases in survival that accompany population aging can best be understood as the result of a complex, dynamic process. Thus, whether increased life is accompanied predominantly by additional healthy or morbid years is not predetermined. What are the implications of this characterization of population aging for geriatric practice? First and foremost, practitioners must recognize their vital role in determining the character of the lengthened lives of the older population. A compression of morbidity is not a foregone conclusion or an inevitable result of increased longevity. There is a large role for medical practitioners in determining the direction of changes in the health status of the older population. Whether extra years of life are healthy and active or disabled and dependent is strongly related to the medical interventions employed by practitioners. A focus in earlier decades on reducing mortality from diseases such as myocardial infarction, kidney disease, and stroke added more years of unhealthy life, as persons survived but remained dependent upon dialysis machines, pacemakers, or other medical technologies. In contrast, efforts aimed at preventing, reversing, and generally slowing the progression of disabling conditions such as diabetes, joint disease, osteoporosis, and arthritis may have contributed to a compression of the morbid period in more recent years.

The dynamics of population aging also suggest an important role for recovery and rehabilitation, even among the very old. Today recovery rates among the disabled geriatric population may be as high as 20% (32). Technologic advances in areas such as bone and joint replacements, new surgical and drug therapies for neurologic disorders such as Parkinson's disease, and advances in stroke rehabilitation all suggest that even greater increases in recovery and rehabilitation may be attainable. Demographers have demonstrated that additional gains in recovery rates would have a profound effect on reducing disability prevalence in the population (27, 33).

Finally, although Fries's compression of morbidity theory suggests that the health of the older population will become more homogeneous as premature mortality is reduced and more persons die of natural causes, the dynamic process of population aging described here suggests that geriatric practitioners will serve an even *more* diverse older population. Other demographic trends will reinforce this trend toward increased heterogeneity. For example, there are substantial racial and ethnic differences in life expectancy and active life in the United States, though as better-educated cohorts age, some of this disadvantage may be reduced (36). Furthermore, even if the health of the older population improves, vast increases in the

sheer number of older Americans with chronic disease and disability are expected between now and 2020, when the peak of the baby boom generation will reach old age. As these compositional changes unfold, meeting the needs of an increasingly large and diverse patient population will certainly pose a challenge to geriatric practitioners.

REFERENCES

1. US Bureau of the Census. Population Projections of the United States by Age, Sex, Race, and Hispanic Origin: 1995 to 2050. Current Population Reports (Series P25–1130). Washington: US Government Printing Office, 1996.
2. National Center for Health Statistics. Report of Final Mortality Statistics, 1995. Monthly Vital Statistics Reports, vol 45, no 11, suppl 2, PHS 97–1120, 1997.
3. Preston H, Himes C, Eggers M. Demographic conditions responsible for population aging. Demography 1989; 26:691–704.
4. Horiuchi S, Preston SH. Age-specific growth rates: the legacy of past population dynamics. Demography 1988; 25:429–441.
5. Preston SH. American Longevity: Past, Present, and Future (Policy Brief 7). Syracuse , NY: Syracuse University Center for Policy Research, 1996.
6. National Center for Health Statistics. Causes of death contributing to changes in life expectancy: United States, 1984–1989. Vital Health Stat 20 1994;23: 94–185.
7. World Health Organization. The Uses of Epidemiology in the Study of the Elderly: Report of a WHO Scientific Group on the Epidemiology of Aging. Geneva: World Health Organization, 1984.
8. Gruenberg EM. The failures of success. Milbank Mem Fund Q Health Soc 1977;55:3–24.
9. Kramer M. The increasing prevalence of mental disorders: a pandemic threat. Psychiatr Q 1983;55:115–143.
10. Fries JF. Aging, natural death and the compression of morbidity. N Engl J Med 1980;303:130–135.
11. Fries JF. The compression of morbidity. Milbank Mem Fund Q Health Soc 1983;61:397–419.
12. Fries JF. The compression of morbidity: near or far? Milbank Q 1989;67:208–232.
13. Walford RL. The extension of maximum life span. Clin Geriatr Med 1985;1:29–35.
14. Manton KG. Epidemiological, demographic, and social correlates of disability among the elderly. Milbank Q 1989;67(suppl 2):13–57.
15. Manton KG. Changing concepts of morbidity and mortality in the elderly population. Milbank Mem Fund Q 1982;60:183–244.
16. Manton KG, Singer B. What's the fuss about compression of mortality? Chance 1994;7:21–30.
17. Myers GC, Manton KG. Compression of mortality: myth or reality? Gerontologist 1984;24:346–353.
18. Rothenberg R, Lentzner HR, Parker RA. Population ag-

ing patterns: the expansion of mortality. J Gerontol 1991;46:S66–S70.

19. Verbrugge M. Longer life but worsening health? Trends in health and mortality of middle-aged and older persons. Milbank Mem Fund Q 1984;62:475–519.

20. Waidmann T, Bound J, Schoenbaum M. The illusion of failure: trends in the self-reported health of the U.S. elderly. Milbank Mem Fund Q 1995;73:253–287.

21. Crimmins EM, Saito Y, Ingegneri D. Changes in life expectancy and disability-free life expectancy in the United States. Pop Dev Rev 1989;15:235–267.

22. Manton KG, Stallard E, Corder L. Changes in morbidity and chronic disability in the U.S. elderly population: evidence from the 1982, 1984, and 1989 National Long Term Care Surveys. J Gerontol 1995;50B4:S194–S204.

23. Haan MN, Selby JV, Rice DP, et al. Trends in cardiovascular disease incidence and survival in the elderly. Ann Epidemiol 1996;6:348–356.

24. Crimmins EM, Saito Y, Reynolds S. Further evidence on recent trends in the prevalence and incidence of disability among older Americans from two sources: the LSOA and the NHIS. J Gerontol 1997;52B2:S59–S71.

25. Manton KG, Corder L, Stallard E. Estimates of change in chronic disability and institutional incidence and prevalence rates in the U.S. elderly population from the 1982, 1984, and 1989 National Long Term Care Survey. J Gerontol 1993;48:S153–S166.

26. Manton KG, Corder L, Stallard E. Chronic disability trends in elderly United States populations: 1982–1994. Proc Natl Acad Sci U S A 1997;94:2593–2598.

27. Rogers A, Rogers R, Belanger A. Longer life but worse health? Measurement and dynamics. Gerontologist 1990;30:640–649.

28. Robine JM, Michel JP, Branch LG. Measurement and utilization of healthy life expectancy: conceptual issues. Bull World Health Organ 1992;70:791–800.

29. Robine JM, Ritchie K. Healthy life expectancy: evaluation of global indicator of change in population health. BMJ 1991;302:457–460.

30. Crimmins EM, Saito Y, Ingegneri D. Trends in disability-free life expectancy in the United States, 1970–1990. Pop Dev Rev 1997;23:555–572.

31. Robine JM, Mathers C, Brouard N. Trends and differentials in disability free life expectancy: concepts, methods, and findings. In: Caselli G, Lopez A, eds. Health and Mortality Among Elderly Populations. Oxford, UK: Clarendon Press, 1996:182–201.

32. Wolinsky FD, Stump T, Callahan CM, Johnson RJ. Consistency and change in functional status among older adults over time. J Aging Health 1996;8:155–182.

33. Crimmins EM, Hayward MD, Saito Y. Changing mortality and morbidity rates and the health status and life expectancy of the older population. Demography 1994; 31:159–175.

34. National Center for Health Statistics. Current estimates from the National Health Interview Survey, United States, 1984. Vital Health Stat 10 1986;156.

35. National Center for Health Statistics. Vital Statistics of the United States, 1990 Life Tables, vol 2, section 6 (PHS 94-1104). Washington: Public Health Service, National Center for Health Statistics, 1994.

36. Land KC, Guralnik JM, Blazer DG. Estimating increment-decrement life tables with multiple covariates from panel data: the case of active life expectancy. Demography 1994;31:297–231.

Health Care Organization and Financing

In the United States the medical and health care of those over age 65 is spread across a variety of delivery systems, often with poor coordination among them. The basis for the financing of medical care of seniors became more straightforward when Medicare was mandated in the 1960s. However, Medicare insurance does not provide complete coverage of all health care. Fragmentation of care and the inflationary consequences of Medicare have led to major political controversy and proposed revisions of social policy related to organization and financing of systems for health care for seniors, as well as for younger Americans. This chapter reviews policy antecedents to the organization and financing of health care for older Americans, describes delivery and financing systems in the United States, highlights organization and financing models in other developed nations, and summarizes major proposed changes, some of which are being piloted.

HISTORICAL BASIS OF U.S. OLD AGE POLICIES

In the United States of the 1800s, recommendations for relief for the needy were based on county-administered programs, primarily in institutional settings. At the onset of this century, industrialized countries were developing social welfare programs to insure against the risks faced by industrial workers. Old age, if it was achieved, was likely to be associated with the health risks of impoverishment, illness, and isolation, in part because of the removal from a rural economy, in which the old tended to remain at least partially employed. The association with impoverishment, illness, and isolation led to inclusion of old age, with accidents and unemployment, as a risk to be addressed by social insurance policy in industrial societies (1). However, the United States lagged Europe in addressing old age dependency, perhaps because the Civil War veterans pension program prevented impoverishment for two thirds of U.S. elders at the turn of the century (2).

Federal Policy for Income Support

By 1910 cohorts that were not eligible for Civil War pensions were more prevalent. With no federal program in place, private-sector and state-sponsored pensions were introduced, with mixed success. Retirement was not mandatory in the United States, as it was in many European countries. However, extant pension and retirement plans supported retirement in the 60s. During this period of high unemployment, a program to legitimize removal of those over 65 from the workforce was welcomed. Income support for those over 65 and some younger disabled workers was enacted in 1935. This Social Security income was funded through mandated employer and employee contributions (Federal Insurance Contributions Act, or FICA). Enactment of the legislation was given impetus by the dire economic conditions of 1929, which convinced even those most resistant to federal social safety programs that some support of basic income was warranted. Health care insurance specific to older Americans was not to come for another 30 years. The compelling demands of World War II (WW II) and resistance to a mandatory big government program are invoked as reasons for the delay (2).

Federal Policy for Illness and Isolation

Age-relevant social policies subsequent to 1935 gained support partly because of increased academic interest (2). Once the risk of old age impoverishment had been addressed by Social Security, attention was turned to the illness and isolation risks of old age. In 1940 the National Institutes of Health were created and instructed to conduct clinical studies on the aged and basic research on senescence. After WW II concerns about poor access to health care facilities for all Americans led to the Hill-Burton program (1946), which provided capital funding for the construction of hospitals and nursing homes. Legislation coordinating housing and aging programs (meals, socialization, personal care, and long-term care) followed incrementally until 1965, when in a glorious burst, Medicare, Medicaid, and the Older Americans Act (OAA) were passed.

Medicare

Medicare was created by Congress in 1965, decades after it was first proposed for the growing numbers of elderly poor and uninsured in this country. It is structured as a health insurance plan for all citizens over age 65 rather than as a means-tested plan. Some younger disabled persons and those with end-stage renal disease are also covered. The actively employed are not eligible for Medicare as the primary insurer until they reach age 70. They are covered by their employer's group insurance until age 70.

Medicare is divided into part A, which covers restricted amounts of inpatient care and acute nursing home or home health services, and part B, which partially covers most physician and outpatient services, durable medical equipment, and a few other services. Medicare part A is financed as a trust account and receives funds primarily from employee and employer payroll taxes. The most recent revision of the tax, which requires Congressional action, was in 1990. The current rates

are 1.45% for both employer and employee up to $125,000 of cash compensation. In addition, patients must pay coinsurance and deductibles, which averaged 6% of elders' per capita income in 1991 (3). Medicare part B is financed as an insurance account funded by premium payments. In addition, deductibles and copayments apply for services. Not all elderly can afford part B (see Elements of Health Care Delivery).

Even for those who are eligible, Medicare parts A and B together do not provide comprehensive health coverage, especially long-term care either in nursing homes or at home. There is limited coverage for nonacute care driven by recovery from acute illness (for instance, rehabilitation in a nursing home after hip surgery) and home monitoring of a few chronic illnesses, such as diabetes. But for the most part, nursing and medical care is restricted to hospital and outpatient settings. Additional coverage gaps are dental and mental health care and outpatient pharmaceuticals. As a result, the average total after-tax proportion of income spent by the elderly on all personal health expenses is now close to 18%, including cost sharing for parts A and B (3). Medicare's annual expenditures were about $178 billion in 1995 (4), constituting more than 17% of the nation's health expenditures. Medicare covers more than 30 million older people and more than 31 million people altogether.

Medicare is administered by the Health Care Financing Administration (HCFA), which develops Medicare's administrative rules and carries out health services research directed primarily toward cost containment and quality. HCFA contracts with entities such as physician review organizations (PROs) to carry out audits related to utilization and quality management. It has active fraud and abuse detection programs, contracts with insurance companies to process claims and provide administrative reports (fiscal intermediaries) and, as the administrator of the largest health insurance program in the country, carries considerable influence in health care policy arenas. HCFA's large claims-based databases have provided the foundation for much health services analysis in recent years. HCFA has reorganized its administrative structure to give formal recognition to its increased emphasis on managed care and continues to explore variations on managed care through its waiver programs (see Subsequent Federal Policy).

Medicaid

Medicaid, while it covers a smaller set of eligibles than Medicare, has broader benefit coverage. It covers preventive, acute, and nursing home institutional care for the poor who are aged, blind, disabled, pregnant, or the parent of a dependent child. It also makes provision for coverage of dental care, prostheses, eyeglasses, prescribed drugs, and intermediate-term care facilities. In the early 1990s, 25 million people were covered, or about 10% of the population.

Medicaid is jointly funded by the federal and state governments through general taxes. The federal government matches state expenditures through rates that vary by each state's selected eligibility threshold of personal income and assets, relative to the federal poverty level. However, the federal and state governments together have set economic eligibility thresholds that exclude about 60% of those below the federal poverty line (3). Paradoxically, Medicaid, while developed as insurance for the poor, is the only public program that covers long-term nursing home care. This has resulted in middle-class seniors spending down assets to qualify for Medicaid's nursing home coverage. Medicaid does not, however, cover community-based long-term care except through waiver programs (see Subsequent Federal Policy).

Medicaid is administered by the states within guidelines established by the federal government. The guidelines cover Medicaid's required services, the minimum level of payments to providers, and eligibility criteria. States may elect to expand services, payments, or eligibility pools, and the federal government will match approved expansions on a scaled basis. HCFA acts as the federal government's program liaison. Medicaid's expenditures in 1994 were more than $129 billion, or about 14% of the nation's health expenditures that year (3).

Older Americans Act

The Older Americans Act (OAA) set as its program goals the facilitation of local assistance for family- and community-based elder care and was the conduit for meals, socialization, personal care, and long-term care programs authorized by Congress. There were no eligibility restrictions for elders, though services were to be targeted to those with the "greatest social or economic need." At enactment and since, the program budget has been much smaller than those for Medicaid or Medicare, so the OAA has far lesser effects.

Subsequent Federal Policy

Following the enactment of Social Security, Medicare, Medicaid, and the OAA there were amendments and revisions, including provisions for new coordinating agencies, legal protections against discrimination for older workers, and block grants to states for programs, often administered through OAA-related agencies. Additional approved services included homemaking, adult day care, transportation, training, employment services, information and referrals, nutrition assistance, protective programs, and health support (2).

Other newer types of legislation have proved important to the organization and financing of health care for seniors. First came the Employee Retirement Income and Security Act (ERISA) of 1974; next was legislation establishing additional national aging research; later came provisions for allowing demonstration programs within Medicare and Medicaid, and latest is legislation dealing with the quality and financing of nursing home care.

ERISA is noteworthy because it has been interpreted by the U.S. Supreme Court to preempt states from regulating self-funded group insurance programs. This has assumed increased importance for cohorts between ages 65 and 70 who are still employed and covered by employer self-insured programs, which are not required to include federally or state-mandated benefits or mandated quality and utilization standards. Also in 1974, the National Institute on Aging was established to bring the medical research agenda for aging into higher priority. Later legislation supported age-related social research via long-term care gerontology centers based in universities.

In 1978, the first of the demonstration program grants for Medicare beneficiaries, the channeling grants program, was passed. The National

Long Term Care Demonstration published its experience with the costs, utilization, and satisfaction of providing nursing and support services for nursing home-eligible patients at home. The findings of the channeling demonstration showed few differences of medical outcome measures but increased administrative and utilization costs when the study group was compared with similar Medicare beneficiaries. Patients and families clearly preferred care at home (5).

In general, demonstration and waiver programs allow for voluntary enrollment of Medicare or Medicaid beneficiaries in programs that expand benefit coverage but set other limits, such as choice of physicians. Goals are usually to reduce costs while promoting continuity, quality, satisfaction, and efficiency. Most of the initiatives must have a waiver from Medicare's rules on open access to care because they limit choice of providers or practitioners. In actuality, HCFA allows disenrollment on a monthly basis. This is more flexible than most employer-sponsored insurance, which usually allows only annual changes between plans if there is a choice of plans. The waiver models are categorized as integrated care, primary and acute care, or long-term care (6), depending on which type or types are included. Waiver programs usually require overall cost neutrality, though most programs hope for cost savings.

Later demonstration and waiver programs included the predecessors to Medicare managed care risk (capitation) contracts, in the early 1980s; social HMOs, in 1985; the Program for All Inclusive Care of the Elderly (PACE), in 1986; Evercare, in 1987; Arizona's Long Term Care System, in 1989; and various other initiatives, such as recent efforts in New York at cluster care for the homebound (7). Pooling of Medicare money with other insurance money has been explored to allow broader benefit coverage, alternative care settings, and alternative service provision.

The Omnibus Budget Reconciliation Act (OBRA) of 1987 and the Medical Catastrophic Care Act (MCCA) in 1988 included significant provisions related to the quality of care in nursing homes and the financing of long-term care. The provisions of OBRA 1987 have resulted in a standardized nationwide database, the Minimum Data Set, reflecting ongoing quality monitoring

and the demographic, social, and health status of nursing home residents. MCCA, funded by a tax on elders, was repealed because of major opposition, leaving long-term care funded by Medicaid and private funds. OBRA legislation of 1994 made it more difficult for persons to transfer assets to others within 3 years of applying for Medicaid, forcing even greater use of personal resources to pay for chronic care.

MODELS FOR HEALTH CARE FINANCE AND ORGANIZATION

The financing solutions to impoverishment, illness, and isolation in the United States are generally described as insurance. Classically, insurance principles hold that the risk of catastrophic financial loss can be ameliorated if the event that creates the loss is unpredictable, uncommon, and very costly and if the cost is spread across many. One of the problems in U.S. health insurance is that on a population basis the events against which it is insuring are common, relatively predictable, and not catastrophically expensive. It has become expected that health insurance will be used for routine care rather than only at times of catastrophe. Thus, Medicare acts more like a national checking account from which expenditures are made on a regular basis than like true insurance. In the United States insured persons are divided into risk pools, sometimes by choice, as when they choose between plans an employer offers, and sometimes by age, as in the case of Medicare. Grouping of insured people into separate pools creates the potential for adverse selection (less healthy, higher cost pools) and its converse, skimming (more healthy, lower cost pools), which have implications for the setting of insurance premiums and for comparisons between groups. Other practical difficulties have arisen as a result of the application of risk pools, but the major current concern in the United States is inflationary cost (8).

Delivery of health care in the United States is done in an increasingly competitive market as opposed to a regulated environment. At times, the United States has taken a national approach to budgeting and planning for health care resources and delivery, most notably in the 1930s and 1940s and in 1974, with the National Health Planning and Resources Development Act. This act produced, in part, a certificate of need (CON) process for approval of new health care facilities, including nursing homes. Many states have retained CON processes for nursing homes, although national planning and regulatory activities were dismantled in the late 1970s and early 1980s.

In contrast to a regulated environment, a true free market requires informed consumers; no artificial constraints on supply, demand, or price; no bias or influence by particularly large buyers or sellers, including governments; and no barriers to entry or exit of the market. The increased emphasis on competition in U.S. health care has generated much controversy about whether health care is a public good or a commodity. The supporters of national insurance argue that a true free market for health care cannot exist and question whether competitive reforms are possible in a system that already has many choices for consumers (9). The supporters of competition point to the valuations that persons make in everyday life, the flexibility of open markets, and the benefits of innovation (9). Comparisons with other developed countries have tended to emphasize the United States as an outlier, with its absence of national health insurance or national health delivery system. This is changing, however, as more countries incorporate competitive features into their health care systems.

Comparison With Countries in Organization for Economic Cooperation and Development

The countries with which the United States is most often compared are part of the Organization for Economic Cooperation and Development (OECD), which includes Australia, Austria, Belgium, Canada, Denmark, Finland, France, Germany, Great Britain, Greece, Iceland, Ireland, Italy, Japan, Luxembourg, the Netherlands, Norway, Portugal, Spain, Sweden, Switzerland, and Turkey. Programs that have not been adopted in the United States but that have been tried in OECD countries include publicly financed health services and national delivery systems for which all citizens are eligible. These approaches may be exclusive or may coexist with private insurance and delivery entities and often with budgeting and

planning systems that use budgets to cap expenditures, limit benefits explicitly (usually through a negotiated process), and match infrastructure with projected need (10). Problems with heavily planned and budgeted systems include stagnation of service delivery and lack of response to new technologies. However, population health statistics, per capita spending, rates of health cost increase, and citizen satisfaction have tended to favor such systems (11).

Closest to a national insurance and delivery system in the United States is the one created for military personnel, in which a full spectrum of care is financed. The Veterans Affairs (VA) plays a similar role for a small segment of elders and has expanded its spectrum of care from acute, rehabilitation, and institutional long-term care to include more outpatient, preventive, and community care (12). Geographic access, however, is limited.

Because health care costs have been rising disproportionately to gross national product in all OECD countries (13), new solutions have been sought even in countries that previously were thought to have cost-controlled but effective systems, such as Great Britain. Market principles have been introduced into Great Britain's centrally planned, publicly financed health system (14, 15). Likewise, many of these countries are being challenged by increases in their elderly population, with the associated additional costs of long-term care. Germany has recently instituted a national compulsory insurance program, the Dependency Insurance Act, to address chronic care dependency needs (16).

ELEMENTS OF HEALTH CARE DELIVERY

Our medical delivery system can address preventive, acute, rehabilitative, chronic disease, and long-term care. Settings include dedicated small offices and larger outpatient clinics, acute-care and chronic-disease hospitals, inpatient and outpatient rehabilitation facilities, long-term care facilities and programs, and seasonal or special settings, such as for vaccination programs and blood pressure screenings. Ownership may be private or public and incorporated as for profit or not for profit. Practitioner staffing may be by physicians or by physicians' assistants and nurse practitioners. Nurse staffing may be by hospital- or college-trained registered nurses or by licensed practical nurses. Health aides provide nursing home and home care, and personal care attendants work in both public and private home care programs. Programs may be voluntary or mandated, stand alone, or be integrated with other levels of care by ownership or by agreement. A host of other settings and caretakers have been encompassed as the definition of health care has expanded beyond what is illness-related to include prevention, well-being, and function.

While health insurance coverage and eligibility dictate access to some settings, there is a considerable degree of choice for most elderly. For instance, an older person may receive hospital care in one or more of the following: community hospitals, academic or specialty hospitals, VA hospitals, or military hospitals. Outpatient care may take place in private offices, federally funded health centers, VA or military clinics, or community clinics. The Indian Health Service is a comprehensive service for eligible citizens but does not restrict its eligibles from seeking care elsewhere.

Coverage of long-term care initially developed an institutional bias because of Medicaid's benefit structure. Waivers for community-based care are now available but tend to be used for younger disabled populations. The states with the longest and best-integrated community-based long-term care programs are, respectively, Arizona and Oregon (6, 17).

Delivery of care in the United States is considered to be highly fragmented because of lack of insurance, uneven availability of facilities or providers (access), and lack of coordination between settings (continuity). While health system planning in the United States has periodically addressed the need for more or for fewer facilities or providers, there has been no successful national commitment to building regional models of primary, secondary, and tertiary care, as is the case in nationalized systems (18).

Because seniors have a higher prevalence of acute and chronic disease, higher hospitalization rates, and more complicated recoveries than younger people, access to care and continuity of care are particularly important. The initial enactment of Medicare helped to address many of the access problems for acute illness of the elderly but offered less for preventive care and very little for long-term care. Recently, coverage for some preventive screening and vaccinations has been added to the benefit package. Long-term care, however, is not part of Medicare coverage, as previously noted.

In addition to insurance coverage for health care, Medicare legislation included funding for graduate medical education to increase the number of physicians available in the general population and, secondarily, to improve access for the elderly. However, there persist some inequities in access related to both insurance coverage and the delivery infrastructure. Medicare part A insures against the costs of hospitalization and covers most seniors in this country. Medicare part B is available to the same seniors and covers outpatient care but requires a monthly premium and a higher level of cost sharing. The unpredictability of the cost sharing, which is driven by outpatient use, is a burden for some seniors. This gap is addressed by insurance that covers the monthly premiums for part B, deductibles, and various other benefits. Gap insurance premiums may come from private insurance or Medicaid insurance or de facto by access to VA facilities. In recent years about 42% of seniors, or 13 million people, own individual Medigap policies; about 13% of seniors, or 3.9 million people, are eligible for both Medicare and Medicaid (19); and about 1.7 million are supported by the VA system, exclusive of other systems (12). An additional 32% of seniors, or 9.6 million people, have coverage in addition to part A through their employers. This leaves 1.9 million elders, or about 6.3%, with no outpatient coverage.

The current geographic distribution of physicians and their willingness to participate in Medicare also play a role in access. Participation in Medicare is usually defined in terms of assignment. Assignment is an administrative agreement through which providers agree to accept a Medicare fee schedule, creating a predictable copayment for patients, as opposed to an open-ended billing arrangement, which may increase financial barriers to care.

ELEMENTS OF FINANCE

The United States spends more on health care services than does any other nation. . . .These expenditures are financed by a complex mixture of public payers (federal, state, and local government), as well as private insurance and individual payments. . . . and charity.

—De Lew, 1992 (13)

Finance is the science of management of public revenues and of the conduct of the public's money matters. Concerns about the rising cost of health care were identified as early as 1970 by finance experts and are attributed in part to the influence of Medicare. When Medicare was enacted in 1965, political compromises were made to enable its passage. One agreement was that Medicare would pay "usual and customary charges." Without a cap, either in the form of price controls or volume controls, this proved to be an open opportunity for inflation. Since Medicare covered more lives than any other single insurer, its policies set a tone in the medical marketplace, and an inflationary spiral was begun. Additional contributors to health care cost increases are believed to be an excess of providers, which generates demand for services disproportionate to need; new technology, which inflates benefit packages; antitrust legislation, which proscribes providers from many kinds of efficient but anticompetitive agreements; and more recently, ever larger for-profit health care organizations, which take dollars out of the health care sector as profits.

The severity of health care inflation up to 1992 led the federal government, through HCFA, to undertake a number of cost-reducing measures. Price controls were attempted in the 1970s, but volume increased. Subsequently HCFA adopted reimbursement systems for Medicare that are driven not by current charges but by other factors. Diagnostic related groups (DRGs) were developed in the late 1970s and early 1980s for quality assessment but were adopted in 1983 for prospective payment to hospitals as a cost-per-case system. The Resource-Based Relative Value Scale (RBRVS) is a new reimbursement system for payments to physicians, implemented from 1992 to 1996 and based on valuations of the resources needed to produce physicians' services. DRGs and RBRVS have been adopted by various state governments and insurers. Coming soon is a new hospital outpatient reimbursement system know variously as ambulatory care groups, ambulatory visit groups, and ambulatory patient groups (20).

Attempts to limit inflation of Medicare's benefit package have resulted in technology assessment criteria for inclusion of new diagnostic and therapeutic technologies. The federal Office of Health Technology Assessment and other technology assessment programs sponsored by the American Medical Association, the American College of Physicians, and Blue Cross and Blue Shield have contributed as well. The Prospective Payment Assessment Commission considers new technologies in hospitals when updating prospective payments to hospitals. Federal and state governments have also sought to constrain expenditures by supporting new models for care under the demonstration and waiver programs described elsewhere.

At present more than 44% of national expenditures for acute and subacute services are paid through government financing. For institutional long-term care services, more than 55% is funded by Medicaid and Medicare, with additional funding through VA programs (3) and the remainder primarily through private dollars rather than insurance. Community-based long-term care is funded through out-of-pocket payments, private insurance, and Medicaid waivers.

To address the coverage gap between Medicare parts A and B and to pay for institutional and community-based long-term care, private insurance expansion has been encouraged as a cost-sharing measure. Despite the drawbacks of health insurance as a model for financing health care, it is familiar to Americans. Because of initial excessive diversity in the policies available for coverage of the Medicare gap, with consequent consumer confusion and rip-offs, in 1990 federal legislation standardized Medigap policies into 10 packages. The packages all include core benefits of part A coinsurance for stays longer than 60 days, part B coinsurance, blood deductibles, and lifetime reserve days. In addition, they may include skilled nursing facility coinsurance, part A deductibles, part B deductibles, part B excess charges, foreign travel, at-home recovery, prescription drugs, and preventive care. The most popular policies include the coinsurance and deductible coverage and foreign travel coverage.

The goals of the Medigap legislation were to facilitate comparisons of policies, preserve choice, promote market stability and competition, and avoid adverse selection. As of 1996 it appeared the goals had been largely achieved (21). Medigap insurance was initially successful, continues to be so, and is less likely to generate consumer complaints since the 1990 legislation. However, as health care costs increase, so do the premiums for the Medigap policies, leading to a classic insurance death spiral in which people with less need for the coverage drop the policy as it becomes more expensive, leaving a pool of persons with higher needs, which becomes more expensive to insure, since the costs cannot be spread as broadly.

Long-term care insurance has been less successful than Medigap insurance. It is postulated that unlike routine health care or even hospitalization, most consumers do not imagine themselves ever using nursing home care. At least, they do not imagine it at the age when buying such insurance would be relatively affordable. As a result the growth in private long-term care insurance is slow. Reported barriers to sales of long-term care insurance include confusion about public coverage, policy elements, and adequacy and uncertainties about the likelihood of needing long-term care (22).

Finally, managed care has been embraced by federal and state governments as a key strategy in controlling costs. Interest in the success of early HMOs at decreasing costs while preserving quality (23) and desperation at the rate of increase of costs have led a dash to newer types of managed care organizations (MCOs) and expectations that they will be equally successful at managing cost and quality. The movement of Medicare beneficiaries to competitive MCOs, or "managed competition," has also received impetus from the failure of the 1993 Health Security Act. In 1995 more than 10% of Medicare beneficiaries were enrolled in MCOs (24), though proportions vary widely, depending on which managed-care market is examined. The South California area, for instance, has about 25% of Medicare managed-care enrollees, whereas Ohio has fewer than 2% (25). Because of the high penetrance of Medicare managed care in California, Arizona, and Florida, the MCOs in those states are being watched closely for indications that managed care is meeting its promise of decreased costs with maintenance of quality. Recent studies have raised concerns about both.

HEALTH CARE REFORM

Despite improvements in access since the advent of Medicare, Medicaid, and OAA, a number of problems in our health care system for old age remain or have developed. These include rapidly increasing costs, insufficient definitions of medical necessity and benefit language (26), persistent tolerance of rationing by lack of access to insurance and variations in benefit coverage, cost shifting, administrative inefficiency, and lack of coordination of care. Unexplained variations in quality of outcomes and intensity of resource use are also noted in our system (27). Patient satisfaction varies as well.

HCFA and other parties have attempted to deal with quality and satisfaction variations by expanding quality and utilization management over many years. HCFA's contract with the various state PROs is now in the "fourth scope of work" and promotes quality improvement activities in a continuous quality improvement or total quality management style. Recently HCFA has committed to developing outcome measures pertinent to its beneficiaries through the Health Plan Employer Data Information Set program, in addition to continuing its established structure and process measures for quality. At present any hospital that is to receive Medicare dollars must be certified by the Joint Commission on the Accreditation of Healthcare Organizations. PROs continue to act as quality and utilization auditors. HCFA is also paying more attention to consumer satisfaction as a basis of comparison for its managed care programs.

By 1992 citizens had become sufficiently concerned about quality, choice, and cost in health care to support proposals for national health care reform. After the election of President Clinton in 1992, his administration undertook a health care reform planning effort that resulted in the fall of 1993 in a proposed Health Security Act. This was a proposal for a national health insurance system, to be administered on a regional basis by a mix of public and private entities. Provisions of the act addressed many of the problems identified earlier in the chapter, but the annual increases in health care costs slowed markedly for commercial insurers from 1992 to 1993. By the fall of 1993, much of the desperation had left the health care reform movement. Insurers, small employers, and other entities that would be most adversely affected mounted a successful countercampaign. However, annual health care cost increases slowed less for government programs, which have tended to cover difficult and high-risk cases via the Medicare and Medicaid populations. As a result, the federal and state governments have continued to be highly interested in cost-moderating initiatives.

As of the summer of 1998, budget reconciliation legislation will decrease the projected increases in the Medicare budget, primarily through cuts to hospitals and physicians. Proposed changes that would have affected taxpayers, such as copayments for home care, were largely rejected by lawmakers. Also rejected or delayed were changes in the reimbursement and billing practices for Medicare part B and projected shifts of payments from surgical to primary care providers. New provisions to modify graduate medical education and related payments were included, as well as revisions in fraud and abuse programs and establishment of managed care risk bearing groups. This regulation, following on the failure of the Health Security Act, fits a pattern of incremental change in U.S. policy (28) rather than radical change. In general, major health care reform is said to be unlikely in the United States because of our heterogeneity as a people, our distrust of government, and an absence of commitment to community (28).

PROJECTIONS

Just before the turn of the century, it seems reasonable to revisit observations regarding old age that were carried into the present century. Demographic projections of increasing numbers of citizens surviving beyond age 65, or even to 85, are well known (29). Less well appreciated is that experience with poverty, illness, and isolation may not carry forward. Recent data on morbidity and dysfunction in old age (29, 30) support Fries's

suggestion in 1980 (30a) that age-related morbidity and mortality might be delayed and the duration of morbidity shortened. Assumptions about a standard retirement age may also be challenged, by both persons and policy initiatives. Data on the stages of life that are most costly are challenging assumptions that those beyond age 85 have the highest costs for acute care (31). Conversely, long-term care costs are highest for this group (32, 33). Continuing interest in support for seniors in the community instead of in institutions is reflected in studies of assisted living, continuing care retirement communities, naturally occurring retirement communities, and other combinations of housing and support services. Many of the staffing, administrative, and service issues faced in the long-term care waiver programs are anticipated to be reproduced in assisted-living programs (34).

What seems clear is that Social Security income, Medicare and Medicaid, as large parts of the federal budget, will continue to drive discussion and revision in the classic elements of health insurance: eligibility, benefits, reimbursement, and financing. Proposals of the past few years have included raising the age of access to benefits, trimming the benefit packages, decreasing reimbursements to providers, increasing taxes, and increasing cost sharing, to name the most obvious. Additional recent measures to decrease demand for care include elimination of funding to train physicians through Medicare's graduate medical education fund and even payments to hospitals *not* to train more doctors.

Money, and especially lack of it, is a known stressor in families and communities. As the United States struggles with its inflationary health care system, predictions of generation wars and entitlement wars (35, 36) may reduce the commitment to address the illness and isolation risks of old age. More explicit rationing of health care is also predicted (37).

Less likely in the near term are attempts to legislate national health insurance or a national health delivery system. With major OECD countries turning from nearly exclusive government sponsorship of their health care systems to introduction of competition, the U.S. tradition of incrementalism in policy making, and the euphoria about the general state of the economy (with a halo effect for all proposals that include competition), a national move from a competitive mode to a regulatory mode is unlikely. However, both the federal government and state governments will continue to explore options for reconfiguring insurance and care packages for Medicare and Medicaid beneficiaries (38).

REFERENCES

1. Hudson RB. The evolution of the welfare state: shifting rights and responsibilities for the old. Int Soc Secur Rev 1995;48:83–97.
2. Koff TH, Park RW. Historical background to aging policy. In: Hendricks J, ed. Aging Public Policy Bonding the Generations. Amityville, NY: Baywood, 1993:45–68.
3. Levit KR, Lazenby HC, Sivarajan L, et al. National health expenditures, 1994. Health Care Financ Rev 1996;17:205–242.
4. Gosselin PG. Trimming medicare. Boston Globe, October 19, 1995.
5. Kemper P, Murtaugh CM. Lifetime use of nursing home care. N Engl J Med 1991;324:595–600.
6. Snow KI, Riley T, Booth M, Fuller E. Managed Care for the Elderly: A Profile of Current Initiatives. Portland, ME: National Academy for State Health Policy, 1993.
7. Hornbrook MC. Improving care and constraining costs: evaluating New York City's cluster care demonstration. Health Serv Res 1996;31:509–513.
8. Iglehart J. The American health care system: private insurance. N Engl J Med 1992;326:1715–1720.
9. Glaser W. The competition vogue and its outcomes. Lancet 1993;341:805–812.
10. Glaser W. Paying the hospital: foreign lessons for the United States. Health Care Financ Rev 1983;4:99–110.
11. Greenwald LM. Meaning in numbers. Health Manage Q 1992;third quarter:6–9.
12. Wilson NJ, Kizer KW. The VA health care system: an unrecognized national safety net. Health Affairs 1997;16:200–204.
13. De Lew N, Greenberg G, Kinchen K. A layman's guide to the U.S. health care system. Health Care Financ Rev 1992;14:151–169.
14. Ham C. Population-centered and patient-focused purchasing: the U.K. experience. Milbank Q 1996;74:191–212.
15. Maynard A, Bloor K. Introducing a market to the United Kingdom's national health service. N Engl J Med 1996;334:604–607.
16. Scheil-Adlung X. Social security for dependent persons in Germany and other countries: between tradition and innovation. Int Soc Secur Rev 1995;48:19–34.
17. McCall N. Lessons from Arizona's Medicaid managed care program. Health Affairs 1997;16:194–199.
18. Grumbach K, Bodenheimer T. The organization of health care. JAMA 1995;273:160–167.
19. Merrell K, Colby DC, Hogan C. Medicare beneficiaries covered by Medicaid buy-in agreements. Health Affairs 1997;16:175–184.
20. Duncan DG, Servais CS. Preparing for the new outpatient reimbursement system. Health Care Financ Manage 1996;50:42–43,46–49.
21. McCormack LA, Fox PD, Rice T, Graham ML. Medigap reform legislation of 1990: have the objectives been met? Health Care Financ Rev 1989;18:157–172.
22. Cohen MA, Kumar AKN. The changing face of long-term care insurance in 1994: profiles and innovations in a dynamic market. Inquiry 1997;34:50–61.
23. Miller RH, Luft HS. Managed care plan performance since 1980. JAMA 1994;271:1512–1519.
24. Wolf LF, Gorman JK. New directions and developments in managed care financing. Health Care Financ Rev 1996;17:1–5.
25. Zarabozo C, Taylor C, Hicks J. Medicare managed care: numbers and trends. Health Care Financ Rev 1996;17:243–250.
26. Eddy DM. Benefit language: criteria that will improve quality while reducing costs. JAMA 1996;275:650–657.
27. Fisher ES, Wennberg JE, Stuker TA, Sharp SM. Hospital readmission rates for cohorts of Medicare beneficiaries in Boston and New Haven. N Engl J Med 1994;331:989–995.
28. Iglehart J. The American health care system: introduction. N Engl J Med 1992;326:962–968.
29. Waite LJ. The demographic face of America's elderly. Inquiry 1996;33:220–224.
30. Manton KG, Corder L, Stallard E. Chronic disability trends in elderly United States populations: 1982–1994. Proc Natl Acad Sci U S A 1997;94:2593–2598.
30a. Fries JF. Aging, natural death, and the compression of morbidity. N Engl J Med 1980;303:130–135.
31. Perls TT, Wood ER. Acute care costs of the oldest old: they cost less, their care intensity is less, and they go to nonteaching hospitals. Arch Intern Med 1996;156:754–760.
32. Kemper P. Case management agency systems of administering long-term care: evidence from the channeling demonstration. Gerontologist 1990;30:817–824.
33. Hoffman C, Rice D, Sung HY. Persons with chronic conditions. JAMA 1996;276:1473–1479.
34. Brown KB. Assisted living: a model of supportive housing. In: Advances in Long Term Care. New York: Springer, 1992.
35. Rockefeller JD IV. The Pepper Commission report on comprehensive health care. N Engl J Med 1990;323:1005–1007.
36. Gist JR. Entitlements and the federal budget: facts, folklore, and future. Milbank Q 1996;74:327–358.
37. Aaron H, Schwartz WB. Rationing health care: the choice before us. Science 1990;247:418–422.
38. Moon M, Holahan J. Can states take the lead in health care reform? JAMA 1992;268:1588–1594.

CHAPTER 55

GILBERT L. WERGOWSKE, PATRICIA LANOIE BLANCHETTE, AND JON PATRICK COONEY

Retirement

Within two years he was dead.

—Robert H. Moser (1)

Despite increasing evidence to the contrary, anecdotes of failure and poor health after retirement continue to dominate the American cultural perception of retirement. The departure from business or public life or the cessation of a long working or professional career is described by the "veteran observer of unsuccessful retirements" quoted above as, "terribly parched and resonating with doom, a dreary prescription for early demise" (1). The main reason for the gloom is that we associate retirement with an end to productivity. That perception must change as the concept of productivity is uncoupled from salaried employment.

In many parts of the world retirement is not an option; people work until incapacity or death. Our concept of retirement at age 65 dates from the government of Kaiser Wilhelm II (1888– 1941), when life expectancy at birth was only 63 years. Life expectancy has greatly increased (2), our workforce has changed, and the very concept of the inevitable correlation of aging and disease is being altered (3). However, the concept of retirement is stagnated because of our cultural ideology venerating work as one's sole source of worth (4). A grudging compromise to the increases in productive life expectancy is the increase in age for mandatory retirement to 70.5 years. Because workers with seniority are more expensive to their employers, however (5, 6), and where younger workers abound, mandatory retirement is apt to continue as a tool to reduce business costs.

ENGAGEMENT WITH LIFE

Continued engagement with life is the key to successful retirement. Older people neither consider themselves old nor are perceived as old as long as they remain productive (7). Formal and informal volunteer activity commonly replaces paid work after age 55 and continues through age 75 or longer. Nearly 40% of people over age 60 report at least 1500 hours of productive activity in the past year (8, 9). As one successful retiree commented, "I didn't retire, I retreaded." Such networking and activity have a protective effect on health (10, 11) and benefit our society tremendously, even though they are not recognized as part of our gross national product. Formal and informal volunteerism in later life must be facilitated, encouraged, and applauded for its benefit to society and to the individual.

Leisure activity is no less important. Because all of us are at risk for chronic illness as we age, it is likely that activities must also change. Flexible coping strategies are the most successful (12). Social support promotes the flexibility required to adjust or replace leisure activities. Those who cease some leisure activity without replacement are at increased risk for adverse health consequences (13). Facilitating continued meaningful leisure activity therefore assumes great importance in promoting health and productivity.

SUCCESSFUL RETIREMENT

Instead of pathologic versus healthy aging, Rowe and Kahn (14, 15) describe successful versus usual aging. This refocusing promotes the concept of a risk-based approach. In their scheme, *usual agers* are "nonpathologic but high risk," while *successful agers* are "low risk and high function." Neither group is considered as diseased. They list three main components for successful aging: low probability of disease and disease-related disability; high cognitive and physical functional capacity; and active engagement with life. Three important dicta emerge from their work. First, intrinsic factors alone do not dominate risk factors for disease in old age. Second, as age increases, the relative contribution of genetic factors decreases and the force of environmental factors increases. Third, *usual aging* characteristics are modifiable. Retirement fits this model very well, as there is nothing innately pathologic or degenerative about retirement.

Many gerontologists have described the increasing health and engagement into the later years as either an extension of the healthy middle years or the "second middle age." Another way to describe the phenomenon is captured in the term "the third age." Rather than describing life stages as youth, middle age, and old age, the life stages are separated into youth, the second age (gaining independence and raising a family), the third age (personal achievement and self-development), and the fourth age (frailty and decline) (16).

However one considers the passage of time and one's life, preparation for transitions and taking things in acceptably small steps is best for adaptation. The pattern of work that is emerging is significantly different now than at the height of the industrial age. Rather than working for 20 to 30 years for the same employer, then breaking cleanly into retirement, a pattern of periods of work followed by periods of transition, retraining, and job changes is more common. Contrary to popular belief, many people in their 60s who are looking for work are looking for full-time rather than part-time employment. The adaptation of the work environment as a result of the Americans with Disabilities Act in 1992 opened new possibilities for people of any age with physical disabilities. People who can plan for transitions, such as leaving full-time employment for contracting or consulting work, have an easier time adjusting. Retirement followed by a rehire at reduced time for the same company is also common, taking advantage of pensions to enable a more focused period of work. Workers suddenly displaced have a much harder time, but most eventually adjust. Older displaced workers have a much harder time finding work and a higher discouraged unemployed rate. Planning for the possibility of losing one's job, saving for such events, is much more healthful. One worker described this nest egg as his "go to hell fund," a cushion to allow job change that also serves as a safety net in case of a business decline.

LOW PROBABILITY OF DISEASE

Studies that concentrate on use of health care services suggest there is no adverse health effect due to ceasing work (17). True, when work-limiting ill health is cited as the reason for retirement, especially early retirement, the probability of death within 2 years of retirement is increased by about 4% (18). However, perceived changes in health after retirement are more often attributable to one or more chronic diseases with onset many years before quitting work (19). Moreover, subjective ratings of poor health in retirement correlate more with depressive symptoms than with physical illness or functional disability (20).

A growing body of evidence suggests that our concept of increased risk of disease and disability with advancing age from an immutable and inevitable genetically determined aging process is incorrect (14). The Swedish Adoption/Twin Aging Study data and other studies suggest that many *usual aging* characteristics are due to lifestyle and other factors that are *age related* but not *age dependent* (21–23). Established risk factors, such as for cardiovascular and cerebrovascular disease, can be modified dramatically with lifestyle interventions (3, 24), and physical function can be improved (25, 26). Additionally, one may argue that it is not the absence of disease but the adjustment to disease that matters. The life of Anna Mary Robertson (Grandma) Moses (1860–1961) exemplifies this argument. Crippled by arthritis and unable to continue her needlework in her 70s, she turned to painting. She had no previous training in art. Not everyone has the exceptional talent of Grandma Moses, but everyone has some kind of talent.

HIGH COGNITIVE AND PHYSICAL FUNCTIONAL CAPACITY

Four of five community-dwelling people over age 65 have at least one chronic health problem (27). Arthritis is the most common. Despite listing a chronic disease, however, 70% of whites and 52% of African-Americans reported themselves to be in "good health" (28). Social isolation and low levels of education and income are consistently related to the perception of poor health and to increased health care costs in retirement and aging studies (29, 30). The overrepresentation of African-Americans in the lower education, lower income, and more isolated groups may explain their lower sense of health. By the time of retirement, even by the time of first employment, the solutions to these particular problems have largely eluded us.

Gall et al. (31) confirm earlier studies that income and voluntary retirement status predict successful retirement in the first few years better than does physical health. Internal locus of control increases the probability of successful long-term adjustment. Satisfaction with health and relationships appeared to peak about a year after retirement. Despite decline in physical status about 6 to 7 years post retirement, health satisfaction remained above preretirement levels (30). In successful retirement, increased freedom and self-direction generate an increase in the perceived control over events, especially for those who did not have high job satisfaction and retired voluntarily as soon as they had the resources (31–34).

Although the prevalence of dementia nearly doubles each decade after age 65 (35, 36), no one has yet proposed that retirement causes dementia, as they have with physical disability. Still, probably no other disease process robs more enjoyment from retirement. Research on the cause and treatment of Alzheimer's disease remains in its infancy, but some clues from aging and dementia research may help us preserve cognitive function in general. First, dementia involves a striking loss of neuronal connections, and the loss of nerve cells not seen in normal aging (37, 38). Second, antioxidants may slow the clinical progression of Alzheimer's disease (39). Multiple studies list education as the strongest predictor of high cognitive function (40), followed closely by regular physical exercise (41, 42). Regular mental exercises throughout life delay the onset of Alzheimer's dementia and are highly recommended for everyone. In retirement, many successful and fulfilling second careers have blossomed, as has completion of college degrees long delayed by the demands of employment and child rearing. But then, are these people retired in the traditional sense?

COMMON PROBLEMS IN RETIREMENT

Most of the major problems in retirement stem from poor planning. Poor financial planning may be based on the misconceptions that the need for income will drop substantially in retirement and that Social Security will be enough (43). Neither is true, and careful early financial planning for retirement is very important. While the mortgage may be paid off, new expenses arise, such as the need to purchase more services or the desire to travel for pleasure or to stay in touch with family. A conclusion of the 1981 President's Commission on Retirement is that to maintain the standard of living, households require 75% of preretirement income. Social Security was never intended to be one's sole income in retirement, yet a large proportion of the elderly have no other source (44). Some retirees are blessed with good pensions, but not all. Those who retired before pension reform laws were instituted may be receiving only a few dollars per month, a return of principal without benefit of the earnings on that retirement principal. The 1974 Employee Retirement Income Security Act (ERISA) established standards for private pension plans, and the Retirement Equity Act of 1984 further improved security with the extension of certain benefits to widows, widowers, and divorced spouses. However, today's very old may have retired before these laws were enacted and have tiny pensions today. Despite a lifetime of working, they depend on Social Security, family assistance, and public support. Public housing and meals programs remain the means of subsistence for many. One example is our patient, a nurse retired after over 30 years of service at a local hospital. Although she worked very diligently, her pension is $34 per month. Old railroad pensions are also very low. One of our patients receives $7 monthly after 30 years of service. Moreover, in today's climate of business downsizing, rightsizing, and outsourcing, fewer can expect to remain with a single employer long enough to accumulate the traditional pension. Despite earlier vesting, as provided for in the Tax Reform Act of 1986, continuous individual financial preparation for retirement, begun early in the work years, is essential for success.

Several societal changes lessen the likelihood that children can be counted on to make up the substantial difference between financial and social needs in old age. First, there has been a delay in starting families, often into the 30s. Parents of those who postpone starting a family find their children struggling at the critical stages of building their own careers and families at the time of their parents' greatest financial need. Also, the national and international job market separates families. For example, one patient has a child in New York, a child in Frankfurt, and a child in Singapore. Which child will be responsible for Mom and Dad, who still live where they were born and don't want to leave?

THE PHYSICIAN'S ROLE

Traditionally, physicians deal with matters of health and disease rather than with social issues, and social services have been inadequate. This condition has led to an eschewing of the medical model in favor of the social model in some circles. Neither is adequate, and an interdisciplinary model has emerged. Consider the case of a frail elder living alone in a third-story walk-up apartment with no local family to monitor her. A neighbor may inquire if she is not seen up and about for a few days. What if she is found on the floor with a broken hip, dehydrated and ill because of a delay in discovery? She may survive surgery but need a nursing home at least temporarily. This is neither solely a medical nor solely a social problem. The social risk was ig-

nored until it became a medical problem. Timely intervention to ensure that she had adequate income, nutrition, and social support might well have averted her nursing home bill which we, the public, complain so bitterly about paying. She might even be volunteering at the local library, leading a children's reading group today, if intervention had occurred earlier. The best outcome will occur if an interdisciplinary model is applied to her plan of care.

Physicians must continue to monitor health and encourage healthful behaviors, especially in view of new research indicating that much of the degeneration we attributed to normal aging is modifiable. However, physicians must also address social concerns. For example, most jobs now require an employment physical examination. Occupational health examinations are required to monitor workers with certain exposures, and a retirement physical examination is often requested. Each work-related encounter presents the physician with an opportunity to advise the worker to be very careful about planning financially for retirement.

Special considerations for medical diagnosis and intervention during any physician-patient encounter include hearing and vision loss, social isolation and depression, and abuse and neglect. While any sensory loss predisposes to frailty, hearing loss may be occult and insidious, mimicking dementia and worsening social isolation. Elders must adjust to social loss, loss of companionship of their coworkers and friends, loss of a spouse, and sometimes loss of children. Meeting new companions and starting new activities usually require considerable encouragement in the face of loss. Failing that, isolation worsens. An inventory of activities and social contacts should be part of the periodic health maintenance visit to the physician. Depression frequently presents atypically in the elderly, but it is eminently treatable. Elders who are abused and neglected may actively conceal their plight for fear of retaliation, further loss of freedom, or fear of institutionalization.

Finally, physicians must be politically and socially active, challenge the conscience of society, and ensure that we get the most for our health care dollar. For indeed the true measure of a society is how it cares for its most vulnerable members.

CONCLUSION

Like baseball, preparing for retirement is played in innings, each with multiple scoring opportunities and hazards. For *successful retirement,* practice, planning, and discipline expand the opportunities and diminish the risk of injury. For *usual retirement,* inadequate practice, poor planning, and lack of discipline limit the opportunities and multiply the hazards. There is nothing intrinsic to retirement or baseball that adversely affects physical or mental health, but it is always nice to have a healthy lead going into the later innings. Even in the last inning of the game, sound advice and thoughtful preparation modify many of the hazards. And because we are the home team, we always get the last at bat.

REFERENCES

1. Moser RH. On retirement. Ann Intern Med 1997;127: 159–161.
2. Portnoi VA. The natural history of retirement. Mainly good news. JAMA 1981;245:1752–1754.
3. Hazzard WR, Bierman EL. Preventive gerontology: strategies for attenuation of the chronic disease in aging. In: Hazzard W, Andres R, Bierman E, Blass J, eds. Principles of Geriatric Medicine and Gerontology. 2nd ed. New York: McGraw-Hill, 1990:167–171.
4. Ekerdt DJ. Why the notion persists that retirement harms health. Gerontologist 1987;27:454–457.
5. O'Connor J. The Fiscal Crisis of the State. New York: St. Martin's Press, 1973.
6. Minkler M. Research on the health effects of retirement: an uncertain legacy. J Health Soc Behav 1981;22:117–130.
7. Kaufman SR. The Ageless Self: Sources of Meaning in Late Life. Madison, WI: University of Wisconsin Press, 1986.
8. Herzog AR, Kahn RL, Morgan JN, et al. Age differences in productive activities. J. Gerontol 1989;44:S129–S138.
9. Herzog AR, Morgan JN. Age and gender differences in the value of productive activities: four different approaches. Res Aging 1992;14:169–198.
10. House JS, Landis KR, Umberson D. Social relationships and health. Science 1988;241:540–545.
11. Seeman TE, Berkman LF, Carpentier PA, et al. Behavioral and psychosocial predictors of physical performance: MacArthur studies of successful aging. J Gerontol 1995;50A:M177–M183.
12. Blalock SJ, DeVellis BM, Holt K, Hahn PM. Coping with rheumatoid arthritis: is one problem the same as another? Health Educ Q 1993;20:119–132.
13. Zimmer Z, Hickey T, Searle MS. The pattern of change in leisure activity behavior among older adults with arthritis. Gerontologist 1997;37:384–392.
14. Rowe JW, Kahn RL. Successful aging. Gerontologist 1997;37:433–440.
15. Rowe JW, Kahn RL. Human aging: usual and successful. Science 1987;237:143–149.
16. Manheimer RJ. The Second Middle Age: Looking Differently at Life Beyond 50. Detroit: Visible Ink Press, 1995.
17. Soghikian K, Midanik LT, Polen MT, Ransom LJ. The effect of retirement on health services utilization: the Kaiser Permanente Retirement Study. J Gerontol 1991; 46:S353–S360.
18. Boaz RF, Muller CF. The validity of health limitations as a reason for deciding to retire. Health Serv Res 1990;25: 361–386.
19. Kremer Y. The association between health and retirement: self-health assessment of Israeli retirees. Soc Sci Med 1985;20:61–66.
20. Mulsant BH, Ganguli M, Seaberg EC. The relationship between self-rated health and depressive symptoms in an epidemiological sample of community-dwelling older adults. J Am Geriatr Soc 1997;45:954–958.
21. Heller D, de Faire U, Pedersen NL, et al. Genetic and environmental influences on serum lipid levels in twins. N Engl J Med 1993;328:1150–1156.
22. Stunkard A, Harris J, Pedersen N, McClearn G. The body mass index of twins who have been reared apart. N Engl J Med 1990;322:1483–1487.
23. Hong Y, de Faire U, Heller D, et al. Genetic and environmental influences on blood pressure in elderly twins. Hypertension 1994;24:663–670.
24. Sticht JP, Hazzard WR. Weight control and exercise: cardinal features of successful preventive gerontology. JAMA 1995;274:1964–1965.
25. Fabre C, Masse-Biron J, Ahmaidi S, et al. Effectiveness of individualized aerobic training at the ventilatory threshold in the elderly. J Gerontol 1997;52A:B260–B266.
26. Buchner DM, Cress ME, de Lateur B, et al. The effect of strength and endurance training on gait, balance, fall risk, and health services use in community-living older adults. J Gerontol 1997;52A:M218–M224.
27. National Center for Health Statistics. Aging America: Trends and Projections. Washington, 1984. Reported in U.S. Senate, Select Committee on Aging.
28. National Center for Health Statistics. Current estimates from the National Health Interview Survey, 1988. National Center for Health Statistics. Vital Health Stat 1989;10:84–114.
29. Bosworth HB, Schaie KW. The relationship of social environment, social networks, and health outcomes in The Seattle Longitudinal Study: two analytical approaches. J Gerontol 1997;52B:P197–P205.
30. House JS, Landis KR, Umberson D. Social relationships and health. Science 1988;241:540–545.
31. Gall TL, Evans DR, Howard J. The retirement adjustment process: changes in the well-being of male retirees across time. J Gerontol 1997;52B:P110–P117.

32. Skinner EA, Connel JP. Control understanding: suggestions for a developmental framework. In: Bates MM, Baltes PB, eds. The Psychology of Control and Aging. Hillsdale, NJ: Lawrence Erlbaum, 1986:35–70.

33. Hoff EH, Hohner HV. Occupational careers, work and control. In: Bates MM, Baltes PB, eds. The Psychology of Control and Aging. Hillsdale, NJ: Lawrence Erlbaum, 1986:207–236.

34. Henretta JC, Chan CG, O'Rand AM. Retirement reason versus retirement process: examining the reasons for retirement typology. J Gerontol 1992;47:S1–S7.

35. White L, Petrovitch H, Ross GW, et al. Prevalence of dementia in older Japanese-American men in Hawaii: the Honolulu-Asia Aging Study. JAMA 1996;276:955–960.

36. Breteler MM, Claus JJ, van Duijn CM, et al. Epidemiology of Alzheimer's disease. Epidemiol Rev 1992;14:59–82.

37. Terry RD, Peck A, DeTeresa R, et al. Some morphometric aspects of the brain in senile dementia of the Alzheimer's type. Ann Neurol 1981;10:184–192.

38. Hyman BT, West HL, Gomez-Isla T, Mui S. Quantitative neuropathology in Alzheimer's disease: neuronal loss in high-order association cortex parallels dementia. In: Iqbal K, Mortimer JA, Winblad B, Wisniewski HM, eds. Research Advances in Alzheimer's Disease and Related Disorders. New York: Wiley, 1995:453–460.

39. Sano M, Ernesto C, Thomas RG, et al. A controlled trial of selegiline, alpha tocopherol, or both as treatment for Alzheimer's disease. N Engl J Med 1997;336:1216–1247.

40. Albert MS, Savage CR, Jones K, et al. Predictors of cognitive change in older persons: MacArthur studies of successful aging. Psychol Aging 1995;10:578–589.

41. Cook NR, Evans DA, Scherr PA, et al. Peak expiratory flow rate and 5–6 year mortality in an elderly population. Am J Epidemiol 1989;130:67–78.

42. Neeper SA, Gomez-Pinilla F, Choi J, Cotman C. Exercise and brain neurotrophins. Nature 1995;373:109.

43. Burkhauser RV, Duncan GJ. Life events, public policy and the economic vulnerability of children and the elderly. In: Plamer JL, Smeeding T, Torrey BB, eds. The Vulnerable. Washington: Urban Institute Press, 1988:55–88.

44. Reno VP. The role of pensions in retirement income. In: Pensions in a Changing Economy. Washington: Employee Benefit Research Institute, 1993:19–32.

CHAPTER 56

PATRICIA LANOIE BLANCHETTE AND JAMES H. PIETSCH

Evaluation of Competence

Clinicians working with older people are often asked for an opinion regarding a patient's competence because clinical and legal situations make the clinician's opinion valuable. Regardless of the thoroughness of the evaluation, however, the clinician gives only an opinion. When competence is contested, a court makes the determination. Common situations in which an opinion is sought include capacity to give informed consent, to make a living will or durable power of attorney for health care decisions, to support the need for a representative payee, to serve as one's own trustee, to make or revoke a will, to make large gifts, or to sell personal property. In giving an opinion regarding capacity, it is important that the clinician not be influenced by the outcome of that opinion. In trying to help the family, the clinician may be tempted to give an opinion without doing a complete assessment or knowledge of the social situation. In addition, the clinician may not understand undue influence or the potential use of the opinion in subsequent legal actions. Clinicians uncomfortable with their skills of assessment should consult another clinician who does this routinely.

Opinions that might impinge upon freedom or self-determination of older persons must never be taken lightly. Clinicians should not feel pressured to participate in such assessments and should participate only if they believe that the request for assessment is appropriate and if they have the time to perform a thorough examination. It is important to seek information about the social situation. They must also be skilled to do so by virtue of training and experience and know the relevant state laws.

TERMINOLOGY
Capacity and Competence

The terms capacity and competence are often used interchangeably. However, capacity refers to the ability of a person to perform a particular function, to make a decision about his or her person or property. Competence traditionally refers to the legal determination of that ability. Specific capacity is sometimes called decisional capacity. However, a person who is decisionally incapacitated in one area is not necessarily globally incapacitated. An adult is presumed to be competent in the eyes of the law unless adjudged incompetent in a court of law. The presumption of competence is based on the principle of autonomy, or self-determination. Therefore, if the term incapacitated is used with regard to a person, it is best to be precise in the use of the language to include "decisionally incapacitated with regard to. . . . "

Specific Capacity and Specific Competence

These terms refer to the ability to perform a particular function, to understand the significant benefits, burdens, risks, and alternatives, and to make and communicate a decision about an issue in question. When people are impaired, they can retain the ability to make informed decisions about some things while lacking the ability to perform more complex functions. Capacity is not like a light with an on-off switch, but more like a lamp on a rheostat, with varying intensities for specific needs. For example, a person may not have the capacity to make an informed decision about a serious medical procedure but be capable of deciding which person they trust to make a proxy decision for them. A person may be capable of making or revoking a will but incapable of understanding the complexities and options of a legal contract. It is common for a clinician to be asked whether a person "is competent." The clinician should reply, "Competent to do what?" That is, evaluation of competence must involve an assessment of the capacity and judgment to perform the specific functions in question.

Who Can Assess Capacity

Although it is usual for psychiatrists, psychologists, and sometimes social workers to be involved in assessing capacity, other clinicians may do equally well with proper training and experience. Psychiatrists usually determine the need for involuntary mental health treatment. Geriatricians, internists, family practitioners, neurologists, and other physicians familiar with this work may offer the additional ability to assess the person's medical status and to give an opinion about the reversibility of incapacity. Transient situations may include the influence of medications and other substances, recovery from serious medical illness, metabolic abnormalities, lingering effects of anesthesia, hyperglycemia or hypoglycemia, hypoxia, or recovery from head injury.

LEGAL FRAMEWORK
Judicial Proceedings

It is important to consider the legal and cultural framework in which competence is adjudicated. In the United States, the principle of autonomy, or individual freedom, is highly valued, balanced by safety and the need to protect citizens against harm to themselves or to others. States and judges vary somewhat interpreting these principles. For example, in some courts, a *guardian* of person or property is typically appointed for someone who is determined to be incompetent, resulting in considerable restrictions on personal freedom and civil rights (1). In other states the court more commonly appoints a *conservator* and strictly limits his or her authority. Alternatives to guardianship are often preferable

(2). In both instances, whether there is a guardian or conservator, a fiduciary relationship is established, and a bond may have to be posted to protect the rights and assets of the incapacitated person.

Determinations of incompetence typically follow a petition that a person cannot adequately care for his or her person or property or poses a danger to the self or others (1). Health care providers may ask attorneys to show them the statutory or other legal basis for declaring someone incompetent. In most instances there is no such evidence, nor is there a court process for a person to request a determination that he or she is competent. Other common situations include the attempt to set aside the making or revocation of a will or reversing a gift, sale, or exchange of personal property based on the retroactive determination of lack of competence at the time of the action. In these instances, experienced clinicians may be asked to evaluate the case of a plaintiff or defendant, expecting that assessment to be refuted by clinicians whose opinions support the opposing view.

DIAGNOSTIC INTERVIEWING AND TESTING
Evaluating Capacity

Capacity is generally thought to be present when a person can (*a*) understand the nature of the situation, act, or problem and available options, including no action; (*b*) understand risks and benefits of the options; (*c*) make a reasoned decision; and (*d*) communicate a decision. The mental capacity needed to make and communicate a reasoned decision varies with circumstances. That is, different levels of ability may be needed to make specific decisions with regard to medical treatment, to execute or revoke a will, or to execute a living will, trust, or power of attorney.

Confidentiality

Any discussions about a person's capacity should be kept confidential. For example, discuss the patient's care with family members or others only with the patient's permission or with those having legal authority to receive the information. Many states have laws delineating surrogacy for an impaired person. As with capacity and competence, it is necessary to understand the legal framework of the clinical interaction. When legal issues are at hand, it is best to work with an attorney who is the advocate for the patient, with specific permission of that person, or under a court order.

Considerations in the Process of Assessing Capacity

The person being interviewed should be made as comfortable as possible and afforded privacy. One should make efforts to maximize the patient's ability to perform, such as favorable selection of time of the day, consideration of hearing or vision loss, good lighting, comfortable positioning, and rest breaks. Aids such as hearing amplifiers and large-print materials should be considered. The patient's preferences and any limits with regard to confidentiality should be determined, explained, and respected. The reason for the evaluation and its possible uses should be explained to the patient with every effort to make the patient understand. Translation should be provided when the patient and evaluator do not have the same primary language, paying particular attention to accent, slang, patois, Creole, and pidgin terms. Furthermore, cultural differences regarding causes and treatments for illness should not be misinterpreted as signs of incompetence (3).

Determination of Baseline Functioning

Previous status is relevant to assessment of current functioning. For example, a patient recovering from an acute medical illness, head injury, delirium, or general anesthesia or under the influence of psychoactive medications may be considerably more impaired than at the baseline. Major social or legal decisions may have to be deferred until it is determined whether significant improvement in cognitive functioning may occur or to enable a search for reversible causes of impairment. It may take 6 to 8 weeks or more for delirium to clear completely.

Meaningful Interview

An interview assessing understanding of the specific nature of the decision in question; a per-

son's ability to make judgments, weigh options, and give personal reasons for the decision; and the ability to communicate this decision are more valuable than indirect assessments, such as standardized tests. The best evidence is the patient's verbatim answers to the examiner's questions. A person's own words in response to a series of pertinent questions will speak most eloquently if capacity to make the decision is questioned in the future. The examiner should document verbatim relevant questions and answers if a person's capacity may later be questioned or if the examination's purpose is to determine specific capacity. For a finding of decisional capacity, the examiner need not agree with the patient's decision but only determine whether the patient understands, can weigh options, applies personal values and life experiences to make a reasoned decision, and can communicate that decision. Serial assessments are particularly helpful whenever possible, especially if the patient's memory is impaired or the clinical situation is changing. A finding of capacity may be validated if a memory-impaired patient reaches the same decision upon subsequent assessments.

Additional History

Depending on the circumstances, history obtained from family, friends, and other health care providers can be very helpful, especially with regard to baseline functioning and rapidity of change. However, the examiner should be careful not to be unduly influenced by persons who have a stake in the outcome of the determination.

Supplementary Assessment

Ancillary assessments may be very helpful. For example, if a question arises about an older person's ability to continue to live alone or to return to independent living, the physician should consider ordering an in-home assessment by an occupational and physical therapist with particular attention to the patient's abilities and independence in activities of daily living. For example, suppose a younger couple moves into a wealthy older woman's home and influences her to spend large sums of money. After visiting, the patient's daughter, who lives at some distance and has not seen the patient for many months, objects to the situation and retains an attorney to secure guardianship of the property. The daughter maintains that the older woman is unable to live independently and is unduly influenced by the younger couple because she depends on them to remain in her own home. The couple maintain that the woman can live independently and has approved the expenditure of large sums, so they deny undue influence. The geriatrician performs a complete physical examination and mental status assessment in the office and orders an in-home assessment by an occupational therapist. The mental status assessment reveals the patient to be seriously cognitively impaired. The occupational therapist determines that the patient is highly unsafe in her own home with regard to simple acts of preparing food, cooking, walking, and bathing. The court may determine the patient incompetent in both personal and financial affairs, may grant guardianship to the daughter, and may order the young couple to repay a large sum of money garnered as a result of undue influence on the patient.

Refusal to Consent to Assessment

The patient may refuse or be unable to cooperate fully or at all with the assessment. The decision whether to proceed with the assessment depends on the clinical and legal situation. If the patient is too ill to participate, a brief report of the interaction with the patient should be documented. If the examiner is doing a court-ordered assessment, the interview may be rescheduled to a time when the patient may be more cooperative. If the patient continues to be uncooperative, the report may contain visual observations, details of the interaction with the patient, and reports of other interviews. However, the report should emphasize that the patient was not cooperative and may not have performed optimally.

Lucid Interval

The concept of fluctuating decisional capacity derives from the example of mental illnesses, such as schizophrenia, in which the patient may have lucid intervals while taking medication or is otherwise improved. Patients with moderate to severe dementia are unlikely to regain decisional

capacity. If capacity appears to fluctuate, the lucid interval and assessment should be thoroughly documented, and the diagnosis of dementia reconsidered.

Mental Status Assessment

The assessment should describe level of alertness, cooperation with the examination, ability to attend to the questioning, physical ability to perform the tasks, speech, use of language, thought content, mood and affect, any delusions or hallucinations, and behavior. It is also important to determine the degree of awareness or insight into impairments, especially with regard to a person's ability to plan or compensate for acknowledged impairments. If there is a specific decision to be made, questions about previous similar decisions, social context, and values concerning the decision should be discussed. The patient's understanding of possible outcomes arising from decisions should be assessed, especially concerning the import of the decision, other persons influencing the decision, concerns about being a burden to other people, religious and cultural beliefs, and promises made to self or others.

Cognitive Testing

Cognitive testing should cover several domains, including orientation, attention, learning, problem solving, short- and long-term memory, and language, especially those that are relevant to the specific capacities in question. No tests are free from the bias of culture or education. However, to the extent possible, the evaluator should use instruments determined to be culturally neutral (4, 5). Evaluation tools or instruments, the actual tests used, should be selected by the clinician to assess both specific capacities in question and general abilities. Using standardized and validated testing instruments is useful primarily for comparing the same person over time and for communicating performance abilities to others. Depending on the reason for the assessment and the extent of disability, tests may range from screens, such as the Mini-Mental State Examination (6), to a battery of neuropsychologic evaluations taking several hours. Various neuropsychologic batteries may be helpful when impairment is mild and to help with specific diagnosis. They permit going beyond a determination of presence or absence of impairment to help determine cause and predict reversibility. The ecologic validity of a test, i.e., a cognitive test's ability to predict actual performance on a daily living task, such as driving or taking medication correctly, should also be considered (7).

Physical and Laboratory Examination

A physical examination in addition to cognitive testing is helpful with diagnosis, determining whether painful conditions may be impinging on attention and suggesting reversibility of the condition. Appropriate laboratory tests, such as hematocrit, oxygen saturation, electrolytes, hepatic and renal function, vitamin B12, red blood cell folate values, thyroid functioning, and serologic tests for syphilis may add to the assessment of possible diagnostic causes of impairment and potential reversibility.

Neuroimaging Studies

While not essential to determine the presence of cognitive impairment, neuroimaging may help to make or eliminate diagnoses such as subdural hematoma, stroke, and brain tumor and help determine causes and potential for reversibility of such impairments.

SPECIAL SITUATIONS
Memory Impairment

Memory impairment by itself does not mean that a person is decisionally incapacitated. Determining decisional capacity in persons with memory impairment depends on specific questions about the issue at hand. Intact capacity is supported by a finding that in repeated sessions the same decisions are made. For example, a patient with short-term memory loss and prostate cancer may be advised by his urologist and oncologist to have an orchiectomy. Because he also has mild to moderate Alzheimer's disease, a geriatrician may be consulted with regard to decisional capacity to give informed consent for the procedure. Upon careful evaluation, the geriatrician determines that the patient does have the capacity to give informed consent. However, the patient may not remember the decision or even his diagnosis from one day to the next. Upon

subsequent daily assessment, he may make the same decision to have the procedure performed. The consistency of his decision, along with family observation of the assessment and previous similar decisions to have surgery, may guide the urologist to proceed with the orchiectomy. The family may be asked to witness that the patient is providing informed consent.

Attention Deficits

Attention deficits are the hallmark of delirium, a possibly reversible cause of incapacity. Delirium is a common experience, such as with high fever, dehydration, inebriation, or opioid pain medication use. One would not wish to make major decisions or calculate one's income taxes in such a state. However, in most people the impairment is transient. Attention deficit may also be present in people who are under a great deal of stress, are very anxious, and hence cannot retain what they are told long enough to make a decision. It helpful for the clinician to be familiar with many methods to test for attention deficit to predict potential for reversibility of impairment, to help with diagnosis, and to assess the validity of other cognitive testing.

REPORTS

The report of competence assessment may contain the reason for the assessment and the source of referral; steps taken to assure an ethical and valid assessment; reports of collateral interviews, with sources noted; assessment of cognitive function covering several domains; performance-based measures; clinical assessment of medical and mental health factors; key findings; potential for reversibility of impairments; and conclusions. It helps to include verbatim quotations of clinician-patient interactions. In legal situations, the clinician should be prepared to provide evidence of training and experience, usually in the form of a curriculum vitae.

REFERENCES

1. Pietsch JH, Lee LH. The Elder Law Hawaii Handbook. Honolulu: University of Hawaii Press, 1998.
2. Kapp M. Alternatives to guardianship: enhanced autonomy for diminished capacity. In: Smyer M, Schaie KW, Kapp MB, eds. Older Adults' Decision-Making and the Law. New York: Springer, 1996:182–201.

3. Buchwald D, Caralis PV, Gany F, et al. Caring for patients in a multicultural society. Patient Care 1994; June:105–123.

4. Teng EL, Hasegawa K, Homma A, et al. The Cognitive Abilities Screening Instrument (CASI): a practical test for cross-cultural epidemiological studies of dementia. Int Psychogeriatr 1994;6:45–58.

5. Teng EL. Cross-cultural testing and the Cognitive Abilities Screening Instrument. In: Yeo G, Gallagher-Thompson D, eds. Ethnicity and the Dementias. Washington: Taylor & Francis, 1996:75–84.

6. Folstein MF, Folstein SE, McHugh PR. "Mini-mental state". A practical method for grading the cognitive state of patients for the clinician. J Psychiatr Res 1975;12: 189–198.

7. Assessment of Competency and Capacity of the Older Adult: A Practice Guideline for Psychologists. Milwaukee: National Center for Cost Containment, Department of Veterans Affairs, March 1997.

CHAPTER 57

PATRICIA P. BARRY AND BRUCE E. ROBINSON

Community-Based Long-Term Care

The concept of long-term care refers to the health, personal, and social services needed to attain and maintain optimal physical, social, and psychologic function by frail and dependent persons with chronic impairments. An implicit goal is also to provide care in the least restrictive environment possible. For recipients, the community is the setting in which they have greatest autonomy; for policy makers, community-based long-term care has the potential to be a cost-effective alternative to institutional care. Services include those necessary to prevent avoidable deterioration of health, treat acute exacerbations of chronic illness, maintain independence to the extent possible, and restore optimal function. Long-term care may involve high-tech medical services or low-tech assistance with activities of daily living. Preventive, diagnostic, therapeutic, rehabilitative, supportive (nonmedical), and health maintenance services may be provided. Personal care and supervision usually include unpaid care by family and friends and paid paraprofessional services.

More than 10 million Americans need some type of long-term care; about 55% of these are elderly (1). Since only about 20% of the elders who require long-term care are in nursing homes, most long-term care is provided in community settings; in addition, approximately 85% of non-institutional long-term care is unpaid, provided by families. Table 57.1 lists sites of care commonly provided in the community.

CARE COORDINATION AND CASE MANAGEMENT

The organization and integration of community-based long-term care consists of as-sessment of the patient, determination of his or her needs, care planning, resource management, coordination, monitoring, and periodic reassessment, usually with a multidisciplinary team of care providers. The care coordinator or case manager acts as an advocate for the patient and provides the links between the patient and family and appropriate community services, facilitating and supporting informal support systems and coordinating the efficient use of services to provide effective and quality care. Although the physician may not have the resources or the inclination to be the case manager, he or she should provide significant supervision of care in the community. Case management may be provided by home care corporations, private consultants, managed-care programs, or other care providers, such as nurses or social workers. The most difficult task for the case manager is to match the needs of the patient with necessary resources.

The first step in evaluation and planning for the long-term health care of frail elderly persons is to obtain and organize information regarding his or her performance of activities of daily living (ADLs), physical health, mental health, socioeconomic resources, and environment. This may be accomplished by use of the coordinated multidimensional, multidisciplinary approach called comprehensive geriatric assessment. The goals of assessment are to improve diagnostic accuracy, guide the selection of interventions to restore or preserve health, recommend an optimal environment, predict outcomes, and monitor clinical change (2). These are often interdependent, so that diagnostic accuracy leads to appropriate interventions and better use of available services,

Table 57.1

Environments for Older Persans[a]

Family home
Retirement community
Continuing-care retirement community
Congregate housing
Adult day care
Adult foster care
Assisted living facility
Special care unit
Nursing home

[a]As one moves down the list, the preference for the lifestyle tends to decline while the availability of and ease of access to services increases.

resulting in improved level of function and optimal placement. In particular, it is important to *target assessment to persons most likely to benefit*, especially those who are frail or at a critical transition point in long-term care. In addition, it is essential to *link assessment with care management and follow-up services* to implement the recommendations. Geriatric assessment is thus part of the *process* of case management, including referral, collection of information, assessment, and development and implementation of a care plan, with periodic reassessment and modification.

A recent meta-analysis of comprehensive geriatric assessment found that both home assessment of community-residing elderly and home assessment of those recently discharged from hospital resulted in significantly greater likelihood that they would remain at home compared with controls (3). A 3-year randomized controlled trial of in-home comprehensive geriatric assessment and prevention education for community-dwelling elderly over age 75 resulted in improved function and reduced chronic nursing home placement in the intervention group (4).

HOME CARE

Home is the setting preferred by most elderly for receiving care. Home care is the provision of equipment and/or services to functionally impaired, disabled, or ill persons in the home. It thus includes health services such as physician house calls, visiting nurses, and other skilled care and social support services such as home-

making, chores, and meals. Home *health* care has been more narrowly defined as the provision of skilled health care services in the home, including medical care. Home health care may be a substitute for either acute hospital care or long-term institutional care, or it may reduce length of stay in either setting. Home health care may be a substitute for outpatient care for persons who are homebound or cannot be transported and may be preventive, diagnostic, therapeutic, rehabilitative, and/or long-term maintenance care.

Functional disability appears to be the most important predictor of the use of home care. Other risk factors that are clearly important but have not been well studied include the availability of informal caregivers or alternative services such as day care or nursing home care and the ability to provide coordinated services (5).

Medicare has paid home health agencies on the basis of reasonable costs. However, after relatively modest growth in the 1980s, Medicare's expenditures for home health care increased rapidly in the 1990s, from $2.4 billion in 1989 to $17.7 billion in 1996 (6) because a larger number of Medicare beneficiaries used the home health benefit and more services were provided to each beneficiary. Increased use of the benefit appeared to be due to several factors: legislation and policy changes that liberalized coverage criteria; transformation of home health care from posthospital to long-term care; and decreased administrative control over the benefit. Plans to move the home health benefit from cost-based reimbursement to a prospective payment system are under consideration but are limited by difficulty in determining an appropriate unit of service.

Specific preventive and assessment programs in the home have been evaluated and demonstrated to be effective (3, 4). Disease prevention in the home includes the traditional medical interventions, home safety considerations, provision of assistive equipment, and attention to family relations, education, and counseling. In addition to assessment, diagnostic home visits can provide important information, and home visits by physicians and/or geriatric nurse specialists may result in identification of problems not detected by primary care physicians in office visits, most often in the areas of psychobehavioral difficulties, safety, caregiver issues, and even new medical problems (7). In particular, a stepwise diagnostic approach is often suitable for a controlled, supportive home environment.

Less is understood about the usefulness of therapeutic and rehabilitative medical care in the home. Sophisticated equipment designed and produced for home use is widely available, including intravenous products and ventilators. In most communities, skilled therapy can be provided, including nursing, physical, occupational and speech therapy, respiratory therapy, counseling, and many others. Many of these interventions should be further evaluated.

Little is known about the efficacy of long-term home medical care, potentially the most important to the frail elderly (8). The strongest predictors for its use are being homebound, needing help with one or more ADLs, being dependent in functional health areas, scoring increased errors on mental status, and having no involvement with social groups (9). The role of physicians in home care is variable and inconsistent, but it includes communication with health care providers, patients and families, authorization of services, and even house calls. The outcomes and costs of physician home visits, as well as how to target services, have not been adequately evaluated. An American Medical Association panel on home care (10) noted several barriers that discourage physician house calls, including poor reimbursement, inefficiency, medical liability issues, and resource limitations. Two physician surveys (11, 12) confirmed the significance of these factors in reducing the likelihood of physician care in the home. Nevertheless, medical and supportive care for chronically ill and functionally disabled patients can be provided in the home as an alternative to long-term institutional care.

The cost-effectiveness of home care in general remains controversial. Provision of comprehensive home care to frail but otherwise unselected elderly apparently does not significantly improve quality of life and rarely decreases costs; thus, current programs serving untargeted populations are unlikely ever to be cost effective. Limitation of services also has the potential to decrease costs, but research regarding the effec-

tiveness of different types of home care is scarce, and as one moves from general home care to specific home health care to home medical care, less information is available. Accumulating evidence supports the utility of providing specific, necessary services in the home to carefully targeted recipients, in a manner similar to the provision of other health care interventions. The difficulty with home care, as with many other services, is the inability to distinguish needs from wants. Conversely, once the commitment is made to supply care in the home, providers must be able to furnish a well-managed, coordinated system of services that minimizes risk and maximizes function.

One critical review surveyed 12 experimental or quasi-experimental studies of home care and found no evidence of a consistent effect on mortality, hospitalization, physical function, or nursing home placement (13). Another review evaluated 16 waiver-financed demonstration projects serving more than 6000 high-risk elderly that substituted comprehensive case management and increased community home services for nursing home care (14). Overall, many of these programs improved quality of life by reducing unmet needs and increasing confidence in receipt of care and satisfaction with life. Although the programs marginally reduced nursing home and hospital costs, overall costs were increased by additional case management and community services. Most subjects, in fact, were not actually at high risk for nursing home placement. One program did, however, reduce costs by targeting only very disabled elderly who had been identified by a state nursing home admission screen (14).

A comprehensive case-managed home care program for 197 elderly who were eligible for admission to a skilled nursing home resulted in increased hospital admissions and Medicare costs, decreased nursing home admissions and Medicaid costs, and decreased overall costs (15). A randomized controlled study of a Department of Veterans Affairs (VA) hospital-based home care (HBHC) program for those with two or more ADL impairments or terminal illness found that although functional status did not improve, both in-hospital and net per person health costs were significantly lower in the HBHC patients, primarily because of fewer acute-care admissions (16). The cost of home care increases markedly with impairment. Since institutional care costs increase only marginally with level of impairment, the result is a break-even point in home care, with home care for the very impaired being considerably more expensive than institutional care. This creates an interesting dilemma, since the level of impairment is frequently used to determine eligibility for home care (17). Therefore, the provision of a broad range of home care services to an unselected population of disabled elders is not likely to reduce costs or to improve quality of life significantly. Targeting of services to a better-selected population at risk is more likely to be efficacious, and provision of more specific services by health care professionals to a carefully targeted population seems even more likely to be beneficial. In particular, the role of physicians in home care should be better understood and, if desirable, should be encouraged.

HOSPICE CARE

In the United States in 1996 an estimated 554,740 deaths were due to cancer (18), an increase of nearly 20% in the previous decade; this number will continue to increase with the aging of the population. Hospice is a palliative and supportive home care system for coordinating the care of these patients at the end of life. Hospice care, provided by a diverse team of professionals, is focused on broad elements of health (physical, mental, social, and spiritual), and offers assistance over longer periods than other Medicare-funded interventions. The goal of care is to support the quality of life of patient and family while eventually accepting a comfortable death at home. The increasing participation of physicians in hospice care requires the acquisition of specific knowledge and skills needed for good care of the dying patient.

Early hospice care arose as a movement to improve the care of the dying through simple palliative and supportive services. Hospice programs tended to reject the technologic and institutional approach that was then prevalent in care of the dying while articulating goals of peace, comfort, and dignity and often depending on philanthropic support and largely volunteer staff. A major development in the provision of hospice services was the authorization of Medicare reimbursement, heavily influenced by the National Hospice Study. From the efforts of participants in this study and the fledgling National Hospice Organization (NHO), the definition of hospice and the structure of hospice services emerged (19). Under Medicare, hospice was funded as a capitated system, with the basic payment for care set by statute (most recently, $90.40 per day in Florida), and the basic outline of the hospice services required set by federal and state guidelines. In 1994, Medicare was the primary payment source for two thirds of hospice patients, and other payers often use Medicare guidelines to set fees and services. Since costs of hospice paid by Medicare recently exceeded $1 billion, it has attracted the attention of those responsible for limiting costs in the overall effort to reduce Medicare expenditures.

Medicare hospice coverage provides supportive care and financial benefits not available in other programs. Home care services do not have to be skilled. No copayments are required, and drugs related to the terminal illness are funded by Medicare. Hospice care is strongly interdisciplinary, with required involvement by nursing and medicine, social service providers, clergy, and volunteers. Only one third of hospice staff are skilled nursing personnel; about 15% are counselors or social workers; and nearly one fourth are home health aides and homemakers who provide services to lessen the family's burden of personal care (20).

The dominant site of hospice care is the home. In fiscal year 1993, 87% of hospice expenditures were for routine home care days, with only 11% of expenditures for inpatient days, suggesting that fewer than 1 day in 20 under hospice care is spent in hospital. Another major difference between hospice and conventional care is the timing of services: hospice care expenditures tend to be relatively level in the last 6 months of life, with providers in the home throughout the terminal period offering supportive services. In contrast, conventional care expenditures are generally lower in periods beyond 3 months prior to death, with dramatic escalation in the last month or two of life because of increased hospital use (21).

The advantages of the hospice benefit in terms of cost to the patient and quantity and diversity of home care provided make it important to refer patients in a timely manner. The most common obstacle to early referral by the physician is the difficulty in determining life expectancy in cancer and other chronic diseases until very near the time of death. All hospice programs have substantial numbers of patients who are not referred until the last week or two of life. Table 57.2 presents the NHO's suggested general criteria for referral to hospice. The NHO recommends that the decision to refer for hospice care and the decision to invoke the Medicare hospice benefit be separated both conceptually and clinically. The Medicare benefit is appropriate when anticipated survival is 6 months or less and when the patient and family agree to a palliative approach to care with a comfortable death as an acceptable outcome.

Although cancer is the most frequent referring diagnosis for hospice care, patients with other diagnoses who meet the criteria of life expectancy and philosophy are also eligible. Terminal patients with far advanced heart, kidney, liver, lung, and neurologic disease are eligible for care, and they constitute an increasing proportion of hospice referrals. The great difficulty in determining prognosis for these diseases has resulted in the development of guidelines for hospice referral (Table 57.3), an attempt to develop some consistency within the hospice industry in standards for hospice eligibility. They also seek to resolve tension between the hospice providers and federal regulators, who have recently begun to challenge admissions and in some cases demand large repayments from hospice organizations for unauthorized care.

Table 57.2

National Hospice Organization General Criteria for Hospice Care

1. Life-limiting condition known to patient and family
2. Selection of treatment goals directed at relief of symptoms
3. Either of the following:
   Clinical progression of disease (disease specific, multiple hospitalizations, or functional decline)
   Severe nutritional impairment related to the disease

ADULT DAY HEALTH CARE

Adult day health care is designed to meet the needs of functionally impaired adults in a community setting, with group interaction and planned programs that are not usually available in the home. Adult day health care centers (ADHCs) provide nursing, social, and a combination of other services, which may include rehabilitation; health maintenance; functional, social, and recreational activities; and a hot meal. The number of ADHCs has increased significantly over the past 20 years, and this growth is expected to continue. Programs vary significantly in the types of services provided, objectives, staffing, characteristics of clients, and cost of care. Many programs are underfunded and underused (22).

ADHCs may be hospital- or nursing-home based or freestanding, are usually nonprofit, and are often subsidized by public or philanthropic funds. Currently no Medicare coverage is available for ADHCs, and Medicaid funding varies by state; some states have none. These centers can offer substantial help to caregivers who wish to maintain a frail older person at home but need relief from the continuous responsibility of care. Clients may attend 1 to 5 days a week; special transportation may be provided within a limited geographic area but is often expensive and requires special equipment. Programs for the day care of persons with dementia are available in many communities; these may provide valuable respite for families and enable such impaired elderly to remain at home.

The VA conducted a large, multicenter randomized controlled trial to determine the effectiveness of its ADHC programs (23). Patients who were offered VA's ADHC services in the first phase of the study had significantly higher average VA health care costs than patients assigned to customary care, with no apparent incremental health benefit to themselves or their caregivers. Whether the results of this VA study are applicable to community ADHCs is not clear but should be evaluated.

In contrast, San Francisco's On Lok program is a successful working model of capitated, risk-based acute and long-term community care of vulnerable elderly with a strong emphasis on

Table 57.3

NHO Guidelines for Prognosis in Chronic Diseases

Condition	Criteria
Heart disease	NYHA IV, EF < 20%, refractory to optimal treatment
Pulmonary disease	Disabling dyspnea, FEV_1 < 30%, frequent emergencies, cor pulmonale, hypoxemia on O_2, hypercapnia
Dementia	Bed or chair bound, ADL dependent, incontinent, unable to communicate, severe medical comorbidity, nutritional compromise
Stroke	Acute phase beyond 3 days: coma, abnormal brainstem response, no verbal response, no withdrawal to pain; dysphagia precluding nutrition when artificial feedings refused; poststroke dementia, Karnofsky score < 50%, nutritional compromise; recurrent aspiration pneumonia, urinary infection, sepsis, decubiti
Renal disease	Meet criteria for transplant or dialysis but refuse; CrCl < 15 mL/min; serum creatinine > 8 mg/dL (6 mg/dL for diabetics)
Liver disease	Not considered for transplant, albumin < 2.5, prothrombin time > 5 sec over control, recurrent variceal bleeding, cachexia, alcohol use; at least one of these: refractory ascites, SBP, hepatorenal syndrome, hepatic encephalopathy, coma

Adapted from Stuart B, Alexander C, Arenella C, et al. Medical Guidelines for Determining Prognosis in Selected Non-Cancer Disease. 2nd ed. Arlington, VA: National Hospice Organization, 1996.
NYHA IV, New York Heart Association category IV; EF, ejection fraction; FEV_1, forced expiratory volume in 1 second; CrCl, creatinine clearance; SBP, spontaneous bacterial peritonitis.

ADHC. The national demonstration Program of All-Inclusive Care for the Elderly (PACE), which is modeled after the innovative On Lok program, consists of the following elements:

1. Nursing home-eligible clients who choose to receive services in the community
2. Integrated funding by capitated Medicare and Medicaid payments, with providers at financial risk
3. Integrated service delivery through ADHCs
4. Case management by multidisciplinary teams

PACE was originally replicated at seven sites from 1987 to 1992; another generation of replications has now developed from the original sites, for a total of 16 sites. Evaluation of the PACE sites has found considerable variation among them, including capitation rates (24). Enrollment has been slower than expected, and all sites have excluded some persons eligible for nursing home placement, suggesting that selective enrollment has occurred. The most important barriers to enrollment are required attendance at ADHCs, financial limitations, and loss of freedom of choice. As sites matured, they have typically become more flexi-

ble in their care plans and have accepted more frail elders.

RESPITE CARE

Respite services provide temporary relief for caregivers, often in an institution, and thus support maintenance of frail elderly in the community. Short stays (usually up to several weeks) in nursing homes provide opportunities for family vacations, trips, and even elective health care procedures or hospitalizations. The VA has urged the development of inpatient respite care programs at its medical centers. In the community Medicaid may provide coverage to eligible persons, and some states have subsidized respite programs. However, the cost of this care, equivalent to nursing home care, is usually the responsibility of the family.

In addition to respite care, some skilled nursing facilities allow short-term admissions for geriatric assessment and rehabilitation, which may improve the elderly person's function and potential for remaining in the community. If this is posthospital care, it may be paid for by Medicare; otherwise, funding is not usually available except in VA medical centers that offer this service.

RESIDENTIAL CARE

Nearly 1.5 million older persons reside in housing that offers additional services in a home-like environment, loosely termed residential care. This sector of the long-term care market is expanding dramatically, driven by various initiatives to reduce nursing home care, the growth of the older population, the diminishing ratio of elderly to community support, and the increasing acceptance by older people of the benefit of such facilities in providing comfort and security with advancing age and disability.

Residential care facilities include a wide range of living environments and support services described by terms such as assisted living facilities, board and care homes, adult foster care, sheltered housing, and congregate housing. The great diversity in designation, regulation, and services from state to state and the lack of uniformity of the models within each group and state lead to difficulty in describing such facilities. Table 57.1 lists common choices available, in increasing order of service availability and amenities. Table 57.4 provides a list of important considerations in choosing a residential setting. The physician should help by identifying present and probable care needs for the next few years to facilitate appropriate matches between facilities and persons.

CONGREGATE HOUSING AND CONTINUING CARE RETIREMENT COMMUNITIES

Neither age-segregated retirement communities nor continuing-care retirement communities (CCRCs) are residential care facilities, but for older persons developing disability, both may offer better access to services than do family homes. Congregate housing is a term for complexes of apartments or homes for a target population (often the disabled or elderly) that often have some additional services. The CCRC is a community offering several levels of care, usually independent living, assisted living, and nursing home care, and with staff and services to support residents through the continuum of sickness and disability. Such facilities often require a sizable entry fee and a monthly maintenance fee, but more are developing as rentals for a straight monthly

Table 57.4

Considerations for Residential Care

Lifestyle
  Attractiveness of environment
  Activities
  Operator-client relations
  Client-client relations
  Meal service
  Client mix (disability level, types)
Physical health support
  Supervision of health care
  Medication administration
  Monitoring (e.g., glucose, blood pressure)
  Availability and training of staff
  On-site health services (physician, nursing)
  Special diets
  Injections
Mental health support
  Level of supervision
  Escape and injury prevention
  Appropriate activities
Functional support
  Housekeeping, laundry
  Transportation
  Personal care assistance (grooming)

fee. Some CCRCs are life-care, which means that after the entry fee and monthly maintenance fee are paid, all necessary services will be provided; this component of the market is shrinking. Most CCRC contracts offer improved access to and financial support for higher levels of service, but each contract must be read carefully with regard to what services will actually be provided and how much financial liability is incurred by the person when assisted living or nursing home care becomes necessary.

CCRCs offer some security that if additional services are needed, they will be available on site. Couples can thus more easily remain together if one person needs additional care that cannot be provided in the home. The higher concentration of older persons may facilitate development of on-site medical and nursing programs for common needs. CCRCs are also an attractive lifestyle choice for some independent older persons, who enjoy the social opportunities of congregate dining and the community activities designed for their age group and interests. CCRCs vary considerably in tolerance for disability within the independent living portion of the facility, attempting to balance the needs of the person with the service capacity of the program and the preferences of the healthier residents for a highly functioning peer group.

ADULT FOSTER CARE

This term is used for small, family-owned group homes that provide room and board with variable levels of personal care and oversight to a few clients unable to care for themselves. More than 60,000 of these are licensed nationwide; some are unlicensed. Most depend on public funds, often state or county welfare payments. The small size of these programs makes visibility low, and locating a bed for an interested patient can be difficult. Limited information on the quality of care suggests that satisfaction of families is high in adult foster care, and for a segment of the population, it provides an effective alternative to nursing home placement (25).

ASSISTED-LIVING FACILITIES

Assisted-living facilities (ALFs) combine the access to services and supervision of the nursing home with the personal control over schedule and space that is usually associated with living at home (26). Consumer preferences and lower costs have led to rapid growth of this segment of the residential care market; it is projected that the number of ALF beds will exceed the number of nursing home beds by 2005.

Services usually include housing, meals, 24-hour emergency monitoring, supervision of medications, socialization with peers, and limited assistance with ADLs. Continence care, more extensive assistance with ADLs, and an environment designed for care of persons with dementia are sometimes also available. Individual states may have several categories of licensure within the ALF designation, requiring different levels of service and permitting varying types of clients. There is no Medicare coverage for ALF care, and Medicaid funding levels are generally low, limiting choices for these clients.

Within a licensing designation, each facility has considerable latitude in program design and choice of clients. State regulations may deter-

mine acceptable clients; in Florida, for example, sufficient independent mobility to evacuate the building in case of fire is a requirement, and inability to maintain continence is considered an indication of need for a higher level of care.

Special care units licensed as ALFs, particularly for Alzheimer's disease and related disorders, are becoming more widely available. These units combine environmental design to maximize freedom and independence with programs specific to the interest and needs of their clients. ALF licensure, staffing, and regulatory requirements are considerably less strict and therefore less expensive than those of nursing homes. The advantage to clients and families is that more money is available to pay for programs and amenities; a concern, however, is the potential for less sophisticated care that results from fewer trained staff and less stringent regulatory requirements. In addition, the needs of residents may exceed the services available, necessitating transfer to a nursing home.

ADVICE TO PATIENTS AND FAMILIES

Awareness of local residential care opportunities and the regulations that affect their ability to care for clients is necessary for advising choice of facility. Physicians can provide unique information on the current and anticipated requirements for medical and nursing services, the course and stability of known chronic diseases, and the identification of special medical needs that must be met for successful care. The goal is to match the finances, preferred lifestyle, and individual requirements, with all important needs met. Some states require a medical evaluation for admission to ALF or adult foster care, which may seek the physician's opinion on the appropriateness of placement and may offer criteria for appropriateness. Patients and families should be encouraged to read the contracts for care with diligence, as staff and marketing materials may well suggest more care than the contract will actually provide. One useful exercise may be to consider the financial implications if one member of a couple needs nursing home care. Identification of services that will be provided by the facility and those that are covered by Medicare can result in better understanding of what is being purchased.

PUBLIC POLICY ISSUES

Unfortunately, studies of community-based long-term care programs have generally failed to demonstrate an effect on mortality, likelihood of nursing home admission, or functional status; such programs also appear to increase use of inpatient and outpatient services and health care costs. For example, an analysis of 32 experimental or quasi-experimental studies of adult day health care, with or without home care, for the provision of community-based long-term care, showed that results varied little despite differences in populations, services, locations, and other factors (27). In nearly all studies that were reviewed, these community-based long-term care programs did not provide a survival benefit or slow the rate of functional deterioration, and costs were actually increased. Satisfaction was improved only in the short term, and most subjects, in retrospect, were not really at risk for nursing home placement, as control group placement rates were low. These findings may result from failure to target the elderly most at risk for nursing home admission, such as those with increased age, dementia, dependency in ADLs, lack of spouse or child, female sex, and poverty. Targeting may improve outcomes, but it requires efforts to improve prediction of risk. To be cost-effective, these programs must aggressively control expenditures, limit services, and constantly focus on avoiding hospitalization.

Although the cost-effectiveness of community-based long-term care has not been established, it is clear that the alternative to such programs, i.e., institutional care for all frail and dependent elderly, is neither feasible, desirable, nor affordable. In the United States the lack of an organized health care system has resulted in a fragmented Band-Aid approach to care of the vulnerable elderly. If instead there were a comprehensive continuum of resources providing services at many levels of care, such services could be targeted to the specific needs of certain elderly as identified by geriatric assessment. Decisions to move from one level of care to another would be determined by the needs of the person.

A comprehensive financial support system that funds flexible and varied programs is essential, since financing for only one or two types of services will result in inappropriate referral to and overuse of these funded programs, as has been the case in the past. Managed-care programs, especially capitated ones, clearly have both the incentive to reduce costs and the flexibility to purchase services that meet individual needs. Such programs for the elderly, especially if they combine Medicare and Medicaid funds, may be able to provide an improved continuum of community-based long-term care in the future.

Adequate reimbursement for physician care in the community must also be provided, and it should take into account the complexity and time-consuming nature of such care. Physicians must increase their involvement in community-based care and their familiarity with services available in their own vicinity to provide the most appropriate care for their patients. Failure to make appropriate referrals may result in inadequate access to services and in unnecessary institutional care. Established relationships with visiting nurses, social service agencies, and case manager services simplify the provision of information and coordination of care for the frail and dependent elderly and help to maintain their quality of life as long as possible.

REFERENCES

1. Feasley J, ed. Institute of Medicine. Best at Home: Assuring Quality Long-Term Care in Home and Community-Based Settings. Washington: National Academy Press, 1996.
2. National Institutes of Health Consensus Development Conference Statement: geriatric assessment methods for clinical decision-making. J Am Geriatr Soc 1988;36: 342–347.
3. Stuck A, Siu AL, Wieland GD, et al. Comprehensive geriatric assessment: a meta-analysis of controlled trials. Lancet 1993;342:1032–1036.
4. Stuck A, Aronow HU, Steiner A, et al. A trial of annual in-home comprehensive geriatric assessments for elderly people living in the community. N Engl J Med 1995;333:1184–1189.
5. Chappell N. Home care research: what does it tell us? Gerontologist 1994;34:116–120.
6. Scanlon WJ. Home Health Cost Growth and Administration's Proposal for Prospective Payment (GAO/T-HEHS-97–92). Washington: General Accounting Office, 1997.

7. Ramsdell JW, Swart JA, Jackson JE, Renvall M. The yield of a home visit in the assessment of geriatric patients. J Am Geriatr Soc 1989;37:17–24.

8. AMA Council on Scientific Affairs. Home care in the 1990s. JAMA 1990;263:1241–1244.

9. Branch LG, Wetle TT, Scherr PA, et al. A prospective study of incident comprehensive medical home care use among the elderly. Am J Public Health 1988;78:255–259.

10. AMA Council on Scientific Affairs. Educating physicians in home health care. JAMA 1991;265:769–771.

11. Boling PA, Retchin SM, Ellis J, et al. The influence of physician specialty on house calls. Arch Intern Med 1990;150:2333–2337.

12. Keenan JM, Boling PA, Schwartzberg JG, et al. A national survey of the home visiting practice and attitudes of family physicians and internists. Arch Intern Med 1992; 152:2025–2032.

13. Hedrick S, Inui T. The effectiveness and cost of home care: an information synthesis. Health Serv Res 1986; 20:851–880.

14. Kemper P. The evaluation of the National Long Term Care Demonstration: 10. Overview of the findings. Health Serv Res 1988:23:161–174.

15. Steel K. Home care for the elderly: the new institution. Arch Intern Med 1991;151:439–442.

16. Cummings JE, Hughes SL, Weaver FM, et al. Cost-effectiveness of Veterans Administration hospital-based home care. Arch Intern Med 1990;150:1274–1280.

17. Blazer D. Home health care: house calls revisited. Am J Public Health 1988;78:238–239.

18. Parker SL, Tong T, Bolden S, Wingo PA. Cancer statistics, 1996. CA Cancer J Clin 1996;46:5–27.

19. McCann BA. Forward. In: Mor V, Greer DS, Kastenbaum R, eds. The Hospice Experiment. Baltimore: Johns Hopkins University Press, 1988.

20. Hospice Facts and Statistics. Washington: Hospice Association of America, January 1995.

21. An Analysis of the Cost Savings of the Medicare Hospice Benefit. Arlington, VA: National Hospice Organization, 1995.

22. Conrad KJ, Hanrahan P, Hughes SL. Survey of adult day care in the United States: national and regional findings. Res Aging 1990;12:36–56.

23. Hedrick SC, Rothman ML, Chapko M, et al. Summary and discussion of methods and results of the Adult Day Health Care Evaluation Study. Med Care 1993;31: SS94–SS103.

24. Branch LG, Coulam RF, Zimmerman YA. The PACE evaluation: initial findings. Gerontologist 1995;35:349–359.

25. Oktay JS, Volland PJ. Foster home care for the elderly as an alternative to nursing home care: an experimental evaluation. Am J Public Health 1987;77:1505–1510.

26. Kane RA, Wilson KB. Assisted living in the United States: a new paradigm for residential care for frail older persons. Washington: American Association of Retired Persons, 1993.

27. Weissert WG, Hedrick SC. Lessons learned from research on effects of community-based long term care. J Am Geriatr Soc 1994;42:348–353.

Institutional Long-Term Care

Long-term care has been defined as "a set of health, personal care, and social services delivered over a sustained period of time to persons who have lost or never acquired some degree of functional capacity" (1). The components of the long-term care system may be grouped as home based, community based, institutional, or mixed.

Many physicians have disdained institutional long-term care and have struggled to define a meaningful medical role in residential care for those with major chronic conditions. Reality contradicts such limited, largely negative impressions. Instead—in an era of an aging American population and major changes in the health care system—institutional long-term care is evolving into a dynamic, diverse component of a revamped approach to personal and health care service delivery.

The objectives of this chapter are to explain the current and future roles of long-term care, discuss the similarities and differences among its various settings and populations, and consider the roles of attending physicians and medical directors in such settings.

THE POPULATION WITH CHRONIC ILLNESSES AND DISABILITIES

The scope of the population served in long-term care has expanded greatly. More elderly persons require or desire some assistance with various aspects of their lives. Also, more persons of all ages require some short- or intermediate-term care after acute episodes of illness or injury. All persons have an identifiable foundation based on three major dimensions: physical, functional, and psychosocial (Table 58.1). The foundation may be impaired because of combinations of developmental, acute or chronic medical, or other problems.

For instance, heart failure may contribute to physical decline and lead to impaired mobility and self-care deficit, which results in difficulty obtaining food, undernutrition or dehydration leading to pneumonia, hospitalization, cognitive impairment, and further functional decline. Or significant cognitive impairment due to cerebrovascular disease may result in self-neglect, leading to worsening of diabetes, increased debility, and social withdrawal.

The scope of support required for those with significant deficits depends on the severity and scope of those deficits and the reversibility of underlying causes. Limited deficits and those due to treatable causes may require limited services. Substantial or long-lasting deficits may require comprehensive support and services delivered periodically or continuously. Table 58.2 summarizes the levels of care for those with chronic illnesses and disabilities. In addition to the many independent persons, the community-based population includes and formal residential long-term care such as assisted living tends to serve predominantly level 1 or 2 persons, while nursing facilities tend to have mostly level 3 and some level 2 persons.

RISK FACTORS FOR INSTITUTIONALIZATION

Much long-term care is given informally by friends and family in the community. However, informal caregivers may reach their limits for various reasons. Factors associated with institution-

Table 58.1

The Three Dimensions of All Human Beings

Dimension	Examples	Examples of Disruptions
Physical	Adequate cellular metabolism; appropriate function of vital organs; fluid, electrolyte, and acid-base balance; structural integrity of musculoskeletal system	Heart failure; stroke; dehydration; fractured hip Frailty resulting from aging and illness
Functional	Ability to perform essential ADLs such as bathing, waste elimination, and eating to maintain adequate physical and social functioning	Inability to eat due to stroke Self-care deficits due to Alzheimer's disease General weakness and dysfunction due to recent major acute medical illness Impaired mobility due to hip fracture
Psychosocial	Capacity to have satisfying personal life experiences Ability to maintain behaviors within socially acceptable boundaries Ability to relate to others in mutually beneficial ways	Physically violent or aggressive behavior due to multiinfarct dementia Difficulty relating to others due to personality disorder Social withdrawal due to depression

alization, including physical, functional, and psychosocial elements, have been identified (Table 58.3). Numerous initiatives have tried to prevent or postpone institutionalization. They include support for home-based activities of daily living (ADLs) and instrumental ADLs (IADLs), aggressive management of chronic disease, home-based health care, comprehensive geriatric assessment while hospitalized, aggressive rehabilitation after acute illness, and broadening of available community-based care and treatment options. There is some evidence to support the value of several of these approaches, although none of them has been consistently validated.

LONG-TERM CARE ENVIRONMENT

Despite the shifts in service sites and approaches to care for impaired elderly, the nursing facility remains the primary site for delivering *institutional* long-term care. Residential facilities emphasize protected living arrangements and minimal to moderate assistance with psychosocial, activity, and personal care needs, and chronic hospitals and subacute care units focus on managing medical problems. Home-based long-term care still is limited by issues of cost and

coordination that may make it unsuitable for many of those with complex needs. Nursing facility care brings together a broad spectrum of increasingly sophisticated and varied around-the-clock personal and health care services.

The term nursing home is still used to refer to the residential side of care received in these settings, but nursing facility is used more often to refer to long-term care facilities meeting eligibility requirements for Medicaid reimbursement that provide long-term care. Under the federal Omnibus Budget Reconciliation Act of 1987 (OBRA '87) regulations, the designation nursing facility replaced former designations of intermediate care facilities and skilled nursing facilities (SNFs). SNF refers to the Medicare skilled facility, emphasizing short-term intensive nursing and medical care after an acute medical illness, usually post hospitalization.

Most nursing facilities offer combinations of personal care, medical, restorative and rehabilitative services, including around-the-clock nursing care, to a mixture of frail impaired elderly and some younger chronically ill and impaired persons. Specialized programs or services may include adult day care, formal dementia units, geri-

Table 58.2

Levels of Care and Service Needs in Those With Chronic Illness and Disability

	Independent	Low CID (Level 1)	Moderate CID (Level 2)	High CID (Level 3)
Health and wellness	Minimal or no active chronic disease Low risk for acute illness or exacerbation of chronic disease Person can recognize and act on risks to life, safety Health care is incidental part of person's life	Minor chronic illnesses or disabilities Low to moderate risk of acute illness or exacerbation of chronic disease Can usually recognize risks to life, safety, but may need help with appropriate action Requires no more than occasional (significantly less than monthly) health care assessments or interventions	Chronic illness or disability causing moderate physical or functional impairments Moderate risk of acute illness or exacerbation of chronic disease Condition changes may require prompt evaluation and intervention Person may not recognize risks to life, safety or health, or be able to obtain appropriate intervention May need regular health care evaluations or interventions	One or more active chronic diseases have caused major functional impairment or require substantial ongoing care and treatment High risk of acute illness or exacerbation of chronic disease Condition changes often require prompt evaluation and active intervention Person may not recognize risks to life, safety; cannot obtain appropriate interventions Health care is essential, regular part of life
Medications	Can take medicines in correct dosages and at correct time with little or no assistance	May require reminders, supervision of medication management	May require administration of medications with monitoring of effectiveness and side effects	May require administration of extensive medication regimen and extensive or frequent monitoring of effectiveness and side effects
Functional status	Little or no significant functional impairment No impairment requires more than occasional minimal support, oversight, intervention	Some ADL deficits, minimal overall disability Impairments may require occasional support or intervention	Impairments in ADLs causing moderate disability Impairments require regular support or intervention Functional impairments may minimally jeopardize patient's health or safety	Impairments in ADLs causing major disabilities Functional impairments may create high risk of health or safety complications

continued

Table 58.2 (continued)
Levels of Care and Service Needs in Those With Chronic Illness and Disability

	Independent	Low CID (Level 1)	Moderate CID (Level 2)	High CID (Level 3)
Psychosocial factors	Behavior is generally socially appropriate and personally adequate Can interpret and react adequately to the world despite any deficits Fluctuations in morale appropriate to situation Can make decisions about health and well-being consistent with history of judgment, education, etc.	May need occasional help to identify and modify behaviors May need occasional help to interpret events and react appropriately to others Emotions and mood occasionally disruptive enough to require minor interventions May need support for decision making about health and well-being but can participate substantially May require help or occasional supervision to function safely	Cognitive-behavioral deficits may affect ADLs more than occasionally, requiring skilled support May be unable to identify and modify inappropriate behaviors May be unable to interpret events and react appropriately to others May need substantial support for decision making about health and well-being or may be unable to participate May require regular help or supervision to function safely	May be unable to identify or modify socially unacceptable behaviors Cognitive-behavioral deficits may regularly or continuously affect ADLs, require substantial skilled support May require extensive supervision for socialization May have frequent fluctuations in mood and emotions requiring complex intervention, support, or evaluation May be unable to participate in decision making related to health and well-being
Social relationships	Social relationships are adequate for person's purposes	May have occasional difficulties in appropriate socialization, which may require support or guidance	May require considerable support and supervision for appropriate socialization	May require extensive supervision for appropriate socialization

CID = chronic illness and disability.

Table 58.3

Factors Associated With Risk of Institutionalization[a]

Use of walking aids
Cognitive deficits
Living alone or with unrelated persons
Lack of social supports
ADL problems, personal care dependency
Poverty
Respiratory or nervous system disorders in men
Musculoskeletal disease in women
Female gender
Poor self-rated health status
IADL limitations
Deficiencies in informal health network

Adapted from Kane RA, Kane RL. Long-Term Care: Principles, Programs, and Policies. New York: Springer, 1987.
[a]Based on review of multiple research studies.

atric assessment, geropsychiatric services, hospice care, pastoral care, postacute care, respite care (short-term stays), and social services.

Primarily because of the high cost of inpatient acute hospital care, hospital stays have been progressively shortened. Many acutely ill persons receive some or all of their medical care outside of a hospital. Nursing facilities and skilled nursing units in various settings now play key roles in providing such care, either after or instead of hospitalization. Other forms of long-term care that provide primarily medical services for persons with chronic functional impairments include chronic disease (long-term) hospitals and freestanding or hospital-based subacute care programs.

Chronic disease (long-term) hospitals care for a mixture of elderly and younger persons needing acute, postacute, and long-term intensive medical and nursing services, ongoing assessments, or specialty services such as chronic ventilator care. Compared with the nursing facility population, the long-term hospital population is typically younger on average, includes more men, and has a greater proportion of trauma and psychiatric illness complicated by medical illness. Few more than 100 long-term hospitals exist in the United States, including for-profit, not-for-profit, and governmental facilities.

Subacute care programs have emerged in the past few years to provide short- to intermediate-term postacute hospital care such as postoperative care, ongoing treatment of the later stages of acute medical illnesses, rehabilitation, and intravenous therapies. Most of these are subunits of SNFs or hospital-based rather than stand-alone facilities. They are licensed at the acute, specialty hospital, or skilled level. Some function primarily as inpatient rehabilitation units, offering intensive short- or intermediate-term goal-oriented rehabilitation services, while others combine medical and rehabilitative services. Subacute populations considerably overlap those in long-term hospitals and inpatient rehabilitation units (2).

Settings and Levels of Care

It is essential to shift the regulatory and reimbursement emphasis from settings to levels of care. Previously, sites and care levels were tightly linked; for instance, hospitals cared for those with acute illnesses and subacute changes, and nursing facilities cared for the elderly with major functional impairments due to chronic conditions but usually did not treat related acute medical conditions. Assisted living began primarily as a residential program for the minimally impaired who needed or desired some assistance with personal care and IADLs (e.g., shopping, cooking, cleaning). People needing care have been transferred readily among these and other sites, and providers have developed comfortable, predictable niches.

However, this approach has been found to be both costly and substantially in conflict with care continuity. In a major transition, the many health and personal care services are available in various settings instead of a few specialized settings. Distinctions among sites are increasingly blurred. Those needing a given level of care may choose from among several sites, and the same site may provide several levels of care.

Many frail and chronically impaired persons, including long-term facility residents, with shifting needs have been receiving a broader spectrum of services at the same site instead of being transferred to other sites for components of their care. More organizations are also combining residential housing, assisted living, and nursing facilities either on the same campus (e.g., continuing care retirement communities), or within the same network to offer a coordinated approach to persons' changing conditions. In addition to physicians, other trained persons are sharing responsibilities for managing both the causes and the consequences of medical illness, including major functional and psychosocial effects.

As a result of these and other changes, nursing facilities have a growing role as geriatric medical centers, providing care not only to their own residents but also for those living elsewhere who need a combination of health and personal care outside the hospital. For instance, it should be feasible with appropriate reimbursement to place assisted-living residents and community-dwelling elderly with various complex or unstable chronic problems or comparatively uncomplicated acute illnesses, in an SNF to identify and manage the various causes (3). Eventually those persons would return to their former settings.

Similarly, many assisted-living settings have expanded their ability to provide functional and psychosocial support often and broadly enough to let the residents avoid or postpone nursing facility care. Some of them offer nursing and other skilled evaluations and treatments. While most assisted-living programs prefer to be viewed as residential rather than institutional, their populations increasingly share many of the characteristics and needs of nursing facility residents.

Consequences of Uncoupling Sites and Levels of Care

As sites and levels of care have become significantly unlinked, it is now more appropriate to view long-term care primarily from the perspective of levels of care and care processes rather than of programs and places. Institutional long-term care consists of a continuum of programs and services delivered across time and among several sites, mostly to elderly but also to some younger adults with significant chronic illnesses and behavioral, cognitive, and functional impairments. A given setting may provide care to a diverse population with a broad range of needs. Several settings may provide similar services to comparable populations. All of the care must be coordinated across these settings.

VARIOUS APPROACHES TO COMMON PROCESSES

Many approaches in various settings have been tried under various program titles to meet the needs of this population, e.g., hospice, palliative care, or terminal care programs for the dying; and dementia special care, closed, or Alzheimer's units for those with advanced dementia. Efforts to understand, regulate, and accredit these providers have taken various forms.

Providers throughout the long-term care continuum should recognize their similarities more than their differences. Closely scrutinizing these programs reveals substantial overlap in all of these settings. Their varying emphasis on different facets of care does not exempt them from identifying and addressing other pertinent conditions. Each program ultimately must ensure performance of the same care processes with a frequency, intensity, and complexity (Table 58.4) that varies with the individual's needs. The program names are less significant than the scope of their care processes and services. Understanding this should enable licensing, regulation, and reimbursement of providers based primarily on levels of care grounded in the needs of those served rather than on the provider's characteristics.

Ultimately providers will differentiate themselves according to their effectiveness and efficiency in assessing and meeting each person's needs. The optimal approach may be a la carte (combinations of services) or a program offering a package of services, such as subacute or nursing facility care. Each provider must be able to offer a broad spectrum of service combinations, associate with others who can supplement those services, or limit the scope of persons they serve. The repeated use of high-intensity, high-cost settings such as hospitals becomes less tolerable as it is recognized that many problems can be detected and prevented before becoming full-fledged medical crises.

For instance, demented persons on special units in assisted-living and long-term care facilities need functional and psychosocial support. But they may also have complications of their medical conditions or medications. Therefore, despite the emphasis on managing functional and psychosocial concerns, the specialized dementia provider

Table 58.4

Care Processes Across the Continuum

Process	Objectives	Key Questions
Assessment	Collect information to enable definition of patient's needs and problems	What must be evaluated to identify causes and define consequences of illness or situation?
Definition of problem	Define person's problems and needs so as to develop appropriate care plan	What are manifestations or consequences of situation?
Cause-and-effect analysis	Relate physical, functional, psychosocial causes of problems and consequences	What causes the situation? To what extent are causes correctable? How would addressing causes affect consequences?
Set care goals and objectives	Define purpose of giving care, criteria to determine when objectives have been met	What are overall goals? How do we know when goal is met? How will specific treatments and services help to reach goals?
Care planning	Create a plan to address problems, including responsibilities of various persons and disciplines, based on recognition of causes and consequences	What specific treatments and services will be rendered? How will we know treatments and services have reached their goals in relation to the overall goal? How will we know when enough specific treatments and services have been provided?
Management of known problems	Identify and implement appropriate treatments to address causes and consequences of problems and risks	What treatment changes are needed? Which treatments should be cause specific, which symptomatic or outcome related?
Management of new problems and complications	Identify and manage new problems and problems that are results of poor health	What new problems or diseases have arisen since admission? What are their causes? How and how urgently should they be managed?
Prevention of nosocomial and iatrogenic problems	Identify areas of high risk and problems that may arise from medications and treatments or from being in a health care facility; institute measures to prevent those problems or manage them if they occur	What are the significant risk factors for this person? What measures should be taken to try to reduce the risks? How can it be recognized when a risk factor becomes an actual problem?
Preparation for completion of treatment course	Identify discharge potential, point at which transfer elsewhere is feasible Plan for discharge and transfer by ensuring appropriate transfer site, follow-up of problems, communication with the patient, family, other caregivers	Who has discharge potential and to what degree? What is a realistic time frame? How to determine that someone is approaching readiness for discharge? What factors are impeding progress toward discharge?

Adapted from Levenson SA. Subacute and Transitional Care Handbook. St. Louis: Beverly-Cracom, 1996.

must also address the physical and medical issues appropriately and in a timely manner. In contrast to nursing facilities, which are expected to have on-site staff who can manage complex combinations of problems, assisted-living providers have the option to obtain such services through outside arrangements. However, if assisted-living providers accept persons with needs and problems comparable with those encountered in nursing facilities, they should expect to be held to the standard of either ensuring comparable care or fully disclosing their limitations.

It is also important to reconsider traditional reimbursement systems that emphasize places and programs over processes. For example, Medicare benefits focus primarily on *where* a person receives care (hospital, SNF, home care) and on specific treatments or services (e.g., hospice care, intravenous lines, suctioning) instead of considering the level of care. Thus, providers tend to emphasize placing people in covered settings and providing reimbursable services while having little incentive to seek less costly alternative settings or to focus on primary, secondary, or tertiary prevention. Several demonstration projects have attempted to show that more all-inclusive care is both beneficial and cost effective (4). Henceforth it is essential to focus reimbursement on the provision of services justified by the condition and needs of persons in any setting qualified to provide that service. An attempt to do this in SNFs through a shift to prospective payment is expected to expand by 1999.

ESSENTIAL PROVIDER CAPABILITIES

To care for persons with illness and disability in any part of the long-term care continuum, providers need specific capabilities to perform relevant care (Table 58.5). For instance, if someone is incapable of understanding and adhering to a complex medication regimen and cannot readily identify related side effects or complications, a provider must be able to administer medications, monitor their effect, and identify their undesirable side effects.

In an evolving care delivery system, sharp separation of the treatment of causes of problems from the management of their consequences is not feasible. Either alone or in combination with others, each provider must determine the optimal approach to both defining and managing a person's needs and problems. They may have to consider cost-effectiveness, the likely effects of proposed treatments on goals and problems, and consequences that are likely to remain after causes are treated. They may also be expected to identify strategies to reduce variation in the provision of care by different persons to those with comparable needs.

FACTORS IN APPROPRIATE CARE AND PLACEMENT

These conceptual shifts in care provision, defining roles of various providers, and methods for determining appropriate placement and reimbursement for care should help establish the foundation for a true care continuum. The settings for this continuum are by now well established, and their roles continue to evolve.

Physicians are vital to implementation of the aforementioned principles. While it is not based solely on medical factors, determining a person's specific need for institutional long-term care or another alternative requires identifying his or her needs and problems, determining an appropriate level of care, and then matching the person to providers. Neither diagnoses (the causes of their problems) nor consequences (such as behavioral or functional disturbances) alone can adequately define a person's needs or care. A sequential approach to making such determinations can be defined (2).

PHYSICIANS' ROLE IN INSTITUTIONAL LONG-TERM CARE

Physicians play an increasingly significant role in the care of institutionalized persons. Chronic and acute disease significantly affects these persons' quality of life, and functional decline attributed to aging is often actually due to treatable conditions (5). While by definition chronic disease cannot be cured, its effects can often be mitigated (6). Also, associated acute medical illnesses may be managed successfully, and undesirable physical and functional complications of acute and chronic illnesses and their treatments (so-called excess disability) may be prevented.

Table 58.5

Provider Capabilities at Various Levels of Care for Those With Chronic Illness and Disability

	Independent	Low CID (Level 1)	Moderate CID (Level 2)	High CID (Level 3)
Provider's capabilities	Facilitate access to appointments; diagnostic, related services; appropriate providers and practitioners	Facilitate, coordinate access to appointments; diagnostic, related services; appropriate providers and practitioners	Ensure access to appointments; diagnostic, related services; appropriate providers and practitioners	Ensure access to appointments; diagnostic, related services; appropriate providers and practitioners
	Address general risk factors for the population	Recognize and address risk factors specific to person	Recognize major functional, psychosocial risk factors, basic medical risk factors specific to person	Recognize, act on most major risk factors specific to person
	Provide occasional limited support, setup, reminders to help compensate for limited functional deficits, psychosocial problems	Identify scope of person's basic problems	Accurately describe, define scope of person's problems	Accurately describe, define scope, likely causes of person's problems in all dimensions
		Relate identified causes of person's functional, psychosocial problems, risks to their deficits where relevant to care	Provide support as needed for deficits in any early loss ADLs, deficits in late loss (eating and toileting) ADLs	Compensate as needed for any number of substantial functional deficits
		Provide occasional or regular support, setup, and reminders to help person compensate for deficits at least in early loss of ADLs (bathing, dressing, grooming, mobility)	Identify likely causes of functional, psychosocial problems, understand relation of medical causes to functional deficits	Provide interventions targeted to causes of problems and risks
				Regularly ensure direct or indirect access to necessary medications and treatments
				Manage complex behaviors of

continued

Table 58.5 (continued)

Provider Capabilities at Various Levels of Care for Those With Chronic Illness and Disability

Independent	Low CID (Level 1)	Moderate CID (Level 2)	High CID (Level 3)
	Facilitate and coordinate access to necessary medications and treatments	Ensure access to necessary medications and treatments	disruption or risk to self or others
	Ensure access to medications and treatments occasionally when person cannot readily get them	Manage periodic behaviors of disruption or risk to self or others	Monitor for active symptoms, condition changes, or significant risks that require skilled interpretation, prompt reporting to a health care practitioner, or other interventions
	Manage occasional uncomplicated behaviors of disruption or risk to self, others	Monitor mildly unstable behavior problem, follow up a medical problem	
	Observe situations not likely to require skilled interpretation or immediate interventions		
	Coordinate services as needed		

CID = chronic illness and disability.

Definable problems such as undernutrition, dehydration, electrolyte imbalance, skin breakdown, and depression occur among institutionalized elderly persons. They are often due to treatable medical causes and may be exacerbated by underlying chronic functional impairments. Also, about 1.5 million infections occur annually in nursing homes, accounting for 54% of the acute medical problems of nursing home residents, 48% of the hospitalizations, and 63% of deaths. Probably many hospital admissions from nursing facilities could be prevented (7). Thus, nursing facility residents need better and more frequent onsite medical attention than in the past.

Clinically, medical expertise centers on making correct diagnoses and choosing and implementing appropriate treatments. For instance, treating possibly reversible cognitive or behavioral disturbances requires expertise in diagnosis, testing, and prescribing and some knowledge of the neuropsychiatric basis of mental function and dysfunction. Or the physician must know that repeated falling may be due to the cumulative hypotensive effects of several medications. No matter where the person lives or is being treated, a repeat faller or high-risk person should be assessed for medical risks or causes unless there is explicit justification for not doing so.

Support from physicians is also needed in areas not directly related to disease management. Physicians make or influence most decisions concerning use of health care facilities and resources. They should be familiar with the services that they order, authorize, or arrange and with the options for programs, agencies, tests, treatments, orders, and care plans that may help accomplish desirable patient-specific goals at the lowest cost.

Consistent with the principle of maximizing independence and avoiding institutionalization whenever possible, the physician should carefully evaluate the need for institutionalization, counsel the family and patient, and suggest options to deliver care and support. For example, the physician can certify the need for therapies; certify and recertify the need for home, institutional, or other care; provide and interpret necessary and appropriate medical information; and provide periodic reports of the patient's medical status and prognosis.

The medical care should also relate to the broader context of the person's care, including the patient's and family's wishes and compliance with care standards (Table 58.6). For instance, decisions about the aggressiveness of managing heart disease in a nursing facility patient should be influenced by considering the potential benefits of improved endurance and the ability to participate in social and personal care activities, in addition to more traditional objective medical criteria such as fewer episodes of angina or improved ejection fraction. Therefore, quality medical care often means optimum, not maximum, medical intervention and treatment.

The primary care physician has an important role in ensuring that the participation and recommendations of medical specialists and of services such as home care or day care are coordinated with other general aspects of the person's medical care. For instance, a surgeon's decision to insert a gastrostomy tube should consider other determinations such as any significant comorbidities and whether such measures may enhance quality of life and are consistent with the patient's values and the patient's and family's wishes.

Attending physicians should work closely with an organization's medical director to support and educate the interdisciplinary health team members and administrative staff and to participate in problem solving to improve the quality of long-term patient care. They should accept and respond to feedback about their practices and their overall performance. Table 58.7 summarizes physicians' clinical responsibilities and Table 58.8

Table 58.6

Desirable Attributes of Long-Term Health Care

Facilitate provision of personal care

Focus on enhancing quality of life

Be flexible, consistent with person's wishes, condition, and prognosis

Attempt to distinguish treatable illness or dysfunction from irreversible effects of aging or progression of chronic disease

Be timely and appropriate when intensive health care intervention is indicated

Table 58.7

Clinical Responsibilities of Physicians in Institutional Long-Term Care

Accurate and timely medical assessments

Careful definition and description of current and potential problems and diagnoses

Establishing of a realistic prognosis

Help in establishing realistic care goals based on assessment and prognosis

Medical orders consistent with conclusions and goals

Managing chronic illnesses to maximize function and personal comfort

Managing acute illness as aggressively as indicated by person's goals, condition, prognosis

Adequate and timely follow-up of effects and complications of medications and treatments

Modifying medication and treatment orders in line with such reassessments

Explaining reasons for various medical decisions

Requesting, using, coordinating appropriate consultation

their other responsibilities in institutional long-term care.

PHYSICIANS' ROLE IN REGULATORY COMPLIANCE

A decade has passed since the passage of the landmark legislation establishing comprehensive federal regulations (OBRA '87) for nursing facilities and SNFs nationwide. These regulations reflect many of the common problems of the chronically ill and functionally impaired of any age group, especially the frail elderly. In many ways, they represent a *standard of care* for this population, albeit one imposed via regulation. Research has established a broader empiric basis for many of these requirements, while other regulatory provisions appear to need further empiric support or modification.

For example, one study demonstrated a difference in incidence of pressure ulcers between high-risk (21-month incidence above 19.3%) and low-risk (21-month incidence below 6.5%) nursing facilities. The major patient-related factors associated with pressure ulcer incidence in high-risk homes were difficulty walking, fecal incontinence, diabetes mellitus, and difficulty in feeding oneself. Factors in the low-incidence

homes were difficulty walking, difficulty in feeding oneself, and male gender (8).

Weight loss is common in nursing facility residents, but its source is often obscure and its management is often governed by habit or opinion. The differential diagnosis of involuntary weight loss is extensive, with cancer, depression, and disorders of the gastrointestinal tract the most common causes. In approximately one fourth of weight loss cases in general, no cause is found despite extensive evaluation and long follow-up. In the majority of cases in which a cause is to be found, history, physical examination, and limited laboratory and radiologic studies reveal it. If an initial evaluation does not identify a cause, careful follow-up rather than undirected diagnostic testing is recommended (9).

In providing care in long-term care facilities, physicians should focus particularly on several themes of the OBRA '87 federal regulations: (*a*) helping determine the highest practicable levels of function for each patient, (*b*) ensuring that treatments are medically necessary, and (*c*) helping to demonstrate that negative outcomes are medically unavoidable. These themes are relevant for all care settings, not just the nursing facility.

Table 58.8

Other Related Responsibilities of Physicians in Institutional Long-Term Care

Be aware of services for patients and families; make needed referrals to facilitate such services

Help persons find and remain in the least restrictive setting compatible with condition and needs

Interpret medical information for patients, families, interdisciplinary team members who provide care and handle clinical, ethical, social, psychologic, functional problems

Support and educate caregivers

Help patients and families have realistic expectations of medical interventions

Help patients and families cope with implications of significant medical illnesses

Help patients gain appropriate access to long-term care programs and services

Ensure that medical and related decision making respects wishes and needs of patients and families

Supporting the Highest Practicable Outcome

Physicians have a critical role in defining a person's needs and problems, the causes of problems and their potential reversibility, and the effect of treating the causes and managing the problems. For instance, many causes of hospitalization are preventable; they relate to conditions such as dehydration and infection that cause signs and symptoms over several days or weeks (10). While not expected to cure chronic medical problems, physicians should try to identify and manage possible medical causes of disabilities or dysfunctions when doing so may improve function and quality of life.

Ensuring That Treatments Are Medically Necessary

Medical necessity means that there is a legitimate reason for each treatment or medication; an effort is made to find the most therapeutic, least risky or harmful treatment alternative; there is monitoring for possible side effects or complications of the treatment; there is some attempt to ensure that potential benefits justify the risks or side effects; and there is periodic reappraisal to show that the treatment or medication is still needed. Physicians have a vital role in each of these areas.

Ensuring That Negative Outcomes Are Medically Unavoidable

Medically unavoidable complications and negative outcomes occur because of unavoidable conditions or characteristics of the patient or because of clear reasons interventions are not desired or appropriate rather than because of process failures or neglect. Demonstrating appropriate intention requires explaining decisions to treat or not to treat significant or potentially significant problems. Otherwise an external reviewer cannot tell whether appropriate process occurred. For instance, one study in a community nursing facility found that weight loss of 5 pounds or more occurred in 19% of subjects; 15% lost 5% of body weight; and 4% lost more than 10% of body weight. Depression accounted for 36% of the weight loss. Other causes included medications, psychotropic drug reduction, swallowing disorders, paranoia, dementia with apraxia, gallstones, obsessive-compulsive disorder, dehydration, and increased energy use resulting from incessant wandering, tardive dyskinesia, and chronic obstructive pulmonary disease (11). However, since the cause of some weight loss cannot be readily identified and since not all weight loss is reversible, the physician should help address avoidable weight loss and identify the likely reasons some significant weight loss is unavoidable or irreversible.

Some of the tactics to achieve medically necessary treatments and avoid preventable negative outcomes include writing medical orders that minimize possibilities for error, misinterpretation, drug incompatibilities, and therapeutic duplication; recognizing and avoiding the sources of iatrogenic illness among the elderly; providing timely and clinically pertinent documentation; and responding rationally rather than defensively to quality assurance discussions and suggestions (12).

PHYSICIANS' PARTICIPATION IN INSTITUTIONAL LONG-TERM CARE

Physicians' presence in long-term care facilities has been sporadic, and the quality of practice has been inconsistent. Long-term and subacute care have not attracted much interest from physicians and until recently have not been the subject of much research. In one such study nursing facilities had on average 8.6 attending physicians, 32 residents per physician, 70% of residents cared for by nonstaff physicians, no daily physician present, and no cross-coverage. Some 43% of facilities had closed medical staffs. Closed staffs were most likely in large facilities and those that had many Medicaid residents, used physician extenders, and had many residents per nurse. Facilities with closed medical staffs reported medical care practice patterns that would be associated with better quality of care (13). Many physicians in nursing facilities have but several patients apiece, and many facilities deal with several dozen or more physicians. Under these circumstances physicians may have little incentive to provide effective care and support, and facilities may be severely challenged to hold such physicians accountable.

Overcoming Obstacles to Fulfilling the Attending Physician's Role

As health care is expanding beyond traditional settings, physicians should recognize and fulfill their roles competently and consistently. The reasons cited by physicians for their relative indifference to long-term and subacute care (e.g., dislike for chronic care medicine, poor reimbursement for visits, perception of too many hassles, including accompanying paperwork, perception of excessive regulatory requirements, and belief in inferior or inadequate care) must be overcome rather than used as the continuing basis for poor or indifferent performance.

The physician's role may be improved if attending physicians take a broader, more orderly approach to fulfilling their functions (Table 58.9), supported by an effective medical director. Generally, experience suggests that even a modest amount of interest and appropriate participation by attending physicians can make a considerable difference in outcomes and care quality.

Table 58.9

A Systematic Approach to Fulfilling Physicians' Functions

Perform an appropriate medical assessment
Define a patient's medical and functional problems
Identify links among diagnoses, between diagnoses and problems
Evaluate patient's overall condition and prognosis
Help establish realistic care goals and expectations
Help establish medical needs
Write pertinent medical orders
Request pertinent support services and consultations
Reduce the effects of chronic illness
Manage intercurrent acute illness with appropriate aggressiveness
Maximize function and quality of life
Provide adequate, timely follow-up until problems are resolved
Periodically reassess care plan and treatments
Modify medical orders periodically according to reassessments
Document medical rationale for decisions to treat or not to treat
Explain medical regimen to staff, patients, families
Understand family resources and expectations

EVOLVING ROLE OF THE LONG-TERM CARE MEDICAL DIRECTOR

The medical director plays a key role in ensuring effective participation of physicians and good overall care quality. Over the past decade the medical director's role in long-term and postacute care has become more visible and much more clearly defined (Table 58.10). Still, the potential benefits of such a physician are often not well understood, and the position may be used ineffectively.

The OBRA '87 regulations expanded the original SNF requirement for a medical director to include nursing facilities. These are the only two long-term care sites where a medical director is required. However, other settings, such as assisted living, home care, and hospital postacute units, that care for persons with complex chronic conditions and functional impairments could also benefit from effective medical direction to improve care and address factors that produce excessive variation in outcomes. Broader provider responsibilities in health-related areas such as comprehensive assessment, prevention of skin breakdown, reduction of hospital use, and appropriate medication use demand additional participation by physicians.

Within regulations, the medical director's role is more implicit (broadly defined with few details) than explicit. In 1988 a consensus was reached about 4 major roles, 9 broad functions, and well over 100 different possible tasks for medical directors (14). Only some of these functions are required by law and regulations, while the remainder represent greater *depth* of medical direction (15).

Medical directors have several core functions, and their role has shifted from advisory to one with more authority and responsibility. The contemporary medical director must play a broad *participatory and leadership* role. This includes the direct supervision of physicians and support for overall systems and process improvements that improve the overall quality of care, e.g., the physical environment, infection control, and employee health (16). Effective physician role modeling has been identified as critical to changing physicians' performance (17). There must be some rules for physicians' practices based on care standards and

Table 58.10

Major Functions of the Medical Director

Participate in administrative decision making; recommend and approve policies and procedures

Organize and coordinate care services of physicians, other professionals

Participate to ensure appropriateness and quality of medical and related care

Participate in development and conduct of education programs

Articulate facility's mission to community; represent facility in community

Participate in surveillance and promotion of health, welfare, and safety of employees

Acquire, maintain, apply knowledge of social, regulatory, political, economic factors affecting care of patients

Provide leadership for research and development activities in geriatrics and long-term care

Help to establish policies, procedures for ensuring that rights of patients are respected

Adapted from Pattee JJ, Altemeier TM. Results of a consensus conference on the role of the nursing home medical director. Ann Med Direct 1991;1:5–11.

guidelines that reflect knowledge about disease management in the elderly and the factors affecting outcomes. Effective leadership is needed to give physicians feedback about improving their practices and coordinating medical care with that of other disciplines. Such efforts are needed to achieve better and more timely compliance by physicians and to reduce excessive variation in practices and outcomes.

LINKS BETWEEN ACUTE AND LONG-TERM CARE

Many nursing facility residents require care of acute medical illnesses, and many nursing facilities are providing short-term postacute care. These persons have or are at risk for complications and acute instability requiring prompt medical interventions. Other persons are being admitted as residents to long-term care facilities soon after a severe acute medical illness.

Demonstration projects (social HMOs, or SHMOs, and Program of All-Inclusive Care for the Elderly, or PACE) have tried to integrate various aspects of care outside of institutional settings. The success or failure of these approaches will influence the roles of institutional providers.

Obstacles to care continuity across settings include regulations, reimbursement, and practitioners' attitudes. Failures of continuity result in redundant, inefficient service and may contribute to avoidable morbidity and mortality. To enable care continuity and to address many of the problems resulting from lack of it, physicians must improve the links between acute and long-term care in areas such as information transfer, coordination of care, and discharge planning (18).

SUMMARY: THE EVOLVING ROLE OF THE LONG-TERM CARE CONTINUUM

The health care and personal care delivery systems are decentralizing; i.e., care is moving from specific sites to which people are sent and instead is being provided in or near their residences. As the long-term care continuum also changes, institutions are becoming the focal point for the longer-term care of more complex persons and for more complex short-term care of many persons based in the community or in long-term care facilities. Many long-term care settings have broadened their capabilities and the scope of their services, but only some of them have sufficiently developed essential systems and processes. Thus there is still a gap between the potential and actual capabilities of many of these providers and their practitioners. The effective use of the long-term care continuum is also inhibited by payers' confusion over its potential and existing skills.

True care integration requires a systematic, coordinated, patient-centered approach. Creating an efficient, effective long-term care system requires emphasizing similarities rather than differences among care recipients and providers and deemphasizing sites and procedures as principal areas for reimbursement or regulatory concentration. It also demands effective participation by physicians and competent medical leadership.

REFERENCES

1. Kane RA, Kane RL. Long-Term Care: Principles, Programs, and Policies. New York: Springer, 1987:4.
2. Levenson SA. Subacute and Transitional Care Handbook. St. Louis: Beverly-Cracom, 1996.
3. Zimmer JG. Needed: acute care in the nursing home. Patient Care 1993;27:59–68.

4. Eng C, Pedulla J, Eleazer GP, et al. Program of all-inclusive care for the elderly (PACE): an innovative model of integrated geriatric care and financing. J Am Geriatr Soc 1997;44:1429–1434.

5. Williamson JD, Fried LP. Characterization of older adults who attribute functional decrements to "old age." J Am Geriatr Soc 1996;44:1429–1434.

6. Five-year findings of the hypertension detection and follow-up program. I. Reduction in mortality of persons with high blood pressure, including mild hypertension. Hypertension Detection and Follow-up Program Cooperative Group. JAMA 1979;242:2562–2571.

7. Council on Scientific Affairs. American Medical Association white paper on elderly health. Arch Intern Med 1990;150:2459–2472.

8. Brandeis GH, Oi WL, Hossain M, et al. A longitudinal study of risk factors associated with the formation of pressure ulcers in nursing homes. J Am Geriatr Soc 1994;42:388–393.

9. Reife CM. Involuntary weight loss. Med Clin North Am 1995;79:299–313.

10. Ouslander JG. Medical care in the nursing home. JAMA 1989;262:2582–2590.

11. Morley JE, Kraenzle D. Causes of weight loss in a community nursing home. J Am Geriatr Soc 1994;42:583–585.

12. Ouslander JG, Osterweil D, Morley J. Medical Care in the Nursing Home. 2nd ed. New York: McGraw-Hill, 1996.

13. Karuza J, Katz PR. Physician staffing patterns correlates of nursing home care. J Am Geriatr Soc 1994;42:787–793.

14. Pattee JJ, Altemeier TM. Results of a consensus conference on the role of the nursing home medical director. Ann Med Direct 1991;1:5–11.

15. Pattee JJ, Otteson O. Medical Direction in the Nursing Home. Minneapolis: Northridge Press, 1991.

16. Levenson SA, ed. Medical Direction in Long-Term Care: A Guidebook for the Future. Durham, NC: Carolina Academic Press, 1993.

17. Greco PJ, Eisenberg JM. Changing physicians' practices. N Engl J Med 1993;329:1271–1274.

18. Fanale J, Levy M. The interface between the nursing home and hospital. J Med Dir 1993;3:38–40.

Sexuality

Contrary to societal beliefs that older adults are asexual, many researchers have documented continuing interest in sexual activity throughout adult life. The range of sexual expression documented is quite broad, with deemphasis on sexual intercourse and an increased interest in touching and other forms of intimacy. When problems with sexuality arise, health care providers must know these issues to help their older adult patients.

Most studies are retrospective or cross-sectional and thus subject to recall bias and cohort effects. Nonetheless, it is well established that sexual activity and interest persist until the end of life, at least in a substantial minority. Kinsey et al. (1) were first to document a decline in sexual activity with age. Perhaps Kinsey's most important contribution (other than establishing sexual behavior as a legitimate area for research) was the finding that sexual activity in men diminishes gradually with age; in other words, there is no age at which activity stops precipitously. Kinsey's companion study of women concluded that the observed decline in women's sexual activity with age resulted from male aging, since the frequency of activities such as masturbation remained constant with age (2).

Pfeiffer et al. (3) at Duke University demonstrated continuing interest in sexuality by older adults in a cohort of men and women who were followed for 10 years. While on average about 40% of women and 60% of men expressed interest in sexuality throughout the decade of observation, reported frequency of sexual intercourse declined significantly for men, from 70 to 25% while remaining almost constant (average 20%) for women. Pfeiffer et al. (4) reported that women ceased sexual activity because their spouse died, became ill, lost interest, or lost potency.

More recent surveys of sexuality in older adults include a national survey of sexuality in married persons (5). In this survey, which included 807 respondents aged 60 or older, about half reported having sex at least once in the past month. Only a quarter of those older than age 75 had had sex in the last month. As earlier studies suggest, the health status of the respondent's partner was related to frequency of sexual relations. One of the most consistently cited predictors of frequency of sexual activity in later life is the frequency of sexual activity in youth (6). This finding also was confirmed in one of the few longitudinal studies of the aging process, the Baltimore Longitudinal Study of Aging (7).

Another recent study of sexual practices in community-dwelling elderly is unique in its inclusion of a very elderly (average age 86) and very healthy cohort. Bretschneider and McCoy (8) conducted an anonymous survey of upper-middle-class residents of California life-care communities. Only residents who did not require any regular medication and had no daily nursing or medical needs were eligible for the study. Sexual thoughts and activity were frequent in this group. Some 70% of men and 50% of women thought about being close or intimate with the opposite sex often or very often; 53% of the men who responded and 25% of the women who responded had regular sex partners. The most frequent sexual behaviors, in order of most frequent to least frequent, for both men and women in this survey were touching their partners, masturbation, and sexual intercourse (8).

There are few studies of sexual beliefs and activities of older gays and lesbians. One small survey of gay men found that 86% of those older than 60 were still sexually active (9). However, these men reported less interest in sex than younger respondents. Level of sexual enjoyment did not vary by age. While it is unclear what effects homosexuality has on a person's ability to age successfully, it appears that integration into the gay community is associated with satisfaction with aging in older gays and lesbians (10, 11).

CHANGES IN SEXUAL FUNCTION WITH AGE

Masters and Johnson described four stages of human sexual response: excitement (also known as arousal), plateau, orgasm, and resolution (12). In men, all four stages change with age. Erections take longer to achieve and may be less full during the excitement stage. Older men may require more direct stimulation to achieve an erection, and they are less likely to achieve erection with visual or psychologic stimulation alone. The plateau phase is usually longer, which may have the positive result of better control of ejaculation. Some older men who lose their erections prior to ejaculation may not be able to regain them. Preejaculatory secretions are reduced or absent. As orgasm nears, the length of time of ejaculatory inevitability is reduced. Orgasm itself is shorter. The force of ejaculation is reduced, sometimes to the extent that semen only dribbles out. However, few older men notice a subjective difference in orgasmic pleasure. During resolution, detumescence and testicular descent occur more rapidly than in young adulthood. Older men also have a longer refractory period following orgasm, often approaching days rather than minutes when younger.

Masters and Johnson (12) also demonstrated changes in sexual function in aging women. These changes are mediated by the decline in estrogen production that occurs with the onset of menopause. At menopause, estradiol production by the ovaries decreases significantly, resulting in increased levels of the gonadotropins, follicle-stimulating hormone, and luteinizing hormone.

The loss of estrogen causes the vagina to become thinner and the uterus to shrink. Breast glandular tissue is replaced by fat. Despite these changes of menopause, recent investigations have failed to find any direct association between hormonal levels and sexual function in menopausal women (13, 14).

All four phases of sexual arousal and orgasm in women are affected by age. During the excitement phase, less vaginal lubrication and less vasocongestion of the genitalia occur than in younger women. The vagina opens less fully, and the labia majora may not flatten and separate. During the plateau phase, less vasocongestion and tenting of the vagina occur, and there is less elevation of the uterus. During orgasm there are fewer uterine contractions (12).

To investigate an older adult's concerns with sexuality, a health care provider must learn to ask a sexual history in a way that is comfortable for both the provider and the patient. At least a few questions about sexual practices or beliefs should be part of the assessment of every new geriatric patient. Even if the patient has no present concerns, this demonstrates to the patient that the provider considers sexuality an area of health like any other and that he or she is willing to discuss this subject. Sexual history also may give the physician valuable information regarding the patient's other problems, such as the effects of medication, or even suggest a previously unknown diagnosis (e.g., chest pain during intercourse may be due to angina) (15). Questions should be asked in a neutral tone and a nonjudgmental fashion.

Areas of investigation, with sample questions, are shown in Table 59.1. The degree to which these areas are pursued varies with the presenting complaint and the patient's level of concern. In addition to questions about the sexual concerns of patients, a history of the patient's overall health should include medication use, previous surgery (especially in the abdomen or pelvis), and chronic diseases, including psychiatric illnesses.

Chronic illnesses are common in the older adult. Chronic diseases can impair sexual function directly, as in the case of diabetes mellitus and its effects on erectile function, or indirectly by causing other symptoms, such as chronic pain

Table 59.1

Sample Questions Regarding Sexuality and Areas of History That May Have to Be Investigated

Initial inquiry for a new patient

 Do you have any questions or concerns about your sex life? *or*

 Are you satisfied with your sex life?

 Are you sexually active with men, women, or both?

For patients with sexual complaints

 Have you lost your desire for sex (with your spouse, with others)?

 How often do you have sex?

 How many partners do you have?

 Are you able to have an orgasm with masturbation?

 How often do you masturbate? Has there been any change in the frequency of masturbation?

 Do you have unsafe sex, especially with anyone who engages in high-risk behavior (e.g., injection drug use, multiple partners)?

 Are you having pain during sex? (If yes) Does it vary with position or type of activity?

 Are you afraid something will happen to your spouse or to you during sex (e.g., a heart attack)?

 How well are you getting along with your spouse?

 Did you have a similar problem when you were younger?

 Have you ever had any surgery, radiotherapy, or other treatment in your pelvic area?

 Are you worried that your disease will affect your sex life?

 Do you have problems with dryness during intercourse (for women)?

 Do you have difficulty with erections being hard enough for intercourse (for men)?

 Do you have difficulty maintaining erections during masturbation (for men)?

(e.g., osteoarthritis) or shortness of breath (e.g., chronic obstructive pulmonary disease). Major depression can result from impaired sexual function or may cause loss of interest in sexual activity. Attention to chronic illnesses, especially as they affect function, may result in improved sexual function as well.

The possibility of sexually transmitted diseases (STDs) is another consideration. Risk factors for STDs include sex with multiple partners, injection drug use, sex with injection drug users, sex with persons who exchange sex for money or drugs,

and blood transfusion during 1978 to 1985. Older adults who are sexually active with multiple partners should be advised to practice safe sex, including using condoms, and should be considered for human immunodeficiency virus antibody screening, rapid plasma reagin screening, and immunization against hepatitis A and B (16).

As in all areas of geriatric practice, adverse drug effects are an important consideration in the evaluation of sexual dysfunction. Both prescription and recreational drugs may cause or contribute to sexual problems in older adults (17). Because most of the evidence linking drugs to sexual dysfunction is poor in quality, clinicians often must make an educated guess as to whether drugs are involved in an individual patient's problem. An empiric trial of a substitute drug or withdrawal of the implicated offender may answer the question.

The drug class most commonly implicated is antihypertensives. Virtually all antihypertensive medicines in use for any length of time have been linked to sexual dysfunction, at least anecdotally. Thiazide diuretics may cause erectile dysfunction and reduced libido, although this is probably rarer than previously thought (17). Another diuretic, spironolactone, more commonly causes sexual dysfunction. This effect probably is mediated through its steroid structure, which mimics sex hormones. Centrally acting sympatholytics, such as clonidine and the rarely used methyldopa and guanabenz, decrease sympathetic tone, impairing erections. Doses of propranolol greater than 160 mg daily were associated with erectile dysfunction in one trial of hypertension treatment, although men more than 65 years old were excluded (18). Peripherally acting antihypertensive drugs such as reserpine and guanethidine also may cause erectile dysfunction. Sexual dysfunction appears to be rare with calcium channel blockers, angiotensin-converting enzyme inhibitors, and peripheral α-adrenergic blockers such as prazosin. Another relevant cardiovascular drug is digoxin, which is structurally similar to sex steroids. It is associated with decreased libido, gynecomastia in men, and erectile dysfunction. Clofibrate and disopyramide also may cause erectile dysfunction.

Psychotropic medicines also are a frequent cause of sexual dysfunction. The monamine oxidase inhibitors, neuroleptics, and tricyclic and heterocyclic antidepressants are the most common offenders. Trazodone, a heterocyclic antidepressant, has been associated with priapism in many case reports. Selective serotonin reuptake inhibitors are associated with reduced libido (19), although this can be difficult to distinguish from the depression for which the drug was prescribed.

Miscellaneous drugs linked to sexual dysfunction include cimetidine, metoclopramide, opioids used chronically, and anticonvulsants. Recreational drugs, including the legally available drugs alcohol and nicotine, are often associated with sexual dysfunction.

ERECTILE DYSFUNCTION

Erectile dysfunction, the inability to achieve or maintain erection of sufficient rigidity or duration to permit satisfactory sexual performance, is the most common form of sexual dysfunction in older men (20). Although it is clear that the prevalence of erectile dysfunction increases with age, this appears to be less the result of aging itself than of the parallel increase in prevalence of chronic diseases that may lead to it, including diabetes, atherosclerosis, hypertension, and prostatic disease. In one study of almost 1300 mostly white men aged 40 to 70, the prevalence of complete erectile dysfunction increased from 5% in men aged 40 to 15% in men aged 70 (21). Current smoking at least doubled the risk of erectile dysfunction among subjects with heart disease and hypertension.

Erections and ejaculations are complex physiologic phenomena that require intact neurologic, vascular, and hormonal systems. Sympathetic impulses originating from T12 through L1 maintain flaccidity through constriction of arteries, arterioles, and sinusoids in the corpora cavernosa. Parasympathetic impulses originating from the sacral spinal cord cause arterial vasodilation in the penis by inhibition of sympathetic tone and by causing release of nitric oxide, a potent smooth muscle relaxant, from endothelium (22). Increased arterial flow engorges the corpora cavernosa and decreases venous drainage, resulting in tumescence. Ejaculation occurs when reflex centers in the cord at L1 and L2 send sympathetic impulses to the vas deferens, which then contract

and expel sperm into the internal urethra. Contractions of the prostate add seminal fluid to form semen. The ischiocavernosus and bulbocavernosus muscles contract, increasing urethral pressure, and semen is expelled (23).

Because atherosclerosis is so common in the elderly, vascular diseases are the most common class that cause erectile dysfunction. Atherosclerosis of the pelvic vessels is especially likely in men with other risk factors for atherosclerosis, such as diabetes mellitus, hypertension, tobacco use, and hyperlipidemia. A venous leak is another form of vascular disease. This occurs when the emissary veins remain patent as arterial flow increases. Ordinarily these veins are compressed against the tunica albuginea by the expanding corpora cavernosa (24). This is thought to be the mechanism of dysfunction in patients with Peyronie's disease, in which a fibrous plaque of unknown cause develops within the penis, distorting the anatomy and pulling the veins open.

Numerous endocrinopathies are associated with erectile dysfunction, but far and away the most common is diabetes mellitus. Erectile dysfunction, which results through a vascular or neurologic mechanism in diabetic men, may even be the presenting symptom. A less common but easily treatable endocrine cause of erectile dysfunction is hypogonadism. Elevated prolactin levels also can cause erectile dysfunction.

Neurologic impairments cause erectile dysfunction through a variety of mechanisms, from peripheral and central neuropathy (e.g., multiple sclerosis and diabetes mellitus) to trauma to central nervous system injury (e.g., spinal cord injury, stroke, dementia). Chronic diseases indirectly may affect the ability to maintain an erection by causing worry over discomfort in either the patient or his partner.

Psychiatric issues that may cause difficulty with erection include depression and bipolar disorder. The drugs used to treat these entities may impair libido and erectile function, further complicating the evaluation of these patients. Some men fall prey to widower's syndrome, in which a previously potent man has difficulty with sexual expression with a new partner after the death of his spouse. Stress may cause erectile dysfunction or may coexist with other causes.

The patient and his partner should be interviewed together, at least initially. The most important types of information to be obtained are (*a*) the concerns of the patient and his partner; (*b*) the quality of their relationship; (*c*) the onset of the problem and whether it was abrupt or gradual; (*d*) the duration, quality, and frequency of erection; and (*e*) changes in libido. The medical history should be reviewed with attention to diseases associated with erectile dysfunction. The physical examination should include a careful search for evidence of hypogonadism, such as gynecomastia, loss of pubic hair, or reduced beard growth. The penis should be examined for sensation, meatal position, fibrosis, and plaques. The scrotum should be palpated for testicular size, hydroceles, and varicoceles. The rectal examination should include sphincter tone and examination of the prostate for size, masses, and tenderness. Evidence of vascular disease, such as diminished pulses or shiny hairless skin over the legs, should be sought. The neurologic examination should include standing and supine pulse rate and blood pressure measurements to assess autonomic function and a sensory examination to exclude neuropathy (25).

Because vascular disease is the most common cause of erectile dysfunction in older men, the arterial supply of the penis should be tested in men without another readily discernible cause. A noninvasive test is the penile-brachial index, or PBI. The PBI is obtained by recording the penile blood pressure by Doppler and comparing it with the blood pressure in the arm. A normal value is greater than 1. An index of 0.75 or below greatly increases the chance that erectile dysfunction is due to vascular disease. Values below 0.65 are considered diagnostic.

Other tests that may be helpful include fasting plasma glucose for diabetic screening, thyroid function tests, including thyroxine and thyroid stimulating hormone, testosterone and luteinizing hormone levels, and prolactin levels. Many experts advocate screening for depression in patients with sexual dysfunction. Neither the stamp test, in which a role of stamps is placed around the penis to see if they are broken by an erection during sleep, nor the more formal nocturnal penile tumescence test appears to be helpful in diagnosing erectile dysfunction in older men (26).

The treatment of erectile dysfunction depends on the cause. Multiple factors may be implicated, so the approach to treatment is often multifaceted. As in any older patient with a new problem, substitution for or discontinuation of possible offending medicines should be considered as a first step. If depression is found to be either the cause or the result of the dysfunction, counseling or drug therapy may be necessary. Diabetic patients should have their glucose control improved, although this may not bring about any immediate improvement. If zinc deficiency is suspected in a diabetic patient or in a patient taking a diuretic, zinc replacement may improve erectile function (25). Hypogonadal patients usually benefit from treatment with parenteral testosterone. Oral therapy should be avoided because it is more widely associated with adverse effects, including elevated lipid levels and hepatotoxicity.

In patients with a vascular component, other strategies may be needed. Smokers should be helped to stop. A trial of pentoxifylline is worthwhile in these cases. The results of vascular surgery have been disappointing in these patients (24). A vacuum tumescence device often helps patients who fail to respond to other therapies or if the cause is primarily vascular. These devices cause erections by producing a vacuum inside a tube that fits over the penis. Once the penis is erect, the tube is removed and a tight band is placed around the proximal end of the penis to maintain the erection. Two drawbacks are that a moderate degree of manual dexterity is required and bruising sometimes results.

Intracavernous injections of papaverine with phentolamine have also been used to produce erections. Response rates average about 60%; the highest response rates occur in patients with a neurogenic cause (21). Injection therapy should be supervised by an experienced urologist because of the possibility of priapism, which in extreme cases requires surgical intervention. Other adverse side effects include bruising, plaque formation, and elevation of liver function tests. Neither drug is approved by the U.S. Food and Drug Administration (FDA) for the treatment of erectile dysfunction.

Patients who do not respond to increasing doses of papaverine and phentolamine can be treated with alprostadil (prostaglandin E_1), which had more than an 80% response rate in clinical trials (20). The FDA-approved indications of this drug (available as Caverject) are erectile dysfunction of vascular, neurologic, psychologic, and mixed causes. Alprostadil appears to be safer than injection therapy with papaverine and phentolamine. The most frequent side effect is penile pain, which is dose dependent and usually subsides with detumescence (20). Prolonged erection and penile fibrosis are infrequent complications. A microsuppository formulation is now available for intraurethral administration (27).

Yohimbine is an α_2-adrenergic blocker that for many years has been used for erectile dysfunction. A randomized placebo-controlled cross-over trial in men with erectile dysfunction of organic cause found no significant advantage of yohimbine over placebo (28). Yohimbine may be more effective in men with impotence of psychogenic or uncertain cause.

Penile prostheses may be used by men who do not respond to drug therapy. Initially hailed as a major advance in the treatment of erectile dysfunction, prostheses are now reserved for those who do not respond to other therapies (24). Rigid, hinged, or malleable rods and inflatable prostheses are available. Inflatable prostheses may not be suitable for patients with arthritis or other diseases affecting dexterity.

Arousal disorders (decreased libido) most often result from hypogonadism, recreational drug use, an adverse drug effect, marital strain, or other psychologic problems. These patients can be treated as described earlier. Absence of emission can be caused by retrograde ejaculation, sympathetic denervation, hypogonadism, or drugs. Retrograde ejaculation may be caused by diabetes or may follow surgery on the bladder neck. Ejaculation also may be impaired by drugs, especially sympatholytic antihypertensive agents, such as guanethidine, guanadrel, and phenoxybenzamine.

SEXUAL DYSFUNCTION IN WOMEN

The most common sexual complaints of older women are vaginal dryness and dyspareunia (painful intercourse), loss of interest (decreased libido), and infrequent orgasm. Many of these problems have their origin in the physiologic changes that occur with menopause. If hormone replacement therapy (HRT) is not begun during menopause, symptoms of vasomotor instability, such as hot flashes and insomnia, affect the majority of women, but these are seldom a problem by the time a woman reaches age 65 (29). With the passage of time, however, the loss of estrogen can cause vaginal atrophy, dryness, and eventually dyspareunia. In a recent systematic survey of British women aged 55 and older, 8% complained of vaginal dryness and 2% had dyspareunia (29).

Just as in men, evaluation of the older woman with a sexual complaint begins with a thorough history. Especially important is the attitude of the patient's partner to her problem. Patients should be asked when the problem began, whether there are any recent changes in health status of the patient or partner, the history of the relationship, and a general sexual history (Table 59.1). The physical examination should focus on signs of any undiagnosed disease that may affect sexuality (e.g., hypothyroidism), the status of any chronic disease (e.g., osteoarthritis), and the pelvic examination. This examination includes visualization of the external genitalia and anus and with a speculum, the vagina and cervix. Evidence of previous surgery or scarring, a cystocele or rectocele, vaginal atrophy, and signs of STDs, such as warts, ulcers, or discharge, should be noted. The speculum examination also permits a cervical smear to be taken from women who have not had adequate screening for cervical cancer (29). A bimanual examination (including a rectal examination) can detect abnormal masses, tenderness, and poor sphincter tone.

Vaginal atrophy and often dyspareunia respond to HRT with estrogen and a progestin. Other benefits of HRT include the prevention of osteoporosis and reduced mortality from cardiovascular disease (30–32). A progestogen should be administered with estrogen in women with a uterus to prevent endometrial cancer. In patients in whom HRT is contraindicated or who are not interested in hormonal therapy, a water-soluble lubricant such as K-Y Jelly is recommended.

Counseling to remind patients of normal changes in sexual function with aging may be helpful as well. Older adults may need permission to experiment with different sexual positions to find more comfortable ones. Other couples may no longer be interested in sexual intercourse but may engage in other forms of sexual expression, such as touching or kissing.

As with older men, a decline in sexual desire can have many causes: marital difficulties, depression, painful intercourse, poor health of the partner, adverse drug effects, chronic illness, or increased prolactin levels. Treatment obviously depends on the cause of the decline. HRT usually improves vaginal dryness and atrophy but does not appear to increase sexual desire directly (33, 34). Testosterone may be useful in some women with decreased arousal.

Both men and women may require referral when sexual dysfunction does not improve under the primary care provider's guidance. Referral may be needed for patients for specialized testing, evaluation of endocrine disorders, for surgery, or for psychiatric evaluation. Therapists who specialize in sexual problems may be helpful when there are serious problems in the marital relationship or if the provider lacks the time or training (25). To obtain the addresses of certified therapists in their state, health care providers should send a self-addressed stamped envelope to the American Association of Sex Educators, Counselors, and Therapists (AASECT), P.O. Box 238, Mount Vernon, IA 52314-0238.

Sexuality is often overlooked by those who care for nursing home residents. Surveys of sexual beliefs in nursing home residents and in nursing home staff show several barriers to residents' sexuality, including lack of privacy or a partner, feelings of unattractiveness, chronic illness, loss of interest, and the attitudes of physicians and staff (35). To counter these problems, privacy can be improved by allowing for conjugal visits and by using do-not-disturb signs. Home visits also can be arranged. Providing access to beauty parlors and barbers helps residents to combat feelings of sexual unattractiveness. Also, nursing home workers may need reminders that older adults may employ forms of sexual expression other than sexual intercourse.

REFERENCES

1. Kinsey AC, Pomeroy WB, Martin CE. Age and sexual outlet. In: Kinsey AC, Pomeroy WB, Martin CE, eds. Sexual Behavior in the Human Male. Philadelphia: Saunders, 1948:218–262.
2. Kinsey AC, Pomeroy WB, Martin CE, Gebhard PH. Sexual Behavior in the Human Female. Philadelphia: Saunders, 1953.
3. Pfeiffer E, Verwoerdt A, Wang HS. The natural history of sexual behavior in a biologically advantaged group of aged individuals. J Gerontol 1969;24:193–198.
4. Pfeiffer E, Verwoerdt A, Wang HS. Sexual behavior in aged men and women. Arch Gen Psychiatry 1968;19:735–758.
5. Marsiglio W, Donnelly D. Sexual relations in later life: a national study of married persons. J Gerontol 1991;46:338–344.
6. Berezin MA. Sex and old age: a further review of the literature. J Geriatr Psych 1976;9:189–209.
7. Shock NW, Greulich RC, Costa PT Jr, et al. Normal Human Aging: The Baltimore Longitudinal Study of Aging. Washington: US Department of Health and Human Services, 1984.
8. Bretschneider JG, McCoy NL. Sexual interest and behavior in healthy 80- to 102-year-olds. Arch Sex Behav 1988;17:109–129.
9. Pope M, Schulz R. Sexual attitudes and behavior in midlife and aging homosexual males. J Homosex 1991;20:169–177.
10. Friend RA. The individual and social psychology of aging: clinical implications for lesbians and gay men. J Homosex 1987;14:307–336.
11. Quam JK, Whitford GS. Adaptation and age-related expectations of older gay and lesbian adults. Gerontologist 1992;32:367–374.
12. Masters WH, Johnson VE. Human Sexual Response. Boston: Little, Brown, 1966.
13. Dennerstein L, Dudley EC, Hopper JL, Burger H. Sexuality, hormones and the menopausal transition. Maturitas 1997;26:83–93.
14. Cawood EH, Bancroft J. Steroid hormones, the menopause, sexuality and well-being of women. Psychol Med 1996;26:925–936.
15. Cheadle MJ. The screening sexual history: getting to the problem. Clin Geriatr Med 1991;7:9–13.
16. Guide to Clinical Preventive Services. Report of the U.S. Preventive Services Task Force. 2nd ed. Baltimore: Williams & Wilkins, 1996.
17. Deamer RL, Thompson JF. The role of medications in geriatric sexual function. Clin Geriatr Med 1991;7:95–111.
18. Adverse reactions to bendrofluazide and propranolol for the treatment of mild hypertension. Report of Medical Research Council Working Party on Mild to Moderate Hypertension.Lancet 1981;2:539–543.
19. Montano CB. Recognition and treatment of depression in a primary care setting. J Clin Psychiatry 1994;55(suppl):18–34.

20. NIH Consensus Conference. Impotence. NIH Consensus Development Panel on Impotence. JAMA 1993;270: 83–90.

21. Feldman HA, Goldstein I, Hatzichristou DG, et al. Impotence and its medical and psychosocial correlates: results of the Massachusetts male aging study. Int J Impot Res 1992;4(suppl 2):A17.

22. Broderick GA. Intravenous pharmacotherapy: treatment for the aging erectile response. Urol Clin North Am 1996;23:111–126.

23. Guyton AC. Textbook of Medical Physiology. Philadelphia: Saunders, 1986.

24. Mulligan T, Katz PG. Urologic considerations in geriatric erectile failure: geriatric sexuality. Clin Geriatr Med 1991;7:73–84.

25. Kligman EW. Office evaluation of sexual function and complaints. Clin Geriatr Med 1991;7:15–39.

26. Kaiser F. Sexuality and impotence in the aging man. Clin Geriatr Med 1991;7:63–72.

27. Intraurethral alprostadil for impotence. Med Lett Drugs Ther 1997;39:31–32.

28. Morales A, Condra M, Owen JE, et al. Is yohimbine effective in the treatment of organic impotence? Results of a controlled trial. J Urol 1987;137:1168–1172.

29. Barlow DH, Cardozo LD, Francis RM, et al. Urogenital ageing and its effect on sexual health in older British women. Br J Obstet Gynaecol 1997;104:87–91.

30. Bellantoni MF. Osteoporosis prevention and treatment. Am Fam Physician 1996;54:986–992.

31. Stampfer MJ, Colditz GA. Estrogen replacement therapy and coronary heart disease: a quantitative assessment of the epidemiologic evidence. Prevent Med 1991;20:47–63.

32. Miller KL. Hormone replacement therapy in the elderly. Clin Obstet Gynecol 1996;39:912–932.

33. Coope J. Hormonal and non-hormonal interventions for menopausal symptoms. Maturitas 1996;23:159–168.

34. Omu AE, al-Qattan N. Effects of hormone replacement therapy on sexuality in postmenopausal women in a Mideast country. J Obstet Gynaecol Res 1997;23:157–164.

35. Richardson JP, Lazur AM. Sexuality in the nursing home patient. Am Fam Physician 1995;51:121–124.

Driving and the Older Adult

In our society, transportation needs are mostly met by the automobile. Demographic changes in our society have resulted in increasing numbers of older drivers (1). It is estimated that by 2050, 39% of drivers will be over age 65 (2). The ability to drive enables elders to maintain a vital link with their communities. Older adults who have stopped driving are at risk for isolation, depression (3), and functional impairment (4). Assisting with transportation needs may result in additional stress on caregivers of older adults. There is a significant societal cost in providing transportation for those who do not drive. Health professionals can play a key role in maintaining or improving driving skills in their older patients. If driving is no longer possible or permissible, clinicians can assist in guiding their patients to other means of transportation.

DEMOGRAPHICS AND CHARACTERISTICS

The demographics of our aging population indicates that the number of older drivers on the road will increase in the next few decades. The increase will likely be due to a combination of factors, including the aging of the population, an increase in the number of women drivers, and an increase in the need to reach destinations by motor vehicles (5). Over the past 10 years the average distance driven per year has increased in all age groups and both sexes, but it still declines with age. The percentage of the population that drives decreases with age (6), presumably because of a variety of reasons including physical frailty, medical illnesses, financial hardships, and perhaps a cohort effect. In addition, older drivers tend to avoid driving at night, in bad weather, during rush hour, and in congested thoroughfares.

The traffic violation rate per licensed driver is high for both the young and old driver (7). Traffic violations in older adults tend to reflect problems with attention and complex traffic situations, such as making left turns, failure to yield, and missing stop or traffic signs. The younger population tends to have high rates of violations for speeding, reckless driving, and driving while intoxicated. The absolute number of crashes that involve older drivers is small compared with that of the rest of the population. However, public safety concerns about the driving performance of this group has been raised by evidence showing a higher crash rate per mile driven for drivers aged 70 or more than in other adult age groups (8). This increase has been attributed to age-related changes in driving skills (9) in addition to various medical illnesses (10).

Dementia has been hypothesized to contribute to this increased crash rate in older adults (11). Evidence for dementia playing an important role in older adult crashes includes an increasing prevalence of dementia of the Alzheimer type (DAT), which doubles every 5 years over age 65 (12), unsafe driving in demented subjects (13, 14), and poorer road skills in subjects with DAT than in elderly controls (15, 16). Driving with dementia may be fairly common. A recent study (17) indicated that 20% of drivers over age 80 who renew their license may have a significant cognitive impairment.

Direct evidence examining crash rates of demented drivers in large population-based studies is lacking. However, studies from tertiary care referral centers and specialty clinics have compared drivers with DAT and controls. Most studies reveal a higher crash rate in drivers with DAT than in controls (18–20), although there is one exception (21). However, many of these studies are limited by a small number of subjects, the use of questionnaire data rather than state recorded data, the lack of appropriate control data, absence of measures of exposure (distance driven per year), failure to document injuries, and lack of information on crash characteristics.

OLDER DRIVERS AT RISK
Motor Vehicle Crashes

Unintentional injury is the third leading cause of death in the United States (22). Each year motor vehicle crashes are associated with more than 40,000 deaths, 500,000 hospital admissions, 5 million injuries, and a cost estimated to be $48.7 billion in lost productivity (23). The prevention of a motor vehicle crash is an appropriate goal for the primary care clinician. Each year older adults are an increasing proportion of the motor vehicle injury problem. Older adults are also more susceptible to injury in crashes than their younger counterparts (8). The federal government recently described the urgent need to identify factors that increase crash risk in this population (24). Many states have or are considering legislation requiring physicians to assist in the identification of unsafe drivers. Improvement in driving skills or identifying unsafe drivers with irreversible medical impairments has a tremendous potential to lower the crash and injury rate for all drivers and pedestrians.

Human error is the most common cause of motor vehicle crashes. However, causes of crashes are not always obvious and may be complex. One study revealed that road user errors were present in 95% of accidents, and 44% of drivers were found to have made perceptual errors (25). Perceptual errors included distraction, lack of attention, incorrect interpretation, misjudged speed and distance, and looked but failed to see. Crashes often result from human error, but causes may or may not be attributable to medical illness, such as visual impairment or alcohol use. There also may be environmental and/or vehicular causes of any

given crash that outweigh the contribution of impairment in driving skill.

Michon (26) described strategic, tactical, and operational aspects of driving that may explain individual differences in performance and play a role in crash causation. Figure 60.1 depicts a model of many factors in causing crashes. The period of time when the motor vehicle (kinetic energy) is no longer under adequate control is referred to as the precrash phase (27). Vehicular factors may determine whether an injury occurs, such as its crashworthiness, the use of seat belts, and the presence and type of airbags. Human factors such as age, bone density, aortic disease, and muscle strength may also help determine the type or extent of injury. A discussion or review of the factors that may result in injury to the occupant (the injury phase) is beyond the scope of this chapter. The interested reader is referred to textbooks on injury control (28).

Older adults have higher rates of crashes at intersections when merging or making turns than do younger adults (29). There are several plausible explanations for these types of crashes. Older drivers may have difficulty in obtaining information in a timely manner because of impaired abilities in visual search or attention. Restricted neck range of motion and impaired visual acuity may further prevent or degrade appropriate sensory input. Impaired ability to assess with accuracy the speed of oncoming traffic or the speed necessary to complete the maneuver may be a problem. Cognitively impaired older adults may forget or simply be unable to scan the environment during stressful driving situations that increase load on working memory. A decrease in lateral eye movement detected in a recent on-the-road driving test and decreases in visual tracking in DAT drivers indicate more impairments in visual search than are found in controls (15). The detection of these impairments and efforts to improve these declines are discussed in the section on assessment of driving skills.

Many diseases that are fairly common in older adults affect driving ability. They include but are not limited to sensory deprivation (30), diabetes (31), seizure disorders (32), dementia (19), stroke

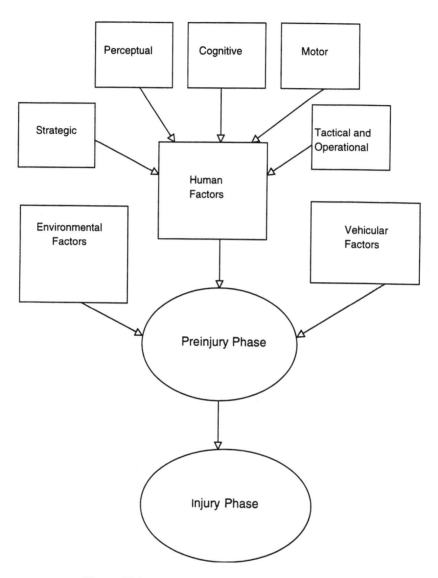

Figure 60.1.   Model of motor vehicle crash causation.

(33), psychiatric disorders (34), cardiovascular disease (35), sleep apnea (36), musculoskeletal disorders (37), and alcohol and drug use (38). Studies have also indicated that drivers whose medical status can change abruptly, as with seizures, diabetes, heart disease, and so on, are at high risk for a crash (39).

Relatively few studies focus on medical conditions as risk factors for motor vehicle crashes in older adults. One study used a case-control approach from a health maintenance organization and compared older drivers injured in crashes with a control group (40). The major medical illness that predicted an increased risk for injury in an automobile crash was diabetes, especially for older diabetics taking insulin or hypoglycemic agents.

The variation in stages of any disease (such as diabetes) with effects on multiple organ systems makes generalizations difficult. The potential for comorbidity is also high, since older drivers may have more than one disease. However, identifying medical illnesses that may increase crash risk is practical and has the potential to be a focus for intervention or treatment. One of the current goals of the American Association of Automotive Medicine (AAAM) is to establish disease severity scales and eventually correlate them to the driving task.

Another approach to index crash risk in older adults is to perform functional and physical assessments (41). With increasing age and age-related disease, studies have documented declines in visual acuity (42), hearing (43), and perceptual response time (44) and an increase in processing time (45). Declines in static visual acuity (46), scotopic and mesopic static acuity (47), motion perception (48), glare recovery time (49), contrast sensitivity (30), dynamic visual acuity (50), visual fields (51), visuospatial skills (52), complex reaction time (53), and selective (54) and divided attention (55) have all been noted to impair driving skills. There is also a decline in the functional visual field, or useful field of view, with age (56). This measure has been correlated with crash data in an older driver population (57). However, measurement of many of these physiologic skills is quite expensive, may require special equipment and intensive training, and is not readily available to most clinicians.

A recent review on the assessment of older drivers suggested that an office-based assessment should focus on static visual acuity, hearing, any arthritis, and dementia (58). One author (59) suggested that physicians are in a unique position to screen older drivers for problems that impair driving abilities, and these should include past crashes or violations, static visual acuity and fields, auditory screening, cognitive screening including mental status examinations, functional status, musculoskeletal screening, sleep disorders, alcohol screening, and a medication review. Motor abilities relevant to driving have been discussed in the literature, and their assessment may include muscle strength evaluated by manual muscle testing and measuring range of motion of the neck and extremities (60). A recent study found that foot abnormalities, fewer blocks walked, and poor design copying on the Mini-Mental Status Examination were associated with an increased risk for a crash in older drivers (61).

Brief physiologic or functional measures appear ideal, since they can be given reliably and cost-efficiently in the outpatient setting. A summary of medical illness and physiologic measures can be found in Table 60.1.

Primary care physicians can play an important role in injury prevention. Physicians must consider teaching their patients to perceive their own vulnerability. An average citizen has a 1:3 chance of sustaining a disabling traffic-related injury during a lifetime of driving. Lay literature such as *Consumer Reports* may be helpful in assessing which vehicles are most crashworthy. Physicians also should know why their patients resist using safety belts; common explanations are physical discomfort, traveling short distances, and too much trouble (62).

Physicians should discuss with adults of all ages the barriers to preventing seat belt use. Risks for avoiding seat belt use include obesity, alcohol use, inactivity, and low income (63). Alcohol is an important risk factor for a crash. Alcohol use in older adults appears to be rising.

Table 60.1

The Primary Care Physician's Role in Assessing Driving Fitness

Functional measures
  Vision
  Hearing
  Reaction time
  Attention
  Visuospatial skills
  Judgment
  Muscle strength
  Joint flexibility
Medical conditions
  Cardiac disease
  Risk for heart attack
  Diabetes
  Pulmonary disorders
  Alcoholism
  Use of sedating medications
  Dementia
  Cerebrovascular disease
  Risk of stroke
  Arthritis
  Visual impairments
  Hearing impairments

Three drinks in an hour for a man or 90 minutes for a women raises the blood alcohol level to.05 g/dL, at which the risk of crash doubles. Car phones have also been noted to double the crash rate in one recent study. Table 60.2 summarizes these important issues. It is suggested that the primary care physician incorporate an injury control approach into the health maintenance practice for older adults.

Cessation of Driving

There is a significant societal cost in providing transportation for those who do not drive. In addition, loss of driving privileges can result in a loss of independence and self-esteem. Unfortunately, there has been minimal effort to improve or maintain driving skills in older adults. Clinical reviews on the assessment of older drivers and research in this area mainly focus on screening methods to identify unsafe drivers, on restricting older drivers, or on license revocation. There is an urgent need to identify older adults at risk for cessation of driving and to develop interventions that can maintain or improve the ability to drive.

Epidemiologic studies have begun to identify older adults who are at risk for cessation of driv-

Table 60.2

The Primary Care Physician's Role in Injury Prevention

Risk factors for not using seat belts
  Obesity
  Smoking
  Alcohol use
  Race
  Low income
  Low education
Health maintenance issues
  Use of safety restraints
  Vehicle in good working condition
  No alcohol when driving
  Obey the speed limit
  Discourage use of cellular phone while driving
  Review medical conditions that may impair driving skills
  Consider refresher course for driving (55 Alive)
  Use safety helmet when riding motorcycle or bicycle

ing. They include those with visual impairment, activity limitations, stroke, Parkinson's disease, arthritis, hip fracture, and memory loss (3, 64). Interestingly, activity limitations were one of the strongest risk factors for cessation of driving (64). In one study, difficulty climbing stairs, the inability to walk half a mile or perform heavy housework correlated with cessation of driving (64). Increasing disability in high-level function is associated with older adults who drive fewer miles (3); important findings in this study indicate that 50% of the subjects with the diseases associated with increased risk were still driving. However, most of the older adults with these diseases who stopped driving did so voluntarily. This indicates that there may be a window of opportunity for intervention and maintenance of driving skill in the frail older adult.

There are many reasons older adults stop driving. Insight into cognitive or physical deficits, pressure from physicians or family, finances, convenience (if others can provide transportation), loss of insurance, or inability to renew a license may result in driving cessation. The health professional may be directly involved in this process. It is important for the clinician to handle this situation in a very professional, sensitive, and understanding manner. A loss of driving privileges is not to be taken lightly. How a physician addresses these issues may have an important effect on the psychologic and physical health of the patient, the acceptance of the decision to stop driving, and the use of community transportation resources.

In the event that the patient must permanently stop driving as a result of a new medical illness, the physician should be certain that the illness is not treatable or reversible and that the illness would place the person or society at an unacceptable risk for a crash. This decision should be discussed openly and the discussion documented in the patient's chart. In the event the patient accepts the physician's advice, it is imperative that alternative modes of transportation be discussed.

Public transportation systems (65) are relatively inexpensive and may have reduced fares for senior citizens. Because of restricted locations, physical limitations, and perhaps psychologic factors, these services are typically underused by older adults. Public mass transit systems may offer special projects such as Call-A-Ride, from Bi-State Development Company in St. Louis. These services provide door-to-door delivery for older adults in a large van, many of which are equipped with lifts. The state may assist in the funding of transportation services. In Missouri, the Older Adults Transportation Service, Inc. (OATS), is operated by a not-for-profit corporation. Local communities, societies, retirement centers, and local church groups may use funds or volunteers to provide transportation to medical appointments, grocery shopping, and socialization.

Patients may refuse to stop driving despite the physician's advice. The physician should make every effort to offer the patient a second opinion or refer him or her for further testing (see the section on ethics, law, and public policy). This discussion should be well documented in the patient's chart. The physician may consider writing a letter to the department of motor vehicles (DMV). If the patient does not have the insight into the illness, the family, DMV, and physician may have to work together to stop the person from driving. Especially in situations such as DAT, these efforts may include removing the car keys, removing the car from the premises, filing down the ignition key, disabling the battery cable, or having the police or revenue department confiscate the driver's license.

ASSESSING DRIVING SKILLS
Assessment by a Clinician

Driving competency may be an issue in an older adult for several reasons. The patient may have insight into the medical impairment and may question his or her own ability to drive safely. In addition, a concerned family member or friend may have observed declining driving skills. The DMV may have identified a concern and referred the person to his or her physician for a driving evaluation. Many older adults continue to work as drivers (e.g., school bus drivers) and may require an annual health examination. Finally, the physician may consider the issue with the onset or recurrence of new symptoms or disease.

Several recent literature reviews suggest some practical approaches to assessing older drivers (58, 59, 66–68). These articles often recommend screens to assess older drivers for functional decline or diseases that may impair driving ability. Screening has been recommended for a history of crashes or violations, static visual acuity and fields, hearing, cognition, functional status, musculoskeletal status, sleep disorders, alcohol use, muscle strength, range of motion, and medication usage. In spite of their common use in clinical settings, the reliability and validity of many of these screens have not been studied with respect to their efficacy in identifying older drivers at risk for a crash or cessation. In addition, there is little evidence to date that indicates the physician can identify the "safe older driver" (58). However, pending further studies, a step-by-step method of assessing the driving ability of older adults appears prudent.

The assessment should begin with the driving history. A checklist of important human, environmental, and vehicular factors can be found in Table 60.3. Obtaining history from another person who has driven with the patient or observed his or her driving may be useful. Inquiries as to any close calls, mishaps, disorientation, or getting lost in familiar areas should raise a red flag. "Do you feel safe riding with the patient?" can also be a useful question. If the answer is no, the interviewer should probe further to ask whether this is a change. If the risky behavior has been noted for years, one might be reluctant to attribute this change to a new medical illness.

Usually the physician assesses older adults because of an onset or recurrence of a medical disorder. Disease states by themselves do not in-

Table 60.3

Driving History

Frequency, length, and reason for trips
Location (city or rural) of trips
Type of roadways
Driving at night, in rush hour, in adverse conditions
Use of a navigator
Any caregivers who drive
Familiarity with roadways
Caregiver's perception of driving skill
Transporting passengers
Crashes, tickets, near misses, lost

dicate the extent of functional impairment. Therefore, it is imperative that the clinician adopt some type of measure of disease severity. For instance, if the driver has a history of congestive heart failure or angina, the New York Heart Association class may be useful. If the patient has cataracts or glaucoma, the measurement of near and far visual acuity in addition to assessment of visual fields and extraocular eye movements is imperative. Drivers with a history of a right-sided cardiovascular accident should be tested not only for a decline in motor strength or coordination but also for cognitive impairment, such as neglect or hemispatial inattention.

Special mention is made of dementing illnesses, which are fairly common in the older adult population. Because of the aging of our driving population, we can expect increasing numbers of drivers with dementing illnesses over the next few decades (69). As described earlier, it is imperative that the clinician perform a comprehensive examination and attempt to find reversible causes for the dementing illness. Additional studies indicate that 50% of drivers with DAT stop driving 3 years after disease onset (14). Although most clinicians agree that moderate to advanced DAT should preclude driving, recent information suggests it may still be safe for some older adults with mild DAT to drive (21). Thus, drivers with early DAT appear to be at risk for driving impairment and driving cessation. The clinician should assess the severity of the dementing illness by using a severity scale such as the Clinical Dementia Rating Scale, a mental status screen score, and/or by measuring specific impairments in memory, judgment, insight, orientation, processing speed, and language. If memory is the only major cognitive impairment detected, driving privileges may be maintained but should be followed closely.

Polypharmacy is common in older adults, and many medications affect driving skills. Most cases of physician liability that involve driving are related to issues such as medication use. Table 60.4 lists some of the common medication classes that either increase crash risk or impair driving skills when assessed by a simulator or road tests. Some medications have been noted to impair psychomotor abilities, but strong evidence of an association with impaired driving skills has not yet been found or studied. These medications should also be prescribed with caution. The clinician is advised to warn a patient of a drug's potential to affect function such as driving or operating heavy machinery and to document this conversation in the medical record. Once the issue of driving competency is raised, the physician does well to perform a medication review and attempt to discontinue any drugs that may contribute to driving impairment. Recently, long-acting benzodiazepines have been associated with increased crash rates (70).

Physicians may be called on to calculate the risk of sudden incapacity for those who drive for an occupation. Older adults already contribute significantly to the workforce and will likely continue to do so. Many older adults are driving moving vans, taxicabs, private buses, school buses, and so on. Employers may want to know the risk of sudden incapacity, such as having a stroke or heart attack while driving the vehicle. The risk of these events can be calculated by simple probabilities (71) and epidemiologic risk factors (72, 73).

Table 60.5 illustrates the probability equation for predicting these events. Table 60.6 indicates the cardiac, stroke, and motor vehicle crash risk profile of a hypothetical 54-year-old man and a 74-year-old man, both school bus drivers. According to a point system for cardiac and cerebrovascular risk factors, the younger driver has 3 times the risk of a sudden incapacitating event as the older driver. The employer, the company,

Table 60.4

Medications That May Impair Driving Skills

Opioids
Benzodiazepines
Antidepressants
Antihypertensives
Hypnotics
Antipsychotics
Antihistamines
Glaucoma agents
NSAIDs
Muscle relaxants
Alcohol

Table 60.5

Probability Equation for the Risk of Sudden Incapacity While Driving

The risk of harm (RH) to other road users posed by the driver with an acute medical event can be estimated by this equation:

$$RH = TD \times V \times SCI \times AC$$

where TD = time driving (percentage), V = type of vehicle driven (1 for a truck, 0.5 for a passenger car), SCI = risk of sudden cardiac death or incapacitation, AC = probability that such an event will result in a fatal or injury-producing accident

---

and/or the clinician ultimately have to decide what is an acceptable risk for the given occupation. However, this example illustrates why age is one of the worst predictors of performance. Age alone should not be the determining factor in driving ability. Functional assessment and the detection of diseases that can impair driving abilities appear to be the most prudent and appropriate methods in approaching these matters.

Once these steps have been taken, the clinician can usually place patients in one of several categories based on their clinical judgment. Many older adults have very mild impairments, in which case recommendations to continue driving privileges are appropriate. Restrictions (driving during the day, avoiding rush hour, avoiding bad weather, slow speeds) can be added if deemed appropriate. If the disease process is thought to be progressive, the physician should reevaluate for driving at regular intervals. For instance, an older diabetic adult driver on insulin should have periodic examinations to detect new organ impairments (retinopathy or neuropathy) to determine whether disease progression interferes with driving.

The disease state may be so severe and irreversible that recommendations to stop driving appear appropriate. However, many persons fall into the gray area. In this case, several other professionals or organizations may help with the evaluation and should be considered as referral sources. The majority of the focus in the literature is on identifying the high-risk older driver (74). More effort should be made to improve or maintain driving skills in older adults (75).

Referral Sources

A driving simulator, if available, is one method to assess driving abilities. Road performance tests are another. There is no nationally accepted standard for road testing. Many road tests are scored subjectively under varying conditions and without measures of reliability or validity. Many testing centers use a car and a driving course that are unfamiliar to the subject. All of these variables make interpretations of these tests difficult. Despite these limitations, road tests have been advocated by several authors as the preferred method to assess driving competency (76, 77). A performance-based road assessment may reveal driving skills that are impaired by a dementing illnesses or frailty (78). This information could be used to clarify how frailty or dementia affect the driving task, to identify drivers at high risk for a crash, and to examine areas that may be amenable to intervention. My preference is to have road tests performed by instructors or occupational therapists with experience in evaluating drivers with medical impairments.

Many diseases can affect cognition in older adults, such as DAT, cardiovascular accident, medication, and Parkinson's disease. Some cognitive deficits are subtle and remain undetected by the primary care physician. Neuropsychologists may determine the severity of any cognitive impairment in domains that pertain to driving. In Alzheimer's disease, impairments in various perceptual and cognitive skills that may affect driving include processing time (79), visual scanning (80), visuospatial deficits (81), spatial vision (82), impaired judgment and insight (83), attention deficits (84), depth perception (85), and visual fields (86). Primary care physicians who do not have the expertise or time to pursue these types of tests may consider referral to a neuropsychologist.

Many occupational therapists are experts in the assessment of driving skills. Most such therapists are based in rehabilitation centers, have access to cars with a dual set of brakes, and perform some type of pre-road testing of visual, cognitive, and motor skills before embarking on a road test. The vehicle assessment of driving skill may be on a closed and/or open course. The therapist may be able to assist in modifications of

Table 60.6

Hypothetical Examples of the Risk of Sudden Incapacitation While Driving[a]

Characteristic	Example 1: 54-Year-Old	Example 2: 74-Year-Old
Age (years)	54 (11, 0)	74 (19, 6)
Sex	Male	Male
Blood pressure	145/86 (3, 7)	110/70 (-1, 1)
Diabetes	No	No
Smoking	Yes (4, 3)	No
Coronary artery disease claudication, congestive heart failure	No	No
History of atrial fibrillation	No	No
Left ventricular hypertrophy	Yes (9, 5)	No
Total cholesterol, HDL	210/36 (1 and 3)	230/41 (2 and 2)
Yearly risk of stroke	2%	6%
Yearly risk of heart attack	4%	2%
Risk of death or injury to other road users	3 in 10,000	1 in 10,000

[a]Assumptions for both drivers: time driving (TD) = 0.25, type of vehicle (V) = 1, and probability that such an event will result in a fatal or injury-producing accident (AC) = 0.02. Numbers in parentheses indicate points for heart attack, stroke.

the patient's vehicle to assist in operation or improve safety.

The physical therapist can be an indispensable member of the driving rehabilitation team. Cerebrovascular disease and muscle atrophy from disuse, arthritis, and parkinsonism are just a few conditions that can affect muscle function or joint range of motion. Recent epidemiologic data on older adult drivers indicate that back pain, arthritis (6), and the use of pain medications (87) are associated with high crash rates. Thus, limitations in muscle strength due to pain or disuse or restrictions in range of motion of joints such as the hands, feet, and neck may play an important role in driving impairment. Improvements in muscle strength and joint function have the potential to improve driving skills. A physical therapist can work on increasing strength and range of motion in the older adult driver, which may maintain or improve driving skills.

Clinicians can advise their patients as to whether their medical illness should preclude driving. However, licensing is determined by the state. Clinicians are often surprised that a medically impaired driver can renew his or her license or pass the state driving test. However, the state DMV often has limited resources or guidelines on how to assess medically impaired drivers. Many

states have forms for the physician to fill out in case the issue of driving safety is raised. States with medical advisory boards may appoint specialists in certain areas to assist in difficult situations.

Many private and public agencies may be able to assist clinicians and older adult drivers in the assessment process. The American Association of Retired Persons (AARP) offers a course for the adult driver over age 55 called 55 Alive. This 2-day course is offered through AARP local chapters. The course reviews age-related changes that can affect driving and suggests how to improve driving skills. Many states offer insurance discounts for senior citizens who take the course. Private driving schools may be available in your local area to assist with evaluation and education of older adults. Table 60.7 lists several agencies that may be helpful for the clinician interested in assessing or improving driving skills in older adults.

ETHICAL, LEGAL, AND PUBLIC POLICY ISSUES

Despite information about the patient's illness, the patient or family may lack insight into the patient's risk for causing injury while driving. Families may feel uncomfortable discussing the issue or may not have the resources or desire

Table 60.7

Resources and Agencies on Older Adult Drivers for Clinicians

Subspecialists in medicine
Neuropsychologists
Occupational and physical therapists
AARP 55 Alive Program
American Association of Automotive Medicine
Transportation Research Board
National Safety Council
Department of Motor Vehicles
Department of Transportation
Insurance companies

to become responsible for the patient's transportation. Revocation of a driver's license may force the patient to move or enter a residential or long-term care facility. Therefore, patients and families do not always comply or agree with the staff's recommendations.

Physicians may simply decide to document this refusal to comply in the chart, as long as the information is given to someone with decision-making capacity. However, this situation may justify a letter to the DMV. This breach of confidentiality is ethically appropriate when performed in the best interest of the patient and the community (7). A general precedent is that physicians have responsibilities to warn their patients if they are at risk for injury (88). A letter to the DMV does not have to state the driver's specific diagnosis; stating the diagnosis could be viewed as a breach of confidentiality without a signed release from the patient. The letter can simply state that there is a concern about the person's ability to drive safely because of an unspecified medical condition. Most state departments call in the driver and require him or her to sign a release of information that allows a dialog between the driver's physician and the DMV. The state ultimately must decide whether someone can remain licensed to drive. Most states have a process that allows for appeals in case the driver wishes to reinstate a revoked license.

Physicians may fear litigation from the patient or family for a breach of confidentiality when they report their concerns to the DMV. However, a physician can be held liable for not reporting a patient's medical condition to the DMV if the driver causes harm in a crash. Thus, the physician may be caught in a double legal bind. The decision to report patients to the DMV varies with personal practices and state requirements. Since the common law and statutes vary among states, legal counsel should guide the evaluation process and determine the regulations that apply for each locality.

Screens for medical impairments during license renewal are unfortunately not consistent across states, despite some evidence that suggests even very brief measures may be beneficial (89). Many states have laws that address specific medical diagnoses. Some require drivers to reveal any medical history such as diabetes or a seizure disorder during license renewal. Many states address certain diseases and require a specific period of stability if the disease becomes active. Recently, some states, including California, have required physicians to report diseases such as Alzheimer's disease to the public health department, which in turn notifies the DMV. The DMV then evaluates the driver, usually by a road test. Some clinicians have expressed concerns that this policy will lead patients to avoid medical care or will put physicians at odds with their patients. The risks, benefits, and cost of this type of approach are unknown.

States vary in their efforts and success in legislating safety. Many laws to improve road safety are crafted and proposed, only to be tabled by special interest groups or placed on low priority by legislators. In Missouri, we are in the third year in attempts to pass a law to identify and address the issues of the medically impaired driver. This law would allow for family members to report unsafe drivers; at present only physicians, judges, and the license renewal staff are allowed this privilege. The law would also establish a medical advisory board, giving it the authority to make decisions. Finally, the law would require a brief cognitive test in addition to the visual test during license renewal.

Very few states are successful in passing age-related restrictions for license renewal. In addition, strong lobby groups such as the AARP oppose age-related legislation that would cause additional burden and focus only on the older driver population. They point to the small number of older drivers who are in crashes and the fact that most older drivers are safe. As discussed previously, age is a poor predictor of performance. Focusing on functional variables and disease states again appears most appropriate for public policy issues. States can require physicians to refer drivers with a specific diagnosis (the mandatory approach). Some states make reporting voluntary and give the physician legal immunity in case of a referral.

FUTURE RESEARCH NEEDS AND CONCLUSIONS

Most research on older drivers focuses on methods to identify the driver who is at risk for a motor vehicle crash, medically impaired, or at risk for driving cessation. The useful field of view should be examined in additional settings to determine whether it is efficacious for a general population of older drivers. This test may be useful as a secondary screen after drivers fail their brief visual or cognitive screen during license renewal. Additional physiologic factors should be studied, because they may help to predict who is unsafe behind the wheel. Research should begin to focus on improving driving skills in frail older adults. More viable treatment options for Alzheimer's disease are becoming available. The effect on driving skills for those in the early stages of the disease may also be a fruitful area for study.

More older adults will be driving in the next few decades. Many will be safe and should not be the focus of intensive testing by primary care physicians or by the DMV during license renewal. However, some older adults have physiologic impairments caused by medical diseases. A comprehensive step-by-step approach appears to be the most appropriate method to assess older adult drivers whose driving competency has been questioned. Many diseases that affect driving can be detected and treated by the primary care physician. Physicians should take an active role in assessing risk of injury in a motor vehicle and driving cessation in their patients. Referral to additional sources may be helpful in the evaluation and treatment process. Empathy, sensitivity, and counseling to discuss alternative methods of transportation are necessary when driving is no longer permissible or possible for the older adult.

REFERENCES

1. O'Neill D. Physicians, elderly drivers, and dementia. Lancet 1992;339:41–43.
2. Malfetti J, ed. Drivers Fifty-Five Plus. Falls Church, VA: AAA Foundation for Traffic Safety 1985.
3. Marottoli RA, Ostfeld AM, Merrill SS, et al. Driving cessation and changes in mileage driven among elderly individuals. J Gerontol 1993;48:S255–S260.
4. Carr D, Jackson T, Alquire P. Characteristics of an elderly driving population referred to a geriatric assessment center. J Am Geriatr Soc 1990;38:1145–1150.
5. Retchin SM, Anapolle J. An overview of the older driver. Clin Geriatr Med 1993;9:279–296.
6. Foley DJ, Wallace RB, Eberhard J. Risk factors for motor vehicle crashes among older drivers in a rural community. J Am Geriatr Soc 1995;43:776–781.
7. Graca JL. Driving and aging. Clin Geriatr Med 1986;2:577.
8. Evans L. Older driver involvement in fatal and severe traffic crashes. J Gerontol 1988;43:S186–S193.
9. Reuben D, Silliman R, Traines M. The aging driver. Medicine, policy, and ethics. J Am Geriatr Soc 1988;36:1135–1142.
10. Waller J. Cardiovascular disease, aging, and traffic accidents. J Chron Dis 1967;20:615–620.
11. Odenheimer G. Dementia and the older driver. Clin Geriatr Med 1993;9:349–364.
12. Jorm AF, Korten AE, Henderson AS. The prevalence of dementia: a quantitative integration of the literature. Acta Psychiatr Scand 1987;76:465–479.
13. Lucas-Blaustein M, Filipp L, Dungan C, Tune L. Driving in patients with dementia. J Am Geriatric Soc 1988;36:1087–1091.
14. Gilley D, Wilson R, Bennett D, et al. Cessation of driving and unsafe motor vehicle operation by dementia patients. Arch Intern Med 1991;151:941–946.
15. Fitten LJ, Perryman KM, Wilkinson CJ, et al. Alzheimer and vascular dementias and driving. JAMA 1995:273;1360–1365.
16. Hunt L, Morris JC, Edwards D, et al. Driving performance in persons with mild senile dementia of the Alzheimer type. J Am Geriatr Soc 1993;41:747–752.
17. Stutts JC, Stewart JR, Martell C. Cognitive test performance and crash risk in an older driver population. Accid Anal Prev 1998;30:337–346.
18. Friedland R, Koss E, Kumar A, et al. Motor vehicle crashes in dementia of the Alzheimer type. Ann Neurol 1988;24:782–786.
19. Drachman D, Swearer J. Driving and Alzheimer's disease: the risk of crashes. Neurol 1993;43:2448–2456.
20. Dubinsky R, Williamson A, Gray C, Glatt S. Driving in Alzheimer's disease. J Am Geriatr Soc 1992;40:1112–1116.
21. Trobe JD, Waller PF, Cook-Flannagan CA, et al. Crashes and violations among drivers with Alzheimer disease. Arch Neurol 1996;53:411–416.
22. Kane R, Ouslander J, Abrass I. Demography and epidemiology. In: Kane R, Ouslander J, Abrass I, eds. Es-

sentials of Clinical Geriatrics. New York: McGraw-Hill, 1984:21.

23. Rice D, MacKenzie E. Cost of Injury in the United States: A Report to Congress. San Francisco: Institute for Health and Aging, University of California, and Injury Prevention Center, Johns Hopkins University, 1989.

24. Research and Development Needs for Maintaining the Safety and Mobility of Older Drivers. Transportation Research Circular 398, May 1992.

25. Sabey BE, Staughton GC. Interacting Roles of Road Environment, Vehicle and Road Use in Accidents. V International Conference of the International Association of Accident and Traffic Medicine, London, 1975.

26. Michon JA. A critical review of driver behavior models: what do we know, what should we do? In: Evans L, Schwing RC, eds. Human Behavior and Traffic Safety. New York: Plenum, 1985:487–525.

27. Introduction to motor vehicle crashes. In: The Injury Fact Book 1992. New York: Oxford University Press, 1992:213.

28. Waller J. A Guide to the Causes and Prevention of Trauma. Oxford: Lexington Books, 1985.

29. Ball K, Owsley C. Identifying correlates of accident involvement for the older driver. Hum Factors 1991:33; 583–595.

30. Shinar D, Schieber F. Visual requirements for safety and mobility of older drivers. Hum Factors 1991;33:505–519.

31. Crancer JA Jr, McMurray L. Accident and violation rates of Washington's medically restricted drivers. JAMA 1968;205:272–276.

32. Hansotia P, Broste SK. The effect of epilepsy or diabetes mellitus on the risk of automobile accidents. N Engl J Med 1991;324:22–26.

33. Wilson T, Smith T. Driving after stroke. Int Rehabil Med 1983;5:170–177.

34. Doege TC, Engelberg AL, eds. Medical Conditions Affecting Drivers. Chicago: American Medical Association, 1986.

35. Waller JA. Chronic medical conditions and traffic safety: review of the California experience. N Engl J Med 1965;273:1413–1420.

36. Findley LJ, Unverzagt ME, Suratt PM. Automobile accidents involving patients with obstructive sleep apnea. Am Rev Respir Dis 1988;138:337–340.

37. Roberts WN, Roberts P. Evaluation of the elderly driver with arthritis. Clin Geriatr Med 1993;9:311–322.

38. Ray WA, Gurwitz J, Decker MD, Kennedy DL. Medications and the safety of the older driver: is there a basis for concern? Hum Factors 1992;34:33–47.

39. Waller J. Physician's role in highway safety. Functional impairment in driving. N Y State J Med 1980;80: 1987–1991.

40. Koepsell TD, Wolf ME, McCloskey L, et al. Medical conditions and motor vehicle collision injuries in older adults. J Am Geriatr Soc 1994;42:695–700.

41. Wallace RB, Retchin SM. A geriatric and gerontologic perspective on the effects of medical conditions on older drivers: discussion of Waller. Hum Factors 1992;34:17–24.

42. Kline D, Schieber F. Vision and aging. In: Birren JE, Schaie KW, eds. Handbook of the Psychology of Aging. 3rd ed. New York: Van Nostrand Reinhold, 1990: 296.

43. Olsho L, Harkins S, Lenhardt M. Aging and the auditory system. In: Birren JE, Schaie KW, eds. Handbook of the Psychology of Aging. 3rd ed. New York: Van Nostrand Reinhold, 1990:332.

44. Olson PL, Sivak M. Perception-response time to unexpected roadway hazards. Hum Factors 1986;28:-91–96.

45. Salthouse T. Speed of behavior and its implications for cognition. In: Birren JE, Schaie KW, eds. Handbook of the Psychology of Aging. 2nd ed. New York: Van Nostrand Reinhold, 1985:400–426.

46. Davison P. Inter-relationships between British drivers' visual abilities, age, and road accident histories. Ophthalmol Physiol 1985;5:195–204.

47. Shinar D. Driver Visual Limitations, Diagnosis, and Treatment. Tech report DOT-HS-5–01275. Bloomington: Indiana University, 1977.

48. Henderson R, Burg A. Vision and audition in driving. Final report DOT-HS-009–1–009. Santa Monica, CA: Systems Development Corp, 1974.

49. Burg A. The Relationship Between Vision Test Scores and Driving Record: General Findings. Report 67–24. Los Angeles: University of California, Los Angeles Department of Engineering, 1967.

50. Burg A. Vision Test Scores and Driving Record: Additional Findings. Report 68–27. Los Angeles: Department of Engineering, University of California, 1968.

51. Johnson CA, Keltner JL. Incidence of visual field loss in 20,000 eyes and its relationship to driving performance. Arch Ophthalmol 1983;101:371–375.

52. van Zomeren AH, Brouwer WH, Minderhoud JM. Acquired brain damage and driving: a review. Arch Phys Med Rehabil 1987;68:697–705.

53. Mihal W, Barrett G. Individual differences in perceptual information processing and their relation to automobile involvement. J Appl Psychol 1976;6:229–233.

54. Avolio B, Kroeck K, Panek P. Individual differences in information-processing ability as a predictor of motor vehicle accidents. Hum Factors 1985;27:577–587.

55. Ponds R, Brouwer W, Wolffelaar. Age differences in divided attention in a simulated driving task. J Gerontol 1988;43:P151–156.

56. Ball K, Beard B, Roenker D, et al. Age and visual search: expanding the useful field of view. J Opt Soc Am [A] 1988;5:2210–2219.

57. Owsley C, Ball K, Sloane M, et al. Visual/cognitive correlates of vehicle accidents in older drivers. Psychol Aging 1991;6:403–415.

58. Reuben D. Assessment of older drivers. Clin Geriatr Med 1993;9;449–459.

59. Underwood M. The older driver: clinical assessment and injury prevention. Arch Intern Med 1992;152:735–740.

60. Marottoli R, Drickamer M. Psychomotor mobility and the elderly driver. Clin Geriatr Med 1993;9:403–411.

61. Marottoli RA, Cooney LM, Wagener DR, et al. Predictors of automobile crashes and moving violations among elderly drivers. Ann Intern Med 1994;121:842–846.

62. Mawson AR, Biundo JJ. Contrasting beliefs and actions of drivers regarding seat belts: a study in New Orleans. J Trauma 1985;25:433–437.

63. Hunt DK, Lowenstein SR, Badgett RG, Steiner JF. Safety belt nonuse by internal medicine patients: a missed opportunity in clinical preventive medicine. Am J Med 1995;98:343–348.

64. Campbell MK, Bush TL, Hale WE. Medical conditions associated with driving cessation in community-dwelling, ambulatory elders. J Gerontol 1993;48;S230–S234.

65. Roper TA, Mulley GP. Caring for Older People. Public transport. BMJ 1996;313:415–418.

66. Wiseman EJ, Souder E. The older driver: A handy tool to assess competence behind the wheel. Geriatrics 1996; 51:36–45.

67. Carr DB. Assessing older drivers for physical and cognitive impairment. Geriatrics 1993;48:46–52.

68. Carr D, Schmader K, Bergman C, et al. A multidisciplinary approach in the evaluation of demented drivers referred to geriatric assessment centers. J Am Geriatr Soc 1991;39:1132–1136.

69. Evans D, Funkenstein H, Albert A, et al. Prevalence of Alzheimer's disease in a community population of older persons: higher than previously reported. JAMA 1989; 26:2551–2556.

70. Hemmelgarn B, Suissa S, Huang A, et al. Benzodiazepine use and the risk of motor vehicle crash in the elderly. JAMA 1997;278:27–31.

71. Stuck AF, van Gorp WG, Josephson KR, et al. Multidimensional risk assessment versus age as criterion for retirement of airline pilots. J Am Geriatr Soc 1992;40: 526–532.

72. Anderson KM, Wilson PW, Odell PM, Kannel WB. An updated coronary risk profile. Circulation 1991;83: 356–362.

73. Wolf PA, D'Agostino RB, Blanger AJ, Kannel WB. Probability of stroke: a risk profile from the Framingham Study. Stroke 1991;22:312–318.

74. Johansson K, Bronge L, Lundberg C, et al. Can a physician recognize an older driver with increased crash risk potential? J Am Geriatr Soc 1996;44:1198–1204.

75. O'Neill D. The older driver. Rev Clin Gerontol 1996;6: 1–8.

76. Donnelly, R, Karlinsky H. The impact of Alzheimer's disease on driving ability: a review. J Geriatr Psychiatry Neurol 1990;3:67–72.

77. Kapust L, Weintraub S. To drive or not to drive: preliminary results from road testing of patients with dementia. J Geriatr Psychiatry Neurol 1992;5:210–216.

78. Fox GK, Bowden SC, Bashford GM, et al. Alzheimer's Disease and Driving: Prediction and Assessment of Driving Performance. J Am Geriatr Soc 1997;45:949–953.

79. Storandt M, Botwinick J, Danziger W, et al. Psychometric differentiation of mild senile dementia of the Alzheimer type. Arch Neurol 1984;41:497–499.

80. Hutton JT. Eye movements and Alzheimer's disease: significance and relationship to visuospatial confusion. In: Hutton JT, Kenny AD, eds. Senile Dementia of the Alzheimer Type. New York: Alan R Liss, 1985:3–33.

81. Teng EL, Chui HC, Schneider LS, et al. Alzheimer's dementia: performance on the Mini-Mental State examination. J Consult Clin Psychol 1987;55:96–100.

82. Nissen MJ, Corkin S, Buonanno FS, et al. Spatial vision in Alzheimer's disease: general findings and a case report. Arch Neurol 1985;42:667–671.

83. Gustafson L. Psychiatric symptoms in dementia with onset in the presenile period. Acta Psychiatr Scand Suppl 1975;257:7–35.

84. Parasuraman R, Nestor P. Attention and driving skills in aging and Alzheimer's disease. Hum Factors 1991;33: 539–557.

85. Olson CM. Vision-related problems may offer clues for earlier diagnosis of Alzheimer's disease. JAMA 1989; 261:1259.

86. Steffes R, Thralow J. Visual field limitation in the patient with dementia of the Alzheimer's type. J Am Geriatr Soc 1987;35:198–204.

87. Tuokko H, Beattie BC, Tallman K, et al. Predictors of motor vehicle crashes in a dementia clinic population: the role of gender and arthritis. J Am Geriatr Soc 1995; 43:1444–1445.

88. Gooden v Tips, 651 S.W.2d 364 (Tex. App.1983).

89. Levy DT, Vernick JS, Howard KA. Relationship between driver's license renewal policies and fatal crashes involving drivers 70 years and older. JAMA 1995;274: 1026–1030.

Accidents in the Elderly

Despite advances in accident prevention, which have resulted in a decline in the accidental death rate over the past 30 years, accidents remain a common cause of death and disability in the older population. Accidents are the seventh leading cause of death in the population aged 65 to 84 and equal diabetes mellitus as the sixth most common cause in those over age 85 (1). The incidence of accident-related death increases with each decade after age 65 (2) (Fig. 61.1).

Falls, motor vehicle accidents, fires, choking, and poisoning are the major causes of accidental death in the elderly, claiming thousands of lives annually (Fig. 61.2). Most nonvehicular accidents occur in the home. Long-term care facilities and hospitals are the sites of fewer than 10% of such deaths.

In addition to the mortality caused by accidents, there is a notable effect on quality of life from accident-induced injury. The best example is hip fractures caused by falls. Not only does the injury directly impair functional capacity, but the fear of falling again often results in restricted activity, whether imposed by the person who fell or by family members. Sometimes the concern for injury may even result in placement of the elderly person in an institution. Fear of an automobile accident also may restrict activity and increase dependence. Accidents such as falls may be markers for overall deterioration in health status of an older adult. Accidental injuries that reduce mobility and functional ability may begin a cascade of consequences that eventually lead to death from other illnesses.

Research into the causes and prevention of accidents leads to insights on interventions to decrease the effects of accidents in the elderly population. Incorporating this knowledge into everyday practice to assess a patient's risk of accidental injury or death can help determine strategies to reduce this risk.

FALLS

Each year one third of community-dwelling elderly persons over age 65 fall (3). The proportion increases to about half by age 80. About half of those who fall do so more than once. Each year more than half the ambulatory residents of extended care facilities fall. The seriousness of falls in the older population is more than just a matter of frequency; the frail elderly are likely to suffer serious injury (4). Falls are the leading cause of accidental death in the population over age 65, accounting for 10,300 deaths in 1993 (2). The number of deaths annually from falls peaks around age 85. Falls are both a marker for and a cause of short-term adverse health outcomes. Only about half of the elderly admitted to a hospital after a fall are alive a year later. Recurrent falls are frequently cited as one reason for admission of previously independent elders to nursing homes.

Fortunately, most falls do not produce serious injury. About 5% of falls result in a fracture or hospitalization, and fewer than 1% result in a hip fracture (5). More common fractures are those of the humerus, wrist, and pelvis. Soft tissue injuries such as hemarthroses, sprains, dislocations, and bruises often require medical attention.

The effect of hip fracture on an older person's health and function is well documented. The effects of other fractures from falls have not been

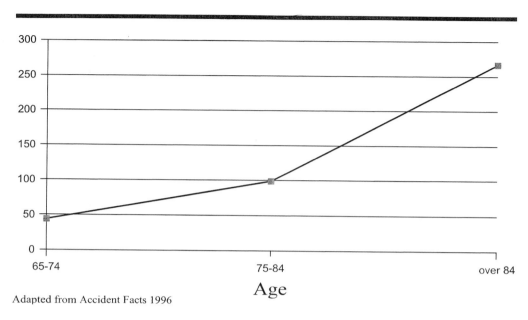

Adapted from Accident Facts 1996

Figure 61.1. Accidental death rate per 100,000 population, 1993. (Adapted from Accident Facts, 1996. Chicago: National Safety Council, 1996.)

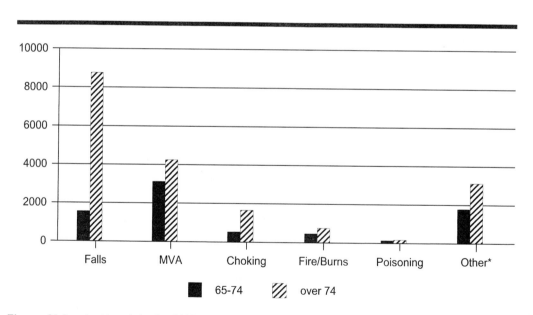

Figure 61.2. Accidental deaths, 1993. "Other" includes medical and surgical complications, air and water transport, machinery, and excessive cold. *MVA,* motor vehicle accidents.

described. Beyond the morbidity and mortality associated with falls is another factor that adversely affects the quality of life of the older person who falls. Fear of falling may cause a restriction of activities, either self-imposed or imposed by caregivers. Half of those who fall report being afraid of falling, and one in four admit to limiting essential activities of daily living at home (6).

Families frequently cite recurrent falling as one reason for admission to nursing homes. Unfortunately, restraints remain the primary means of preventing frequent falls in nursing homes. Although restraints may decrease the number of falls, they have been shown to do more harm than good; they insult the older person's dignity; and they should be avoided (7).

Causes of Falls

Falls result from a complex interaction of intrinsic and environmental factors (3, 8, 9). About 40% of falls involve some type of interaction with an environmental hazard. About 10% are related to acute medical illness, such as pneumonia or congestive heart failure, although some classify these as multifactorial. Another 5% result from an overwhelming intrinsic event such as a stroke or syncopal event. Attempts to devise uniform classifications for the causes of falls in the elderly have proved the task difficult. The interactions of the elderly person, activity, and environmental factors may vary with each event.

Intrinsic Risk Factors

The intrinsic risk factors that predispose the older person to falling comprise multiple diseases and disabilities superimposed on the physiologic changes of aging. Maintaining an upright posture and walking are complex acts requiring the integration of a number of systems. Dysfunction in one system may affect the functioning of other systems, increasing the risk of falling.

Within the nervous system, conditions affecting the central integrative function, the special senses, and peripheral sensory function can contribute to falls (10, 11). With normal aging, reaction time is slowed, primarily because of prolonged integrative function in the central nervous system. Diseases that impair this central sensory integration and response, such as Parkinson's disease, stroke, and dementia, have been associated with an increased incidence of falls (12).

Vision is also an important factor in balance and walking (13, 14). With normal aging there is a decrease in the amount of light transmitted to the retina. Light-dark adaptation is slow, glare is not well tolerated, and both near and peripheral vision decline. Cataracts, glaucoma, and di-

abetic retinopathy can intensify these limitations. Bifocal lenses may heighten the risk of falls in circumstances such as descending stairs.

Whether presbycusis is accompanied by an age-related change in vestibular function is unclear. However, a number of conditions common in the elderly are well known to affect balance. Benign positional vertigo is common in the elderly, as is exposure to aminoglycosides, furosemide, and other ototoxic agents.

Proprioception appears to decline with age; one of three elderly patients have a clinically detectable abnormality of position sense. There is evidence that the cervical spine has an important role in maintaining balance. Proprioceptive abnormalities resulting from cervical spondylosis due to underlying arthritis may affect the balance.

Conditions affecting the musculoskeletal system, especially the lower extremities, may impair stability and increase the likelihood of falling. Some elderly patients have a weakness in ankle dorsiflexion, which may explain their propensity to fall over backward with minimal displacement (14). Other common conditions affecting the muscles and joints, such as myopathies, strokes with hemiparesis, and arthritis, also may contribute to the risk of falling. Osteoarthritis of the knees often results in quadriceps weakness, and weakness of the hip musculature and quadriceps is a significant factor in falls. Foot disorders, such as hammer toes, bunions, painful calluses, and nail deformities, can pose significant problems in gait, particularly when they are compounded by inappropriate footwear.

A number of other conditions have been implicated as causative factors in falls. Several age-related physiologic changes predispose the elderly to orthostatic hypotension. The use of medications such as diuretics, antihypertensives, and antidepressants may contribute to orthostasis. Diseases resulting in abnormalities of autonomic nervous system function, such as diabetes mellitus and Parkinson's disease, can also lead to orthostasis. Although orthostatic hypotension is less common than previously thought and its role as a cause of falls is disputed, it should be considered as a contributing factor when the fall occurs while the person is in the act of standing up or after a meal (15).

Medications play a significant role in falls among the elderly. Most frequently implicated are benzodiazepines, either long acting or in high doses; antidepressants; and phenothiazines (16, 17). Other medications, such as diuretics, antihypertensives, and cardiac medications, may also contribute to falling. Recent studies fail to show an association of alcohol consumption with falls and injury (18). These studies may have been limited, however, by the use of self-report of alcohol consumption and underrepresentation of heavy drinkers in the study population (19). The role of alcohol in recurrent falls remains under study. One in ten elderly persons suffers from depression, which has been associated with an increased risk of falls independent of the effect of medication. The increased risk may be due to a lack of attention to environmental hazards, a decline in general health associated with depression, or a desire to injure oneself.

Finally, cardiorespiratory diseases, metabolic disorders, or other systemic illnesses may compromise the complex functions responsible for stability. Medications used to treat these conditions may further increase the risk of falling.

Activity

Most falls among both community and institutionalized elderly occur during routine daily activities that involve only mild to moderate displacement. Modest regular physical activity might be assumed to increase strength, endurance, coordination, and balance, thereby reducing the chance of falling. However, this higher level of activity results in an increased number of opportunities to fall and thus a higher rate of falls (3).

Environmental Factors

Most falls by community-dwelling elderly occur in the home, and about half involve an environmental hazard (3, 6, 9, 20). Approximately 10% of falls are on stairs, usually because they are poorly lighted or not equipped with handrails or because of visual impairment or bifocal lenses. Descending stairs appears to be more difficult, especially for elderly women, than ascending stairs. Most falls at home are caused by tripping. Pets, furniture, electrical cords, and even grandchildren have been implicated. Other frequently cited household hazards include slippery floors, loose throw rugs, doorway thresholds, stepladders, and slippery bathtubs. Finally, because visual perceptual problems are common in the elderly, distracting optical patterns on stairs, escalators, and floor coverings may also pose a threat.

Evaluation

The purpose of evaluation is to identify risk factors that can be modified. Because the likelihood of falling increases with the number of risk factors, correcting even a few of them can significantly reduce the risk of falling (21). A careful history, a complete medical examination, and an assessment of gait and balance are the key elements. Because falls are a common underreported problem in the elderly, clinicians should include asking about falls as part of the routine review of systems (22, 23).

Patients may be vague about the history. They may say that they tripped over something or just went down. Additional history from a third party is helpful but usually is more available in the hospital or nursing home than in the home. Clinicians should elicit information about what the patient was doing at the time of the fall and any associated symptoms he or she may have had preceding and following the fall. Specific questions are useful: Did the fall follow a change in position from sitting to standing? Did the patient have dizziness or syncope at the time of the fall? Was there pain or weakness in one or both extremities? Finally, the clinician should perform a careful review of medications, with special attention to drugs associated with falls, such as benzodiazepines, antidepressants, and phenothiazines. A general medical history identifies chronic diseases, such as diabetes, Parkinson's disease, and arthritis, that increase the likelihood of falling.

The complete physical examination should give special emphasis to the neurologic and musculoskeletal systems. Although the relation between postural hypotension and falls remains controversial, supine and standing blood pressure at 1 and 5 minutes should be measured.

The neurologic examination should include a formal assessment of the patient's mental status using an instrument such as the Folstein Mini-Mental State Examination, a test of visual acuity, and an evaluation of lower-extremity strength and sensation, including touch, proprioception, and position sense. Increased muscle tone or cogwheeling should be noted. Cerebellar function should also be tested. The musculoskeletal system should be examined for conditions such as arthritis of the hip or knees or foot problems, which can hinder walking. The remainder of the physical examination should identify systemic diseases that may compromise a function of the systems involved in gait.

Balance and gait should be assessed with a series of maneuvers that replicate the usual tasks required in the activities of daily living. Two simple tests of balance and gait are easily administered in the office. The get-up-and-go test and the performance-oriented assessment of mobility entail observing position changes and common maneuvers such as reaching up, turning, and bending over (24). Gait is observed for initiation, step height, length, continuity and symmetry, speed, path deviation, and turning. This is accomplished by having the patient get up from a chair, walk a distance at a usual rapid pace, and return to the examiner. At that time balance may be assessed by observing the patient react to an external nudge, stand with eyes closed, reach up, bend over, and turn the neck from side to side. After the patient completes these maneuvers, the examiner observes the patient sitting in the chair without using the hands. If the patient uses an assistive device such as a cane, the assessment should be done with and without the aid. The assistive device should be evaluated for proper function and safety.

The role of laboratory and diagnostic studies has not been rigorously assessed. Generally recommended are complete blood count, electrolytes, glucose, blood urea nitrogen, creatinine, urinalysis, and thyroid function tests, with further testing as indicated by the history and physical examination (25). A chest radiograph and resting electrocardiogram may be reserved for those in whom a cardiopulmonary problem is suspected. Patients with syncope and palpitations or pulse irregularities warrant Holter monitoring, but it should not be a routine part of the diagnostic workup (26). Electronystagmography may be helpful in cases of true vertigo.

Typically this evaluation reveals multiple risk factors possibly contributing to the fall. Once they have been identified, a systematic approach to modifying them should begin. As they are resolved, new factors may emerge, creating the need for continual reassessment of risks for falling.

Prevention

Interventions aimed at reducing fall-related injury should address patient, environment, and activities. The Frailty Injuries: Cooperative Studies of Intervention Techniques (FICSIT) trials have shown that short-term exercise (10 to 36 weeks) can reduce falls and fall-related injuries (27). Shorter and less intensive interventions have proven to be less successful (28). Motivated persons should be encouraged to participate in appropriate exercise programs. For others, it is reasonable to attempt to reduce the number of contributing risk factors without creating new ones. For example, the treatment of depression, a known risk factor for falls, should be weighed against the use of tricyclic antidepressants, another known risk factor. The use of a cane or walker may be helpful at times, but such devices may also contribute to falls if used incorrectly.

A number of home hazard checklists have been developed to help older persons make their homes safer. Many hazards can be eliminated by proper lighting, hand rails and grab bars, non-slippery floor surfaces, and removal of obstacles. High-risk areas such as bathrooms and stairs should have special attention. However, older persons often are reluctant to make even small changes in their environment. Careful education with follow-up by a home health nurse, physical therapist, or occupational therapist can help improve compliance with recommendations.

Patients should also be counseled to avoid clearly hazardous and probably unnecessary activities such as climbing on ladders, stools, or chairs, and walking on ice. However, activities that improve strength, flexibility, and endurance, such as regular exercising and climbing stairs, should be encouraged. It is important for the patient to try to achieve a balance between excessive concern about falls and the need to maintain mobility and functional independence.

MOTOR VEHICLE ACCIDENTS

Elderly drivers account for a minority of injuries from motor vehicle accidents. Drivers over age 65 do, however, have a higher crash rate per miles driven than the general population. The rate of involvement in a fatal accident per 100,000 drivers is lowest for the age group 65 to 74; for those over 75, the rate is about equal to that of the age group 25 to 34 (2). The low rate is due mainly to the fact that older drivers drive fewer miles. When the fatality rate is adjusted for miles driven, 70-year-old drivers have 3 times the rate of fatal accidents as 20-year-olds have. As the population ages, the increase in older drivers is likely to result in an increased number of accidents. In 1993 motor vehicle accidents accounted for 7,350 deaths in persons over age 65, making them the second leading cause of accidental death in older Americans.

The increase in frequency of motor vehicle accidents probably results from a combination of the normal physiologic changes of aging and the chronic medical conditions prevalent in this population. Medications with central nervous system effects, including benzodiazepines, tricyclic antidepressants, and antihistamines, that have the potential to impair driving ability are commonly used in this population (29).

A number of physiologic and pathologic changes associated with increased age result in a decline in vision as one ages. Visual acuity, visual field, and night vision all decline, and light-dark adaptation is delayed (30). Visual perceptual changes interact closely with cognitive function. Visual attention and mental status may account for as much as 20% of the increased accident rate among older drivers (31). Among persons with dementia of the Alzheimer's type, performance on information-processing measures, specifically the switching of specific attention, divided attention, and sustained attention, are impaired in the early stages of the disease and may contribute to the increased accident risk (32).

In a study of the effects of age on motor function, participants were found to initiate and execute movements more slowly and with less precision as they age (33). Specific medical conditions such as hip disease also affect driving ability. Multiple conditions that impair activities of daily living also may adversely affect driving ability. Despite these changes, road test skills appear to be well preserved in the healthy elderly population (34). However, the relation between road test performance and accident rates has not been established. Further studies are needed to assess road test performance by elderly persons with single or multiple medical impairments and to determine correlations between road test performance and motor vehicle accidents (35).

Pedestrian Accidents

Of the 7350 deaths from motor vehicle accidents in 1993, about 1500 involved pedestrians. One-third more pedestrian deaths occurred in the age group over 75 than in the age group 65 to 74. Despite the observation that older pedestrians are the safest age group at intersections, standing the farthest away from traffic, appreciating the greater risk of injury at night, and exercising appropriate safety precautions, the majority of vehicular pedestrian deaths among the elderly occur at intersections (36). Decreased walking speed and the older person's difficulty in judging vehicle velocity may be factors. Only 5% of the elderly over age 70 can walk fast enough to cross safely at many intersections controlled by traffic lights, and one fourth of older pedestrians are unable to cross a typical busy urban intersection safely (37). Decreased peripheral vision and hearing, along with an increased reaction time, may also raise the risk. An investigation of traffic-related injuries to the elderly found that about half the injuries resulted from falls with no vehicular involvement (38). Many of the falls involved ice and snow, but high curbs also presented a problem. These nonvehicular hazards may distract the person from attending to traffic. Rates of injury are also higher in areas that have substantial business and commercial traffic.

Driver-Related Accidents

Elderly occupants of motor vehicles in accidents accounted for almost 4800 deaths in 1993. More than 90% occurred during the daytime and more than 90% involved two or more vehicles. More than 60% occurred at intersections, where timed perceptual decisions are crucial. Elders who are in a vehicular accident are at increased risk for injury and death, despite the fact that they tend to drive large cars and thus presumably have protection in an accident.

FIRES AND BURNS

When death from complications of medical and surgical procedures is excluded, death from fire is the fourth leading cause of accidental death in people over age 65. Some 1200 elders died of fire and burns in 1993. The majority of deaths were among those over age 75 (Fig. 61.2). About 90% of these occurred at home. Flame burns account for most burns in the elderly and scalds, about 20% (39). Burn rates for men tend to decrease with age, but they remain relatively constant for women. However, the mortality rate rises with age despite recent improvements in survival after burns. The elderly account for 12% of the overall population but almost 30% of fire deaths (40). Older African-Americans have 5 times the residential fire death rate of whites, and men have a higher rate than women. In part because of regulations requiring fire-resistant clothing for infants and young children, 80% of deaths from burning clothing are in the elderly. In fact, 27% of the female patients admitted to one burn center had been burned by clothing ignited during cooking (41).

Baux's formula, which equates burn mortality with the additive factors of burn surface area and the patient's age, was reaffirmed in 1984 despite recent improvements in the survival of elderly burn patients (42). However, early aggressive surgical treatment in one burn center improved survival from 37 to 52% over 10 years (43). The hospital length of stay of surviving patients was reduced by almost half. Another center reported an 80% overall survival rate for elderly burn patients and a 67% rate for patients over age 75 (44). In this group, mortality rate correlated with the patient's age, burn size, any inhalation injury, number of complications of care, and fluid resuscitation requirements but not with the number of preexisting medical problems. Aggressive surgical intervention was also used in this group, although others have questioned this approach.

Mortality data alone suggest that aggressive care for elderly patients with burn injuries is justified. But what about the quality of life after discharge? Studies of older burn victims have shown that most survivors return home, although about half require some assistance (45). About a fourth of those over age 75 require admission to a nursing home following discharge from a burn center, but only about 5% overall require institutionalization (46, 47). There is no difference in death rate of survivors in comparison with the normal population (48).

Prevention of fire and burn injuries requires an appreciation of the factors that may predispose the elderly to injury and death. In residential fires the elderly are prone to mental and physical conditions that impair ability to escape. Problems with vision, hearing, cognition, and mobility all may contribute. Burns from clothing fires may occur more frequently because of decline in overall physical condition, decreased sense of smell, arthritic hands, a weak grasp, and decreased reaction time. Many elderly have difficulty dropping to the floor and rolling, which is the recommended maneuver to extinguish burning clothes. Although the elderly realize the potential for tap water scald burns in their homes, few believe that exposure to hot-only tap water at temperatures common in many homes could cause a scald burn in 30 seconds or less. Furthermore, in one study previous victims of tap water scald burns had not lowered the settings of their hot water thermostats (49).

Cigarette smoking and excessive alcohol consumption play a well-recognized role in residential fires. Some 15% of those over 65 smoke, and 12% consume more than five alcoholic drinks per day. Continued efforts to promote smoking cessation and responsible alcohol use will decrease burn injuries in addition to promoting overall health. The use of fire-resistant upholstery and bed linens is increasing. Making fire-resistant clothing available to older persons as well as to infants would also be helpful. The development of a self-extinguishing cigarette is technically feasible but unlikely given the financial state of the tobacco industry.

By 1985, 74% of U.S. homes had smoke detectors, but the homes of older people and the poor were less likely to have them. Households without smoke detectors have a 50% higher risk of fire-related fatality than homes with smoke detectors. The early warning provided by a smoke detector may be especially important to an older person with impaired mobility.

Other preventive measures include lowering the hot water temperature to less than 120°F, preferably to about 110°; using stoves with front- or side-mounted controls; using microwave ovens instead of stoves; keeping fire extinguishers convenient and charged; ensuring that elderly persons are familiar with the use of fire extinguishers and have an escape plan in the event of fire and that they practice fire drills regularly.

POISONING

Poisoning is a significant problem in the elderly population, accounting for more than 500 deaths per year, or 13% of poisoning deaths in the United States. Most result from medications and most are unintentional (50). Confusion, dementia, mistaken identity of medications, and placing medicines in a container with an incorrect label all may contribute to this problem. The elderly are more vulnerable to toxicity and death from drugs because changes in body composition and renal and hepatic functioning affect pharmacokinetics. Underlying diseases, especially cardiovascular disease, also increase the risk of death from medication overdose. The elderly tend to be on multiple medications, both prescription and over the counter. Errors in taking medicines increase when three or more are prescribed.

Cardiovascular drugs account for about 40% of the deaths from medications, 3 times the frequency of the next category, analgesics, antipyretics, and antirheumatics (2). Other implicated agents are oral hypoglycemics, psychotherapeutics, and theophylline. In addition to death, adverse consequences of medication poisoning include falls, accidents, confusion, and hospital admissions.

Physicians should carefully counsel their older patients about use of medicines. Patients should be cautioned not to place medicine in a container other than the one in which it was dispensed, with the exception of organized daily dispenser systems. Medicines should be stored separately from household cleaners and chemicals. The physician should assess the literacy status of the older patient and take extra time to explain instructions to those who have difficulty reading. Large-type labels should be used on prescription bottles. In addition to carefully explaining a drug's effects, side effects, and precautions, the physician should frequently question the patient about adverse effects. Monitoring drug levels is important, especially digitalis levels and prothrombin times for patients on warfarin. Patients should be encouraged to bring their medicines to each office visit for review, and attempts should be made to discontinue medications whenever possible.

CHOKING

Accidental ingestion or inhalation of objects or food resulting in suffocation from obstructed respiratory passages is a common but little-studied problem in the elderly. Some 2200 elderly patients choked to death in 1993. About 200 fatal choking incidents occur each year in nursing homes and extended care facilities (51). A number of factors may contribute to death by choking in the older population. Cognitive impairment, swallowing disorders from cerebrovascular accidents or Parkinson's disease, and ill-fitting or absent dentures all may play a role (52). The use of psychotropic medications or alcohol may increase the risk of aspiration. In long-term care facilities, inadequate supervision during mealtime may result in aspiration of food. It is important that staff in such facilities be trained in appropriate first aid, such as the Heimlich maneuver. Further study of this significant cause of mortality in the elderly is needed.

REFERENCES

1. Vital Statistics of the United States 1990. Hyattsville, MD: US Department of Health and Human Services, 1994.
2. Accident Facts, 1996. Chicago: National Safety Council, 1996.
3. Tinetti ME, Speechley M, Ginter SF. Risk factors for falls among elderly persons living in the community. N Engl J Med 1988;319:1701–1707.
4. Sattin RW, Huber DA, DeVito CA, et al. The incidence of fall injury events among the elderly in a defined population. Am J Epidemiol 1990;131:1028–1037.
5. Nevitt MC, Cummings SR, Hudes ES. Risk factors for injurious falls: a prospective study. J Gerontol Med Sci 1991;46:M164–M170.
6. Nevitt MC, Cummings SR, Kidd S, Black D. Risk factors for recurrent nonsyncopal falls: a prospective study. JAMA 1989;261:2663–2668.

7. Rubenstein LZ, Josephson KR, Robbins AS. Falls in the nursing home. Ann Intern Med 1994;121:442–451.

8. Lipsitz LA, Jonsson PV, Kelly MM, Koestner JS. Causes and correlates of recurrent falls in ambulatory frail elderly. J Gerontol Med Sci 1991;46:M114–M122.

9. Robbins AS, Rubenstein LZ, Josephson KR, et al. Predictors of falls among elderly people: results of two population-based studies. Arch Intern Med 1989;149: 1628–1633.

10. Masdeu JC, Wolfson L, Lantos G, et al. Brain white-matter changes in the elderly prone to falling. Arch Neurol 1989;46:1292–1296.

11. Richardson JK, Ching C, Hurvitz ED. The relationship between electromyographically documented peripheral neuropathy and falls. J Am Geriatr Soc 1992;40:1008–1012.

12. Koller WC, Glatt S, Vetere-Overfield B, Hassanein R. Falls and Parkinson's disease. Clin Neuropharmacol 1989;12:98–105.

13. Felson DT, Anderson JJ, Hannan MT, et al. Impaired vision and hip fracture: the Framingham Study. J Am Geriatr Soc 1989;37:495–500.

14. Lord SR, Clark RD, Webster IW. Physiological factors associated with falls in an elderly population. J Am Geriatr Soc 1991;39:1194-1200.

15. Jonsson PV, Lipsitz LA, Kelley M, Koestner J. Hypotensive responses to common daily activities in institutionalized elderly: a potential risk for recurrent falls. Arch Intern Med 1990;150:1518–1524.

16. Kerman M, Mulvihill M. The role of medication in falls among the elderly in a long-term care facility. Mt Sinai J Med 1990;57:343–347.

17. Sorock GS, Shimkin EE. Benzodiazepine sedatives and the risk of falling in a community-dwelling elderly cohort. Arch Intern Med 1988;148:2441–2444.

18. Nelson DE, Sattin RW, Langlois JA, et al. Alcohol as a risk factor for fall injury events among elderly persons living in the community. J Am Geriatr Soc 1992;40: 658–661.

19. Carson JE. Alcohol use and falls. J Am Geriatr Soc 1993;41:346 (editorial).

20. DeVito CA, Lambert DA, Sattin RW, et al. Fall injuries among the elderly. J Am Geriatr Soc 1988;36:1029–1035.

21. Rubenstein LZ, Robbins AS, Josephson KR, et al. The value of assessing falls in an elderly population: a randomized clinical trial. Ann Intern Med 1990;113:308–316.

22. Campbell AJ, Borrie MJ, Spears GF, et al. Circumstances and consequences of falls experienced by a community population 70 years and over during a prospective study. Age Ageing 1990;19:136–141.

23. Cummings SR, Nevitt MC, Kidd S. Forgetting falls: the limited accuracy of recall of falls in the elderly. J Am Geriatr Soc 1988;36:613–616.

24. Tinetti ME, Williams TF, Mayewski R. Fall risk index or elderly patients based on number of chronic disabilities. Am J Med 1986;80:429–434.

25. Rubenstein LZ, Robbins AS, Schulman BL, et al. Falls and instability in the elderly. J Am Geriatr Soc 1988;36: 266–278.

26. Rosado JA, Rubenstein LZ, Robbins AS, et al. The value of Holter monitoring in evaluating the elderly patient who falls. J Am Geriatr Soc 1989;37:430–434.

27. Province MA, Hadley EC, Hornbrook MC, et al. The effects of exercise on falls in elderly patients: a preplanned meta-analysis of the FICSIT Trials. JAMA 1995;273: 1341–1347.

28. Hornbrook MC, Stevens VJ, Wingfield DJ, et al. Preventing falls among community-dwelling older persons: results from a randomized trial. Gerontologist 1994;34: 16–23.

29. Ray WA, Gurwitz J, Decker MD, Kennedy DL. Medications and the safety of the older driver: is there a basis for concern? Hum Factors 1992;34:33–47.

30. Klein R. Age-related eye disease, visual impairment and driving in the elderly. Hum Factors 1991;33:521–525.

31. Owsley C, Ball K, Sloane ME, et al. Visual/cognitive correlates of vehicle accidents in older drivers. Psychol Aging 1991;6:403–415.

32. Parasuraman R, Nestor PG. Attention and driving skills in aging and Alzheimer's disease. Hum Factors 1991;33: 539–557.

33. Stelmach GE, Nahom A. Cognitive-motor abilities of the elderly driver. Hum Factors 1992;34:53–65.

34. Carr D, Jackson TW, Madden DJ, Cohen HJ. The effect of age on driving skills. J Am Geriatr Soc 1992;40:567–573.

35. Carr D, Schmader K, Bergman C, et al. A multidisciplinary approach in the evaluation of demented drivers referred to geriatric assessment centers. J Am Geriatr Soc 1991;39:1132–1136.

36. Harrell WA. Perception of risk and curb standing at street corners by older pedestrians. Percept Mot Skills 1990;70:1363–1366.

37. Hoxie RE, Rubenstien LZ. Are older pedestrians allowed enough time to cross intersections safely? J Am Geriatr Soc 1994;42:241–244.

38. Sjogren H, Bjornstig U. Injuries to the elderly in the traffic environment. Accid Anal Prev 1991;23:77–86.

39. Ostrow LB, Bongard FS, Sacks ST, et al. Burns in the elderly. Am Fam Physician 1987;35:149–154.

40. Gulaid JA, Sacks JJ, Sattin RW. Deaths from residential fires among older people, United States 1984. J Am Geriatr Soc 1989;37:331–334.

41. Turner DG, Leman CJ, Jordan MH. Cooking-related burn injuries in the elderly: preventing the "granny gown" burn. J Burn Care Rehabil 1989;10:356–359.

42. Jerrard DA, Cappadoro K. Burns in the elderly patient. Emerg Med Clin North Am 1990;8:421–428.

43. Slater AL, Slater H, Goldfarb IW. Effect of aggressive surgical treatment in older patients with burns. J Burn Care Rehabil 1989;10:527–530.

44. Saffle JR, Larson CM, Sullivan J, Shelby J. The continuing challenge of burn care in the elderly. Surgery 1990; 108:534–543.

45. Larson CM, Saffle JR, Sullivan J. Lifestyle adjustments in elderly patients after burn injury. J Burn Care Rehabil 1992;13:48–52.

46. Hammond J, Ward CG. Burns in octogenarians. South Med J 1991;84:1316–1319.

47. Keys TC, Moresi JM, Deitch EA. Thermal injury in the elderly: the limited need for nursing home care. J Burn Care Rehabil 1989;10:494–531.

48. Manktelow A, Meyer AA, Herzog SR, Peterson HD. Analysis of life expectancy and living status of elderly patients surviving a burn injury. J Trauma 1989;29:203–207.

49. Adams LE, Purdue GF, Hunt JL. Tap-water scald burns: awareness is not the problem. J Burn Care Rehabil 1991;12:91–95.

50. Klein-Schwartz W, Oderda GM. Poisoning in the elderly: epidemiological, clinical and management considerations. Drugs Aging 1991;1:67–89.

51. Saunders LD, Green M, Doebbert G, et al. Mortality from unintentional injuries in California, 1985. West J Med 1989;150:478–483.

52. Ekberg O, Feinberg M. Clinical and demographic data in 75 patients with near-fatal choking episodes. Dysphagia 1992;7:205–208.

Acute and Chronic Care of the Elderly: Minimizing Iatrogenic Illness

For many clinicians care of the frail elderly patient is complicated not only by multiple often severe comorbidities but by the fear of doing harm while providing that care; many of the usual kinds of care provided for a younger patient may harm the older adult. Given that the elderly account for one third of hospital discharges and nearly half of inpatient days, it is essential that models of inpatient care for older persons be based on sound geriatric principles. In addition, the rate of hospitalization is highest among those over age 85 (1, 2). Errors of omission and commission should be important targets for risk reduction.

Any illness or impairment that results from a therapeutic intervention, a diagnostic procedure, or a failure to provide appropriate care can be viewed as iatrogenic. Not surprisingly, these occur most commonly in older patients. This is a result of a combination of factors. Age-related physiologic changes and decline in organ function account for many of the adverse reactions to medications and surgery and further contribute to declines resulting from untreated illness. The simple fact is that elderly patients have more comorbidities than younger ones. This increased exposure to medical interventions increases the risk for adverse consequences of care. Finally, combined social and psychologic conditions common among older patients play a significant and sometimes overriding role in choices about care and decisions about where care is to be provided.

AVOIDING IATROGENESIS IN GERIATRIC SYNDROMES
Polypharmacy: Medication Use, Misuse, and Overuse

Attention to reducing errors in medication use can significantly improve the care of older patients. Some 90% of Americans over age 65 take at least one prescription medication daily, and most take two or more (3). A number of factors contribute to this. On average, older people have more chronic medical problems than others. Elderly patients seek relief for common symptoms and ailments, often using nonprescription drugs and sometimes pursuing care from several physicians. The result may be overuse of medications. Of all of the areas under a clinician's purview, a patient's drug regimen is often most malleable. The geriatrics approach to polypharmacy, a highly individualized and continually updated medication plan that aims to limit iatrogenic complications, can also serve as a successful model of care generalizable to many medical issues.

Drugs and the Effects of Aging

The overall effects of a drug in an older adult depend on age-related changes in pharmacokinetics and pharmacodynamics. The results of these changes in elderly patients are generally prolonged activity, a variable (usually increased) drug effect, and an increase in the incidence of drug toxicity and adverse drug reactions (4). Aging commonly results in increased adipose tissue, decreased lean body mass, and a reduction in total body water. These can cause significant changes in drug levels and duration of action, increasing the risk of toxic effects. Table 62.1 contains examples of these changes and their effects. Being mindful of the how aging can affect the metabolism of drugs may reduce iatrogenic consequences of drug use in the older adult.

Adverse Drug Reactions

Symptoms commonly seen as a result of an adverse drug reaction include confusion, nausea, decreased balance, change in bowel pattern, and sedation. These common generic symptoms can be mistaken for other illnesses, and occasionally other medications are added to treat these symptoms. This increases the likelihood of a drug-drug interaction and additional side effects. The reported incidence of such adverse reactions is 2 to 10% in younger adults and rises to 20 to 25% in elderly patients. Its estimated that 3 to 10% of hospital admissions for elderly patients are due to adverse drug effects (5). Advanced age, female gender, low body weight, hepatic or renal insufficiency, polypharmacy, and a history of drug reactions are all associated with an increased risk of adverse drug reactions.

Optimal Medication Use

Although changes related to aging contribute to adverse drug reactions, it is conceivable that the likelihood of the elderly having an adverse drug reaction is simply due to the increased exposure to medications (6–9). Reducing the num-

Table 62.1

Aging Physiology: Medication Effects

Age-Related Changes	Possible Effects
Increased adipose tissue	Marked increase in $T_{1/2}$ of lipid-soluble drugs, e.g., benzodiazepines, barbiturates
Decrease in serum albumin by 15–20%, other plasma proteins (worsened by liver disease, acute or chronic illness)	High concentrations of digoxin, theophylline, phenytoin, warfarin; toxicity when drug displaced from protein-binding site by a second drug; free drug levels (not total) increased
Decreased lean body mass and muscle; Na/K ATPase	Increased digoxin levels
15% decrease in total body water (exacerbated by diuretics)	Increased concentrations of alcohol, lithium, cimetidine, digoxin
Elevated α_1-acid glycoproteins (acute phase reactant increased during inflammation, e.g., rheumatoid arthritis)	Decreased unbound (active) levels of lidocaine, propanol, due to increased binding
Decline in hepatic blood flow (45% reduction by age 65)	Major reduction in first-pass metabolism
Slow cytochrome P450 enzyme reactions with decline in phase I hepatic catabolism	Prolonged activity of diazepam, alprazolam (lorazepam, oxazepam, triazolam unaffected; no active metabolites)
Renal blood flow down 40%, renal function declines steadily (great variation)	Serum creatinine not reliable for renal function, even in normal range; higher levels of renally cleared drugs: aminoglycosides, digoxin, procainamide, vancomycin, lithium
Decreased adrenergic receptor response	Less bradycardia with β-blockers
Increased receptor response	Benzodiazepines: sedation; opioids: increased analgesia, respiratory suppression; warfarin: increased anticoagulation; increased anticholinergic effects on CNS, heart, bowel, bladder

ber of medications prescribed has been shown to decrease the likelihood of adverse drug reactions (10). Whenever an older patient has a change in condition or an acute illness, it is essential to consider whether a medication can be blamed. Virtually any medication can be the primary cause of a new symptom or loss of function. Alternatively, a patient's medicines can worsen the effects of an illness by contributing to cognitive and functional impairments.

How many drugs are too many is probably the wrong question, given the high degree of variation among older patients' health problems. What medicines does this patient really need may be more appropriate. Periodic review of a patient's medication list is an essential component in preventing iatrogenesis. Each medicine should be considered in terms of continued necessity, possible interactions, and risk-benefit ratio. Every additional medicine must be given similar scrutiny. Whenever there is a change in a person's condition, this kind of review is needed to assess for a drug's role in the underlying illness or its presentation, potential for excess dis-

ability, and likelihood of subsequent need. For example, in a patient who has had a massive stroke, the continued use of preventive medications such as aspirin and lipid-lowering agents may become much less important than measures to relieve comfort. Cost considerations are no small concern for most older patients, and the list of medicines must be viewed with affordability in mind, especially when adding more drugs. A clinician should be aware that withdrawing a medication carries the same risk as adding one: drug cessation can make the patient better or worse or have no effect at all. Table 62.2 contains some simple advice to assist in decisions about the use of medications in the older patient.

Delirium

Delirium, also known as acute confusional state, is a general disorder of cerebral metabolism and neurotransmission resulting in neuropsychiatric manifestations such as confusion, sleepiness, and agitation. Delirium is reported in 11 to 24% of older adults upon admission to the hospital and develops in another 5 to 35% of patients. Studies

Table 62.2

Practical Prescribing in the Elderly

Make a diagnosis before initiating drug therapy. Avoid treating symptoms empirically.

Establish a *therapeutic goal* or end point. Pick clear goals (e.g., duration of use, target blood pressure). Measure cognitive and functional status before treatment.

Consider *nondrug therapies* (behavior management, physical therapy for osteoarthritis, fiber and daily walks for constipation, calcium and daily walks for osteoporosis, exercise for almost everything).

Consider *when to avoid preventive medicines* (aspirin, warfarin, antihypertensives). After a major change in status, the goal may change from prevention to symptom relief or comfort care.

Consider *underlying physiologic defects:* renal insufficiency, congestive heart failure, dementia, alcoholism.

Take a *drug history.* Have patients *brown bag* their drugs to office visits. Ask about *nonprescription* drug use. Team up with pharmacy for details on refills or actual usage.

Start low. Start with small doses (e.g., *50 or 25% of usual dose* as a good estimate) to avoid toxicity. Use the lowest effective dose.

Go slow. Dose increases should be smaller and more widely spaced than usual. Consider weekly increments where possible.

Periodically review the medication list. *Discontinue* temporary use medications that are still being taken and others that are no longer needed. Check for *interactions.* Consider *dose reductions* where possible.

Simplify medication schedules to maximize compliance. Aim for *once to twice daily* dosing.

Suspect *a drug as the cause of any decline* in function or cognitive loss (confusion, falls, incontinence, inability to perform activities of daily living).

Discuss *why a medicine is being used, drug and nondrug* alternatives, *consequences* of noncompliance, common *adverse reactions,* and *what to do if they occur.* Provide this in a *written format.*

Become familiar with a few drugs *and stick with these (learn geriatrics dosing, expected effects).*

that used patient self-report of symptoms had an overall incidence of 58%, suggesting underrecognition. Not surprisingly, the incidence rises with age and degree of illness. However, this common condition is frequently unrecognized or misdiagnosed, especially in the elderly. After controlling for confounding factors, studies consistently find prolonged hospitalizations, impaired physical function, and an increased need for home care or institutionalization among delirious patients. In addition, the delirious patient may have difficulty understanding the plans for care, participating in rehabilitation, and giving consent for proposed procedures. The observed increase in short-term morbidity and mortality in the hospitalized older patient appears to depend more on advanced age and the severity of illness than on delirium. Therefore, delirium may be an indicator of severity of illness or disorders of grave prognosis.

Treatment of the underlying disorder usually produces rapid improvement of the delirium. However, there is increasing evidence that the symptoms of delirium are not transient but often persist, even with appropriate treatment. In a study of 125 elderly inpatients, only 4% showed complete resolution of the symptoms of delirium by the time of discharge. By 3 and 6 months after hospital discharge, only 21% and 18% respectively had resolution of all new delirium symptoms. Indeed, long and perhaps permanent memory impairment is common in subjects who have had delirium, persisting in up to 55% of those affected. Delirium may therefore be a harbinger for dementia rather than a cause.

Delirium is common in the hospitalized elderly, and therefore, all hospitalized elderly patients require careful evaluation and monitoring. The clinician must remain vigilant for evidence of inattention, deterioration in mental status, disorganized thinking and speech, and diminished alertness in all older patients. Serial or repeated assessments reduce the likelihood of missing the often transient and fluctuating symptoms.

Recognizing persons at risk for delirium can improve recognition of delirium itself and thereby reduce unnecessary complications. Of the many risk factors for the development of delirium, advanced age is associated with the highest risk. Elderly patients may be susceptible to delir-

ium as a result of physical changes associated with normal aging. As described earlier, these changes can lead to higher free (active) drug levels and toxicity. Consequently, dosages of medications that would be considered therapeutic in younger adults may be too high for elderly patients and cause toxic side effects in the form of delirium. Medications whose metabolism can be effected by changes in hepatic and renal function, such as many of the medications used for pain control and sleep disturbances, may therefore precipitate delirium. Abrupt withdrawal of certain medications can also predispose to delirium. Finally, decreases in cortical brain cells, acetylcholine storage, and muscarinic receptor plasticity associated with normal aging reduce neurologic reserve and increase the risk of delirium in the elderly, especially with the use of anticholinergic medications.

Alcohol intoxication and withdrawal are common causes of delirium but are often not suspected in the elderly. Agitation, anxiety, insomnia, tremors, and nausea may be mistakenly attributed to other causes when delirium is not considered. Many medications are thought to contribute to the development of delirium, most importantly neuroleptic and opioid use, postoperative meperidine, and long-acting benzodiazepines and anticholinergic drugs. Medications not commonly considered in association with anticholinergic effects, such as cimetidine, prednisolone, and theophylline, can actually produce significant anticholinergic toxicity, resulting in attention and memory impairment. Although it is not clear whether sensory deprivation (e.g., vision and hearing impairment, beds in rooms without windows), sensory overload (e.g., intensive care units), sleep deprivation, or transfer to an unfamiliar environment can cause delirium directly, these factors contribute to and aggravate delirium in the elderly.

Management of delirium in the elderly has three components: (*a*) identifying and treating the underlying causes, (*b*) using nonpharmacologic measures to ameliorate symptoms, and (*c*) initiating pharmacologic treatment for control of severe agitation and behavioral dyscontrol associated with delirium. Since delirium can result from any number of causes, determining the cause of a patient's delirious state often entails tests and procedures that themselves can cause further adverse effects. The cumulative effect may be a multifactorial decline in function. Nonpharmacologic interventions include maximizing the safety of the environment and providing psychosocial support. Environmental changes include enhancing the patient's ability to interpret the environment appropriately. Avoiding the stimulus overload in a loud and busy unit and the stimulus deprivation of an isolated, dark, windowless room are advisable. Family members can reassure the patient, provide reorientation, and reduce anxiety and agitation.

For the agitated patient whose medical care and safety are at risk (e.g., removing intravenous lines or respiratory equipment), antipsychotics can be beneficial. Haloperidol (Haldol) is the preferred antipsychotic because it is potent and has few anticholinergic and hypotensive side effects. Benzodiazepines are also employed in the management of delirium to sedate the agitated patient. When agitation is associated with sedative-hypnotic withdrawal, a benzodiazepine such as lorazepam, which has few, if any, active metabolites, is the treatment of choice. To minimize the risk of adverse effects, these agents should be reduced and eliminated once behavior symptoms are controlled or the reason for use has passed.

Given the link between severity of illness and the onset of delirium, it remains unclear whether delirium can be prevented per se. Nevertheless, identification of the elderly who are at high risk (Table 62.3), minimization of medications (especially anticholinergics, sedative-hypnotics, and opioids), early recognition and treatment of illnesses, and close management of chronic illnesses (e.g., heart failure) are necessary components of preventive care. Specific nursing interventions (e.g., preoperative discussions about delirium, reorientation, increased nursing continuity) reduce the incidence of delirium after surgery. Prevention of serious illness in frail elders by immunizations for influenza and pneumonia and close management of chronic illnesses such as congestive heart failure are important ways of reducing the risk of delirium. Establishment of family and community support systems (e.g., home health services, day

Table 62.3
Risk Factors for Delirium

Baseline cognitive impairment
Depression
Dementia
Alcoholism
Male gender
Parkinson's disease
Age > 70 years
Poor premorbid functional status
Vision impairment
Severe illness
Multiple comorbid diseases
Cerebrovascular disease (primarily stroke)
Fracture on admission
Symptomatic infection
Total knee arthroplasties
Cardiac and noncardiac thoracic surgery
Aortic aneurysm surgery
Laboratory abnormalities: markedly abnormal
   preoperative serum sodium, potassium, calcium,
   chloride or glucose levels, high blood urea nitrogen-
   creatinine ratio, leukocytosis, alkalosis, hypoxemia,
   hypoalbuminemia

care) can be used for early detection of delirium and ease the return to the more familiar home environment following an illness.

Dementia

Cognitive impairment and dementing illness affect 25 to 50% of adults over age 80 (11–14). Unfortunately, this condition may be undetected, unknown, or unrecorded in patients admitted to a hospital. Whether or not it is present in a person's medical history, dementia is important. A person with cognitive impairment who undergoes a total knee arthroplasty may have a difficult recovery because of memory problems. For those with moderate dementia, day-to-day carryover of instructions in physical therapy may be severely limited. Success of the procedure itself may be in peril as a result of a patient's inability to remember repeated admonitions from nursing staff about the need to ask for help when trying to stand or walk. Falling while trying to use the toilet in the middle of the night may undo all of the delicate repair work just performed, as well as causing further injuries.

Nutritional problems frequently arise among demented patients. Although hyperphagia infrequently accompanies dementia, anorexia and weight loss are much more common, especially following an illness or surgery (15–17). The well-recognized risks of premorbid undernutrition include impaired wound healing, pressure sores, and prolonged hospitalizations. Impaired oral intake after an illness or surgery may further jeopardize successful recovery. Early identification of those at risk is therefore important.

Delirium commonly affects demented adults hospitalized for any type of illness. This can significantly prolong or delay recovery. In addition, clinicians must be aware that adults with dementia and delirium have limited abilities to understand and solve problems. Therefore, the issue of informed consent in these cases often is problematic. As a result, reliance on caregivers and family for the appropriate direction of care becomes essential. In fact, the very goals of treatment can change drastically during a hospitalization. A previously well older adult with mild cognitive impairment who has a stroke after a hip replacement may become so severely incapacitated that family members must decide about hospice care for end-of-life treatment. Indeed, establishing the plan of care for the demented patient after hospitalization can be one of the most difficult problems. Identification of responsible caregivers, determination of their ability to performed the required services, and assessment of the need for subacute or long-term care are common areas of concern for patients with dementia or any chronic illness and their families.

Functional Impairment

As a result of pain, fatigue, and generally feeling unwell, elderly patients who require hospitalization for illness or surgery often prefer to remain in bed. However, sustained bed rest quickly leads to cardiac and muscular deconditioning and predisposes patients to pressure sores and constipation. In addition, falls related to orthostatic hypotension and imbalance from loss of neuromuscular tone are a significant risk.

Among community residents over age 80, 20% need help in bathing and 10% need help for transferring and using the toilet (18–20). Functional status is more likely to decline in this group of frail elders than in younger patients. The use of physical restraints such as belts, jackets, and limb restraints, in addition to bed rails and geriatric chairs, requires intense scrutiny. Although such devices may be necessary for brief use when dictated by safety reasons, their effectiveness for other uses is far from established. In fact, the use of physical restraints is more likely to lead to injuries such as falls or pressure ulcers than to prevent them, and restraints may contribute to problem behaviors because of their psychologic effects. Deaths by strangulation have also occurred (21). Psychoactive drugs such as neuroleptics and anxiolytic agents can be used as chemical restraints for safety purposes, but they are highly associated with injuries from falls, and they contribute to delirium, further delaying rehabilitation and prolonging hospitalization (22, 23). Intravenous lines and indwelling bladder catheters can also function as de facto restraints, and their use should be considered with this in mind.

Avoiding iatrogenic illness and preventing unwanted complications of hospitalization or long-term care necessarily entail an aggressive approach to optimizing mobility. Put simply, patients respond best when they are trained to move as much as possible, as early as possible, unless limited by safety or severity of illness. In the intensive care setting, passive range of motion and turning the patient from side to side every 2 hours (24) can contribute mightily to limiting the development of pressure sores and contractures. As recovery ensues, mild to moderate strengthening exercises, promotion of sitting and standing, and monitored walking must be encouraged as early as illness allows. Physiatrists, physical and occupational therapists, and nursing staff can provide many of these services. Their evaluations can also add significant input to decisions on posthospital care needs.

Increased mobility is useful for behavior management as well. For the demented patient, scheduled walking can provide strengthening and orientation. When the demented adult is awake late at night, it can be useful to have that patient placed in a geriatric chair in the hallway so the patient and the nurses can watch each other. This can be useful, because many isolated patients with dementia call out, yell, become agitated, or wander because of sensory deprivation or fear, isolation, or confusion about where they are (25, 26). Or they may simply be bored. This can be a useful way of avoiding unnecessary physical and chemical restraints.

Eyeglasses and hearing aids can promote mobility. Loss of these sensory inputs may contribute to the patient's desire to remain in a bed or chair, for a patient may feel unsure or unsafe with less than optimal vision and hearing. Therefore, it is necessary that a patient have his or her eyeglasses at hand and that these are used for all appropriate activities, including walking and going for tests or procedures. Similarly, use of a patient's own hearing aids can provide essential auditory cues and increases the patient's ability to participate in decisions about care. It is wise for a practitioner to make available a portable amplifying device (headphones with a small amplifier) for interviews and patients' use. This can correct some of the misinformation and lack of understanding that occur when an older adult has unmodified presbycusis. When sensory deficits are combined with a dementing illness, the effect on behavior can be disastrous (27). Therefore, augmenting sensory input by whatever means available can be an important preventive measure.

Finally, many older adults wear dentures or partial replacements. These often become misplaced or forgotten on transfer to hospital or long-term care center. For some patients, nutrition can be enhanced by having those dentures available (28). However, other patients do not use their dental prosthesis for reasons of comfort, fit, or personal preference.

A SYSTEMS APPROACH

The most common iatrogenic illnesses recognized among older hospitalized patients are adverse drug reactions, complications of diagnostic and therapeutic procedures, fluid and electrolyte disorders, infections, and falls and other trauma (29–34). For some, complications beget other complications, so that an individual patient may have a series of insults as a result of a single error. Many clinicians have patients who have had this kind of cascade of decline. Prevention of ia-

trogenic illness among hospitalized older patients may require a new approach.

It may be useful to borrow techniques that the business community uses to address similar problems. Modifying the behavior of a single physician or other practitioner is certainly one approach. This method is usually based on educating individual practitioners or improving one's competence in certain surgical procedures. Institutional and governmental bodies often oversee medical practice, using hospital accreditation, nursing home surveys, and reviews of opioid prescribing practices. Although these may be useful end points in themselves, the mechanisms for determining compliance are not necessarily directed at or successful in reducing iatrogenic illness in older adults. In addition, these efforts are often punitive, shifting attention away from patient care and favoring crossing the t's and dotting the i's to meet regulatory requirements.

Business practice has embraced several new systems of management designed to reduce quality problems and improve efficiency. Several areas of medical care have aspects that at first glance appear to be unrelated to such business models, but on further review these medical system problems can indeed be seen to benefit from a nontraditional approach. This is not to suggest that medical care is a product but rather recognizes the human qualities of medical care teams. Management of these processes recognizes the significant likelihood of error, miscommunication, misunderstanding, and acts of omission. These are recognized as an expected part of most human interactions, affecting the practices of all medical care teams from clinic to hospital to nursing home.

The use of a business model in the management of human behavior among health care entities may best be applied to certain systems and procedures. A strong focus on a chosen goal is more likely to be successful than some overarching attempt to change an entire institution. However, the input, vision, and active engagement of corporate leaders are essential to the success of these endeavors. Such a systems approach can be applied to numerous quality-of-care problems, including such issues as polypharmacy, delirium care, restraint reduction, management of falls, and handling of the dementia patient.

Over the past 20 years business management theory has undergone many changes, often in response to the specific economic problems of the times. Some of these management approaches can rightly be termed fads, while others seem to take on an absurdly cultlike atmosphere, as any follower of the comic strip *Dilbert* can affirm. Company employees who have suffered under programs that valued style over substance may thus be cynical about future attempts at improvement. Nevertheless, an expedient view of the use of any business management practice in the health care field should be the simple question, does this work? The demand for results should shape the plan for change from the outset, much as the hypothesis shapes the research methods in scientific studies.

Quality Improvement

W. Edwards Deming, a statistician, first broached the topic of continued improvement in quality control by combining planning, scientific study, and measurement in an atmosphere typified by an involved workforce and responsive leadership. As is well known, these methods were thought to be instrumental in the rise of the Japanese economy but were not incorporated into American business management until the 1980s. Joseph M. Juran modified this concept of statistical quality control methods into a more comprehensive method, total quality management (TQM). Under TQM, previously rank-structured organizations learn to involve all job levels in the management of the organization. Problems are dealt with at the lowest appropriate organizational level to increase efficiencies. This means that areas of concern and avenues for improvement become the responsibility of all employees, roles previously reserved for supervisory and administrative staff (35).

The principles of quality management center on setting goals and tracking measurable objectives. In this matter, all parts of the institutional system (whether this be production of a product or provision of services) come under intense and constant scrutiny. This differs in design and philosophy from the older-style approach of quality assurance, which merely measures the end result of any process (35). As such, quality management

requires that all levels of an organization participate in the process, involving high-level leaders and point-of-service workers. Goals are set and progress and outcomes are monitored by following measurable objectives. These results are continuously reviewed, creating a sort of feedback loop in which changes beget results that are analyzed, prompting further refinements. In this manner, quality can perhaps continuously improve (35).

Health Care and Management Theory

For most clinicians and health care organizations, the implications for a systems approach to patient care are significant. Lessons learned from the business world suggest that simply relying on persons alone to fix certain problems or improve targeted practices is insufficient and almost certain to fail. In short, it is becoming more apparent that for many quality-of-care issues, improvement is not a *people problem* but a *systems problem* (36). That is, methods designed to "fix" individual physicians' behavior to improve the quality of care are not likely to succeed. This is not because health care workers are unmotivated, ineducable, or uncaring, but rather that the very systems and procedures under which they function are often designed to allow or even favor undesired outcomes, albeit unwittingly.

Poor system design creates "accidents waiting to happen." The concept of systems failure as the underlying cause of errors has not been widely accepted in the practice of medicine. Rather, technical efforts at error reduction have focused on persons and episodes, using training, exhortation, rules, and sanctions to improve performance errors. . . . Error. . .experts reject this approach, noting that it is more effective to change the system as a whole. (37)

The primary objective among physicians and other practitioners is good patient care. For the elderly, this entails not only reduction in morbidity and mortality associated with care but improvement in functional status and quality of life wherever possible. To attain these goals, systems must be designed to produce success, and progress should be continuously assessed along the way. Such ongoing reviews result in modified outcomes, and the tracking of selected processes consequently lead to changes in strategy. Among TQM purists, there is no real end point. Further change and continued improvement are always possible. However, given the increasingly limited resources available for care of the elderly, achieving certain targets may be acceptable.

Clinical practice guidelines are a simple tool of quality management to promote preventive care issues such as smoking, hyperlipidemia, vaccinations, hypertension, pain control, and management of congestive heart failure, to name a few. The *Guide to Clinical Preventive Services* (38), first published in 1989 by the U.S. Preventive Services Task Force, and guidelines published by the Agency for Health Care Policy and Research (39) provide evidence-based medicine approaches to provision of preventive and chronic care services. This sort of best-practices approach is an essential tool in the quality management approach to health care.

For care of the older patient, setting goals and measurable objectives can be applied not only to preventive care issues such as reducing risk of heart attacks and strokes but also to geriatrics-specific targets such as the management of incontinence, reduction in falls and traumatic fractures, appropriate shortening of hospital stays through early recognition and management of delirium and mobility problems, and increasing outpatient identification of dementia and depression in older adults who are at risk. Selection of the particular area of concern depends on the demographics of the population being served and on the type of organization in question. Greatest success may be found initially by "picking the low-hanging fruit" (40). Selecting practice areas in your community known to be error prone or ripe for improvement is likely to be successful, increasing the chances for success with subsequent endeavors. Physicians and administrative leaders can identify areas of greatest concern, but all affected parties should be engaged in the process. Once a project is identified, measurable goals are established. These should be demonstrably understood by those who will provide the care or institute the changes, as it is these workers who will be providing the ongoing measurements of benchmarks and outcomes necessary for feedback and continuing assessment.

Target outcomes vary greatly. Large institutions and health maintenance organizations may choose areas such as the appropriateness of certain procedures, reduction of unwanted or unnecessary procedures, institutionwide risk reduction, or the availability and timeliness of physician visits. Assessment of customer satisfaction in the larger health care organization is really not much different from that of the non-health care market. A public-health approach to TQM might select targets such as the appropriateness of use of new technologies for the elderly (e.g., angioplasty devices), education initiatives such as increasing awareness of cognitive impairment issues, or increasing provision of necessary immunizations. In all of these examples, the processes should be similar, requiring that persons responsible for attaining these goals feel ownership of these problems, accept responsibility for the implementation of the planned strategies, and have real power to stay involved and make changes where appropriate.

Intellectual Capital

Management of information is a primary concern of quality management. For the health care industry, recent improvements in information technology hold promise to remedy some of the more difficult problems in elder care. Knowledge is the primary ingredient of medical care. It is not merely the patents, procedures, pharmaceuticals, skills, or technologies that are available, but the clinician's own body of knowledge that determines the kind of care an older patient may receive. As a result, managing that knowledge—finding intellectual capital, storing it, sharing it, and increasing it—has become one of the most important tasks of those who care for older patients. A working definition of intellectual capital in medicine might be the sum of everything everybody in a health care organization knows that gives it a competitive or quality edge and can be captured so that it can be described, shared, and exploited (41). For elder care, the limited physical and human resources available demand arrangements that are ever more valuable. Management of knowledge entails the use of the background expertise, and relations among clinical assistants, desk personnel, nurses, and their older patients can be an extremely valuable source of ideas for reforming processes. When a particular aspect of care should be improved, e.g., reducing medication errors, intellectual capital management encourages contributions from every person involved in the system. This human capital can rightly become more devoted to activities that result in innovation, and intellectual capital grows when the organization uses what people know and when information is widely available to the organization.

It becomes important, then, to identify what people know and who knows it (41). Recognizing skills often goes beyond job titles. For example, one or two nurses on a particular hospital shift may be recognized by their peers to excel in the care of the confused older adult. From the standpoint of intellectual capital, it is important for the larger organization to be aware of this expertise and exploit it. That is, if one strategy for a hospital is to reduce episodes of delirium or their adverse effects (morbidity and mortality), attention must be paid to these nurses' knowledge about care of these persons. Such information can be shared with the rest of the institution. Such a process can be used in determining best practices for many kinds of care in older patients.

Avoiding iatrogenesis, when approached from a systems standpoint, demands the involvement of the entire institution. Knowledge must be shared to develop competencies across many locations of care (e.g., nursing floors, long-term care wings, outpatient clinics). In this sharing of knowledge, health care workers can be bound by a common set of problems and the pursuit of solutions in a community of practice (41). Communities of practice are engaged in the continuous processes of knowledge transfer and innovation. But to succeed, the larger organization must recognize their presence, provide the necessary resources for continued learning, and furnish the overall strategy or vision behind it.

For the task of reducing iatrogenic problems, concepts of knowledge management, intellectual capital, and communities of practice can take several forms. Communication among members of an organization can be fostered by the simple use of an internal web page, an intranet. This web page can serve several functions. For example, ongoing projects can be identified so that all employees are aware of the existing strategies. This avoids duplication of effort. People involved in similar projects might then be able to tap the experience gained by the persons involved in one project and apply it to their own. Whether the goal is to reduce the formation of pressure sores, limit the number of falls, or smooth the transition to home care, projects listed on a web page can allow for e-mail or bulletin board employee input of ideas and suggestions, taking advantage of knowledge and skills that would have been unknown or unused previously.

Such an intranet can serve as a directory of knowledge (41), a guide to the accumulated knowledge of the organization and its members, and a record of lessons learned. To become an asset, this intellectual capital requires such management. Care protocols, process descriptions, and identification of areas of expertise are possible with this kind of technology. Given the high turnover rate common to long-term care facilities, it seems useful to make accumulated staff experience available to the newcomer, if only to reduce the learning curve. Common topics such as appropriate skin care in the nursing home can be addressed in such a fashion. The identification of what works is often best known to some of these workers but is lost when they move on to other jobs or facilities (41).

When this kind of knowledge can be tapped and placed on an intranet, it becomes available for all. For much of medicine there are insufficient data to justify specific detailed protocols of care, but general guidelines can be developed for many medical problems. For example, it might be helpful for doctors and nurses caring for an older patient with chronic obstructive pulmonary disease who has just undergone a knee replacement to have available on an internal web site simple case descriptions of prior similar patients. Brief descriptions of what went right and what went wrong allow other team members to benefit from this knowledge and do the job better next time or risk "losing the recipe" (41). Medical content on the World Wide Web has expanded at an astounding rate since 1990. Textbooks, journals, reviews, and guidelines are all available, giving valuable information on many medical issues. Access to this external knowledge can provide significant added expertise for use on an internal web page. However, care must be taken to use reliable sources when searching medical web sites, as there are numerous pages containing unproven and misleading information.

SUMMARY: CASE EXAMPLES

These methods may sound well and good as business theory, but how would such management techniques work in the real world? Can the theories of quality management and intellectual capital play a significant role in the care of patients? The answer is not blind implementation of some new business program or new software but recognition that the information and knowledge people use in the care of elderly patients is as important as any glucometer, temperature probe, or blood pressure cuff reading. Moreover, this special knowledge can be managed more productively. A couple of case examples may illustrate this point.

Case 1

The leaders in a long-term care facility determine that a particular area of concern is reduction in medication errors. Persons representing all aspects of care at the facility work on the planning process. The administrator, director of nursing, physician, pharmacist, licensed practical nurse, and nursing assistant all provide input. An egalitarian format is appropriate to encourage participation from workers not traditionally charged with this level of responsibility. This kind of involvement is essential because the identification of problem areas in the delivery of medication to the elderly nursing home patient is likely to be best known by those providing the direct service.

The entire process of medication delivery is scrutinized in detail. How medicines are obtained, packaged, and distributed to the resident is described. Errors or potential errors along this path often become evident when this process is examined. A simple tracking mechanism is instituted, so that accurate data regarding medication errors are recorded. Recognizing the human desire to avoid blame for mistakes, accurate, detailed reporting of all incidences must be promoted as an institutionwide goal. However, this is likely to require changes in punishment and incentive systems to avoid interfering with reliable data collection. The process undergoes frequent reexamination, using the results of measurements from points along the path of the delivery of the medications. This process does not end but has as its goal continuous improvement. This does not mean that there will be no errors or that reduction in total number of errors is likely to improve beyond a certain point but that once an acceptable steady state is achieved, attention can be turned to other desired targets. Revisiting of the original goal should occur on a periodic or scheduled basis.

Case 2

A medium-sized clinic run by the local hospital wishes to reduce admissions for congestive heart failure (CHF) to win a managed-care contract for their Medicare recipients. This can be viewed as a project in reducing iatrogenic complications, since rehospitalization for heart failure can be viewed as physician dependent; i.e., the medical system has some control over its occurrence. Therefore, it is a proper goal of a quality management team and can be seen as contributing to reduction in iatrogenic complications of care. A systems approach might include a general overview of the entire care of an older patient with CHF. Included would be all personnel who can affect the care of these patients: the nurse, the administrator, the social worker, the dietitian, the home health care worker, the outpatient physician, the inpatient physician, and desk personnel. Several issues come to light. It is important to search medical literature for known risk factors for readmission for CHF (dietary indiscretion, medication noncompliance, incomplete understanding of the disease by the patient, insufficient treatment for prior episodes, new or unrecognized disorders contributing to CHF) (42, 43).

Individual team members can be solicited for their views on what is contributing to relapses or readmission in their own community. These answers can be very specific for a certain location, depending on the unique interplay of forces of care in a particular community. One could even consider walking a patient through a typical admission, discharge, outpatient checkup, and readmission scenario to picture the things that may contribute to repeated admissions. This kind of brainstorming technique, when occurring in an open and unimpeded environment, can greatly facilitate each party's understanding of the other's work life and how they interrelate and depend on each other in caring for patients.

Next, a goal might be established and the path to that goal laid out. An example might be to aim for a 10% reduction in hospital readmissions within 3 months of discharge. The particular changes in care plan that must be undertaken to accomplish this are detailed. Use of research findings on reducing CHF readmissions can shorten considerably the group's time investment, since they do not have to reinvent the wheel. Patient education, strict dietary compliance, optimal medical regimens, case management, and scheduled physician and home health care reassessments have been proved successful (42, 43). Baseline data on the current process and its readmission rate are collected. Then the particular target data are gathered in a simple workable format to facilitate compliance. Review of the data and assessment of progress against planned benchmarks must occur at scheduled intervals. What works is kept, and what does not work is discarded. The process can be updated periodically or when new information becomes available (e.g., scientific reports, new technologic advances, improved surveillance techniques).

Ideally, the process itself is kept in some form on a widely accessible internal web page. This way, individual team members can track progress along with the select few data gatherers. This provides the necessary sense of team spirit or belonging essential to any such project. In addition, this web page can solicit comments from involved personnel so that problems can be identified at the earliest point and new ideas presented along the way. Finally, after what is judged to be successful implementation, a brief case study description of the process can be added to this project's web site so that future projects can use it as their database. Again, this allows building on experience and keeps an organization from losing the recipe.

CONCLUSION

It may be obvious to the reader that this format can be applied across many organizational levels. It can be used, for example, by the public health sector in managing large populations to achieve desired targets of reduced iatrogenesis, such as improved pneumococcal vaccination, influenza prophylaxis, early stroke care, or promotion of the use of advance directives. Although it is certainly true that a proper role of the physician in reducing iatrogenic complications in their older patients is to improve one's own knowledge of care of the elderly, this is really only the starting point. Attention to the physiology of older adults, the proper uses of medications, the risks associated with hospital and outpatient care of the elderly, and keeping abreast of best practices and care guidelines remain important goals for any practitioner. A broader based systems approach may be more successful and efficient, and less burdensome than one relying on individual practitioners' behavior (36, 37). In addition, it takes advantage of the valuable experience of health care workers at all points of patient interaction, rather than wasting or disregarding this resource, as often happens. Quality management techniques, reengineering, and other such methods are merely tools. They require leaders who have a vision of the appropriate care of older persons and the desire to implement any resulting strategies to achieve those goals. Otherwise, the parties involved view the process as a waste of time and make any future attempts less likely to succeed.

From TQM to just-in-time manufacturing and on to the more recent trends such as reengineering and business transformation, businesses seem to have moved from fad to fad seeking solutions to chronic business problems. Nevertheless, it is important to recognize that larger businesses, such as health maintenance organizations and hospital chains, have employed these very techniques to create strategies aimed at proving the bottom line of these companies. The disease management method, clinical pathways, the use of gatekeepers, and formulary restriction are examples of quality improvement methods that have changed the delivery of health care, affecting the elderly American population to an ever-increasing degree. Many of these strategies are directed at lowering costs, and it is yet unclear what the effect on society as a whole will be (36, 44). Nevertheless, it is clear that these kinds of tools can be similarly useful when the desired improvements involve care more than cost.

Certain persons or organizations may wonder whether this kind of investment in time, personnel, and resources is in their best interest. However, it can be argued that the likelihood of success in reducing iatrogenesis for the older patient may be significantly less when the primary plan for improvement depends on changing individual practitioners' behavior. As the multimillion dollar diet industry clearly demonstrates, changing behavior is extremely difficult. Even when improvement does occur, backsliding into old behaviors is often the norm. A systems approach offers wise use of the most important resources in the health care field: its workers. Furthermore, it may be simpler and more effective to modify protocols of care in a hospital or nursing home than to attempt to achieve similar levels of compliance by educating 300 individual physicians, hoping they will all fully integrate desired improvements in care. In the search for improvements and the quality of care, the physician and administrator would be wise to consider their use for targeted care issues.

REFERENCES

1. Creditor MC. Hazards of hospitalization of the elderly. Ann Intern Med 1993;118:219–223.
2. US Senate Special Committee on Aging. Aging America: Trends and Projections. Washington: US Government Printing Office, 1988.
3. Moellar JF, Mathiowetz NA. Prescribed Medications: A Summary of Use and Expenditures by Medicare Beneficiaries. National Medical Expenditure Survey Research Findings 3 (DHHS (8HS) 89–3448). Rockville, MD: National Center of Health Services Research and Health Care Technology Assessment, 1989.
4. Montamat SC, Cusack BJ, Vestal RE. Management of drug therapy in the elderly. N Engl J Med 1989;321:303–309.
5. Chrischilles EA, Segar ET, Wallace RB. Self-reported adverse drug reactions and related resource use: a study of community-dwelling persons 65 years of age and older. Ann Intern Med 1992;117:634–640.
6. Cadieux RJ. Drug interactions in the elderly: how multiple drug use increases risk exponentially. Postgrad Med 1989;86:179–186.
7. Nolan L, O'Malley K. Prescribing for the elderly: 1. Sensitivity of the elderly to adverse drug reactions. J Am Geriatr Soc 1988;36:142–149.
8. Gurwitz JH, Avorn J. The ambiguous relation between aging and adverse drug reactions. Ann Intern Med 1991;114:956–966.
9. Karmour I, Dolphin RG, Baxter H, et al. A prospective study of hospital admissions due to drug reactions. Aust J Hosp Pharm 1991;21:90–95.
10. Lamy PP. Adverse drug effects. Clin Geriatr Med 1990; 6:293–307.
11. Beard CM, Kokmen E, O'Brien PC, Kurland LT. The prevalence of dementia is changing over time in Rochester, Minnesota. Neurology 1995;45:75–79.
12. Gallo J, Reichel W, eds. Handbook of Geriatric Assessment. Rockville, MD: Aspen, 1988:117.
13. Patterson CJ. Detecting cognitive impairment in the elderly. In: Goldbloom RB, Lawrence RS, eds. Preventing Disease: Beyond the Rhetoric. New York: Springer-Verlag, 1990.
14. Skoog I, Nilsson L, Palmertz B, et al. A population-based study of dementia in 85-year-olds. N Engl J Med 1993; 328:153–158.
15. Hope RA, Fairburn CG, Goodwin GM. Increased eating in dementia. Int J Eat Disord 1989;8:111–115.
16. Grey GE. Nutrition and dementia. J Am Diet Assoc 1989;89:1795–1802.
17. Bucht G, Sandman P. Nutritional aspects of dementia, especially Alzheimer's disease. Age Ageing 1990;19: S32–S36.
18. Fried LP, et al. The epidemiology of frailty: the scope of the problem. In: Perry HM, Morley JE, Coe RM, eds. Aging, Musculoskeletal Disorders and Care of the Frail Elderly. New York: Springer, 1993:3–16.
19. US Senate Special Committee on Aging: Aging America: Trends and Projections. Washington: US Government Printing Office, 1992:144.
20. Kovar MG, Hendershot G, Mathis E. Older people in the United States who receive help with basic activities of daily living. Am J Public Health 1989;79:778–779.
21. Tinetti ME, Liu WL, Ginter SF. Mechanical restraints use and fall-related injuries among residents of skilled nursing facilities. Ann Intern Med 1992;116:369–374.
22. Schor JD, Levkoff SE, Lipsitz LA, et al. Risk factors for delirium in hospitalized elderly. JAMA 1992;267:827–831.
23. Marcantonio ER, Juarez G, Goldman L, et al. The relationship of postoperative delirium with psychoactive medications. JAMA 1994;272:1518–1522.
24. Panel for the Prevention and Prediction of Pressure Ulcers in Adults. Pressure Ulcers in Adults: Prediction and Prevention. Clinical Practice Guideline 3 (AHCPR 92–0047). Rockville, MD: US Department of Health and Human Services, Public Health Service, Agency for Health Care Policy and Research, 1992.
25. Cohen-Mansfield J, Werner P, Marx MS. Screaming in nursing home residents. J Am Geriatr Soc 1990;38:785–792.

26. Bridges-Parlet S, Knopman D, Thompson T. A descriptive study of physically aggressive behavior in dementia by direct observation. J Am Geriatr Soc 1994;42:192–197.

27. Carlson DL, Fleming KC, Smith GE, Evans JM. Management of dementia-related behavioral disturbances: a nonpharmacologic approach. Mayo Clin Proc 1995;70:1108–1115.

28. Reuben DB, Greendale GA, Harrison GG. Nutrition screening in older persons. J Am Geriatr Soc 1995;43:415–425.

29. Steel K, Gertman PM, Crescenzi C, Anderson J. Iatrogenic illness on a general medical service at a university hospital. N Engl J Med 1981;304:638–642.

30. Jahnigen D, Hannon C, Laxson L, Laforce FM. Iatrogenic disease in hospitalized elderly veterans. J Am Geriatr Soc 1982;30:387–390.

31. Schroeder SA, Marton KI, Strom BL. Frequency and morbidity of invasive procedures: report of a pilot study from two teaching hospitals. Arch Intern Med 1978;138:1809–1811.

32. Hanson LC, Weber DJ, Rutala WA, Samsa GP. Risk factors for nosocomial pneumonia in the elderly. Am J Med 1992;92:161–166.

33. Leape LL, Brennan TA, Laird N, et al. The nature of adverse events in hospitalized patients. Results of the Harvard Medical Practice Study II. N Engl J Med 1991;324:377–384.

34. Lefevere F, Feinglass J, Potts S, et al. Iatrogenic complications in high-risk, elderly patients. Arch Intern Med 1992;152:2074–2080.

35. Walton M. The Deming Management Method. New York: Perigee Books, 1986:55–95.

36. Herzlinger RE. Market-Driven Health Care: Who Wins, Who Loses in the Transformation of America's Largest Service Industry. Reading, MA: Addison-Wesley, 1997:172.

37. Leape L, Bates DW, Cullen DJ, et al. Systems analysis of adverse drug events. ADE Prevention Study Group. JAMA 1995;274:75–76.

38. Guide to Clinical Preventive Services. Report of the U.S. Preventive Services Task Force. 2nd ed. Baltimore: Williams & Wilkins, 1996.

39. AHCPR Publication. Rockville, MD: Agency for Health Care Policy and Research.

40. Micklethwait J, Woolridge A. The Witch Doctors. New York: Times Books, 1996:151.

41. Stewart TA. Intellectual Capital: The New Wealth of Organizations. New York: Doubleday/Currency, 1997:11–13, 66–68.

42. Senni M, Redfield MM. Congestive heart failure in elderly patients. Mayo Clin Proc 1997;72:453–460.

43. Seager LH. Congestive heart failure: considerations for primary care physicians. Postgrad Med 1995;98:127–137.

44. O'Shea J, Madigan C. Dangerous Company: The Consulting Powerhouses and the Businesses They Save and Ruin. New York: Times Books, 1997:164–182.

CHAPTER 63

RICHARD SORCINELLI, ROSEMARY JOHNSON-HURZELER, JOHN W. ABBOTT, DOUGLAS THISTLE, AND FREDERICK A. FLATOW

Management of the Dying Patient: Hospice, A Life Force

Hospice has turned an eternal secret into a living principle—that what's truly important is life lived richly, deeply, and meaningfully, for as long as life lasts. Dignity, family, comfort and caring are hospice—an idea whose time has come.

A hospice patient

As expertise in palliative care continues to grow in the United States, the need for hospice care will extend beyond its original boundary of the cancer patient who is near death. Although care of the dying is labor intensive and resource consumptive, statistically hospice care affects only a small number of patients. In 1995 only 14.8% of the 2.4 million dying patients in the United States were cared for by hospice (1). Optimal hospice and palliative care programs to address pain and suffering in the dying have been vastly underused and undervalued by both the public and health care professionals in America. Approximately a quarter of a million patients in the United States die each year in need of hospice care (2). The aged, frail and debilitated with chronic, progressive illnesses, and those afflicted by end-stage vital organ diseases and acquired immunodeficiency syndrome (AIDS) now fall within the purview of hospice ministrations. In the face of dehumanizing technology, hospice care offers hope and attentive personal treatment for the myriad problems that will continue to beset the aged for whom the benefits of curative medical intervention are dwindling. (Some 71%

of hospice patients are over age 65. The ages of the remaining 25% of the hospice population range from childhood through middle age (2).)

WHY HOSPICE CARE?

Profound technologic advances in the past 4 decades have emphasized diagnostic investigation and aggressive interventions focused on cure as opposed to care of the whole person. Increased life span and general well-being due to these medical advances have also been accompanied by degenerative chronic diseases of the elderly, with debilitating symptoms and ultimate death. As a result, families and health care professionals face difficult decisions regarding the use of high-tech life-support measures. These dilemmas are heightened in the care at the end of life.

To ensure that patients admitted to Medicare-reimbursed hospitals, nursing homes, and home care agencies are informed of their legal options to refuse cardiopulmonary resuscitation (CPR), ventilator support, and any other unwanted life-support measure, Congress passed the Patient Self-Determination Act (PSDA) in 1991. Persons can designate a proxy, or decision maker, and are encouraged to communicate with family, proxy, and physician about their wishes in the event that the patient is incapable of making his or her own health care decisions.

Societal and professional denial of death as a valuable, important, and inevitable passage in life's journey is a significant barrier to health care planning. Direct, candid communication among the primary physician, other specialists, the patient, family members, and designated decision maker that reflects the patient's wishes, values, and beliefs about treatment decisions and terminal care is necessary but often does not take place at all.

Finally, approximately 60% of the 2.4 million deaths in the United States still occur in the acute-care setting, and 20% die in extended-care facilities (1). The Robert Wood Johnson Foundation-funded SUPPORT project revealed in 1995 that most study patients dying in the acute-care setting were in moderate to severe pain during the last 3 days of life, and 38% spent their final 10 days on life support in an intensive care unit. Some 49% of dying patients who had requested a do-not-resuscitate (DNR) order did not have one at the time of death. Furthermore, 30% of the families of dying patients lost all of their savings to the high cost of treatment at end of life (3). Today, one of the greatest dissatisfactions among those who are gravely ill is the care they receive during the final phase of their life (4–9).

The contemporary focus on physician-assisted suicide and legalization of euthanasia is seen by many as an outgrowth of the medical profession's failure to meet the needs of the dying (10). In 1997 the Supreme Court found that the Constitution did not contain any fundamental right to hasten death by having a physician's assistance with suicide. It also held that the well-established right to refuse treatment is not only very different from assistance with suicide but that it is worthy of constitutional protection. Ethically and legally, withholding and withdrawing treatments that are invasive, undesirable, and not beneficial to the patient are not acts of physician-assisted death or euthanasia. Rather they are acts that respect individual autonomy and privacy.

The major barriers to hospice and palliative care programs are cultural, ethical, educational, technologic, financial, bureaucratic, and regulatory. As a result, referrals are often made too late for the patient and family to benefit fully from optimal hospice and palliative care services. Although palliative care is not a routine aspect of academic medicine because of lack of education, research, and funding, increased media and pub-

lic attention to care at the end of life generates continued interest and promotes development of palliative care and hospice services for optimal end-of-life treatment in hospitals, at home, and in long-term care facilities.

WHAT IS HOSPICE CARE?

Although all good hospice care is palliative, not all palliative care qualifies as hospice care. It is necessary to define both terms, as they are used interchangeably in the literature. Hospice care entails interdisciplinary support and skilled care for persons in the last phases of incurable disease so that the dying may live as comfortably as possible. Hospice recognizes dying as a normal part of life and focuses on maintaining the quality of remaining life; it neither hastens nor prolongs death. Hospice care embraces the belief that with appropriate care and a caring community sensitive to their needs, patients and their families may attain a degree of mental and spiritual preparation for a death that is satisfactory to them (11).

According to the World Health Organization (WHO), palliative care is the active total care of patients whose disease may not respond to curative treatment. The goal of palliative care is to achieve the best possible quality of life for patients and their families. It affirms life and regards dying as normal while emphasizing relief from pain and other distressing symptoms, integrating the physical, psychosocial, and spiritual aspects of patient care, offering a support system to help the patient live as actively as possible until death, and helping family members cope during the patient's illness and in their bereavement (12).

Timing and points of entry to hospice and palliative care are key distinctions. Admission criteria for Medicare- and Medicaid-funded hospice programs require that the patient no longer be pursuing curative treatment, that a physician's written prognosis be 6 months or less of remaining life, and that the majority of care be delivered in the home. In contrast, palliative care can be initiated in the acute care setting earlier in the disease process, while the patient is still receiving aggressive curative treatments, including radiotherapy and chemotherapy. This allows the patient to benefit from skilled symptom management and supportive services.

Hospice care is distinguished from palliative care in that hospice care is rendered at the end of the palliative care spectrum and remains the appropriate option when the burden of treatment outweighs the benefit to the patient (13). It should be part of a seamless progression of services delivered to patients with advanced irreversible illness. From its roots as a social movement, hospice has nurtured the evolution and maturation of palliative care (14).

The first recognized hospice program in the United States was established in Connecticut in 1974, influenced by Dame Cicely Saunders' program and advanced techniques for managing pain and suffering at St. Christopher's Hospice in London. The Connecticut Hospice developed principles envisaged as the framework of a philosophy designed to respond to the needs of dying patients and their families (Table 63.1).

The national hospice movement has grown explosively since then, and there are now more than 2000 Medicare-certified hospice programs throughout the United States (2), in part because of heightened sensitivity to the needs of the dying and their families and recognition that 40% of Medicare moneys expended in the last year of life are spent in the last month of life and that hospice care is cost effective. It was noted in 1995 that there is a saving of $1.52 for every $1 spent on hospice care and a further saving in the last month

of life, owing to substitution of cost-effective home care days for more costly inpatient days (1, 2, 15).

Since 1983 the following essential components of hospice care under the federally funded Medicare Hospice Benefit (16) have determined conditions of compliance for program development, operations, and quality assurance:

- Care provided by an interdisciplinary team
- Care delivered predominantly in the home (more than 80%)
- 24-hour availability of intermittent skilled nursing visits for pain and symptom control
- Participation of the primary physician and the family in care plan development
- Patient and family as the unit of care
- Social services counseling and chaplain core services for patient and family
- Physical, occupational, and nutritional services as needed
- Home health aide services for personal care; homemaker services
- Specially trained and supported volunteers for direct and administrative services
- Coverage of 95% of cost of medications for palliation
- Medical equipment and supplies necessary for terminal care
- Contracted pharmacy services with 24-hour availability
- Bereavement follow-up service for a full year after the death

Hospice is the appropriate option when the burden of treatment outweighs the benefit to the patient. It should be part of a seamless progression of services to patients with advanced irreversible illness. The techniques that have been learned from 25 years of hospice development are applicable to the care of a broader segment of the population approaching death; this chapter addresses the specific needs of elderly patients with irreversible illness. Hospice care is well suited to the needs of elderly patients because it addresses all dimensions of their lives.

WHO NEEDS HOSPICE CARE?

Patients appropriate for hospice care have diagnosed terminal illness with a limited life ex-

Table 63.1

Ten Principles of Hospice Care

Patient and family are regarded as the unit of care.

Services are physician directed and nurse coordinated.

Emphasis is on control of symptoms (physical, sociologic, spiritual, psychologic).

Care is provided by an interdisciplinary team.

Trained volunteers are an integral part of the team.

Services are 24 hours a day, 7 days a week, on call, with emphasis on availability of medical and nursing skills.

Family members receive bereavement follow-up.

Home care and inpatient care are coordinated.

Patients are accepted on the basis of health needs, not on ability to pay.

There are structured systems for staff support and communication.

pectancy. Terminal illness, however, is difficult both to define and to diagnose. Prognoses of advanced cancers are often easier to predict than other life-limiting diseases, such as AIDS and end-stage cardiac, hepatic, pulmonary, renal, or neurologic diseases. As a result, errors in prognosis are common and can lead to overstated life expectancy, which may partially explain very short and declining lengths of stay for hospice patients (1).

Patients with nononcologic diseases often have other known probable causes of death, such as multiple organ failure or persistent recurrent infection, in addition to their primary diagnosis. Also, a patient may have multiple medical problems, none of which may individually amount to a terminal diagnosis but when taken together indicate a terminal condition. The National Hospice Organization has published medical guidelines for determining prognosis in selected noncancer diseases to aid clinicians with prognostication (17). The prognosis of terminal illness therefore depends on clinical judgment combined with objective assessment of the natural history of the disease; treatments and response to date; performance status; thorough physical assessment, including neurologic and orthopaedic; and knowledge of the psychology and sociologic factors of the patient, family and physician.

The conventional definition of terminal prognosis, a life expectancy of 6 months or less, with written certification of this prognosis by the primary physician is a requirement for admission to Medicare and Medicaid hospice programs. The decision no longer to pursue curative interventions is addressed, as hospice offers palliative rather than curative treatment and interventions. Although not required for admission, treatment decisions such as DNR are explored in conjunction with the patient's values, preferences, and goals for care. According to the physician's input, knowledge of the disease process, therapeutic options, and discussion with patient and family, an advanced-care team may help to determine when the goals of care should change from life-prolonging to comfort.

The bench mark of a prognosis of 6 months or less came into existence in 1983 as part of the parameters established for the Medicare hospice benefit (18), which benefit served as a reimbursement model and helped to define the essential components of hospice care. There are few data in the medical literature to enable accurate predictions, so prognostication depends on clinical judgment combined with the psychologic and sociologic factors of the patient, family, and physicians.

The admission criteria for cancer diagnoses at the Connecticut Hospice are (*a*) proven diagnosis of cancer (biopsy and/or diagnostic radiology); (*b*) documentation of advanced disease; (*c*) symptoms related to disease progression or treatment side effects, including but not limited to pain, respiratory distress, nausea, vomiting, skin impairment, impaired elimination, weakness and fatigue, confusion, delirium, seizures, altered nutritional status; and (*d*) decline in performance and functional status. These criteria are flexible and based more on reasonable goals of care than on time frames. A prognosis of less than 6 months is more easily established in cancer patients when objective assessments of the natural history of the malignancy, treatment and response to date, and most important, performance status are considered. Prognostication in noncancer illnesses can be more difficult.

MANAGEMENT OF THE HOSPICE PATIENT

Optimal management and care of the hospice patient requires the comprehensive skills of an interdisciplinary team of health care and other professionals consisting of physicians, nurses, pharmacist, social worker, pastor, artists, and dietitian or nutritionist; also extensive use of trained volunteers. Care is directed not only to the patient with irreversible illness but also to the family, and it continues for the family during the period of bereavement.

Treatment of hospice patients, whether inpatient, respite, or home care, is directed at improving or maintaining comfort. As a rule, no aggressive diagnostic or therapeutic approaches are employed. Brief inpatient stays may be appropriate for some patients for control of acute pain or other symptoms, such as dyspnea, confusion, anxiety, incontinence, constipation, diarrhea, nausea, and vomiting, which can be best addressed in the hospital through close observation, continuous monitoring, and careful titration of medication.

Pain, one of the most feared and best-remembered symptoms of chronic and terminal illness, requires expert attention. Assessment and communication skills are paramount, as is solid knowledge of pharmacologic and nonpharmacologic interventions. Ongoing professional education, supervision, interdisciplinary communication, documentation, accuracy, and continuous quality improvement are critical to this process. Once pain and other somatic symptoms are controlled, attention can be directed toward the emotional, psychologic, spiritual and other needs of the patient and family.

Role of the Physician

The medical director may serve as physician for patients who do not have a primary care physician. The primary responsibility for directing care lies with the primary physician, preferably one with whom the patient has a long-term relationship. Physicians are called on to offer not only clinical expertise but awareness of and sensitivity to the patient's and family's issues and concerns.

Although hospice nurses prepare and teach patients about life-support measures and treatment decisions, it is primarily the physician's responsibility to initiate discussion about the prognosis and the burdens or benefits of various treatments. Early candid discussion about advance directives and teaching patients and families about the place of palliative and hospice care in the continuum of care can assist patients and families with difficult but important decisions and avoid inappropriate high-tech care.

Time spent with the patient and family in the preterminal and terminal phases of disease, addressing their issues, concerns, and questions candidly and compassionately, is critical, as dying is a tremendous transition, a period of uncertainty and loss for both the patient and family. With meticulous attention to symptom palliation, comprehensive interdisciplinary support, and good coordination of care and comfort across settings, this period may also produce personal growth, reconciliation, closure, and a peaceful death.

Callahan (19) defines a peaceful death, i.e., a death without unnecessary suffering, neither hastened nor delayed, and ultimately not deformed by technology, as a reasonable goal of medicine.

Role of the Interdisciplinary Team

The hospice care team, together with the medical director and the primary physician, work together to assure that all of the patient's and family's needs and goals of care are addressed and met, to the fullest extent possible, using a team approach and the patient- and family-centered model. The team director's role is to coordinate the interdisciplinary effort to develop and communicate the individualized care plan for each patient and family. Skilled hospice nurses are expert in assessing and addressing pain and other symptoms of terminal illness, recognizing that pain is not limited to the physical domain but encompasses psychologic, emotional, spiritual, and existential dimensions. The plan of care is never static, as the patient's condition may change rapidly and require frequent intervention and team collaboration.

Licensed social workers address financial and bureaucratic issues and emotional and psychosocial dimensions of dying, and they work with children in the home. Chaplains are available to address spiritual issues, regardless of a person's or family's religion, and may assist in funeral preparations and other rituals of death. Trained and supervised home health aides assist with personal care. The ancillary services of pharmacists, artists, physical and occupational therapists, and dietary services augment and support team efforts to provide comprehensive care.

After undergoing extensive training, the hospice volunteer may serve as a companion offering respite and help with errands or trips to the doctor's office or as a resource and administrative support to the program. Federal requirements for hospice care are that 5% of care hours be rendered by volunteer staff (16). The bereavement coordinator supervises the bereavement services for the family, children, and the community. Supportive services are available for staff and volunteers also.

Culturally sensitive and superior holistic care is a prudent goal for terminal care in any setting.

The diverse perspectives and skills of the hospice interdisciplinary team can contribute to more thoughtful insights; assistance with appropriate health care, personal planning, and decision making; and increased awareness of patient and family needs.

Appropriate accreditation and licensure requirements, business and hiring practices, orientation and ongoing training programs, and staff and volunteer support services are necessary to ensure quality assurance, compliance, and improvement.

General Inpatient Care

The nursing care plan is the infrastructure for involvement of all other disciplines, such as social work, pastoral care, arts, diet, and volunteers. The interdisciplinary team assesses each patient to develop a care plan aimed at maximizing physical and psychologic comfort. A thorough assessment of the patient's physical status looks also at how the illness has affected the patient's roles, lifestyle changes, and relations with the family and the community as well as the ways the death will affect the family. From the time the patient is admitted to the hospice program one must anticipate the bereavement needs of the family. Patients may be admitted to a contracted acute care hospital or a skilled nursing facility-level hospice residence for short-term acute management of symptoms that cannot be managed in the home, such as intractable pain, nausea, vomiting, or seizures. Team members continue to be involved, communicating the patient's plan of care to the staff of the facility to ensure continuity of care, avoidance of unwanted interventions, and timely discharge planning.

Levels of Care

The four levels of reimbursable care under the Medicare hospice benefit (16) are routine home care, skilled continuous nursing in the home for short-term acute symptom management to prevent hospitalization, short-term hospitalization for acute symptom management, and respite care for brief periods of relief for the family. Reimbursement for hospice services under Medicaid, HMOs, and other private insurance plans often models the Medicare hospice benefit.

Routine Home Care

Most hospice care is delivered in the home. For some, home is a house or apartment. For others it is an extended-care facility, nursing home, or assisted-living community. As needs increase, community residences are being developed to offer a homelike environment to hospice patients who do not have a home or a primary caregiver. The role of the family as primary provider of care, the community with diverse values and religious beliefs, and the absence of institutional structure contribute to the challenges and richness of opportunity for appropriate community-centered end-of-life care. As such, support and education of the family are essential to care of the patient, and each discipline's skilled assessment, compassion, and communication are necessary in any setting.

In home care the interdisciplinary team enters the home at the invitation of the patient and family as "guests" at a unique, special time in the life of the patient and family. As with inpatient hospice clinical practice, each patient and family is assessed by the interdisciplinary team, and a plan is developed with input from each discipline to meet the patient's and family's needs. Nursing assessment is crucial in home care. The nursing assessment of the patient's clinical status is critical because the physician depends on this information either to continue the hospice plan or to change it. This requires exquisite clinical description by the nurse. The nurse describes a pattern of signs and symptoms that create a picture, including observation and description of lung sounds, heart sounds, vital signs, sputum if needed, and changes in turgor. Nurses must anticipate the progression of a disease process and determine the needs in advance to avoid crises.

The challenge of home care is the fact that it is being delivered at home by family members and informal caregivers who must be taught how to care for this patient in conjunction with home health aides and skilled nursing. This is a great challenge for many patients and their families who have no medical background. The accomplishment of these caregiving objectives is a major factor and comfort in grieving.

The nursing role includes support of all caregivers. Family caregivers must not only be taught how to care for the patient but also receive affirmation and praise for their sensitivity and the care they render. The partnership of family members and the hospice team facilitates the role of family and friends as caregivers. This exchange of support is a critical element of hospice care. In the last analysis, however, patients become the teachers, teaching caregivers how to live.

Continuous Care

Patients with acute symptoms such as those described earlier may require brief periods of skilled nursing care at home, usually 1 to 3 days, to monitor and stabilize acute pain and escalating symptoms and avoid hospitalization.

Respite Care

The burden on families and informed caregivers can be a tremendous responsibility as well as tremendously gratifying. Family members may need respite to go to a distant event, such as a wedding, graduation, or funeral. Intended to offer the stable patient a brief stay (up to 7 days) in a contracted hospital or nursing home, the patient's hospice plan of care is overseen by the hospice team and the staff in the respite setting.

SPIRITUAL DIMENSIONS OF HOSPICE CARE

Theologian Dorothee Soelle, in her classic text on suffering, pointed out two very important components of suffering: perceived powerlessness and perceived meaninglessness. It is in that struggle against powerlessness, the struggle to find meaning in our lives, that so much important work is done at end of life (20). The power of life review and the personal narrative to this most personal and profound part of life's journey are critical for the dying and their families. Spirituality plays an important role in this coming to know. It does not relieve us of suffering; rather, it gives us a framework in which to do the work, with guidance and encouragement, if we are willing. Readings, spiritual prayers, rites, and sacraments may be helpful to some.

Much has been written about the isolation of the dying, avoidance by friends and families who don't know what to say and by health care professionals who think they no longer have anything to offer. This work in process requires excellent listening skills, respect for the person, reflection, and empathic awareness of the situation, as the patient lives it and tells it. The fact that human life has spiritual dimensions becomes acutely evident as the end of life approaches. Many patients want to bring spiritual feelings to the fore. A major component of pain is spiritual (21) (Table 63.2).

The resources a hospice pastoral caregiver can bring to the patient and family depend, of course, on the spiritual dynamics that motivate a partic-

Table 63.2

Ten Aspects of Spiritual Pain

Abandonment	A feeling of being forgotten by God
Anger	May be directed toward God or people
Betrayal	Similar to abandonment but with an extra valance
Despair	Being without hope; having nowhere to turn
Fear, dread	What does death mean? What will it bring? Where? May be directed toward the process of dying or toward what comes afterward
Guilt	Self-recrimination, feelings of having left undone things that should have been done, or having done what should not have; a sense of death as deserved punishment
Meaninglessness	A feeling that life is without purpose, has no fundamental meaning
Regret	Sadness associated with irreversibility, of dreams that must remain unfulfilled, of a deeper painful wish or longing for what cannot be
Self-pity	Why me? Why should I be in this condition?
Sorrow, remorse	Profound sadness, likely to be associated with impending separation from loved ones

ular person. Every religious value system has corresponding sources of spiritual strength. In the Christian context some of these are forgiveness, God, hope, prayer, presence, rites, and trust (22). Many persons must face spiritual issues if death is to occur with any kind of equanimity.

Symptom Management

The Connecticut Hospice identifies pain, nausea, vomiting, confusion, dyspnea, restlessness, and impaired elimination as the most common symptoms among the hospice patient population. Fatigue is another major symptom among the dying. And finally, undiagnosed and untreated depression is a significant factor in care of the terminally ill, with the highest incidence in the elderly (23).

Pain

Pain management is the key to successful hospice for patients and their families. The International Association for the Study of Pain defines pain as "[a]n unpleasant sensory and emotional experience associated with actual or potential tissue damage, or described in terms of such damage. Pain is a complex experience that is always subjective based on input that is both sensory (body) and emotional (cognitive processing and learned). It may or may not be associated with actual tissue damage. The approach to its management must include assessment of both nociceptive and psychologic processes" (24).

Untreated pain is one of the most dehumanizing symptoms of terminal disease. The basis of good pain management entails the development of a relationship of trust that conveys respect, interest in your patient's report of pain, its location and types (bone, visceral, somatic), and what factors escalate it and relieve it. Suffering can be relieved along with pain, making the process physically more gentle, although it is beyond our power to cure the underlying condition. Pain is an emergency, and no one should live or die in pain. The barriers to effective pain management (25, 26) include the following:

- Societal barriers
  —Failure to distinguish between legitimate and illegitimate use of opioids
  —Fear of addiction
  —Cultural pressure to prescribe opioids by customary practice rather than by pharmacologic principles
  —Irrational and detrimental practice of reserving opioids until death is imminent
- Physician barriers
  —Knowledge gaps in pain management and symptom control
  —Misconceptions regarding pain management
  —Regulatory barriers and scrutiny
- Patient barriers
  —Reluctance to report pain
  —Fear that pain signifies advancing disease
  —The desire to be a "good" patient and not bother the physician with complaints of pain
  —Concern about unmanageable side effects

For example, a hospice home care patient with advanced cancer of the colon tolerated a lot of pain because he felt that he had not been a good person and that he deserved the pain. For this patient, spiritual issues had to be addressed before physical pain could be relieved.

Many patients and health care providers fear loss of control and heightened somnolence induced by the medications. Patients develop tolerance to the sedating effects of opioids and are relieved when reassured that the sedative effects are short-lived. Careful titration and reassessment are critical, as is education about the realistic aspects of pain control. Unwarranted fears of addiction or tolerance and predictable side effects with planned palliative measures should be discussed. Many hospice patients resume a higher level of activity, complete a project, attend an important event, or return to work once pain is relieved.

In another case, a patient whose profession and life was engineering and mathematics could not think clearly enough on morphine to do the work he wanted to do. A fentanyl patch allowed him enough clarity to spend 4 hours a day working without forfeiting pain relief, and he regained a sense of control.

The basis of good pain management is the belief in the patient's complaint of pain. A careful pain history must be obtained through assessment of psychologic and social factors confounding the patient's expression of pain (25–

32). Some strategies call for journal keeping, with documentation of medication use, breakthrough doses, and concrete data as well as subjective descriptions and notations of pain.

Opioid analgesics, such as morphine and fentanyl, and nonsteroidal anti-inflammatory drugs (NSAIDs), such as Trilisate, are the major classes of analgesic drugs for patients with moderate to severe pain. Opioids are effective and easily titrated, and they have a favorable benefit-to-risk ratio (12). Morphine is the most commonly used because of its availability in a variety of dosage forms and its well-characterized pharmacokinetics and pharmacodynamics. There is no standard or ceiling dose of morphine; the correct dose is the dose that relieves the pain. This dose varies from patient to patient, but as long as side effects are minimal, opioids can be given safely in escalating doses until pain is relieved. The majority of hospice patients tolerate oral long-acting morphine preparations with short-acting MSO_4 concentrate for breakthrough pain. Transdermal delivery systems work well for patients with bowel obstruction or other difficulties in administering and receiving oral analgesia. Steroids may be used in patients with brain tumors.

Although little research has been done on pain in the elderly, the elderly should be considered at risk for undertreatment of pain because of inappropriate beliefs about their pain sensitivity, pain tolerance, and ability to use opioids. Elderly patients, like other adults, require aggressive pain assessment, management, and reassessment of persistent pains. Constipation must be aggressively treated with an active prevention protocol.

A recent study on relief of pain in oncology patients demonstrated that 42% were undertreated for pain. Equally disturbing was the finding that patients over age 70 were at increased risk for undertreatment of pain. Unwarranted concerns on the physician's part about causing addiction, hastening death, or incurring legal liability were noted, but these factors should not create a barrier to the optimal care of the dying and relief of their pain (29).

The elderly are more sensitive than other populations to the analgesic effects of opioids, with higher peak effect and longer relief (30). Because of metabolic and excretion changes, the elderly,

especially those who are opioid naive, are particularly sensitive to the sedating and respiratory effects of opioids. Therefore, long-acting drugs such as methadone may be contraindicated. Meperidine is never indicated in chronic pain treatment because of its short duration of action (2.5 to 3.5 hours) and its toxic metabolite, normeperidine, which can cause central nervous system excitation and lower the seizure threshold.

The most frequent symptom of bone metastases is pain, although 25% of patients have no symptoms. Pain is usually dull, aching and local to the area of involvement, although patients may have multiple sites of bone metastases. Complications include pathologic fractures, hypercalcemia, and spinal cord compression. Radiotherapy is an effective palliative intervention; it can also relieve pain due to nerve root or soft tissue infiltration. NSAIDs as adjuvants to opioids offer excellent palliation of bone pain.

Tricyclic antidepressants (amitriptyline, nortriptyline, desipramine) and certain anticonvulsants (phenytoin, carbamazepine, and gabapentin) have been useful in the pharmacologic management of neuropathic pain, the hardest pain to manage. Tricyclics are most effective for burning pain. Anticonvulsants work best for shocklike, lancinating pain. Treatment may commence with low doses (amitriptyline 10 to 25 mg at bedtime) and increase slowly in elderly and debilitated patients. This approach takes advantage of the sedating effects of the drug when insomnia is a problem and prevents falls due to orthostatic hypotension (31).

When the confused or demented have difficulty communicating their pain to health professionals, they often receive weak opioids or nonopioids because their caregivers mistakenly believe that they cannot tolerate opioid agents (31). If nonopioids alone are ineffective, it is necessary to commence treatment with low doses of short-acting opioids in combination with nonopioids and monitor and escalate rapidly until optimal pain relief is achieved. Frequent communications with the patient, family, and caregivers are essential to monitor the results, side effects, and response.

Pain often is not assessed when elderly patients grimace, moan, or cry out when turned or subjected to painful dressing changes or other therapies, because this is considered normal behavior and not an expression of pain. Behavioral observation is necessary to anticipate and prevent unnecessary pain and suffering. Often a hospice patient receives an additional opioid rescue dose for breakthrough pain approximately 45 minutes before receiving care or a dressing change. Other issues such as incontinence, comfort care, and urinary retention should also be addressed.

The WHO defines addiction as psychologic dependence and craving for the mood-altering effects of a drug and an overwhelming involvement in obtaining the drug for nonmedicinal purposes. Patients treated chronically with opioids can develop tolerance and become physically dependent on opioids, but fewer than 0.1% become psychologically dependent (32). Physical dependence describes the body's adaptation to the opioid. It is characterized by withdrawal syndrome if the drug is stopped abruptly or an antagonist is administered.

Tolerance describes the lessening effect of a stable dose over time. Tolerance to the respiratory depression and sedative effects of opioids develops quickly, and patients with persistent severe pain may tolerate monumental dosages of opioids without respiratory compromise. Tolerance and physical dependence should not be confused with psychologic addiction. Patients with a history of substance abuse tolerate even larger doses of opioids before they achieve optimal control.

In addition to sound pharmacologic interventions, nonpharmacologic methods of pain management include alternative therapies such as guided imagery, music, massage, meditation, self-expression with art and drawing, acupressure, and therapeutic touch. Although not well researched in elderly populations, measures such as physical therapy, transcutaneous electrical nerve stimulation (TENS), repositioning or splinting a painful extremity, application of heat or ice, and massage may be helpful also.

For pain management, the regimen must be kept as simple as possible, with the fewest possible medications administered by the easiest route. Adjuvants, such as NSAIDs, are used according to the patient's type of pain. Pain management requires that the physician do the following:

- Perform a careful medical and in particular neurologic examination and review the results of diagnostic tests. Do not fail to evaluate the extent of disease.
- Manage the pain during the assessment to facilitate the diagnostic workup.
- Diagnose the mechanism and cause of pain, then outline and initiate a therapeutic approach.
- Provide around-the-clock medication administration as well as rescue doses for breakthrough pain.
- Increase the routine dose of the patient's analgesic if 3 or more rescue doses of medication were needed during the preceding 24 hours.
- Write for a range in dosage to avoid any delay in administration.
- Assess pain continuously with treatment.
- Quantitate pain according to a numeric, descriptive, or pictorial scale.
- Remember that in general physicians tend to underestimate the patient's perception of pain (32).

The single most important rule of thumb for control of pain, nausea, depression, and many other symptoms is to anticipate events. First treat the symptoms with appropriate medication, and then use regular dosing to prevent symptom recurrence. This approach provides many secondary psychologic and physical benefits for the patient and the family (e.g., reduces anxiety, promotes sleep, increases mobility) (31).

ALTERNATIVE ROUTES OF OPIOID DELIVERY. While the oral route is preferred, it is occasionally necessary to consider a transdermal, sublingual, buccal, rectal, parenteral (including portable subcutaneous or intravenous patient-controlled analgesia), inhalator, or spinal route. Advantages of and indications for topical analgesics are convenience, long-term use, confusion, difficulty swallowing, and reluctance to use injections early in the pain management regimen. Intractable neuropathic pain may necessitate consideration of intraspinal nerve blocks and epidural administration of opioids. The elderly and the dying should be evaluated carefully for benefit versus burden. In the elderly, as in other populations with chronic pain, the simplest dose schedule and least invasive modalities should be used first.

ADDITIONAL PAIN-RELIEVING MODALITIES. Radiotherapy is the most effective modality for bone pain and is also useful in relieving pain due to nerve root or soft tissue infiltration. It can help alleviate obstruction and control hemorrhage. Radiopharmaceuticals can address metastatic bone pain (prostate or breast cancer) in a patient who does not respond to standard palliative interventions. Strontium-89 is a local injectable source of radiation that has proved useful in the treatment of bone pain.

The literature demonstrates that pain in the hospice population is not completely controlled but that 90% of pain is adequately eased in most hospice settings. For example, a patient with splanchnic bed involvement, retroperitoneal pain low in the abdominal pelvis presents complicated issues. The occasional patient returns to the hospital to have a splanchnic alcohol block. Neuropathic pain is the hardest to control. It does not respond well to the opioids without significant sedation, so the adjuvants are used.

DOSAGE RANGES. The Agency for Health Care Policy and Research *Clinical Practice Guidelines for the Management of Cancer Pain* (31) is an invaluable resource for clinical practitioners in skilled management of chronic pain. Included are assessment tools, specific dose ranges for children and the elderly, and pharmacologic and nonpharmacologic modalities. A simple, well-validated, effective method for ensuring rational titration of cancer pain therapy has been defined by the WHO (12). This approach, based on the concept of an analgesic ladder, is found to be effective in 95% of patients with cancer and more than 75% who are terminally ill. The five essential components in the WHO approach to drug therapy for cancer pain are the following:

- By the mouth
- By the clock
- By the ladder
- For the individual patient
- With attention to detail

The first step is the use of acetaminophen or aspirin or another NSAID. When pain persists or increases, add an opioid, such as oxycodone or codeine, to the first drug. Next use higher doses of opioids. Opioids and NSAIDs have dosage ceilings; use separately, not to exceed maximum dosages. Pain that is persistent or moderate to severe requires higher doses or increased potency of opioids (12).

Nausea and Vomiting

As with other side effects, it is important to determine the cause of nausea and vomiting. Ondansetron is often used for cancer chemotherapy, lorazepam and cannabinol, for anticipatory nausea. Prochlorperazine is used prophylactically by mouth in long-acting tablets every 12 to 24 hours, as needed, or by rectum every 4 to 6 hours, to control nausea and emesis. Chlorpromazine is used for hiccups and severe nausea and vomiting in hospice patients. Another neuroleptic, haloperidol, is available in liquid form for patients who cannot tolerate tablets. In addition to its antiemetic effect, it has a mild tranquilizing effect. It is helpful to administer antiemetics on a fixed schedule once symptoms are under control. Meclizine or hydroxyzine is useful for nausea and vomiting related to motion. Scopolamine transdermal patch is now available for motion sickness.

Confusion

Confusion and delirium are common in advanced or terminal disease. Confusion may be related to direct effects of disease progression (such as brain metastasis) or the indirect effects of progressive disease, such as electrolyte imbalance, metabolic encephalopathy, infection, or paraneoplastic syndromes, and side effects to treatment. The following may be appropriate treatment for the elderly: general supportive treatment, such as hydration; symptomatic treatment with a benzodiazepine (lorazepam, with a short half-life and no active metabolite); a neuroleptic (or both a benzodiazepine and a neuroleptic if symptoms are not controlled) (35); haloperidol (less sedating); or a phenothiazine when sedation is required.

Dyspnea

Dyspnea is common and very distressing to hospice patients and their families. It may worsen as the patient approaches death because of slowing mucociliary apparatus, leading to the death rattle. Scopolamine transdermal patches are a noninvasive and effective means for control of end-stage secretions. The approach to treatment of dyspnea begins with consideration of suspected causes, such as known disease, acute or superimposed disease, cancer-induced complication, effect of cancer therapy, and terminal slowing of the mucociliary system. Once this is done, the risk-benefit ratio of therapeutic interventions and the life expectancy of the patient are considered. The final decision regarding treatment should rest with the patient. For many terminally ill patients, oxygen, opioids, corticosteroids, and benzodiazepines remain the treatment of choice. Begin with oral immediate-release morphine sulfate (MSIR) 2.5 to 5 mg every 4 hours unless the patient is already taking morphine for pain control at a higher dose. The dose may be increased by a third to a half daily if three or more rescue doses were needed during the preceding 24 hours. Parenteral or rectal suppository morphine may be used if the oral route is not available. Nebulized morphine may be used if sedation becomes a problem. Nebulized morphine use is based on the rationale that morphine can affect local receptors in the bronchioles and affect shortness of breath without the systemic and side effects of systemic morphine.

Depression, Anxiety, and Restlessness

Depression is a common element in the elderly and in those living with terminal disease. Approximately 25% of patients with cancer have severe depressive symptoms, with the prevalence up to 75% with advanced disease (34). Depression can be treated with low doses of a tricyclic antidepressant, such as amitriptyline at bedtime. Antidepressants, used alone or in combination, may also be helpful in treating pain. The tricyclics may have a coanalgesic opioid-sparing effect independent of mood.

Restlessness and psychiatric symptoms in terminally ill patients with pain should be viewed initially as a consequence of untreated pain. The management of specific disorders such as depression, delirium, and anxiety in patients with terminal disease requires assessment of mental status, drug interactions, and disease progression. Consider urinary retention or constipation.

Injectable drugs are rarely used in home hospice palliative cares. A benzodiazepine, lorazepam, is used frequently for anxiety and restlessness, and diazepam can be given orally (crushed tablets) or as an enema. On rare occasions, fewer than 5%, terminal pain is not adequately relieved with these modalities. Patients may require sedation for intractable pain, in particular tumors of the brain and spinal cord.

Impaired Elimination

All patients routinely taking opioids have constipation, so they take a laxative as a matter of course.

Impaired Nutritional Status

While it has been well established in law, ethics, and medicine that patients have a right to refuse treatments that are invasive and unwanted, withholding artificial feedings and hydration continue to be a troubling issue for patients, families, and health care providers. Questions about starvation and dehydration are common in caring for the dying. Numerous studies show that terminally ill patients generally do not get hungry, and those who do need only small amounts of food for alleviation, not artificial feeding or hydration. Thirst and dry mouth are relieved with ice chips, and excellent oral hygiene for comfort is taught to family members. Human physiology may explain the relative comfort of patients in the final stages of dying. Caregivers, patients, and families need to know that loss of normal appetite is to be expected in the dying and does not contribute to any suffering.

SUPPORT FOR DYING

The term actively dying describes signs and symptoms that the body is preparing for the final stage of dying. Typically these signs include coolness, changes in skin color, increased sleepiness and lack of response, disorientation, incontinence, decrease in urine output, decrease in desire for fluid or food, congestion, and changes in breathing. Actively dying patients withdraw emotionally and decrease social contact, then withdraw physically. Patients may appear withdrawn and are selective as to whom they want to be with and who performs their care.

Families are reminded that the last sense to go is hearing and that they may want to say final good-byes. Occasionally a family member expresses feelings and lets the dying person know that it is all right to go, that they and other family members will take care of each other. Occasionally a spiritual adviser says prayers at the bedside with family and close friends.

The Connecticut Hospice uses a publication, *Information for Family Members: Commonly Asked Questions About Dying* (35), as an adjunct to discussion with family members to explain the physiology of dying and the specific signs and symptoms that are evident as the body is preparing for the final stage of life. Common physical, neural, and emotional changes are explained, as are the signs that death has occurred. Families are informed of what will happen after the death regarding verification of the death, announcement, care of the body, funeral arrangements, and so on. This is often done in advance so that a family is prepared for the process and understands the natural history of various disease processes and the signs and symptoms. Patients ask, "What can I expect?" Hospice caregivers use this opportunity to describe the things that typically occur, the indicators to watch for, and the interventions that can be used.

Indications for terminal sedation include poor pain control, which affects 10% of patients. It may be necessary to give enough morphine to sedate the patient in order to control the pain. Sedation is an accepted side effect at the end of life, as it is for a surgical or traumatic event.

NEW INITIATIVES

Many medical know-hows, what-fors, and know-whens help us with the never-finished business of medical management of a therapeutic response to disease and symptoms of disease. Although the goals for the patient may change, the person does not have to change his or her physician. The value of the attending physician to continue to treat through the various phases of illness must not be underestimated. This continuity breeds trust and support for the choices the patient must make to stay in control of his or her life. There are two new initiatives in this area. The first is a broad, overarching new approach to advance directives called Physician Assisted Living (PAL). The second is CanSupport Care.

Physician Assisted Living

Opinion surveys conducted in 1995 and 1996 by the Hospice Institute brought to light the need for a public information initiative that promised patients choice by heightening awareness of the hospice option. This initiative would enable consumers to consider and commit to writing their preference for hospice care before they face the complex issues that arise when serious advanced illness is diagnosed. On September 24, 1997, this initiative, known as Physician Assisted Living, was begun. With all of the advances in the care of patients, the many failures in the provisions of end-of-life care have been striking. Although in some circumstances we simply do not know the right actions on behalf of patients, all agree with compassionate attention and comfort to those who are dying. Connecticut's Physician Assisted Living is an exemplary program providing a means and framework for coordinated planning by all concerned in the best interest of the dying patient. The physician can create the best possible setting to provide responsive, supportive, and compassionate care.

It is hoped that by demonstration of this new advance directive in Connecticut and by educating physicians, nurses, social workers, and pastors of acute care hospitals, the directive will be used throughout the country, enhancing and promoting the welfare of all patients. Connecticut has provided a grant to set up in hospitals related interdisciplinary team training programs called Train the Trainer.

CanSupport Care

CanSupport Care is a disease management home care program initially designed for patients with cancer but eventually for persons with other disease as well. It is a new effort to help patients with cancer early in their disease and throughout all the phases of it. Patients may enter CanSupport Care while participating in clinical trials. Once a patient is admitted to the program, the care is managed by case managers of CanSupport

The Refocus Zone

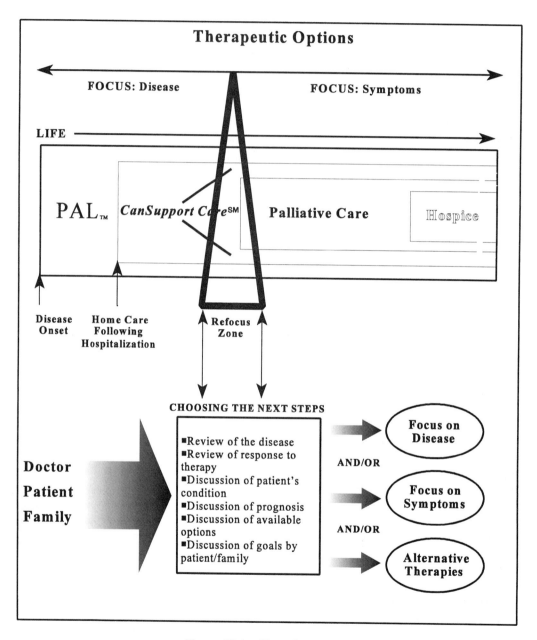

Figure 63.1.   The refocus zone.

Care in collaboration with oncologists, gerontologists, family members, and a particular management care organization. Throughout the program, patients continue appropriate treatment of their disease in addition to typical home care such as nursing, social work, and various forms of therapy. The program also offers the expertise of an oncologic team, telenursing (a service in which registered nurses answer patients' questions 24 hours a day on camera), transportation to doctors' offices, and counseling. The program also includes the new CarePhone technology, which boosts confidence and safety of caregivers at home. Treatment plans are always developed to meet and match lifestyles. These trials, now going on in Connecticut, compare patients coming to a program such as this early in disease progression with those using the traditional approaches. Its hypothesis is that early entry into supportive care will result in a higher quality of life or perhaps a longer life.

Figure 63.1 depicts how these new initiatives work, with the central theme being the refocus zone. Just before entering this zone the physician must be prepared to deal with all of these issues by answering the following questions:

- What do this patient and family understand?
- What do this patient and family want?
- What degree of futility is there?
- What and how severe are the patient's symptoms?
- What is the tempo of progression over the past few weeks or months?
- Can I anticipate how the patient will die?
- What are reasonable goals?
- Could I make this patient worse by whatever I do?
- What do I do if the patient and family disagree with my recommendation?
- What are the specific ways to involve the patient and family in decision making?

CONCLUSION

The success of hospice care in the United States is a triumph of the human spirit over the many forces of technology and modern medicine that deny death. Hospice care calls on physicians to support patients and families through the penultimate chapter of their lives and ultimately through the moment of death. The proliferation of hospice programs and the explosion of palliative care and hospice-related literature (see the bibliography) attest to the importance of hospice care and its emerging status as a medical specialty.

Society has become sensitized to the values of hospice, that no person should die alone or in pain. This concern has been addressed through a new initiative beginning in Connecticut, Physician Assisted Living, which proposes amendment to living will statutes allowing for advance election of hospice care as a part of the development of a living will. The Connecticut attorney general has launched an administrative process to distribute a form to consumers, creating awareness of hospice care long before diagnosis of terminal illness.

When irreversible illness is diagnosed, hospice is the appropriate early intervention. Hospice care empowers patients not to be dehumanized. Among many other things, hospice caregivers offer patients and their families a sacred space for struggling with the joy and pain of the human experience. Often in the midst of chaos, members of the hospice team use their diverse gifts to help patients and their families embrace emerging forms of authentic creativity. In the delicate movement of the intimate and ultimate life change, that which is often described as holy, full of mystery, and infinite, reveals itself through the life patterns, relationships, and essence, or soul, of the patient. It is hard to imagine accompanying someone on a more meaningful life journey than this one (36).

REFERENCES

1. Hospice fact sheet. Arlington, VA: National Hospice Organization, July 1996 (http://www.nho.org//facts.htm).
2. Hospice Facts and Statistics 1996. Washington: Hospice Association of America, 1996:6.
3. A controlled trial to improve care for seriously ill hospitalized patients. The study to understand prognoses and preferences for outcomes and risks of treatments (SUPPORT). The SUPPORT Principal Investigators. JAMA 1995;274:1591–1598.
4. Good care of the dying patient. Council on Scientific Affairs, American Medical Association. JAMA 1996;275:474–478.
5. Randal J. Preparing for life's end: do health professionals need more training? J Natl Cancer Inst 1997;89:15–16.
6. ABIM End-of-Life Patient Care Project. Identification and Promotion of Physician Competency. Cambridge, MA: Harvard Medical School, 1995:1–6.
7. Schonwetter RS. Care of the dying geriatric patient. Clin Geriatric Med 1996;12:253–265.
8. Greipp ME. SUPPORT study results—implications for hospice care. Am J Hosp Palliat Care 1996;13:38–39.
9. Field MJ, Cassel CK, eds. Approaching death: improv-

ing care at the end of life. Executive Summary, Committee on Care at the End of Life, Institute of Medicine. Washington: National Academy Press, 1997.

10. Vacco v Washington. United States. 117 S. Ct. 2293, 2298, 1997.

11. Standards of a Hospice Program of Care. Arlington, VA: National Hospice Organization, 1993.

12. World Health Organization. Cancer Pain Relief and Palliative Care. Technical Report Series 804. Geneva: WHO, 1990.

13. Conant L, Lowney A. The role of hospice philosophy of care in nonhospice settings. J Law Med Ethics 1996; 24:365–368.

14. Byock I. Ethics from a hospice perspective. Am J Hosp Palliat Care 1994;11:9–11.

15. Lewin-VHI, Inc. An analysis of the cost savings of the Medicare hospice benefit. In: Hospice Facts and Statistics 1996. Washington: Hospice Association of America, 1996:6.

16. Medicare Conditions of Compliance. 418.70. 42 U.S.C. 1395 (dd) et seq.

17. National Hospice Organization. Medical Guidelines for Determining Prognosis in Selected Non-Cancer Diseases. Arlington, VA: National Hospice Organization, 1995.

18. U.S.C. Section 1965 et seq.

19. Callahan D. The Troubled Dream of Life: Living With Mortality. New York: Simon & Schuster, 1993:41.

20. Cassell EJ. Recognizing suffering. Hastings Cent Rep 1991;21:24–31.

21. Abbott JW. Hospice Resource Manual for Local Churches. Spiritual Pain and Spiritual Growth: Ten Aspects of Spiritual Pain. New York: Pilgrim Press, 1987:21.

22. Abbott JW, ed. Hospice Resource Manual for Local Churches. Pilgrim, OH: Pilgrim Press, 1988.

23. Cherny NI, Coyle N, Foley KM. The treatment of suffering when patients request elective death. J Palliative Care 1994;10:71–79.

24. Tollison CD, Satterthwaite JR, Tollison JW, eds. Handbook of Pain Management. 2nd ed. Baltimore: Williams & Wilkins, 1994:3.

25. Rousseau P. Hospice and palliative care. Dis Mon 1995; 41:779–842.

26. Doyle D, Hanks G, McDonald N, eds. Oxford Book of Palliative Medicine. Oxford, UK: Oxford University Press, 1993.

27. Deleted in proof.

28. Enck RE. A review of pain management. Am J Hosp Palliat Care 1992;8:6–9.

29. Cleeland CS, Gonin R, Hatfield AK, et al. Pain and its treatment in outpatients with metastatic cancer. N Engl J Med 1994;330:592–596.

30. Kaiko RF. Age and morphine analgesia in cancer patients with post-operative pain. Clin Pharmacother 1980; 28:823–826.

31. Agency for Health Care Policy and Research. Management of Cancer Pain. Clinical Practice Guideline 9 (AHCPR 94–0592). Rockville, MD: US Department of Health and Human Services, Public Health Service, Agency for Health Care Policy and Research, 1994.

32. Portnoy RK. Chronic opioid therapy in nonmalignant pain. J Pain Symptom Manage 1990;5:S46–S62.

33. Stiefel F, Fainsinger R, Bruera E. Acute confusional states in patients with advanced cancer. J Pain Symptom Manage 1992;7:94–98.

34. Bukberg J, et al. Depression in hospitalized cancer patients. Psychosomat Med 1984;46:199–212.

35. Information for Family Members: Commonly Asked Questions About Dying. Brandford, CT: Connecticut Hospice, 1992.

36. Abbot JW. Nuances, The Soul of Hospice. Branford, CT: Connecticut Hospice, 1997.

BIBLIOGRAPHY

Abyad A. Palliative care: the future. Am J Hosp Palliat Care 1993;10:23–28.

Alspach G. Caring when curing is no longer possible. Crit Care Nurse 1996;16:12, 15.

Appleton M. Hospice medicine: a different perspective. Am J Hosp Palliat Care 1996;13:7–9.

Austin C, Cody C, Eyres P, et al. Hospice home care pain management: four critical variables. Cancer Nurs 1986; 9:58–65.

Baack CM. Nursing's role in the nutritional care of the terminally ill: weathering the storm. Hosp J 1993;9:1–13.

Baines M. Intestinal obstruction. Cancer Surv 1994;21:227–235.

Bergevin P, Bergevin R. Recognizing depression. Am J Hosp Palliat Care 1995;12:22–23.

Bergevin P, Bergevin R. Recognizing delirium in terminal patients. Am J Hosp Palliat Care 1996;13:28–29.

Berry P, Ward S. Barriers to pain management in hospice: a study of family caregivers. Hosp J 1995;10:19–33.

Berry Z, Lynn J. Hospice medicine. JAMA 1993;270:221–222.

Bohnet N. Hospice concepts in home care. Caring 1996;15: 44–50.

Bone R. Hospice and palliative care. Dis Mon 1995;41:769–842.

Bradshaw A. The spiritual dimension of hospice: the secularization of an ideal. Soc Sci Med 1996;43:409–419.

Byock I. Patient refusal of nutrition and hydration: walking the ever-finer line. Am J Hosp Palliat Care 1995;12:8.

Christakis NA, Escarce JJ. Survival of Medicare patients after enrollment in hospice programs. N Engl J Med 1996; 335:172–178.

Cooke MA. The challenge of hospice nursing in the 90's. Am J Hosp Palliat Care 1992;9:34–37.

Corless IB. Dying well: symptom control within hospice care. Annu Rev Nurs 1994;12:125–146.

Davis C, Hardy J. Palliative care. BMJ 1994;308:1359–1362.

Dawson N. Need satisfaction in terminal care settings. Soc Sci Med 1991;32:83–87.

Dobratz J. The life closure scale: a measure of psychosocial adaptation in death and dying. Hosp J 1990;6: 11–15.

Dobratz M. Analysis of variables that impact psychological adaptation in home hospice patients. Hosp J 1995;10: 75–88.

Dudley J, Smith C, Millison M. Unfinished business: assessing the spiritual needs of hospice clients. Am J Hosp Palliat Care 1995;121:30–37.

Emanuel E. Cost savings at the end of life: what do the data show? JAMA 1996;275:1907–1914.

Emanuel EJ, Emanuel LL. Economics of dying: the illusion of cost savings at the end of life. N Engl J Med 1994;330: 540–544.

Eng M. The hospice interdisciplinary team: a synergistic approach to the care of dying patients and their families. Holistic Nurs Pract 1993;7:49–56.

Fainsinger R, Miller M, Bruera E, et al. Symptom control during the last week of life on a palliative care unit. J Palliat Care 1991;7:5–11.

Feuz A, Rapin C. An observational study of the role of pain control and food adaptation of elderly patients with terminal cancer. J Am Diet Assoc 1994;94:767–770.

Fifeld M. Relieving constipation and pain in the terminally ill. Am J Nurs 1991;7:18–23.

Gordon A. An interdisciplinary team approach toward death education. Am J Hosp Palliat Care 1996;13:21.

Gordon M, Singer PA. Decisions and care at the end of life. Lancet 1994;17:52–60.

Greipp ME. Decisions to utilize hospice—pilot study results. Am J Hosp Palliat Care 1996;13:27–30.

Grey R. The psychospiritual matrix: a new paradigm for hospice care giving. Am J Hosp Palliat Care 1996;13:19–25.

Gurfolino V, Dumas L. Hospice nursing: the concept of palliative care. Nurs Clin North Am 1994;29:533–546.

Herth K. Engendering hope in the chronically and terminally ill: nursing interventions. Am J Hosp Palliat Care 1995; 12:31–39.

Higginson I. Palliative care: a review of past changes and future trends. J Public Health Med 1933;15:3–8.

Hogan J. Seeking a better way to die. Sci Am 1997;276:100–105.

Hohl D. Patient satisfaction in home care/hospice. Nurs Manag 1994;25:52–54.

Holden C. Nutrition and hydration in the terminally ill cancer patient: the nurse's role in helping patients and families cope. In: Gallagher-Allred C, Amenta MO, eds. Nutrition and Hydration in Hospice Care. Binghamton, NY: Haworth, 1993.

Home-health and hospice care—United States, 1992. MMWR Morb Mortal Wkly Rep 1993;42:820–824.

Infeld D, Crum G, Koshuta M. Characteristics of patients in a long term care hospice setting. Hosp J 1990;6:1–2.

Jackson A. Source of knowledge. Nurs Times 1995;91:55–57.

Johnson Hurzeler R, Barnum E, Klimas S, Michael E. Hospice care. In: Harris MD, ed. Handbook of Home Health Care Administration. Gaithersburg, MD: Aspen, 1997:782–789.

Khoo D, Hall E, Motson R, et al. Palliation of malignant intestinal obstruction using octreotide. Eur J Cancer 1994; 30A:28–30.

Kliska J. Hospice: beyond boundaries. Conn Med 1994;58: 349–352.

Lamberts S, Van Der Lely A, De Herder W, Hofland L. Octreotide. N Engl J Med 1996;334:246–249.

Long MC. Death and dying and recognizing approaching death. Clin Geriatr 1996;12:259–268.

Manion J. Cancer pain management in the hospice setting. Minn Med 1995;78:25–28.

McCann R, Hall W, Groth-Juncker A. Comfort care for terminally ill patients: the appropriate use of nutrition and hydration. JAMA 1994;272:1263–1266.

McMillan SC, Mahon M. A study of the quality of life of hospice patients on admissions. Cancer Nurs 1994;17:52–60.

McMillan SC. Pain and pain relief experienced by hospice patients with cancer. Cancer Nurs 1996;19:298–307.

Meares CJ. Terminal dehydration: a review. Am J Hosp Palliat Care 1994;11:10–14.

Melvin T, Ozbek IN, Eberle DE. Recognition of depression. Hosp J 1995;10:39–46.

Miles SH, Weber EP, Koepp R. End of life treatment in managed care: potential and peril. West J Med 1995;163: 162–305.

Millison M. The importance of spirituality in hospice work: a study of hospice professionals. Hosp J 1990;6:63–65,78.

Millison M. A review of the research on spiritual care and hospice. Hosp J 1995;10:3–18.

Moinpour C, Polissar L. Factors affecting place of death of hospice and nonhospice cancer patients. Am J Public Health 1989;79:1549–1551.

Morgan A, Lindley C, Berry J. Assessment of pain and patterns of analgesic use in hospice patients. Am J Hosp Palliat Care 1994;11:13–19, 22–25.

O'Callaghan CC. Pain, music creativity and music therapy in palliative care. Am J Hosp Palliat Care 1996;13:43–49.

O'Sullivan Maillet J, King D. Nutritional care of the terminally ill adult. In: Nutrition and Hydration in Hospice Care. Binghamton, NY: Haworth, 1993.

Paton L. The Sacred Circle: a conceptual framework for spiritual care in hospice. Am J Hosp Palliat Care 1996;13: 52–56.

Paton L, Wicks M. The growth of the hospice movement in Japan. Am J Hosp Palliat Care 1996;13:26–31.

Praill D. Approaches to spiritual care. Nurs Times 1995; 91:55–57.

Prigerson H. Determinants of hospice utilization among terminally ill geriatric patients. Home Health Ser Q 1991; 12:81–112.

Randal J. Preparing for life's end: do health professionals need more training? J Natl Cancer Inst 1997;89:15–16.

Raudonis B. The meaning and impact of empathic relationships in hospice nursing. Cancer Nurs 1993;16:304–309.

Reichel W, ed. Care of the Elderly: Clinical Aspects of Aging. 4th ed. Baltimore: Williams & Wilkins, 1995:647.

Robinson B, Pham H. Cost effectiveness of hospice care. Clin Geriatr 1996;12:417–428.

Schonwetter R. Care of the dying geriatric patient. Clin Geriatr 1996;12:253–265.

Seale C. A comparison of hospice and conventional care. Soc Sci Med 1991;32:147–153.

Sheahan P. Psychological pain and care. Nurs Times 1996; 92:63,66,68.

Snyder JR. Therapeutic touch and the terminally ill: healing power through the hands. Am J Hosp Palliat Care 1997;14:83–87.

Sontag MA. A comparison of hospice programs based on Medicare certification status. Am J Hosp Palliat Care 1996;13:32–41.

Spence R. Nutrition in hospice care. Caring 1988;7:50–51.

Stjernsward J, Colleau S, Ventafridda V. The World Health Organization Cancer Pain and Palliative Care Program. Past, present, and future. J Pain Symptom Manage 1996;12:12–14.

Storey P. What is the role of the hospice physician? Am J Hosp Palliat Care 1992;9:4–5.

Storey P. Symptom control in advanced cancer. Semin Oncol 1994;21:748–753.

Thalbuber W. Overcoming physician barriers to hospice care. Minn Med 1995;78:25–28.

Tierney J, Wilson D. Hospice versus home health care: regulatory distinctions and program intent. Am J Hosp Palliat Care 1994;11:14–19, 22.

Turner K, Chye R, Aggarwal G, et al. Dignity in dying: a preliminary study of patients in the last three days of life. J Palliat Care 1996;12:7–13.

Van der Poel C. Ethical aspects in palliative care. Am J Hosp Palliat Care 1996;13:49–55.

Von Gunten CF, Twaddle ML. Terminal care for noncancer patients. Clin Geriatr Med 1996;12:349–358.

Von Gunten CF, Von Roenn JH, Johnson-Neely K, et al. Hospice and palliative care: attitudes and practices of the physician faculty of an academic hospital. Am J Hosp Palliat Care 1995;12:38–42.

Watt K. Hospice and the elderly: a changing perspective. Am J Hosp Palliat Care 1996;13:47–48.

Wholihan D. The value of reminiscence in hospice care. Am J Hosp Palliat Care 1992;9:33–35.

Willert M, Beckwith B, Holm J, Beckwith S. A preliminary study of the impact of terminal illness on spouses: social support and coping strategies. Hosp J 1995; 10:35–48.

Willis W. Hyperalgesia and allodynia: summary and overview. In: Willis WE, ed. Hyperalgesia and Allodynia. New York: Raven, 1992:1–11.

Wilson S. The family as caregivers: home hospice care. Fam Community Health 1992;15:71–80.

Zerwekh J. A family caregiving model for hospice nursing. Hosp J 1995;10:27–44.

Spiritual Aspects of Aging

In the past 100 years medicine has largely diverged from its historical roots in many cultures as a facet of religion. This divergence of the role of religion from the medical sciences started with the theory of evolution formulated by Charles Darwin, when the role of the church lost authority to the material basis of science and medicine. It marked the beginning of the modern schism between science and religion; in the 16th century it was considered heresy for science to question the will of God.

The scientific paradigm (proof) has elevated physicians in modern society to a position of control over the lives of their patients in which the role of religious paradigm (faith) is largely ignored in favor of pharmaceutical and/or surgical intervention for reducing the life-threatening effects of disease or biologic disabilities. The religious and spiritual paradigm of healing has emerged in Western medicine in the past decade. Prayer for healing in the elderly is considered to be an important component of medical intervention (1, 2).

BACKGROUND

In what is now the United States, the first European contacts with shamans of the native American tribes led to calling them medicine men, or those who ministered to the members of the tribe and acted as spiritual guides for protection against the hazards of life (3). The origin of the complementary nature of spirituality and medicine is seen in the etymologic sources of the word holy, which derives from the Germanic and Old English *halen,* or healing.

Reflection on our own past lives has made us aware of the role of spirituality or more specifically religion as an ever-changing feature of the relation between our lifestyles and the value systems that we live by. However, a distinction should be made between spirituality and religion. Spirituality is an awareness of personal identity in relation to a higher power within the surrounding cultural environment. The hazards implicit in the local climate, availability of food, reproductive potential, and disease all confer an element of anxiety about our limited control over these conditions. The mystical visualization of a deity who has the power to overcome these threats and to protect us from harm becomes part of our personal view of existence. Religion is the socially derived acceptable behavior in a specific cultural group framed within an organization's construct of God and the related history of spiritual insights recorded in scriptures or passed on through oral tradition. In practice the expression of spirituality and religious tradition are considered to be synonymous.

The role of religion is largely determined by personal attitudes, i.e., acceptance, ambivalence, or rejection, which are developed and expressed within societal norms. The person living in any religious tradition develops a relative sense of compassion and self-interest based on experience, and that sense affects his or her mental and physical welfare during aging (4).

STAGES OF SPIRITUAL MATURATION

As we age, reminiscence of our actions in youth leads to various emotional attitudes toward religion. These can be interpreted as feelings of guilt or of comfort depending on the religious tradition or secular persuasion developed during the formative years. In Western society spiritual life can be divided into three broad time frames. The first 3 decades are a period of maturing our value systems in the context of our culture, testing them against the social environment, and using the values that best benefit survival within societal norms. The second 3 decades are a time of using intrinsic skills and values to develop a stable environment for raising children, guiding them in the religious tradition that we have found useful in our own lives, and adapting to changes that arise from technologic developments. The remaining decades are a period of declining societal productivity with retrospection on the spiritual implications of our earlier lifestyles and their effect on those around us. It is in this third phase of life that we reflect on the role of experience in the religious and philosophical attitudes that we have used and the ways they prepare us for mortality.

To obtain a picture of a person's spiritual attitudes in the mature years it is useful to define the spiritual developmental profile that precedes this period. Among several theories for the development of spiritual sensitivity in humans, Koenig (5) subdivided spiritual lives into five stages of development.

First Stage

In the first stage, birth to 2 years old, the first images of God are external and identified with the actions of the mother. If she is loving and caring, the child's image reflects that. The basic behavior is trust, comfort, and dependence. The mother's attitude to the child is conditioned by the hormonal changes of pregnancy, which facilitate her bonding to it.

Second Stage

The second stage, 2 to 6 years, is when the child internalizes the image of God. It is idealized in the mother's behavior, which the child mimics to please her. God can be seen as loving or judgmental, with an influence that becomes more powerful as the guiding role of the parent or parents is seen to be more fallible and prone

to mistakes. Clergy and other authorities, especially teachers, tend to become god figures.

Third Stage

The third stage, 6 to 12 years, is when the notion of evil and the devil create anxiety; the image of God as a controlling entity still resembles that of parents and teachers. Prayer becomes meaningful as a feeling of trust in a protective God. It is a time of rituals such as the rites of passage of confirmation and bar mitzvah, which affirm a decision to follow God within a specific religious tradition.

Fourth Stage

During the fourth stage, 13 to 29 years, adolescence begins at the onset of puberty with the emotional and identity changes that culminate in a more mature image of God. There may be acceptance, rejection, or ambivalence, and it may be influenced and modified more by peer pressure than by the parents. The person stabilizes within a tradition of faith (obedience) or creates a different personal faith developing to a higher level of relation with God than pure obedience. In this stage faith either integrates with or overcomes intellectual quandaries of belief.

Fifth Stage

The fifth stage is from age 30 to the end of life. Here life experiences such as joy, pain, and suffering impinge on our image of God to refine it and make it more relevant to our own reality. In this context a violent person who is kind to another is generally considered to be more spiritually mature than an affluent person who neglects his obligations to his family (5). Behavioral stereotyping in a negative sense requires an awareness of the many psychosocial components that contribute to such an assessment so that effective spiritual understanding may enhance communication (6).

After age 70, remorse and repentance come into play in relation to redemption. Repentance and forgiveness can diminish the anxiety that arises from guilt or disobedience and regenerate the trust and comfort of earlier stages of faith. This can lead to a renewed outlook on life in relation to others and a positive acceptance of death. Such spiritual renewal may transcend the most debilitating disease and is recognized in the elderly as a personal equanimity beyond expectations for their circumstances.

PSYCHOBIOLOGIC COMPONENTS OF SPIRITUALITY

Belief in God to enhance physical healing has long been used in many human cultures. More recently, Benson and Friedman (7) pioneered the study of the biologic basis of spirituality to describe the nature of physical healing induced by mental means, usually in the form of prayer or meditation. They coined the term relaxation response for these biologic effects primarily because of its antistress and restorative influence. It is analogous to the placebo effect in medical therapy, which is well documented (7, 8). This effect is expressed in the patient as a belief in the therapeutic value of a procedure that will favor a positive result; it occurs independently of a known curative effect, such as the action of antibiotics toward bacterial infections. It can be induced by an innocuous substance, such as saline solution, given to a patient with a positive mental attitude to allow the beneficial effect to occur. Turner et al. (9) suggest that stress reduction methods to diminish anxiety may account for some of the placebo effect. Conversely, disbelief in the effectiveness of a known therapeutic procedure may diminish its value. The healing qualities of the placebo effect are similar to those seen in the spiritual belief systems of many religions, and modern medical practice is slowly returning to this mode of intervention despite longstanding doubts about its value. This is true especially for the treatment of chronic pain. The utility of spiritual intervention in treating chronic pain is defined by Caudhill and Friedman (10) as a form of psychotherapy and couched in terms of cognitive restructuring. To clarify its value for patients, they defined the dimensions of acute and chronic pain in functional terms as follows.

Acute Pain

Acute pain is characterized by short duration, a known cause, responsiveness to opioids and other analgesics, central endorphin suppression, temporary functional disruption, and mental anxiety.

Chronic Pain

Chronic pain lasts longer than 6 months. It has a vague cause, possibly a defect in pain perception pathways. It is characterized by diminished response to acute pain therapy and loss of functional capacity for an indefinite period.

To overcome the debilitating effects of chronic pain, meditation to manage anger, anxiety, and depression is more effective than pharmaceutical intervention, more so in spiritually inclined persons than in those without religious beliefs (11). Religions with a meditative component of mental control of bodily processes, as found in Far Eastern traditions, are likely to be more effective in controlling chronic pain disorders, since the practice of meditation favors this outcome (12). In Western religions the spiritual approach to healing by means of meditation could be valuable if physicians provided more support for such methods (13).

AGING, PRAYER, AND HEALING

After age 60 physical problems become more common and disabling, whereas spiritual awareness becomes more focused. This may lead to a decline in overt religious activities (attendance at church, mosque, synagogue, or temple) and more prayer (14). Intrinsic spirituality (prayer) is likely to be found in elder conservative or orthodox believers, whereas extrinsic religiousness (church activity) tends to arise from sociopolitical motives in 30- to 60-year-olds (15). Ethnic diversity can influence this orientation. For example, Native Americans, African-Americans, and Native South Americans have more intrinsic than extrinsic qualities to their belief systems, as seen by their use of drums, dance, and icons in festive rituals (15). Stress and illness in the later years are more likely to be tolerated through prayer and social religious involvement, which is more prevalent in African-Americans than in other American ethnic groups (16). Group participation in prayer and Bible reading by religious elders also benefits them by raising morale during illness and may reduce recovery time (16).

The effectiveness of prayer to facilitate healing has shown that faith is a valuable adjunct to conventional therapy in primary care (3). The stress and anxiety of severe disease can be eased by the use of prayer, and coping is positively associated with both age and the severity of the illness (11). In a longitudinal study of religion and aging Blazer and Plamore (17) found that religious ritual and happiness were positively correlated and increased with age. In terminally ill cancer patients, religious meaning and the strength of belief reduced the fear of death; other factors, such as low pain levels and close family support, also contributed to its reduction (18). Intrinsic spirituality was found to protect against the fear of dying in the elderly, and close family enhanced survival (19).

The body of evidence on the beneficial effect of spiritual belief on the health status and mortality of the elderly strongly suggests that spiritual intervention in physical and psychiatric health care can be a powerful therapeutic measure in clinical practice (20). Since a large number of the elderly in the United States are likely to be institutionalized or hospitalized in their final years, symptoms of spiritual distress should be recognized and addressed. Spiritual distress in clinical care scenarios has been defined by Maas et al. (21). Its signs include the following array of symptoms and interventions (21).

Causation

Spiritual distress may be caused by physical disability and terminal disease. Loss of a spouse or other close family member may also distress the spirit, as may hospital barriers to religious practice and health care providers who oppose the patient's beliefs.

Symptoms

The patient in spiritual distress questions the meaning of life, suffering, and existence. He or she may question the value of life extension, especially if in chronic pain. Such persons commonly claim abandonment by God, are unhappy, and regret their past. Some have thoughts of suicide.

Intervention

Interventions for a patient in spiritual distress include prayer with a pastor, caregiver, or family, meditation, socialization with friends and family, and compassionate and uplifting communicative care.

When institutionalized persons who are religious are depressed, the level of spiritual comfort can be raised by providing them with religious icons, such as crosses or menorahs; religious music (hymns, chants); religious art or nature scenes, and prayers. With patients in the latter stages of terminal disease, compassionate care by both physicians and health care personnel should include comfort and solace. When death is clearly imminent, the limitations of and options for life extension by technologic intervention should be compassionately and truthfully discussed with patients and their families. In these cases spiritual enhancement may be more comforting.

SUMMARY

Intervention by the physician on a compassionate religious level with the aged and physically impaired is found to have beneficial health effects independent of surgical or pharmaceutical therapy. Spiritual therapy has roots in the biologic actions associated with the placebo effect and can be amplified by the use of meditative and/or cognitive restructuring methods to improve the outcome of chronic diseases such as chronic pain, cardiovascular disease, and asthma. Physicians' awareness of the spiritual needs of the elderly can diminish the anxiety and depression associated with physical disability and terminal disease in the course of normal human aging. Spiritual distress of normal and cognitively impaired elderly can be alleviated by means of rituals associated with specific religions (hymns, prayers, and icons) to which the person responds at an emotional level. The acceptance of death as a nonthreatening feature of life requires a compassionate relationship between the patient, physician, and other health care personnel to allow for spiritual comfort at the end of life.

REFERENCES

1. Foglio JP, Brody H. Religion, faith and family medicine. J Fam Pract 1988;27:473–474.
2. King DE, Sobal J, DeForge BR. Family practice patients' experiences and beliefs in faith healing. J Fam Pract 1988;27:505–508.
3. Matthews DA. Religion and spirituality in primary care. Mind Body Med 1997;2:9–19.
4. Smith H. The Illustrated World's Religions. San Francisco: Harper Collins, 1994:40–41.

5. Koenig HG. Aging and God. New York: Haworth, 1994.

6. Swinton J, Kettles AM. Resurrecting the person: redefining mental illness: a spiritual perspective. Psychiatric Care 1997;4:118–121.

7. Benson H, Friedman R. Harnessing the power of the placebo effect and renaming it "remembered wellness." Annu Rev Med 1996;47:193–199.

8. Benson H, McCallie DP Jr. Angina pectoris and the placebo effect. N Engl J Med 1979;300:1424–1429.

9. Turner JA, Deyo RA, Loeser JD, et al. The importance of placebo effects in pain treatment and research. JAMA 1994;271:1609–1614.

10. Caudhill MA, Friedman R. Psychology and physiology of pain as related to spiritual healing practices. II. Conference on Spirituality and Healing in Medicine, Boston, December 15–17, 1996 (abstract).

11. Koenig HG. Use of religion by patients with severe medical illness. Mind Body Med 1997;2:31–36.

12. Rapgay L. Buddhist spiritual healing practices. II Conference on Spirituality and Healing in Medicine, Boston, December 15–17, 1996 (abstract).

13. Culver M, Kell M. Working with chronic pain patients: spirituality as part of the treatment protocol. Am J Pain Manag 1995;5:55–61.

14. Levin JS. Religious factors in aging, adjustment and health: a theoretical overview. In: Enright RB Jr, ed. Perspectives in Social Gerontology. Boston: Allyn and Bacon, 1994:217–225.

15. Barrow GM. Aging, The Individual and Society. New York: West, 1996:112.

16. Hooyman NR, Kiyak HA. Social Gerontology: A Multidisciplinary Perspective. Boston: Allyn and Bacon, 1993:369.

17. Blazer D, Plamore E. Religion and aging in a longitudinal panel. Gerontologist 1997;16:82–85.

18. Gibbs HW, Achterberg-Lawlis J. Spiritual values and death anxiety: Implications for counseling with terminal cancer patients. J Counsel Psychol 1978;25:563–569.

19. Zuckerman DM, Kasl SV, Ostfeld AM. Psychosocial predictors of mortality among the elderly poor. Am J Epidemiol 1984;119:410–423.

20. Larson MD, Milano MG. Making the case for spiritual interventions in clinical practice. Mind Body Med 1997;2:20–30.

21. Maas M, Buckwalter K, Hardy MA. Nursing Diagnoses and Interventions for the Elderly. Reading, MA: Addison-Wesley, 1991:598.

Ethical Issues and the Elderly Patient

CHAPTER 65

LAURENCE B. McCULLOUGH, JILL A. RHYMES,
THOMAS A. TEASDALE, AND NANCY L. WILSON

Preventive Ethics in Geriatric Practice

Every physician in geriatric practice by now is well aware of the many ethical issues that physicians, patients, families, institutions, and society confront in the care of elderly patients. These range from such dramatic four-alarm issues as physician-assisted suicide (1–5) and the withholding of nutrition from terminally ill patients (1, 2) through less dramatic but still stressful issues such as deciding about long-term care (6) to mundane issues such as whether elders with cognitive impairments should continue to drive or whether the elder with long-term care needs should continue to live alone (7). These and the many other ethical issues and conflicts in geriatric practice receive a great deal of attention in the literature.

This literature focuses almost exclusively on the *resolution* of ethical conflict in the care of geriatric patients. As a consequence, the *prevention* of ethical conflict in geriatric practice has been neglected in the literature and therefore as a clinical skill. Ethical conflicts are intellectually engaging, especially the four-alarm ones. But they are also stressful for physicians, patients, families, and institutions. It will be far better for all of these parties, especially elders and their family members, for physicians and health care professionals to prevent ethical conflicts more effectively. The purpose of the four chapters in this section of the book is to introduce the physician to ethically justified, clinically applicable strategies of preventive ethics in geriatric practice, with emphasis on the crucial topics of long-term care decision making, advance directive decision

making, and the use of a clinically powerful adjunct to advance directives, the Values History (see Chapters 67 and 68).

This chapter begins with a definition of ethics and its basic concepts and terms. This is the basis for consideration of the two main topics of this chapter, preventive ethics in the physician-patient relationship and preventive ethics for dealing with health care institutions, including managed care organizations (MCOs). Because of their importance and prominence in the geriatrics literature, ethical issues in health care policy affecting the elderly and in research with elderly subjects are also considered.

ETHICS: DEFINITION, CONCEPTS, AND TERMS

Ethics is the disciplined study of morality. Descriptive ethics uses the methods of the qualitative and quantitative social sciences to identify the actual moral beliefs and practices of persons, groups, institutions, and society. Descriptive ethics provides important data that serve as the starting point for normative ethics, including normative geriatric ethics (8). Normative ethics uses the methods of philosophical analysis and argument to define morality. The chapters in this section are concerned with normative ethics (henceforth, simply ethics) in the context of health care. Normative ethics in the context of health care has come to be known as bioethics (9).

Bioethics in geriatric practice, a subspeciality of both geriatrics and bioethics, concerns morality in the physician-patient relationship, for health care institutions, and for society in matters of health care policy. The focus of this chapter is mainly on the first two, with particular attention to strategies for preventive ethics in geriatric practice.

Behavior and Character

Morality concerns the beliefs and practices of people about both behavior and character toward other people, institutions, society, other life forms, and inanimate objects. Ethics inquires into ethically justified behavior. Ethics asks about behavior two questions: what ought we do and what ought we not do.

Ethics is also concerned with ethically justified character: whether we are disposed to be concerned primarily with the interests of others and to act primarily for the sake of their interests rather than always our own. Character is an especially important consideration for the morality of physicians and health care professionals. Character is addressed in terms of the virtues and vices (10). Virtues are traits of character that blunt mere self-interest so that one can identify and routinely protect and promote the interests of others. Vices are traits of character that unleash mere self-interest, so that one ignores or even fails to identify the interests of others, much less serve their interests. Ethics asks about character two questions: what character traits ought to be cultivated as virtues and what character traits ought to be avoided as vices.

Managing Moral Pluralism

In the United States, as in many other countries, we live in a pluralistic society, perhaps the most pluralistic society in the world. There are many sources of morality in a pluralistic society, including law, historical experience and traditions, religious beliefs, professional education and training, personal experience, professional consensus, authorities and experts, and institutional policies and practices. Sometimes the disagreement among the sources of morality in a pluralistic society runs very deep, as it does, for example, on the subject of physician-assisted suicide. The competition among these sources of morality grows more pronounced for bioethics in an international context. Within and across nations there is a striking variety of views on bioethical issues (9, 11).

Ethical Analysis and Argument: Methods of Ethics and Bioethics

Because of the actual and potential disagreement among the many sources of morality in a pluralistic society, no one source or combination of them can be *the* source of morality upon which ethics and bioethics are reliably based (12). Bioethics requires methods that transcend these competing sources of morality. Over the centuries philosophy has developed well-tested and reliable methods to achieve this ambitious goal. These methods are ethical analysis and argument. Ethical analysis aims to identify the nature of ethical issues and conflicts. Ethical argument requires that reasons guide and ground moral judgment and decision making.

Intellectual Criteria for Ethical Analysis and Argument

Ethics relies on analysis and argument that proceed according to intellectual criteria for rigorous thought and judgment and requires one to submit to the intellectual discipline required by such criteria. That discipline requires that one go where ethical analysis and argument take one, not where gut feelings or personal opinion take one. Gut feelings and decisions based on them should not be confused with ethics. Disciplined ethical analysis and argument can develop accounts of morality that can command respect from all, regardless of the particular sources of morality that shape or influence each person. These criteria are clarity, consistency, coherence, applicability, and adequacy.

Clarity requires that basic concepts and terms be provided clear meanings and that relevant distinctions are drawn. Consistency requires that once terms are clarified, they are used with the same meaning throughout an argument. Consistency also applies to argument and requires that reasoning be free of contradiction and not violate logical rules. That is, arguments should reach their conclusions as a matter of logic. Coherence also applies to argument, requiring that premises fit together into a related set that as a whole produces the conclusion. Bioethics is not an ivory tower enterprise. On the contrary, bioethics must be applicable to the actual clinical and social situations that prompt moral concerns on the part of physicians, patients, families, institutions, and society. Bioethics must also be adequate: ethical analysis and argument and the results must be applicable in the future, especially to novel or unforeseen situations. Preventive ethics in geriatric practice, institutional policy, and research uses the ethical analysis and argument to frame reliable judgments.

Competing Accounts

Because bioethics emphasizes rigorous ethical analysis and argument that conform to these criteria and because of the inherent complexity of human behavior and institutions, bioethics often produces more than one rigorous account of what morality in geriatric health care ought to be. This is the case especially for issues of considerable controversy, such as physician-assisted suicide. This feature of bioethics should be seen as an advantage in the clinical setting. Ethical conflict can be avoided if from the outset physicians follow ethical analysis and argument where they lead and identify all ethically justified responses to complex and challenging issues such as withholding nutrition from an elderly patient with advanced dementia. Ethical conflict can also be avoided in clinical situations in which the world does not always cooperate with our well-thought-out attempts to manage it, such as when the extubated patient who was expected to die begins unexpectedly to breathe on his or her own. It is therefore very useful to have in place ethically justified strategies so that if the first one fails, others can be rapidly implemented. The basic approach of this and the next three chapters is to develop preventive ethics and management strategies that emphasize a flexible, practical approach to ethical issues that the physician will confront in the care of elderly patients.

That there can be competing well-made ethical analyses, arguments, and judgments underscores the fact that the results of bioethics are rarely final or certain and therefore are rarely immune to criticism. Rather than aiming at certainty (which is of-ten impossible), bioethics aims at reliability. In this respect, ethical reasoning is like clinical reasoning. The latter is far more frequently marked by differing degrees of probability than it is by certainty. Nonetheless, well-made rigorous clinical reasoning and judgments are reliable in the sense that physicians, patients, institutions, and society may act on them with confidence. So, too, for well-made clinical ethical judgments. This and the next three chapters aim to provide the physician with clinical strategies for preventive ethics and managing ethical issues and conflicts that are based on well-made judgments.

PREVENTIVE ETHICS IN THE PHYSICIAN-PATIENT RELATIONSHIP

Obligation to Protect and Promote the Patient's Interests

To be moral, not simply contractual and entrepreneurial, the physician-patient relationship must be other-directed, from the physician to the patient (for the most part) and from the patient to the physician. The physician's primary concern should be to serve the patient's interests, with the physician's own interests in a systematically secondary status. It has been a staple of the history of Western medical ethics at least since the 18th century that the physician's primary ethical obligation is to serve the patient's interests (13). If the physician is to produce effective clinical judgment, decision making, and behavior, he or she must be committed to discerning and fulfilling this basic ethical obligation. An account of morality for physicians therefore starts with the virtues that make the obligation to serve the patient's interests a way of life for physicians (14).

Four Fundamental Virtues

Four virtues are fundamental to the physician-patient relationship (14, 15). These virtues direct the physician's attention primarily to the patient's interests and as a rule away from the physician's interests and motivate him or her to protect and promote the patient's interests as a matter of routine in clinical practice.

Two virtues direct the physician's primary attention to the patient. The first virtue is *self-effacement,* the willingness routinely to put aside personal, economic, and social differences that should not count in the care of patients. The goal of self-effacement is to prevent the physician's interests from becoming his or her primary focus of concern, causing the patient's interests to slip from view. The second virtue is *self-sacrifice,* the routine willingness to risk one's other relationships, health, and even life as required in the appropriate care of patients. Self-effacement and self-sacrifice blunt the physician's understandable inclination to focus on himself or herself and turn the primary concern and attention to the interests of the patient.

Two virtues motivate the physician to serve the interests of the patient in clinical practice. *Compassion* is willingness to acknowledge and respond to relieve the suffering and distress of others. Compassion has an intellectual component, the capacity to know when a patient is in pain, suffering, or distressed. Compassion also has a motivating and behavioral component; it moves the physician to relieve the patient. *Integrity* is the willingness to form and adhere to rigorous, well-made clinical ethical judgments— following the five criteria we have discussed— about how to protect and promote the interests of the patient. Competence is thus a component of integrity. This is crucial in medicine because of the enormous power that physicians can wield in the care of patients (16). Integrity therefore requires the physician to act within and not exceed the competencies of medicine to serve the patient's interests. Integrity is also the source of satisfaction that comes from practicing medicine with a commitment to excellence. Compassion and integrity move the physician to protect and promote the patient's interests according to the highest intellectual and moral standards.

The moral demands of these virtues have limits. One of the central questions of the ethics of physicians is therefore what ought to count as justified limits to the obligations generated by these four virtues. In particular, physicians have legitimate self-interests that they are justified in taking into account and sometimes protecting, thus setting limits on these four virtues. Legitimate self-interest, a controversial category in contemporary bioethics (15, 17), includes the three following sorts of interests of physicians. The first are the requisites for providing good pa-

tient care, such as adequate rest and time to study and reflect. The second are obligations to others than patients, such as spouse, children, and friends. This includes a reasonable income, i.e., enough to meet these obligations. The third are activities beyond medicine in which the physician finds meaning and coherence in life. Unless a compelling case can be made for them, other forms of self-interest of physicians should be regarded as mere self-interest and thus do not justifiably limit the obligations generated by the virtues of a physician.

Consider the ethics of physician-assisted suicide. It is a clinical reality that some forms of pain or suffering relief for seriously ill or dying patients work only at the price of compromising the patient's quality of life. Many patients reasonably judge such losses to be unacceptable. One form of suffering, serious pain that attacks the patient's dignity and humanity, is traded for another, obtunded consciousness that destroys the relationships that make the patient's life meaningful. Compassion requires the physician to acknowledge the patient's unavoidable suffering in such circumstances and to relieve it. The only means of relief seem to be those that will cause the patient to die quickly of a cause other than the illness. It is therefore a matter of ethical obligation for the physician, on the basis of the virtue of compassion, to provide the means for such patients to commit suicide and even to administer the means directly for patients who are physically unable to do so for themselves but are competent to request such assistance. Thus, physician-assisted suicide cannot be ruled out ethically by the virtue of compassion, a disturbing conclusion.

Beneficence and Respect for Autonomy in Clinical Judgment and Practice

The four fundamental virtues of the physician direct and motivate his or her moral obligation to serve the interests of the patient. But how to do so for each particular patient? This question is addressed by the principles of beneficence and respect for autonomy. These two principles translate into clinical judgment and practice the general obligation to protect and promote the patient's interests by making this general obligation applicable to an individual patient. The key to doing so is the recognition that there are two perspectives on the interests of the patient: (*a*) that of medicine, translated into judgment by the principle of beneficence; and (*b*) that of the patient, translated into judgment by the principle of respect for autonomy (15, 18).

Beneficence

The ethical principle of beneficence requires the physician to act so that the consequences for the patient of the physician's behavior are reliably expected to be a greater balance of goods over harms as those goods and harms are understood from a rigorous clinical perspective. This is the most ancient of all ethical principles of bioethics (19).

Beneficence emphasizes the benefit of the patient, not the avoidance of harm, as the primary consideration. That is, *primum non nocere,* or first do no harm, is not the primary meaning of beneficence. First do no harm occurs nowhere in the Hippocratic texts, for example. Indeed, its historical origins are unknown. A version of the principle of non-malfeasance (13), it is not a first principle of bioethics, because if it were modern medicine would have to cease its work. Virtually none of what medicine, geriatric medicine especially, offers patients is free of harm. Because medicine is fundamentally oriented to benefiting patients *on balance,* beneficence is the primary ethical principle, with nonmaleficence a limiting principle: when the physician is doing only harm to the patient, which can sometimes happen, he or she ought to stop it.

To employ the principle of beneficence reliably in clinical judgment the physician should be able to do the following. First, the physician identifies the clinical goods to be sought and the clinical harms to be avoided. The clinical goods and harms of beneficence-based clinical judgment can be identified by use of professional competencies. The goods that the health care professions are competent to seek for patients are the prevention of premature or unnecessary death and the prevention, cure, or amelioration of disease, injury, handicap, and unnecessary pain and suffering. Death is premature when it occurs before life expectancy is up. Death is un-

necessary when it can be prevented at an ethically justified cost in terms of iatrogenic pain, suffering, injury, disease, handicap, or effect on quality of life. Pain and suffering are unnecessary when they do not produce any of the other goods of beneficence; they are harms to be avoided.

Second, the physician reaches rigorous judgments about which courses of intervention or nonintervention are reliably expected to produce a greater balance of goods over harms and thus serve the interests of the patient to some reasonable degree. Beneficence-based clinical judgment typically identifies a range or continuum of responses that serve the patient's interests, rather than just one. The physician should avoid the language of best interests as taken to mean that beneficence-based clinical judgment routinely identifies *the only response* that is in the patient's interest. One of the principal sources of paternalism in the clinical setting is failing to see alternatives that are justified in beneficence-based clinical judgment.

The goods and harms to which beneficence-based clinical judgment can speak are limited by professional competencies. Physicians, as health care professionals, are capable of addressing some but not all human goods. This feature of beneficence-based clinical judgment is crucial for understanding religious objections by patients to certain forms of medical interventions, such as the refusal of blood products by Jehovah's Witnesses. Members of this faith community value their health and life, but they value more their steadfast obedience to God's commands, which they understand to include the prohibition of blood products. Medicine is not competent to determine whether this hierarchy of values is reasonable, inasmuch as medicine, as a science-based secular profession, can claim no competence in theologic matters (15, 20). Failure to appreciate the limits of beneficence-based clinical ethical judgment sets up the physician for egregious forms of paternalism, such as waiting until a Jehovah's Witness patient who has refused blood products lapses into unconsciousness and then administering them.

Respect for Autonomy

The principle of respect for autonomy requires the physician to act so that the consequences for the patient of the physician's behavior are reliably expected to be a greater balance of goods over harms *as those goods and harms are understood from the patient's perspective.* That is, each patient has personal values and beliefs and can form preferences on the basis of them. This is true of geriatric patients, as it is of any other adult patient. Respect for autonomy translates the patient's perspective on his or her interests into clinical ethical judgment.

To employ the principle of respect for autonomy reliably the physician first provides an adequate amount of information to the patient or the surrogate about the patient's condition; about all medically reasonable options for its management, including watchful waiting; and about the benefits and risks of each management strategy, including watchful waiting. It is important that the physician identify and correct mistaken or false beliefs of the patient about these matters. This disclosure requirement renders unethical gag orders used explicitly or implicitly by MCOs.

Second, the physician elicits from the patient or the surrogate values and beliefs of the patient relevant to the task of evaluating the condition and management options. That is, the patient needs cognitive understanding of the consequences of various management strategies and evaluative understanding of their worth or importance from the patient's perspective (21). This is an especially important consideration in advance-directive decision making (see Chapters 66 and 67). As with beneficence-based clinical judgment, the goal is to identify the full range or continuum of management strategies that protect and promote the interests of the patient to some reasonable degree according to the patient's own values.

INFORMED CONSENT AS A PREVENTIVE ETHICS STRATEGY

When the principles of beneficence and respect for autonomy are properly used in clinical judgment and practice, clinical decision making becomes a process of negotiating management strategies on the common ground created by identifying all issues of beneficence and autonomy. This should be the goal of the informed consent process, not the largely meaningless bureaucratic ritual epitomized in the request to "go get the consent" (22). When this occurs, informed consent is neglected as the basic strategy of preventive ethics in geriatric practice. In the absence of a meaningful informed consent process, creating a common ground between beneficence-based and autonomy-based clinical ethical judgment will happen rarely and only by accident.

We propose a nine-step informed consent process (23). Hereafter in this chapter "informed consent" refers specifically to this nine-step process. Although this number of steps may at first appear to be burdensome, they are necessary for creating synergy rather than conflict between beneficence-based and autonomy-based clinical judgment. With practice this process can be achieved over a series of routine encounters with patients. These steps begin with the recognition that the geriatric patient needs enough information to participate meaningfully in the informed consent process and that the patient may need or welcome assistance in this process. The steps are as follows:

1. The physician begins by eliciting from the patient what he or she believes about the condition, its diagnosis, options for managing it, and the prognosis under each alternative.
2. In a respectful and supportive fashion the physician identifies and corrects errors or incompleteness in the patient's fund of knowledge. (This does not require that the patient be provided a complete medical education.)
3. The physician explains his or her clinical judgment about the patient's condition and all medically reasonable options, including watchful waiting.
4. The physician helps the patient, as needed or requested, to develop as complete as possible a picture of the condition and options, including watchful waiting. This is cognitive understanding.
5. The physician helps the patient, as needed or requested, to identify his or her relevant values and beliefs.
6. The physician, as needed or requested, helps the patient *in a nondirective* fashion to evaluate alternative management strategies in terms of the patient's values and beliefs. This is evaluative understanding.

7. The patient is asked to identify which alternatives are consistent with his or her values and beliefs: to express value-based preferences.
8. The physician makes a recommendation, based on the clinical judgment expressed in step 3 and the patient's preferences expressed in step 7.
9. A mutual decision about managing the patient's condition is reached.

Disagreement should be negotiated by repeating the steps.

Patients' Obligations in Informed Consent

This approach to informed consent assumes that the physician-patient relationship is a genuine partnership (24). At the very least, this implies some mutual obligations. In short, patients have obligations, too. Historically the obligations of patients to their physicians were a staple of medical ethics (25). Only recently has this subject begun to receive attention again (26, 27).

Informed consent makes explicit reference to the patient's cognitive and evaluative understandings of his or her condition and options for managing it. At the very least, this requires that the patient attend to what the physician has to say. Moreover, when matters are serious—as they are when the patient's interests are at risk for being harmed in far-reaching and irreversible ways, such as with aggressive management of stage IV heart failure—the patient owes the physician a level of serious attention and due consideration of the benefits and risks of management options. That is, the patient owes it to the physician to be serious when matters are serious, such as in cases of chronic debilitating diseases, life-threatening events, and terminal illnesses.

Morality in the physician-patient relationship therefore entails a genuine partnership, mutual obligations, and a commitment on the part of the physician to strategies that prevent ethical conflict when possible and managing it well when it does occur. Informed consent can be used to prevent ethical conflict by reaching mutually agreed-upon decisions, complemented with a willingness to negotiate to manage ethical conflict.

Informed Consent and Diminished Decision-Making Capacity

Patients with diminished decision-making capacities pose special challenges to the physician in geriatric practice, given the significant rates of dementing disorders and other factors that can adversely affect an elderly patient's decision-making capacity, such as disorientation caused by hospitalization. Decision-making capacity is variably reduced, even in a single patient over time, a clinical phenomenon that it well appreciated in geriatrics. This means that the patient's capacity to give informed consent is variably affected.

The patient should be presumed, legally and ethically, to be capable of informed consent. The variable ways in which decision-making capacity can be reduced should not by themselves be taken as evidence that the patient cannot give informed consent. Clinical signs of variably reduced decision-making capacity should alert the physician to the fact that the patient may require extra assistance, especially with steps 4 to 6. That assistance should be undertaken to ameliorate reduced capacity to make a decision. That is, in addition to standard evaluations of the patient's mental capacities (e.g., Mini-Mental Status Examination), the informed consent process itself should be used as an evaluation tool. Patients must be given sufficient opportunity to show themselves capable of informed consent, especially by exercising evaluative understanding.

Failure to do so may lead to inappropriate labeling of patients as having lost decision-making capacity. This, in turn, may lead to unnecessary failure to respect the autonomy of such patients to the extent that their autonomy can be exercised in informed consent. The risk of such failure can be compounded by reliance on standard mental status evaluation instruments (including those validated for geriatric patients), because in our view these instruments are not adequate to evaluate a patient's capacity for evaluative understanding. The capacity for informed consent by the patient must be tested by the nine-step process. If the patient cannot participate, even with vigorous assistance from the physician, especially in steps 4 to 6, the patient can reliably be regarded as having sufficiently reduced decision-making capacity that someone else must make decisions for the patient. An adequate attempt has been made to improve decision-making capacity and that attempt has failed to bring the patient up to a threshold of substantial autonomy.

Two Standards for Surrogate Decision Making

Two standards have been proposed as guidelines for surrogacy in these circumstances. The first is that the surrogate decision maker should as far as possible make the decision that the patient would have made if he or she could. This is called substituted judgment (28). Attempts to elicit the patient's values and beliefs in step 5 can be a valuable adjunct to this process. The surrogate decision maker should be taken through the nine steps of informed consent. In the course of step 5 the surrogate should be asked to identify the patient's values and beliefs and in steps 6 and 7 to identify all of the options consistent with the patient's values and beliefs. The surrogate should then and only then be asked which alternative is preferable. Failure to carry out steps 6 and 7 sets up the physician for conflict if the surrogate's preferred alternative is reliably thought to be unreasonable to the physician. The chances that this will occur are greatly reduced by first asking the surrogate to identify all alternatives consistent with the patient's values and beliefs and then asking the surrogate for a preference.

Sometimes neither the surrogate nor anyone else knows what the patient's relevant values and beliefs might be. (Regularly practicing informed consent as a preventive ethics strategy over time greatly reduces the chances of this occurring.) In that case the surrogate decision maker should be asked to make a decision according to the second standard, namely a decision that seems most in accord with a reasonable perspective of the patient's interests. This is the best interests standard (28). Again, to prevent ethical conflict, the surrogate decision maker should be asked to identify all reasonable alternatives in steps 6 and 7 and to give serious consideration to the physician's recommendation made in step 8.

The basic clinical strategy of preventive ethics in geriatric practice should by now be clear. The physician should seek always to avoid either-or

decisions in the thinking of patients, surrogate decision makers, and his or her own thinking. The physician should ask himself or herself whether the patient's or the surrogate's preference expressed in steps 6 and 7 is reasonable in beneficence-based clinical judgment and assume the burden of proof that it is not. In short, preventive ethics habitually seeks to create common moral ground with patients and surrogate decision makers.

Case Study

A 68 year-old man had wet gangrene in his left foot secondary to poor vascularization, a complication of his many years of diabetes mellitus. The patient resisted surgical management because as a Jehovah's Witness, he wanted to avoid the need for blood products. His team negotiated with him a plan of vigorous intravenous antibiotic therapy, which failed to improve his condition, and he was at risk for systemic infection and death, facts of which he was fully aware. When presented with the option of surgical management, the patient indicated that this would be acceptable provided that no blood products were administered.

His request caused consternation among some members of his team, and the patient was told that surgery could not be done safely without blood products, at which point the patient refused the surgery and asked that antibiotic treatment continue. The medical student on the team took it upon herself to ask the chief surgical resident if surgery without blood products was a reasonable option. The chief resident thought that surgery was certainly a higher risk without blood products but not high enough to be regarded as unreasonable. The patient would have to understand that the surgery would be performed as quickly as possible, that blood products would not be administered, and that his refusal of blood products would increase his risk of both death and postoperative morbidity. The student took this information back to her team and then to the patient, who consented to surgery without blood products. The surgery (below-the-knee amputation) was successful and the patient was discharged for rehabilitation and preparation for a prosthesis.

PREVENTIVE ETHICS AND HEALTH CARE INSTITUTIONS

The physician-patient relationship is affected by institutional third parties that own or manage the resources consumed in the care of patients. These resources are no longer owned solely by patients and their physicians. The owners include private entities, mainly the employers or former employers of patients and patients' spouses, and local, regional, state, and federal governments. Medicare and Medicaid are major government payers for medical care and long-term care, respectively, for geriatric patients. Privately and publicly owned resources are managed by both private and public institutions of health care. Moreover, providers of health care, including both physicians and institutions, increasingly find that they are expected to finance the health care of patients, such as by completing and submitting paperwork for Medicare beneficiaries and covering losses incurred when payment does not cover costs. These changes, which have resulted in a complex pattern of ownership and management of health care resources, have an important ethical implication: neither the physician nor the patient has an overriding right to the use of privately and publicly owned health care resources. There are limits on the use of health care resources and considerable dispute about where those limits should be set.

The Principle of Justice

Disputes about the management of health care resources are managed under the ethical principle of *justice*. In general, the ethical principle of justice requires persons and institutions to render to each person what is due him or her. The task is to identify reliably and with sufficient justification what counts as due someone. There have been many responses to this complex task in the history of Western philosophy; there are competing ethical theories of justice, no one of which can claim final authority or supremacy over the others (the fond hopes of advocates of particular philosophical theories of justice to the contrary notwithstanding).

Substantive and Procedural Justice

Against this disputed background, however, it is possible to make two important distinctions and apply them in the clinical setting to guide the physician's response to the institutional management of resources at the bedside. The first distinction is between *substantive justice* and *procedural justice*. Substantive justice concerns what the outcome of the distribution process ought to be, i.e., *who* ought to get *what* as due to him or her. Procedural justice concerns the distribution process itself, i.e., how the decision-making *process* about scarce resources ought to be conducted. There is far more agreement among philosophical theories of justice about procedural justice than there is about substantive justice. Basically, procedural justice requires that the interests of all affected parties be meaningfully taken into account in decisions about how to manage institutional resources.

Horizontal and Vertical Distribution of Health Care Resources

The second distinction concerns issues of justice in health care. On the one hand, there are ongoing disputes about whether to provide universal access to some basic, decent minimum of health care resources. This has been termed the horizontal distribution of health care resources (29). This is the level of the policy debates about a right to health care and the appropriate response to such a right by public and private owners and managers of health care resources. This will be considered in detail in the next section.

On the other hand, there are disputes in the clinical setting about bedside allocation of institutional resources according to intensity of intervention. This has been termed the vertical distribution of health care resources (29). This is the level of debates in the clinical setting about how much to provide for a particular patient when provision of high-intensity care for that patient may well distort both vertical and horizontal distribution of resources, affecting the interests of other patients, institutions, payers, and society.

Bedside Vertical Distribution of Health Care Resources

Recently, Morreim (29) made a proposal for the bedside vertical distribution of health care resources. Morreim argues that instead of a single standard of care we should distinguish a standard of medical expertise from a standard of resource use. The physician can be held to a standard of beneficence-based judgment about the interests of patients, Morreim argues, whether or not there are resources to implement such clinical judgment. By contrast, the physician, she argues, cannot be required to confiscate resources not owned by either the physician or the patient, such as by hoarding resources for his or her own patients. The physician can and ought to be held, Morreim maintains, to a standard of reasonable advocacy for vertical distribution of resources for his or her patient. That advocacy must take into account the legitimate interests of institutions, their moral fiduciary obligations to patients, and the obligations of patients.

The Legitimate Interests of Institutions

A new feature of bioethics has emerged as a permanent part of its future. The institutional owners and managers of health care resources have legitimate interests concerning the use of such resources, and those owners and managers are not inevitably ethically obligated to risk harm to their legitimate interests to provide care to particular patients.

The Moral Fiduciary Obligations of Institutions

At the same time institutions that provide health care have beneficence-based and autonomy-based obligations to their patients. Traditionally, provider institutions such as clinics and hospitals have been understood to be bound by an obligation to serve the interests of their patients, just as physicians have been. Like physicians, provider institutions can usefully be considered the moral fiduciaries of their patients. They are primarily to be concerned with the interests of patients and only secondarily with their own interests. A central ethical issue in the management of health care institutions concerns how to prevent and manage ethical conflicts between the institution's moral fiduciary obligations to its patients and its legitimate interests, such as fiscal stability.

Patients' Obligations

Patients have ethical obligations in the allocation of institutional resources, although this topic has received little attention in the literature on justice and health care. These obligations have two sources. The first source of patients' obligations is found in the distinction between what might be called the negative and positive exercises of autonomy, or negative and positive rights (30). Negative rights are understood in ethical theory to be rights to be left alone, especially when no one else's legitimate interests are at risk. Respect for autonomy is strongest in the case of such negative rights, creating a very heavy burden of proof for paternalism, i.e., interfering with negative autonomy for purely beneficence-based reasons. Positive rights are understood in ethical theory to be claims on others for their resources or resources held in common in society. Most of the resources consumed in health care are not owned by the patient. Thus a patient's positive right to institutional resources, even when it is exercised as the outcome of informed consent, is properly subject to limits. That is, institutions and society have legitimate interests in the ownership and management of health care resources that limit the positive exercise of the patient's autonomy to consume those resources. The patient therefore has an ethical obligation to take account of and respect those legitimate interests.

The second source of patients' obligations is found in what we term the obligations of the prudent saver. Americans have created a patchwork quilt of private entitlements (Medicare, Medicaid, Veterans Affairs, military medicine, Champus, city and county hospitals and clinics) through private health insurance and public entitlements to health care. None of these entitlements, however, is an entitlement to *everything*. All private insurance plans include covered and noncovered benefits, deductibles, and copayments. Public plans are also limited and also can have deductibles and copayments. In short, patients are expected to pay for some of the costs of health care. This requires patients to have been and to be prudent savers for such costs.

This is a difficult obligation for many persons, especially elders with modest income and little or no savings, perhaps because they lived from paycheck to paycheck for many years. It may be unrealistic to think of such persons—and there are many tens of thousands who are Medicare beneficiaries and qualified veterans—as prudent savers. Yet they come into the care of physicians and institutions who have fiduciary beneficence-based obligations to them. It may not be fair to physicians, institutions, and society to expect them to pay for health care for those who are not prudent savers. Yet, as fiduciaries of patients, physicians and institutions have an ethical obligation to provide adequate care, care that at least meets beneficence-based clinical judgment about what is in the patient's interest.

Four Steps of Reasonable Advocacy

Preventive ethics strategies in dealing with health care institutions, including MCOs, must take into account such matters of substantive justice as the vertical distribution of institutional resources, the legitimate interests of the institution, the moral fiduciary obligations of the institution, and the patient's obligations to the institution, including whether the patient should be regarded as a prudent saver. In response to this moral complexity we propose a preventive ethics strategy that draws on Morreim's proposal that the physician act as a reasonable advocate for the patient. Four steps are involved in executing this strategy.

First, reasonable advocacy requires that the physician be able to demonstrate through informed consent that a proposed management plan is in the patient's interest and that the plan is reliably expected to benefit the patient. Clinical impressions about what is marginally beneficial are a weak basis upon which to advocate for patients. There is no right on the part of the patient to intervention that is not expected to be beneficial and no moral fiduciary obligation on the part of the institution to provide it. Not all denials of payment by MCOs, therefore, are unethical.

Second, reasonable advocacy requires that the physician identify how the institution's legitimate interests will be affected and be able to argue that risks to those interests are ethically justified in a particular case. The latter condition is more readily satisfied when the outcome of non-intervention for the patient in *beneficence-based* clinical judgment is very grave, such as failure to prevent unnecessary death or permanent, serious disability. This aspect of reasonable advocacy presumes that the institution in question has a clear understanding of its legitimate interests. This is usually not the case, however, especially in poorly capitalized and poorly managed MCOs. Thus a crucial element of preventive ethics in dealing with health care institutions is to foment ongoing discussion within the institution about its mission and legitimate interests and to teach MCOs, in particular, about their fiduciary obligations to take financial risks to meet the well-documented beneficence-based needs of their patients.

Third, reasonable advocacy does not include the simple assertion that the patient always comes first. There was once a time when provider institutions were understood in terms of the "purest beneficence" in their obligation to expend resources on their patients (31). The need for institutions to attend to and take reasonable measures to protect their legitimate interests makes "My patient always comes first" ethically irresponsible. Physicians should incorporate economic discipline into clinical judgment so that finite resources are appropriately managed to protect all of the patients for which an MCO is responsible.

Fourth, the physician should challenge institutional policy that prohibits placing the legitimate interests of the institution at risk. When institutions do so, they put their moral fiduciary obligations systematically in second place to their economic and other interests. They may be free to do so, but only if they explicitly abandon their image as a moral fiduciary of patients. Part of preventive ethics in dealing with provider institutions is to call them back constantly to their moral fiduciary obligations, especially for patients who were not or cannot be prudent savers. Doing so creates the common moral ground for negotiating vertical access for one's patients to institutional resources. Both for-profit and not-for-profit MCOs are at risk for losing sight of their moral responsibilities. Physicians should not hesitate to undertake the moral instruction of MCO managers when it is required to meet the well-documented beneficence-based needs of patients.

ETHICAL ISSUES IN GERIATRIC HEALTH CARE POLICY

There are two main ethical issues in health care policy. The first concerns allocation of resources. The second concerns research with elderly subjects.

Allocation of Geriatric Health Care Resources

There is a voluminous literature on the subject of allocation of geriatric health care resources. There is also growing awareness among practicing physicians of ethical issues in geriatric health care policy (32). These issues are at some remove from the clinical setting of geriatric practice, but decisions about them by federal, state, and local governments will have both direct and indirect effects on geriatric practice.

Any discussion of geriatric health care policy must begin by acknowledging that the elderly enjoy a statutory entitlement to largely hospital-based, physician-oriented services. It is important to underscore that contrary to public rhetoric about this entitlement, Medicare does not meet the health care needs of all older Americans. For example, older Americans and their families bear considerable cost for Medicare-reimbursed outpatient services (not a trivial concern with the shift toward outpatient and same-day procedures that once entailed hospitalization) and for services that Medicare is not designed to cover, such as family-provided home care. Medicare also provides a large indirect subsidy to children and grandchildren of elders; these descendants might otherwise as a matter of moral and, in many states, legal obligation have to use their own money to pay for hospital and physician services. So the elderly are an advantaged population when it comes to medical care (33), as are, indirectly, their children. Only mandatory veterans, perhaps, enjoy a comparable advantage. Elderly mandatory veterans are thus especially advantaged.

Much of the ethical debate has centered on whether horizontal and vertical access to health care resources can be justifiably limited on the basis of age. Kapp (34) astutely pointed out that age discrimination is a curious worry about a government that already discriminates in favor of old age and that already pays for generous medical services to the elderly. The arguments of those such as Callahan (35) and Daniels (36) tend to abstract from these political realities, calling into question the applicability of their ar-

guments that age discrimination is ethically justified. Their arguments, however, help to underscore the apparent unraveling of public support for the Medicare program.

Jecker (37) raised an important issue, namely the disproportionate effect on women of attempts to limit access to health care on the basis of age. These effects, she argues, must be analyzed under the principle of justice in the larger context of gender-based discriminatory practices in our society. This will become a more important consideration for long-term care policy as we come to terms with the disproportionate number of elderly women in this population.

Any debate about allocation of geriatric health care resources leads to competing conclusions about how horizontal and vertical distribution of health care resources ought to be accomplished through public policy. This is because of the competing accounts of substantive justice in the history of Western philosophy. That competition has been going on for 2500 years and shows no signs of convergence on a single, final theory of substantive justice. Thus, efforts by the federal government to encourage Medicare beneficiaries to enroll in MCOs are not, in principle, unethical.

Ethical debates about geriatric health care policy and the political resolution of those debates should be viewed against the implications of this intellectual background. There are several. First, proposals about the substantive justice of geriatric health care policy must be argued. Simple advocacy for the elderly as if ethical analysis and argument were not required should not command intellectual respect, much less automatic assent. Second, physicians have something to contribute to this debate, namely a perspective on the substantive justice issues afforded by their own experience and ethical commitments. An individual physician can speak at meetings and in the literature, and organizations of physicians have spoken and will continue to speak to the issues. Third, any political resolution of ethical debate will be fragile. This is because a political resolution will vote into law one or more but not all views on substantive justice. The "losing" positions will not have their intellectual force diminished one iota, and their voices will continue to be heard. As experience is gained with policy resolutions of particular problems such as Medicare's home care services and as the ethical debate continues, support for that political resolution can weaken. Indeed, we should expect it to weaken. This is just what is happening with Medicare and to a lesser extent with Social Security. As citizens, physicians therefore must attend to the ethical debate, contribute to it and to the formulation of political resolutions, and be prepared to keep their shoulders to the wheel, for this is a never-ending task. The problems are chronic, inherently controversial, and thus can at best be managed well but not solved once and for all.

Ethical Issues in Research With Elderly Subjects

There is already a considerable body of law reflecting consensus on the ethics of research with human subjects. Because of the abuse of human subjects of research by governments, including that of the United States, and by institutions and investigators, federal regulations of research on human subjects place an unswerving emphasis on respect for the autonomy of the subject, the need to justify the research on scientific grounds, and the need to protect vulnerable populations from more than minimal risk.

This understandable caution poses ethical challenges for researchers in geriatric medicine and health care, particularly for research on patients with diminished or lost decision-making capacity and on nursing home residents. There is a compelling need for increased scientific knowledge and clinical skills to care for the ever-growing numbers of such patients. Yet such patients often cannot consent or refuse to participate in research, and they are often vulnerable by reason of frailty compounded by life in the nursing home. Sachs and Cassel (38) argued that despite these problems, appropriate guidelines for the protection of elderly subjects of human research can be devised.

CONCLUSION

The literature of geriatric ethics, like the literature of bioethics generally, continues to develop. Philosophical methods with a track record in bioethics, such as that employed here, which is based on both virtues and principles, will con-

tinue to be refined. At the same time, bioethics will be enriched by the contributions of philosophical methods new to the field. For example, communitarian ethics emphasizes the importance of the commons, the resources that a family, a community, an institution, or a nation holds in common and holds that "tragedies of the commons," the ethically unjustified overuse of commonly held resources, ought to be prevented. This has important unexplored implications for the use of critical care units by elderly multiply morbid patients. The physician should be alert to these developments in the literature of geriatric ethics.

REFERENCES

1. American Geriatrics Society Public Policy Committee. Voluntary active euthanasia. J Am Geriatr Soc 1991;39: 826.
2. American Medical Association Council on Ethical and Judicial Affairs. Decisions near the end of life. In: Code of Medical Ethics Reports of the Council on Ethical and Judicial Affairs of the American Medical Association. Chicago: American Medical Association, 1991:49–63.
3. Teno J, Lynn J. Voluntary active euthanasia: the individual case and public policy. J Am Geriatr Soc 1991;39: 827–830.
4. Jecker NS. Giving death a hand: when the dying and the doctor stand in a special relationship. J Am Geriatr Soc 1991;39:833–835.
5. Watts DT, Howell T. Assisted suicide is not voluntary active euthanasia. J Am Geriatr Soc 1992;40:1043–1046.
6. McCullough LB, Wilson NL, eds. Long-Term Care Decisions: Ethical and Conceptual Dimensions. Baltimore: Johns Hopkins University Press, 1995.
7. Kane RA, Caplan AL, eds. Ethical Issues in the Everyday Life of Nursing Home Residents. New York: Springer, 1990.
8. McCullough LB, Wilson NL, Teasdale TA, et al. Mapping personal, familial, and professional values in long-term care decisions. Gerontologist 1993;33:324–332.
9. Reich WT, ed. Encyclopedia of Bioethics. 2nd. ed. New York: Macmillan, 1995.
10. Pence G. Virtue theory. In: Singer P, ed. A Companion to Ethics. Cambridge, MA: Basil Blackwell, 1991:249–258.
11. Lustig BA, Brody BA, Engelhardt HT Jr, McCullough LB, eds. Regional Developments in Bioethics: 1989–1991. Bioethics Yearbook II. Dordrecht: Kluwer Academic, 1992.
12. Engelhardt HT Jr. The Foundations of Bioethics. 2nd ed. New York: Oxford University Press, 1996.
13. Beauchamp TL, Childress JF. Principles of Biomedical Ethics. 4th ed. New York: Oxford University Press, 1995.
14. McCullough LB, Chervenak FA. Ethics in Obstetrics and Gynecology. New York: Oxford University Press, 1994.

15. McCullough LB. The physician's virtues and legitimate self-interest in the physician-patient contract. Mount Sinai J Med 1993;60:11–14.

16. Brody H. The Healer's Power. New Haven, CT: Yale University Press, 1992.

17. Pellegrino ED, Thomasma DL. The Virtues in Medical Practice. New York: Oxford University Press, 1993.

18. Beauchamp TL, McCullough LB. Medical Ethics: The Moral Responsibilities of Physicians. Englewood Cliffs, NJ: Prentice-Hall, 1984.

19. Baker R. The history of medical ethics. In: Bynum WF, Porter R, eds. Encyclopedia of the History of Medicine. London: Routledge, 1994:848–883.

20. Engelhardt HT Jr. Bioethics and Secular Humanism: The Search for a Common Morality. Philadelphia: Trinity Press International, 1991.

21. White BC. Competence to Consent. Washington: Georgetown University Press, 1996.

22. Wear S. Informed Consent: Physician Beneficence and Patient Autonomy. Dordrecht: Kluwer Academic, 1992.

23. McCullough LB. An ethical model for improving the physician-patient relationship. Inquiry 1989;25:454–465.

24. Veatch RM. The Patient as Partner. Bloomington, IN: Indiana University Press, 1987.

25. American Medical Association. Code of medical ethics. Proceedings from the national convention 1846–1847. In: Baker R, ed. The Codification of Medical Morality, vol 2: Anglo-American Medical Ethics and Medical Jurisprudence in the Nineteenth Century. Dordrecht: Kluwer Academic, 1995:65–87.

26. Benjamin M. Lay obligations in professional relations. J Med Philos 1982;10:83–105.

27. Meyer MJ. Patients' duties. J Med Philos 1992;17:541–555.

28. Brock D, Buchanan A. Deciding for Others. Cambridge, UK: Cambridge University Press, 1989.

29. Morreim EH. Balancing Act: The New Medical Ethics of Medicine's New Economics. Washington: Georgetown University Press, 1995.

30. McCullough LB, Chervenak FA. Limits on refusing treatment. Hastings Cent Rep 1991;21:12–18.

31. Percival T. Medical Ethics. Baltimore: Williams & Wilkins, 1927.

32. Williams ME, Connolly NK. What practicing physicians in North Carolina rate as their most challenging geriatric medicine concerns. J Am Geriatr Soc 1990;38:1230–1234.

33. Feder J. Health care and the disadvantaged: The elderly. J Health Polit Policy Law 1990;15:259–269.

34. Kapp MJ. Rationing health care: will it be necessary? Can it be done without age or disability discrimination? Issues Law Med 1989;5:337–366.

35. Callahan D. Setting Limits: Medical Goods in an Aging Society. New York: Simon & Schuster, 1987.

36. Daniels N. Am I My Parents' Keeper? An Essay on Justice Between the Young and the Old. New York: Oxford University Press, 1988.

37. Jecker N. Age-based rationing and women. JAMA 1991;266:3012–3015.

38. Sachs GA, Cassel CK. Biomedical research involving older human subjects. Law Med Health Care 1990;18:234–243.

CHAPTER 66

LAURENCE B. McCULLOUGH, NANCY L. WILSON,
JILL A. RHYMES, AND THOMAS A. TEASDALE

Long-Term Care Decision Making

Long-term care has been defined as a "range of services that address the health, personal care, and social needs of individuals who lack some capacity for self-care" (1). Long-term care decision making is occasioned by physical, mental, or social changes that result in a loss of function such that the elder, family members, friends, or physician believes that the services of others are required to supplant self-sufficiency (2). Long-term care decisions thus concern nearly all aspects of a person's daily life (3, 4). Often many decisions must be made over time. Family members are usually intimately involved and play several roles, including caregiver and decision maker (5). The physician is often not involved when the dyad of elder and family member make a decision about long-term care, such as for the elder to move in with a family member after the death of a spouse (6, 7). The physician frequently becomes involved after the elder and family are well into the decision-making process, e.g., after an acute event such as a fall. Such decision making operates under many constraints, including personal finances, limits on family members' ability or willingness to provide care, state and federal regulations, and the bureaucracies of public and private institutions that deliver or administer services (8, 9).

Physical, social, and mental changes that prompt a decision about long-term care have ethically significant consequences (10). This chapter provides a values-oriented approach to informed consent as a preventive ethics strategy in making decisions about long-term care.

First, we provide an ethical analysis of long-term care to distinguish it from acute care. Second, we discuss the physician's role in the decision with emphasis on the physician as a good-faith mediator of a values-laden informed consent process. Third, we briefly consider empiric research concerning the values of decision makers and the ethical implications of it. Fourth, we describe a process of informed consent that adapts the preventive ethics strategy of Chapter 65 to long-term care decision making. Fifth, we discuss decisions about long-term care in the context of nursing homes. Sixth, we consider long-term care decisions regarding elders with dementias.

ETHICALLY DISTINCTIVE FEATURES OF LONG-TERM CARE

Long-term care differs from acute care in important ways. Hofland (11) notes that acute care typically addresses well-defined problems and well-defined options for managing them. Long-term care is more ambiguous, with problems less well defined and options therefore more resistant to clear definition. Acute care involves mainly clear-cut problems: the patient has a fractured hip or congestive heart failure of a specific stage. Put more precisely, the patient has or is thought to have an anatomic or physiologic abnormality. Pathophysiology is the province of the health care professions, medicine in particular. Thus, a built-in feature of acute care is that the physician rather than the patient has the intellectual basis for naming the patient's problem and identifying clinically effective ways to manage it. This dependence on physicians to name and help us manage our problems when we are patients in acute-care settings is one of the sources of the power of physicians over patients. These forms of power cannot usually be shared with the patient, although decision making should be shared (12).

The physician's power is exercised in an institution with resources for the diagnosis and management of acute problems. Physicians, not patients, control access to these resources, another source of the physician's power in the acute care setting. The physician's power is exercised within a hierarchy in which the physician writes orders that other professionals or technologists carry out. Physicians recommend management strategies to patients, even strongly, but no longer issue orders to patients to which compliance is to be prompt and implicit, as was expected in 19th-century American medical ethics (13).

An important implication of the physician's role in acute care, especially in the hospital, is that patients depend on their physicians. One court has stated that patients have an "abject dependence" on their physicians (14). This kind of dependence drains power from the patient, and the necessity to obtain informed consent can be understood as a response to enhance the patient's autonomy.

In summary, in the acute care setting the physician possesses the power to name the problem. The physician is thus the chief ontologist, undertaking diagnostic workups to place the patient's reality into the appropriate pathophysiologic category. (Ontology is the philosophical study of categories of reality.) The patient cannot perform this role because the patient lacks the relevant knowledge. The physician controls access to institutional resources and so enjoys significant power. The informed consent process and increasingly, third party payers and managers function as significant counterweights to the physician's power. The patient's pathophysiology and the response of physicians and health care institutions to it have significant implications for the patient in other spheres of life and for others in the patient's life, but these are implications of acute care.

Long-term care differs sharply in all three respects. First, the elder may not be a patient at all. He or she is usually living in the community, getting along more or less well enough with life. The physical, mental, or social changes that are occurring may not be seen as problems by the elder, even though family members or the physician may see them as problems. In short, there is no chief ontologist in long-term care decision making. For example, an older woman living alone may regard herself as quite capable of taking care of herself, yet her daughter notices that her mother's nutritional status seems to be deteriorating. *Competing realities*—for *both* the elder's problem and for the caregivers' problems—constitute the defining feature of long-term care decision making. Competing realities are a major source of ethical conflict within that process. Moreover, even when the reality is agreed upon, its significance may not be. An elder and family members may disagree about how risky it is for the elder, recovering from the effects of a severe fall at home, to continue to live at home alone.

Second, the resources that might be marshaled in response to a situation that is agreed to be a problem are not under the sole control of the physician. This is because most of the resources consumed in long-term care in the United States are those of the so-called informal caregivers, the elder's moral intimates: spouses, children, stepchildren, in-laws, neighbors, and friends. These persons and the elder do not occupy a hierarchy. As Jecker pointed out, their relationships constitute tangled and often inchoate webs of obligations (15).

Moreover, the informal caregivers do not stand in hierarchic relationships to physicians or institutions that deliver formal long-term care. In short, no one issues orders to anyone except in institutional settings such as the nursing home. Requests, recommendations, compromise, and negotiation are the tools of decision making in long-term care (16). The exercise of autonomy in this context is less dramatic than it is in end-of-life decisions (see Chapters 67 and 68). Rather, the physician's concern should be with the everyday exercise of autonomy (17) and with the potentially corrosive effect on autonomy of nursing home routine (18).

Third, the psychosocial spheres of the elder's life are an essential, not extraneous, to long-term care decision making. This is because the elder's problem, while it may be occasioned by mental or physical change, is occasioned just as often by social change, such as the death of a spouse or a child being transferred out of town. Loss of self-sufficiency is frequently a social phenomenon in the life of the elder and his or her moral intimates, not a medical one. Relocating to receive care or accepting assistance with daily tasks may have a profound effect on an elder's identity and opportunity to perform cherished social roles.

In summary, long-term care decision making involves competing realities and competing interpretations of realities. There can be disagreement about whether multiple mental, physical, or social changes that reduce self-sufficiency in activities of daily living have occurred and, when they have occurred, whether they should count as problems. There is no chief ontologist, even when the elder is a patient. The power to name the problem is thus contested, not settled as it is in the acute care setting. Second, the power to command resources in response to a long-term care problem (once it is agreed to be such) is widely diffused among the elder, informal and

formal caregivers, and institutions. Because of the large role that they play, informal caregivers are a major long-term care resource and important decision makers with the elder and the physician. The obligations of family members and their legitimate interests are essential to deciding whether they ought to serve as such a resource. Third, long-term care is inherently biopsychosocial. Indeed, long-term care decision making—with its competing realities, essentially temporal character, and shifting cast of participants—may best exemplify the biopsychosocial model in health care and social services.

PHYSICIAN'S ROLE

The physician's roles in this complex decision-making context are several. In our research we have identified a number of roles played by the physician in long-term care decision making (Table 66.1). For present purposes the most important of these roles is the *good faith mediator* of a decision-making process that is often well along by the time the physician becomes involved in it.

A good faith negotiator resists becoming an unquestioning advocate for any one party. In particular, the physician should beware being en-

Table 66.1

Roles of the Physician in Long-Term Care Decision Making

Physician-educator	
Formal Caregiver	Provide medical care and plan medically appropriate diagnostic tests and clinical management
Educator	Communicate diagnoses and prognoses; discuss care needs; provide information about long-term care resources in the community
Gatekeeper	Authorize access to appropriate agencies, payment schemes, etc.
Counselor	
Historian	Remember and remind elder and family of elder's course, previous decisions, and results of those decisions
Mediator	Counsel elder and family via nondirective assistance with decisions. As neutral party seek win-win outcome to prevent and manage ethical conflict between elder and family and between elder/family and community agencies and institutions
Advocate	
Advocate	For management that is reliably judged to be in the elder's interest medically
Surrogate	Stand-in for other participants in decision making when necessary
Lawgiver	Directing a course of action

listed by family members in carrying out decisions in which the elder was not involved. At the same time, being an uncritical advocate of the elder's autonomy overlooks morally legitimate limits that family members may want to place on their caregiving role and responsibilities.

VALUES

In short, long-term care decision making is a complex and unavoidably *value-laden* process. Indeed, the process is mainly about negotiating the practical implications of each participant's value commitments, commitments of which he or she (the physician included) may be unaware. The physician's preventive ethics role is to bring these values to the surface in the search for a common ground, because the search for a common ground of values is the defining feature of preventive ethics in clinical practice. That is, long-term care decision making ought to be a process in which the evaluative understanding (the assessment of options on the basis of one's values) of each party is as explicit as possible. The option can be an emotionally wrenching or even guilt-laden and therefore potentially divisive dispute between elders and family members over options, such as whether the elder stays at home or goes to the nursing home. Focusing on options in the absence of participants' underlying values sets up those participants for ethical conflict by obscuring from their view their common ground of values. This outcome is a disservice to elders and their families. Recent research into the values of participants in long-term care decision making indicates that informed consent aimed at a common ground of values as the basis for long-term care decision making is a realistic, practical clinical role for the physician to pursue.

This research emphasizes the importance of values in long-term care decision making. One focus is on what the values, beliefs, and behavior of people ought to be, i.e., normative ethics. This is true particularly regarding the implications of the ethical principle of respect for autonomy (19, 20). Normative studies have also been concerned with the values held by family members, particularly the value of filial obligation, which is the obligation of adult children to care for their frail

elderly parents or parents-in-law (15, 21). A second focus of research on long-term care decision making is on descriptive ethics, empiric studies of the values of elders and family members (22–27) and of the values held by health care professionals (28–30).

A recent empiric study mapped the self-reported values of the three most common participants in the long-term care decision-making process: elders, involved family members, and health care professionals (31). In mapping the personal, familial, and professional values in long-term care decisions, three questions were addressed:

1. What values do participants in long-term care decision making report retrospectively as relevant to the process? These values constitute a map for long-term care decision making.
2. How frequently are various values reported by elders, family members, and health care professionals as relevant to the process of deciding about long-term care?
3. How common and how different are the values held by elders, involved family members, and health care professionals?

Older people who had changed their living situation and/or started receiving help with personal care because their capacity for self-care was reduced were identified. Equivalent numbers of persons who had made one of five care arrangements during the preceding month were included: (*a*) remained at home with the addition of paid help; (*b*) moved in with a relative or acquaintance to receive help; (*c*) began attending adult day care; (*d*) entered congregate housing with services; or (*e*) entered a nursing home. These settings were chosen to reflect the fact that most functionally disabled elders with long-term care needs do not live in institutional settings. Older people who had made changes for reasons not related to functional needs were excluded, as were those with significant cognitive or communication problems. The total sample analyzed consisted of 23 interview sets: 24 elders including one married couple, 23 family members, and 13 professionals, for a total of 60 interviews subjected to qualitative data analysis.

The sampled elders' ages ranged from 70 to 94, which is consistent with that of a long-term care population. The elders interviewed were predominantly white (96%) and included an equal distribution of men and women. Their mean educational level was high, and a substantial percentage were in the middle- or high-income range. The older people interviewed most often identified a family member (82.6%) and someone of another generation (82.6%) as most closely involved in their decision. The long-term care decisions ranged proportionately over a wide range of options, most of them in community-based settings.

The 23 family members or friends ranged widely in age, their mean age of 57 reflecting this caregiving population (32). Before the decision was made, all but 4 of the 23 family members or friends had been providing either direct assistance or financial help to the older person. Clearly, changes in elder care or residence would influence the lives of these family members or friends. The professionals included both medical and social service practitioners who were experienced in geriatric and long-term care. In contrast to the elders, most family members, friends, and professionals reported previous personal experience with long-term care decision making.

A semistructured instrument was used to standardize the interviews and provide interviewers with questions useful in probing for additional information. Data analysis proceeded according to accepted methods of qualitative investigation (32), beginning with a descriptive analysis of the respondents, followed by content analysis of the interview transcripts. Large numbers of specific values were identified for elders (348 specific values), family members and friends (398 specific values), and professionals (241 specific values). These were consolidated in two further steps: grouping into generic values and into categories of values. The goal was to produce a clinically useful map that represented the respondents' values.

This qualitative analysis resulted in a values map of manageable size that includes categories of generic values of elders, family members, friends, and professionals. Table 66.2 lists the main categories of values of each of these groups according to frequency of response. The generic values of elders within these categories are broad in scope, ranging from the general to the quite specific. For elders, generic values range from maintaining self-image to being safe from personal and property crime. For family members or friends, generic values range from preparing for the elder's future to minimizing job conflict. For professionals, generic values range from independence for the elder to getting physical therapy or rehabilitation for the elder. The values map reflects multiple decisions that involve all aspects of a person's daily life for a long time.

Table 66.2

Categories of Generic Values of Elders, Family Members or Friends, and Professionals

Values of Elders	Values of Family Members	Values of Professionals
Environment	Care	Care
Identity	Security	Health
Relationship	Psychologic well-being	Relationship
Care	Caregiver burden	Psychologic well-being
Health	Relationship	Quality of environment
Caregiver burden	Quality of environment	Respect for the elder
Finances	Respect for the elder	Caregiver burden
Security	Health	Elder involvement in decision making
	Finances	Finances
	Caregiver benefits	
	Filial responsibilities	
	Elder identity	

When *all* values were considered, commonalities and differences emerged. For the sample as a whole, 31 (86%) of the elders' generic values were also identified by family members or friends. For the sample as a whole, 42 (82%) of family members' or friends' generic values were also identified by the elders. Of the professionals' generic values, 25 (66%) were also identified by both elders and family members or friends and 7 (19%) were identified by either elders or family members or friends.

This study was subject to several limitations. Because of its retrospective nature, it may be influenced by recall bias or the avoidance of cognitive dissonance. The values expressed, especially those of the elder and family members, may have been influenced by the fact that both parties were interviewed after they had some experience with the long-term care decision they had made. It cannot be determined, therefore, whether the commonalities of generic values and categories of generic values were functions of the long-term care decision-making process or something that participants bring to the process. Nonetheless, the high rates of commonality strongly support a preventive ethics approach to long-term care decision making. Although the sample is large for a qualitative study (60 interviews), the sample does not represent all participants in long-term care decision making, because its size is limited to 23 decisions and because it lacks racial and economic diversity.

Two observations about the general features of the values map are in order. First, when one compares the top three categories by frequency of response of values for each group of respondents, some interesting differences emerge. For elders, these top-listed values concern environment, identity, and relationship. For family or friends, they are care, security, and psychologic well-being. For professionals, the values are care, physical health, and a tie between relationship and psychologic well-being. Given the high percentage of physicians among the professionals, their emphasis on health-related values was not surprising. The lower frequency of these values among elders and family members or friends may reflect an assumption that health concerns had already been addressed or it may reflect a priority of other values. These data suggest that there is a potential for conflict among competing values but that there is considerable commonality of values, particularly between elders and their family members. A preventive ethics approach to long-term care decision making seeks to avoid conflicts among competing values.

This study also indicates that the physician must be attentive to the fact that elders may have values and priorities in long-term care decision making that are not health related. Elders expressed values related to identity, for example, more often than values concerned with physical and mental health—in contrast to the frequency of health-related generic values expressed by the professionals. How to balance these two may well be a central preventive ethics task of the long-term care decision-making process.

INFORMED CONSENT

The informed consent process described in Chapter 65 can be effectively adapted to long-term care decision making. In implementing this process as a good-faith mediator, the physician should keep in mind the main implications of the preceding discussion.

First, the participants in long-term care decision making may or may not agree on the nature of the elder's and the family's situation. An attempt should be made by the physician to have participants reach as much agreement as possible on the nature of the situation. If that attempt fails, decision making should proceed for each description of the elder's situation. Competing descriptions do not always have to result in different long-term care plans for the elder.

Second, the physician should appreciate that he or she can order only institutional, hierarchic resources. The family members and other involved informal caregivers are acting from a sense of obligation, tempered and limited by legitimate interests on their part—especially other obligations in their lives and their concern for other family members, such as teenage children. These constraints must be identified and taken into account.

Third, the elder and family members are exercising their autonomy in an everyday, undramatic fashion (17). This exercise of autonomy concerns the details of daily living, such as activities, access to personal possessions, visits with family and friends, and so on. This is true especially in the nursing home (18) (discussed later in the chapter). Their values can be at stake, therefore, in subtle ways that should be elicited.

Fourth, the nursing home is frequently described as a total institution. In particular, its corrosive effect on the autonomy of elders and the sense of obligation on the part of family members should not be underestimated (18).

Fifth, the inherently psychosocial nature of long-term care decision making means that this process is necessarily value laden. Thus, the primary concern of the physician should be to assist elders and family members articulate their evaluative understanding and to express preferences for managing the elder's situation in terms of their values.

Sixth, the physician can expect that some values are held in common between elders and their families, although their rankings of those values may differ. The physician should also beware his or her own understandable tendency to give priority to health-related values. Elders and families may not do so.

With these considerations in mind, the decision about long-term care can be undertaken with ethical justification in a stepwise process that reflects the informed consent process described in Chapter 65. The goal is to prevent the ethical conflict that can occur in the absence of an ethically justified, orderly approach to the decision that explicitly includes identification of and reflection on values.

A VALUE-BASED PREVENTIVE ETHICS APPROACH TO LONG-TERM CARE DECISION MAKING

This nine-step process is designed to prevent ethical conflicts over decisions about long-term care. In it the physician acts as good-faith mediator.

1. *Defining the elder's situation.* The physician initiates the process by eliciting from the elder and from involved family members (of other informal caregivers) what they believe the elder's situation to be, the options that are available to manage it, and the prognosis under each option. An attempt should be made to reach agreement on the facts of the elder's condition, a view that neither underestimates nor overestimates the elder's capacities and the care burden those capacities imply for family members.

2. *Participants' fund of knowledge.* In a respectful and supportive fashion the physician corrects factual errors or incompleteness in the elder's or family members' fund of knowledge through providing information directly or—this is important—linking elders and families with knowledgeable professionals in the community. The elder and family members may not be aware of all long-term care services for which the elder is eligible. Also, sometimes family members have steered the elder toward one option and not informed the elder about others. Family members should be alerted in advance that informed consent requires the physician to provide the elder and them with full information. This is one of the first duties of the physician as good-faith mediator.

3. *The physician's judgment.* The physician provides and explains his or her clinical judgment about the elder's situation and available management strategies, including watchful waiting. The physician should give particular attention to the elder's functional capacities, how they might be improved or strengthened, and their long-term prognosis. The physician should emphasize that options should be considered as subject to trials. They may not work; the elder may not accept them; the family may not accept them; the elder's situation may change. Time limits for such trials and markers of success and failure should be established, if possible.

4. *Cognitive understanding.* The physician should work with the elder and the involved family members to help them develop as complete as possible a picture of the elder's situation and *all* of the available management strategies, including watchful waiting. Watchful waiting in this context includes a trial of the elder continuing with his or her present living

arrangement with an agreement from the elder to a frank appraisal of the success of this strategy and its effects on family members.

5. *Participants' values.* The physician works with the elder and family members to help them identify their relevant values. The categories of values in Table 66.2 may be mentioned to elders and family members who have difficulty in expressing their values. Some persons do not have a powerful values-oriented vocabulary, and the physician's task is to help them express their concerns clearly.

6. *Evaluative understanding.* The physician helps the elder and family members *in a nondirective fashion* to evaluate long-term care options, including a trial of present arrangements, in terms of their values. As a good-faith mediator, the physician should not take sides in this process but should listen for values held in common and for value differences and help elders and families appreciate both their commonalities and differences.

7. *Value-based preferences.* The elder and family members are asked to identify which long-term care arrangements are consistent with their values. The goal should be for both the elder and the family members to consider and identify all options that are consistent with their values. Doing so maximizes the chance that an agreement can be reached.

8. *The physician's recommendation.* The physician makes a recommendation based on the clinical judgment expressed in step 3 and the elder's and family members' value-based preferences expressed in step 7. It is reasonable to expect the elder and family members to take account of the physician's judgment, either about the health-related aspects of each option or about areas where agreement has emerged in the previous steps.

9. *The management plan.* A mutual decision about managing the patient's situation is reached— or is not. In that case the task of the elder and family members is to respect each other's values, understand why they disagree, and seek to manage their disagreement. This nine-step process will have to be repeated as the elder's situation changes or the arrangement is found not to be satisfactory to the elder or family

members. Long-term care decisions are seldom made once and for all.

LONG-TERM CARE DECISIONS IN THE NURSING HOME

This strategy can be used for the full range of long-term care decisions, including nursing home placement as the outcome of the process. Once the elder and family have made a decision for the nursing home, decision making continues. This point is worth emphasizing, because as Agich (17) pointed out, the elder's autonomy is very much at stake in the day-to-day decisions in nursing home life, because autonomy is expressed in these day-today decisions. The day-to-day ethical issues in the life of nursing home residents have been discussed in a volume edited by Kane and Caplan (9). The physician should be attentive to such mundane exercises of autonomy as phone privileges, roommate selection, and opportunity for spiritual growth. The physician should take advantage of the nursing home's staff's day-to-day knowledge of the elder to identify what is important to the elder, especially those with dementing disorders and diseases. As Agich argues, there can still remain in the midst of dementia ethically significant expressions of autonomy, such as going into a stairwell for peace and quiet (17).

Instead, as Lidz et al. (18) have documented, the nursing home as a total institution corrodes the elder's autonomy. In this setting the physician's role is appropriately an advocate for the elder's autonomy in the sense described in Chapter 65. A responsible advocate recognizes ethically justified limits on the exercise of an elder's autonomy when those limits are grounded in the institution's clear sense of its fiduciary obligations to the elder and its legitimate interests. The physician should work with nursing home administrations to create an environment in which the nursing home is not so systematically corrosive of the elder's autonomy. Lidz et al. (18) call into question nursing home policies that excessively favor considerations other than autonomy. For example, they point out that too much regard for bodily safety can lead to use of restraints that undermine autonomy, making the elder worse off. Patients with different cognitive abilities, they suggest, should not be routinely mixed together, inasmuch as this erodes the abilities of those with the least cognitive loss. In short, the physician can enhance the elder's autonomy in the nursing home by obliging the nursing home to review its policies and practices with a view to whether they enhance or undermine autonomy of residents.

LONG-TERM CARE DECISION MAKING REGARDING ELDERS WITH DEMENTIA

Elders with mild and even moderate dementia may be capable of participating in the informed consent process. As noted in Chapter 65, the best way to determine whether the elder with mild or moderate dementia can participate is to attempt the informed consent process. The same strategy should be employed in making decisions about long-term care for elders with dementia. They should not be presumed, by virtue of a diagnosis of dementia, to be incapable of participating in the decision. An important area of future research in long-term care decision making concerns the capacity of elders with dementia to participate in the process, especially in the identification and expression of their values and evaluative understanding.

We recommend that when the elder cannot participate, the substituted judgment standard described in Chapter 65 be employed to guide decision making. The goal should be to identify the patient's relevant values so that those values can shape the nine-step decision-making process. Family members are an important source of information about the elder's values. The physician's experience and discussions with the elder may also be a source for identifying the elder's values. Family members should be supported in the identification of reasonable limits on their obligation to provide long-term care for the elder. This is an especially important consideration for long-term care for demented elders, given the considerable emotional, physical, and spiritual demands that caring for such elders can impose on their family members. Family members, especially frail spouses, siblings, or adult children, are not obligated to sacrifice themselves endlessly in the care of a loved one. The physician may with ethical justification recommend that family members consider limiting their obligations to provide care, especially when the burden of caregiving has compromised the health of family members.

REFERENCES

1. Kane RA, Kane RL. Values and Long-Term Care. Lexington, MA: Lexington Books, 1982:4.
2. McCullough LB. Long-term care for the elderly: an ethical analysis. Soc Thought 1985;11:40–52.
3. Kane RA, Kane RL. Long-Term Care: Principles, Programs, and Policies. New York: Springer, 1987.
4. Pelaez M, David D. Training professionals to enhance autonomy in long term care. Gerontologist 1991;31 (suppl):71.
5. High DA. A new myth about families of older people? Gerontologist 1991;31:611–618.
6. Gold DT. Late-life sibling relationships: does race affect typological distribution? Gerontologist 1990;30:741–748.
7. Horowitz A, Silverstone BM, Reinhardt JP. A conceptual and empirical exploration of personal autonomy issues within family caregiving relationships. Gerontologist 1991;31:23–31.
8. Dunkle RE, Wykle ML, eds. Decision Making in Long-Term Care: Factors in Planning. New York: Springer, 1988.
9. Kane RA, Caplan A, eds. Ethical Conflicts in the Management of Home Care: The Case Manager's Dilemma. New York: Springer, 1993.
10. McCullough LB, Wilson NL, eds. Ethical and Conceptual Dimensions of Long-Term Care Decision Making. Baltimore: Johns Hopkins University Press, 1995.
11. Hofland B. Introduction. Generations 1990;14:(suppl) 5–8.
12. Brody H. The Healer's Power. New Haven: Yale University Press, 1992.
13. American Medical Association. Code of Medical Ethics. Proceedings From the National Convention 1846–1847. Chicago: American Medical Association, 1848:83–106.
14. Canterbury vs Spence 464 f. 2d 772, 785 (D.C. Cir. 1972).
15. Jecker N. The role of intimate others in medical decision making. Gerontologist 1990;30:65–71.
16. Moody HR. Ethics in an Aging Society. Baltimore: Johns Hopkins University Press, 1992.
17. Agich GJ. Autonomy in Long-Term Care. New York: Oxford University Press, 1993.
18. Lidz CW, Fischer L, Arnold RM. The Erosion of Autonomy in Long-Term Care. New York: Oxford University Press, 1992.
19. Collopy BJ. Autonomy in long-term care: some crucial distinctions. Gerontologist 1988;28:(suppl)10–17.
20. Collopy BJ. Ethical dimensions of autonomy in long-term care. Generations 1990;14(suppl):9–12.
21. Selig S, Tomlinson T, Hickey T. Ethical dimensions of intergenerational reciprocity: implications for practice. Gerontologist 1991;31:624–630.

22. Wetle TT, Levkoff S, Wikel JC, Rosen A. Nursing home resident participation in medical decisions: perceptions and preferences. Gerontologist 1988;28:(suppl)32–38.

23. Sabatino CP. Client rights, regulations and the autonomy of home care consumers. Generations 1990;14:(suppl)21–24.

24. Wetle TT, Crabtree B. Balancing safety and autonomy: defining and living with acceptable risk. Gerontologist 1991;31:237 (abstract).

25. Kivnick HQ. Client values: perceptions, preferences, and what difference do they make? Gerontologist 1991;31:237 (abstract).

26. Farran CJ, Keane-Hagerty E, Salloway S, et al. Finding meaning: an alternative paradigm for Alzheimer's disease family caregivers. Gerontologist 1991;31:483–489.

27. Kane RA. Type and frequency of ethical issues facing publicly subsidized case managers in long-term care. Gerontologist 1991;31:237 (abstract).

28. Kaufman SR, Becker G. Content and boundaries of medicine in long-term care: physicians talk about stroke. Gerontologist 1991;31:238–245.

29. Eustis NN, Fischer LR. Relationships between home care clients and their workers: implications for quality care. Gerontologist 1991;31:447–456.

30. McCullough LB, Wilson NL, Teasdale TA, et al. Mapping personal, familial, and professional values in long-term care decisions. Gerontologist 1993;33:324–332.

31. Stone RS, Catetera GL, Sangl J. Caregivers of frail elderly: a national profile. Gerontologist 1987;27:616–626.

32. Patton MQ. Qualitative Evaluation and Research Methods. 2nd ed. London: Sage, 1990.

CHAPTER 67

LAURENCE B. McCULLOUGH, DAVID J. DOUKAS,
WARREN L. HOLLEMAN, AND REBECCA B. REILLY

Advance Directives

Most physicians who treat older patients know what advance directives are: the living will and the durable power of attorney for health care. While conceived and introduced into American medicine as legal instruments to effect and protect patient's choices about end-of-life care, advance directives can also serve as preventive ethics tools for the physician caring for patients at the ends of their lives. This is the case particularly when advance directives are well understood by all parties: the physician, the patient, the patient's family, the physician's professional colleagues, and health care institutions, particularly hospitals and nursing homes. This chapter provides an ethically justified, practical approach to the use of advance directives to anticipate and prevent the ethical conflicts that can occur in association with them.

Accordingly, the legal development and ethical significance of the living will and durable power of attorney are explained first. Then some of the ethical conflicts that can be associated with advance directives are considered. Finally, a stepwise preventive ethics approach to advance directives in clinical practice is presented.

LEGAL DEVELOPMENT AND ETHICAL SIGNIFICANCE OF ADVANCE DIRECTIVES

Advance directives have become so commonplace in the thinking of most physicians, though not yet in their practices, that we sometimes forget the legal and ethical rationales for them (1). These origins are important because they help the physician to appreciate both the power and the limitations of these legal documents.

Legal Right of Self-Determination

The story begins at the turn of the century, in the common law of informed consent, which developed as part of malpractice law. In a landmark case decided by the highest court of the State of New York in 1914, *Schloendorff versus Society of New York Hospital,* Justice Cardozo applied the fundamental legal doctrine of self-determination to informed consent: "Every person of adult years and sound mind has the right to determine what shall be done to his body, and a surgeon who performs an operation without the patient's consent commits an assault" (2). The only exception that the New York Court of Appeals allowed was for emergencies: the patient's life is in immediate peril and there is no time in which to obtain consent. The point of informed consent as a legal requirement has been clear since *Schloendorff.* Each adult patient is presumed competent and as such has the right to control what is done or not done for him or her. Consent may be granted or withheld entirely according to the patient's values and preferences.

Legal Right of Privacy

The story continues with the well-known ruling of the United States Supreme Court on abortion in 1973. *Roe versus Wade* (3) and cases that preceded it established that there is a constitutional protection of privacy and that this constitutional protection extends to the physician-patient relationship. Privacy creates a zone or area of thought, speech, and behavior into which the government may not intrude unless there is compelling reason to do so. Privacy thus creates a zone of noninterference around the physician-patient relationship into which the state may not intrude without sufficiently compelling reasons. The burden of proof is on the state because there is a presumption in favor of privacy. The state may, for example, intrude into privacy to protect life of the individual (out of a paternalism known as *parens patriae*, the state as one's parent) or of others (e.g., to protect them from serious harm).

The interest of the state in protecting life is based on the Fourteenth Amendment to the United States Constitution, which prohibits the taking of life, liberty, or property of persons without due process of law. The state may also intrude into privacy when criminal matters are at stake. (In *Roe* the Supreme Court found that the fetus is not a person in the meaning of the term in constitutional law and so is not accorded protection by the Fourteenth Amendment before viability. Hence, abortion before viability is a protected exercise of a privacy right by the pregnant woman in consultation with her physician.)

When the case of Karen Ann Quinlan, known as *In Re Quinlan* (4) reached the Supreme Court of New Jersey, the court had the tools of legal self-determination (expressed through informed consent) and of privacy with which to analyze and decide the case. The latter becomes more prominent. Ms. Quinlan suffered two prolonged episodes of anoxia of unknown origin, was resuscitated by a rescue team, was hospitalized, and subsequently was in a persistent vegetative state. Inasmuch as she was an adult, her father petitioned the court for guardianship of her person for the purpose of requesting that ventilatory support be discontinued. He understood that if his request was granted, his daughter would most likely die rather than breathe on her own. The lower courts denied his request, but the Supreme Court of New Jersey granted it.

Portions of that court's reasoning are crucial to the physician. The court first asked itself, in effect, if it could decide this case on the basis of informed consent and legal self-determination. If Ms. Quinlan had made statements that effectively refused such things as ventilators later, those earlier statements should bind her physicians in the present. That is, self-determination could be exercised in advance, in the form of informed refusal of life-prolonging intervention. In Ms. Quinlan's case the New Jersey court took the view that her prior statements were not specific enough to count as advance informed refusal. In doing so, the court seemed to imply that clear, specific statements by competent adults in advance of becoming incompetent might indeed be binding.

The court then turned to the constitutional right of privacy, based on *Roe* and cases that had preceded it in the federal courts, as well as the New Jersey state constitution's provisions on the right to privacy. Three reasons, based on compelling state's interests, for justified state intrusion into privacy were considered and rejected by the New Jersey Supreme Court.

The first was the state's legitimate interest in the preservation of life, based in the Fourteenth Amendment. Privacy would have to give way before a compelling interest in the preservation of Ms. Quinlan's life. Did the state have such an interest? No, reasoned the court, because Ms. Quinlan's prognosis was very poor and her treatment was very invasive. Her prognosis was considered to be very poor because she was not expected to recover to a cognitive, sapient state. The treatment was considered to be very invasive because she was receiving 24-hour intensive nursing care, ventilatory support, intravenous antibiotics, a catheter, and a feeding tube.

The court's second consideration was the ethical integrity of medicine. Would it be an unconscionable violation of medical ethics to disconnect Ms. Quinlan's ventilator? No, the court reasoned, because there were already arguments in the medical literature that it is not the physician's ethical obligation to preserve life without exception.

The court's third consideration was whether discontinuation of her ventilator would involve either Ms. Quinlan's physicians or her hospital in criminal behavior. No, the court reasoned, because withdrawal of the ventilator would not constitute killing. She would die of irreversible respiratory failure secondary to massive, irreversible central nervous system injury. Thus, this was not a matter of suicide or homicide. The court added that even if homicide were involved, it would not be unlawful given the collapse of the state's compelling interest in preserving the life of a patient who is in persistent vegetative state.

Ms. Quinlan's privacy rights thus prevailed in the court's reasoning. There was one remaining problem to address. She could not exercise those rights herself. To be meaningful, the court reasoned, her rights would have to be exercised *for* her. The court satisfied itself only that Mr. Quinlan was a conscientious and trustworthy agent for his daughter and therefore should be allowed to exercise her rights for her.

Contrast Between the Rights of Self-Determination and Privacy

Here emerges a crucial dimension of the constitutional right of privacy. Each of us retains the right to privacy despite even the irreversible loss of the capacity to make our own decisions. Others can exercise our privacy rights for us, because (like Mr. Quinlan) they are trustworthy, not necessarily because they would exercise our privacy rights as we would. The logic of self-determination as the basis for advance decision making about life-prolonging intervention would require instead that others exercising one's right exercise it as one would oneself as closely as possible. This distinction becomes clear in other cases, such as *Satz versus Perlmutter* (5), in which the Florida District Court of Appeals affirmed the right of self-determination of any competent adult patient to refuse any medical intervention, even if his or her life would end as a result. *Satz* makes it clear that self-determination is a far more powerful right than the right of privacy, because no interest of the state is presumably stronger than a citizen's legal right of self-determination. In summary, the common law of refusing intervention, even when death is the expected result, is based on an interesting admixture of privacy and self-determination.

The Living Will

The *Quinlan* case was followed rapidly by legislation to codify into statute the common law right to refuse—in advance of incompetency and terminal illness—life-prolonging intervention for terminal illness. Living wills typically cannot be used to request treatment, only to refuse it, although some states do allow requests for intervention via the living will. In 1976 California was the first to enact natural death legislation, and now

almost all states have legislation providing for living wills by statute (6). These statutes are based on an amalgam of legal principles—not well worked out in the statutes—of self-determination, privacy, and the state's compelling interest in preserving life.

Self-determination is obviously the basis of the right to project into the future a binding decision to refuse medical intervention. But the limitation to terminal illness and other end-stage conditions, such as permanent unconsciousness, of most living will statutes or natural death acts, as they are known in some states, reflects a right to privacy tempered by the state's interest in the preservation of life. In addition, many states exclude application of living wills to pregnant women, a provision that clearly reflects an interest in preserving life. (As far as we know, no legal challenge to that exclusion has been reported in those states.)

The state's compelling interest in the preservation of life is even more obviously expressed in the provision for revocation of the living will. Typically, only competent adult patients may execute a living will, but statutes make no provision for *competently* revoking a living will. Anyone may revoke a living will at any time by tearing it up or verbally negating it. This provision of living will statutes makes sense only on the assumption that the statute expresses the state's compelling interest in preserving life when in doubt.

Living will statutes also provide criminal and civil immunity for physicians and institutions who carry out a valid living will in which no malpractice occurs. We know of no reported cases challenging this protection anywhere. This indicates very wide acceptance of living wills in society. The purpose of this provision is to prevent family members from using threat of a suit for wrongful death to override the patient's living will.

Living will legislation has evolved since 1976. Initially, the definition of terminal illness in legislation applied to classic instances, such as late-stage cancers. Ironically, the initial definitions of terminal illness did not include what is now termed permanent vegetative state, Ms. Quinlan's diagnosis. Some states' definitions of terminal illness now reflect this evolution toward a broader scope of diagnoses. Physicians should know the definition of terminal illness and other medical conditions under which the statute can be invoked in their jurisdiction. The federal government recognizes the living will in Veterans Affairs (VA) institutions. The VA policy includes permanent vegetative state as a terminal illness.

The living will, then, is an expression of informed refusal before the patient is terminally ill as defined by relevant statute (or VA policy) and has lost decision-making capacity. Loss of decision-making capacity is a clinical judgment to be made according to prevailing standards. No adjudication of incompetence by a court is required by living will statutes or VA policy.

States vary according to whether the patient's declaration or living will must be written. In addition, states vary on whether a written or oral declaration must take a particular form. Almost all states allow the patient to list and attach explicit treatment refusals to a living will. In addition, most states provide for the exercise of the rights to refuse for patients without living wills, usually by family members listed by priority. Physicians should know the provisions of the relevant state statute and VA policies and procedures.

Durable Power of Attorney for Health Care

As experience was gained with living wills, a concern arose that the scope of informed refusal was not broad enough. Sometimes the patient is not terminally ill but also not competent, and it was questioned whether the patient would want aggressive management. Usually the patient is represented by family members. While it has long been customary to ask family members for permission to treat or not in such cases, the legal sanctions for this custom were indeed scant.

For many years common and statutory law allowed for power of attorney, the assignment of certain of one's legal powers to others, such as to dispose of jointly owned property in the absence of one of the owners. Power of attorney does not persist beyond that person's loss of decision-making capacity. A simple power of attorney is by definition not durable. Hence, the durable power of attorney was invented precisely to permit the conveyance of one's legal powers to an-

other upon one's loss of capacity to make decisions. The durable power of attorney for health care permits the conveyance to the agent or proxy of one's powers to make health care decisions upon loss of decision-making capacity. As with living wills, the loss of decision-making capacity is a clinical judgment, to be made in accordance with prevailing standards. Adjudication of incompetence by a court is not required. A durable power of attorney can be used to request or refuse treatment, giving this legal instrument greater scope and power than the living will in most jurisdictions.

The legal rationale of durable power of attorney is clearly founded in self-determination. Some states, however, have legislated limits on situations in which the agent may exercise powers of decision making, including pregnancy, involuntary admission to a psychiatric facility, and the authorization of electroconvulsive shock therapy. As far as we know there is no reported case of legal challenge, especially for wrongful death, against a physician or hospital who has let a patient die under the instructions of an agent or proxy holding a legally valid durable power of attorney.

The Living Will and Durable Power of Attorney for Health Care Contrasted

For a durable power of attorney to take effect, *only the loss of decision-making capacity* is required. There is no requirement, as there is in living wills, that the person also be terminally ill. There are other important differences between the living will and the durable power of attorney. The living will can typically be used only to refuse life-prolonging intervention. The durable power of attorney can be used just as informed consent can be used, either to *request or refuse* any intervention. The living will stands alone as representing the patient's preferences, whereas a durable power of attorney is carried out by the patient's agent or proxy. The living will presupposes that the patient knows what is to be withheld. The agent holding durable power of attorney is supposed to know what options are available to manage the patient's condition, as well as the patient's values and preferences to the extent possible.

THE PATIENT SELF-DETERMINATION ACT

The final piece of the legal puzzle is the federal Patient Self-Determination Act of 1990, which took effect in December 1991 (7). A parallel policy for VA institutions took effect in 1992. This statute grew out of the case of Nancy Beth Cruzan of Missouri, decided by the United States Supreme Court in 1990 (8). Cruzan was in a severe automobile accident that left her in a permanent vegetative state, and she was supported by gastrostomy tube feedings. Her parents requested that this life support be discontinued because previous conversations with her indicated that this is not what Cruzan would have wanted.

The original trial court agreed that the state's clear and convincing standard of evidence (75% probability of correctness) was satisfied by the evidence of Cruzan's prior statements. On appeal to the Missouri Supreme Court, this decision was reversed on the grounds that this evidentiary standard had not been met. The matter was appealed to the U.S. Supreme Court, challenging Missouri's evidentiary standard as an unconstitutional infringement on the rights to privacy and self-determination. A majority of the court (expressed in several opinions) held that Missouri's evidentiary standard was not unconstitutional. One opinion adopted the legal right of informed refusal "for the purposes of this case," an ambiguous endorsement of the doctrine of informed consent in these matters as it has developed in the common law of the various states.

The effect of the court's ruling was that Missouri and New York, at the time the one other state with a provision for clear and convincing evidence about prior statements and preferences, could retain it. Since that time, similar evidentiary standards have been upheld in Michigan and Delaware. The Supreme Court did not require the states to set such a standard for evidence about the prior wishes of persons without living wills or durable power of attorney. After the Supreme Court decision, the case was reheard, her parents' original request was granted, and the attorney general of Missouri declined to appeal the new decision.

In 1990 Senator John Danforth of Missouri introduced to Congress the Patient Self-Determination Act which was attached to the Omnibus Budget Reconciliation Act of that year (7). This law aims to reduce the number of situations in which patients do not have advance directives by requiring HMOs and institutions that receive federal moneys to notify their patients on admission (or enrollment in the case of HMOs) about their rights under relevant state law to execute an advance directive. The law also requires that the medical record document whether or not the patient has an advance directive. In addition, patients are to be notified about their general rights of informed consent. Finally, among other provisions, the law requires hospitals to have policies on these matters, to notify patients that there are such policies, to describe those policies to patients, and to teach the professional staff and community of the institution about advance directives. Physicians should know the policies and practices of the institutions in which they provide care to geriatric patients.

The physician should *not* assume that the Patient Self-Determination Act solves the problem of patients not having advance directives (9, 10). The main weakness of this federal law is that discussions with newly admitted patients may be hindered by such factors as time constraints, distractions, disorientation, fear, pain, serious illness, or diminished cognitive capacity and no requirement that the institution obtain copies of a patient's advance directives if they exist. This law would not have helped Cruzan because it will not help any patient who arrives at the emergency department of a hospital having lost decision-making capacity. This law also invites bureaucratization into the admissions process and thus invites the physician to assume that others have had adequate discussions with patients. To prevent this failure of communication, physicians should understand that they bear primary responsibility for discussing advance directives with patients in the *outpatient* setting and for anticipating and seeking to prevent ethical conflicts in association with advance directives in the inpatient setting. Geriatricians practicing in hospitals have an especially important role in preventing bureaucratization from circumventing adequate discussion with patients about advance directives.

ETHICAL PROBLEMS WITH ADVANCE DIRECTIVES

Despite their many benefits, advance directives have highlighted and in some instances created ethical problems for physicians, patients, and their families. These problems are now well enough understood that they can be anticipated and prevented in the clinical setting.

One problem is that physicians are reluctant to ask patients their preferences regarding end-of-life care. This reluctance may be due to fears of offending the patient, time constraints, or the physician's own discomfort with the subject of death. Patients want to discuss these matters but many wait for physicians to initiate the discussion. One study of patients who had not discussed end-of-life preferences with their physicians indicated that 68% wanted the physician to raise the issue and that only 11% did not. In all age groups, most patients considered it important for physicians and patients to discuss this matter, regardless of the patient's health (11–13).

Also, patients may not realize that not having advance directives may be harmful to their interests. In the absence of advance directives, decisions abhorrent to the patient may be made. In addition, decisions may not be made by persons who know that patient well, whom the patient trusts, or who have the patient's interests at heart. The patient's family sometimes disagrees over how to manage the patient's condition. Sometimes no family members are available. In these situations the physician or the person assigned by the institution must make a judgment, which can be difficult when the physician is not acquainted with the patient's values and preferences. In one study in which patients were asked their preferences regarding end-of-life care and their physicians were asked what treatments they thought their patients preferred, the physicians' accuracy was no greater than chance would have predicted. This result is particularly alarming, given that the overwhelming majority of patients (90%) expected their wishes to be represented accurately by their physicians (14).

The living will lacks specificity. Typically statutes refer to the withdrawal of mechanical or other artificial means of support. Emanuel and Emanuel (15) proposed the medical directive and

Emanuel (16), the health care directive (16) to address this problem. These documents, however, involve multiple scenarios and many decisions. The clinical applicability of such documents is limited by their cumbersome and complicated nature. Doubts have also been raised about their clinical adequacy (17). These points, in our judgment, are well taken: the lack of specificity must be addressed without abandoning utility and simplicity.

Proxy decision makers vary in their ability to reflect the patient's preferences. Researchers presenting decision-making scenarios to patients and their proxies found that in many of the scenarios almost as many proxies got it wrong as got it right (11, 12, 18, 19). The physician should advise the patient to select a person or persons who know the patient well and who have the equanimity, wisdom, and courage to make appropriate decisions in stressful situations. Incidentally, the physician should also advise the patient to pick one or two alternative agents for durable power of attorney for health care in case the first-named agent is not available. The physician should not assume concordance between proxy decision makers and the patient's preferences.

One reason that the proxy often does not know the patient's wishes is that the patient did not discuss the matter with the proxy or provide written instructions. One ethical challenge raised by advance directives, then, is the physician's obligation to attempt to persuade patients to communicate to the proxy their preferences, beliefs, and values regarding suffering, pain, death, and end-of-life care. In some cases the patient may decline to provide instructions out of trust and deference to the agent. This is certainly a valid exercise of the patient's autonomy. Patients may not provide instruction because they do not want to address the questions involved, preferring to leave these matters to their agents. Finally, the patient may not provide instruction because the statutory language or institution's forms do not provide the opportunity for doing so. Many standard documents used to designate durable power of attorney for health care contain space for instructions but sometimes this space is very small. The VA policy provides an entire form specifically for this purpose.

Patients may write instructions or make oral statements in association with a living will or durable power of attorney that strike the physician as unreasonable, inappropriate, or producing substandard care. These may be requests either for or against treatment. Aggressive management does not make sense in all cases any more than watchful waiting always does. A particularly troublesome situation is caused when the patient's agent requests that "everything be done" for a patient who has suffered severe and irreversible brain damage. To respond accordingly would require the physician to provide care that conferred no benefit and perhaps harm on the patient and certainly a harm to other patients who might have benefited from more appropriate use of scarce medical resources.

This was precisely the situation confronted by the physicians caring for Helga Wanglie (20, 21), who elected to seek resolution through the hospital ethics committee and, unsuccessfully, the court in response to a request from the patient's husband that everything be done. Such solutions seldom satisfy any of the parties involved. It is far better to address these problems with patients before they lose their capacity to decide, before medical crises arise, and before ethical conflicts become refractory (22). The physician should review the patient's living will and instructions to the agent, and if any unreasonable or inappropriate requests are found, discuss them with the patient without delay. Such discussion might reveal that the request is rooted in the patient's anxiety, depression, guilt, religious fear, financial uncertainty, or a failure in the physician-patient relationship such as miscommunication or mistrust. If the physician addresses these underlying problems preventively, i.e., consistently with respect for the patient's autonomy, the patient may be persuaded to alter the inappropriate request.

Patients and their families sometimes overstate what their religious convictions require of them in preventing death. The Western religious traditions, which include Judaism, Christianity, and Islam, view human life as sacred and view failure to show reverence for human life as the most egregious of sins. Thus in the Western religious traditions there is a strong taboo against suicide. In Dante's *Inferno,* canto 13, for example,

people who committed suicide are considered worse than murderers, worse even than serpents. Some patients and families feel obligated to insist on aggressive management until the moment of death, believing that anything else constitutes suicide. The physician can help terminally ill patients and their families by reminding them of the limits of medical science and of human life as well. Failing to "do everything" is not the equivalent of suicide or murder if nothing will extend life or if extending life only artificially prolongs the moment of death. Refusals to accept death at this stage may be rooted less in religious factors than in psychologic factors such as denial or guilt or in misunderstandings caused by the physician's failure to communicate that death is imminent. The physician who addresses these factors preventively prepares patients and their families to face death. If religious objections persist, the physician should consider consulting the patient's religious adviser, who can address the patient's religious fears about death and attempt to clear up any theologic misperceptions about the sinfulness of accepting death. Such consultations sometimes reveal that the religious adviser misunderstood the seriousness of the patient's illness and has been inappropriately advising the patient to fight the illness. Once the physician and religious adviser are on the same wavelength, there is much greater likelihood that they can together help the patient and family face death.

The physician's professional colleagues may have difficulty with particular strategies for permitting patients to die, in particular the withdrawal of nutritional support. Some take the view that withdrawal of nutritional support is tantamount to murder and suicide, that the cause of death is starvation rather than the illness itself, and that nutrition and hydration are not medicines but ordinary sustenance. Justice Scalia articulated such a view in the *Cruzan* decision (8), and Ms. Quinlan's parents expressed a similar view in their decision to continue providing nutrition to their daughter after withdrawing her from ventilatory support, despite receiving the permission of Roman Catholic theologians to withhold nutrition and fluids (23). The courts that have examined this matter, however, have uniformly ruled that nutritional support is the same as any other nursing or medical intervention and that its withdrawal is, like that of a ventilator, not a killing, thus extending the reasoning of the *Quinlan* court (24–26).

The patient's family and loved ones may object to the patient's decisions as expressed in advance directives. The worst time for conflict about such matters is after the patient has lost decision-making capacity. It is far better to help patients identify and deal with potential problems within their family before those decisions are to be implemented, and give the family time either to accept them or at least respect them. If this approach fails, however, the physician is legally and morally obligated to honor the patient's living will despite the objections of the family. We have unfortunately encountered situations in which the physician shirked this responsibility. The expressed wishes of the patient are to be respected by all parties, and the physician has an important role in teaching family members, particularly by setting an example of respect for the patient's wishes and encouraging and expecting recalcitrant family members to follow the example. The findings of the SUPPORT study, that living wills are sometimes not implemented by physicians, is particularly disturbing in this respect (9, 10).

An advance directive is not a physician's order. When advance directives apply, they must be translated directly into physician's orders that reflect and implement the patient's preferences. These orders should be explicit, comprehensive, and well publicized among appropriate professional staff and colleagues: no professional caring for the patient should have any doubt about just what is and is not to be done when life-threatening events occur. The SUPPORT study underscores the need for such orders to make advance directives clinically effective (9, 10, 27). Institutional policy can play an important role in preventing this problem (28).

The physician's obligations do not end with writing orders for nonaggressive management. There are substantive ethical obligations to the dying and their families. The patient is owed respect for dignity and appropriate management of pain, symptoms, and suffering. The family is owed assurance and support that the patient's wishes are being carried out and that therefore

everything that ought to have been done was done in a professional and caring manner. In this way, family members are given good memories of their loved one to sustain them in their loss. In addition, appropriate end-of-life care may prevent requests for physician-assisted suicide.

Some patients, families, and physicians have misconceptions about the applicability of living wills to reversible illness and injuries in which death is not imminent. Some persons may be afraid to sign a living will for fear that aggressive management will be withheld in acute nonterminal situations. The physician should assure such patients that the living will applies only to terminally ill patients. Some patients make too strong and general a statement, such as "I don't want ever to be put on machines." The physician should inform such patients that there are situations in which a trial of mechanical support may save their life and return them to their previous state of health and quality of life or something close to it.

There is potential for abuse by proxy decision makers and other family members or friends who might benefit from a premature death or a prolonged life. For example, family members have been known to request that patients in a permanent vegetative state be kept on life supports not to benefit the patient but to benefit themselves, perhaps by continuing to receive pension checks. The physician should be willing to challenge proxy decision makers who appear to be acting from interests other than those of the patient. If individual confrontations fail to uphold the patient's interests, the physician should involve the institution's ethics committee and if necessary, the courts. One safeguard against such abuse in some jurisdictions is that family members, heirs, and creditors are not allowed to witness the signing of the durable power of attorney for health care.

A PREVENTIVE ETHICS STRATEGY FOR ADVANCE DIRECTIVES

These ethical conflicts usually occur because the physician waits too long to consult the patient about decision making or fails to translate advance directives into explicit orders in a timely fashion. Such decisions should be discussed well in advance of hospitalization or admission to a nursing home. If the patient is willing, the family should also be involved, so that they know, understand, respect, and support the patient's decisions. Institutions' administrations can encourage this process. In the clinic in which Holleman serves as consultant, a letter explaining advance directives is given to all patients as they sign in with the receptionist (Fig. 67.1). Advance directives are displayed in the waiting room, the nurses' station, and the examining rooms. Records of conversations and copies of advance directives are part of the patients' charts.

For patients who make it to the hospital or nursing home without advance directives, the response of the physician's institutions to the Patient Self-Determination Act should not be presumed to be sufficient. Decision making can be initiated during discharge planning in anticipation of readmission. Discussion of advance directives with all elderly patients—in the outpatient setting, at discharge planning, and at

admission—should be regarded as the ethical standard of care. Too many ethical conflicts occur because physicians are not initiating conversations with geriatric patients about advance directives. The primary clinical task, therefore, is to prevent such conflicts, particularly the ones we have discussed.

We propose a 10-step preventive ethics strategy for advance directives (Table 67.1). This strategy is based on years of addressing ethical conflicts and recognizing that they are often preventable. These steps take time, but they are cost effective because they save time and prevent stress and ethical conflicts for patients, families and loved ones, institutions, and society. In addition, they are likely to conserve financial and medical resources by reducing the amount of aggressive management provided to terminally ill patients.

First, the physician and patient should engage in a sensitive but honest discourse about the values that underlie the patient's health beliefs and preferences about end-of-life care. Chapter 68,

---

Dear Patient:

On December 1, 1991, a new law, the Patient Self-Determination Act, went into effect. Under that law, if you are admitted to a hospital for any reason, you will be asked if you have an advance directive. If not, you will be provided information about advance directives and encouraged to write one. There are several types of advance directives, but the ones most commonly used are called durable power of attorney for health care and living will (or directive to physicians).

A durable power of attorney for health care enables you to specify in advance the person you wish to make medical decisions for you, should you become seriously ill and unable to communicate.

A living will, or directive to physicians, tells your doctors how you want to be treated should you lose your ability to communicate. If, for example, you suffered a severe stroke or a serious head injury from which you were not expected to recover, would you want to be kept alive on a breathing machine? Or would you prefer simply to be kept comfortable and allow nature to take its course? You can indicate such preferences through the use of a living will.

Thinking about these things is not easy, but the best way to assure that your wishes are honored is to express them in advance. As physicians at the Baylor Family Practice Center we encourage all patients, regardless of your age or health status, to take the time to consider advance directives. We suggest that, instead of waiting until you are admitted to a hospital, that you do it now. We hope you will discuss this matter with your loved ones and with your family physician at your next visit. *Materials are available from the brochure rack in the reception area or from your nurse.*

As your family physicians our goal has always been to serve you as best we can. You can help us serve you by expressing your wishes clearly.

Sincerely,
Your Baylor Family Physicians

Figure 67.1. Sample letter concerning advance directives.

Table 67.1

A Preventive Ethics Strategy for Advance Directives

1. Explore the patient's core values and beliefs regarding end-of-life care, using the Values History (Chapter 68).
2. Describe interventions used to respond to life-threatening events.
3. Explain the different types of advance directives (living will and durable power of attorney for health care) and review completed patients' directives for inconsistencies or unreasonable preferences.
4. Be wary of using the term withdrawing "care."
5. Ask patients if anyone in their family may have problems with their preferences, and address family members' concerns.
6. Involve a religious adviser when appropriate and with the patient's consent.
7. Ask yourself whether any colleagues have objections to the patient's preferences and address colleagues' concerns.
8. Ask where the patient keeps originals of advance directives, record directives in patient's chart, and distribute copies to relevant parties.
9. When the advance directives apply clinically, write an order that expresses and implements the patient's preferences. These orders should always address pain and symptom relief and maintenance of dignity.
10. Insist that compliance with physicians' orders implementing advance directives become part of the definition of quality and are measured in the total quality management process.

on the Values History, provides a structured clinical approach to these conversations.

Second, the patient should be provided with a frank description of the kinds of intervention that are used in aggressive management of life-threatening events, especially critical care interventions. The physician should briefly but accurately describe such interventions as intubation and support by mechanical ventilation, cardiopulmonary resuscitation, admission to the critical care unit, and the administration of medication, fluid, and nutrition by peripheral and central lines as well as nasogastric and percutaneous endoscopic gastrostomy tubes. Both the short- and long-term consequences should be discussed, including the probability of implementing the patient's preferences given the patient's present and future expected health status. Patients with chronic diseases should appreciate that life-threatening events usually accelerate the process of decline, and aggressive management followed by survival usually leaves the patient with a lower baseline than before the event.

It is especially important that the concept of trial of intervention be discussed with the patient. Increasingly, aggressive management is undertaken as a trial to determine whether it will benefit the patient and is stopped if it becomes clear that it is no longer doing so. Recent research in-

dicates that patients who want aggressive management accept the concept of a trial and prefer it over "always doing everything" (29). In particular, the physician should explain to the patient and the patient's family that admission to the intensive care unit is a trial of intervention. Indeed, such a trial is usually necessary because it is quite difficult to predict which patients will benefit from intensive care admission.

Third, the physician should explain advance directives to geriatric patients (30), and describing the two forms of advance directives, their purposes, and the conditions in which they take effect. The living will can typically be used by patients only to refuse treatment in advance of both terminal illness (as defined in relevant state law or VA policy) and reasonable clinical judgment that they have lost the capacity for making their own decisions. The physician should be clear with the patient about whether applicable law of living wills defines permanent vegetative state as a terminal illness. If it does not, the patient is well advised to consider executing a durable power of attorney explicitly to cover this possibility.

The durable power of attorney for health care can be used by patients to assign to someone else, the patient's agent or proxy, the power to make decisions for them when in reasonable clinical judgment they have lost the capacity to make their own decisions. In some jurisdictions the patient need not also be terminally ill, as is the case for living wills. If relevant statutes exclude certain conditions or procedures (e.g., electroshock convulsive therapy), these exclusions should be made clear to the patient.

The physician should review the patient's durable power of attorney. If these instructions are unclear, unreasonable, or difficult to implement, this should be explained so that patients can clarify their intentions and preferences. For example, a request that everything be done may not make sense for a patient who is surely dying despite aggressive management that results, on balance, only in unnecessary pain and suffering. Such an outcome is justifiably regarded as unreasonable in beneficence-based clinical judgment, and this should be explained to the patient. All alternatives should be reviewed so that the patient's preferences do not later lead to conflict with beneficence-based judgment. If the patient persists in providing instructions that the physician finds unreasonable to the point of inability in conscience to carry them out, the physician should seek consultation from the institutional ethics committee. If that is unsatisfactory, the physician should consider referring the patient to a colleague willing to carry out those instructions and withdraw from the patient's care (22).

Any conversations between the patient and the agent to which the physician is witness should be recorded in the patient's chart. This record can serve as an important reference point later, when particular decisions need to be made.

Both the living will and the durable power of attorney for health care should be reviewed for instructions that might lead to clinically contradictory courses. Conflicts (e.g., between having a living will and an instruction on the durable power of attorney to "do everything") should be pointed out and the patient's preference for the management of such conflict elicited. The patient should be asked to draft new documents if necessary, and the physician should record such preferences in the patient's record.

Fourth, the physician should beware of ever using the language of withdrawing or withholding "care." *Care* for patients, especially for patients who are dying, should never be withdrawn. All patients remain members of the moral community until their deaths. Caring for patients includes diligent attention to and management of unnecessary pain and protection of the patient's dignity (31). The patient's suffering can be alleviated by addressing such symptoms as nausea, dyspnea, and shortness of breath.

Fifth, patients should be asked whether they anticipate that anyone in the family may have concerns, problems, or objections regarding the decisions in their advance directives. For example, a patient may prefer to name an adult son or daughter as agent rather than the spouse, especially if the spouse has cognitive impairment. The patient's spouse may be unaware of this preference. The physician should offer the patient the opportunity to meet with family members so that these preferences and decisions can be explained. The physician can point out that family members have an ethical obligation to respect the patient's choices. Adult children, especially, should be made aware of and should avoid role reversal, taking over decision making as if the patient were a child and the adult children, the parents.

Sixth, many patients make health care decisions on the basis of their religious beliefs, traditions, and convictions (32). Patients often turn to religious advisers for help in making decisions about advance directives. When they do, the religious adviser should not be offering advice in a vacuum. With the patient's permission, therefore, the religious adviser should be provided with the information described in steps two and three of this process. In addition, the physician should be aware that most faith communities do not make it obligatory to resist death at all costs. Rather, moral theologic views tend to recognize limits to what medicine can and should accomplish. Some patients are not aware of this and so overestimate what their faith requires of them. If a patient or a religious adviser insists that his or her faith requires that everything be done, this should be discussed frankly, apprising them of the prospects of success and the cost in unnecessary morbidity, pain, and suffering to the patient and family. The religious adviser should be asked to consider carefully all of the clinical information that he or she now has and reconsider the advice earlier given to the patient or the patient's family.

Seventh, physicians should ask themselves and inquire among colleagues, especially nurses and trainees, whether any one has concerns, problems, or objections to the patient's advance directives. Some may object to withdrawal or withholding of nutrition as a form of killing by starvation.

There are two responses to this sort of objection. If the patient is being supported by interventions besides nutritional support (e.g., a ventilator, antibiotics, or pressor drugs), one or more of these may be discontinued to allow the patient to die comfortably. This response is very useful in the case of patients on multiple life supports, because it does not require that colleagues participate in what they may judge in conscience to be killing by starvation. The second response applies when nutritional support is the main or sole intervention that is preventing the patient's death. This is frequently the case for patients in a permanent vegetative state. Not everyone accepts the explanation that death subsequent to discontinuation of nutritional support is caused by metabolic decline and immune system failure secondary to irreversible central nervous system injury or disease. As noted earlier, at least one member of the United States Supreme Court, Justice Scalia, does not, and those who share his opinion may be correct. This view should therefore be regarded as reasonable and should be respected. Such a view, however, cannot be allowed to stand in the way of implementing advance directives, because there is no conclusive argument that withdrawal or withholding of nutrition must be regarded as killing by starvation in all cases. Individual clinicians who agree with Justice Scalia must respect the patient's preference as also being reasonable. They can in conscience withdraw from the patient's case, but they are not free to block the implementation of an advance directive.

Eighth, ask patients where they keep originals of their advance directives and who has copies. The physician, with the patient's consent, should be sure that there are copies of the patient's directives in the patient's office records, the hospital records, the nursing home's records, and with family members. In particular, the physician

should be certain that the emergency department of the patient's hospital has copies of these directives.

Ninth, having undertaken the previous seven steps, the physician is in a position to write an order that implements the patient's advance directives. The physician's orders should be comprehensive and clear. The goal is this: no professional with responsibility for the patient, upon reading the orders, should be unclear or uncertain in any way about what should and should not be done in a life-threatening event. These orders should be readily accessible in the patient's chart, e.g., as a face sheet.

Tenth, the completion of end-of-life treatment orders should be reviewed by institutions as part of their total quality management and continuous quality improvement processes. Such review can improve on the shortcomings identified in the SUPPORT study (9, 10).

As noted earlier, there are serious beneficence-based and autonomy-based obligations to dying patients. Chief among these are adequate pain and suffering control and maintenance of dignity. Hence, the physician's orders should in all cases address protection of dignity and the management of the patient's pain, symptoms, and suffering.

Seriously ill patients can tolerate high doses of analgesics if the level is titrated appropriately (33, 34). Proper pain and symptom management reduces the risk of suicide among seriously ill patients (35). Proper titration of pain medication also minimizes the risk of mortality from aggressive pain and symptom management. The patient's death is acceptable in beneficence-based judgment. Quality assurance mechanisms should be extended to cover review of pain and suffering management for dying patients, so that these matters can be addressed openly and with institutional sanction. Quality assurance in this matter is essential, given that physicians continue to undertreat pain despite recent advances in pain management (34, 36).

CONCLUSION

Executing an advance directive is a weighty matter. In effect, the patient is making decisions about how he or she will die and be remembered by loved ones. Such decisions are obviously freighted with religious beliefs and moral values. Recognition of the importance of discussing values related to advance directives has led investigators to develop an adjunctive document known as the Values History. Because of its clinical importance, the Values History is discussed separately in Chapter 68.

REFERENCES

1. President's Commission for the Study of Ethical Problems in Medicine and Biomedical and Behavioral Research. Deciding to Forego Life-Sustaining Treatment: A Report on the Ethical, Medical, and Legal Issues in Treatment Decisions. Washington: US Government Printing Office, 1983.
2. Schloendorff v Society of New York Hospital. 211 NY 125, 126, 105 N.E. 92, 93, 1914.
3. Roe v Wade. 410 United States Reports 113, 1973.
4. In Re Quinlan. 70 NJ 10, 1976.
5. Satz v Perlmutter. 362 S.2d 160, Florida District Court of Appeals, 1978.
6. Wolf SM, Boyle P, Callahan D, et al. Sources of concern about the patient self-determination act. N Engl J Med 1991;325:1666–1671.
7. The Patient Self-Determination Act. 42 U.S.C. Sections 1395 cc and 1396 a suppl, 1991.
8. Cruzan v Director, Missouri Dept. of Health. 111 L Ed 2d 224, 110 SCT 2841, 1990.
9. A controlled trial to improve care for seriously ill hospitalized patients. The study to understand prognoses and preferences for outcomes and risks of treatments (SUPPORT). The SUPPORT Principal Investigators. JAMA 1995;274:1591–1598.
10. Teno JM, Lynn J, Wenger N, et al. Advance directives for seriously ill hospitalized patients: Effectiveness with the Patient Self-Determination Act and SUPPORT investigation. J Am Geriatr Soc 1997;45:500–507.
11. Lo B, McLeod GA, Saika G. Patient attitudes to discussing life-sustaining treatment. Arch Intern Med 1986;146:1613–1615.
12. Emanuel LL, Barry MH, Stoeckle JD, et al. Advance directives for medical care: a case for greater use. N Engl J Med 1991;324:889–895.
13. Edinger W, Smucker DR. Outpatients' attitudes regarding advance directives. J Fam Pract 1992;35:650–653.
14. Seckler AB, Meier DE, Mulvihill M, Paris BEC. Substituted judgment: how accurate are proxy predictions? Ann Intern Med 1991;115:92–98.
15. Emanuel LL, Emanuel EJ. The medical directive: a new comprehensive advance care document. JAMA 1989;261:3288–3293.
16. Emanuel L. The health care directive: learning how to draft advance care documents. J Am Geriatr Soc 1991;39:1221–1228.
17. Sachs GA, Cassel CK. The medical directive. JAMA 1990;263:1069–1070.
18. Uhlmann RF, Pearlman RA, Cain KC. Physicians' and spouses' predictions of elderly patients' resuscitation preferences. J Gerontol Med Sci 1988;43:M115–M121.
19. Zweibel NR, Cassel CK. Treatment choices at the end of life: a comparison of decisions by older patients and their physician-selected proxies. Gerontologist 1989;29:615–621.
20. Miles SH. The case of Helga Wanglie: a new kind of "right to die" case. N Engl J Med 1991;325:511–515.
21. Rie MA. The limits of a wish. Hastings Cent Rep 1991;21:24–27.
22. Doukas DJ, McCullough LB. A preventive ethics approach to counseling patients about clinical futility in the primary care setting. Arch Fam Med 1996;5:589–593.
23. Beauchamp TL, Childress JF. Principles of Biomedical Ethics. 4th ed. New York: Oxford University Press, 1994.
24. In re Conroy. 486 A.2d 1209 NJ, 1985.
25. Bouvia v Superior Court. California Reporter, 225 Cal. Rptr. 297. Cal.App.2 Dist., 1986.
26. Brophy v New England Sinai Hospital, Inc. 398 Mass. 417, 498 N.E.2d 626, 1986.
27. Teno JM, Licks S, Lynn J, et al. Do advance directives provide instructions that direct care? J Am Geriatr Soc 1997;45:508–512.
28. Emanuel LL, Barry MJ, Stoeckle JD, et al. Advance directives for medical care: a case for greater use. N Engl J Med 1991;324:889–895.
29. Reilly RB, Teasdale TA, McCullough LB. Option of trial in advance directives. Gerontologist 1992;32(special issue 2):69.
30. Markson L, Clark J, Glantz L, et al. The doctor's role in discussing advance preferences for end-of-life care: perceptions of physicians practicing in the VA. J Am Geriatr Soc 1997;45:399–406.
31. Wanzer SH, Federman DD, Adelstein MD, et al. The physician's responsibility toward hopelessly ill patients. N Engl J Med 1989;320:844–849.
32. Grodin MA. Religious advance directives: the convergence of law, religion, medicine, and public health. Am J Public Health 1993;83:899–903.
33. Foley KM. Diagnosis and treatment of cancer pain. In: Holleb AI, Fink DJ, Murphy GP, eds. American Cancer Society Textbook of Clinical Oncology. Atlanta: American Cancer Society, 1991:555–575.
34. Ogle KS, Warren D, Plumb JD. Pain management in advanced cancer. Prim Care 1992;19:793–805.
35. Foley KM. The relationship of pain and symptom management to patient requests for physician-assisted suicide. J Pain Symptom Manage 1991;6:289–297.
36. Solomon MZ, O'Donnell L, Jennings B, et al. Decisions near the end of life: professional views on life-sustaining treatments. Am J Public Health 1993;83:14–23.

CHAPTER 68

DAVID J. DOUKAS AND LAURENCE B. McCULLOUGH

Assessing the Values of Elders Toward End-of-Life Care: The Values History

Advance directives were developed over the past two decades to enhance the autonomy of patients in making end-of-life treatment decisions. In this chapter we argue that these decisions are ultimately based on values. The two legally recognized advance directives are the living will and durable power of attorney for health care (Chapter 67). Despite their laudatory intent, these instruments fall short of their goal of being autonomy enhancing because they fail to identify the values of patients that justify and give meaning to treatment decisions. Because advance directives do not legally require physicians and surrogate decision makers to discuss the patient's underlying values, a valuable opportunity to understand the reasoning and concerns underlying the patient's treatment decisions is lost. The preventive ethics approach to this clinical problem in end-of-life care is to use the Values History, a supplementary advance directive instrument to the living will and the durable power of attorney for health care (1–6).

The Values History enhances the patient's autonomy in two important ways that go beyond conventional advance directives: (*a*) it encourages discussion between the patient and the physician about the patient's values regarding end-of-life treatment; and (*b*) it facilitates a detailed informed consent process about the patient's reasoning concerning treatment preferences. This two-phase approach allows for and encourages the use of standard advance directives, complemented by a discussion of values

and values-based preferences that provides a rich context for determining what the patient wants in the event of incapacity. The rationale for this approach rests on normative and empiric findings that informed consent may be weakened without a values discussion and is strengthened by its inclusion (1, 2). The discouraging data from the SUPPORT study about the failure to prepare and implement advance directives underscore the need for this preventive ethics approach to advance directives (7, 8).

THE PATIENT SELF-DETERMINATION ACT

Following the U.S. Supreme Court decision in the Cruzan case, Congress enacted the Patient Self-Determination Act of 1990 (PSDA) to facilitate and encourage teaching patients about advance directives (9). The PSDA mandates that all Medicare- and Medicaid-funded health care institutions (e.g., hospitals, hospice, home health agencies, and health maintenance organizations [HMOs]) inform patients of their rights regarding informed consent and refusal of care and about advance directives under applicable state laws (10). As a result of the PSDA, patients are supposed to be routinely told about informed consent and refusal, the living will, and the durable power of attorney for health care. However, the opportunity to prepare a living will or durable power of attorney on admission to such a facility is far less than optimal, because of the severity of illness often required for hospital admission and because some patients are in a medical state preventing consent. The SUPPORT data question the success of the PSDA as an autonomy-enhancing remedy. Moreover, the PSDA does not remedy recognized problems with advance directives (1, 11).

The living will and durable power of attorney for health care can meet important needs by allowing patients to make decisions about medical intervention prospectively. However, each of these advance directives is flawed, requiring supplementation if physicians are to use them to best effect. The living will is vague in describing the treatments the patient has refused (11, 12). This ambiguity has led to misinterpretation of the living will because of its lack of detail (11, 12). Not surprisingly, physicians' interpretations of living wills can dictate the judgment about the document's validity in particular circumstances (12). This variation may help to explain the SUPPORT study finding of uneven implementation of advance directives.

The durable power of attorney for health care is another legal instrument created with good intent. It empowers an agent to make decisions for a patient based on the patient's preferences when the patient lacks the capacity to do so. It may also fall short, for it is limited by the extent to which the agent and patient confer about the patient's values and explicit treatment preferences (1, 13).

Both the living will and durable power of attorney ask the patient to make decisions about end-of-life care without exploring and discussing the values upon which such decisions are based. Indeed, physicians can fulfill their legal obligations under the PSDA without the values underlying those preferences ever being discussed. This practice is ethically problematic because both documents have an implied values-laden emphasis on patients' preferences about end-of-life care. Neither advance directive, however, attempts to articulate a detailed inventory of the patient's values. This is because neither advance directive legally requires the physician to discuss the patient's values prospectively (14, 15). The PSDA does not require a physician to participate in its execution (one of the main weaknesses of the law) and applies only to one outpatient setting, the HMO. With the PSDA, the

physician need not have any involvement in the patient's medical decision making in signing a living will or durable power of attorney for health care. Patients may be spoken to or just given written materials on advance directives by non-health care personnel such as admission clerks. Some questions arise regarding how well informed is the consent:

- Does the patient understand the document?
- Has the patient carefully reviewed his or her own values regarding end-of-life care?
- Has the patient carefully considered relevant treatment options?
- Has the patient considered how he or she envisions dying?
- Has the patient discussed his or her values about family involvement and burden?
- Has the patient considered aggressiveness of treatment and pain control?
- Will the physician be able to translate the patient's preferences into orders for care?

EXPLORING THE PATIENT'S VALUES

The limitations of the living will and durable power of attorney for health care led us and our colleagues (1–5) to develop a value-based advance directive instrument called the Values History. While appointing an agent and preparing a living will are important health care planning steps, they are not clinically adequate for assuring that the patient's preferences will be respected when he or she is incapacitated. The need to respect these preferences has been established by the SUPPORT study (7, 8). The patient's values and beliefs help the physician to understand the basis upon which these advance directives were executed by the patient. These values can clarify the reasoning of these directives to the patient's family and physician while also allowing for elaboration of the reasoning behind specific treatment preferences. These values give greater meaning to a standard advance directive, greatly increasing their clinical utility.

Documenting the patient's values brings context to these preferences. In several studies the values in the Values History have been empirically evaluated with regard to specific medical interventions (6, 16, 17). There are significant correlations between patients' values and selection of medical therapies that they would wish to forgo if they were terminally ill. In a study of three generations of families, subjects expressed concerns about avoiding therapies that could burden their family members (16). Similarly, in an outpatient population there was a significant correlation of preferences of forgoing all forms of end-of-life therapy with concerns about family distress (6). In a study of HIV-infected men, concerns about their own physical pain and burden and the desire to be able to communicate with a willing physician who would implement their wishes had paramount importance (17). These findings represent evidence supporting the claim that knowledge of patients' values can help physicians interpret the patient's medical preferences when the patient can no longer participate in decision making. This approach allows for greater flexibility by heightening awareness of the reasoning behind attitudes toward certain treatments. The values and expressed preferences in the Values History can assist the physician in writing orders when the need arises. The SUPPORT study points to the frequent failure to write such orders, a problem that the use of the Values History may begin to correct.

The Values History also is different from, and enhances the function of, the living will and durable power of attorney for health care, in that trials of intervention can be articulated for specific treatments (18). The patient can decide prospectively that an intervention can be attempted, then stopped, according to the patient's choice, either after a specific time or when reasonable medical judgment shows that it is not expected to benefit the patient. The concept of trials of intervention is important in critical and long-term care, replacing the all-or-nothing approach (19). Critical care management is increasingly undertaken as a trial of intervention to determine whether continuing it will benefit the patient. The patient should understand that in contemporary critical care, an admission to the intensive care unit is itself a trial of intervention. Such a trial is undertaken in the absence of the patient's refusal because it is quite difficult to predict which patients will and will not benefit from intensive care admission. Existing advance directives do not address such clinical realities, but the Values History does. The Values History is a helpful embellishment to standard advance directives by being more explicit about limits of therapy in medical care that the patient has articulated. Recent research indicates that patients understand the concept of a trial of intervention and prefer it to always doing something (20). Trials of intervention also facilitate finding common ground between the patient's and the physician's values. Identifying common ground of values is the core of preventive ethics.

COMPONENTS OF THE VALUES HISTORY

The Values History (Fig. 68.1) contains two parts: the values section, which identifies values, and the directive section, which articulates preference statements based on the patient's values. The introductory section of the Values History explains its function as an appendix to advance directives. Almost all jurisdictions and Department of Veterans Affairs (VA) policy allow specific statements about the patient's preferences to be added to a living will as well as the durable power of attorney for health care, when their intent is in concordance with the advance directive. The reader is directed to review local law or policy in this regard.

The values section begins with two statements. The patient is asked which is more important to him or her, length of life or quality of life. This query is essential as an initial point to discussing future health care because critical care for seriously ill patients often involves a trade-off between lengthening life and maintaining its quality. This question allows and encourages patient and physician to discuss aggressiveness of health care, as well as its risk, morbidity, and the need for pain control. The patient is asked about his or her own evaluation of length of life versus quality of life. The patient is then asked to identify specific end-of-life values that are most important to him or her. The physician is encouraged to discuss the patient's values at length to facilitate elaboration or the addition of other values that more completely reflect the person's concerns or beliefs.

The directives section elicits treatment direc-

The Values History

Patient Name: _____

    This Values History serves as a set of my specific value-based directives for various medical interventions. It is to be used in health care circumstances when I may be unable to voice my preferences. These directives shall be made a part of the medical record and used as supplementary to my living will and/or durable power of attorney for health care for those medical circumstances identified in these documents.

I. VALUES SECTION

    There are several values important in decisions about end-of-life treatment and care. This section of the Values History invites you to identify your most important values.

    A. Basic Life Values

        Perhaps the most basic values in this context concern length of life versus quality of life. Which of the following two statements is the most important to you?

        _____ 1. I want to live as long as possible, regardless of the quality of life that I experience.

        _____ 2. I want to preserve a good quality of life, even if this means that I may not live as long.

    B. Quality of Life Values

        There are many values that help us to define for ourselves the quality of life that we want to live. The following list contains some that appear to be very important. Review this list (and feel free either to elaborate on it or to add to it) and circle those values that are most important to your definition of quality of life.

        1. I want to maintain my capacity to think clearly.

        2. I want to feel safe and secure.

        3. I want to avoid unnecessary pain and suffering.

        4. I want to be treated with respect.

        5. I want to be treated with dignity when I can no longer speak for myself.

        6. I do not want to be an unnecessary burden on my family.

        7. I want to be able to make my own decisions.

        8. I want to experience a comfortable dying process.

        9. I want to be with my loved ones before I die.

        10. I want to leave good memories of me to my loved ones.

        11. I want to be treated in accord with my religious beliefs and traditions.

        12. I want respect shown for my body after I die.

        13. I want to help others by making a contribution to medical education and research.

        14. Other values or clarification of values above:

II. DIRECTIVES SECTION

    Some directives involve simple yes or no decisions. Others provide for the choice of a trial of intervention. Initials/Date

    _____ 1. I want to undergo cardiopulmonary resuscitation.

    _____   TRIAL to determine effectiveness using reasonable medical judgment.

    _____   NO

Why?

    _____ 2. I want to be placed on a ventilator.

    _____   YES

    _____   TRIAL for the TIME PERIOD OF _____

    _____   TRIAL to determine effectiveness using reasonable medical judgment.

    _____   NO

Why?

    _____ 3. I want to have an endotracheal tube used in order to perform items 1 and 2.

    _____   YES

    _____   TRIAL for the TIME PERIOD OF _____

    _____   TRIAL to determine effectiveness using reasonable medical judgment.

    _____   NO

Why?

(continued)

Figure 68.1.   The Values History. (Reprinted with permission from Doukas D, McCullough L. The Values History: the evaluation of the patient's values and advance directives. J Fam Pract 1991;32:145–153.)

_____ 4. I want to have total parenteral nutrition administered for my nutrition.
_____ YES
_____ TRIAL for the TIME PERIOD OF _____
_____ TRIAL to determine effectiveness using reasonable medical judgment.
_____ NO
Why?

_____ 5. I want to have intravenous medication and hydration administered; regardless of my decision, I understand that intravenous hydration to alleviate discomfort or pain medication will not be withheld from me if I so request them.
_____ YES
_____ TRIAL for the TIME PERIOD OF _____
_____ TRIAL to determine effectiveness using reasonable medical judgment.
_____ NO
Why?

_____ 6. I want to have all medications used for the treatment of my illness continued; regardless of my decision, I understand that pain medication will continue to be administered including narcotic medications.
_____ YES
_____ TRIAL for the TIME PERIOD OF _____
_____ TRIAL to determine effectiveness using reasonable medical judgment.
_____ NO
Why?

_____ 7. I want to have nasogastric, gastrostomy, or other enteral feeding tubes introduced and administered for my nutrition.
_____ YES
_____ TRIAL for the TIME PERIOD OF _____
_____ TRIAL to determine effectiveness using reasonable medical judgment.
_____ NO
Why?

_____ 8. I want to be placed on a dialysis machine.
_____ YES
_____ TRIAL for the TIME PERIOD OF _____
_____ TRIAL to determine effectiveness using reasonable medical judgment.
_____ NO
Why?

_____ 9. I want to have an autopsy done to determine the cause(s) of my death.
_____ YES
_____ NO
Why?

_____10. I want to be admitted to the intensive care unit for my medical care, if necessary.
_____ YES
_____ NO
Why?

_____11. For patients in long-term care facilities or receiving care at home who experience a life-threatening change in health status: I want 911 called in case of a medical emergency.
_____ YES
_____ NO
Why?

Figure 68.1. (_continued_)

_____ 12. OTHER DIRECTIVES:
I consent to these directives after receiving honest disclosure of their implications, risks, and benefits by my physician, free from constraints and being of sound mind.

_____   _____
Signature   Date

_____
Witness

_____
Witness

13. PROXY NEGATION:
I request that the following persons NOT be allowed to make decisions on my behalf in the event of my disability or incapacity:

_____
_____
_____

_____   _____
Signature   Date

_____
Witness

_____
Witness

14. ORGAN DONATION:
Specific State Version Inserted Here
15. DURABLE POWER OF ATTORNEY FOR HEALTH CARE AND LIVING WILL:
Specific State Versions Inserted Here

Figure 68.1. (*continued*)

tives from the patient in light of those values and beliefs. The goal of this two-part approach is to encourage the physician and patient to discuss the use of medical treatments at the end of life. This interchange may be valuable to the patient by clarifying his or her values (21). The physician, in turn, can better respect the patient's autonomy by helping to remove constraints that could hinder the informed consent process (21). There are two goals of this values discourse: First, to clarify the patient's personal and value-based reasons for consenting to or refusing treatment; and second, to augment physicians' understanding of these values and preferences so that they can later implemented in the form of physician's orders. The Values History helps both physicians and patients by reducing the ambiguities of the living will and durable power of attorney for health care and catalyzes conversations on end-of-life care. Accomplishing these goals enables the physician to write orders for the patient's management on the basis of the patient's values.

The Values History's directive section begins by considering treatment preferences in acute-care situations, such as consent for or refusal of cardiopulmonary resuscitation (CPR), ventilator use, and endotracheal tube use. Next it elicits preferences regarding chronic care, including the use of intravenous fluids, enteral feeding tubes, total parenteral nutrition, medication, and dialysis. During this phase the physician explains the treatment modalities, their beneficial effects, short-term and long-term consequences, and possible short-term and long-term harms in the context of terminal illness, irreversible coma, and permanent vegetative state (as described in the patient's living will or durable power of attorney for health care). During conversations on the consequences of discontinuing treatment, the patient should be reassured that the administration of medications for symptom relief (including treatment for pain, nausea, and shortness of breath) will not be withheld if indicated for the patient's comfort. Patients should be assured that when appropriately administered, analgesia does not significantly increase the risk of death and that any incremental risk of death is ethically and legally acceptable in good medical practice, everyday moral judgment, and religious traditions.

For all of the directives except CPR, the patient may choose intervention (unless it is futile), a trial of intervention (limited either by time or by medical judgment), or no intervention. With CPR, the patient may choose either a trial of intervention to determine medical effectiveness or refusal. With all other therapies, if no benefit of the therapy is apparent, the patient may also decide that after a set time trial the intervention should be discontinued. A time-limited trial is concrete and preferred for patients who wish parameters to be explicit. The patient can alternatively decide to have a treatment continued so long as it benefits him or her in the physician's best medical judgment. Benefit-based trials are predicated on a significant level of trust between the patient and physician. Benefit-based trials require the physician to allow adequate time for a therapy to determine whether continued benefit is reasonably to be expected before stopping it. The physician should explicitly discuss the parameters of a benefit-based trial with the patient. Benefit-based trials more accurately convey how the agent in a durable power of attorney for health care may approach intervention in an unforeseen future medical condition.

The Values History also offers several unique directives: refusal of intensive care unit (ICU) care, request for autopsy, a directive to exclude a specific person from decision making, and "do not call 911" for patients in long-term care facilities or home care (22). The blank at the end of the directive section allows consent, refusal, or trials of intervention for other specific procedures not otherwise addressed (e.g., specific types of surgery). The Values History concludes with consent for organ donation (to be attached in a form as required by local jurisdictions).

SPECIAL CONSIDERATIONS

Writing and using advance directive orders for patients in nursing homes, patients electing to die at home, and for surgery involves special considerations and requires further discussion. For nursing or home care patients, the order not to call 911 avoids all forms of aggressive management, such as resuscitation equipment and personnel trained to use it.

This directive may meet some institutional resistance if a nursing home has a defensive perception of death. Some managers of nursing homes and emergency medical teams may resist the order not to call 911. This challenge has been met in several jurisdictions with legislation allowing for do-not-resuscitate (DNR) orders at home. The reader is encouraged to pursue this avenue for further documenting orders not to call 911. In the absence of such legislation, the physician's response should be the following. First, there is no risk of lawsuit against the nursing home, given that we know of no lawsuits against physicians or hospitals that have implemented valid advance directives. Besides, legislation of these statutes typically grants civil immunity. Second, the nursing home can and should develop policies that respect and implement living wills. This process is instructive for the institution's personnel and leadership and is required by the PSDA. Third, death subsequent to an advance directive implemented by an order not to call 911 is acceptable because it respects the patient's autonomy.

For patients receiving home health care, there have been other proposals about using orders not to call 911 (20). However, there are several difficulties with this strategy. First, medical orders are usually written to be implemented by health professionals, not family members. The physician has no authority over family members. A family member may panic or frankly refuse to allow such an order, triggering the emergency medical services (EMS) system. Second, family members may justifiably limit their obligations, including the obligation to care for the loved one dying at home (23). Some family members may reasonably judge the care burdens of doing so to be beyond their physical, emotional, or financial capacities.

A patient does not have an unlimited autonomy-based positive right to impose unreasonable care burdens on other family members. Writing an order not to call 911 without a mutually respectful discussion of the sense of family members' obligations and their thoughtful sense of limits on those obligations sets up the physician, the patient, and the family for an ethical conflict. This conflict can be prevented by discussing with family members the care burdens and identifying home health services, such as hospice, for which the patient may qualify, that reduce those burdens to a reasonable level. Family members also need to know that ambulance crews in jurisdictions without home DNR orders usually employ full resuscitation protocols in response to all 911 calls, although this practice is beginning to change. Families can avoid this outcome by taking the patient to the hospital when medical needs arise but before an emergency. The physician can write orders addressing how the patient should be managed in the emergency department. Discharge planning from any hospitalization is an opportune time to write such readmission orders. The physician should work with emergency department colleagues to facilitate such orders and work toward hospital policies supporting their use.

Patients with advance directives may require surgery to reduce their pain and suffering. The patient may be a reasonable risk for surgical management. From a surgeon's point of view, the problem with DNR orders is that administration of anesthesia or intraoperative technique can result in life-threatening events from which the patient has a reasonable probability of recovering to enjoy the benefits of the surgery. It makes little beneficence-based clinical sense to let the patient die of reversible iatrogenic events when the patient is reliably expected to benefit from the surgery. Such reasoning underlies why surgeons and anesthesiologists argue for suspending DNR orders during surgery despite autonomy-based arguments to the contrary. Surgeons and anesthesiologists in some institutions have responded with policies requiring DNR suspension in the perioperative period. Resistance on the part of surgeon and anesthesiologist to a patient's or physician's wanting to maintain the DNR order may prevent the surgery, causing unnecessary suffering.

Discussions between the physician, surgeon, and patient can obviate ethical conflict on perioperative DNR orders. The physician should be prepared to present a clear statement of the patient's problem and why the operation is expected to address that problem. The patient's surgical risk should be frankly appraised. The physician should negotiate with the surgical team to define the period of suspension. The physician should be aware of surgeons' understandable sensitivities about responsibility and accountability for surgical mortality rates. The physician and the surgical team should collaborate with their institutions and payers to ensure that death subsequent to surgery and reinstatement of the DNR order is an acceptable form of postoperative mortality.

METHOD OF USE

The implementation of the Values History can be accomplished in seven steps (Table 68.1). If the patient consents, family members can be part of this process. In those cases, the patient's family and specifically the agent holding the durable power of attorney for health care should receive a copy of the completed Values History. Any misconceptions should be clarified at a meeting of family members, health care surrogate, patient, and physician. Such discussions of the patient's values and end-of-life preferences help avoid misunderstanding should the patient become unable to communicate. These conversations between the patient and family members can facilitate the resolution of conflicts on health care goals for the patient.

A Values History can be completed by a patient over several visits, which has two advantages over precipitous consent to other advance directive instruments (24, 25). The Values History is intended to be used in a reflective and introspective process by the patient, so that decisions are made thoughtfully over time. With an ongoing conversation, the physician can distribute the time required for these discussions during several medical visits, given the lack of insurance or Medicare reimbursement for such counseling. Values statements would be discussed during initial visits. Specific treatment directives would be discussed subsequently, concentrating on interventions that are most pertinent to the patient's medical problems.

These discussions help prevent future attempts by family members and others to interfere with implementation of the patient's value-based pref-

Table 68.1

A Method of Communication Using the Values History

1. Upon the patient's execution of either the living will or durable power of attorney for health care, the physician explains that critical care sometimes extends life while lowering its quality and discusses the patient's fundamental value judgment on quality of life versus length of life regarding aggressive medical management and end-of-life care.
2. The physician discusses the values section of the Values History and invites the patient to consider and express priority for length versus quality of life.
3. The physician reviews the patient's quality-of-life values with the patient. The patient selects the values most important to him or her while exploring others.
4. The patient and physician discuss the various therapeutic options in the directive section, using the patient's values as a framework.
5. The physician helps facilitate the consent process:
   a. Shapes the process in relation to known values of the patient
   b. Explores other values that may emerge in the process
   c. Clarifies for the patient inconsistencies between values and directives in a nonpaternalistic fashion by removing reversible constraints to consent
   d. Discusses treatment options in terms of the patient's known diseases, disorders, high-risk activities, and genetic propensities
6. Other specific preferences concerning surgery and calling 911 from home or the nursing home, proxy negotiation, and organ donation should be discussed.
7. The directives individually should be initialed and dated. The complete Values History should be signed by the patient, dated and witnessed, with *copies* placed in the medical chart (doctor's office, hospice, or extended-care facility). The original should be placed in a readily available place in the patient's home that is known to family and friends.

---

erences. We urge that the completed Values History be reviewed with the patient every 6 to 12 months, especially if there is a significant change in the patient's health. In this way, changes in values or preferences that may occur over time can be discussed and documented. Orders can be updated as necessary.

CONCLUSION

The Values History is a clinical instrument intended to be used in conjunction with the living will and the durable power of attorney for health care. We propose that the Values History enhances respect for the patient's autonomy more than either of these advance directives without it. The Values History is therefore a powerful supplementary document that can add clarity, meaning, and clinical utility to advance directives while also facilitating the patient's conversation on end-of-life care with family and physicians. The patient and the physician have a tool of considerable power to articulate the patient's values and preferences regarding end-of-life care, so that orders that honor these preferences can be written.

REFERENCES

1. Doukas DJ, Reichel W. Planning for Uncertainty: A Guide to Living Wills and Other Advance Directives for Health Care. Baltimore: Johns Hopkins University Press, 1993.
2. Doukas DJ, McCullough LB. The Values History: the evaluation of the patient's values and advance directives. J Fam Pract 1991;32:145–153.
3. Doukas DJ, McCullough LB. Assessing the Values History of the aged patient regarding critical and chronic care. In: Gallo J, Reichel W, eds. Handbook of Geriatric Assessment. Rockville, MD: Aspen, 1988:111–124.
4. Doukas DJ, Lipson S, McCullough LB. Values history. In: Reichel W, ed. Clinical Aspects of Aging. 3rd ed. Baltimore: Williams & Wilkins, 1989:615–616.
5. Doukas DJ, McCullough LB. Truthtelling and confidentiality in the aged patient. In: Reichel W, ed. Clinical Aspects of Aging. 3rd ed. Baltimore: Williams & Wilkins, 1989:609–615.
6. Doukas DJ, Gorenflo DW. Analyzing the Values History: an evaluation of patient medical values and advance directives. J Clin Ethics 1993;4:41–45.

7. A controlled trial to improve outcomes for seriously ill hospitalized patients. The Study to Understand Prognoses and Preferences for Outcomes and Risks of Treatment (SUPPORT). The SUPPORT Investigators. JAMA 1995;274:1591–1598.

8. Teno JM, Lynn J, Wenger N, et al. Advance directives for seriously ill hospitalized patients: effectiveness with the Patient Self-Determination Act and the SUPPORT intervention. J Am Geriatr Soc 1997;45:500–507.

9. Doukas DJ, Brody H. After the Cruzan case: the primary care physician and the use of advance directives. J Am Board Fam Pract 1992;2:201–205.

10. Omnibus Budget Reconciliation Act of 1990. Public License 101–508 §§4206, 4751.

11. Wolf SM, Boyle P, Callahan D, et al. Sources of concern about the patient self-determination act. N Engl J Med 1991;325:1666–1671.

12. Eisendrath S, Jonsen A. The living will: help or hindrance? JAMA 1983;249:2054–2058.

13. Wanzer S, Adelstein J, Cranford R, et al. The physician's responsibility toward hopelessly ill patients. N Engl J Med 1984;310:955–959.

14. Emanuel EJ. A review of the ethical and legal aspects of terminating medical care. Am J Med 1988;84:291–301.

15. Tomlinson T, Howe K, Notman M, Rossmiller D. An empirical study of proxy consent for elderly persons. Gerontologist 1990;30:54–64.

16. Doukas DJ, Antonucci TA, Gorenflo DW. A multi-generational assessment of values and advance directives. Ethics Behav 1992;2:51–59.

17. Doukas DJ, Gorenflo DW, Venkateswaran R. Understanding patients' values (letter). J Clin Ethics 1993; 4:199–200 .

18. Wear S. Anticipatory ethical decision-making: the role of the primary care physician. HMO Pract 1989;3:41–46.

19. Civetta J, Taylor R, Kirby R, eds. Critical Care. Philadelphia: Lippincott, 1988.

20. Reilly R, Teasdale T, McCullough LB. Option of trial in advance directives. Gerontologist 1992;32:69.

21. Ackerman T. Why doctors should intervene. Hastings Cent Rep 1982;12:14–17.

22. Stollerman G. Decisions to leave home (editorial). J Am Geriatr Soc 1988;36:375–376.

23. Jecker NS. The role of intimate others in medical decision making. Gerontologist 1990;30:65–71.

24. Scissors K. Advance directives for medical care (letter). N Engl J Med 1991;325:1255.

25. Forrow L, Gogel E, Thomas E. Advance directives for medical care (letter). N Engl J Med 1991;325:1255.

Index

Page numbers in *italics* denote figures; those followed by a t denote tables.